PHYSIOLOGY
OF SMALL AND LARGE
ANIMALS

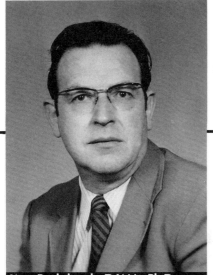

Yves Ruckebusch, D.V.M., Ph.D.
(1931–1989)

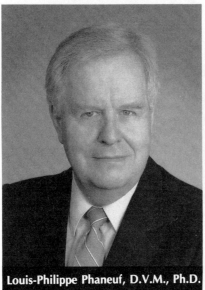

Louis-Philippe Phaneuf, D.V.M., Ph.D.

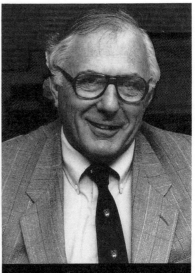

Robert Dunlop, D.V.M., Ph.D.

PHYSIOLOGY OF SMALL AND LARGE ANIMALS

Yves Ruckebusch, D.V.M., Ph.D. (deceased)
National Veterinary College
Toulouse, France

Louis-Philippe Phaneuf, D.V.M., Ph.D.
College of Veterinary Medicine
University of Montreal
St. Hyacinthe, Quebec, Canada

Robert Dunlop, D.V.M., Ph.D.
College of Veterinary Medicine
University of Minnesota
St. Paul, Minnesota, U.S.A.

B.C. Decker, Inc. • Philadelphia • Hamilton

Publisher

B.C. Decker Inc
One James Street South
11th Floor
Hamilton, Ontario L8P 4R5

B.C. Decker Inc
320 Walnut Street
Suite 400
Philadelphia, Pennsylvania 19106

Sales and Distribution

United States and Puerto Rico
Mosby–Year Book Inc.
11830 Westline Industrial Drive
Saint Louis, Missouri 63146

Canada
Mosby–Year Book Ltd.
5240 Finch Ave. E., Unit 1
Scarborough, Ontario M1S 5A2

Australia
**McGraw-Hill Book Company Australia
Pty. Ltd.**
4 Barcoo Street
Roseville East 2069
New South Wales, Australia

Brazil
Editora McGraw-Hill do Brasil, Ltda.
rua Tabapua, 1.105, Itaim-Bibi
Sao Paulo, S.P. Brasil

Colombia
Interamericana/McGraw-Hill de Colombia, S.A.
Carrera 17, No. 33-71
(Apartado Postal, A.A., 6131)
Bogota, D.E., Colombia

Europe
McGraw-Hill Book Company GmbH
Lademannbogen 136
D-2000 Hamburg 63
West Germany

France
MEDSI/McGraw-Hill
6, avenue Daniel Lesueur
75007 Paris, France

Hong Kong and China
McGraw-Hill Book Company
Suite 618, Ocean Centre
5 Canton Road
Tsimshatsui, Kowloon
Hong Kong

India
Tata McGraw-Hill Publishing Company, Ltd.
12/4 Asaf Ali Road, 3rd Floor
New Delhi 110002, India

Indonesia
Mr. Wong Fin Fah
P.O. Box 122/JAT
Jakarta, 1300 Indonesia

Italy
McGraw-Hill Libri Italia, s.r.l.
Piazza Emilia, 5
I-20129 Milano MI
Italy

Japan
Igaku-Shoin Ltd.
Tokyo International P.O. Box 5063
1-28-36 Hongo, Bunkyo-ku,
Tokyo 113, Japan

Korea
Mr. Don-Gap Choi
C.P.O. Box 10583
Seoul, Korea

Malaysia
Mr. Lim Tao Slong
No. 8 Jalan SS 7/6B
Kelana Jaya
47301 Petaling Jaya
Selangor, Malaysia

Mexico
**Interamericana/McGraw-Hill de Mexico,
S.A. de C.V.**
Cedro 512, Colonia Atlampa
(Apartado Postal 26370)
06450 Mexico, D.F., Mexico

New Zealand
McGraw-Hill Book Co. New Zealand Ltd.
5 Joval Place, Wiri
Manukau City, New Zealand

Portugal
Editora McGraw-Hill de Portugal, Ltda.
Rua Rosa Damasceno 11A-B
1900 Lisboa, Portugal

South Africa
Libriger Book Distributors
Warehouse Number 8
"Die Ou Looiery"
Tannery Road
Hamilton, Bloemfontein 9300

Singapore and Southeast Asia
McGraw-Hill Book Co.
21 Neythal Road
Jurong, Singapore 2262

Spain
McGraw-Hill/Interamericana de Espana, S.A.
Manuel Ferrero, 13
28020 Madrid, Spain

Taiwan
Mr. George Lim
P.O. Box 87-601
Taipei, Taiwan

Thailand
Mr. Vitit Lim
632/5 Phaholyothin Road
Sapan Kwai
Bangkok 10400
Thailand

United Kingdom, Middle East and Africa
MacGraw-Hill Book Company (U.K.) Ltd.
Shoppenhangers Road
Maidenhead, Berkshire
SL6 2QL England

Venezuela
Editorial Interamericana de Venezuela, C.A.
2da. calle Bello Monte
Local G-2
Caracas, Venezuela

NOTICE

The authors and publisher have made every effort to ensure that the care recommended herein, including choice of drugs and drug dosages, is in accord with the accepted standards and practice at the time of publication. However, since research and regulation constantly change clinical standards, the reader is urged to check the product information sheet included in the package of each drug, which includes recommended doses, warnings, and contraindications. This is particularly important with new or infrequently used drugs.

Physiology of Small and Large Animals

ISBN 1-55664-136-2

Library of Congress catalog card number: 89-50928

YVES RUCKEBUSCH
(1931–1989)

On Saturday, December 16, 1989, a cerebral hemorrhage quietly ended the life of Yves Ruckebusch. Ten months earlier, he had survived a cardiac arrest and had been granted a reprieve without cerebral anoxia. He credited his so-called second life to the rapid and persistent cardiorespiratory reanimation performed by his research collaborator, Dr. Charles H. Malbert, who had mastered this emergency technique in the military service. After prolonged hospitalization, much of it in the intensive care unit, he was recuperating and learning to use his indomitable energy with some restraint. A week before his death, he had participated actively in a meeting on a subject he was closely associated with—substances acting therapeutically or helpful for animal production (SATHAP; *SITAPA, or substances d'intervention thérapeutique et d'aide aux productions animales*).

An only child, he was born on December 1, 1931, and raised on a farm in northern France, on the Flemish-Belgium border. The war years of his youth had imprinted him with a deep humanitarian trait and a firm belief in international cooperation. Benevolent, with a keen sense of humor and without affectation, he always responded to the quest for knowledge and enjoyed the company of colleagues. Eventually, most foreign visitors would sign his guest-book and come to his home to share a hospitable dinner prepared by his gracious scientist-wife, Michele Ruckebusch-Cordier. In contrast, his agrarian upbringing had endowed him with a capacity for practical and efficient work, which was fed by a phenomenal and dedicated energy. For instance, convinced that English was essential for publication of his research outside of France, he would arrange for Anglophone colleagues to review one or several of his manuscripts during the course of a visit in Toulouse. The drafts, dutifully prepared before their arrival, also served to update them on the current research of the laboratory. Besides provoking relevant questions, the exercise led to a friendly exchange of ideas, in his open-door office, over a cup of coffee obtained from an ever-present coffee pot.

Although modest, in spite of his scientific fame and influence, Yves Ruckebusch was grateful for the recognition granted by colleagues from all parts of the world. On the walls of his office were honorary degrees from the University of Ghent, the University of Liège, and the University of Montreal, and the certificate of honorary membership of the European Association for Veterinary Pharmacology and Toxicology, as well as a memento photograph from a group of American veterinary pharmacologists, some of the marks of esteem shown by the scientific community.

These lines aim at remembering Yves Ruckebusch, a man who will be missed by his colleagues and friends all over the world. The work of Professor Ruckebusch, his important contribution to fundamental research in gastrointestinal physiology and pharmacology, is in itself a memorial. Knowledge in the field of gastrointestinal science will continue to progress and undoubtedly will undergo evolution, but we are confident that his scientific legacy will not be lost to posterity.

Physiology is the experimental science par excellence
of all sciences; that in which there is least to be learnt
by mere observations, and that which affords the
greatest field for the exercise of those faculties
which characterize the experimental philosopher.

Thomas Henry Huxley

(1825–1895)

FOREWORD

Physiology of Small and Large Animals is designed to serve as a textbook for students of both veterinary medicine and animal science and as a reference text in comparative physiology. It examines the functions of body cells, and the integrated physiological mechanisms that are required to control growth, maintenance, production, reproduction, and behavior of the major species of domestic animals.

Physiology is the science that describes the normal functions and activities of living organisms. Most of the basic functions necessary to life are common to all animals, although adaptations to diet and environment cause marked differences among the various groups of animals, and even between closely related species. Yet, most physiology texts focus on human physiology and on only those characteristics of other species that are assumed to have direct application. *Physiology of Small and Large Animals* covers our present understanding of physiological mechanisms from the combined results obtained in a variety of species. Therefore, special attention is given to the various strategies adopted for assimilation and utilization of nutrients, excretion of waste material, metabolism, thermoregulation, reproduction, and the neurohumoral control of these processes.

Early chapters deal with basic cellular physiology and lead into discussions of the specialization of cells for various functions, and their incorporation into tissues, organs, systems, and the animal as a whole. Each system of the body is described, with the liberal use of illustrations and explanations of their functions, interactions, and neuroendocrine control. Close attention is given to similarities and differences among species. It includes many aspects of physiology relevant to managerial and veterinary practices.

The authors of this text have a wealth of combined experience in research and teaching on these subjects. Professor Ruckebusch's research has given us a great deal of the current knowledge of species variations in the neurohumoral regulation of motor activity in the digestive tract. He has clarified some of the changes in gastrointestinal motility associated with periods of digestion, interdigestion, and sleep. His sudden death, in December 1989, took from us a dedicated and productive scientist who will be sorely missed by all who benefited from his contributions and friendship.

Professor Dunlop's research is associated with the problems of metabolic disorders in ruminants. He has served as head of the Department of Physiology and Pharmacology, College of Veterinary Medicine, University of Saskatchewan, Saskatoon, Canada; as founding dean of veterinary colleges in Uganda (Makerere University) and Western Australia (Murdoch University); and as dean of the College of Veterinary Medicine at the University of Minnesota. His worldwide experience adds considerable insight as to the importance of physiology in the training of students in veterinary medicine and other animal sciences. Professor Phaneuf, a long-time editor of the *Canadian Veterinary Journal,* served as the driving force in the development of this text. He has extensive experience in the teaching of physiology and pharmacology at the Faculty of Veterinary Medicine, University of Montreal, Saint-Hyacinthe, Quebec, Canada. He has the distinction of having been the last graduate student to receive a Ph.D. under Professor H.H. Dukes, at Cornell University. He is now serving as President of the World Association of Veterinary Physiologists, Pharmacologists, Biochemists, and Toxicologists, an affiliate of the World Veterinary Association.

Physiology of Small and Large Animals will be especially useful for teachers and students in veterinary medicine and in the animal sciences related to agriculture and companion animals. Its use can be broadened also to zoologists and to others who require information on comparative physiology and on the adaptations of animals to diet and to environment.

C. Edward Stevens

Associate Dean
Research and Graduate Programs
North Carolina State University
College of Veterinary Medicine
Raleigh, North Carolina

ACKNOWLEDGMENTS

Completion of this book would not have been possible without the endorsement and encouragement of the successive administrations of the veterinary colleges of the University of Montreal in Saint-Hyacinthe, Quebec, Canada, headed by deans Roy and Larivière, and of the National Veterinary College in Toulouse, France, headed by directors Lautié and Ferney, as well as acting Vice President for the Health Sciences C. Perlmutter, and Dean Thawler, at the University of Minnesota.

We are indebted to many colleagues for reading chapters and contributing time and ideas: from Physiology and Pharmacodynamics, at Toulouse, C.H. Malbert and P.L. Toutain, as well as A.M. Merritt (University of Florida, Gainesville) and C. Crichlow (University of Saskatchewan) during their sabbaticals; from Animal Anatomy and Physiology, at Saint-Hyacinthe, C.B. Delorme and N. Larivière; from Research Center on Animal Reproduction, at Saint-Hyacinthe, R.G. Cooke, A. Goff, R.H.F. Hunter, and C. Price; from Medicine, at Saint-Hyacinthe, Y. Couture and P. Guay; and from the University of Minnesota, in Minneapolis, F. Halberg.

We owe much to the librarians Ms. Serraz (Toulouse) and Mr. Jetté (Saint-Hyacinthe), and Ms. Carlson (St. Paul), for their assistance with interlibrary loans and for their leniency toward our hoarding of unbound and bound journals.

We are grateful to Ms. Costes and Mr. Maliguoy (Toulouse), and Mr. Demers and Ms. Tellier (Saint-Hyacinthe) for their dedicated artistic skill and clerical expertise.

Finally, we convey our deepest gratitude to Mr. Walter S. Bailey, president of B.C. Decker, Inc., Publisher, for his confidence in us, and to Ms. Gina Scala, the project editor, for her kind and efficient professional guidance.

CONTENTS

GENERAL PHYSIOLOGY

CHAPTER 1

CELLULAR LIFE CYCLE—CELL GROWTH AND REPRODUCTION

General physiology studies the general principles of mechanisms that govern the vital processes of life in organisms. In simple as in complex living organisms, the cell is the functional unit (Fig. 1–1). Each cell has the capacity for metabolism, growth, reaction to stimuli, and reproduction. Within this miniature living organism, chemical reactions occur to contribute to the global function of the complex organism.

The life cycle of a cell extends from mitosis of origin to mitosis of division. Cellular individuality of a new cell begins with the mitosis that prepares its existence and ends with the mitosis that eventually divides it into two identical daughter cells. Ninety-five percent of the life of the new, or daughter, cell is spent in interphase, which immediately follows the mitosis of inception (Fig. 1–2).

In types of derepressed cells (e.g., cells of bone marrow, of gut epithelium, and of germinal layer of skin), reproduction is rather rapid, and the cell life cycle may last only 10 to 30 hours. In some other types of cells (e.g., smooth muscle), repression or inhibitory control slows reproduction for many years. In nerve cells and striated muscle cells, reproduction is repressed and does not occur at all, and the cell life cycle extends over the entire lifetime of the animal.

This chapter deals with some functional events that occur throughout the life cycle of daughter, or new, cells, especially during interphase (resting state) and immediately before mitosis (reproductive state).

INTERPHASE, OR GROWTH AND DIFFERENTIATION PHASE OF THE CELLULAR LIFE CYCLE

The nucleus of a new cell operates as a control center for all cell activities. This nucleus is equipped with a full complement of genetic information—the germ line, or germ plasm, made of deoxyribonucleic acid (DNA), which passes from generation to generation via the germ cells. Each nucleated cell of the animal body contains the same set of genes that is found in the fertilized ovum from which the animal body was formed. The new cell usually uses only part of this genetic message to grow, to differentiate, and to function as a specialized adult cell. The genetic message is normally maintained in a repressed state; that is, some genes remain inactive or unexpressed. Derepression and activation of selected portions of the genetic message are brought about by a variety of hormones and other agents such as enzymes (Fig. 1–3).

Period of Rapid Cell Growth

Immediately after their formation, the small daughter cells begin a period of rapid growth. In cells reproducing rapidly, this period may occupy as much as 35 percent of the total cell life cycle. Rapid cell growth is characterized by accelerated formation of ribonucleic acid (RNA), extensive protein synthesis, and proliferation of nucleoplasm and cytoplasm.

Cell size is determined primarily by the amount of DNA in the nucleus, since DNA regulates the RNA in the cytoplasm and the extent of protein synthesis. Growth factors not tied to production of DNA cause growth and increase the production of differentiation factors. Cytosine arabinoside, used in cancer studies, would act against growth factors (Fig. 1–4). Fully differentiated cells are thought to secrete autocrine substances, which inhibit both the growth and the reproduction of the cell of origin. Cells treated experimentally with colchicine are made to increase their nuclear DNA content and to grow proportionately larger.

Growth of cells in vitro requires the presence of growth factors, adequate physical space, and absence of autocrine secretions (i.e., the cells' own secretions).

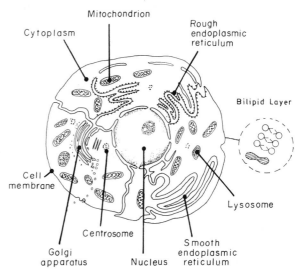

Figure 1–1 The cell is the smallest unit of living matter that can function independently. Its cytoplasm contains several organelles (mitochondria, rough and smooth endoplasmic reticulum, Golgi apparatus, lysosomes, and secretory vesicles) and is limited by semipermeable membranes (plasma membrane and nuclear membrane).

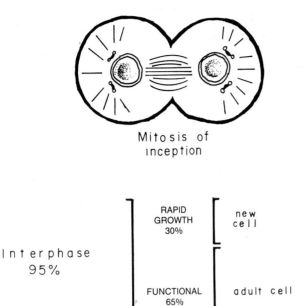

Mitosis of
inception

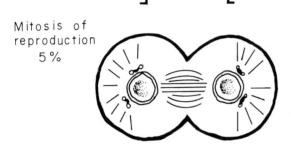

Interphase
95%

Mitosis of
reproduction
5%

Figure 1-2 Representation of the major events in the life cycle of daughter cells from initial mitosis of inception, or origin, to their ultimate mitosis of reproduction. Interphase, which begins with a rapid phase of growth and differentiation leading to a functional adult cell, is the longest part of the life cycle of new cells (95 percent). Mitosis of reproduction accounts for only 5 percent of the cell life cycle.

Cell Protein Synthesis

The cytoplasm of a daughter cell produces two types of proteins, *structural* (organelles, membranes) and *functional* (enzymes, factors, hormones). During the cell growth period, production of both types of proteins is necessary to lead the new cell eventually to differentiation and adulthood. Once the cell is adult, its protein production is usually limited to enzymes (i.e., functional proteins). Occasionally, structural proteins are also formed by adult cells to repair minor cell structural wear and tear or damage.

During the period of cell growth, the nucleolus (nucleic organelle for storage of ribosomal RNA) enlarges. This reflects the increase in the nuclear production of RNA that occurs from detached strands of DNA, which are used as templates. Ultimately, three types of RNA, with different roles in protein synthesis, reach the cytoplasm: *messenger RNA* (mRNA), which carries the genetic code (contains the codons) into the cytoplasm; *transfer RNA* (tRNA), which transfers amino acids (AAs) to the ribosomes and carries the anticodons; and *ribosomal RNA* (rRNA), which is the part (60 percent) of the ribosome where protein molecules are assembled and formed.

Proteins formed in the ribosomes of the granular endoplasmic reticulum are glycosylated (glycoproteins) and folded. Most of those originating from ribosomes in the cytosol are free proteins (Fig. 1-5). Proteins produced in nerve cell bodies are transported along the axon (axoplasmic transport) to the boutons (axon terminals).

Proteins are secreted or excreted from the cells by exocytosis in vesicles formed by the Golgi apparatus. The entry of calcium ions in the cytosol favors fusion of the vesicular membrane with the plasma membrane. Usually, about 1 hour elapses between initiation of synthesis and exocytosis of proteins. Most proteins are synthesized as larger proteins (precursors) from which polypeptide sequences are cleaved off (Fig. 1-6). The large proteins that are precursors of hormones are called *preprohormones* and *prohormones*. For example, prepro-opiomelanocortin (265 AA) formed in the adenohypophysis yields melanocyte-stimulating hormones (alpha-MSH, 33 AA, and beta-MSH, 17 AA) and adrenocorticotropic hormone (ACTH, 39 AA).

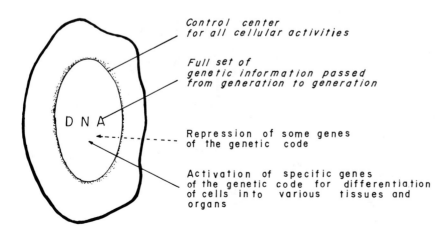

Control center
for all cellular activities

Full set of
genetic information passed
from generation to generation

Repression of some genes
of the genetic code

Activation of specific genes
of the genetic code for differentiation
of cells into various tissues and
organs

Figure 1-3 Control of the differentiation of cells occurs by partial activation and repression of the control center (nucleus) for all protein synthesis (i.e., of the genetic potential in the nucleus).

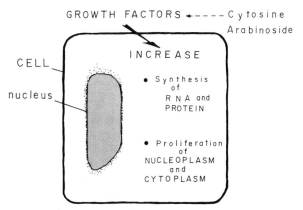

Figure 1–4 Protein synthesis mechanism is activated by reaction of hormones or growth factors with plasma membrane receptors during the early interphase period of rapid growth.

Some hormones induce protein synthesis (structural and functional) in their target cells. Steroid hormones, from the gonads or the adrenals, enter the cells and bind to specific receptors in the cytoplasm. This receptor-steroid complex eventually reaches the nucleus to derepress or to activate genes for the ribosomal synthesis of structural (glands, smooth and striated muscle cells) and enzymatic (anabolic effect) proteins. Thyroid hormones act differently, since tri-iodothyronine (T_3) and thyroxine or tetraiodothyronine (T_4) activate genetic synthesis of functional proteins (enzymes) by binding directly to receptors in the nucleus of many types of cells for several days (Fig. 1–7). By mechanisms yet unknown, insulin and growth hormone (GH) also increase protein synthesis by ribosomes.

Many antibiotics (e.g., chloramphenicol, streptomycin, neomycin, cycloheximide, tetracycline, puromycin, chloroquine) act by inhibiting protein synthesis in cells. Useful antibiotics selectively limit antiproteogenesis to bacteria without affecting animal cells. Puromycin inhibits protein synthesis in both bacterial and animal cells and is a poor therapeutic tool. Diphtheria toxin is the reverse of a good antibiotic; it does not affect bacteria but inhibits proteogenesis in animal cells.

Control of Intracellular Metabolic Activities

The vast differences in the intracellular functions and activities of the various cells are regulated by genetic and enzymatic mechanisms. These control systems maintain the proper proportions and quantities of the numerous organelles and cellular constituents in cells with different morphology and functions.

Without exception, the cells in an animal have identical

Figure 1–5 Morphologic and functional intermediaries for synthesis of proteins, RNAs, which are controlled by DNAs, are responsible for the genetic code, the transport of AAs, and the assembly of proteins (structural and functional) in the ribosomes.

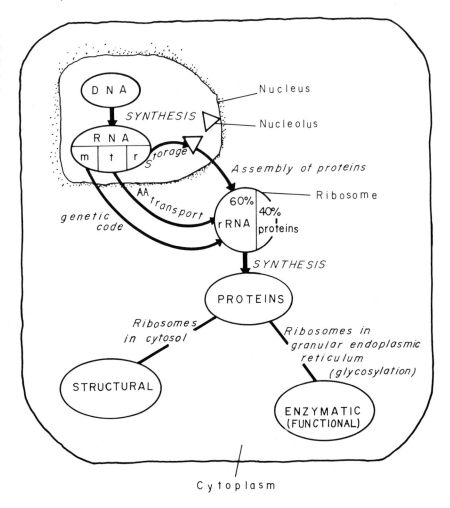

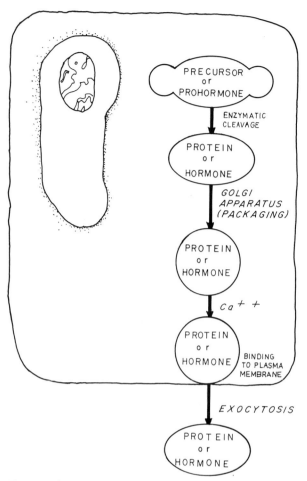

Figure 1–6 Large proteins (prohormones or precursors) formed in the ribosomes usually undergo enzymatic cleavage and shed some polypeptides. The Golgi apparatus then packages the hormones or proteins into vesicles. Afterward, calcium ions in the cytoplasm cause these vesicles to fuse with the plasma membrane in preparation for exocytosis, or emiocytosis, of the proteins into the extracellular fluid.

strands of DNA carrying the same genes (30,000 to 100,000 genes). Their functional and morphologic diversities are the result of differentiation (i.e., the repression or the activation of different genes by intracellular genetic regulatory—promotor, repressor, activator—proteins). This concept of differentiation would encompass all the theories about the means used by cells to change their characteristics to form the various organs and tissues of the animal body. Some differentiation factors cause maturation of cells (e.g., inductors of macrophages and granulocytes) by binding to DNA and by activating genes. These intracellular genetic regulatory proteins, or differentiation factors, operate primarily to control the concentrations of intermediary substrates of carbohydrate, lipid, and protein metabolism.

Differentiation factors are reported to change the expression of the genetic effects of oncogenes (mutation-provoking substances). Some substances (retinoid derivatives of vitamin A, interferon) induce differentiation of cancer cells into normal cells. Other substances that have been used for

their effects on tumors are dimethyl sulfoxide (DMSO), derivatives of vitamin D_3, methotrexate, and teleocidins (indol alkaloid tumor promoters).

Enzymes involved in intracellular biochemical syntheses are also controlled by inhibitors and activators. Inhibition is usually by a substance, formed after the action of a series of specific enzymes, that neutralizes the first enzyme of the system. This negative feedback mechanism regulates the intracellular concentrations of vitamins and of substances related to nucleotide and protein syntheses (purine and pyrimidine bases, AAs).

Activation of enzymes often coincides with the inhibition of other enzymes. The control system operates by negative feedback either to stop synthesis of enzymes provided in excessive amounts or to activate synthesis of enzymes present in low or deficient concentrations. For example, during the synthesis of DNA and RNA, as the adequate level of purine bases is reached, the purine-producing enzymes are inhibited, and the enzymes for the synthesis of pyrimidine bases are activated. Events are reversed when the pyrimidine bases are at their peak concentrations: their enzymes are inhibited and those for synthesis of purine bases are aroused.

MITOSIS, OR REPRODUCTIVE PHASE OF THE CELLULAR LIFE CYCLE

Mitosis, with its stages (prophase, prometaphase, metaphase, anaphase, and telophase), is a prelude to the end of the life cycle of the daughter cells of a preceding mitosis. During late interphase, mitosis-provoking events are brought about by mechanisms still unknown. Initiation of the cell division process is preceded by a higher rate of synthesis of proteins and of DNA to replicate the chromosome code of somatic or of reproductive cells. A general model, applicable to all cells able to divide, involves the action of an enzyme, protein kinase C. This enzyme reacts with diacylglycerol in the presence of calcium ions and adenosine triphosphate (ATP) to phosphorylate proteins and to activate cell division (synthesis of proteins and DNA).

The sequence proceeds as follows: Plasma membrane receptors are activated by growth factors or hormones. Triphosphoinositol in the cytoplasm and diacylglycerol in the plasma membrane are produced by hydrolysis (inhibited by lithium) of an inositol derivative (phosphatidylinositol phosphate) by phospholipase and calcium ions. From the endoplasmic reticulum (an enormous bag with numerous infoldings) triphosphoinositol liberates calcium ions, which bind to calmodulin in the cytoplasm. Finally, diacylglycerol (with calcium ions and phosphatidylserine) activates protein kinase C, which makes the cytoplasm alkaline by adding sodium ions in exchange for hydrogen ions, which are extruded at the plasma membrane.

Diacylglycerol can be replaced by phorbol esters (tumor-promoting agents, or TPA), which are mitogenic substances (i.e., they increase cell divisions). Diacylglycerol also antagonizes triphosphoinositol, and thus prevents liberation of calcium ions from the endoplasmic reticulum (Fig. 1–8).

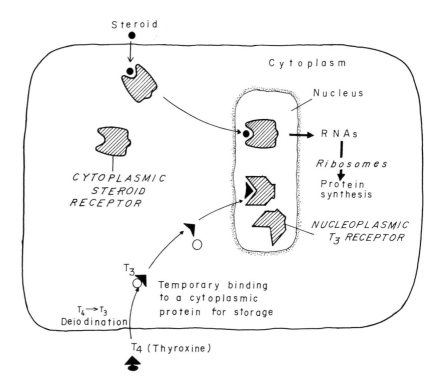

Figure 1–7 Hormones may penetrate the plasma membrane to activate protein synthesis by different means. Steroid hormones form a steroid-receptor complex that enters the nucleus to activate DNA for synthesis of enzymatic proteins. T_4 undergoes cytoplasmic deiodination to T_3, that attaches directly to a nucleoplasmic receptor for proteinogenesis. Some T_3 may bind temporarily to a protein, which then acts as a reservoir of T_3.

Figure 1–8 Model of sequence of intracellular events leading to cell division after stimulation of plasma membrane receptors by growth factors and/or hormones. Activation of protein kinase C is achieved by formation of diacylglycerol from phosphatidylinositol diphosphate. Formation of inositol triphosphate (IP$_3$) results in liberation of calcium ions (Ca^{++}) from the endoplasmic reticulum.

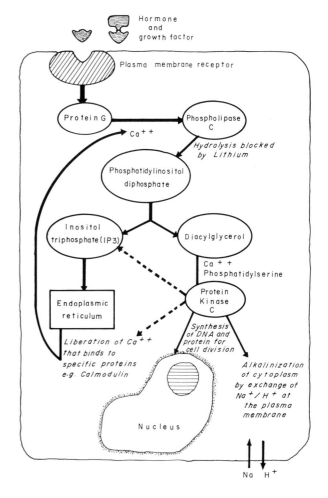

CHAPTER 2

BODY FLUID COMPARTMENTS

The two principal liquid compartments of the organism, the intracellular and the extracellular fluids (ICF, ECF), have different volumes, chemical compositions, and relations with the organism. The intracellular fluid is relatively stable, without important changes in composition and volume. Conversely, owing to its numerous subdivisions, the ECF is relatively unstable compared with the ICF. Dynamic differences are found in plasma of arterial and of venous blood, in lymph, and in interstitial fluid. This chapter presents the various fluid compartments and the dynamics of ECFs.

LIQUID COMPARTMENTS OF THE BODY

Total body water changes with age and adiposity. It represents about 57 percent of the body mass in an adult animal and may be as much as 75 percent in neonates. Tissues of older or of obese animals may contain as little as 45 percent total water.

The water of the body is distributed between the 100 trillion (10^{12}) cells and the ECF. The composition of the liquid in each cell is variable but similar enough to consider these trillions of small compartments as a whole, the ICF. The fluid outside the cells, the ECF, can be divided into transcellular fluid, interstitial fluid, and blood plasma.

The transcellular fluids are separated from the plasma by another epithelium beside that of the capillary endothelium. Cerebrospinal fluid (CSF), aqueous and vitreous humors, serous fluids of the potential cavities, synovial fluids, secretions in the alimentary canal, and urine in the genitourinary tract are considered transcellular fluids.

Measurement of Body Fluid Volumes

Total body water may be calculated by euthanizing an animal and drying the whole animal to measure the loss of mass. Blood volume has been evaluated merely by bleeding an anesthetized animal to death and measuring the volume delivered from the circulatory system. This method is inaccurate for measuring blood volume: because of clotting and of vasoconstrictor mechanisms a large quantity of blood remains in the vessels. Both of these invasive techniques are inconvenient and require killing the animal.

Several indirect methods that are noninvasive, nondestructive, and repeatable on the same animal are available to measure total body water, extracellular volume, and plasma volume. The basis of each is the fundamental concept of dilution (Fig. 2–1). A known quantity of marker, a dye or a xenobiotic compound, when added to the fluid in a reservoir of unknown volume, diffuses into the fluid of the entire

reservoir. By measuring the concentration of the marker in an aliquot of the fluid in the reservoir, the volume of the marker-fluid mixture in the reservoir can be calculated. The formula is:

$$\text{Volume (mL)} = \frac{\text{Amount of substance injected}}{\text{Concentration of substance/mL}}$$

Total Body Water

To determine total body water, the marker to be added (injected) must diffuse into both ICF and ECF. After several hours, tritiated water meets this requirement. By accounting for normal losses (urine and insensible evaporative losses by skin and lungs) of tritiated water, and applying the formula of the dilution principle to its plasma content, the average total body water is about 57 percent of the total body mass.

Other marker compounds suitable for measurement of total body water are heavy water (^2H_2O with deuterium, or ^2H), antipyrine, sulfanilamide, thiourea, and urea. Because of variations in the results, values found with these markers are usually reported with their identification (total water thiourea) for easier comparisons.

Extracellular Fluid of the Body

For measuring the volume of ECF by the dilution technique, the ideal marker must not diffuse across the cell membrane. Low-diffusing marker substances such as radioactive sodium, radioactive chloride, radioactive bromide,

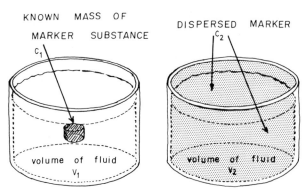

KNOWN MASS OF MARKER SUBSTANCE

DISPERSED MARKER

Figure 2–1 Concept of the dilution technique for measuring the fluid volume of a reservoir. A known amount of marker substance added to reservoir diffuses into the entire reservoir. After equilibrium, a measure of the concentration of the marker per millimeter of marker fluid is used to calculate the volume of the reservoir.

thiocyanate ion, thiosulfate ion, inulin, and sucrose have been used to evaluate extracellular volume. Because results vary from substance to substance, reference is made not to the extracellular volume but to the space occupied by a specific substance (e.g., sodium space, thiocyanate space). Mean values are about 22 percent of body mass.

Intracellular Fluid of the Body

The volume of fluid inside the cells cannot be determined by the dilution technique. It is found by subtracting ECF from total body water. ICF is 35 percent of body mass; in other words:

% Total body water (57%) − % ECF (22%) = 35%

Blood Plasma Volume (Intravascular Extracellular Volume)

A dye (T-1824, also called Evans' blue) that combines almost immediately with plasma proteins and remains within the intravascular fluid is commonly used to measure plasma volume by the dilution technique. The amount of dye injected is divided by the concentration found in the plasma after 10 min of mixing; the result is usually near 4.6% of body mass, or 46 mL/kg (Table 2–1). Accordingly, the plasma volume of a 20-kg dog is about 46 mL × 20 kg = 920 mL. The capillary beds of the different tissues vary in permeability to plasma proteins.

Interstitial Fluid

There is no direct method for measuring interstitial volume. Any substance that penetrates into the interstitial fluid also spreads to all portions of the ECF. The interstitial fluid volume can be approximated by subtracting the plasma volume from the ECF volume. Usual values are about 17 to 18 percent of body mass.

Blood Volume

A substance suitable for measuring blood volume must disperse throughout the blood and remain in the intravascular system. Substances used to determine blood volume either bind to plasma proteins (vital dye, radioactive iodine) to yield plasma volume, or combine with red blood cells (radioactive elements: ^{32}P, ^{59}Fe, ^{51}Cr) to yield erythrocyte volume. In addition, the hematocrit (Hct), or packed cell volume (PCV in L/L), must be measured by centrifuging a column of blood that has been treated with an anticoagulant (heparin or ethylene*di*amine*tetra*acetate [EDTA]). The formulas for calculating blood volume are as follows:

Starting with plasma volume:

$$\text{Blood volume (mL/kg)} = \frac{\text{Plasma volume (mL/kg)} \times 1.0}{1.0 - \text{PCV (L/L)}}$$

Starting with erythrocyte volume:

$$\text{Blood volume (mL/kg)} = \frac{\text{Erythrocyte vol. (mL/kg)} \times 1.0}{\text{PCV (L/L)}}$$

For example, in a 20-kg dog, with a plasma volume of about 920 mL and a PCV of 0.40 L/L, the calculated blood volume would be:

(920 × 1.0) ÷ (1.0 − 0.40)
or 920 ÷ 0.60 = 1,533.4 mL blood per 20 kg
(i.e., 1,533.4 ÷ 20 = 76.7 mL blood per kilogram)

Blood volume values for adult animals are about 50 mL per kilogram for pigs, 60 mL per kilogram for ruminants, 70 to 80 mL per kilogram for small animals, and 100 mL per kilogram for horses (Table 2–2). A corrective factor, which varies with the species, should be applied to raw PCV values to correct for trapped plasma.

TABLE 2–1 Representative Values for Plasma Volume in Animals

Animal	Plasma Volume (mL/kg)
Cat	46.5
Cow	36.5
Chicken	
Chick	87
Adult	46
Dog	49.8
Goat	54
Horse	
Saddle	52
Thoroughbred	62
Work	43
Pig	
Sucking	65
Weaned	47
Rat	29
Sheep	51

TABLE 2–2 Representative Values for Blood Volume in Animals

Animal	Blood Volume (mL/kg)
Cat	66.7
Chicken	
Chick	120–95
Adult	65
Cow	
Beef	57
Dairy	60
Dog	88
Goat	70
Horse	
Saddle	77.5
Thoroughbred	107.5
Work	67.5
Pig	
Sucking	100–70
Weaned	70–35
Rat	45
Rabbit	67.5
Sheep	60

COMPOSITION OF BODY FLUIDS

Major components of plasma, interstitial fluid, and ICF are expressed in millimoles per liter (mmol/L) or micromoles per liter (μmol/L) in preference to milliequivalents per liter (mEq/L) as an expression of concentration. The index of osmotic effect is stated in milliosmoles per liter (mOsm/L). In terms of mass, nonelectrolytes and protein particles are larger than ions. Large particles account for 60 percent of the mass of constituents dissolved in the interstitial fluid, for 90 percent of those in plasma, and for 97 percent of those in ICF (Fig. 2–2). The mass per volume of fluid of nondiffusible particles has little importance, since a molecule of protein such as albumin (70,000 daltons) has the same osmotic action as a molecule of glucose (180 daltons).

ICF contains large quantities of potassium and phosphate, and moderate amounts of magnesium and sulfate. It stores large amounts of proteins, four times as much as the plasma, but it is poor in sodium and chloride and is almost without calcium.

Both interstitial fluid and plasma hold large amounts of sodium and chloride and reasonably large quantities of bicarbonate but little potassium, calcium, magnesium, phosphate, sulfate, and organic anions. Plasma contains four times more nondiffusible ions (7.3 g protein) than interstitial fluid (1.8 g).

Total osmotic pressure is identical in the ICF and interstitial fluids of the body—about 300 mOsm per liter, or more exactly 280 mOsm per liter after correction for intermolecular attraction. A small (1.5 mOsm per liter) but important additional osmotic pressure is present in the blood plasma, or

intravascular ECF. In the ECFs (interstitial and plasma), 80 percent of the total osmotic pressure is due to sodium and chloride ions. In the ICF 50 percent of the total osmotic pressure depends on potassium ions (Fig. 2–3).

The *oncotic pressure* of blood plasma, the small additional osmotic pressure of 1.5 mOsm per liter found in the intravascular ECF, is due to the plasma proteins. It is also called *colloid osmotic pressure* and is different from total osmotic pressure. On the basis that 1 mOsm per liter gives an osmotic pressure of 17.0 mm Hg, its value can be calculated as 26 mm Hg. In the body fluids, oncotic pressure represents 1/200 of the total osmotic pressure of all the dissolved substances exerting an osmotic pressure at the cell membrane. Even if it is only a weak osmotic force, oncotic pressure plays a very important role in the maintenance of plasma and interstitial fluid volumes. A nondiffusible molecule reduces the net diffusion of water (osmosis). The osmotic pressure at the capillary membrane, a force opposite to net water diffusion, is thus related to the concentration of nondiffusible molecules.

Osmotic Equilibrium in Body Fluids

The tremendous osmotic pressures at equilibrium on each side of the cell membrane displace water and diffusible particles at the slightest osmolal upset. The general concept is that at equilibrium both ICFs and ECFs reach identical osmolality.

When a cell is exposed to a hypoosmolal solution, net water diffusion (osmosis) occurs from the outside to within the cell. At the same time, particles move from the cytoplasmic to the extracytoplasmic side of the membrane and increase the osmolality of the ECF. The cell becomes dilated and the ICF diluted until osmolal equilibrium is attained (Fig. 2–4).

Conversely, when the cell is placed in a hyperosmolal fluid, water is displaced from the cell, and particles from the ECF invade the cytoplasm. At equilibrium, the process leaves the cell smaller (crenated) and the ICF more concentrated.

Osmometry

Osmotic pressure can be determined with an instrument (cryoscope, osmometer) that measures precisely (±0.001° C) the freezing point (i.e., the change from a liquid to a solid) in supercooled biological fluids. One mOsm per liter water lowers the freezing point by 1.858 millidegrees C and increases osmotic pressure by 17 mm Hg. By common usage, osmotic pressure is directly proportional to the freezing point.

An accepted physiological convention qualifies a fluid as isotonic, hypertonic, or hypotonic to plasma according to its effect on erythrocyte size. An *isotonic* fluid (osmolality approximating 9 g sodium chloride per liter), often called a physiological solution, does not change the volume of erythrocytes. A *hypertonic* fluid decreases the size of erythrocytes, and a *hypotonic* fluid increases the size of

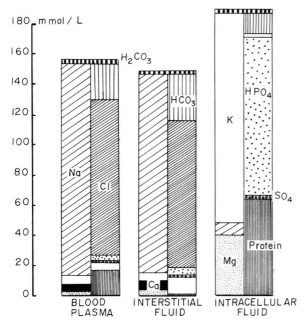

Figure 2–2 Histogram of general concentrations of substances found in plasma, in interstitial fluid, and in intracellular fluid (concentrations are expressed in milli*moles* per liter).

CONSTITUENTS
mOsm/L

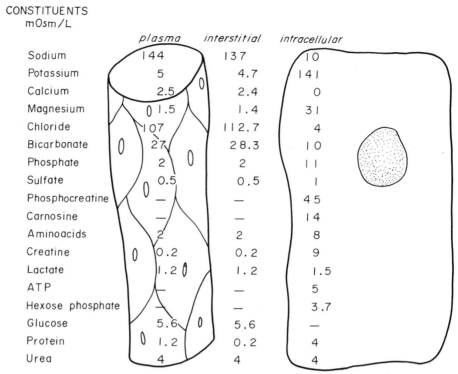

	plasma	interstitial	intracellular
Sodium	144	137	10
Potassium	5	4.7	141
Calcium	2.5	2.4	0
Magnesium	1.5	1.4	31
Chloride	107	112.7	4
Bicarbonate	27	28.3	10
Phosphate	2	2	11
Sulfate	0.5	0.5	1
Phosphocreatine	—	—	45
Carnosine	—	—	14
Aminoacids	2	2	8
Creatine	0.2	0.2	9
Lactate	1.2	1.2	1.5
ATP	—	—	5
Hexose phosphate	—	—	3.7
Glucose	5.6	5.6	—
Protein	1.2	0.2	4
Urea	4	4	4

Figure 2–3 Conceptual concentrations of the constituents of body fluids (plasma, interstitial fluid, and intracellular fluid, with milli-*osmoles* per liter as an expression of osmotic pressure).

erythrocytes. A very hypotonic fluid not only dilates but ruptures erythrocytes, a process called *hemolysis*. The liberated water-soluble protein, hemoglobin, colors the fluid red.

In heparinized blood, minimal and maximal individual resistance (*fragility of erythrocytes*) can be evaluated with a battery of saline solutions of different strengths (0.0 to 0.9 percent sodium chloride). Aliquots of 0.1 mL blood gently shaken with 2 mL of each test solution and centrifuged after 10 minutes are examined for hemolysis. Normally, hemolysis begins in 0.6 percent sodium chloride concentration and is complete at 0.2 percent (Fig. 2–5).

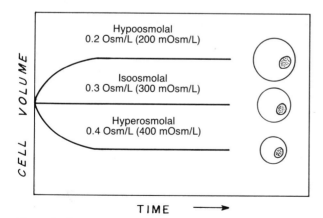

Figure 2–4 Cellular volume variation according to the hypo-, iso-, and hyperosmolality of the surrounding fluids.

CHANGES IN VOLUMES AND COMPOSITION OF BODY FLUIDS

Rapid, equivalent, and bidirectional exchanges of water and electrolytes occur between plasma, interstitial, and intracellular fluids. Volumes and composition of body fluids remain unchanged during these passive transfers. Simultaneously, also without affecting the volumes of the body fluids, unidirectional net flow of small molecules occurs (1) from plasma to interstitial and then to intracellular fluid, for substances useful to cells, such as glucose, and (2) from cells to interstitial fluid and then to plasma, for catabolic products such as carbon dioxide. Net changes in body fluid volumes are evaluated according to two fundamental principles: (1) osmolality of ICF and ECF is altered for only a few minutes after an upset in either of the fluid compartments; and (2) osmolalities due to particles in each liquid are unchanged unless an osmotic substance crosses the cell membrane or is lost or gained by one of the fluids. Volumes of ECF and ICF are modified by ingestion or intravenous infusion of water or electrolytes, dehydration, or excessive sweat.

Ingestion or Injection of Water

ECF becomes hypotonic after water is ingested or injected into the body. In a few minutes, by osmosis, this water reaches the cytoplasm, dilates the cells, and equally dilutes the ECF and ICF. The theoretical effects of giving 10 L of water to a 70-kg pig can be calculated (Table 2–3).

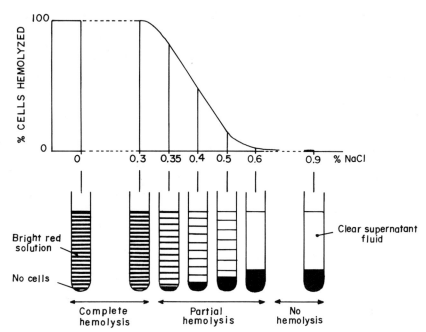

Figure 2–5 The fragility or resistance of erythrocytes to hemolysis. The percentage of lysed erythrocytes increases as the sodium chloride (NaCl) solution becomes more hypotonic. Hemolysis of normal red cells starts at 0.5 percent NaCl (minimal resistance, or maximal fragility) and is complete by 0.3 percent NaCl (maximal resistance, or minimal fragility).

Addition of Hypertonic Solution

A hypertonic solution, administered orally or injected, raises the osmolality of the ECF and moves water from the interstitial fluid to the plasma and from the cell to the interstitial fluid. The process is best illustrated by an example in which 2 L of 10 percent glucose ($100 g \div 180 g \times 2 L \times 1,000$ mOsm/L or 1,111 mOsm) is given intravenously to a 70-kg pig (Table 2–4). Preinjection fluid volumes are 39.9 L ($70 \times 57\%$) for total fluids, 15.4 L ($70 \times 22\%$) for ECF, and 24.5 L ($39.9 - 15.4$ L) for ICF.

From these calculations, it can be seen that the transient increase in extracellular volume ($20.95 - 15.4 = 5.55$ L) is made at the expense of 3.55 L ($24.5 - 20.95 = 3.55$ L) of intracellular water.

Dehydration in an Animal Body

Dehydration (i.e., loss of water from ICF and ECF) is a serious problem in disorders of the alimentary, respiratory, and urinary systems. Anorexia, excessive insensible evaporation (skin and lungs), or diuresis reduces ECF, but almost immediately intracellular water passes outside the cell to equilibrate osmolalities. These changes are the reverse of those seen above after water administration.

TABLE 2–3 Theoretical Effects of Oral Administration of 10 L Water to a 70-kg Pig

Fluid	Initial State	Immediate Effect	At Equilibrium
Total*			
Volume (L)	39.9	49.9	49.9
Osmolality (mOsm/L)	300	?	239.9
Global osmoles (mOsm)	11,970	11,970	11,970
Extracellular†			
Volume (L)	15.4	25.4	19.3
Osmolality (mOsm/L)	300	181	239.9
Global osmoles (mOsm)	4,620	4,620	4,630
Intracellular‡			
Volume (L)	24.5	24.5	30.6
Osmolality (mOsm/L)	300	300	239.9
Global osmoles	7,350	7,350	7,340.9

* Total water: $70 \times 57\% = 39.9$ L
† Extracellular water: $70 \times 22\% = 15.4$ L
‡ Intracellular water: $39.9 - 15.4 = 24.5$L

TABLE 2–4 Theoretical Effects of Intravenous Administration of 2 L of 10 Percent Glucose (Hypertonic) to a 70-kg Pig

Fluid	Preinjection	Postinjection	Equilibrium
Total			
Volume (L)	39.9	41	41.9
Osmolality (mOsm/L)	300	?	311
Global osmoles (mOsm)	11,920	13,031	13,031
Extracellular			
Volume (L)	15.4	17.4	20.95
Osmolality (mOsm/L)	300	329.4	311
Global osmoles (mOsm)	4,620	5,731	6,515.5
Intracellular			
Volume (L)	24.5	24.5	20.95
Osmolality (mOsm/L)	300	300	311
Global osmoles (mOsm)	7,350	7,350	6,515.5

The degree of dehydration of an animal is assessed by physical examination of elasticity of a skin fold, depth of the eyes in the skull, and moisture and temperature of the oral mucosa. Slight dehydration (5 percent of body mass) is mostly marked by an inelastic skin fold (5 seconds is required for a fold of skin to return to normal), but the eyes are not sunken and the oral mucosa is moist and warm. In moderate dehydration (7 to 8%), a skin fold persists for between 5 and 10 seconds, the eyes are sunken in the orbit, and the oral mucosa is sticky. Severe dehydration (>10%) is signaled by a skin fold lasting more than 10 seconds, by very sunken and softened eyes, and by a dry and cold oral mucosa.

Excessive Loss of Electrolytes

Simple sodium chloride deficiency can result from excessive sweating, a syndrome seen in racehorses in hot climates. The effects on body fluids are similar to those of administration of water: swelling or dilation of cells, and dilution of ECF and ICF.

Vomiting also leads to a loss of water, sodium, chloride, and some hydrogen, all components of gastric secretions. Diarrhea (an increase in fecal water excretion) results from a disruption of the secretion-absorption balance in the gut. The secretion processes overwhelm the absorption capacity of the large intestine and cause an excessive loss of anions (chloride and bicarbonate), cations (potassium), and water in the feces. The net result is a loss of electrolytes from the ECF, which becomes hypotonic and hypovolemic. Cells swell as fluid flows into them and further decreases extracellular volume.

DYNAMICS OF EXTRACELLULAR FLUIDS

Continuous transfer of particles occurs between the various portions of the ECFs, but the volumes of plasma and interstitial fluid remain constant. This section deals with the dynamics of these exchanges and the mechanisms of the microcirculations that control volumes of plasma and lymph.

Microcirculation of Blood

The structures for the microcirculation of blood are arterioles, metarterioles, capillaries, venules, muscular venules, and arteriolovenular shunts. The capillaries, the smallest vessels, have a diameter about the size of erythrocytes (6 to 7 μm). At any moment, at least 5 percent of the blood volume is in the 10^9 capillaries of the animal organism. The number of capillaries is not identical for all tissues. The mean number of capillaries is approximately 1,400 per cubic millimeter or gram of average tissue; it can be only 300 to 1,200 per cubic millimeter in skeletal muscle and may reach 2,000 to 2,500 per cubic millimeter in heart, kidney, brain, and endocrine or exocrine glands. The surface of an animal at rest

represents about 30 mm² per cubic millimeter or gram of tissue. During exercise, this surface can increase three- or fourfold. The capillaries act as areas for exchange of particles (ions and molecules) between plasma and interstitial fluid, through diffusion operations mostly, and through filtration (ultrafiltration in the glomeruli of the kidney).

Physiological Anatomy of Blood Vessels

Arterioles subdivide gradually into metarterioles (30 μm in diameter) and capillaries (8 to 12 μm), which converge into venules (12 to 25 μm), and the latter into muscular venules (30 to 60 μm). A shunt, or thoroughfare vessel, between arteriole and venule is present and can short-circuit blood from the capillary bed (Fig. 2–6). The mean length of a capillary is about 0.1 mm but varies owing to branching and interconnection.

Vasomotion (i.e., vasodilation or vasoconstriction) at metarterioles and muscular venules is under the control of the craniosacral (parasympathetic) part of the autonomic nervous system and of humoral agents (e.g., histamine and bradykinin). In resting tissues, blood flows mostly through the thoroughfare vessels, and most capillaries are collapsed. Oxygen autoregulates the perfusion in tissues: a deficiency causes dilation, whereas abundance results in collapse.

Vasodilation and vasoconstriction account for the variations in the number of capillaries perfused during a unit of time and for changes in the perfusion volume in a given capillary. Many capillaries may be perfused simultaneously in tissues that require fast metabolic regulations (heart, muscles, glands) and in those that must adjust rapidly to the needs of the organisms (gastrointestinal tract, kidney). In a given capillary, vasomotion can create successive periods of dilation and collapse (Fig. 2–7). Circulation of blood in the capillaries is thus intermittent and not continuous.

In the microcirculation, blood flows slowly (0.7 cm per second) in an almost nonpulsatile manner except at the

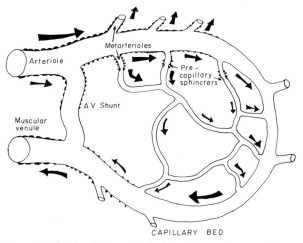

Figure 2–6 Terminal vascular bed showing arteriovenous shunt, precapillary sphincters, and other vessels with vasoconstrictive ability.

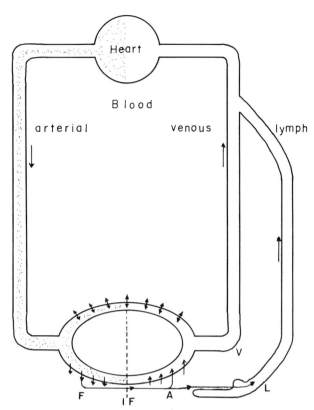

Figure 2–7 General pattern for the return to the heart of both blood and lymph. F, filtration; IF, inhibition of filtration; A, reabsorption into venules (*V*) and lymphatics (*L*).

arteriole. Transit time of blood in capillaries, from the arteriolar end to the venular end, is about 1.2 seconds. Contraction and relaxation of precapillary sphincters account for the sluggish stop-and-go movement of capillary blood flow. The hydrostatic pressure associated with cardiac action decreases from 45 mm Hg in the arterioles to 30 mm Hg in the capillaries and is only 15 mm Hg in the venules. Intravascular pressure is lower than 10 mm Hg in liver capillaries and higher than 80 mm Hg in the capillaries of the renal glomeruli. The hydrostatic pressure in the interstitial fluid is negligible.

Intravascular hydrostatic pressure is the driving force responsible for filtration through the intercellular cement substance (calcium proteinate) of the thin capillary wall (1 μm). The capillary endothelial cement would have the same function as the channels or pores of membranes (i.e., to allow the passage of water and solutes from or to plasma and interstitial fluid; Fig. 2–8).

Exchanges Between Blood Plasma and Interstitial Fluid

Capillary walls seem to have two types of transport systems, one for "small" molecules and another for "large" ones. Very small solutes, including small ions and most

metabolites, readily pass through small pores, which vary in size but have an average radius of about 3 nm. The severely restricted transfer of large molecules, i.e., those exceeding 20,000 daltons, enables them to exert an osmotic force across the capillary wall to maintain fluid balance. These larger molecules must use a different system that either involves larger pores, which are very few per surface unit, or an active transport via cytoplasmic vesicles.

Owing to the tight junctions between the cells, the capillary endothelium behaves like a membrane permeable to small particles but impermeable to large and abundant protein particles of the intravascular ECF. These plasma proteins exert an osmotic pressure of about 25 mm Hg (the *oncotic pressure,* or *colloid osmotic pressure*), which tends to cause fluid movement from the extravascular to the intravascular spaces. Only a very small amount of proteins (1.5 g per 100 mL in muscles, 2 g per 100 mL subcutaneously, 4 g per 100 mL in the gut, 6 g per 100 mL in the liver) cross the capillary wall by vesicular transport, reach the interstitial fluid, and enter the lymph. Other substances (oxygen, glucose, carbon dioxide) pass through the epithelial wall by diffusion and by filtration.

Diffusion, which occurs in both directions (outward from the capillaries: water, oxygen, glucose; into the capillaries: water, carbon dioxide) across the capillary endothelium, is quantitatively more important. Total water diffusion can be 15,000 times the total filtration of water (i.e., 240,000 mL per minute versus 16 mL per minute). Diffusion is the result of kinetic motion of molecules. In a fluid, because collisions are more frequent when the number of like particles is higher, substances diffuse down their concentration gradient, i.e., in the direction of the fluid containing a smaller number of particles. If the particles encounter a semipermeable membrane (with pores), their movement is impeded according to the sizes of the particles and of the pores.

FICK (1855) defined the phenomenon of diffusion in an equation, which states that the rate of linear diffusion of quantity, n, in time, t, or (dn/dt), is equal to the concentration gradient, dc/dx (where c is concentration, and x is direction) multiplied by the specific diffusion coefficient of the substance, D, in cm²/sec, and the cross-sectional area A:

$$dn/dt = (dc/dx)\ DA$$

The free diffusion coefficient is inversely proportional to the square root of its molecular mass.

Lipid-soluble substances can diffuse through the entire area of the capillary wall surface, but lipid-insoluble substances can only pass through the aqueous channels of intercellular pores. The radial size of these pores is in the range of 3 to 4.5 nm.

LANDIS, PAPPENHEIMER, and RENKIN have characterized the restricted diffusion of lipid-soluble molecules from the capillary beds of perfused cat hind limbs. The diffusion of solutes with a mass up to 10,000 daltons or so is only moderately restricted. Solutes with masses above 10,000 daltons are severely restricted in their diffusion.

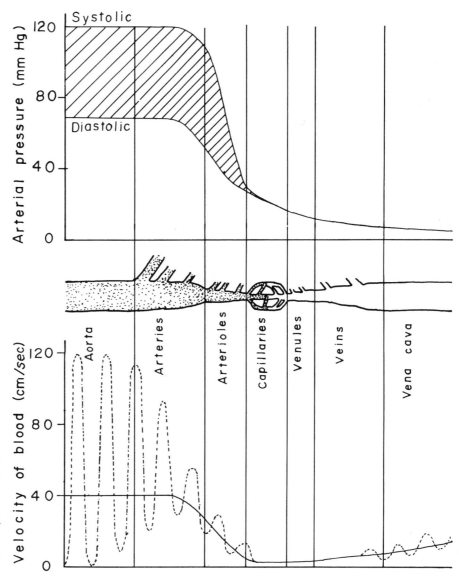

Figure 2–8 Changes in hydrostatic pressure and flow as blood progresses through the systemic circulation. The mean velocity fluctuates in the arteries and arterioles during cardiac systole and diastole. In the capillaries, the flow of blood is constant. In the large veins, blood flows with some slight fluctuations.

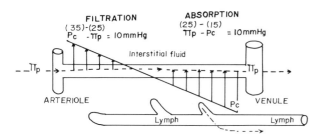

Figure 2–9 Transfers from or into the capillary bed due to progressive lowering of the hydrostatic pressure (P_c) from the arteriolar (35 mm Hg) to the venular (15 mm Hg) ends. The oncotic pressure (Π_p) remains constant (25 mm Hg).

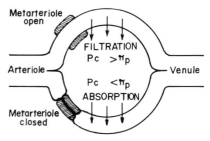

Figure 2–10 Filtration versus osmotic absorption according to perfusion or collapse in the capillary circulation by vasoconstriction of metarterioles.

Filtration is a process that forces fluid through a permeable membrane, or endothelium, because of a difference of pressure between the two sides. Filtration across capillary walls occurs when the hydrostatic pressure in the vessels is greater than that in the interstitial fluid. This hydrostatic pressure gradient must also be greater than any inwardly directed osmotic force (oncotic pressure) that opposes filtration.

Since the oncotic pressure of plasma (Π_p), or the net osmotic pressure of the plasma proteins (colloids), is opposed to the hydrostatic pressure of blood plasma (P_p), transfers occur according to the algebraic sum of these forces. At the arteriolar end of capillaries, *filtration* occurs as hydrostatic pressure of blood in capillaries (P_c) exceeds Π_p. Conversely, at the venular end, as Π_p exceeds P_c, there is *absorption*.

Theoretically, four pressures are implicated in the transfer of water and particles of solutes (Fig. 2–9): hydrostatic pressure of blood in the capillaries (P_c), hydrostatic pressure of interstitial fluid (P_{int}), oncotic pressure of plasma proteins (Π_p), and oncotic pressure of interstitial fluid (Π_{int}):

$$(P_c - P_{int}) - (\Pi_p - \Pi_{int})$$

As P_{int} and Π_{int} are negligible, they are usually disregarded as factors influencing the normal exchanges of water and particles of solutes in most tissues. It should be noted that P_{int} amounts to 30 mm Hg in the kidney. Also, Π_{int} can be increased considerably by local production of bradykinin, histamine, and substance P, which make the capillary wall more permeable to proteins. Filtration of 0.5 percent of the plasma in capillaries occurs when P_c exceeds Π_p. Reabsorption by osmosis happens at the venular end, as Π_p exceeds P_c (Fig. 2–10).

Compared with total osmotic pressure of plasma (about 7.5 atmospheres, or $760 \times 7.5 = 5,700$ mm Hg), plasma oncotic pressure, or colloid osmotic pressure, is very small (only 25 mm Hg). Plasma proteins do not participate equally in the production of oncotic pressure. The smaller albumin molecules (70,000 daltons) contribute more particles per unit of mass than the larger globulin molecules (100,000 to 450,000 daltons).

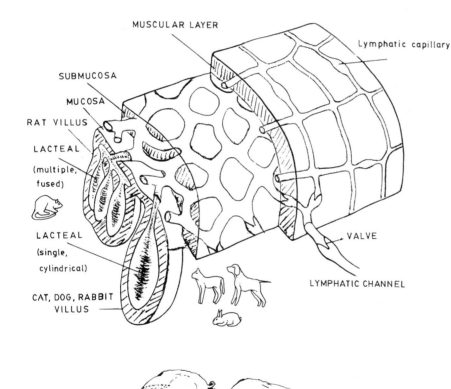

Figure 2–11 **A,** Illustration of the independent lacteal-mucosal-submucosal and myenteric lymphatic systems, which converge into larger lymphatic vessels containing valves. **B,** Cutaneous projection of the areas where interstitial fluid drains into the thoracic lymph duct and into the right lymph duct.

Influence of Vasomotion on Blood Hydrostatic and Plasma Oncotic Pressures

Vasomotion at the metarterioles controls the volume of blood perfused into the capillaries and also the occurrence of either filtration or absorption in the circuit. In an open blood capillary, the hydrostatic pressure, which is higher than the oncotic pressure ($P_c = 35 > \Pi_p = 25$), causes filtration to occur. Oncotic pressure is nearly at a constant value in the entire capillary, but in a collapsed capillary it is higher than the hydrostatic pressure ($P_c = 15 < \Pi_p = 25$), and it produces absorption.

Venular capillaries have 50 percent more surface for maximal absorption. A volume of about 0.4 to 0.8 mL per liter of fluid filtered into the interstitial liquid is not absorbed and must be returned to the blood by the lymphatic system. About 30 percent of the total circulating plasma proteins, mostly leaked in the interstitial fluid of the intestine and liver, are reabsorbed via the lymphatics. Blood and lymph circulate in separate closed systems of conduits from the heart to the tissues and back to the heart. Some of the interstitial fluid enters the lymphatics to return ultimately to the blood.

Lymphatic System

Lymph

The lymphatic vessels carry lymph, a fluid different from tissue fluid. Lymph is transparent or slightly opalescent, contains a clear portion, a varying number of leukocytes, chiefly lymphocytes, and a few erythrocytes. It has less serum globulin, albumin, and fibrinogen than blood but more water, electrolytes, and sugar. Its plasma protein content is variable according to the tissue drained: 15 percent of plasma protein level in muscles and 30, 50, and 80 percent, respectively, in pulmonary, intestinal, and hepatic lymph. It clots at a much slower rate than blood, releasing lymph serum. During the postprandial period of digestion, lymph from the digestive system (chyle) has a high fat content (chylomicrons, alpha-lipoproteins in dogs and cats, beta-lipoprotein in rabbits).

The volume of lymph returned to the bloodstream is more abundant in ruminants than in carnivores. Generally, the daily volume of lymph brought back into the general circulation is nearly equal to the plasma volume. In a 15-kg dog a large infusion of fluid (2 L) has a lymphagogic effect, increasing the amount of lymph tenfold. As much as 50 percent of the plasma protein may be recovered by lymph. Assuming that thoracic duct lymph contains 5 g of protein per liter and that lymph flow is about 4 L per day, some 10 to 20 g of plasma protein would be reabsorbed daily.

On its return to blood, lymph passes through at least one lymph node, which adds lymphocytes and stops xenobiotic substances and foreign organisms that may have gained access to interstitial fluid. Lymph nodes are absent in fowl and pigeons, which have lymphoid tissue in several organs to compensate (bone marrow, bursa of Fabricius, spleen, thymus).

Lymph Channels

Blind-ended lymph capillaries (15 to 25 μm) are about twice the diameter of blood capillaries. Lymph capillary walls are thinner and more porous to proteins than blood capillaries and more able to mop up large proteins and dry up the interstitial space or tissue. In the intestine, independent systems of lymphatic capillaries exist in the lacteal-mucosal-submucosal and in the muscle layers. Each villus of the small intestine has a single cylindrical lacteal (cats, dogs, rabbits) or several lacteals (rats). Lymphatic capillaries from each independent system converge to form larger lymphatic vessels, which join the great veins in the cervicothoracic area. These larger lymphatic vessels have smooth muscles in their wall, have numerous one-way valves, and penetrate one or more lymph nodes. Interstitial space or tissue caudad to the diaphragm and the left side of an animal's body drains into the thoracic lymph duct (on convex surface of the liver); the rest of the body (right side of the head, neck and thorax, and right foreleg) is served by the right lymph duct (Fig. 2–11).

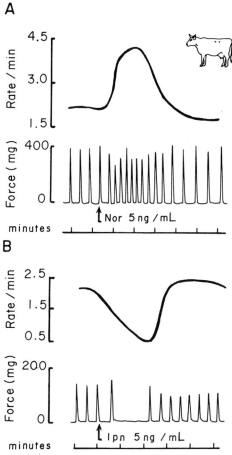

Figure 2–12 Intrinsic rate and strength of bovine smooth muscle in lymphatics in vitro. **A**, Norepinephrine (*Nor*; 5 ng per milliliter) increases the rate of contraction and slightly decreases the strength of smooth muscles in bovine lymphatics. **B**, Isoproterenol (*Ipn*; 5 ng per milliliter) lowers the rate and weakens the intrinsic contractions of bovine lymphatics.

Flow of Lymph

The flow of lymph is primarily due to the combined action of *intrinsic* (*essential*) and *extrinsic* (*accessory*) factors. Intrinsic factors are one-way valves and rhythmic myogenic activity of smooth muscles in the walls of the lymph vessels. In sheep, intrinsic pulsatile pressure patterns occur in all lymphatics. Intrinsic mechanisms for lymph transport are also a normal feature of bovine mesenteric lymphatics. On isolated bovine lymphatics, norepinephrine (alpha-receptor agonist) increases the rate but decreases the strength of smooth muscle activity, whereas isoproterenol (beta-receptor agonist) slows the frequency of the rhythmic smooth muscle contractions (Fig. 2–12).

Accessory (extrinsic) factors that act to compress the lymph channels are tissue pressure (muscles), arterial pulsation, and intraabdominal and intrathoracic pressure variations associated with respiration. Extrinsic factors appear to be important in the propulsion of lymph in the dog's thoracic duct. With exercise, lymph flow increases by 3 to 14 times.

Pressure inside the lymph vessels pulsates (2 to 20 per minute) from a few millimeters to 25 cm water, and the frequency of the pulsations increases with the pressure. At rest, lymph pressure usually approximates venous pressure, and it fluctuates with respiration and heart action (2 to 3 cm water). A differential pressure of 1 to 2 cm water exists at each valve. In a resting dog, lymph pressure in the thoracic duct is about 10 cm water and can be as high as 15 cm water; in the leg, it varies from 3 to 12 cm water (higher near the toe).

The homeostatic functions of the lymphatic system are threefold: (1) substances (proteins, macromolecules) leaked out of blood capillaries and not reabsorbed into the bloodstream at the venular end are reabsorbed to prevent their osmotic effect and a rise in interstitial pressure; (2) materials (proteins, lipids) that have entered the interstitial fluid in the liver, intestine, and kidneys are transported into the bloodstream; (3) large proteins (enzymes) such as lipase and histaminase are transferred from their cells of origin into the general circulation.

Edema

Edema is an abnormal increase in interstitial fluid volume. It may result from (1) increased P_c due to arteriolar dilation, venular constriction, or increased venous pressure (heart failure, incompetent valves, venous obstruction, effect of gravity, increase of total extracellular volume); (2) decreased Π_p because of decreased plasma protein level (starvation edema) or accumulation of osmotically active substances in the interstitial fluid; (3) increased blood capillary permeability caused by histamine, bradykinin, or substance P; or (4) inadequate lymph flow.

Lactation in cows and ewes increases the mammary flow rate of blood, interstitial fluid, and lymph. As gestation usually proceeds during lactation, the mass of the fetus on the abdominal floor gradually compresses the afferent lymph vessel where it leaves the inguinal canal, causing edema. Also, in heifers with incompletely developed mammary veins, edema of the udder results from inadequate venous return and inability of the lymphatics to remove the large amounts of interstitial fluid that form at this time.

CHAPTER 3

FUNDAMENTAL PROPERTIES OF LIVING ORGANISMS—HOMEOSTASIS

The cells of tissues and organs have to perform one or several specific functions. It is essential to understand the exchanges between the cells and their liquid environment before attempting to study the functions of organs.

HOMEOSTASIS AND EXTRACELLULAR FLUID

About 55 to 60 percent, or nearly two-thirds, of the total mass of an animal is water (Fig. 3–1), which is mostly inside the cell, the *intracellular fluid* (ICF). About one-third of the total body water is distributed in the spaces between cells and the transcellular compartment; this is the *extracellular fluid* (ECF). The French physiologist Claude Bernard (1813–1878) first conceived of the ECF as the immediate environment of living cells. In this concept, the ECF is used as an intermediary source of their nutrients and as a receptacle for their waste products. The survival of cells requires that the composition of ECF remain within limits. Bernard postulated that the animal must have mechanisms to maintain relatively constant the composition of this ECF or internal environment, a concept he termed *"la fixité du milieu intérieur."*

Important variations in the components of ECF must be avoided. Any cell of the organism is able to survive in vitro only if it is suspended in a liquid medium that has approximately the components and physical conditions of the ECF (i.e., a physiologic solution).

Claude Bernard tested objectively the validity of the dry mouth theory of thirst by analyzing the urge to drink in animals. In his *Leçons de physiologie expérimentale appliquées à la médecine"* (1856), he described experiments in the horse and the dog which led him to prove that oral-pharyngeal dryness is not the ultimate cause of thirst. He showed that the dehydrated horse or dog with an open esophageal (horse) or gastric (dog) fistula continues to drink until completely exhausted, although its mouth and throat are bathed with water continuously drained out during drinking. When the fistula is closed, the ingested water is absorbed, and thirst is rapidly quenched.

The importance of thirst as one of a series of regulatory mechanisms tending to preserve *la fixité du milieu intérieur* received much attention later, after it had been shown that "osmoreceptors" in the brain regulate the intimate relation that exists between the urge to drink and the osmolality of the internal environment.

Most of the organs contribute to the control of one or many constituents of ECF. An American physiologist, Walter Bradford Cannon (1871–1945), coined the term *homeostasis* for the maintenance of constant conditions in the ECF or internal environment by the integrated actions of the various organs of an animal.

CONCEPT OF HOMEOSTASIS IN LIVING ANIMALS

The concept of homeostasis implies that the performance of organs depends on the operation of their individual cells, which in turn requires a relatively stable ECF. The organs and their cells perform specific roles to help maintain homeostasis, or a constant internal environment. A *dynamic state* of homeostasis, seen in young animals during growth when the mass of animals and the relative importance of some organs increase at a characteristic rate for the species, is called *homeorrhesis*. A *steady state* of homeostasis results from the work of the different systems of organs with specific functions in the animal (e.g., respiratory, circulatory, digestive, urinary, endocrine, and nervous).

The *respiratory system* brings oxygen from the environment into the alveolar air and then from the alveoli into the blood for transport to other parts of the ECF. Thus the proper level of oxygen is supplied to cells for their activity. Carbon dioxide, produced continuously by cells, is taken up by the ECF and returned to the alveoli via the venous blood. The lungs also constantly eliminate carbon dioxide from alveolar air into the expired air.

The *circulatory system* carries blood, its plasma that is a part of the ECF, throughout the animal organism to exchange water and dissolved substances between blood and parts of the ECF adjacent to cells, and to keep the ECF in constant motion. At no time is a portion of the ECF isolated more than a few seconds to a minute without mixing itself with other ECF and undergoing diffusion or exchange.

The *digestive system* provides for absorption of nutrients and ions. After mechanical and chemical treatments, these substances are extracted from food, passed into the blood and/or lymph capillaries, and then carried to other parts of the ECF as nutrients for cells.

The *endocrine system* is usually associated with long-term adaptation. The endocrine system operates through hormones with endocrine, paracrine, or autocrine effects (Fig. 3–2). The endocrine system, which is regulated by negative feedback from the target cells, participates in reactions of the intermediary metabolism involved in production of enzymes for the conversion of nutrients and ions, their absorption from the intestine, and their utilization as nutrients of benefit to cells. Once the cells have used the metabolic

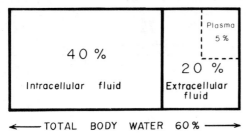

Figure 3-1 Distribution of total body water between the ICF (40 percent) and ECF (20 percent). Plasma is a compartment of ECF.

energy and structural molecules of these substances, the animal body deals with their residues. Some metabolites may be rejected by biliary secretion or excretion (biliary salts), with the possibility of subsequent reabsorption, thereby creating an enterohepatic cycle. Many residues in the blood plasma are directed to the *urinary system* for elimination.

Fundamentally, the *nervous system* provides immediate, short-term, rapid adaptation for protection of the internal environment (e.g., withdrawal reaction to pain) in its almost utopian constancy for survival of cells. The nervous system also enables the animal to touch, taste, smell, hear, and see,

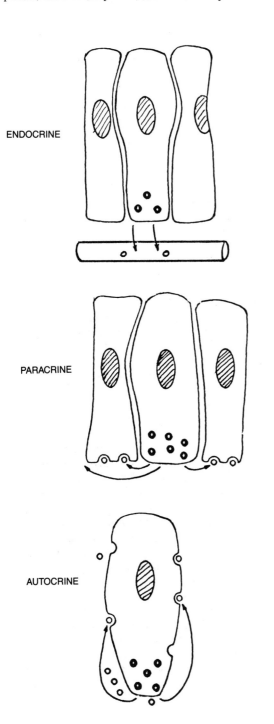

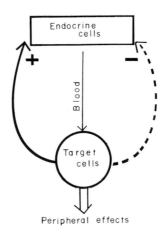

Figure 3-2 **A,** Possible types of effects of a hormone (e.g., somatostatin, or somatotropin-releasing inhibitory factor [SRIF]) produced in the hypothalamus, on distant target cells through plasma (endocrine effect), on neighboring cells (paracrine effect), and on the secretory cell itself (autocrine effect). **B,** Hormonal negative feedback from target cells, which influences the inhibition (———) or stimulation (———) of the secretion of a hormone by endocrine cells.

to guide the search for or selection of food, and to react to danger.

Innate nervous and endocrine mechanisms guide behavioral adaptations to the environment, leading to seasonal and circadian rhythms that involve neuroendocrine "clocks." Through the hypothalamus, a part of the nervous system that develops differently in male and female animals, the nervous and the endocrine systems are joined into the *neuroendocrine system*. This system produces chronobiologic changes in functions or behavior in response to seasonal modifications in temperature and daylight. Cycles of hormone output or production reappear at regular intervals. Reproductive or estrous cycles recur at seasonal, monthly, or weekly intervals. Circadian cycles are repeated at about 24-hour periods, whereas some nycthemeral cycles depend on succession of day and night. Some outputs of hormones are pulsatile, at nearly hourly intervals. Seasonal functional adjustments may be metabolic (lipid deposits in raccoons and bears, hibernation in squirrels, hyperthyroidism, and growth of hair) or behavioral (herd migration in nordic animals, such as caribous).

HOMEOSTATIC MECHANISMS

An important part of physiology deals with the regulatory mechanisms of homeostasis. The maintenance of the constancy of the internal environment requires the collaboration of all tissues, organs, and systems.

Over centuries, important parts of the concepts about physiological regulation have accumulated. *Hippocrates* (*ca* 460–*ca* 360 BC): living beings are self-maintaining, self-renewing, and self-repairing. *Aristotle* (384–322 BC): constituent structures serve special functions in securing continuity of the body. *Descartes* (1596–1650): irritations arouse responses both acquisitive and defensive that preserve the body. *Newton* (1642–1727): stability characterizes living systems as it does nonliving ones. *Lavoisier* (1743–1794): regulation consists in governed exchanges of substances. *Weber* (1795–1878): nerve impulses mediate regulatory activities. *Muller* (1801–1858): specific sense qualities supply the information to which responses follow.

For teaching purposes, the functions of the various systems of an animal's economy can be considered as units of the overall homeostatic mechanisms. Some of these homeostatic units are communications between cells, origin of substances in ECF, elimination of residues or metabolites from ECF, and transfer of ECF.

Communication Between Cells

Communication between cells requires (1) a message, (2) means to convey that message, (3) means to receive that message, and (4) means to understand and respond to that message. In general, the messages between cells are in the form of chemical substances (hormones, neurosecretions of neurotransmitter or neuropeptide, growth factors, negative growth factors or chalones). The chemical substances released from the signaling cells are transported to the recipient cells either through a fluid medium (e.g., synaptic space for neurotransmitters, bloodstream for hormones) or through direct physical contact (e.g., direct space-mediated diffusion). These messages are received by specialized membrane receptors, which activate some intracellular second messenger (nucleotides, calcium ions) mechanisms. In the nucleus, these second messengers cause synthesis of specific proteins.

Hormones are cellular secretions that may exert endocrine effects on remote target cells, paracrine effects on neighboring cells, or autocrine effects on the cell of origin itself (Fig. 3–2). On the basis of their composition, hormones can be classified as amines or amino acids, polypeptides or proteins, steroids, or prostaglandins.

Neurosecretions are produced by neurons to communicate over short distances (200 nm or less). Neurotransmitters are small molecules (e.g., glycine, glutamine, gamma-aminobutyric acid [GABA], norepinephrine, dopamine, acetylcholine) associated with neural tissues. Neuromodulators are polypeptides of various lengths (e.g., substance P, cholecystokinin [CCK], and vasoactive intestinal peptide [VIP]) that may be associated with nonneural tissues. Growth factors are peptides (e.g., erythropoietin, epithelial growth factor [EGF]) that influence cell (erythrocyte) and tissue growth by acting locally or on remote targets in the manner of hormones. Chalones act to reduce or suppress cell or tissue proliferation.

Between adjacent cells, direct chemical signals may be transmitted through special contact areas of the plasma membranes (e.g., tight junctions and gap junctions). In some epithelia (e.g., renal proximal tubules, intestine, and gallbladder) the tight junctions are permeable, or "leaky," to some substances, which can thus transfer from the apical to the basolateral aspects of the plasma membranes. At gap junctions, direct connection channels link adjacent lateral plasma membranes (e.g., smooth muscle cells, cardiac muscle cells) to propagate chemical signals, unless closed by excessive cytoplasmic calcium ions.

In an animal, coordination and integration of all cellular activities by intercellular communications from near or distant tissues or organs are provided by the nervous and endocrine systems. Neurons connected by nerve fibers to effectors (muscles, glands) allow rapid, almost immediate adjustments, which occur to protect the internal environment from sudden external or atmospheric changes (e.g., increase in blood supply in a rabbit's ear when swabbed with or dipped into warm water). As a general rule, neural mechanisms regulate muscular and secretory activities, whereas endocrine mechanisms complement the nervous system and control the rate of metabolic activities.

Major Differences Between Extra- and Intracellular Fluids

The compositions of the fluids inside and outside the cells differ greatly. ECF contains many sodium, chloride, and bicarbonate ions together with the major nutrients—

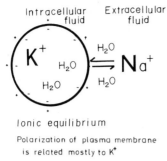

Intracellular fluid   Extracellular fluid

Ionic equilibrium

Polarization of plasma membrane
is related mostly to K⁺

Figure 3–3 Major cations in biologic fluids: potassium (K^+) is predominant inside the cell, whereas more sodium (Na^+) is present outside the cell. Mostly because of the levels of K^+_i (inside the cell) and of K^+_o (outside the cell), the plasma membrane is polarized as per Nernst equation (-60 mV $\times$ K_i/K_o). In the resting cell, the extracytoplasmic side of the plasma membrane is electropositive, and the cytoplasmic side is electronegative.

oxygen, glucose, fatty acids, and amino acids. It also transports carbon dioxide from the cells to the lungs and other cellular substances to the kidneys or liver to be excreted.

ICF holds a great quantity of potassium, magnesium, and phosphate ions but contains very few sodium and chloride ions (Fig. 3–3).

Origin of Substances in Extracellular Fluid

Nutrients reach the ECF through homeostatic mechanisms of the respiratory and the digestive, or gastrointestinal, systems, which are assisted by the striated muscles used for inspiration, prehension and mastication of food, and locomotion. The presence of oxygen in ECF results from alveolocapillary exchanges between alveolar air and venous blood in the perialveolar capillaries of the pulmonary (right heart) circulation.

A considerable portion (about 20 percent) of the peripheral arterial blood expelled from the left heart goes into the blood vessels of the digestive system. Gastrointestinal blood flow increases after feeding. This blood contributes to passage of water and substances into the digestive secretions (saliva, gastric, pancreatic, biliary, and intestinal juices), which are later almost entirely reabsorbed. Absorption of nutrients (hexoses, fatty acids, and amino acids) happens at the apical plasma membrane of cells (enterocytes) covering the villi of the small intestine. Once the nutrients have actively or passively crossed the basolateral plasma membrane of the enterocytes, they are channeled by portal vessels to the liver for chemical changes for use (catabolism) or storage (anabolism) (Fig. 3–4). Coincident with salivation, striated muscle activity is also involved during mastication of prehension, an important mechanical digestive process of herbivorous animals. In ruminants, an additional mastication of rumination (chewing the cud) must be considered an essential element for the liberation of nutrients from food (digestion). Considerable physical energy is expended during locomotion in search of herbage on pastures by herbivores and of prey by carnivores.

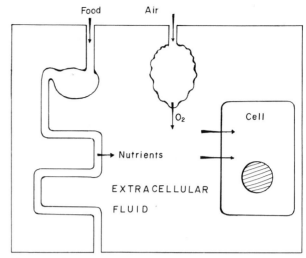

Food   Air

O_2

Cell

Nutrients

EXTRACELLULAR FLUID

Figure 3–4 Cell nutrition and oxygenation occur through the intermediary pathway of ECF.

Elimination of Substances from Extracellular Fluid

During metabolic processes, cells pour into the ECF substances that are unwanted (residues) or useless. Their elimination occurs through the combined efforts of various organs: lungs, kidneys, and liver. During their passage through the lungs, the red blood cells (erythrocytes) take up oxygen and unload carbon dioxide in exchange. This carbon dioxide, the most abundant residue of cell metabolism to enter the ECF, diffuses from the venous blood into alveolar air and is then expelled into atmospheric air during the expiratory phase of respiration. Arterial blood plasma passing through the kidneys undergoes glomerular ultrafiltra-

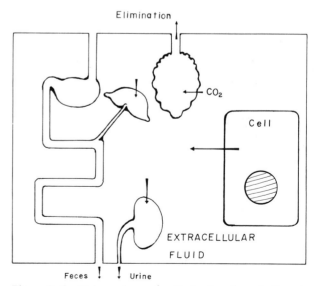

Elimination

CO_2

Cell

EXTRACELLULAR FLUID

Feces   Urine

Figure 3–5 Major pathways for elimination of metabolic residues and carbon dioxide resulting from catabolic activities in the cells.

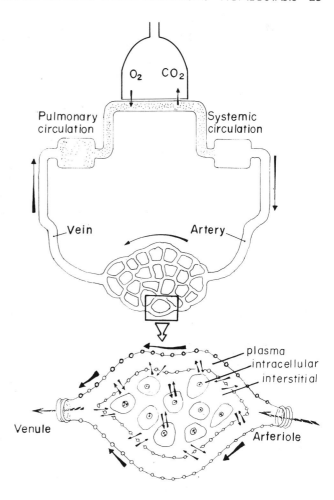

Figure 3–6   Intravascular transport of ECF occurs in two separate circuits, or circulations, where identical global blood flow is provided at different hydrostatic pressures. The arterial pressure in the systemic circulation is much higher (about five- to sevenfold) than in the pulmonary circulation. The contents of the ECF are modified in the pulmonary circulation (gain of oxygen, with loss of carbon dioxide) and at the periphery of the systemic circulation (gain of carbon dioxide and metabolites, with loss of oxygen and nutrients).

tion. Substances useless or superfluous to the cells of the organism are not reabsorbed, and some are even excreted or secreted by the tubular cells. Useful substances, such as glucose and amino acids, are entirely reabsorbed from the primary urine (glomerular filtrate) progressing in the tubules of the nephron. Recovery of water and ions varies according to endocrine homeostatic mechanisms (antidiuretic hormone [ADH], parathyroid hormone [PTH], and aldosterone). Biliary excretion of natural metabolites (bilirubin from hemoglobin of erythrocytes, residues from steroid hormones) or of xenobiotic substances (e.g., barbiturate, bromsulphalein) is also a homeostatic excretory mechanism (Fig. 3–5). Some of the components of bile (e.g., bile salts) are reabsorbed in the ileum and recirculated in a continuous biliary-enterohepatic cycle.

Transfer of Extracellular Fluid

The ECF of blood (plasma) reaches the various parts of the animal body in two phases (Fig. 3–6). The first trans-

port phase of the intravascular ECF is by circulation in the closed cardiovascular system. About 1 minute is required to pump the entire volume of blood (cells and plasma) into the peripheral vascular circuit. During physical exercise, the blood flow accelerates by a factor of up to five, depending on the severity of the exercise. An equivalent quantity of blood always circulates, at a lower hydrostatic pressure, in the pulmonary circuit, where blood plasma is relieved of some carbon dioxide while the red cells are replenished with oxygen.

The second phase of ECF transfer results from movement of blood plasma from the blood capillaries (intravascular) into the extravascular (intercellular, or interstitial) fluid. In a few seconds, as blood plasma traverses the porous capillaries, a continuous exchange (filtration-diffusion) of liquid is established between the intravascular and extravascular ECF. This constant mixing of ECF ensures a stable composition to the fluid surrounding cells and the elimination of carbon dioxide.

CHAPTER 4

MOVEMENT OF PARTICLES ACROSS PLASMA MEMBRANES

Homeostasis is maintained by avoiding sudden changes in the composition of the interstitial (intercellular) and intravascular (blood plasma) portions of the extracellular fluid (ECF). The plasma membranes of cells contribute to homeostasis by regulating the transfers of particles between the intracellular fluid (ICF) and the ECF. In cells grouped to form epithelial boundaries of the ECF, different mechanisms exist for passage to and fro of particles at the apical and basolateral parts of the plasma membrane. This chapter presents some functional characteristics of plasma membranes of cells in general and of apical and basolateral plasma membranes of some epithelial cells.

PLASMA MEMBRANE OF THE CELL

The plasma membrane separates ICF from ECF. It may be considered as an organ that supervises and operates the transport of substances into and out of cells, (i.e., from or into the ECF). It accomplishes this with electrochemical changes.

The characteristic structure of the cell membrane is of fundamental importance for understanding its more important dynamic functions. Some of these important functions are (1) constant bidirectional transfer in and out of cells to maintain cell health and prevent cell death; (2) ionic transfers to maintain a difference in electrical potentials between its inner and outer surfaces and to generate the membrane potentials; and (3) modulation of metabolic activity by means of hormone receptors on its outer surface.

Structure of Plasma Membranes

Plasma membranes, the envelopes of cells, are thin (7.5 to 10 nm), quasifluid, elastic structures. Their composition is largely of proteins (55 percent), lipids (42 percent: phospholipids 26 percent, cholesterol 13 percent, and others 3 percent), and carbohydrates (3 percent).

Lipid Barrier

The fundamental structure of biologic membranes is a lipid bilayer, which is a permeability barrier breached only with carriers. The lipids found in membranes are amphipathic; that is, one end of the molecule is hydrophobic (insoluble in water or lipophilic) and the other end is hydrophilic (water soluble or lipophobic). The phosphate radical of phospholipids and the hydroxyl radicals of cholesterol are hydrophilic and are described as being polar because they are capable of carrying an electric charge. The hydrophobic, or nonpolar, region consists of the hydrocarbon chain of fatty acids. In a typical plasma membrane lipid, two fatty acid molecules are chemically linked to a glycerol backbone, which is attached to a polar head consisting of phosphate, often carrying a charge, to form a phospholipid (Fig. 4–1).

The lipophilic portions (tails), attracted by each other, align themselves to form the center of the plasma membrane. The hydrophilic portions (heads) orient themselves at the inner (cytoplasmic) and outer (extracytoplasmic) surfaces of the plasma membranes (Fig. 4–2). The fluidity and the transport ability depend largely on structural changes determined by the relative proportion of unsaturated fatty acids.

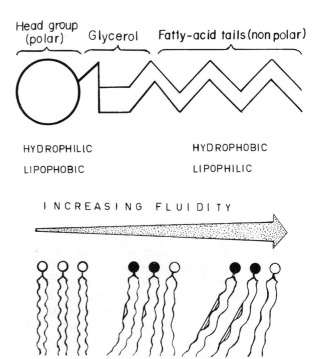

Figure 4–1 Top panel, Phospholipid structural unit of the plasma membrane with polar and nonpolar regions. The lipophilic nonpolar fatty acid tail region, physically incompatible with water-soluble substances, acts as a lipid barrier to such ions and molecules. The hydrophilic polar head region is on the inner and outer sides of the plasma membrane. **Lower panel,** The presence of unsaturated fatty acid tails (●) increases the fluidity of the plasma membrane and the rate of transfer across the membrane. Units with two double-bond fatty acids are more fluid than those with one double bond. Tails with saturated fatty acids (○) are less fluid and permeable.

EXTRACYTOPLASMIC

SURFACE

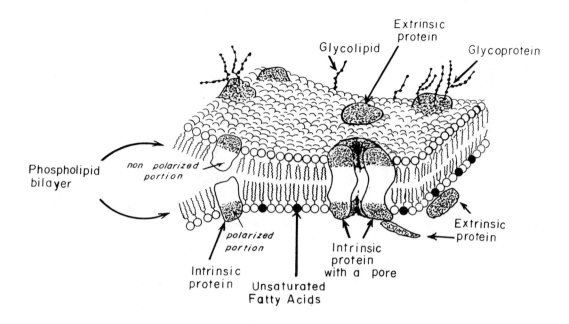

CYTOPLASMIC

SURFACE

Figure 4–2 Biphospholipid structural model of the plasma membrane, with more unsaturated fatty acids on the inner, or cytoplasmic, surface. The intrinsic proteins form pores or channels perforating the plasma membrane. The extrinsic proteins are on either the inner or the outer surface of the plasma membrane. Carbohydrates, always present on the outer surface, are bound to lipids (glycolipids) or proteins (glycoproteins).

Phospholipids with unsaturated fatty acids are predominant at the cytoplasmic surface of the plasma membrane and cause an asymmetry in the bilayer of lipids.

At physiological temperatures, in phospholipids consisting only of saturated fatty acids, the tails are aligned in a rigidly stacked crystalline array, which limits fluidity and transport rapidity in the plasma membranes. In phospholipids that have both saturated and unsaturated fatty acids, the alignment is less orderly and the plasma membrane is more fluid. The double bonds of unsaturated fatty acids give rise to structural deformations that interrupt the rigid order of tails of saturated fatty acids (see Fig. 4–1).

In plasma membranes rich in unsaturated fatty acids, transport can proceed at a rate 20 times faster than in membranes that have few unsaturated fatty acids. Predominance of unsaturated fatty acids in some plasma membranes is a necessary adjustment in cells of organs that normally function at lower temperatures. For example, the legs of a reindeer show a temperature gradient: the highest temperature is near the body, and the lowest near the hooves; to compensate for this situation, the cells near the hooves have membranes whose lipids are rich in unsaturated fatty acids. A homeostatic resistance to freezing is needed to keep blood flowing in arctic fishes in cold sea water. A special plasma lipoprotein, rich in unsaturated fatty acids, provides kinetic effects that lower the freezing point of blood in these fishes.

In this fluid mosaic model of the membrane, lateral interchange of phospholipids is frequent. Conversely, polar phospholipids at the cytoplasmic and extracytoplasmic surfaces can change places mutually (flip-flop) only on rare occasions (Fig. 4–3). The lipid barrier is impermeable to water and water-soluble substances. Lipid-soluble substances (oxygen, carbon dioxide, and alcohols) penetrate this central portion of cell membranes.

Proteins

Between 10 and 20 percent of the volume, or about 40 to 70 percent of dry mass, of cell membranes is made up of a variety of protein molecules. Unlike lipids, the proteins of the plasma membrane are not distributed in arrays and differ widely in numbers and in molecular mass.

On the basis of their relation to the lipid matrix, plasma membranes have two types of proteins: (1) integral, globular, or intrinsic, and (2) peripheral, or extrinsic. Globular proteins penetrate or pierce both layers of lipids and appear on either or both inner (cytoplasmic) and outer (extracytoplasmic) surfaces of the plasma membrane. Peripheral

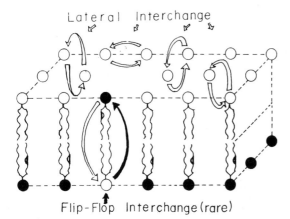

Figure 4–3 Lateral and transversal displacements of phospholipid units occur in the lipid bilayer of the plasma membrane. Through rarely occurring flip-flops, some units with unsaturated fatty acids can be transferred from the inner to the outer surfaces, and vice versa.

proteins, which are mostly water-soluble enzymes, are attached either to globular proteins on the cytoplasmic surface or to the polar region of lipids on the inner or outer surface of the plasma membrane.

Like lipids, the proteins of the plasma membrane are amphipathic. The nonpolar, lipid-soluble region of proteins is embedded in the part of the membrane containing the nonpolar fatty acid tails of the phospholipids. The polar, water-soluble region of the proteins is on either the inner or the outer surface of the plasma membrane. The diversity in composition and in location of proteins accounts for the variety of types of plasma membranes and of connections (tight junction; belt-, spot-, or hemidesmosomes; and gap junctions) between plasma membranes.

Total protein asymmetry (i.e., a complete difference between the cytoplasmic and extracytoplasmic portions of plasma membrane proteins) is essential for proper functioning. Lateral displacements of proteins in the fluid-lipid matrix occur without change in functional asymmetry. However, flip-flop changes of proteins cannot take place without interfering with asymmetry, and thus with function.

Water-soluble peripheral proteins are easily separated without disrupting the membrane; thus they are called *extrinsic proteins*. Isolation of globular proteins is difficult and cannot be done without rupturing the cell membrane; thus they are called *intrinsic proteins*.

Functions of Intrinsic Proteins. Intrinsic proteins act as membrane receptors able to recognize (specificity), activate, and firmly attach (affinity) hormones (polypeptides and amines) to the cell membrane. In the presence of ions, integral proteins may activate membrane enzymes such as adenylate cyclase (Fig. 4–4), which catalyzes the transformation of adenosine triphosphate (ATP) into cyclic adenosine monophosphate (cAMP).

Globular proteins form membrane pores or channels (up to 0.8 nm), which may represent about 1/1,500 of the total surface of the membrane. The size of pores is reduced by an excess of calcium ions in nerve cells and would be increased by antidiuretic hormone (ADH) in collecting tube cells of the kidney. The inner surface of plasma membrane pores is electrically charged. Water-soluble particles of very small size (water, urea, sodium, potassium) pass through these plasma membrane pores with relative ease.

Carbohydrates

Carbohydrates are bound to either lipids or proteins on the extracellular surface of plasma membranes. Glycopro-

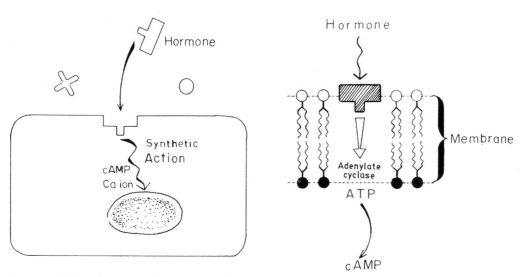

Figure 4–4 Left panel, Intrinsic proteins function as receptors with specificity and affinity for polypeptide hormones to activate nuclear syntheses. **Right panel,** Adenylate cyclase (extrinsic protein on the inner surface of the plasma membrane) is activated to react with ATP to produce cAMP. With adequate calcium ions, this second messenger stimulates specific synthetic activities in the nucleus of the target cell.

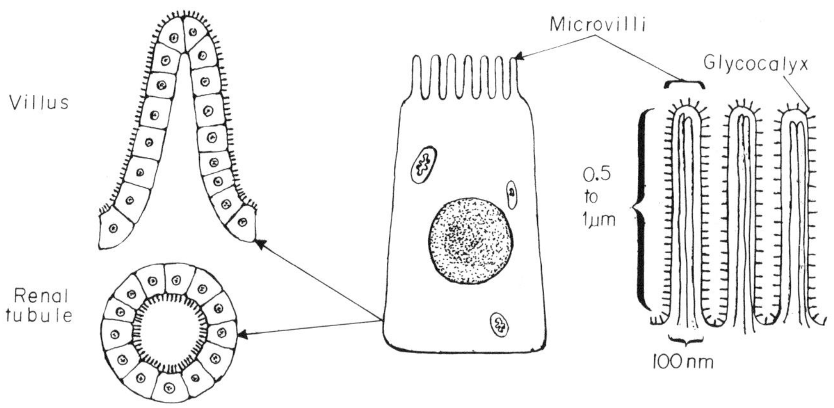

Figure 4–5 Carbohydrates unite with lipids and proteins to form microvilli and glycocalyces. These glycolipids and glycoprotein layers supply enzymes to the outer surface of the plasma membranes of enterocytes and of cells of the renal tubules and offer a protective coat to the apical plasma membrane of these cells.

teins and a few glycolipids form a filamentous layer, fuzz coat, cell coat, or glycocalyx 5 to 20 nm (200 nm in intestinal microvilli) thick. The cell coat protects against proteolytic enzymes, facilitates adsorption of substances (proteins, nucleic acids, viruses), and contributes to aggregation of several plasma membranes to form a tissue (Fig. 4–5).

PASSIVE TRANSPORT MECHANISMS IN PLASMA MEMBRANES

Transport of substances across plasma membranes occurs through two major processes: passive transport, or diffusion, and active transport. *Diffusion* is the continuous free movement of ions and molecules in a liquid solution or in a gas. It occurs without expenditure of energy, as in a "downhill" process, from a concentrated to a diluted medium. *Active transport* refers to the passage through a plasma membrane of a particle bound to a carrier and implies expenditure of energy. It involves "uphill" movement from a diluted to a concentrated medium.

Diffusion

Diffusion of a substance across a plasma membrane can result from liposolubility; loose binding, or adsorption to a lipid-soluble carrier; and access through pores in plasma membranes.

Liposolubility

Gas molecules of small size (oxygen, carbon dioxide) have little interaction with solvents and easily cross the lipid barrier and the water-soluble part of the plasma membrane. Transfers occur at random inward and outward (F_i and F_o), but the net flow of particles (F_n) (i.e., the algebraic sum of F_i and F_o) is from the concentrated to the diluted area (Fig. 4–6).

Other substances (alcohols, steroids, fatty acids) that are dissolved in the lipid part of the membrane continue their random movements through the more viscous protein-lipid

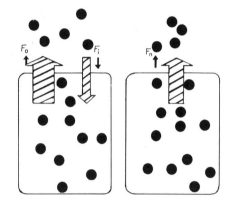

NET FLOW OF PARTICLES (F_n) = Algebraic Sum of Inward (F_i)

and Outward (F_o) Flows

Figure 4–6 Random diffusion transfers on both sides of the plasma membrane. The algebraic sum of inward flow (F_i) and outward flow (F_o) gives the net flow (F_n) of particles across the plasma membrane.

layer at a slower pace. Liposolubility is essential for this kind of passive transport.

Binding to a Lipid-Soluble Carrier

Lipophobic substances (glucose, amino acids) can overcome the lipid barrier of the plasma membrane by binding to a lipophilic protein carrier for *facilitated diffusion* (Fig. 4–7). These particle-specific carriers, which are limited in numbers, can be saturated (all tied up) when the number of particles is excessive. Plasma membrane receptors can also be blocked by chemically similar particles (competitive inhibition); for example, D-galactose blocks the facilitated diffusion of D-glucose. Such carrier-mediated transport from an area of greater concentration of particles into an area of lesser concentration of the same particles does not require or dissipate energy. In many instances, facilitated diffusion involving protein carriers of the plasma membrane is increased by hormones (e.g., insulin accelerates the facilitated diffusion of glucose into muscle cells).

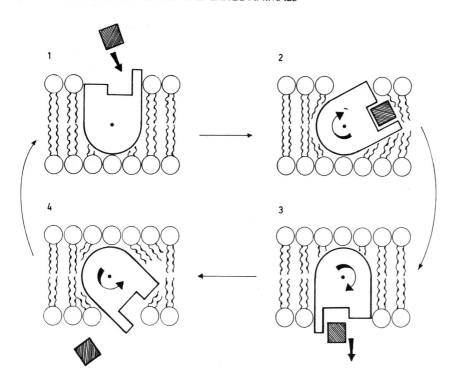

Figure 4–7 Diagrammatic view of facilitated diffusion by binding a lipophobic substance to a lipophilic carrier to cross the lipid barrier of the plasma membrane. 1, Hydrophilic substance (black square) is fixed on the lipophilic carrier. 2, The lipophilic carrier penetrates the lipid barrier (clockwise rotation). 3, The hydrophilic substance is separated from the lipophilic carrier and released into the cytoplasm. 4, The lipophilic carrier returns (counter-clockwise rotation) to the cocked state on the extracellular side of the plasma membrane.

Modalities of facilitated diffusion include coupled facilitated diffusion and exchange diffusion. In the *coupled facilitated diffusion* process, two substances are coupled to the lipophilic carrier to move them across the plasma membrane without expenditure of energy (Fig. 4–8). D-Glucose, L-amino acids, di- and triglycerides, some vitamins, and (in the ileum) bile salts are organic particles often coupled to sodium for carrier-facilitated passive absorption. For example, L-alanine can be taken up at the apical plasma membrane of enterocytes (cells of the intestinal mucosa) by coupling with sodium on a protein carrier. As a result of coupled facilitated diffusion, the concentration of alanine in cytoplasm may be as great as six times the ECF content. The energy for this nonenergetic transport mechanism at the apical area is provided by active transport of sodium at the basolateral area of the plasma membrane of the enterocyte.

Exchange diffusion, the other modality of facilitated transport, occurs in erythrocytes. In exchange diffusion, each introduction of a molecule of galactose into the erythrocyte requires the extrusion of a molecule of glucose (Fig. 4–9).

Penetration Through Plasma Membrane Pores

Pores or channels in plasma membranes also help to move water-coated particles to and from the cytoplasmic fluid and ECF from an area of higher concentration to one of less concentration. Cation channels have been recognized for sodium and potassium, which enter plasma membranes through fast channels, and for calcium ions, which ingress through slow channels (10 to 20 times slower than sodium channels). The transfer of anions occurs through chloride channels.

The *sodium channels,* which are about 10 times more abundant than potassium channels, are better known. On the basis of 70 sodium channels per square micrometer, the sum of their surface would be about 1/100,000 that of the membrane surface. The sodium channels admit hydrated particles of sodium (i.e., a sodium ion and four molecules of water, 0.5 nm diameter). Hydrated potassium particles (about 0.4 nm) can also penetrate the sodium channels of plasma membranes, but these channels are 12 times more permeable to sodium than to potassium particles. Sodium channels are blocked by tetrodotoxin and by the calcium channel blockers.

Potassium channels are for passage of hydrated particles of potassium (i.e., a potassium ion and two molecules of water, <0.4 nm). In some cells of the nervous system, the intracellular penetration of hydrated chloride particles (<0.4 nm) may occur with an outflow of hydrated potassium in the *chloride channels.*

Calcium channels in plasma membranes control the entry of calcium ions into cardiac muscle cells (sinoatrial and atrioventricular nodes) and into vascular smooth muscle cells. Calcium blockers are drugs (nifedipine, verapamil, diltiazem) absorbed in the small intestine that interfere with the entry of calcium ions into cells for cardiac contraction and for vasoconstriction of vessels, which is greater in arteries than in veins. Because these slow calcium channels also allow ingress of sodium into these cells, they are frequently called *calcium-sodium channels.* Other calcium channels, which regulate release of calcium ions from cytosolic stores of skeletal muscle cells, are not affected by these calcium blockers used to dilate arteries and reduce cardiac conduction and contraction.

Water is not an inert molecule. At physiological tem-

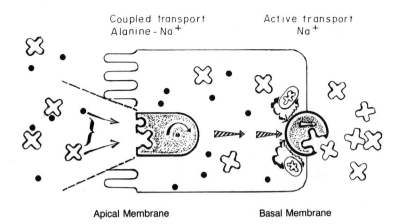

Figure 4–8 Coupled facilitated diffusion (absorption) at the apical plasma membrane of the enterocyte, with active transfer (extrusion) of sodium ion at the basolateral area of the plasma membrane.

perature (37° C), one molecule of water, by means of its hydrogen bonds, adheres to as many as four other molecules of water, to form an aggregate about 0.3 nm in diameter. Dissolved ions and molecules also interact with water to become hydrated. Water is attracted to form a spherical layer, which increases the size of ions and molecules.

Phenomena Associated with Diffusion Across Plasma Membranes

By diffusion through a plasma membrane or its channels (pores), substances pass both inward and outward. A final net flow in one direction results from differences on both sides of the membrane in quantities of particles (osmolality and osmolarity). The phenomena of osmosis, osmotic pressure, and generation of electrical potentials (i.e., diffusion potentials) are related to diffusion.

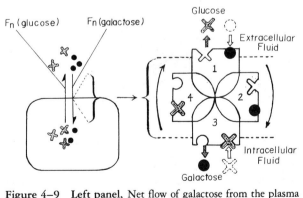

Figure 4–9 Left panel, Net flow of galactose from the plasma into the erythrocyte after a net flow of glucose into the blood plasma. **Right panel,** Diagram of this exchange-diffusion modality of facilitated diffusion in the erythrocyte. *1,* Extracellular fixation of galactose on the lipophilic carrier after extrusion of glucose. *2,* Transfer of galactose into the lipid barrier of the erythrocyte. *3,* Intracellular liberation of galactose followed by intracellular fixation of glucose. *4,* Transfer of glucose through the lipid barrier prior to its extrusion into the plasma.

Osmosis, or Net Flow of Water

Osmosis is the net flow of water across a semipermeable membrane (permeable to water only) separating two solutions of equal volumes but of unequal concentrations. The net flow of water is linked to the difference in strength or the concentration gradient. The excess number of particles in the concentrated solution (i.e., the relative decrease in water) causes a compensatory flow of water from the diluted to the concentrated side of the semipermeable membrane. After a while, equilibrium is reached so that the solutions on both sides of the membrane have the same number of particles per volume of solution (they are isoosmolal) but have different volumes. The volume of the solution that was concentrated at the outset of the experiment is now greater because of a net gain, or flow, of water, and the relative excess of particles per unit of volume is no longer present.

Osmolarity and Osmolality as Indices of Quantity of Particles in a Biologic Fluid. The quantity of particles (ions and molecules) in a solution is expressed in osmoles per *liter* of solution (*osmolarity*) or per *kilogram* of solvent (*osmolality*). When water is the solvent, because 1 L has a mass of 1 kg, osmolarity and osmolality are identical. When plasma is the solvent, a minor difference exists, as the mass of 1 L of plasma is slightly higher than 1 kg, but this slight difference between osmolality and osmolarity is usually ignored.

One osmole (Osm) represents the number of particles in either (1) the molecular mass (weight) of a nonionized (nonelectrolyte) substance (e.g., glucose 180 g, urea 60 g) or (2) the molecular mass of an ionized (electrolyte) substance divided by the number of free ions (e.g., sodium chloride 58.5/2 or 29.8 g). A solution with 1/1,000 Osm in 1 L water has an osmolality or osmolarity of 1 mOsm per liter. The osmolality of ECF and ICF is about 300 mOsm, or 0.3 Osm, per liter.

Osmotic Pressure, or the Force to Counteract Osmosis

The pressure required to prevent osmosis, or the net flow of water into the more concentrated of two solutions

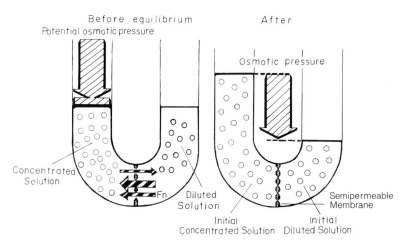

OSMOTIC PRESSURE =
FORCE PREVENTING OSMOSIS

OSMOSIS = NET FLOW OF WATER

Figure 4–10 Representation of the concepts of osmotic pressure and osmosis. **Left panel,** Osmotic pressure is the force preventing osmosis (the net diffusion $[P_n]$ of water) through a semipermeable membrane from a diluted to a concentrated solution. As osmotic pressure is a potential pressure, it is best represented by a system before equilibrium, where both diluted and concentrated solutions separated by a semipermeable membrane are of equal volumes. **Right panel,** After equilibrium both solutions are of equal concentrations, but the volume of the previously diluted one is reduced, whereas the volume of the formerly concentrated one is increased. A net flow of water (osmosis) occurred from the diluted solution to the concentrated one. The osmotic pressure is the total difference in centimeters between the height of water in the columns. Cm water is then converted into mm Hg (1.36 cm water = 1 mm Hg).

separated by a semipermeable membrane, is called *osmotic pressure.* As this definition is not easily visualized, the concept of osmotic pressure is usually illustrated by a system at equilibrium (i.e., where osmosis has already occurred). Then, the solutions are isoosmotic, or isotonic, but a greater volume of fluid is in the column that contained the concentrated solution before equilibrium of the system. Conversely, the diluted part of the system contains less water, and that column is shorter. The osmotic pressure, measured as the difference in the height of the two columns, is expressed in hydrostatic pressure units (mm Hg; Fig. 4–10).

Osmotic Pressure of ECF. At 38° C, a solution of 1 Osm per liter plasma (intravascular ECF) has an osmotic pressure of 19,300 mm Hg. As the osmolality of ECF is about 0.3 Osm per liter, the osmotic pressure of plasma is calculated as 0.3 Osm × 19,300 = 5,790 mm Hg.

Diffusion Potentials in Resting Plasma Membranes

The ECF content of certain ions differs from the concentration found in ICF. For example, ECF usually carries about 140 mmol per liter sodium and 4 mmol per liter potassium, and the ICF holds approximately 14 mmol per liter sodium and 140 mmol per liter potassium. As a result, these ions tend to diffuse constantly—sodium into the cell and potassium outside the cell (Fig. 4–11).

In a resting cell, because of these differences in ion concentrations, an electrical membrane potential is created between the inside and the outside of the plasma membrane. The resting polarity of the plasma membrane is electronegative (anion) on its inner side and electropositive (cation) on its outer side.

With the *Nernst equation* and the knowledge of their inside ($cation_i$) and outside ($cation_o$) concentrations, a theoretical resting membrane potential (*Nernst potential*) can be computed for each major univalent electrolyte (sodium[+],

potassium[+]). It indicates that the diffusion of sodium into and potassium from the cytoplasm accounts for most (70/90) of the resting plasma membrane potential. The smaller remaining part (20/90) is contributed by active transport mechanisms.

Nernst equation:
$$\text{Millivolts} = -60 \times \log (cation_i/cation_o)$$

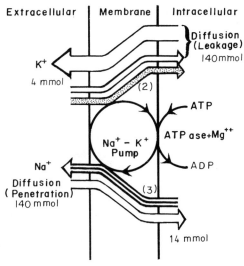

Figure 4–11 Diagrammatic overview of the continuous passive and active process of transfer of sodium and potassium at the plasma membrane. Passive diffusion or penetration of sodium occurs from the ECF into the ICF, and passive diffusion or leakage of potassium from the ICF into the ECF. Active pumping of three sodium ions outside the cell and of two potassium ions inside the cell occurs simultaneously. Since the sodium-potassium pump always leaves some potassium ions outside the cell, the polarity of the surfaces of the plasma membrane is positive on the outside and negative on the inside. A membrane potential of about −90 to −70 mV also exists between both surfaces of the plasma membrane.

With the sodium data—14 mmol per liter (inside) and 140 mmol per liter (outside)—the Nernst potential is

$$-60 \times \log 14/140 \text{ or}$$
$$-60 \times \log 0.1 \text{ or}$$
$$-60 \times 1 = -60 \text{ mV}$$

(which is lower than the usual resting potential of the plasma membrane (-70 to -90 mV).

With the potassium data—140 mmol per liter (inside) and 4 mmol per liter (outside)—the Nernst potential is

$$-60 \times \log 140/4 \text{ or}$$
$$-60 \times \log 35 \text{ or}$$
$$-60 \times 1.54 = -92 \text{ mV}$$

(which is slightly higher than the usual resting potential of the plasma membrane (-70 to -90 mV)

ACTIVE TRANSPORT MECHANISMS IN PLASMA MEMBRANES

Energy-dependent systems are required to displace ions (e.g., sodium, potassium) or minute amounts of fluids against a concentration gradient across the cell membrane.

Active Transport of Sodium and Potassium

To counteract the continuous diffusion and leakage of sodium and potassium through the plasma membrane, a sodium-potassium pump is in constant operation. At each cycle, it simultaneously removes three sodium ions from the ICF and returns two potassium ions from the ECF. It also contributes to creating a part of the resting plasma membrane potential. These sodium and potassium transfers are both uphill actions that require energy. The process is energized from enzymatic hydrolysis of intracellular ATP by a magnesium-dependent ATPase. A bidirectional carrier protein is also involved. It operates from the intracellular to the extracellular border for sodium and from the extracellular to the intracellular margin for potassium.

Active Transport of Minute Quantities of Fluid or Solid

Intermittent mechanisms of plasma membrane transport have been observed by electron microscopy. They occur for the incorporation or extrusion of very small quantities of substances that cannot otherwise cross the plasma membrane. These specialized active transport mechanisms are termed endocytosis and exocytosis.

Endocytosis at Plasma Membranes

Through the process of *endocytosis,* a part of the plasma membrane can incorporate minute granules (proteins, pep-

tides) or very small volumes of liquid from the ECF if they are near the extracytoplasmic surface. The two main types of endocytosis are pinocytosis and phagocytosis.

Pinocytosis (cell drinking), a form of endocytosis seen with the electron microscope, is the capture of microvolumes of liquid from the proximal ECF. The substances to be ingested are adsorbed in an invagination of the outer surface of the plasma membrane and cause a surface tension reaction. With an expenditure of energy, the outside edges around this invagination proliferate, surround, and engulf the target material within a vesicle, or pinocytic vacuole, 100 to 200 nm in diameter. The membrane of the vesicle and the plasma membrane then fuse. The area of fusion breaks down, pinching off the vesicle inside the cell and leaving the plasma membrane intact. In the cell, the membrane around a pinocytic vacuole may fuse with a lysosome, mixing the hydroxylases with the contents (proteins, nucleic acids, glycogen) of the vesicle (Fig. 4–12).

Receptor-mediated endocytosis also occurs at distinctive plasma membrane structures called clathrin-coated pits, with the production of coated vesicles (receptosomes) in the cytoplasm. These receptosomes do not fuse with lysosomes but transfer their contents (lipoproteins, insulin, viruses, nerve growth factor, epidermal growth factor) to the Golgi complex or adjacent endoplasmic reticulum.

Phagocytosis (cell eating) is a type of endocytosis visible under the light microscope. Large particles (microorganisms, fragments of cells) near the extracytoplasmic surface are ingested by special cells (granulocytes, macrophages) as a defense mechanism. Phagocytic cells extend pseudopods, cytoplasmic extensions, to encircle the target and incorporate it. Phagocytosis requires calcium ions and energy.

Exocytosis at Plasma Membranes

Also called emiocytosis (cell vomiting) and reverse pinocytosis, *exocytosis* is the ejection of material, usually secretory granules (100 to 350 nm), from a cell into the ECF. The secretory granules migrate from their site of synthesis to the Golgi complex and there are grouped into microvesicles, which reach the cytoplasmic surface of the plasma membrane. The latter then evaginates to liberate the secretory granules into the ECF (Fig. 4–12). Acetylcholine, chylomicrons, and insulin are examples of substances secreted by exocytosis. Exocytosis requires calcium ions and energy.

Cytopemphis, or Vesicular Transport

Cytopemphis, or vesicular transport, is a mechanism that uses coated vesicles to convey protein across *endothelial cells* of capillary walls. By endocytosis the proteins are first transferred out of the capillary lumen, through the apical surface of endothelial cells, and into their cytoplasm. This is followed by exocytosis from the cytoplasm at the basal or interstitial area of the plasma membrane of the endothelial cell.

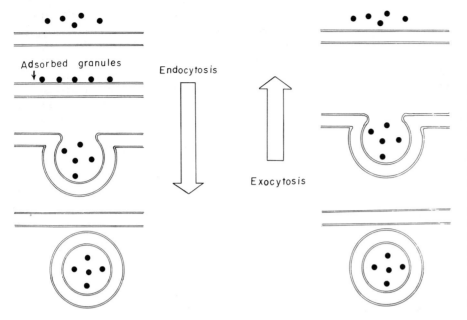

Figure 4–12 The active transport by endocytosis and exocytosis, seen only with electron microscopy are almost mirror images of each other. With *endocytosis,* granules or fluids are circumscribed in a micropouch, or microinvagination, on the outer surface of the plasma membrane, then completely encircled in a vesicle, which is finally released into the cytoplasm. With exocytosis, the Golgi apparatus packages secretory granules into a vesicle, which fuses with the inner surface of the plasma membrane and is then emptied at the outer surface into the ECF.

JUNCTIONS BETWEEN PLASMA MEMBRANES

Besides fixing the inner and outer limits of cells, plasma membranes interact with each other at junctional structures. The junctions are different between blood cells, neurons, and cells in tissues.

Junctions between Plasma Membranes of Blood Cells

Blood cells—erythrocytes and leukocytes—do not have formal associations. Erythrocytes move independently in the plasma, sometimes forming loose aggregations (rouleaux). The erythrocytes of the horse have a propensity to aggregate, form rouleaux, and sediment rapidly. Leukocytes have very pliable plasma membranes that readily form cytoplasmic extensions, or pseudopods, to surround target substances for phagocytosis. Because of the plasticity of their plasma membrane, leukocytes cross vascular endothelium by *diapedesis* (i.e., by infiltrating through "pores" or clefts between endothelial cells) to reach most parts of the ECF.

Junctions between Plasma Membranes of Neurons

At their input (dendrites) and at their output (axon), neurons, or nerve cells, have junctions called *synapses.* Some neuromuscular junctions (an axon contacting muscle cells) are called end-plates and are regarded as specialized synapses.

Junctions between Plasma Membranes of Tissue Cells

The junctions between plasma membranes of cells that form tissues are usually tight junctions, desmosomes, or gap junctions. In general terms, tight junctions and desmosomes tie cells together and give strength and stability to tissues. Gap junctions allow transfer of ions and molecules between adjacent cells (Fig. 4–13).

Tight junctions, or *zona occludens,* surround the apical margins of cells in epithelial structures (intestine, renal tubules, choroid plexus). From each cell, ridges of lipids adhere tenaciously to obliterate part of the intercellular space of adjacent cells. Besides tying the cells together, tight junctions act as a barrier to the movement of particles, from the apical to the basolateral sides of the plasma membranes or from the apical side of the epithelium to the basolateral aspect. They also prevent backflow from the basolateral to the apical areas. Some epithelia (e.g., hepatic sinusoid, small intestine, proximal tubule, gallbladder) are more "leaky" to particles than others. Others (stomach, urinary bladder) have tight junctions where leakage and backflow do not occur.

Desmosomes, or *maculae adherens,* are thickenings of the plasma membranes of two adjacent cells with cytoplasmic fibrils. A filamentous material occupies the intercellular space between the two thickenings. *Belt desmosomes* (intermediate zones, or zonula adherens) are bands linking epithelial cells just below and parallel to their tight junctions. The cytoplasmic fibrils or filaments contain actin and are able to contract. *Spot desmosomes* are small, buttonlike points of attachment that have been likened to spot welds, and their cytoplasmic filaments are thicker and not contractile. The

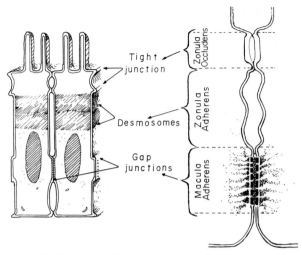

Figure 4–13 Types of junctions between adjacent plasma membranes. Tight junctions and desmosomes bind cells together tightly and provide greater stability to tissues. Gap junctions provide for immediate internal exchanges between cytoplasm of adjacent cells.

intercellular space between spot desmosomes is wider than normal (30 nm versus 25 nm). *Hemidesmosomes* attach the basal plasma membrane of epithelial cells to connective tissue.

Gap junctions have a narrow intercellular space (3 nm) and connect portions of the lateral plasma membranes of adjacent cells. Each connection has a 2-nm channel, which is directly lined up with the channel of a connection in an adjacent cell. Gap junctions allow low-resistance intracellular movement of ions or neurotransmitters of molecular weights under 800 daltons (e.g., hexoses, amino acids) from one cell to the next (without entering the ECF). The diameter of the connection channel is reduced or closed by an increase in intracellular calcium ions. Gap junctions form an electrical synapse or electrically connect one plasma membrane to the other and thus permit rapid propagation of electrical activity (action potentials) between neighboring smooth muscle fibers or cardiac muscle cells.

CHAPTER 5

BIOELECTRICAL PHENOMENA OF THE PLASMA MEMBRANE

Electrical potentials exist across all cell membranes in the animal body, but the homeostatic mechanism of electrogenesis is not identical in all cells. It has been studied extensively in excitable cells of the nervous system, smooth and striated muscles, and exocrine glands. Cardiac electrogenesis, which is associated with normal function or life, can be replaced by a cardiac pacemaker. The use of this device is indicated when either the rate or the conduction of the sinoauricular or of the atrioventricular nervous cells becomes irregular. This chapter presents the elements of the fundamental electrical phenomena of plasma membranes—resting potential and action potential. It also introduces particular action potentials associated with sensory mechanisms (e.g., postsynaptic, evoked, generator, receptor, and microphonic potentials).

ELECTRICAL POLARIZATION

Electrical polarization of the plasma membrane, with outer positivity and inner negativity, is due to an imbalance of ions (mostly potassium and sodium) that can cross the membrane. Resting membrane potential is maintained mostly by continuous passive diffusion of potassium ions, which pass across the polarized membrane 50 to 100 times more easily than sodium ions, and partly by constant operation of the sodium-potassium pump. As the quantity of potassium that diffuses out of the cell exceeds the amount that the sodium-potassium pump can return inside, the excess positive ions line up on the outside surface of the plasma membrane (Fig. 5–1). Since the cytoplasm contains a large number of anions (organic phosphates, and sulfates, and proteins), which cannot diffuse across the plasma membrane, the captive anions line up on the inner side of the plasma membrane. The inside negativity, combined with the great diffusibility of potassium in the sodium and potassium pores or channels, contributes to recall potassium cations from the outside and brings some assistance to the sodium-potassium pump.

RESTING POTENTIAL

By convention the potential on the positively charged outside of the cell is considered as zero and the potential on the negatively charged inside is expressed as a negative value in millivolts (mV). Resting membrane potential is best demonstrated with capillary glass microelectrodes on a giant axon from a nerve cell of a squid (*Loligo*), a crab (*Carcinus*), or a cuttlefish (*Sepia*). One microelectrode is placed into the cytoplasm or the axon of the giant neuron, and the other remains in the extracellular fluid (ECF). The membrane potential of a resting cell, or the resting potential, thus measured, is usually in the range of −70 to −90 mV but can vary from −5 to −100 mV, with the type of cell (Fig. 5–2).

ACTION POTENTIAL

The onset of cellular activity (tension or secretion) is instantly preceded by a change from a resting plasma membrane potential to an action potential on the plasma membrane. For a very short period (<2 milliseconds [ms] in most cells and about 200 ms in heart muscle cells), the polarization of the plasma membrane is reversed; that is, it is depolarized in relation to the resting potential. The inside surface becomes electropositive and the extracellular surface is now electronegative. The electrical potential goes from −90 mV to +45 mV, as diffusion permeability is changed in favor of sodium ions, which can diffuse inside the cytoplasm with thousandsfold greater ease (Fig. 5–3).

Within a few thousandths of a second, the considerable inflow of sodium into the cell is brought to a sudden halt, and almost simultaneously a massive outflow of potassium occurs from the cytoplasm. This corresponds to the *spike*

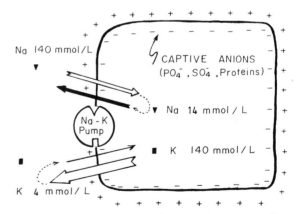

Figure 5–1 Electrical polarity of the resting plasma membrane, with positivity on the outer surface and negativity on the inner one. This situation results from an excess of potassium ions in the ECF as each cycle of the sodium-potassium pump extrudes three sodium ions from the cytoplasm but recalls only two potassium ions. Also, the plasma membrane is impermeable to some organic anions, which line the inside surface.

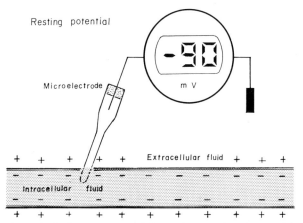

Figure 5–2 Measurement of the resting membrane potential, which is in the range of −90 to −70 mV, with a glass microelectrode inserted into the giant axon of a squid nerve cell.

potential (i.e., the maximal intensity of the action potential) or depolarization, which initiates activity of a cell or transmission of a signal in a nerve fiber or neuron.

Repolarization

During the momentary reversal of polarity on the plasma membrane the process of *repolarization* begins. As plasma membrane permeability to potassium (through potassium channels) increases, diffusion of potassium ions from the inner to the outer membrane surface occurs in priority. With repolarization, the electrical membrane potential is gradually lowered to resting potential or sometimes to a level lower than the resting potential (i.e., hyperpolarization).

The successive changes in polarity can be seen and recorded with the oscilloscope, when an electrical stimula-

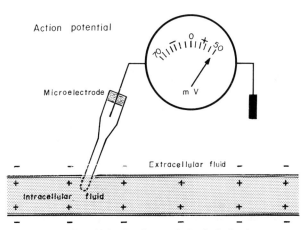

Figure 5–3 Depolarization (hypopolarization) of a plasma membrane, where the polarity of each surface is temporarily reversed (negativity outside and positivity inside) because of changes in the permeability of the lipid barrier. A massive inflow of sodium ions followed by one of potassium ions accounts for this reversal of polarity, an action potential that is associated with cellular activity.

tion (harmless, quantifiable, and repeatable) is applied to a nerve trunk. A *monophasic* action potential occurs when the *positive electrode* is put *inside* the nerve trunk (giant axon of the squid) and the *negative* one *outside*. As it is difficult to place the positive electrode inside an ordinary nerve, a *diphasic* action potential is obtained when *both* electrodes are on the *exterior* of the nerve trunk (Fig. 5–4). The first deflection is downward, since only the first electrode is depolarized and the second one is still electropositive. The second deflection is upward because depolarization has reached the second electrode but the first electrode is already repolarized.

Positive Feedback During Depolarization and Repolarization

When the plasma membrane shows resting potentials, the sodium and potassium channels are operating only partially; the latter are slightly more permeable than the sodium channels. The channels are almost closed to sodium and potassium ions because of minute polypeptide gates near the inner surface of the lipid barrier. The sodium channels have *activation gates*, which open when the membrane potential

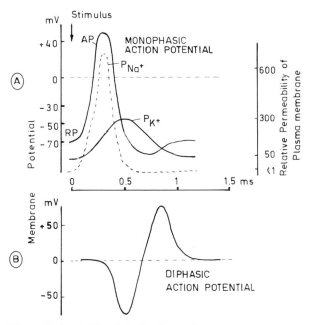

Figure 5–4 **A,** Electrical stimulation of a giant axon, or a nerve trunk. A *monophasic potential* results when the positive electrode is in the structure, and the negative electrode is outside. The inactive, or resting, potential (RP) is about −70 mV, and the plasma membrane is 50-fold more permeable to K^+ than to Na^+ ions. The stimulus increases the permeability to Na^+ (PNa^+) by more than 500-fold, causes a transient (<1 msec) inrush of Na^+ into the cell, and depolarizes the cell to about +40 mV (action potential [AP]). Repolarization overshoots the RP value (hyperpolarization) as K^+ outrush through K^+ channels that open for less than 1 ms to raise PK^+ by 6-fold. An efflux of Cl^- occurs to correct quickly the overshoot. **B,** If both electrodes are outside, the AP is *biphasic*, as it passes first by the negative and then by the positive electrode.

becomes less negative or rises to a threshold, and *inactivation gates,* which close when the membrane potential further decreases its negativity. Similar voltage-regulated gates exist for potassium channels and calcium channels.

Partial depolarization is started by a gradual opening of the activation gates of the sodium channels. The process is amplified by positive feedback (i.e., partial opening brings complete opening). The transfer of sodium across the membrane then increases by 5,000 times and large quantities of sodium are admitted into the cell. At that moment, the membrane is 20 to 30 times more permeable to sodium than to potassium. The electrical polarity is reversed and reaches +40 to +50 mV.

Repolarization begins when sodium no longer enters (i.e., at maximal depolarization). The inner positive polarity repels sodium, and at the same time the inactivation gates of the sodium channels close. Then the gates of the potassium channels are rapidly opened, also by a positive feedback mechanism. The inner surface positive polarity pushes potassium ions into the potassium channels and out of the cells. Arrival of potassium on the outside gradually reestablishes the resting polarity (i.e., electrical positivity on the outside and negativity on the inside of the plasma membrane).

The gates of the sodium channels are less efficient when there is a lack of calcium ions, and leakage of sodium leads to continued depolarization. The operating mechanisms of sodium and potassium channels can be selectively inhibited by tetrodotoxin (TTX) applied outside the cell, for the sodium channels, or tetraethylammonium (TEA) applied inside the cell, for potassium channels.

Characteristics of Action Potentials

The genesis of action potentials is an all-or-nothing event: it occurs only if the intensity of the stimulus reaches the threshold. Subliminal stimuli cannot cause action potential depolarization.

On traces recorded at high speed, a rather long period of hyperpolarization, called the *positive afterpotential,* follows the depolarization-repolarization phase. On a slower recording, the rapid narrow zone of depolarization is called a *spike potential,* and the term is used when referring to a nerve impulse. A portion of gradual and less acute repolarization near the resting potential, called the *negative afterpotential,* precedes the positive afterpotential (Fig. 5–4).

Propagation of Action Potential

The depolarization (spike potential) generated by an effective electrical stimulation of a nerve fiber travels both ways, only in that fiber and without decrement in amplitude. Repolarization starts from the same point and spreads likewise (Fig. 5–5).

The velocity of spike potentials increases with the diameter and myelination of the nerve fiber (e.g., 120 m per second for a 20-μm diameter fiber, and 60 m per second for a 10-μm fiber). Myelin, a fatty substance around axons of

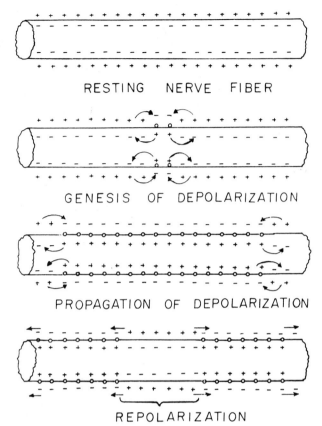

RESTING NERVE FIBER

GENESIS OF DEPOLARIZATION

PROPAGATION OF DEPOLARIZATION

REPOLARIZATION

Figure 5–5 Propagation of the action potential, or the depolarization, generated on a resting nerve fiber by an effective stimulus. The depolarization spreads in both directions. Repolarization follows, starting from the site of the initial stimulus or depolarization.

some neurons which acts as an insulating sheath, is periodically interrupted at nodes of Ranvier. At these gaps in the myelin sheath, the plasma membrane is 500 times more permeable than elsewhere. Spike potentials can jump from one myelin gap to another, a process called *saltatory conduction* (Fig. 5–6).

BIOELECTRICAL POTENTIALS RELATED TO SENSORY MECHANISMS

The basic functional unit of the nervous system must have at least two neurons. The first one has receptors, which act as transducers to receive and to transform a source of physical or chemical energy into spike potentials. These modulations in the electrical polarity of the plasma membrane are propagated on its axon toward the second neuron. This second neuron, separated from the first one by a synaptic cleft, is in synaptic relation with an effector organ (gland, muscle). Several bioelectrical phenomena of depolarization occur during operations of this basic functional nerve unit. Depolarizations are seen at activation of receptors on the plasma membrane of the first neuron, of conduction in axonal plasma membranes, and of synaptic plasma mem-

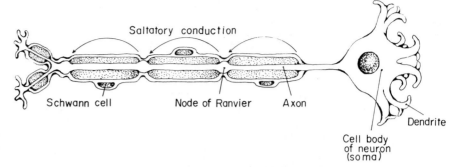

Figure 5–6 Conduction of depolarization from the dendrites (afferent pathways) to the soma (nerve cell) out of the cell on an axon with a myelin covering and to the presynaptic boutons. The saltatory conduction, jumping from one node of Ranvier in the myelin to the other, is faster than conduction on the axon.

brane junctions between axon₁ and neuron₂, and axon₂ and effector.

Generator and Receptor Potentials on Plasma Membranes

Generator potential is a generic term for a local electrical phenomenon, nonpropagated and of variable intensity, caused by an effective stimulation (electrical, photic, thermal, chemical, or mechanical) of a receptor or transducer. Extremes of mechanical, thermal, and chemical energy are encoded by high-threshold transducers called nociceptors (Table 5–1). Graded, local generator potentials on postsynaptic membranes are termed postsynaptic potentials. Generator potentials in the fluids of dendrites, which are transmitted with decrement just as in an electrical cable, are called electrotonic potentials.

Effective stimulation of receptors alters the permeability of the plasma membrane to univalent ions (sodium and potassium) and decreases the negativity of the resting potential (i.e., causes a hypopolarization). As the generator potential continues to decrease and reaches a threshold, it abruptly engenders a single *receptor potential* (i.e., depolarization). The number of receptor potentials is directly related to the intensity of the stimulus. These single or multiple disturbances or receptor potentials, propagated in an all-or-

TABLE 5–1 Receptors or Transducers at the Origin of Generator or Receptor Potentials in Plasma Membranes of Neurons

Chemical stimulus
    Chemoreceptors in carotid bodies and in aortic bodies
    Chemoreceptors for taste
    Olfactory receptors
    Osmoreceptors
Mechanical stimulus
    Hair cells in cochlear canal and skin
    Mechanoreceptors of deep tissues (free and specialized nerve endings), joints, and skin
    Stretch or tension receptors of muscle and tendon
    Visceral pressure receptors
Photic stimulus
    Photoreceptors (cones and rods) of retina
Thermal stimulus
    Thermoreceptors for cold and warmth

nothing fashion in the axon of a receptor neuron, are called nerve impulses, spike potentials, or signals.

Cochlear microphonic and *summating potentials* are generator potentials resulting from stimulation of receptors or transducers, in this case the outer and inner hair cells in the organ of Corti. They show no threshold and spread electrotonically with decrement in the tissues surrounding the cochlea.

> The *cochlear microphonic potentials* originate from pushing or bending of the outer hair cells against the tectorial membrane when a sound stimulus is applied. They simulate the effect of a microphone to convert acoustic energy into sinusoidal electrical energy, and are a tool for analyzing inner and middle ear function. Microphonic potentials, which are not affected by anesthesia, cold, and fatigue, decrease in level after death but persist for hours.

> *Cochlear negative summating potentials,* or cochlear summating potentials, originate from pulling the inner hair cells from the tectorial membrane. They are continuous as long as the acoustic stimulus is maintained, and have the opposite polarity to microphonic potentials.

Postsynaptic Plasma Membrane Potentials

Synapses are junctions between neurons that provide a one-way propagation of action potentials (spike potentials) from axons to neuron (soma), dendrite, or an axon of another neuron (Fig. 5–7).

Their functional anatomy requires that they have a presynaptic terminal knob, or bouton, a synaptic cleft of about 20 nm, and a postsynaptic membrane. Every bouton contains microvesicles of either excitatory (e.g., acetylcholine, norepinephrine, substance P, glutamate) or inhibitory (e.g., glycine, dopamine, enkephalin, serotonin, gamma-aminobutyric acid [GABA]) transmitter (Fig. 5–8).

Each spike potential reaching the bouton causes a number of vesicles to spill their content into the synaptic cleft. Calcium ions are needed for the vesicles to rupture. Excitatory transmitters increase the permeability of the postsynaptic plasma membrane to sodium and potassium and generate an *excitatory postsynaptic potential* (EPSP) or a hypopolarization of the plasma membrane (Fig. 5–9). Release of inhibitory transmitter modifies the permeability of the postsynaptic membrane to potassium and chloride but not to

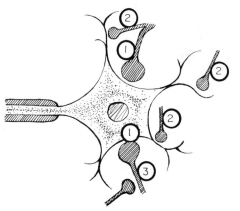

Figure 5–7 Types of synaptic junction in nerve tissues. *1*, Between axon and nerve cell (soma); *2*, between axon and dendrite; *3*, between two axons.

sodium. To produce an inhibitory postsynaptic potential (IPSP), potassium moves rapidly from inside the membrane or chloride enters the cytoplasm. Both these transfers create an excess of inner negativity, or a *hyperpolarization*, with respect to the resting membrane potential (Fig. 5–9).

Evoked or Slow Potentials on the Plasma Membrane of Cortical Neurons

Evoked, or slow, potentials are sensory signals directed to specific surfaces of the brain and recorded in experimental animals. They are used to define the topography of functional sensory areas (e.g., vision, smell, hearing, and somesthesia, or body awareness).

The characteristic response in anesthetized animals is a surface-positive wave followed by a small negative wave

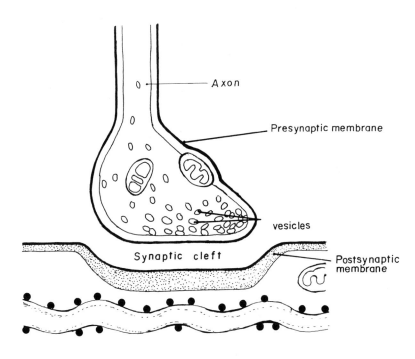

Figure 5–8 Synaptic junction showing its function as one-way valve to direct the action potential from the presynaptic to the postsynaptic membrane. The neurotransmitters contained in the microvesicles are released in the synaptic cleft to modify the permeability of the postsynaptic membrane.

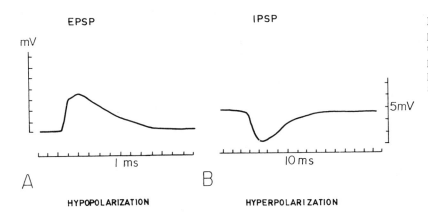

Figure 5–9 Generator potentials on the postsynaptic membrane are either (A) excitatory postsynaptic potentials (EPSPs; hypopolarizing, less negative) or (B) inhibitory postsynaptic potentials (IPSP; hyperpolarizing, more negative).

EVOKED CORTICAL POTENTIALS

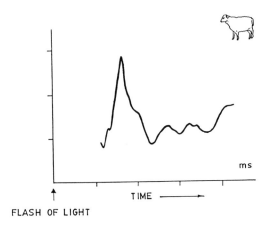

ms

↑
TIME ——→

FLASH OF LIGHT

PERIPHERAL ELECTRICAL CARDIAC POTENTIALS

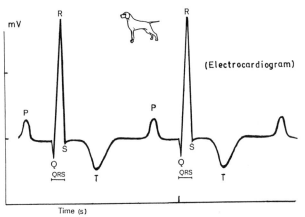

(Electrocardiogram)

Time (s)

Figure 5–10 **Top panel,** Visual evoked potential recorded from subcutaneous needle electrodes placed on the midline of the scalp of a sheep. One electrode is on the occipital crest and the other between the eyes (ground on the vertex, midway between the two electrodes). The stimulus is a flash of light. **Bottom panel,** Recording in a dog of the global changes in potentials produced by the cardiac muscle cells during two cardiac cycles. The electrodes are on the limbs (negative on the right limb, positive on the left limb; i.e., standard bipolar limb lead II). They receive electrical forces transmitted to the periphery by the conductive tissue fluids. These electrical signals are generated during the successive depolarizations and repolarizations of the muscle cells of the atria and ventricles. The P wave is related to the atria, the QRS complex represents ventricular depolarization (mostly of the more muscular left ventricle), and the T wave is associated with ventricular repolarization.

(primary evoked potential) and then by a larger and longer positive-negative deflection (diffuse evoked secondary response). The primary evoked potential is highly localized, whereas the diffuse secondary evoked response is diffused over most of the cortex. In an unanesthetized sheep, an indifferent (neither pleasant nor unpleasant) stimulus such as a single flash of light produces a widespread and prominent diffuse secondary evoked potential (Fig. 5–10). Evoked potentials are associated with sensory input. They are different from the spontaneous electrical potentials of origin still unknown that are obtained by electrocorticography (ECoG) or electroencephalography (EEG).

Peripheral Recording of the Depolarization Complexes of Heart Muscle

During the cardiac cycle, global activity of the heart muscle produces electrical complexes (P, QRS, T), which can be recorded at the surface of the body (Fig. 5–10). A record, over time, of these voltage changes by means of plate or needle electrodes placed at set points over the body surface is referred to as an electrocardiogram (ECG).

REFERENCES FOR SECTION I

Bessis M, Weed RI, Eblond PF. Red cell shape. New York: Springer-Verlag, 1973.

Bettger WJ, McKeehan WL. Mechanisms of cellular nutrition. Physiol Rev 1986;66:1.

Fick A. Uber Diffusion. Ann Physik 1855;94:59.

Fox CF. The structure of cell membranes. Sci Am 1972;226:31.

Garty M, Benos DJ. Characteristics and regulatory mechanisms of the amiloride-blockable Na⁺ channel. Physiol Rev 1988;68:309.

Mitruka BM, Rawnsley HM. Clinical biochemical and hematological reference values in normal experimental animals. New York: Masson, 1977.

Ozawa S, Sand O. Electrophysiology of excitable endocrine cells. Physiol Rev 1986;66:887.

Rasmussen H, Barrett PQ. Calcium messenger system: an integrated view. Physiol Rev 1984;64:938.

Renkin EM. Transport of large molecules across capillary walls. Physiologist 1964;7:13.

Strain GM, Olcott BM, Hockett LD. Electroretinogram and visual-evoked potential measurements in Holstein cows. Am J Vet Res 1986; 47:1079.

Unthank JL, Bohlen HG. Lymphatic pathways and role of valves in lymph propulsion from small intestine. Am J Physiol 1988;254:G389.

Van Driessche W, Zeiske W. Ion channels in epithelial cell membranes. Physiol Rev 1985;65:833.

RESPIRATORY, CARDIOVASCULAR, AND RENAL FUNCTIONS

The chapters of this section may be considered as the expected companions of the chapter on body fluids, since they deal with the mechanisms stabilizing the volume and composition of the internal fluid environment of the body.

As gas exchangers, the *lungs* eliminate some of the carbon dioxide formed during the metabolism of nutrients and maintain the concentration of bicarbonate at less than 30 mmol per liter. Breathing movements promote the transfer of oxygen from the atmosphere into the blood, and in ruminants they contribute to recycle methane from the reticulorumen to the blood. Within definite limits of pressure and flow, the *cardiovascular system* distributes blood to and collects it from all parts of the body through an enormous network of viscoelastic tubes. The heart pump provides the energy, through one-way valvular action, to maintain the pressure and flow gradients. The *kidneys,* which constitute less than 0.5 percent of the body mass, are generously perfused by 20 percent of the cardiac output. They achieve conservation of sodium and water and assist in maintaining the concentration of bicarbonate ions under 30 mmol per liter. With the lungs, the kidneys are responsible for acid-base balance.

Nonrespiratory, or cellular, lung functions, hemodynamics of vital organs (brain, heart, and liver), and renal endocrine functions all represent advances in the understanding of body homeostasis. They will be discussed in a chapter preceding the more traditional concepts of respiratory, cardiovascular, and renal physiology.

CHAPTER 6

NONRESPIRATORY FUNCTIONS OF THE RESPIRATORY SYSTEM

On the basis of morphologic and functional features, the airways and vessels of mammalian lungs can be visualized as elements grouped into three zones—conducting, transitional, and respiratory (Fig. 6–1).

The *conducting zone* includes trachea, bronchi, terminal bronchioles, connective tissue, and main branches of the pulmonary artery and vein (10 percent of total lung volume). The *transitional zone* is composed of the respiratory bronchioles and alveolar ducts (30 percent of total lung volume). The *respiratory zone* contains the alveoli and associated blood capillaries (60 percent of total lung volume).

The conducting and transitional zones are mostly branching airways and blood vessels to humidify, filter, and distribute oxygen-rich air to the respiratory unit. They also provide pathways for elimination of excess carbon dioxide from the alveolar air and for reabsorption of methane from eructed reticulorumen gases.

The respiratory zone is the site of gas exchanges between alveolar air and blood. The functional respiratory units of the lungs are the alveoli and the network of capillaries in their walls. Before any exchange of gases (oxygen, carbon dioxide, and in ruminants, methane) occurs, several barriers must be crossed (Fig. 6–2).

These six alveolus-blood barriers are formed by surfactant or tensioactive film, a thin layer of basal aqueous fluid (hypophase), alveolar epithelium and basement membrane, capillary basement membrane and endothelium, blood plasma, and membrane of the erythrocytes.

The ultimate unit for gas exchange in the mammalian lung is the alveolus, a thin-walled cavity with an open side. The alveolar wall is formed by cells surrounding a dense network of anastomosing capillaries, which have an average diameter of 8 to 15 μm. The three mechanical barriers between air and blood are the alveolar epithelium, which serves to maintain the integrity of the air chamber; the interstitium with collagen and elastic fibers; and the endothelial (capillary) lining, which confines blood within channels of the pulmonary and peripheral circulations.

Squamous epithelial cells cover about 90 percent of the entire alveolar surface, although they account for only 10 percent of the total cell population by number. Following injury, these type I cells can be replaced by type II cells, which then differentiate into type I cells. At alveolar corners, granular cuboidal pneumocytes (type II cells, corner cells) produce a layer of surfactant 10 to 20 nm thick, which reduces the surface tension of small alveoli in the mammalian lung. The essential protective function of continually removing dust particles that have gained access to the alveoli is performed by another important type of cells, the alveolar phagocytes.

The smooth muscle layer of the interstitium persists in the finest bronchioles and even in the alveolar ducts to protect the alveoli from noxious vapors by varying the resistance to air flow. In the horse, under some conditions it can also lead to asthma-type problems such as heaves. Pulmonary capillaries act as a chemical sieve for mixed venous blood in the pulmonary artery. The endothelium of pulmonary capillaries also changes specifically the biologic activity of many circulating vasoactive substances (e.g., angiotensin I).

This chapter presents four aspects of nonrespiratory lung functions: pulmonary surfactant, defense mechanisms, interstitium, and metabolic activities.

PULMONARY SURFACTANT

Pulmonary surfactant, a phospholipid-protein complex that lines the alveoli and perhaps the small airways of the lungs, forms a 0.1- to 0.2-μm film, which is thicker near type II (cuboidal or granular) alveolar epithelial cells. These type II cells, commonly called pneumocytes II, have microvilli on their surface and contain many organelles (mitochondria, endoplasmic reticulum, Golgi complex, multivesicular bodies) and oxidative enzymes (Fig. 6–3). Their characteristic lamellar bodies store a merocrine secretion (the *surfactant*) rich in dipalmitoyl lecithin (DPL) that is extruded onto the alveolar surface.

Macrophages, which are normal components of the alveolar mechanical barrier, may also generate surfactant. In addition, Clara cells in the bronchioles synthesize the surfactant film lining these small airways. These nonciliated, secretory cells also have microvilli, a developed system of organelles, and large granulations.

Pneumocytes II give very little support to the alveolar wall, but are metabolically very active. Following injury to the alveolar wall, pneumocyte II cells rapidly proliferate and differentiate into type I (squamous) alveolar cells, that is, they become structural cells of the alveolus that are more resistant to injury. They may also secrete a variety of enzymes (e.g., phosphatidic acid phosphohydrolase). They are thought to control the electrolyte composition, by absorption and secretion, of the alveolar subphase. This evanescently thin aqueous layer is between the alveolar epithelial cells and the surface film; its total volume in man is 20 mL.

In large animal species the total amount of surfactant in the lungs is estimated at about 4 mL. Chemically, it is made up of electrolytes, mucopolysaccharides, lipoproteins, phospholipids, and proteins. Major components of phospholipids consist mainly of DPL and saturated fatty acids.

Recognized functions of surfactant are (1) maintaining proper humidity of the alveolar wall; (2) providing a constant

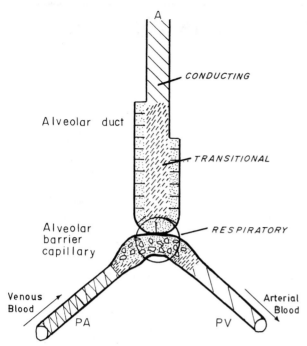

Figure 6-1 Diagram of the organization of the airways (*A*) and blood vessels (*P*) in the respiratory system. Conducting and transitional zones are only pathways for gases. Exchanges of gases occur in the respiratory zone containing alveolar air and blood capillaries. The capillary of the pulmonary artery (*PA*) brings mixed venous blood from the pulmonary circulation, and the pulmonary vein (*PV*) capillary carries arterial blood toward the peripheral circulation.

essential factor for easier pulmonary elastic recoil and reducing the work of breathing during passive expiration; (3) stabilizing the alveoli by lowering the surface tension at the air-liquid interface, or decreasing the tendency of small alveoli to collapse and fuse into larger alveoli at expiration; (4) resisting infiltration of capillary and interstitial fluids

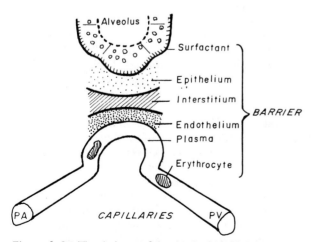

Figure 6-2 The six layers of the alveolus-blood barrier separating alveolar air in the mammalian lung from hemoglobin of the erythrocytes.

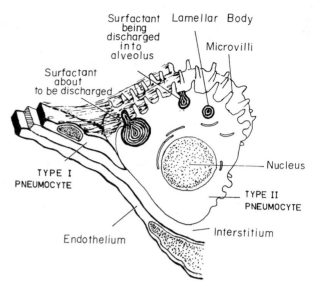

Figure 6-3 Electron microscopic diagram of a type II epithelial cell producing alveolar surfactant, the dipalmitoyl lecithin, which reduces the surface tension in alveoli and decreases their tendency to collapse. Morphologic highlights are microvilli and numerous lamellar bodies in the cytoplasm; the surfactant is discharged into an alveolus.

into the alveoli; and (5) emulsifying very small inhaled particles that may have reached the alveoli and thus facilitating their phagocytosis by macrophages.

Surfactant is not useful during fetal life. Its synthesis late in the prenatal period can be accelerated by maternal administration of glucocorticoids or thyroxine. Alveolar cells (pneumocytes II, macrophages, Clara cells) have steroid cytoplasmic receptors that activate nuclear processes leading to an increase in production of surfactant (Fig. 6-4). Secretion or excretion of surfactant is also increased by oxygen poisoning or by pilocarpine or epinephrine.

Conversely, the cellular output of surfactant is lowered by atropine, by colchicine, and by vinblastine. In cattle, reticulorumen formation of 3-methylindole (3MI) from L-tryptophan in herbages causes a loss of surfactant by promoting the transformation of type II alveolar cells into hypertrophied type I cells. Inactivation of surfactant by aspirated or transudated liquid or experimentally by detergent brings on alveolar instability and atelectasis. Loss of surfactant produces a "stiff lung" that requires greater muscular effort for pulmonary ventilation or increases the work of breathing, lowers pulmonary compliance (lung distensibility), and eventually causes pulmonary edema. Bilateral vagotomy reduces the surfactant film and causes atelectasis and the appearance of stiff lungs, as in respiratory distress syndrome or hyaline membrane disease.

Neonatal respiratory distress, a decrease in lung compliance (stiff lung) due to deficient synthesis of surfactant, occurs in piglets and foals:

"Barkers" is a descriptive term applied to foals and piglets with neonatal respiratory distress. The term "wanderer" is given to foals that survive the respiratory neonatal

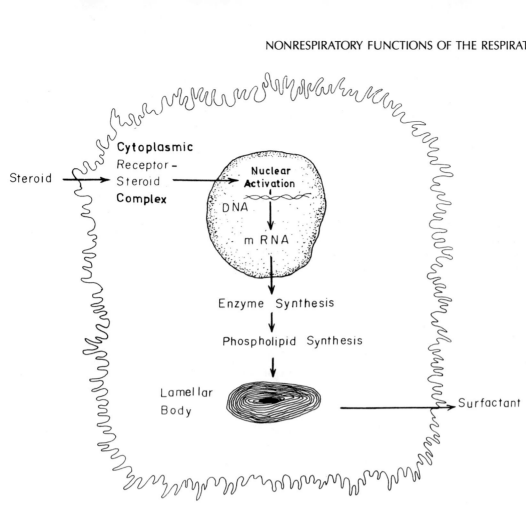

Figure 6–4 Lipid-soluble glucocorticoids diffuse across the plasma membrane to combine with specific receptors in the cytoplasm. The receptor-steroid complex then reaches the nucleus and syntheses of enzymes and phospholipids occur. Surfactant is stored in lamellar bodies and the merocrine secretion is delivered into alveoli.

distress but have brain damage and exhibit an aimless behavior with lack of a normal sense of fear.

Surfactant has a half-life of 15 hours in small laboratory animals and 48 hours in man. It is removed from the alveoli and airways by pinocytosis by cellular components of the alveolar wall, (e.g., pneumocytes I, alveolar macrophages) and by flowing up the conducting airways in the continuous surface film to be evacuated by the mucociliary defense system.

DEFENSE MECHANISMS OF THE AIRWAYS

Before entering the trachea, air must pass into the nares, nasopharynx, pharynx, and larynx to be heated to body temperature and saturated with water vapor. Although the normal airway is through the nares and nasopharynx, air passing through the open mouth is warmed and humidified in the remaining part of the respiratory conducting zone.

Earliest workers in the field of nonventilatory lung function were physiologists of the 19th century who introduced various solutions into the lungs and assessed their rates of absorption.

Gabriel COLIN'S treatise in 1856 includes reference to experiments in which water vapor, ether, chloroform, turpentine, and iodine were instilled into the lungs of horses. His edition of 1873 describes the much quoted experiment in which 25 L of warm water were tipped down the trachea of a horse over a period of 6 hours with no effect other than a deepening of respiration. Trace of excess fluid could not be found in the lungs at necropsy.

In 1857 Claude BERNARD observed that a solution of cyanide placed in the upper airway of a dog is without ill effect while the animal lies on its back, but is lethal within 7 to 8 minutes when the cranial end is lifted, demonstrating the high permeability of the alveoli to this highly lipid-soluble substance.

LAQUEUR, in 1921, with experiments prompted by the damaging effects of phosgene ($COCl_2$, a derivative of chloroform, or $CHCl_3$), noted that while instilled water rapidly disappeared from the lung, normal saline persisted for some time, and 1 molar solution (hypertonic) of sucrose caused pulmonary edema and hemoconcentration.

During inspiration, the upper esophageal sphincter (UES) normally closes to prevent movement of air into the esophagus, although negative esophageal pressures approximate those in the intrapleural space. During recovery from prolonged anesthesia, this function may be impaired, allowing air to pass into the esophagus during each inspiration, and gastric distention may follow.

Aerosol is a term for a fine dispersion in the ambient air of solids or liquids that remain airborne for a substantial amount of time. Many pollutants (carbon dioxide, sulfur oxides, hydrocarbons, nitrogen oxides, particles) exist in this form. Toxic gases are usually disposed of in the nasopharynx, with a contribution of tears from the eyes, which enter the nasal cavity via the nasolacrimal duct.

Defense reactions to invasion by particles in aerosols involve deposition of particles, clearance of deposited particles, and immunologic responses. *Deposition* refers to trapping of particles in the respiratory tract. *Clearance* is the process of removing deposited particles. *Retention* is the difference in time between deposition and clearance.

Deposition of Particles of Aerosols

The deposition of particles depends chiefly on their size. Three patterns of deposition are recognized: impaction for larger ones, sedimentation for medium-sized ones, and diffusion for the smallest (Fig. 6–5).

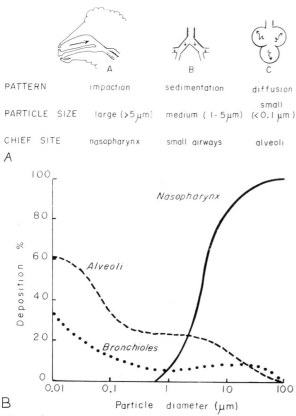

Figure 6–5 Deposition of particles from aerosols. **A,** Patterns of deposition; impaction, sedimentation, and diffusion with the main sites, which are related to particle size. **B,** Percentage of deposited particles in nasopharynx, bronchioles, and alveoli. The largest particles remain in the nasopharynx, 30 percent of the smallest ones settle in bronchioles, but more (60 percent) manage to reach the alveoli.

Impaction refers to the tendency of large particles (100 percent of those 20 μm in diameter, 95 percent of those larger than 5 μm, and 50 percent of those 1 to 5 μm) to fail to turn the corners of the nasopharynx. As a result, these particles impinge on the mucus-coated surfaces. Once a particle strikes the sticky surface, it is trapped and not released into the air stream.

Sedimentation is the gradual settling of 0.5 to 3 μm particles due to their mass, slower air flow, narrower air passages, and sudden changes of direction of air stream. It takes place extensively in the small airways, including the terminal and respiratory bronchioles.

Diffusion, the random movement of particles as a result of their continuous collisions with gas molecules, occurs only with very small particles (<0.1 μm in diameter). Deposition after diffusion takes place chiefly in small airways and in alveoli, where the distances to the wall are least.

Most of the small (0.5-μm) particles inhaled are not deposited at all but are exhaled with the next expiration. During their passage in the air stream, some may enlarge by aggregation or by hygroscopic action and increase their tendency toward deposition. The rate of ventilation affects the patterns of particle deposition of aerosols. Bradypnea (slow, deep respiration) facilitates the penetration of particles in the airways and the deposition by sedimentation and diffusion. Exercise causes faster air flow and favors the deposition of particles by impaction.

Clearance of Deposited Aerosol Particles

Two distinct *clearance mechanisms* remove aerosol particles that have been deposited in the airways; the *mucociliary,* or *mucociliary escalator, system;* and the alveolar *macrophages.*

Mucociliary System for Clearance of Deposited Aerosol Particles

The airways are covered with a mucous film for protection against dryness resulting from repeated passage of air. Mucus, a slimy, complex, sticky mixture of water, electrolytes, and special bronchial mucoproteins, is normally produced from several sources: transudation from plasma, serous and mucous secretions by submucosal glands situated deep in the bronchial wall, and secretion of cells on the bronchial surface epithelium (goblet, serous, and Clara cells).

Both serous and mucous cells of the bronchi are under the control of the parasympathetic autonomic nervous system. Anticholinergics (e.g., atropine) reduce but do not entirely inhibit bronchial secretions. Cholinergic drugs (e.g., pilocarpine) and electrical stimulation of the vagus nerve increase bronchial secretions. Sympathomimetic agents (e.g., isoproterenol) do not affect the bronchial secretions of most species, but in the cat and the dog they increase the size of the submucosal glands and the number of secreting cells. Infection produces bronchial submucosal hypertrophy in the pig. Mucokinetic agents influence the secretion of bronchial glands and increase the ciliary action. They act either directly (e.g., iodides, glyceryl guaiacolate) or indirectly via a gastropulmonary reflex through the vagus nerve. A mucolytic agent, acetylcysteine, administered by nebulization (fine liquid spray) ruptures the disulfide bridges of bronchial mucoprotein, and thus reduces the viscosity of mucus.

In the dog, the mucous film contains about 4 percent protein, is about 10 to 20 μm thick, and has two layers: a superficial, 1- to 2-μm *gel* layer, which is relatively tenacious, viscous, and efficient at trapping deposited particles, and a deeper *sol,* or aqueous, layer (periciliary liquid), which is less viscous and provides a medium in which cilia can move easily (Fig. 6-6).

A ciliated epithelium lines the airway except in alveoli, respiratory bronchioles, vocal cords, epiglottis and oropharynx, crypts of lymphoid masses, the olfactory area, and between the rostral ends of the nasal turbinates and the nostrils. In the respiratory tract, the major function of cilia is to transport mucus. Even when cilia are not present, as in the olfactory area, the mucus is dragged along by the pull of cilia on the mucous sheath covering adjacent areas.

Each ciliated cell has about 150 to 300 cilia (about eight per square micrometer of surface). A cilium is 6 to 7 μm long and 0.150 to 0.200 μm in diameter and is composed of 10 doublets of ciliary filaments, or microtubules, arranged in a circle of nine doublets about a special central doublet, which is responsible for ciliary motility. Dynein (for *dyn*amic prot*ein*) arms are ratchet structures that move one tubule over the other in a doublet of adjacent ciliary filaments, and are believed to generate the movements of cilia (see Fig. 6-6).

Cilia beat continuously in a synchronized fashion at about 600 and 1,200 times per minute or approximately 10 to 20 times per second. Cilia move rapidly on the forward stroke (one-fourth of the contraction time) as rigid rods; their tips strike the bottom of the gel layer and propel the mucus toward the mouth. The back stroke, or recovery phase, is slower (three-fourths of the contraction time), and the cilia are flexed to move entirely within the less viscous sol layer of mucus (see Fig. 6-6). Sympathomimetic influence increases ciliary activity, whereas parasympathomimetic influence decreases it. Immotile cilia with defective mucociliary transfers have been reported in dogs.

Throughout the tracheobronchial tree and the nasopharynx, mucus is continuously being carried toward the

Figure 6-6 **A,** Drawing of an electron micrograph of a cross-section of a cilium with the 10 microtubule doublets and the two dynein arms on each doublet. **B,** Movements of cilia in the periciliary fluid in the forward stroke and the back stroke. **C,** Mucus, produced by mucous glands and goblet cells, consists of a thin, superficial gel layer, which traps inhaled particles, and a deeper aqueous layer, called sol, or periciliary liquid. Mucus is propelled by continuous rhythmic activity of cilia.

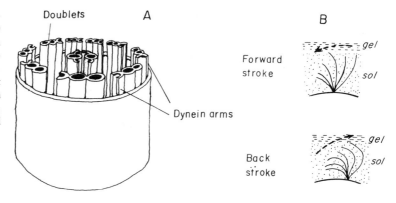

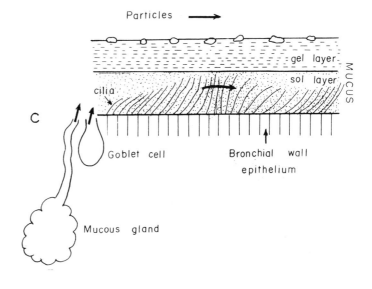

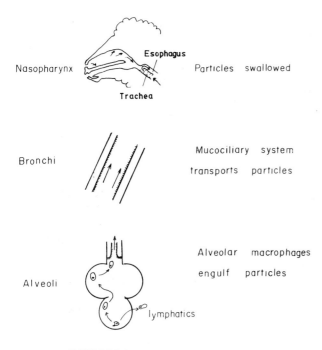

CLEARANCE OF DEPOSITED PARTICLES

Figure 6–7 Inhaled particles deposited on the surface of the airways are moved by the mucociliary escalator system and swallowed after reaching the pharynx. Particles in the alveoli are phagocytosed by alveolar macrophages, which then migrate by mucociliary escalation or escape via lymphatics.

orifice of the esophagus and unconsciously swallowed (Fig. 6–7). Mucus progresses at a rate of about 0.5 mm per minute in small bronchi, increasing orad to some 5 to 20 mm per minute in the trachea. Excess production of mucus may cause hawking—frequent attempts to clear the throat—accompanied by swallowing of mucus and air.

Alveolar Macrophages for Clearance of Deposited Aerosol Particles

Alveolar Macrophages. Macrophages (sometimes called histiocytes) on the alveolar wall and in the interstitium are mobile, phagocytic, and rich in lysosomes and lysozymes. Of medullary origin, or the result of mitosis in mature residents in the interstitium, alveolar macrophages actively adhere to respiratory structures and are the predominant phagocytic cells of the respiratory tract. As such, they usually outnumber neutrophils by a factor of two or three and constitute about 70 percent of cells lavaged from the normal lung. By comparison with other animal species, cattle have relatively fewer resident alveolar macrophages and lower levels of lysozymes.

The number (10^6 per gram of lung) and the phagocytic and bactericidal activity of alveolar macrophages are increased by biochemical antioxidants, secretory immunoglobins (IgA) and immunologic factors (e.g., IgG, complement factors C3a and C4a, lymphokines from T lymphocytes), and carbon dust. Conversely, the motility and

functions of alveolar macrophages are reduced by viral infection, dehydration, chilling, hypoxia, metabolic acidosis (starvation), uremia, oxidizing gases (O_2, O_3, SO_2, NO_2), and substances that increase the level of cyclic adenosine monophosphate (cAMP) (e.g., ethanol, histamine, methylxanthine, prostaglandin E, cholera endotoxin, beta-sympathomimetics, and glucocorticoids). Excessive phagocytosis of inorganic particles (silicate, asbestos, or glass fibers) destroys macrophages. The half-life of alveolar macrophages in vivo is about 4 days, but they can live several months in tissue culture.

Particles deposited in the alveoli cannot be handled by the mucociliary escalator system owing to the absence of cilia in the alveoli and must be engulfed by macrophages. After ingesting foreign substances, macrophages either migrate to the bronchi, where they load onto the mucociliary escalator, or leave the lung in the lymphatics or possibly the blood. When the burden of particles is very large or toxic, macrophages migrate through the bronchial epithelium and pass into the interstitium. The inactivated particles may remain there for some time; most are held in lymph nodes, but some are brought into the general circulation and may be seen in the spleen, the liver, or subpleural spaces. The secretion products of alveolar macrophages are summarized in Table 6–1, and the functions of alveolar macrophages are outlined in Table 6–2.

Clearance and Retention of Deposited Particles by Alveolar Macrophages. Alveolar particles taken up by the macrophages and the mucociliary system are cleared in about 24 hours. For particles that have passed to the interstitium, clearance occurs within 1 to 14 days. A period of 3 months is required for migration of particles from the alveoli to the subpleural spaces.

Toxic inorganic particles (e.g., silicates) are handled differently. They cause liberation of lysosomes from the

---

TABLE 6–1 Secretion Products of Alveolar Macrophages

Enzymes: Lysozymes, esterases, catalase, proteinases (elastase, collagenase, plasminogen activators)
Factors: B lymphocyte, T lymphocyte, plasma cell, cytolytic, colony-stimulating (PMNs, macrophages), leukotrienes
Low-molecular-weight molecules: Prostaglandins, peroxide
Proteins: Complement, interferon

TABLE 6–2 Functions of Alveolar Macrophages

Function of defense against microorganisms
  Cellular immunity
  Humoral immunity
  Phagocytosis (primary mechanism)
  Synthesis of interferon
Nondefensive functions
  Scavenging of cells, particles, and toxins
  Synthesis of catalase, collagenase, elastase
    Fibroblast-activating factor
    Peroxide
    Plasminogen activator
    Prostaglandins

macrophages and start a chain of inflammatory reactions that leads to fibrosis of pulmonary tissue. The process is auto-regenerating as the particles are not eliminated. Other substances (alcohol, virus, ozone, nitrogen dioxide) prevent macrophages from acting as cleaners, decrease their bactericidal power, and favor development of infection.

Deposited bacteria are not eliminated but are killed on the spot by macrophages. Bactericidal activity is due mostly to extremely rapid synthesis of hydrogen peroxide and of a free radical of superoxide in the membrane of macrophages. Lysosomes and proteinases (plasminogen activators) also contribute to the bactericidal action of macrophages.

Immunologic Reactions

A special local immunologic system, bronchus-associated lymphoid tissue (BALT), exists in the lung to limit the penetration of inert or living antigens. This secondary defense mechanism is brought into action to support the primary defense mechanism, alveolar macrophages. A cellular and humoral defense system, it consists of leukocyte infiltration, complement system, and chemical mediators (leukostatic factors, lymphokines, and lymphocyte factor). According to their importance, immunologic reactions can support nonspecific defense mechanisms, can cause hyperimmunization, and can be the cause of respiratory problems such as allergic rhinitis. *Humoral immunity* is provided by the *tracheobronchial part,* and *cell-mediated immunity* is produced in the *interstitial-alveolar-mediastinal part.*

Humoral Immunity

The humoral immunity in the upper airway is provided by abundant secretory IgA (sIgA; 200 mg per deciliter versus 30 mg per deciliter in bovine serum) generated by lymphoepithelial organs. Its immunologic portion is produced by plasmocytes derived from *B lymphocytes* in the bronchioles. The secretory component, a glycoprotein that joins the two groups of four light and heavy polypeptide chains by disulfide bridges (Fig. 6–8), originates from the mucous cells of the bronchial epithelium. This secretory piece probably protects IgA against proteolytic enzymes in the mucus. Other immunoglobulins (IgG and IgM), present in low concentrations, are mostly transudated from plasma. IgA neutralizes virus, agglutinates microorganisms, and prevents attachment of virus or bacteria to the respiratory mucosa. When this barrier of defense is insufficient, lymphocytes and macrophages are mobilized.

Cell-Mediated Immunity

Cell-mediated immunity in the bronchoalveolar region is achieved by increased local formation of specialized, mobile, and recirculating *T lymphocytes.* These cells, not usually present in the bronchoalveolar film, may represent 80 percent of the lymphocytes in blood. In response to antigens (microorganisms, parasites, spores, fungus) or organic dusts (pollen, feathers), T lymphocytes produce and release lym-

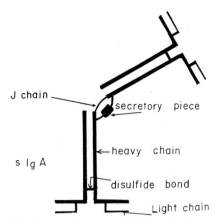

Figure 6–8 Secretory immunoglobulin A (sIgA), a dimer immunoglobulin of mucosal surfaces and of mucus of the upper airways, which contains two monomer IgA subunits as well as two extra polypeptide chains—secretory component and J chain.

phokines. These lymphokines prepare macrophages and their antibacterial or antiviral secretions (interferon, lysosome, complement) to react immunologically mostly with IgG and IgM instead of IgA as in the upper airway and to dispose of inhaled particles. IgE-mediated allergic reactions in cats and dogs (e.g., allergic rhinitis) can occur when IgE (reaginic antibodies) on the surface of mast cells reacts with seasonal antigens (pollen).

NONRESPIRATORY FUNCTIONS OF THE PULMONARY INTERSTITIUM

The interstitium, long considered a simple connective tissue, has complex functions. Besides being a part of the wall structure of large vessels and bronchi and connecting alveoli and capillaries, it contains 40 percent of the total cells of the lungs. Some of these cells have contractile proteins that can cause contraction of the alveolar tissue and formation of folds in the capillaries, hindering the progression of erythrocytes and slowing blood flow. Contractile interstitial cells can influence the ventilation-perfusion ratio of the alveoli. The interstitium has two components, collagen and elastic fibers.

A change in the nature of collagen associated with an excess of its production increases the rigidity of the lung (pulmonary fibrosis). The problem seems to be related to lymphokines generated by T lymphocytes. Reduced resistance to stretching, loss of elasticity, and destruction of alveoli occur in pulmonary emphysema. The problem seems to be associated also with an excessive production of proteolytic enzymes (collagenase and elastase) by alveolar macrophages and neutrophils, or a deficiency in alpha$_1$-antitrypsin. These enzyme dysfunctions disturb the equilibrium between synthesis and lysis of protein components (collagen and elastin) of collagen and elastic fibers.

Rumen lactobacilli transform L-tryptophan in herbages into indoleacetic acid and 3MI, which are absorbed in the general circulation. In the pulmonary circulation, 3MI is altered to a pneumotoxic metabolite by enzymes in the Clara cells. This substance has a lytic effect on type I alveolar cells and increases the number of macrophages and neutrophils in the alveoli (excess elastase). Ultimately type II cells are transformed into hypertrophied type I cells (epithelialization, fetalization, or adenomatosis), and loss of surfactant causes a respiratory distress syndrome with interstitial edema and emphysema. The 3MI from lush regrowth in pasture (atypical interstitial pneumonia, AIP, or fog fever), and 4-ipomeanol in moldy sweet potato (*Fusarium solanae*), are two of many plant agents toxic to cattle. Others, still to be chemically identified, occur in purple mint (*Perilla frutescens*), stinkwood (*Zieria arborescens*), and rapeseed and kale (*Brassica* species).

Somewhat like the capillaries in the alveolocapillary wall, which have a thin and thick wall, the interstitium is not of uniform thickness. On the thin side of the alveolar capillary, where gas exchanges occur, the interstitium is simply epithelial basement membrane fused to endothelial basement membrane (Fig. 6–9). On the thick side of the capillary, the interstitium has some fibrils of collagen and accommodates to exchanges of fluids across the endothelium. Fluids leaving the capillaries move within the thick interstitium of the alveoli and track to the perivascular and peribronchial interstitium containing lymphatic capillaries. The alveolar wall is devoid of lymphatic capillaries, but loose interstitial tissue performs in a similar way. Interstitial edema may result from oxygen toxicity, from drugs (e.g., nitrofurantoin), and from rumen metabolites of L-tryptophan.

METABOLIC ACTIVITIES OF THE RESPIRATORY TISSUES

The lung acts as a metabolic filter on the general venous circulation in much the same way that the liver does on the splanchnic, or portal venous, circulation. Important quantitative anabolic and catabolic reactions occur to regulate natural and xenobiotic (exogenous) substances. These metabolic activities can protect the heart and brain from chemical insults.

This remarkable efficiency is related to the large surface of the alveolocapillary membrane, the great quantity of blood flowing in the pulmonary capillaries as a thin film, and the variety of enzymes produced by endothelial cells of the respiratory membrane. It is estimated that the lungs have $3 \cdot 10^8$ alveoli and that each alveolus may have 1,000 or more capillary segments 8 to 15 μm in diameter.

Within intact lung capillaries, enzymes are partitioned so that some have access to circulating substrates and others do not. Owing to the large number of *caveolae intracellulares* (pinocytic or plasmalemmal vesicles) and to the extensive meshwork of projections, the surface of endothelial cells may be considerably greater than the frequently cited figure of 70 m^2. Enzymes on the surface of the pulmonary endothelial

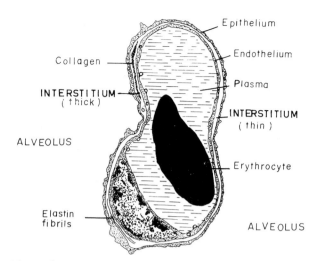

Figure 6–9 Electron micrograph diagram of an alveolocapillary wall with the thin and thick interstitium containing collagen and elastin fibers. The interstitium of the respiratory membrane also serves for lymphatic drainage. ($\times 6,000$)

cells of these small vessels can almost instantly (in less than the capillary transit time of 2 seconds) hydrolyze angiotensin I, kinins (e.g., bradykinin), and adenosine tri-di-, and monophosphate (ATP, ADP, AMP) (Fig. 6–10). Some blood-borne substances are identified and captured by receptors on the membrane surface, then taken into the cytoplasm of endothelial cells via an active transport mechanism for either anabolic (e.g., formation of cAMP from ATP) or catabolic (e.g., serotonin, norepinephrine, and prostaglandins of the E and F series) reactions.

Endothelial cells of the respiratory membrane are paradoxical. They eliminate certain prostaglandins (A and F), and they synthesize and release prostaglandins I_2 and E_2 (PGI$_2$ and PGE$_2$). The synthesis of the inhibitor of platelet aggregation, prostacyclin, or PGI$_2$, is an important function in maintaining the fluidity of pulmonary and arterial blood. In a rabbit that is pregnant or has been given progesterone, PGE$_2$ synthesis is tripled, presumably to aid in suppression of tissue injury or in its resolution.

Pulmonary endothelial cells participate also in the metabolism of chylomicrons through the action of a lipoprotein lipase. These chylomicrons reach the endothelial cells directly from the digestive tract via the thoracic duct and the mixed venous blood. The lung's capacity to control and limit blood loss is provided mainly by thromboplastin, or tissue factor, which originates from the endothelial cells.

Nerve terminals in the lungs produce vasoactive intestinal peptide (VIP) and substance P. These neuropeptides have different effects: VIP relaxes pulmonary smooth muscles, and substance P contracts the smooth muscles of the airways.

Drugs such as heparin and some antibiotics are absorbed by the lungs. In the bovine, after intratracheal injection (2 mL per kilogram right on the most ventral aspect in

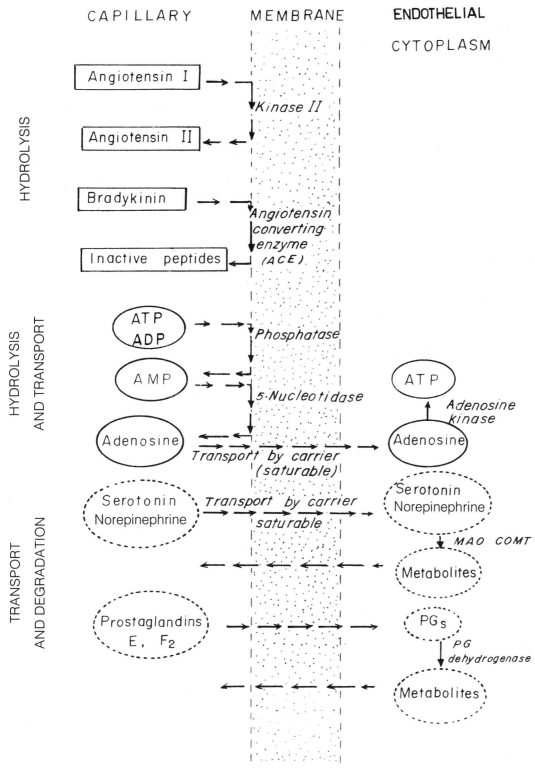

Figure 6–10 Metabolic reactions of hydrolysis, and of transport and degradation on natural blood-borne substances through enzymes in endothelial cells of the alveolocapillary membrane.

the upper third of the cervical trachea), equivalent doses of antibiotics are absorbed more rapidly than from intramuscular or subcutaneous injection sites. Higher and more rapid serum antibiotic concentration peaks are obtained with penicillin, ampicillin, tylosin, oxytetracycline, and chloramphenicol. For lack of a drug reservoir at the site of administration, the serum concentration of these antibiotics declines more rapidly. Conversely, chloramphenicol sodium succinate, dihydrostreptomycin, and neomycin sulfate are absorbed less rapidly by the lungs.

REFERENCES

Afzelius BA, Carlsten J, Karlsson S. Clinical, pathologic, and ultrastructural features of situs inversus and immotile-cili syndrome in a dog. J Am Vet Med Assoc 1984;184:560.

Boat TF, Cheng PW. Biochemistry of airways mucus secretion. Fed Proc 1980;39:3067.

Bowden DH. The alveolar macrophage. Environ Health Perspect 1984;55:327.

Breeze R. Structure, function, and metabolism in the lung. Vet Clin North Am (Food Anim Pract) 1985;1:219.

Fantone JC, Hunkel SL, Ward PA. Chemotactic mediators in neutrophil-dependent lung injury. Annu Rev Physiol 1982;44:283.

Gillis CN. Pharmacological aspect of metabolic processes in the pulmonary microcirculation. Annu Rev Pharmacol Toxicol 1986;26:183.

Liggitt HD. Defense mechanisms in the bovine lung. Vet Clin North Am (Food Anim Pract) 1985;1:347.

Nelson R. Measurement of tracheal mucus transport rate in the horse. Am J Vet Res 1983;44:1165.

Nodel JA, Davis B. Parasympathetic and sympathetic regulation of secretion from submucosal glands in airways. Fed Proc 1980;39:3075.

Pfannkuch F, Blumke S. What's new in lung physiology—Pulmonary vessel regulation/nonrespiratory metabolic lung functions. Pathol Respir Pract 1985;180:718.

Rooney SA. Lung surfactant. Environ Heath Perspect 1984;55:205.

Ryan JW, Ryan US. Metabolic functions of the pulmonary vascular endothelium. Adv Vet Sci Comp Med 1982;26:79.

Schiefer B, Jayasekara MU, Mills JHL. Comparison of naturally occurring and tryptophan-induced bovine atypical interstitial pneumonia. Vet Pathol 1974;11:327.

Van Golde LMG, Batenburg JP, Robertson B. The pulmonary surfactant system: biochemical aspects and functional significance. Physiol Rev 1988;68:374.

Ward PA. Host defense mechanisms responsible for lung injury. J Allergy Clin Immunol 1986;78:373.

CHAPTER 7

MECHANICS OF RESPIRATION

Respiratory mechanics is concerned with the study of the forces operating during the cyclic inflation and deflation of the lungs during breathing. Movements of the lungs and rib cage—the respiratory structures—are caused by the active forces of respiratory muscles and by the passive forces of the elastic recoil of the respiratory structures themselves. The forces applied by the rib cage muscles are spent in overcoming opposing forces: the elastic recoil of the respiratory structures and the resistance to flow of gas in the large and small airways. This chapter presents major concepts of the physics of the respiratory movements, the methodology used in respiratory mechanics to measure elastic recoil forces of the lung and of the rib cage, and airway resistance in animals. Aspects of pulmonary ventilation and of respiratory evaporative cooling in animals are also discussed.

PHYSICS OF RESPIRATORY MOVEMENTS (INSPIRATION AND EXPIRATION)

Subatmospheric Pressure in the Pleural Space

The parietal pleura lines the rib cage, which encloses the visceral pleura covering the lungs. The lungs and rib cage, both elastic respiratory structures, are separated by a narrow space (5 to 10 μm in cats), the *pleural space* (interpleural or intrathoracic), which contains only a thin layer of fluid (about 2 mL) dispersed over a large surface area. This fluid film between the pleurae prevents separation but allows lateral displacement (sliding) of the two pleural sheets. It also causes adhesion of both pleurae, for transmission of the active and passive forces from rib cage and lungs, and helps keep the lungs closely applied to the chest wall (Fig. 7–1).

Elastic recoil pressure of the rib cage, Pst(cw), which tends to spring the ribs outward, and elastic recoil pressure of the lung, Pst, which tends to collapse the lungs, interact and equilibrate to produce a subatmospheric pleural pressure, Ppl, in the pleural space. This relative intrathoracic vacuum causes the lungs to dilate and the rib cage to be pulled inward. During inspiration, the intrathoracic pressure decreases (from about −2.5 to −6 mm Hg) with the expansion of the rib cage. Conversely, during expiration, the negative Ppl returns to its initial or preinspiration level (i.e., passes from about −6 to −2.5 mm Hg) and also returns the lung dilation to a resting level. When the rib cage is surgically opened, loss of the intrathoracic partial vacuum (then Ppl = Pв, or atmospheric pressure) causes the lungs to collapse because of Pst, and the rib cage to expand outward because of Pst(cw).

The action of breathing is analogous to the operation of a pair of bellows (LEONARDO da VINCI, 1452–1519). The lung movement in a living dog was observed through a pleural window by VESALIUS (1514–1564).

In 1804, REISSEISEN (1773–1828) won the first prize from the Berlin Akademie for his discovery of the bronchial smooth muscles with the aid of only a hand lens. The respiratory vagal innervation was found by VOLKMANN, who showed that stimulation of the vagus nerve of a dead animal produced an expiratory puff sufficient to blow out a candle (1844).

INFLATION AND DEFLATION OF THE LUNG DURING A RESPIRATORY CYCLE

Inspiration

Inspiration, or admission of a volume of air (tidal volume) into the airways, is an active process in most animal species. Contraction of the inspiratory muscles increases intrathoracic volume and renders the pressure in the pleural space more negative. During the inspiration phase of quiet breathing, pleural pressure is reduced from about −2.5 to about −6 mm Hg (Fig. 7–2), and the lungs are forced into additional expansion to admit a tidal volume. The pressure in the conducting and transitional airways then becomes slightly less than atmospheric pressure, and air flows into the lungs.

Movement of the *diaphragm* in quadrupeds accounts for nearly all the changes in intrathoracic volume during quiet inspiration. Attached around the rib cage and arching over the liver, the diaphragm moves backward when it contracts, causing an expansion of the abdominal cavity and a higher abdominal pressure (Fig. 7–3). In the horse, the distance of this diaphragmatic movement is about 20 cm, but it may be as much as 80 cm during deep inspiration. The reduced intrathoracic pressure would tend to pull the rib cage inward if the other inspiratory muscles were inactive (as in an anesthetized animal).

The other major inspiratory muscles are the *external intercostal muscles,* which run obliquely between ribs. When the external intercostals contract, the ribs pivot as if hinged at the rachis and increase the transverse diameter of the thoracic cage. The parallel expansion of the rib cage and abdomen is caused by simultaneous contraction of the external intercostals and of the diaphragm muscles.

Contraction of the diaphragm by electrical stimulation of a phrenic nerve was first recorded by Duchenne (1807–1875).

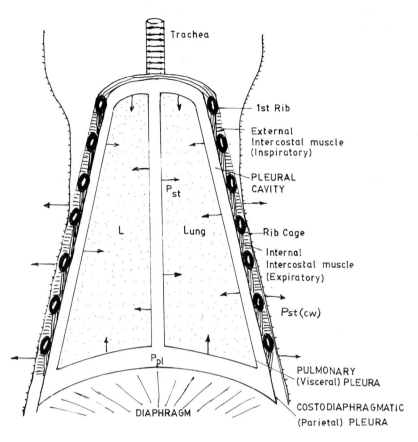

Figure 7–1 Longitudinal section of the thorax in animals. In the thoracic cavity, the lungs exert an inward elastic recoil pressure, Pst, which interacts with the outward elastic recoil of the rib cage, Pst(cw). These forces equilibrate to create the subatmospheric pleural pressure (Ppl<PB) in the virtual space. A film of fluid allows sliding of the pleurae but ensures their adhesion to each other. During inspiration, the rib cage cavity is expanded by contraction of diaphragm and external intercostals. Expiration is passive in eupnea. Internal intercostals are involved during active expiration.

Expiration

In most species, during quiet breathing, *expiration* is passive (i.e., muscles are not used to return the rib cage to its resting volume). Passive expiration, initiated at the end of inspiration, occurs through the elastic recoil of the respira-

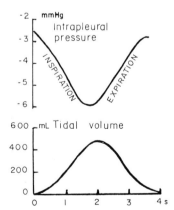

Figure 7–2 During inspiration, Ppl gradually declines from −2.5 to −6 mm Hg. Similarly, during expiration, Ppl returns to its preinspiration level. The entire tidal volume of air is admitted during active inspiration and is expelled during passive expiration. At the beginning of inspiration and end of expiration, air does not flow into or out of the upper respiratory tract.

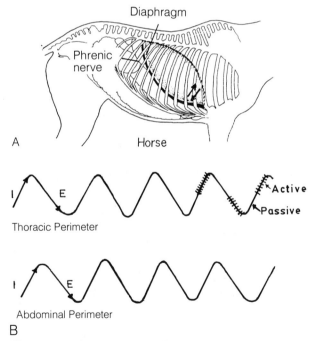

Figure 7–3 A, Arrangement of the diaphragm in quadrupeds. Contraction of the diaphragm increases the capacity of the rib cage and compresses the abdominal organs. Relaxation during expiration has the opposite effect. **B,** The origin of respiration is diphasic in the horse. Both inspiration and expiration begin as passive events and end as active events. Changes in the perimeters of the thorax and the abdomen occur in parallel.

tory structures (lungs and rib cage). These passive forces pull the rib cage and the lungs back to their resting position and volume. Duration of expiration is slightly longer than inspiration ($T_I < T_E$). Curves of the difference in volume divided by the difference in pressure (dVL/dPpl) for inspiration and expiration are different and not overlapping (hysteresis). Higher volume difference values are measured during expiration than during inspiration (Fig. 7–4).

In the normal horse at rest, inspiration and expiration are both diphasic. Normal equine inspiration starts as a passive event but becomes an active process with participation of the diaphragm and external intercostals. Equine expiration also begins passively and changes into an active process involving the abdominal muscles. Part of the energy spent during the end of active inspiration and expiration is momentarily stored and immediately returned as passive energy to initiate the succeeding expiration and inspiration (see Fig. 7–3B).

On exercise and during forced maneuvers involving the abdominal press (i.e., closure of the glottis followed by an active expiration attempt—coughing, vomiting, defecation), the expiratory muscles contract. The major muscles used for this type of active expiration are those of the *abdominal wall*. Their contraction raises intraabdominal pressure and pushes the diaphragm craniad into the rib cage, thus reducing its volume. The *internal intercostal muscles* are also expiratory structures. Contraction of the internal intercostals pulls the ribs caudad, ventrad, and inward, thus decreasing both the craniocaudal and the lateral dimensions of the rib cage. In the dog, spontaneous quiet expiration is an active process rather than a passive one. The abdominal muscles, the transversus abdominis more than the external oblique (obliquus externus abdominis) and triangularis sterni (transversus thoracis), are involved to varying degrees according to the posture of the body and the head.

Anesthetized horses placed in a lateral or supine posture manifest a reduction in lung volume and an increase in asynchronous ventilation. Those changes are reversed by moving the horse to a prone posture.

METHODOLOGY IN STUDYING RESPIRATORY MECHANICS IN ANIMALS

Methods of measuring parameters of respiratory movements in uncooperative animals can be classified as static and dynamic. Static methods yield descriptive measurements of a limited number of respiratory parameters. Dynamic methods, which provide continuous (integrated or summated) measurements, permit computer analysis of the data and computation of derived or theoretical parameters.

Static Methods in Animal Respiratory Physiology

Without the cooperation of the animal, the static methods give descriptive data on the frequency and duration of each respiratory cycle and the amplitude of the movements of the rib cage. In an anesthetized or trained animal, the volume of air inhaled and exhaled and the oxygen consumption may also be measured.

Excursions of the thoracic wall, synchronous with inspiration and expiration movements, can be recorded with devices that measure or reflect changes in rib cage perimeter. Analyses of these traces give descriptive information on the type of respiration (thoracic, abdominal), on the frequency (f) and amplitude of respiratory movements, and on the duration and pattern of inspiration–expiration–pause. Similar information can be obtained, either with *thermistors* that detect temperature changes in air going in and out at the nares, or with *impedance pneumography,* which records variations in impedance between two cutaneous or subcutaneous electrodes placed on each side of the thorax.

In laboratory animals (mice, rats, guinea pigs, rabbits), respiratory frequency can be measured by *body plethysmography.* The animal is placed in an airtight container with controlled air intake and outlet, and extremely small pressure variations caused by inspiration (increase) and expiration (decrease) are recorded.

Figure 7–4 In eupnea, differences in the dV/dP curves as inspiration and expiration form a hysteresis loop. At the same Ppl, the volume curves do not overlap but indicate that a greater volume of air is in the lung during expiration than during inspiration (e.g., at −4 Ppl, pulmonary volume is 55 mL at inspiration and 350 mL at expiration). The resting volume (Vr) is usually identical with the FRC, or air volume remaining in the lung, after a normal expiration. Friction of air in the respiratory tract is one of the contributing factors to this hysteresis loop.

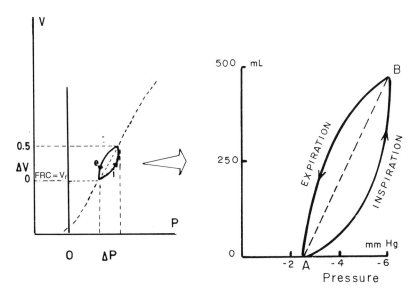

Auscultation of the respiratory tract for breath sounds can serve to evaluate respiratory rate and respiratory movements. At the level of the constriction of the glottis, vibrations of each column of inspired air produce (extrathoracic) *normal breath sounds.* These breath sounds are loudest over the larynx, trachea, and base of the lung (airways >2 mm in diameter) and progressively quieter as distance from the glottis increases. The quietest areas of the lung are those over the diaphragm, that is, farthest from the glottis, where the small (<1- to 2-mm diameter) tubes do not conduct sounds. Louder physiologic breath sounds, resulting from faster air flow, are heard when respiratory rate and depth increase with exercise, excitement, or high environmental temperature. Normal breath sounds have been wrongly termed alveolar sounds, vesicular sounds, bronchial sounds, and bronchovesicular sounds. Besides being archaic, these terms are unjustified, since these normal breath sounds disappear after a tracheotomy, which creates a bypass for air caudad to the glottic constriction of the upper airway. Breath sounds are difficult if not impossible to hear in obese animals and in noisy field conditions. In the horse, two peak flows at inspiration and expiration produce biphasic breath sounds.

Recording *spirometers,* which measure input and output of gas at inspiration and expiration, are also used in anesthetized animals and in animals trained to wear a gas mask or a mouthpiece appropriate to their anatomy and size (Fig. 7–5). The results of spirometry provide information on the volume of gas inspired and expired (V_TI and V_TE) and the minute volume ($\dot{V} = f \times V_T$). It can also be used to measure oxygen consumption ($\dot{V}O_2$) and to give an indication of metabolic activity (e.g., preprandial, postprandial). For example, a pig requires less than 60 minutes after a meal to increase its respiratory frequency and its oxygen consumption.

Dynamic Methods in Animal Respiratory Physiology

In uncooperative animals, the standard and reference technique for evaluating pulmonary mechanics requires the measurement of pleural pressure (Ppl) and volumes of air flow during one or a few cycles of respiratory movements. Pleural pressure is estimated from caudal esophageal pressure (Pes, pressure inside the thoracic portion of the esophagus) and air flow ($\dot{V}$) with a pneumotachograph. Ppl is measured with a balloon catheter or an open-tipped fluid-filled catheter introduced into the esophagus. A local anesthetic is sprayed on the oropharynx, and the outside of the catheter is covered with an anesthetic paste. The balloon or the open tip is positioned orad to the lower esophageal sphincter and connected to differential transducer to record the changes of Pes = Ppl. An airtight mask containing a pneumotachograph and a flow transducer to record air flow ($\dot{V}$), which is electronically integrated to yield tidal volume (V_T), is put on the animal. The dynamic lung compliance (CLdyn) at zero flow and

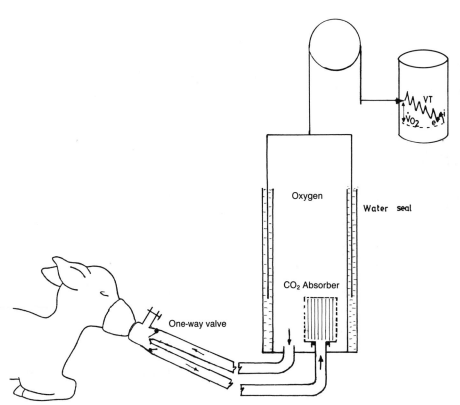

Figure 7–5 Spirometry in trained or anesthetized animals. Through a mask of appropriate size (or a tracheal catheter, if the animal is anesthetized), the animal first breathes outside air until adapted to the instrumentation. Then the valve is closed, and breathing is from and into an oxygen reservoir that has accessories to record inspiration and expiration. Carbon dioxide is absorbed on soda lime, and the amount of oxygen consumed can be computed from the recording. This method yields information on f, V_T, $\dot{V}$, and $\dot{V}O_2$.

single-point lung resistance (RL) are derived from $\dot{V}$, VT, and Ppl. Other parameters and indices (ratios of parameters) of respiratory mechanics at inspiration and expiration are also possible, for example, f, VTI, VTE, TI, TE, total breath duration (TT), $\dot{V}$I, $\dot{V}$E, mean inspiratory flow (VTI/TI), inspi-

ratory duty cycle (TI/TT), peak and midtidal inspiratory and expiratory gas flow (PIF, PIF50, PEF, PEF50), and tidal breathing flow–volume loop (TBFVL; Fig. 7–6). In the horse, temporary tranquilization (xylazine) may be required to facilitate instrumentation.

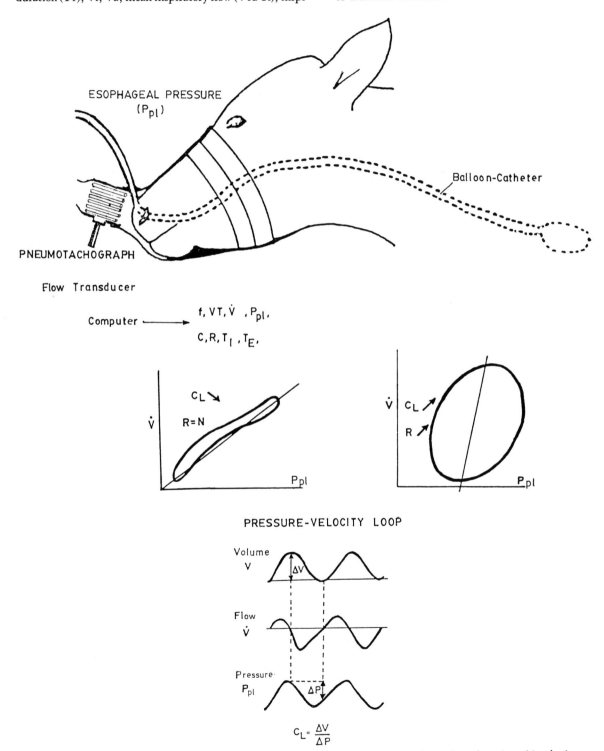

Figure 7–6   In anesthetized, uncooperative, tranquilized, or trained animals pneumotachography and esophageal intubation are used to obtain dynamic parameters of f, VT, $\dot{V}$, and Ppl. From recordings of these values, dV, dP, and dV/dP or Cl can be calculated. With a computer, the relation between flow ($\dot{V}$) and Ppl can be followed and visualized as a pressure-velocity loop.

A pneumotachograph is a mechanical resistance (a wire mesh screen, an orifice, or a bundle of narrow tubes as in the Fleisch design) placed in the air stream, usually incorporated into a face mask. A pressure difference, proportional to flow rate, is sensed by a differential pressure transducer and transformed into a visible signal (oscilloscope) or recorded on a polygraph. This signal can also be integrated to yield flow-volume loop, or, when related to Ppl, it can give volume-pressure curves.

Bipolar electromyography of the respiratory muscles is used to define the instant and the importance of their contractions during the inspiratory or expiratory phase of breathing. The muscle potentials are detected with fine wires implanted in the muscles (laryngeal abdominals, external intercostals) or with intraesophageal electrodes mounted on the balloon catheter, which is brought into contact with tissues near the diaphragm. In resting or anesthetized animals, the glottis is more widely open during inspiration than during expiration.

PULMONARY VENTILATION IN UNCOOPERATIVE ANIMALS

The amount of air that moves into the lungs with each inspiration (or the amount that moves out with each expiration) is called the tidal volume (V_T, or V_{TI}, or V_{TE}). Tidal volume and respiratory frequency (f) are the only respiratory parameters easily measured in trained animals or in anesthetized uncooperative animals (Table 7–1). From their values, the volume of air entering or leaving the respiratory tract per minute (i.e., the minute respiratory volume during inspiration ($\dot{V}I$) or expiration ($\dot{V}E$), can be calculated

$$(\dot{V} = V_T \times f = L/min)$$

Breathing frequency shows an inverse correlation to body mass (f = 70 × $kg^{0.25}$), suggesting that animals with a high metabolic rate have a higher pulmonary ventilation (see Table 7–1). In contrast, the volume of tidal air is related to body mass. V_T (mL) = 7.69 × $kg^{1.04}$ formulates this general concept, and empirically V_T is estimated at 10 mL per kilogram in small animals and 8 mL per kilogram in large animals.

The frequency of breathing (f) in a horse tends to lock in with that of stride frequency, one for one at gaits above a walk (canter, gallop, trot). During galloping $\dot{V}I$ is between 10 and 15 L per minute, whereas f can rise to as high as 150 per minute. This means that $\dot{V}T$ enters and leaves the respiratory system five times each second, with an average flow rate of 50 to 75 L per second (peak flow can be 90 L per second or higher). The ventilation of a racing thoroughbred exceeds 2250 L per minute.

The amount of air inspired or expired per minute ($\dot{V}I$ or $\dot{V}E$) is about 13 L per square meter in a normal calf with an average body mass of 59 kg (the body surface area according to Brody's formula: $S(m^2) = 0.12 \ kg^{0.56}$). Small animals consume more oxygen per unit of tissue than large animals to maintain their body temperature at 38° C. For example, bats consume almost 100 times as much oxygen per kilogram per minute as elephants. Pulmonary ventilation and lung perfusion are considered functional adaptations, whereas the morphologic adaptation of the lung volume and of the alveolar exchange area is a mechanism to satisfy the supply of oxygen. Alveolar diameter, but not lung volume (about 8 percent of the volume of the body), is inversely correlated to metabolic rate. The higher the metabolic rate, the smaller is the alveolar diameter, thus increasing the exchange area markedly (Fig. 7–7).

TABLE 7–1   Resting Respiratory Rate, Tidal Air, Minute Volume, and Functional Residual Capacity in Some Animals

Animal	Mass (kg)	f (breaths/min)	V_T (mL/kg)	$\dot{V}$ L/min/kg	FRC (mL, BTPS)
Calf	155	25	9.7	0.24	3,400
Cat	2.95	26	11.9	0.30	66
Cow (adult)	490	30	7.3	0.22	15,000
Dog	22	24	11.4	0.30	609
Goat	32	19	9.7	0.18	
Guinea pig	0.52	90	7.4	0.64	4.8
(neonate)	0.082	58	5.8	0.41	
Hamster (neonate)	0.0064	78	8.8	0.42	
Horse	475	12	14.1	0.17	18,000
Kitten	0.3	42	14.6	0.66	
Lamb (neonate)	4.4	50	10	0.50	
Monkey	2.68	40			87.5
Mouse	0.03	120			0.3
(neonate)	0.0017	130	8.8	1.15	
Pig	30	26	9.2	0.24	
Piglet	1.2	36	11.7	0.42	
Pony	274	24	9.9	0.24	
Puppy	0.3	30	4.5	0.46	
Rabbit	2.4	39	6.6	0.26	11.3
(neonate)	0.08	70	9.9	0.70	
Rat	0.25	97			1.6
(neonate)	0.007	97	9.5	0.92	
Sheep	42	19	8.2	0.16	1,350

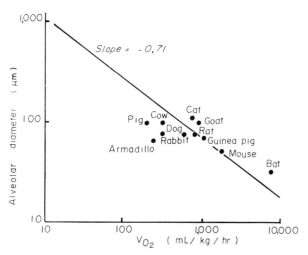

Figure 7–7 Logarithmic plot of mean alveolar diameter as a function of oxygen consumption in some animals.

Other pulmonary ventilation indices can be measured by spirometry in cooperating human subjects. In uncooperative animals these measurements are not possible. An experimental avenue is through body plethysmography with an anesthetized small animal such as a cat or dog. In a body plethysmograph, an animal can be subjected to negative and positive pressures on the thorax to generate or simulate partial or maximal forced inspiration and expiration. The air inspired during maximal inspiratory effort in excess of the tidal volume is termed the *inspiratory reserve volume* (IRV), or the volume of air that can be inspired from the end of a normal inspiration. The additional volume of air expelled by an active expiratory effort following passive expiration is termed the *expiratory reserve volume* (ERV). The air that remains in the lungs after a maximal expiratory effort is called the *residual volume* (RV). The space occupied by air that does not participate in exchanges with blood in the pulmonary vessels is the respiratory *dead volume* (VD).

The *summation of adjacent respiratory volumes* (e.g., VT + ERV or VT + IRV, or IRV + VT + ERV) leads to formation of another term, *capacity* (Fig. 7–8).

Expiratory capacity (EC) and *inspiratory capacity* (IC) refer to the tidal air volume plus expiratory reserve volume (EC = VT + ERV) and inspiratory reserve volume (IC = VT + IRV), respectively. The *vital capacity* (VC), about 80 percent of the total lung capacity, is the greatest amount of air that

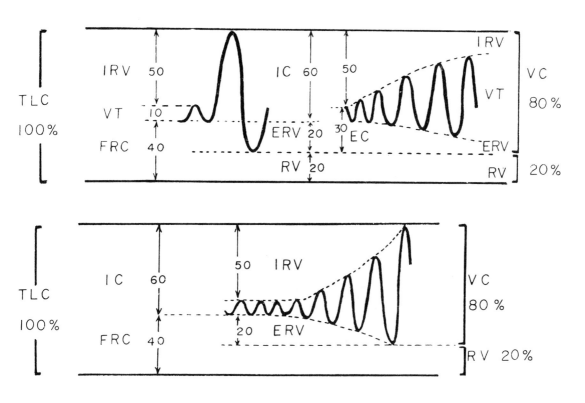

PULMONARY VENTILATION

Figure 7–8 Didactic concept of subdivisions of TLC, assuming reserve volume as 20 percent. Vital capacity (80 percent) includes IRV (50 percent), VT (10 percent), and ERV (20 percent). By combining adjacent volumes into capacity terminology, IC = IRV + VT = 60 percent; EC = ERV + VT = 20 percent; FRC = RV + ERV = 40 percent. The potential volume of VT can also be visualized as an expanding value gradually borrowing from IRC and ERC with a limit reached at VC.

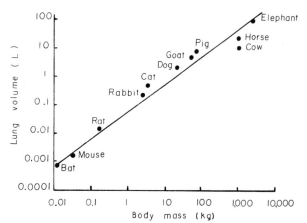

Figure 7–9 Logarithmic plot of lung volume as function of body mass in some animals.

can be expired after a maximal inspiratory effort; VC (IRV + VT + ERV) is an index of pulmonary function in humans. Total lung capacity (TLC) is the sum of all the volumes (TLC = RV + ERV + VT + IRV = 100 percent), and is related to body mass (Fig. 7–9). The *functional residual capacity* (FRC) is the quantity of air remaining in the lung at the end of a normal expiration (FRC = RV + ERV = about 40 percent of TLC). In most animals, FRC corresponds to the elastic equilibrium volume, where expiration ends and from which active inspiration is initiated (i.e., the relaxed lung volume [Vrx] or resting volume [Vr] in the lung = FRC). In the diphasic inspiration of the horse, passive inspiration is initiated below the Vr and active inspiration starts above the Vr. FRC is proportionally greater in large animals than in small animals (e.g., 1.35 L in a 63-kg sheep and 15 L in a 514-kg cow; see Table 7–1). This obviously helps to reduce fluctuations in alveolar and arterial oxygen during breathing. During artificial ventilation, more time is required for alveolar air mixing. A higher blood perfusion of the lung is obtained in small animals, as cardiac output ($\dot{Q}$ = milliliters of blood per kilogram per minute) increases from large animals (80 in cattle) to small animals (120 in dog, 240 in bat).

Limited Effects of Unilateral Pneumonectomy

After unilateral pneumonectomy in puppies and rabbits of 10 weeks, the remaining lung grows to approximately the same mass and volume as that of both lungs of control animals. Alveolar proliferation, rather than alveolar enlargement, has the major role in this regeneration, which requires about 3 weeks. Functionally, differences do not exist in TLC, but RV and FRC are increased because of discordance between the shape of the lung and the thorax. Airways of pneumonectomized rabbits are lengthened in accordance with the increase in lung volume. Maximal expiratory flow of air in pneumonectomized rabbits is 70 percent that of normal animals.

PHYSICS OF BREATHING

Ramification, Velocity of Air, and Resistance in the Airway

During breathing, air flows to and from the nonrespiratory zones (conducting and transitional) and the respiratory zones. The airways, made up of a series of branching tubes, ramify into about 23 generations of narrower, shorter, and more numerous conduits. Of the 23 generations of divisions from the trachea to the alveoli, the first 16 are in the conduction zone, the next three are in the transitional zone, and the last four are in the respiratory zone. Total cross-sectional surface, which is without much change in the first 10 generations, increases gradually to over 100-fold near the 17th generation and suddenly expands to more than 500-fold in the respiratory zone (Fig. 7–10).

Velocity and Air Flow in the Airways

During inspiration, the velocity of air decreases as it enters smaller airways, which collectively add up to a large total cross-sectional area (divergent flow). The bulk flow of air gradually slows as the cumulative cross-sectional surface of the airways increases. As a result of the extremely rapid increase in the combined cross section of the airways in the respiratory zone, the velocity of air becomes very slow (Fig. 7–10), which allows gas exchanges to occur by diffusion. Velocity increases during expiration, as air leaves the bronchial tree of the respiratory zone and heads toward the smaller cross-sectional surface of the conducting zone (convergent flow).

The air flow is turbulent in the trachea and large bronchi, because of the rapid velocity of air in these larger airways. The gas molecules move in all directions with complete disorganization of the stream lines. The net motion of air is due to the bulk flow. In the smaller airways air flow is laminar (i.e., the stream lines are parallel to the sides of the tubes). Gas in the center of the tube moves two times faster than the average velocity, whereas the gas molecules on the sides are slowed down by friction with the walls. Consequently, the velocity front has a parabolic instead of a flat shape.

Airway Resistance

Airway resistance (Raw), the reciprocal of airway conductance (Gaw), varies with lung volume and flow rate. *Total resistance* (RT, or RRS), also known as *pulmonary resistance* to distinguish it from airway resistance (Raw), refers to the sum of lung resistance (RL) and rib cage resistance (Rcw). Upper airway resistance is minimal at large lung volumes and increases during deflation. The major part of airway resistance (Raw) seems located in the upper portion (nasopharynx, glottis, trachea, large bronchi), and in the fourth to ninth branching generations of the lower portion of the respiratory tract. Nose breathing has twice the Raw of mouth

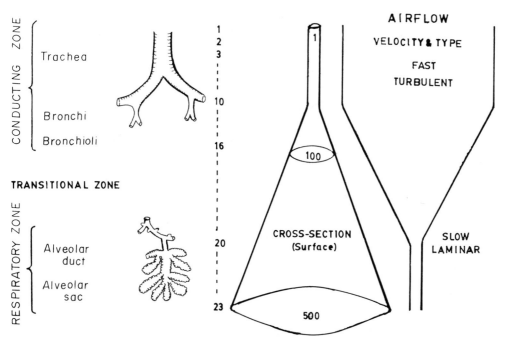

Figure 7–10 Diagrammatic representation of branching of airways into 23 generations. The first 16 generations are in the conducting zone, the next three are in the transitional zone, and the remainder are in the respiratory zone. As ramification occurs, the cross-sectional area increases, mostly after the 10th generation. At the 16th generation, the relative increase in cross-sectional area is 100 fold and it reaches about 500 fold at the 23rd generation. Air flow, rapid and turbulent in the upper airways, gradually decelerates in the deep conducting and transitional zones and becomes slow and laminar in the respiratory zone.

breathing. The peripheral airways (<2 mm in diameter) account for only 20 percent of Raw. Only extensive narrowing of the small airways increases Raw (e.g., bronchoconstriction [Raw × 3] by aging, ozone, nitrogen dioxide, smoke, histamine) and accumulation of secretions (bronchiolitis, allergy, irritants). Raw is higher when the preceding expiration is deep (i.e., down to RV instead of ending at FRC or Vr).

When the lungs are full, the smaller airways dilate because radial traction of elastic tissue in adjacent alveolar septa is greater than constriction due to smooth muscle. At the resting volume of the lungs (end of expiration) these airways are almost closed.

Parasympathetic stimulation increases resistance in the peripheral airways (Rp) more than in the central airways (Rc). Sympathetic regulation also predominantly influences Rp. Adrenergic stimulation can inhibit half the increase in resistance produced by vagal stimulation or excitation, by rendering the smooth muscle less sensitive to constrictive cholinergics. Propranolol, a beta-adrenergic blocker, enhances the stimulating effect of vagal stimulation on airway resistance by two- to fourfold, because it sensitizes the smooth muscle to the action of the parasympathetic constrictors. The constrictor effect of histamine is on the extremely peripheral airway resistance (Rp).

During strong inspiratory efforts, greater degrees of lung inflation are obtained, but the flow becomes more turbulent and lung volume no longer enlarges proportionately to the changes in intrapleural pressure. Factors interfering with distribution of air to alveoli increase the work required for breathing (Fig. 7–11).

Most of these factors are negative and tend to inhibit distribution of air to certain areas. They are offset to a certain extent by the presence of collateral ventilation. These connections, by anastomoses between adjacent small bronchioles and between adjacent alveoli, allow some drift of air into alveoli when the airways serving the alveoli in question are closed or obstructed.

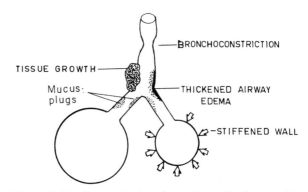

Figure 7–11 Factors that interfere with the distribution of air into the peripheral airways increase both the peripheral resistance (Rp) and the work of breathing.

The frictional resistance to inflow of gas contributes to the hysteresis loop resulting from plotting intrapleural pressure changes against lung volume changes. These measurements during inspiration and expiration produce two different curves instead of two superimposed straight lines (see Figs. 7–4 and 7–12).

Pulmonary perfusion is altered by local disruption of the blood vessels (e.g., emphysema) or by obliteration of vessels by fluid, fibrosis, or air (e.g., pneumothorax alters pulmonary perfusion). Pulmonary vessels compensate for irregularities in ventilation by responding in a manner opposite to that of systemic vessels. Vessels in the pulmonary circulation constrict instead of dilating in response to a reduction in blood oxygen tension or a fall in blood pH as a consequence of a rise in carbon dioxide tension. Blood perfusion is then reduced in the lung areas with decreased ventilation. During intense exercise in racing horses, bronchiolar obstructions may cause asynchronized ventilation among regions of the lungs. This may lead to fluctuations in alveolar pressures, and to ruptures in the capillaries (with epistaxis).

DYNAMIC COMPLIANCE AND RESISTANCE OF THE LUNGS

Dynamic compliance of the lungs and lung resistance are two parameters of respiratory mechanics derived from measurements of esophageal pressure, air flow, and tidal volume.

Compliances of the Lungs, Rib Cage, and Respiratory System

Compliance of the respiratory system (CT, or CRS), or total compliance, is the sum of the compliance of the lung (CL) and of the compliance of the chest wall (Ccw), or rib cage. Measurement of the dynamic compliance (CLdyn) and dynamic resistance (RLdyn) of the lungs with the pneumotachograph and esophageal pressure is the standard technique, requiring five to 10 respiratory cycles. It is the method against which all newer techniques are compared for reproducibility and precision.

Two newer methods that use the pneumotachograph claim to be less invasive by measuring mouth or buccal pressure (Pb) instead of esophageal or pleural pressure. Pb is obtained during brief (<1 second) occlusion of the pneumotachograph either at end-expiration or at end-inspiration. The end-expiration occlusion method yields dynamic inspiratory compliance (CRSdyn) and dynamic resistance (RRSdyn) of the respiratory system. The end-inspiration occlusion method gives static chest wall compliance (CCWst) in addition to static respiratory system compliance (CRSst) and static respiratory system resistance (RRS pass, or RRSst). The results obtained with these new methods have a high coefficient of variation.

Dynamic and Static Compliance of the Lungs

Lung compliance, or extensibility, is a measure of the ease with which the lungs can be expanded. It reflects only the elastic recoil forces of the lungs and not those associated with air flow. It is expressed as the changes in transpulmonary pressure coinciding with changes in the volume of air entering or leaving the lungs (i.e., change in volume per unit change in pressure [dV/dP]) in milliliters per centimeter of water. Since it increases with the size of the lungs, which increase with body mass, lung compliance may be expressed in milliliters per centimeter of water per kilogram of body weight (mL/cm H_2O/kg) to permit comparison of small and large lungs (Table 7–2).

Dynamic compliance of the lung (CLdyn) can be measured during resting breathing (and during hyperpnea in neonatal lambs) at no-flow points when no air flows into or out of the lungs (end-inspiration or -expiration). At that moment, all the muscles are relaxed, and pleural pressure equals the static recoil pressure of the lungs.

CLdyn is reduced by stiffness of the lungs due to expansion (near TLC), engorgement with blood when the pulmonary venous pressure increases, alveolar edema (some alveoli cannot inflate), atelectasis (collapsed alveoli), or fibrosis. The dynamic compliance of the lungs increases with aging and with emphysema.

The hysteresis and CLst or dV/dP can also be determined by measuring changes in transpulmonary pressure (Ppl) upon passive inflation and deflation of excised lungs mounted in an experimental bell (Fig. 7–12).

Lung recoil is the result of two factors: *tissue elasticity* (the integrated elastic characteristics of all tissue elements in the alveolar walls: elastic and collagen fibers, vascular and alveolar epithelia) and *surface tension* (the force with which a surface tends to minimize its area). After saline lavage of excised lungs, the volume-pressure curve reflects only the lung elastic recoil, because lavage has removed surfactant and eliminated the surface tension force (see Fig. 7–12).

The surface tension of the alveoli varies with the presence of surfactant in the fluid lining them. The molecules of this phospholipid surface agent are spread apart as alveolar size increases during inspiration but move together during expiration, thus adjusting surface tension during expiration. If the surface tension is not kept low when the alveoli become smaller during expiration, they collapse in accordance with the equation of Laplace (P = 2T/R). In spherical structures such as the alveoli, the distending pressure (P) is 2 times the tension (T) divided by the radius (R); if T is not reduced as R is reduced, the tension overcomes the distending pressure.

In neonatal respiratory distress (hyaline membrane dis-

TABLE 7–2 Lung and Chest Compliance in Anesthetized Animals

Animal	Compliance (mL/cm water) Lung	Chest Wall	Tidal Volume (mL)
Cat	13.30	13.4	34.0
Dog	63.00	32.0	140.0
Guinea pig	1.30	3.6	3.7
Mouse	0.05	0.3	
Rabbit	6.00	9.4	15.8
Rat	0.40	1.4	
Sheep	70.00	—	273.0

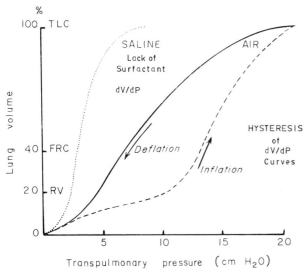

Figure 7–12 Volume-pressure curves of excised normal lungs inflated with air. The curves relating pressures and volumes at inflation (inspiration) and deflation (expiration) are different because of surface tension of the lungs. After saline lavage, the surface tension of the lungs is reduced because of a lack of surfactant, and the pressure-volume curve measures approximately the elasticity of the lung tissue.

ease) due to surfactant deficiency, surface tension in the lungs is high and in many areas the alveoli are collapsed (atelectasis). Similar changes associated with surfactant deficiency occur in animals that have undergone cardiac surgery, during which an oxygenator pump is used and the pulmonary circulation is interrupted. Low levels of surfactant are seen in bilaterally vagotomized guinea pigs and in some abnormalities following occlusion of a main bronchus, occlusion of one pulmonary artery, and long-term inhalation of pure oxygen (oxygen poisoning).

Static Compliances of the Respiratory System and the Chest

In the resting animal, static compliance of the respiratory system (CRsst) and static rib cage compliance (CCwst) may be determined by integration of data obtained by the end-inspiratory obstruction method. This procedure monitors the mouth pressure (Pb) instead of the pleural pressure and interrupts expiration for 0.5 second to elicit the expiratory Hering-Breuer reflex (indicated by a plateau in the Pb).

Dynamic Compliance of the Respiratory System

By interrupting breathing in the pneumotachograph at end-inspiration, results (VT, Pm, air flow) can be integrated to calculate dynamic inspiratory compliance or dynamic compliance of the respiratory system (CRsdyn).

Resistance of the Lungs and Respiratory System

Similarly to compliance, resistance can be computed from pressure values (Ppl or PM) and results from the pneu-

motachograph (VT and air flow). Resistance is expressed in centimeters of water per liter per second per kilogram of body weight and can be static or dynamic.

Dynamic resistance of the lung (RLdyn) is derived from Ppl and VT and air flow values at rest or during hyperpnea. Eupneic dynamic resistance of the respiratory system (RRsdyn) is smaller than RL because it also contains the resistance of the wall of the chest (Rcw). RRsdyn is calculated from PM and pneumotachographic values preceding the end-expiratory occlusion. Eupneic static resistance of the respiratory system (RRspass) is extrapolated from PM and pneumotachographic results just before end-inspiratory occlusion.

EVAPORATIVE COOLING BY THE RESPIRATORY TRACT

In addition to the essential function of gas exchange, the respiratory systems of sheep, cattle, pigs, and dogs are used for evaporative cooling. By rapidly replacing moist air over the evaporative surfaces of the nasal passages or the mouth with dry fresh air, panting triples evaporative heat loss in a hot environment. Rapid shallow panting in ruminants and pigs is caused by activity of the diaphragm. The flow of air is almost confined to the respiratory passages, as these animals keep their mouths closed most of the time while panting. In intense heat, rapid shallow panting is preceded, in ruminants but not in pigs, by a slower and deeper open-mouthed panting associated with more movements of the thorax (internal intercostal muscles).

When a sheep becomes hot, it initially pants at a frequency of 150 to 180 breaths per minute. The frequency is resonant, as the decrease in Ppl is in phase with air flow, whereas Ppl is usually lagging behind air flow. This panting is alternated with short periods of normal respiration, and, as the heat load for the sheep is increased, the proportion of time spent panting increases. During panting, the tidal volume is small (about 50 mL) but sufficient for alveolar ventilation (i.e., normal levels of oxygen and carbon dioxide are maintained in the alveoli, and only the dead space [air not reaching the alveoli] ventilation increases; Fig. 7–13). For a more intense heat load, the above pattern of panting changes to a different type in which the mouth is open and breathing is slower and deeper. This second-stage panting is a sign of distress in which evaporative heat loss is maximized at the expense of lowered alveolar carbon dioxide pressure and blood pH (alkalemia). At 15° C, a 90-kg pig has a VT of 790 mL and f of 15 and vaporizes 0.6 g water per minute. By raising the ambient temperature to 30° C, VT is reduced by 50 percent (i.e., 385 mL), f is increased sixfold (90), and water vaporization is increased fivefold (3 g per minute).

The dog also controls its body temperature in the face of elevated environmental temperature by panting, thus allowing water to evaporate from the mucous membranes of the tongue and upper respiratory tract. A flow current of air is created, with inspiratory air entering the nose and expiratory air preferentially leaving by the mouth. The efficiency of the

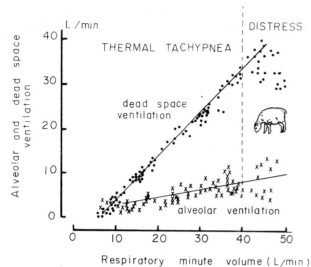

Figure 7–13 During thermal tachypnea, the increase in respiratory minute volume ($\dot{V}$) reflects a higher alveolar ventilation and much greater dead space ventilation. More heat is transferred to the air, which does not contribute to gas exchange.

system is improved by the rate at which panting occurs. Extra heat generated by the muscular work involved in panting is avoided by panting at a resonant frequency of the lungs and thorax. Since the lungs and thorax have elastic properties, they tend to expand and contract with a minimum of external work.

REFERENCES

Abraham WM, Watson H, Schneider A, King M, Yerger L, Sackner MA. Noninvasive ventilatory monitoring by respiratory inductive plethysmography in conscious sheep. J Appl Physiol 1981;51:1657.

Amis TC, Kurpershoek C. Tidal breathing flow-volume loop analysis for clinical assessment of airway obstruction in conscious dogs. Am J Vet Res 1986;47:1002.

Art T, Lekeux P. Respiratory airflow patterns in ponies at rest and during exercise. Can J Vet Res 1988;52:299.

Bartlett DJ, Respiratory functions of the larynx. Physiol Rev 1989;69:33.

Bouhuys A. The physiology of breathing. New York: Grune & Stratton. 1977:p.352.

Clark WT. Dynamic pulmonary compliance as a measurement of lung function in dogs. Vet Rec 1977;101:497.

Curtis RA, Viel L, McGuirk, Radostits OM, Harris FW. Lung sounds in cattle, horses, sheep and goats. Can Vet J 1986;27:170.

Davis GM, Coates AL, Dalle D, Bureau MA. Measurement of pulmonary mechanics in the newborn lamb: a comparison of three techniques. J Appl Physiol 1988;64:972.

Goulden BE, Barnes RG, Quinlan TJ. The electromyographic activity of intrinsic laryngeal muscles during quiet breathing in the anaesthetized horse. NZ Vet J 1976;24:157.

Inoue H, Ishii M, Fuyuki T, Inoue C, Matsumoto N, Sasaki N, Takishima T. Sympathetic and parasympathetic nervous control of airway resistance in dog lungs. J Appl Physiol 1983;54:1496.

Kiorpes AL, Bisgard GE, Manohar M. Pulmonary function values in healthy Holstein-Friesian calves. Am J Vet Res 1978;39:773.

Knowlen GG, Hamlin RL, Rice DA. Evaluation of flow-volume curves generated by forced-expiratory spirometry in anesthetized dogs. Am J Vet Res 1987;48:1390.

Koterba AM, Kosch PC, Beech J, Whitlock T. Breathing strategy of the adult horse (*Equus caballus*) at rest. J Appl Physiol 1988;64:337.

Lekeux P, Hajer R, Breukink HJ. Pulmonary function testing in calves: technical data. Am J Vet Res 1984;45:342.

Mortola JP. Dynamics of breathing in newborn animals. Physiol Rev 1987;67:187.

Musewe VO, Gillespie JR, Berry JD. Influence of ruminal insufflation on pulmonary function and diaphragmatic electro-myography in cattle. Am J Vet Res 1979;40:26.

Sorenson PR, Robinson NE. Postural effects on lung volumes and asynchronous ventilation in anesthetized horses. J Appl Physiol 1980;48:97.

Veit HP, Farrell RL. The anatomy and physiology of the bovine respiratory system relating to pulmonary disease. Cornell Vet 1978;68:555.

West JB. Respiratory physiology. 3rd ed. Baltimore: Williams & Wilkins, 1985:183.

Yee NM, Hyatt RE. Effect of left pneumonectomy on lung mechanics in rabbits. J Appl Physiol 1983;54:1612.

CHAPTER 8

ALVEOLAR VENTILATION

In temperate climates, air inspired by an animal is heated and humidified to body temperature in the conducting zone of the airways. In eupnea, animals breathe through the nose, which has an extensive vascular plexus in the nasal mucosa to warm the inspired air and saturate it with water vapor. The efficiency of this air conditioning system can be demonstrated in a dog breathing ambient air at $-40°$ C. This air is successfully saturated with water vapor and warmed to body temperature ($38°$ C) before it enters the trachea. Mouth breathing, which is easier since 50 percent of the total resistance to air flow is in the nose, is used during exercise.

Heating expands the volume of inspired air by about 5 to 10 percent according to the formula

$$V_{BT} = V_{AT} \frac{(273 + \text{body temperature})}{(273 + \text{ambient temperature})}$$

where V_{BT} is volume body temperature, and V_{AT} is volume ambient temperature.

Water added to saturate the atmospheric air dilutes the inspired air by adding a fractional concentration and a partial pressure of water vapor. In the mixture of tracheal humidified air, each of the other gases undergoes a reduction of its fractional concentration (F) and of its partial pressure (P). (Table 8-1).

The dilution is calculated from the difference in the fractional concentration of water vapor in tracheal and atmospheric air:

$$(F_{H_2O} \text{ trach} - F_{H_2O} \text{ atm})/100$$

The F and P of each gas is then:

$$F_{trach} = F_{atm} \times 100 - (F_{H_2O} \text{ trach} - F_{H_2O} \text{ atm})/100$$

$$P_{trach} = P_{atm} \times 100 - (F_{H_2O} \text{ trach} - F_{H_2O} \text{ atm})/100$$

The water vapor fractional concentration (F_{H_2O}) and partial pressure (P_{H_2O}) increase with temperature (Table 8-2).

TABLE 8-1   Dilution of Atmospheric Air by Water Vapor During Its Passage in the Conducting Airways

Gas	Atmospheric Air P (torr)	Atmospheric Air F (%)	Tracheal Air P (torr)	Tracheal Air F (%)
Carbon dioxide	0.3	0.04	0.3	0.04
Nitrogen	597	78.55	562.9	74.08
Oxygen	159	20.92	149.9	19.72
Water	3.7	0.5	47	6.2
Total	760	100.0	760	100.0

TABLE 8-2   Partial Pressure of Water Vapor at Various Body Temperatures

°C	torr
37.0	47.1
37.2	47.6
37.4	48.1
37.6	48.6
37.8	49.2
38.0	49.7
38.2	50.2
38.4	50.8
38.6	51.3
38.8	51.9
39.0	52.4
39.2	53.0
39.4	53.6
39.6	54.2
39.8	54.7
40.0	55.3

The volume of alveolar ventilation depends on the respiratory rate and on the tidal volume (V_T), both of which are related to body mass. For identical minute volumes ($\dot{V}_I$ or $\dot{V}_E$), alveolar ventilation volume is greater at the lowest respiratory rate and at the largest tidal volume (Table 8-3).

About 66 percent of the volume of the humid inspired air in the upper airways comes into contact with the respiratory membrane and is involved in alveolar ventilation. The volume of air remaining in the conducting zone of the respiratory tract and not contributing to respiratory gas exchanges is termed the *anatomical dead space,* or *anatomical dead volume* (V_{Dan}). The volume of air reaching the alveoli (V_A) is equal to the tidal volume less the volume of the anatomical dead space (i.e., $V_A = V_T - V_{Dan}$). On a minute volume basis, $\dot{V}_A = (V_T - V_{Dan})f$, or $\dot{V}_A = V_T \times f \times 66$ percent.

This chapter presents the concepts of anatomical and alveolar dead spaces, which form the physiological dead space. It also discusses the relationship between alveolar ventilation and alveolar perfusion, the composition of alveolar air, the exchanges between tracheal and alveolar air, and the modifications of alveolar air under low, normal, and high atmospheric pressure.

TABLE 8-3   Changes in Minute Alveolar Ventilation in Relation to Respiratory Rates and Tidal Volumes

$\dot{V}$	V_T	f	V_D	$\dot{V}_D$	$\dot{V}_A$
12,000	1,200	10	200	2,000	10,000
12,000	400	30	200	6,000	4,000
12,000	200	60	200	12,000	0

ANATOMICAL AND ALVEOLAR DEAD SPACES

The sum of the anatomical and alveolar dead spaces constitutes the physiological dead space.

Anatomical Dead Space

The anatomical dead space can be defined from a morphologic and from a functional aspect. *Morphologic anatomical dead space* is the volume of the conducting airways (those not lined with alveoli), and it usually excludes the supralaryngeal airways. It is measured from plastic or plaster casts of the airways. *Functional anatomical dead space,* also known as *series dead space,* is the volume of inspired gas that does not mix with alveolar gas, i.e., that retains the composition of humidified inspired air. It can be measured with difficulty, in cooperative animals, by Fowler's technique, which requires a quick nitrogen gas analyzer. Very few determinations of functional anatomical dead space are reported in animals—dog, 150 mL; cow, 380 mL; giraffe, 1,600 mL—but these vary with body size.

Since gas exchanges in the respiratory system occur only in the alveoli, the gas within the rest of the respiratory system is not available for gas exchange with pulmonary capillary blood. The volume of the anatomical dead space is directly correlated, as is lung volume, with body mass. Most of the anatomical dead space is in the upper airways and trachea, where few volume changes take place, even in disease. Anatomical dead space comprises about 30 to 60 percent of the tidal volume, and its level increases with aging. In a resting sheep with a tidal volume of about 400 mL, only the first 250 mL of the air inspired with each breath mixes with the air in the alveoli; the last 150 mL occupies the dead space. Conversely, with each expiration, the first 150 mL of expired gas is occupying the dead space, and only the last 250 mL is gas that had contact with the alveoli.

Because of the stable anatomical dead space, the volume of air reaching the alveoli of a sheep (alveolar ventilation, VA) breathing 8 L per minute is influenced by the frequency and the amplitude of respiration. Rapid, shallow respiration produces much less alveolar ventilation than slow, deep respiration at the same respiratory minute volume (Table 8–4).

Alveolar Dead Space

Alveolar dead space, or *parallel dead space,* is a (virtual) volume of inspired gas that mixes with gas in alveolar spaces but takes no part in alveolar gas exchanges. Alveolar dead space may be the entire volume of air in a well-ventilated and nonperfused alveolus or a portion of the air volume that does not take part in gas exchange in partially perfused alveoli. This respiratory-inactive alveolar volume of air must be *added to the anatomical dead space to give the physiological dead space, or total dead space.* In health, the anatomical and (total) physiological dead space are about the same; there is very little "wasted" alveolar ventilation.

Alveolar dead space (VDA) is closely linked to alveolar gas exchange and is calculated by subtracting the anatomical dead space (VDan) from the physiological dead space (VD):

$$VDA = VD - VDan$$

Physiological dead space is the volume of gas that is inspired and expired but takes no part in gas exchanges in the alveoli. It is calculated with Bohr's equation, assuming that $PaCO_2 = PACO_2$, since the latter quantity is more easily measured.

$$\frac{V_D}{V_T} = \frac{PaCO_2 - \bar{P}ECO_2}{PaCO_2}$$

VT is the tidal volume, $PaCO_2$ is the partial pressure of arterial carbon dioxide, and $\bar{P}ECO_2$ is the average partial pressure of carbon dioxide in the entire expired air. Partial pressures of gases are expressed as *torr* (1 torr = 1 mm Hg).

In pulmonary disease there is gross imbalance of ventilation and perfusion. Then alveolar dead space may account for 100 percent of tidal volume, especially if the animal is exhibiting rapid shallow respiration. In such circumstances, the animal is doing little more than shunting air in and out of its conducting airways. This situation is not incompatible with life, largely by virtue of the single fact that gases pass along the airway with a parabolic front edge rather than a flat front. Sufficient gases from the apex of the parabola may diffuse into the alveoli to meet minimal requirements for life. Nonetheless, a pattern of rapid shallow respiration should always be regarded with caution, especially when a large physiological dead space may exist. A high oxygen concentration in the inspired air enhances the diffusion of

TABLE 8–4 Alveolar Ventilation under Constant Minute Volume but Varying Respiratory Rates and Depths of Respiration

Respiratory rate (f)	30	20	10
Tidal volume (VT) in mL	266.7	400	800
Minute volume (f × VT = V̇E) in L/min	8,000	8,000	8,000
Alveolar ventilation (VT − VD) f in L/min	3,500	5,000	6,500
	(266.7−150) 30	(400−150) 20	(800−150) 10
Outcome (− or + mL)	−1,500	Normal	+1,500

oxygen into the alveoli but does not assist in the elimination of carbon dioxide. A tracheotomy, which greatly reduces the anatomical dead space, may be life saving.

RELATIONSHIP BETWEEN ALVEOLAR VENTILATION AND PERFUSION

For optimal transfer of oxygen and carbon dioxide, the minute alveolar ventilation ($\dot{V}A$) and the minute alveolar perfusion ($\dot{Q}A$), or cardiac output ($\dot{Q}$), should be about equal, and the ratio of $\dot{V}A$ to $\dot{Q}$ near 1. Small laboratory animals have matched ventilation and perfusion throughout their lungs. Lungs of large animals have mismatched ventilation and blood flow in the dorsal, caudal, and ventral areas, the ventilation-perfusion ratio increasing from the dorsocaudal to the ventral region. Alveoli in the upper dorsum of the lung, well ventilated but poorly perfused, are considered as part of the functional, or alveolar, dead space.

The PAO_2-$PACO_2$, $\dot{V}A$:$\dot{Q}$ diagram (Fig. 8–1) is used to present a conceptual form of the variations of the ventilation:perfusion ratio.

At a $\dot{V}A$:$\dot{Q}$ ratio between 0.8 and 1, alveolar ventilation occurs normally, and $PACO_2 = 40$ torr, $PAO_2 = 100$ torr. When the ratio $\dot{V}A$:$\dot{Q}$ equals infinity, the well-ventilated alveoli are not provided with proper perfusion and gases cannot be exchanged between the alveoli and blood capillaries. In this situation, alveolar air equilibrates with inspired air and $PACO_2 = PICO_2 = 0$; $PAO_2 = PIO_2 = 149$ torr. $\dot{V}A$:$\dot{Q}$ equal to 0 indicates proper alveolar perfusion but failure in alveolar ventilation. This situation usually is the result of an obstruction in small airways. Alveolar air then equilibrates with the partial pressures of gases in the incoming pulmonary artery (venous blood) (i.e., $PACO_2 = P\bar{V}CO_2 = 45$ mm Hg; $PAO_2 = P\bar{V}O_2 = 40$ torr. Alveoli in

the ventral part of the lungs commonly have low ventilation-perfusion ratios and are prone to be unstable and to collapse. Those ventral airways and alveoli are often poorly expanded, since secretions are inclined to collect there because of gravity.

Because of the effect of gravity against the low pulmonary blood pressure (mean or $\bar{x}$:15 mm Hg), blood fails to reach and irrigate capillaries of alveoli in the dorsal and caudal regions of the lung (Fig. 8–2A). Improper perfusion of capillaries in the dorsal pulmonary circulation is also caused by excessive dilatation and higher flow of blood in the vessels in the ventral region of the lung (Fig. 8–2C). Alveolar blood perfusion is intermittent in the capillaries of the intermediate region of the lung, which alternately open and collapse with the systolic (25 mm Hg) and diastolic (10 mm Hg) pressures (Fig. 8–2B).

COMPOSITION OF ALVEOLAR AIR

Because of variations in the $\dot{V}A$/$\dot{Q}$ ratio, the composition of alveolar air is not uniform. Inspired air and alveolar air in the dorsal region of the lung, usually with a high ventilation:perfusion ratio, tend to be identical; that is, they have a low PCO_2 and high PO_2. In contrast, alveolar air in the ventral region of the lung, where there is hypoventilation in relation to perfusion, is likely to reflect the blood gases and to have a low PO_2 and high PCO_2.

Alveolar air is rejected at the very end of expiration (i.e., after expulsion first of air in the anatomical dead space [VDan]) and then of a mixture of dead space air and of alveolar air (Fig. 8–3).

Like air velocity and intrapulmonary pressure, the composition of air changes dynamically during the expiratory phase of pulmonary ventilation. At first the partial pressure

Figure 8–1 Diagram of the PO_2-CO_2-VA/Q concept explaining the importance of matching alveolar ventilation and alveolar perfusion. The normal ventilation : perfusion ratio is between 0.8 and 1 (B). A higher ratio (A) indicates inadequate perfusion (vasoconstriction, embolism) and a tendency for gases in alveolar air to equilibrate with gases in inspired air. This usually occurs in the dorsal part of the lung, which is prone to insufficient blood irrigation by the weak pressure of pulmonary circulation. A lower ventilation : perfusion ratio (C) points to a deficiency in the ventilation and a probable obstruction in the small airways or the alveoli. The alveolar gases equilibrate with the venous blood gases. This situation is more prominent in the ventral parts of the lungs, which are more easily obstructed by fluids and secretions.

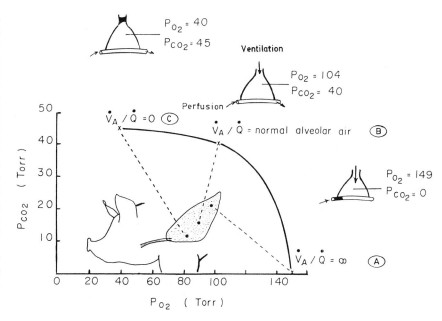

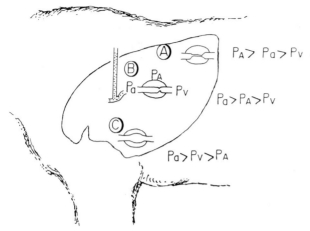

$P_A > P_a > P_v$

$P_a > P_A > P_v$

$P_a > P_v > P_A$

Figure 8–2 Perfusion of alveolar capillaries in different regions of the lungs of large animals. **A,** The capillary pressure is lower than the alveolar pressure, the vessel is collapsed, the alveolus is not perfused, and gas exchange is impossible. The column of blood is heavy enough to counteract and overcome the weak hydrostatic force of pressure in the pulmonary circulation. **B,** Capillary pressure is higher than alveolar pressure and perfusion occurs during systole. During diastole, perfusion fails as the capillary pressure becomes too low. **C,** Both arteriolar and venular capillary pressure are higher than alveolar pressure. Ventilation is maximal but could be increased to match the excessive perfusion.

of oxygen and of carbon dioxide of the anatomical dead space air are similar to those of humidified atmospheric air. Then there is a period when partial pressures are equilibrated, first predominantly with anatomical dead space air and later mostly with alveolar air. The end-phase of (forced or active) expiration contains only alveolar air. The average composition of alveolar and expired air is given in Table 8–5. The composition of alveolar air is also modified during the inspiratory phase of breathing (Fig. 8–4).

TABLE 8–5 Partial Pressures and Fractions of Average Alveolar and Expired Air

	Alveolar Air		Expired Air	
Gases	P (torr)	F (%)	P (torr)	F (%)
Carbon dioxide	40	5.3	27	3.6
Nitrogen	569	74.9	566	74.5
Oxygen	104	13.6	120	15.7
Water	47	6.2	47	6.2
Total	760	100.0	760	100.0

EXCHANGES BETWEEN TRACHEAL AND ALVEOLAR AIR

At the end of expiration, the amount of gas remaining in the lung is the functional residual capacity (FRC). Grossly, it is about four times the tidal volume, which is correlated with body mass ($V_T = 7.69 \text{ kg}^{1.04}$, or 8 mL per kilogram in large animals, 10 mL per kilogram in small animals). The last part of the tidal volume (end-expiration), which contains only alveolar air, is not expelled but occupies

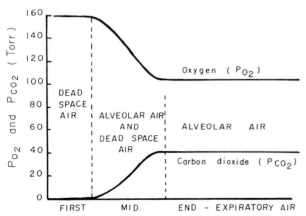

Figure 8–3 Variations in the oxygen and carbon dioxide partial pressures in expired air saturated with water vapor. The initial pressures reflect the displacement of air from the anatomical dead space, which is without loss of oxygen and gain of carbon dioxide. The air pouring out during the intermediate part of expiration has gradually less oxygen and more carbon dioxide. Stable gas pressures are reached with extrusion of alveolar air.

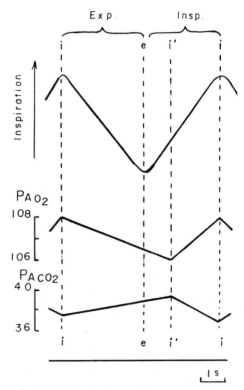

Figure 8–4 Oscillations in the partial pressures of oxygen and carbon dioxide in alveolar air during expiration and inspiration. At the beginning of inspiration (*e* to *i'*) the decrease in oxygen and the increase in carbon dioxide both continue momentarily because of alveolar reentrance of alveolar air that filled the anatomical dead space at the end of expiration. The remaining part of inspiration (*i'* to *i*) shows an influx of oxygen and a dilution of carbon dioxide. Expiration (*i* to *e*) indicates a loss of oxygen and a gain of carbon dioxide in the alveolar air.

the anatomical dead space (30 to 60 percent of VT) and is reinspired with the next inspiration. This explains that at initiation of inspiration, alveolar partial pressure of oxygen is further lowered a little, whereas the partial pressure of carbon dioxide still increases (see Fig. 8–4).

The usual rate of renewal of the alveolar air, or the alveolar ventilation, is thus about 16.5 percent, about one-sixth of the FRC as calculated from

$$V_A = V_T - V_{Dan}$$

$$\frac{V_a}{FRC} \text{ OR } \frac{0.66\ V_t}{4\ V_t}$$

In hypoventilation, when alveolar ventilation is small relative to the metabolic rate, carbon dioxide accumulates, and the alveolar carbon dioxide tension can exceed the normal value of 40 torr. This state of hypercapnia, or hypercarbia, resembles respiratory acidosis.

Conversely, in hyperventilation, the alveolar ventilation is excessive in relation to the metabolic rate. In this situation, a loss of carbon dioxide occurs, and the alveolar carbon dioxide tension is reduced below the reference value of 40 torr. This state of hypocapnia, or hypocarbia, simulates respiratory alkalosis.

Influence of Gas Pressure in Ambient Air

Alveolar ventilation is modified considerably by changes in the partial pressure of gases in the atmospheric air (i.e., low and high atmospheric pressure conditions).

Low Atmospheric Pressure Conditions

An animal suddenly introduced into a chamber without oxygen (e.g., 100 percent nitrogen or 100 percent carbon dioxide) loses consciousness within seconds and soon dies. This principle is used by humane organizations for mass euthanasia of unwanted animals. Sudden decompression in a pressurized aircraft (partial pressures suddenly going from those at 3,000 to those at more than 10,000 m) would have a similar effect on animal passengers or cargo.

Above 3,000 m altitude the atmospheric air oxygen tension is not sufficient to prevent hypoxemia. To be suitable for living freight, aircraft flying above this altitude must provide compressed air to simulate the air at a lower altitude to maintain an alveolar oxygen tension near 100 mm Hg. Animals that are grazed seasonally at high altitudes develop compensating mechanisms within 15 days after exposure to chronic low atmospheric pressure conditions. The adaptation brings a rise in f, VA, and VE or VI accompanied by lower PaO_2, $PaCO_2$ and $\dot{V}O_2$. Erythrocyte parameters are also increased (e.g., hemoglobin and erythrocyte packed cell volume), whereas plasma volume is decreased.

High Atmospheric Pressure Conditions

High atmospheric pressure conditions are now of academic interest only, but they were important when horses and mules served in hyperpressurized cofferdams, or caissons, during underwater construction of foundations and piers. Under water, atmospheric pressure increases by 76 torr per meter. The higher partial pressures cause an excess of gases to dissolve in tissues. Return to normal pressure must

Figure 8–5 Partial pressures and fractional concentrations of alveolar gases at 6,000 m, sea level, and 10 m under water. PAH_2O always remains unchanged (47 torr), but FAH_2O is halved under water and more than doubled at high altitude. The changes in the fractional concentrations of the other gases are not as dramatic as the pressure changes at low or high atmospheric pressures.

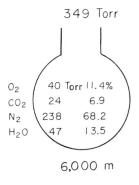

349 Torr

O₂	40 Torr	11.4%
CO₂	24	6.9
N₂	238	68.2
H₂O	47	13.5

6,000 m

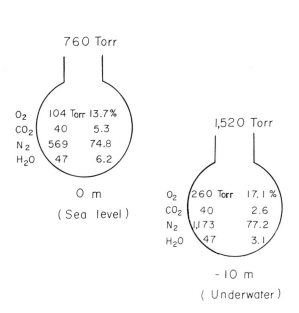

760 Torr

O₂	104 Torr	13.7%
CO₂	40	5.3
N₂	569	74.8
H₂O	47	6.2

0 m
(Sea level)

1,520 Torr

O₂	260 Torr	17.1%
CO₂	40	2.6
N₂	1,173	77.2
H₂O	47	3.1

–10 m
(Underwater)

be progressive to release gases from tissues slowly and avoid their sudden release, which causes air embolism (bends, or caisson disease). Alveolar tensions and fractional concentrations of gases change under low, normal, and high atmospheric pressure conditions (Fig. 8–5).

REFERENCES

Amis TC, Jones HA, Hughes JMB. A conscious dog model for study of regional lung function. J Appl Physiol 1982;53:1050.

Guyton AC. Textbook of medical physiology. 7th ed. Philadelphia: WB Saunders, 1986.

Orr JA, Bisgard GE, Forester HV, Rawlings CA, Buss DD, Will JA. Cardiopulmonary measurements in nonanesthetized, resting ponies. Am J Vet Res 1975;36:1667.

Otis AB. Quantitative relationships in steady-state gas exchange. In: Fenn WO, Rahn H, eds. Handbook of physiology. Section 3. Respiration. Vol 1. Washington, DC: American Physiological Society, 1964.

Rahn N, Farhi LE. Ventilation, perfusion, and gas exchange—the VA/Q concept. In: Fenn WO, Rahn H, eds. Handbook of physiology. Section 3. Respiration. Vol 1. Washington, DC: American Physiological Society, 1964.

West JB. Respiratory physiology. 3rd ed. Baltimore: Williams & Wilkins, 1985.

Willoughby RA, McDonel WN. Pulmonary function testing in horses. Vet Clin North Am (Large Anim Pract) 1979;1:171.

CHAPTER 9

ALVEOLOCAPILLARY TRANSFER OF OXYGEN AND CARBON DIOXIDE

Normal breathing involves lung expansion, which increases the total number of molecules in the lungs. A process fundamental to life is the blending of freshly inspired air with air already inside the lung. This is achieved by convection, or bulk flow of gas into the lung, and molecular diffusion.

The relative contributions of the two mechanisms (convection and diffusion) are intimately related to lung geometry. The initial part of the tracheobronchial tree has high linear velocities and short transit times. In that area of the airways, axial transport by molecular diffusion is negligible in comparison with that by convection. In the lung periphery, the large cross-sectional area of the bronchial tree causes slower linear velocities and is more favorable for transport by molecular diffusion than by convection (Fig. 9–1). At the periphery of the tracheobronchial tree, turbulent molecular transport by convection progressively diminishes until in the alveoli gases is almost stagnant, and lamellar gas transport is totally by diffusion.

Oxygen and carbon dioxide are transferred between tracheal air and alveolar air by convection, without any sharp separation front. The mechanical action of the heart is of some importance during this mixing by convection.

In a given alveolus, gases are considered to be perfectly mixed by a molecular exchange mechanism, which ideally would equalize gas concentrations. Molecular diffusion, which is without net transport of matter, causes molecules in the inspired fresh gas to move toward the alveolocapillary membrane during each breath. Also, with alveolar gas tensions (PA), diffusing capacity of the lung (DL), and differences in mixed venous and arterial gas tensions (P$\bar{v}$ – Pa), diffusion influences gas exchange at the alveolocapillary membrane (Fig. 9–2). Exchanges between alveolar air and blood are different for each gas. Nitrogen, an inert gas, is merely dissolved in plasma. Oxygen constantly leaves the alveolar air to combine with blood hemoglobin. Carbon dioxide enters alveoli from blood, which carries this gas by various means (e.g., bicarbonate ions, carbamino binding to hemoglobin, and dissolved in blood plasma). This chapter presents some characteristics of the respiratory membrane and the transfer processes of carbon dioxide from blood to alveolar air and of oxygen from alveolar air to blood.

ALVEOLOCAPILLARY MEMBRANE

The 300×10^6 polyhedral alveoli of the lung are lined by a thin wall encasing a "sheet" of flowing blood, which circulates in a multitude of capillary vessels about 8 μm in diameter (Fig. 9–3A). The structures separating alveolar air and blood plasma collectively make up the alveolocapillary, or respiratory, membrane. It includes surfactant, alveolar epithelium and basement membrane, interstitium, and basement membrane and capillary endothelium (with pinocytic vesicles) (Fig. 9–3B).

Its thickness is from 0.2 to 0.6 μm, and it represents a surface of about 1 m^2 per kilogram of body mass. The separation of alveolar air and blood by only 0.5 μm explains the swiftness of respiratory exchanges. Under normal resting conditions, the partial pressures of gases in blood and alveolar air equilibrate in 0.8 second. During exercise equilibrium is reached in only 0.5 second, as the respiratory surface is increased, additional lung capillaries open, and some increase their diameter to carry more blood.

Interstitial edema increases the thickness of the respiratory membrane and lowers its efficiency for gas exchange. Pulmonary emphysema has the same effect, as it decreases the functional surface of alveoli and the number of capillaries available for respiratory exchanges.

Diffusing capacity of a gas through the alveolocapillary membrane, measured in milliliters per minute per mm Hg, varies directly with its diffusion coefficient. The diffusion coefficient for carbon dioxide is 20 times that of oxygen.

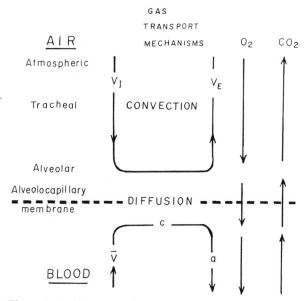

Figure 9–1 Transport and mixing of gases by convection in the initial part and by diffusion in the peripheral part of the tracheobronchial tree.

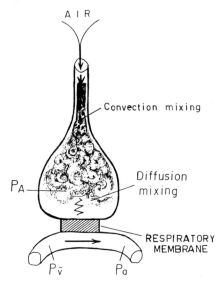

Figure 9–2 Factors that influence gas exchange at the alveolo-capillary membrane. P_A, gas tension in alveoli; *diffusion mixing,* molecular diffusion; D_L, diffusion capacity of the lung; $P\bar{v}$, gas tension in mixed venous blood; P_a, gas tension in arterial blood.

Accordingly, since the diffusing capacity through the respiratory membrane is about 21 mL per minute per mm Hg (torr) for oxygen, that of carbon dioxide is expected to be 20 times higher, about 420 mL per minute per mm Hg (torr).

TRANSFER OF CARBON DIOXIDE

Mixed venous blood arrives at the arterial end of capillaries of the respiratory membrane with a carbon dioxide tension ($P\bar{v}CO_2$) of 45 torr. Across the respiratory membrane, it is confronted with an alveolar carbon dioxide tension (P_ACO_2) of 40 torr. This slight pressure gradient of 5 torr, aided by a diffusion coefficient 20 times that of oxygen, is sufficient to move carbon dioxide almost instantly from blood to alveolar air (Fig. 9–4). As a result, venous-end capillaries of the respiratory membrane, carrying arterial blood, have a carbon dioxide tension (P_aCO_2) identical to that of alveolar air 40 torr.

The carbon dioxide removed from blood to alveolar air (about 420 mL per minute per torr) comes from three main sources. The action of carbonic anhydrase of erythrocytes on plasma bicarbonate ions contributes about 70 percent of the carbon dioxide; the dissociation of carbaminohemoglobin adds another 15 to 25 percent; and the carbon dioxide dissolved in plasma accounts for only 5 to 10 percent of carbon dioxide. In erythrocytes, the HCO_3 anions, produced by catalytic dehydration of H_2CO_3, are removed from the red cells into plasma only if replaced by chloride anions from plasma, which are shifted into the cells (chloride shift). The carbon dioxide remaining in the arterial blood is mostly in bicarbonate (Fig. 9–5).

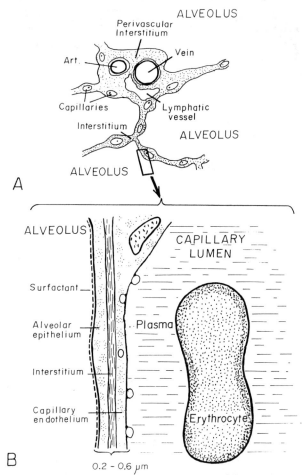

Figure 9–3 **A,** Organization of the alveolocapillary membrane. **B,** Structures separating alveolar air and plasma: surfactant, alveolar epithelial cytoplasm and basement membrane, interstitium, basement membrane, endothelial cell cytoplasm, and membrane with pinocytic vesicles.

Under normal resting conditions, about 4 mL of carbon dioxide is carried from the tissues to the lungs in each deciliter of blood. This amount of carbon dioxide has much influence on the acid-base balance of body fluids. Ordinarily, arterial blood has a pH of 7.4, and incoming venous blood is slightly less alkaline (pH, 7.36). The difference of 0.04 pH unit is due to acquisition of carbon dioxide. The reverse happens in the pulmonary circulation when carbon dioxide is removed from blood to the alveolar air.

Removal of carbon dioxide from the blood depends mostly on the action of carbonic anhydrase in erythrocytes. Administration of an inhibitor of carbonic anhydrase (e.g., acetazolamide) almost doubles the carbon dioxide tension in mixed venous blood and causes a state of acidosis. On an identical scale, dissociation curves for total carbon dioxide and total oxygen differ greatly (Fig. 9–6). The slope of the carbon dioxide curve is steeper and more linear than that of oxygen.

In animals, two parallel dissociation curves exist for

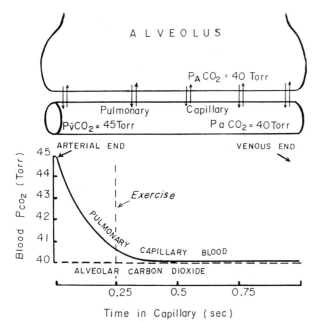

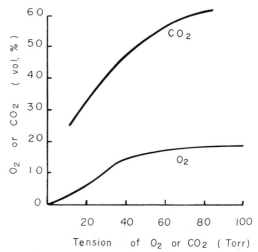

Figure 9–6 Dissociation curves of carbon dioxide and oxygen, using the same volume percent scale, to outline the steeper slope of the carbon dioxide.

Figure 9–4 Changes in carbon dioxide tension along the pulmonary capillary. During exercise, the time available for carbon dioxide diffusion across the blood-gas barrier is reduced.

carbon dioxide, an upper one for venous blood and a lower one for arterial blood (Fig. 9–7). Oxygenation of hemoglobin, in the mixed venous blood at the distal arterial end of the pulmonary capillary, tends to displace carbon dioxide from blood according to a composite of these two curves. Called the Haldane effect, this approximately doubles the amount of carbon dioxide released from the blood in the lung. Conversely, at the periphery, the Haldane effect doubles the pickup of carbon dioxide from tissues to blood.

The Haldane effect is due to the stronger acidity of hemoglobin after it is oxygenated. The increased acidity of

hemoglobin raises the hydrogen ion content in extracellular fluids and erythrocytes. These hydrogen ions combine with the blood bicarbonate ions to form carbonic acid, which then dissociates, and carbon dioxide is released from the blood. The stronger acidic hemoglobin has less tendency to fix carbon dioxide onto carbaminohemoglobin, but favors displacement and release of much of the carbon dioxide bound to carbaminohemoglobin.

A small portion of the two separate carbon dioxide dissociation curves (see Fig. 9–7) is operative between the carbon dioxide tensions of 40 and 45 torr. Point A on the upper curve indicates that at 45 torr of carbon dioxide

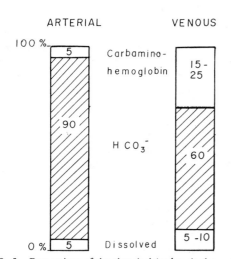

Figure 9–5 Proportions of the chemical (carbaminohemoglobin and bicarbonate) and dissolved forms of carbon dioxide in arterial and mixed venous blood.

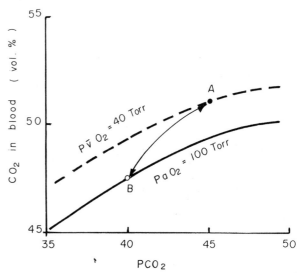

Figure 9–7 Portions of the carbon dioxide dissociation curves when the oxygen tension is 100 and 40 torr. The double-pointed arrow represents the Haldane effect on the delivery and absorption of carbon dioxide.

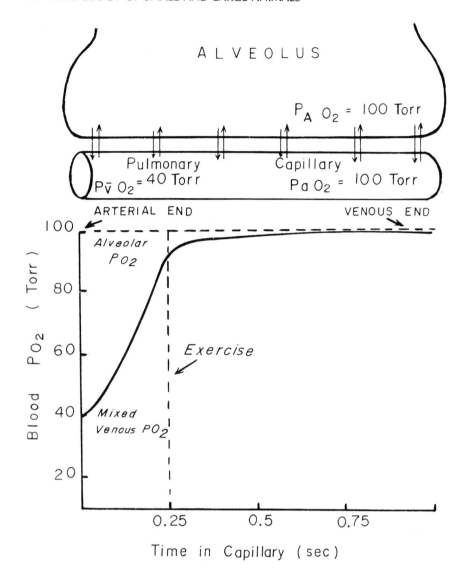

Figure 9–8 Changes in oxygen tension along the pulmonary artery. During exercise, the contact time available for oxygen diffusion across the respiratory membrane is slightly reduced.

tension, 52 volumes percent carbon dioxide combine with blood. On entering the lung, the oxygen tension increases from 40 to 100 torr, and the carbon dioxide dissociation curve is changed from the venous (upper) one to the arterial (lower) one. At point B, blood carbon dioxide is lowered to 48 volumes percent instead of 50 volumes percent, as it would have been if the carbon dioxide dissociation curve had not changed from the upper to the lower one.

CAPTURE OF OXYGEN

In the lungs, oxygen diffuses across the alveolocapillary barrier in 0.25 second, either in the resting state or during exercise (Fig. 9–8). During exercise the contact time across the alveolocapillary barrier is slightly reduced, but ventilation of dorsal and caudal parts of the lung is increased, more capillaries are open for perfusion, and both alveoli and capillaries are more dilated.

An oxygen tension gradient of 60 torr is initially created by the 100 torr in the alveoli and the 40 torr in the venous blood. In less than a third of the time required to transit the length of the capillary, equilibrium is reached. The venular end of the capillary receives arterial blood with an oxygen tension of 100 torr. Usually, the pulmonary veins receive 98 to 99 parts of blood fully oxygenated in the alveolocapillary system, and one to two parts of partially oxygenated blood, which comes from the left ventricle instead of from the right ventricle. It is returning to the left atrium via the pulmonary vein, but has avoided the respiratory (alveolocapillary) membrane by going through the bronchial circulation. Some of its oxygen has already been spent (about 5 torr) to nourish the pulmonary structures, and it has accumulated a small burden of carbon dioxide from the lung tissues.

Each 100 mL of arterial blood contains about 20 mL of oxygen. Most of this oxygen is associated with hemoglobin (99.7 percent), but a small quantity (0.003 per deciliter per torr, or 0.3 percent) is in solution.

REFERENCES

Engel L. Gas mixing within the acinus of the lung. J Appl Physiol 1983;54:609.

Mauderly JL. Effect of age on pulmonary structure and function of immature and adult animals and man. Fed Proc 1979;38:173.

Mauderly JL, Hahn FF. The effects of age on lung function and structure of adult animals. Adv Vet Sci Comp Med 1982;26:35.

Paiva M, Engel LA. Theoretical studies of gas mixing and ventilation distribution in the lung. Physiol Rev 1987;67:750.

West JB. Respiratory physiology, the essentials. 2nd ed. Baltimore: Williams & Wilkins, 1982.

CHAPTER 10

REGULATION OF RESPIRATION

Respiration is primarily an automatic process that continuously adjusts alveolar ventilation to meet body demands for oxygen and eliminate the excess carbon dioxide in blood. It regulates and maintains normal gas concentrations in blood. Also, the respiratory regulating system modifies breathing during drinking, deglutition, and regurgitation (in ruminants) to protect the body from accidental aspiration of liquid or solid material. Breathing must also be integrated with incidental animal activities such as coughing, barking, thermal polypnea, postural control, and exercise.

To meet these changes, breathing is controlled by both humoral and neural mechanisms. The humoral, or chemical, regulation is responsive to the metabolic requirements of the body, and the neural regulation modifies the rate and depth of breathing to fit the needs of the moment.

Like many physiological systems, the structures for respiration form a closed-loop control system operating with *feedback* and *"feedforward"* regulatory strategies. The components of such a regulatory system are *communication channels* (blood, nerves), the *central controller* (inspiratory and expiratory cells), receiving incoming messages from *sensors* (mechano- and chemoreceptors) and generating outgoing signals to *effectors* (inspiratory and expiratory muscles). In a feedback strategy, perceived changes in the regulated variable compel the central controller to generate forcing functions that oppose those changes (e.g., an excess of carbon dioxide in blood acts on the central controller to accelerate alveolar ventilation to bring blood carbon dioxide to a normal level). A feedforward strategy, used in combination with feedback, informs the central controller to generate a corrective command that anticipates changes in the regulated variable (e.g., alveolar ventilation increases abruptly at the onset of exercise before any changes in blood gas concentration). The concept of feedback may be represented as a triangular closed-loop system or as a cybernetic block diagram in which boxes represent the information-processing subsystems (Fig. 10–1).

The *inspiratory muscles*—diaphragm and external intercostals—are the major effector components of the respiratory system. Eupneic expiration, which is the result of rib cage and lung elasticity, is usually passive. The internal intercostals and abdominals are *expiratory muscles* activated only during exercise. Electromyography of respiratory muscles, using surface or needle electrodes for the intercostals and abdominals and an intraesophageal electrode for the diaphragm, may be used to record individual muscle function. Respiratory muscle paralysis (induced by curare or insufficient central controller drive) is also reflected by a decrease in the amplitude of esophageal or pleural pressure oscillations.

Sensors for respiratory regulation are chemoreceptors and mechanoreceptors located within the ventral medulla oblongata (or brainstem) and arterial walls, airways, lungs,

and rib cage. These receptors send neural messages to the central controller, or respiratory center, located in the brainstem. The respiratory center is a collection of interconnected neurons sending rhythmic nerve signals to mostly effector inspiratory muscles. Within limits, the central controller is also influenced by subordinate controller neurons in the cortex and in the rostral pons (pneumotaxic center). The major communication channels are the vagus nerves, which transport afferent and efferent signals, the glossopharyngeal nerves, and the phrenic nerves. The afferent nerve messages from the sensors travel in the vagus and glossopharyngeal nerves, which both end in the nucleus tractus solitari (NTS) near the respiratory center. The phrenic nerves transmit efferent motor impulses from the respiratory center to the diaphragm, and the vagus nerves carry effector signals to the lungs.

This chapter presents the controllers and sensors of the respiratory regulating system. It also discusses the means used to adjust the rate of alveolar ventilation and to coordinate the repeated respiratory cycles with the demands.

THE INTRINSIC RESPIRATORY CENTER

The respiratory neurons are widely dispersed groups of neurons located bilaterally in the reticular substance of the medulla oblongata and of the more rostral pons (Fig. 10–2). In its dorsomedial aspect, the medulla contains neurons of the NTS, also referred to as the dorsal respiratory group (DRG) of *inspiratory* neurons (see Fig. 10–3). The ventrolateral aspect of the medulla holds neurons of the nucleus retroambigualis (NRA), also referred to as the ventral respiratory group (VRG) of *expiratory* neurons, which also have some *inspiratory* neurons. Some nonrespiratory neurons (glossopharyngeal and vagal motor neurons) are found in the neighboring nucleus ambiguus (NA) of the ventrolateral aspect of the medulla. The cranial pons encloses the pneumotaxic center (nucleus parabrachialis medialis, or NPBM).

Medullary Neurons that Cause Rhythmic Inspiration and Expiration

The location of respiratory neurons in the brainstem is approximated by surgical transections of the spinal cord in anesthetized cats or rabbits (see Fig. 10–2). A section caudal to the medulla oblongata (section A) eliminates the motor impulses to the rib cage and diaphragm. A section caudal to the origin of the phrenic nerve (section B) abolishes only the function of the intercostals. Removal of the brain rostral to the pons (section C) does not stop the respiratory

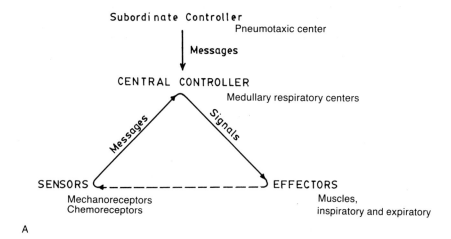

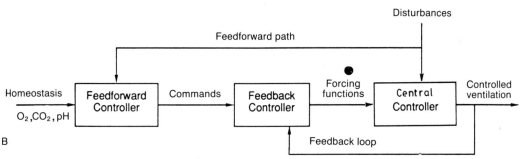

Figure 10-1 **A,** General organization of the regulatory system for respiration. Sensors send neural messages to the central controller, which may also receive other messages from a subordinate controller. The central controller translates these messages into signals (commands, forcing functions) to the effectors. Some changes in the effectors are inhibitory feedback signals to the sensors. **B,** The concepts of feedforward and feedback control strategies are illustrated in this cybernetic representation of the elements of the system regulating respiration. Any disturbance in pH, carbon dioxide, or oxygen content of blood is sent to the central controller for correction by a feedback loop. The feedforward strategy intervenes only when direct cortical messages are sent to the central controller in anticipation of some future need.

rhythm. Respiration even continues if the medulla is transected longitudinally down the midline.

Respiratory responses are obtained by implanting microelectrodes in the interior of the brainstem and stimulating it with repetitive electric shocks. From the microstimulation responses, functional areas have been mapped and types of respiratory neuron groups have been defined (Fig. 10-3). The respiratory neurons are within the reticular formation of the medulla oblongata, caudal to the level of entrance of cranial nerve VIII and dorsal to caudal olivary nuclei. The respiratory medullary neurons are grouped into two functional divisions: a dorsomedial inspiratory group (with some inspiratory activity) and a ventrolateral expiratory group.

In anesthetized cats or rabbits, stimulation of the neurons in the inspiratory area causes the mouth to open wide, the nares to dilate, and the tongue to retract. The muscles involved in spontaneous deep inspiration then contract maximally, and the volume of air inspired may be as much as 10 times the normal tidal air. Contraction of inspiratory muscles may be maintained until the animal dies of asphyxia. Repetitive stimulation of the expiratory center produces and maintains expiration by active contraction of expiratory muscles and by inhibition of inspiratory muscles. Alternating stimulation of these two centers produces coordinated respiratory movements, which can be readily controlled in rate and depth (Fig. 10-4). Simultaneous stimulation of the two centers leads to inspiration, indicating that the inspiratory center is dominant.

The major concentration of inspiratory neurons (DRG) is located in the ventral portion of the NTS, which is the termination site of afferent fibers traveling in cranial nerves IX (glossopharyngeal) and X (vagus) (Fig. 10-5). The DRG may be the initial intracranial processing station for many reflexes that affect respiration. The abundant interconnections within the nucleus appear to provide the basis for a system of neuronal self-excitation, which would explain the progressive increase in phrenic nerve activity seen during inspiration. The NTS is made up of three types of inspiratory neurons: early-burst, late-peak, and postinspiratory. The DRG also may be the site of origin of the rhythmic respira-

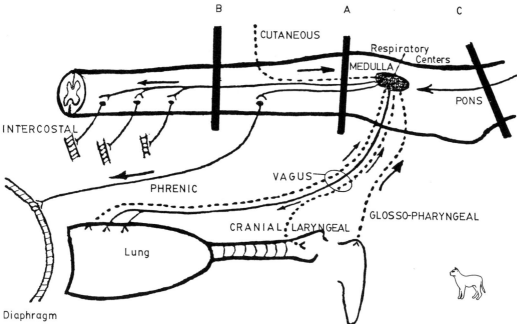

Figure 10–2 Neural mechanism of respiration. A medullary respiratory center receives impulses from incoming nerves from skin, lungs, larynx, and pharynx and generates nerve impulses to muscles (diaphragm, intercostals, abdominals) and lungs. Transection of the brainstem below the vagi abolishes inspiratory signals to the intercostals and the diaphragm (**A**). A section below the origin of the phrenic nerves causes paralysis of the intercostals (**B**). A section in the upper pons produces little modification of breathing (**C**). The superior laryngeal branch of the vagi, the sensory nerve of the larynx, is responsible for an inhibition of respiration and forced expiratory acts (cough). Stimulation of the glossopharyngeal nerve (deglutition) causes instant arrest of respiration. Stimulation of cutaneous nerves (pain) causes deep inspiration.

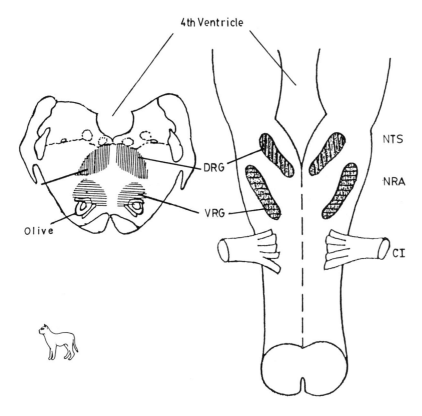

Figure 10–3 Organization of the respiratory center in the cat. Cross section and longitudinal section of the medulla oblongata shows the dorsal position of the DRG (dorsal respiratory group) of neurons, or dorsomedial inspiratory neurons, in the NTS (nucleus tractus solitari), and the VRG (ventral respiratory group), or ventrolateral expiratory (with some inspiratory) neurons, in the NRA within the reticular formation.

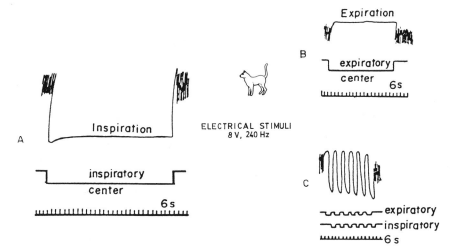

Figure 10–4 Respiratory responses produced by stimulation of the respiratory centers with repetitive shocks (8 volts, 240 Hz). **A,** Stimulation of the inspiratory center produces inspiration. **B,** Stimulation of the expiratory center produces expiration. **C,** Alternate stimulation of the two centers produces corresponding inspiration and expiration.

tory drive to the VRG (a population of both inspiratory and expiratory neurons located in the NRA) and to many spinal respiratory motor neurons.

The VRG neurons, in the NRA, have phrenic motor nucleus arborizations (i.e., they stimulate inspiration by contraction of the diaphragm). They also project to distant sites and drive either spinal motor neurons going to expiratory muscles (primarily intercostals and abdominals) or auxiliary muscles of respiration (pharyngeal, laryngeal) innervated by the vagus nerves.

Intracellular recordings from respiratory neurons in the brainstem have not yet defined the nature of the cellular mechanism involved in respiratory rhythmogenesis. It may be that rhythmic respiratory activity requires the presence of continuous (tonic) or intermittent (phasic) excitatory inputs. The respiratory oscillations would be the result of reciprocal inhibition of interconnected networks of neurons. Many pharmacologic substances affect the central control mechanisms, and depression of respiration by general anesthetics and other drugs is a common veterinary clinical problem.

Fine Tuning of Breathing by the Pontile Pneumotaxic Center

The pneumotaxic center (NPBM) is a subordinate controller that transmits impulses from the cranial pons to the medullary inspiratory area. These impulses modulate or "fine tune" the output of inspiratory signals (see Fig. 10–5). The role of the pneumotaxic center in regulating normal breathing is less crucial than was once thought.

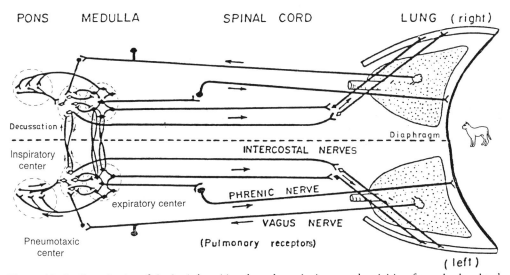

Figure 10–5 Organization of rhythmic breathing depends on the integrated activities of two closely related neural mechanisms: the medullary inspiratory center and the mechanoreceptors in the vagus nerves. The medullary inspiratory center distributes nerve impulses to the various spinal and cranial motor nuclei that innervate the inspiratory muscles to initiate and to coordinate their contractions.

Destruction of the pneumotaxic center produces a slower, deeper pattern of breathing in anesthetized animals. With bilateral vagotomy, the pattern of breathing becomes *apneustic* (inspiratory gasping). Chronic feline preparations with bilateral vagotomy and pneumotaxic destruction breathe apneustically when anesthetized but resume eupneic breathing when awake. This suggests that the function of the pneumotaxic center is more to tune the respiratory pattern than to cut off the inspiration. The pneumotaxic center is no longer thought to affect the rate of breathing by switching off inspiration to initiate expiration and limiting the duration of inspiration or shortening the entire respiratory cycle.

Apneusis is a function of the reticular activating system rather than that of an apneustic center in the caudal pons.

In a decerebrate animal transection of the brainstem at a level that preserves the junction of the caudal pons with medulla oblongata results in continuous repetitive discharge of impulses from the inspiratory center, causing inspiratory gasping, or apneusis. It now seems that apneusis is a functional state involving the *reticular activating system* rather than the action of an apneustic center. Facilitation of inspiration and production of apneusis appear to be related to the activity of the reticular activating system and are separate from the basic respiratory rhythm production, which occurs in the medulla.

ACTION OF MECHANICAL AND CHEMICAL RECEPTORS ON RESPIRATION

The intrinsic respiratory center is modulated by inputs from mechanoreceptors and chemoreceptors. The mechanoreceptors are in the nasal and upper airways, the lungs (stretch, irritant, and juxtacapillary receptors), the muscles and tendons in the rib cage (proprioceptors), the skin (pain, temperature), and the arteries (baroreceptors). Chemoreceptors are located in the brainstem (central) and in arteries (peripheral).

Mechanoreceptors

Mechanoreceptors in the Nasal and Upper Airways

Stimulation of receptors in the nasal and upper airways produces reactions concerned with protection and reanimation of the respiratory system. Receptors in the *nasal airways* respond to foreign matter by the protective reflex of *sneezing* with the objective of expelling the xenobiotic substance from the airway. The sneezing reflex begins with a deep inspiration, brief closure of the glottis with contraction of the expiratory muscles, coinciding with an abrupt forced blast of air through the nose.

In the cat, the *sniff reflex* is used to demonstrate that the activity of the medullary expiratory neurons is easily inhibited by weak activation of inspiratory neurons. Slight stimulation of the receptors in the cat's *nasopharynx* with a fine wire

elicits a brief burst of activity in the inspiratory neurons with a marked and prolonged inhibition of the expiratory neurons.

The *upper airways* possess receptors with afferent fibers traveling in the trigeminal and olfactory nerves. These receptors are sensitive to mechanical stimulation and chemical agents. In an unanesthetized animal, stimulation of these receptors brings reflex *apnea* and *bradycardia*. In the rabbit, reflex apnea and bradycardia are easily demonstrated, as they follow the first breath of air containing *ether, ammonia, cigarette smoke,* or *formaldehyde* (Fig. 10–6).

Receptors in the larynx and trachea also respond to mechanical and chemical stimulation by causing reflex *coughing, bronchoconstriction,* and *hypertension*. Like sneezing, coughing starts with a deep inspiration; the glottis is then briefly closed to build up pressure and abruptly opened to let a violent blast of air escape through the mouth. During light general anesthesia or insufficient local anesthesia, mechanical stimulation of the upper airways during attempts to insert an endotracheal or esophageal catheter may provoke an insurmountable laryngeal spasm.

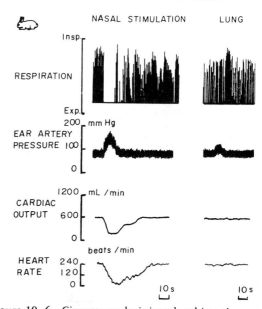

Figure 10–6 Cigarette smoke is introduced into the nose of an unanesthestized rabbit breathing through a tracheostomy and into the tracheostomy inlet (lung). Nasal stimulation causes respiration to stop, ear blood pressure to increase markedly, and cardiac output and heart rate to decrease. Trigeminal afferents are the primary source of the nasal respiratory and circulatory disturbances. Olfactory afferents cannot initiate the respiratory and circulatory disturbances but weakly potentiate the apnea induced by trigeminal stimulation. Arterial baroreceptor mechanisms contribute to the evoked bradycardia. Arterial chemoreceptor mechanisms do not contribute to the circulatory effects but act to terminate the induced apnea. The lung stimulation (pulmonary irritant receptors) accelerates ventilation and produces a slight increase in ear arterial pressure. The afferent impulses travel in the vagi.

Philtrum Acupuncture Point for Respiratory Reanimation. Stimulation of cutaneous and subcutaneous receptors in the area of the nasal philtrum is one of the steps in emergency cardiopulmonary resuscitation. Borrowed from acupuncture, the procedure uses hypodermic needle implantation and manipulation at a site on the nose or planum nasale (acupuncture point GV26, or Governing Vessel 26, or Renzhong), to activate the medullary respiratory centers. Localization of GV26 varies according to species (e.g., a single point near the philtrum in dogs, cats, and horses [in the center of a hair tuft], a triple point near the junction of the hairless nose with the hairy skin in pigs and cows; Fig. 10–7).

Types of Lung Receptors

The three classes of lung receptors (pulmonary stretch, irritant, and juxtacapillary) have different properties and reflex effects. Their afferent messages to the inspiratory neurons travel in nerve fibers incorporated in the vagus nerves. Respiration remains rhythmic, although slower and deeper, after section of the vagus nerves and abolition of the signals from all three types of pulmonary receptors.

Pulmonary stretch receptors within the smooth muscle layer of extrapulmonary airways (bronchi and bronchioles) are activated by distention of the lungs and adapt slowly to a continuous stimulus. Their activation augments bronchial transmural pressure and produces the *Hering-Breuer reflex*. Afferent impulses of overdistention, carried in large myelinated fibers traveling in the vagus, reach the inspiratory neurons to reflexly shorten the duration of inspiratory time (TI) and promote expiration. During the Hering-Breuer reflex, expiratory apnea and a stronger contraction of the expiratory muscles occur. This reflex increases the rate of respiration because it shortens the period of inspiration (i.e., lowers the ratio of inspiratory time to total time of an inspiratory-expiratory cycle [TI/TT]). If lung overdistention is produced during the first 75 percent of the normal TI, expiratory time (TE) is lengthened, whereas TE is shortened if the stimulation is in the last 25 percent of inspiration. The pulmonary stretch receptors are important in terminating lung inflation (inspiration) in anesthetized animals with intact vagi, but the excess volume required to activate the reflex is not the same at the onset and at the end of inspiration. When applied during early inspiration, a bigger stretch, or tidal volume, is needed to inhibit the inspiratory

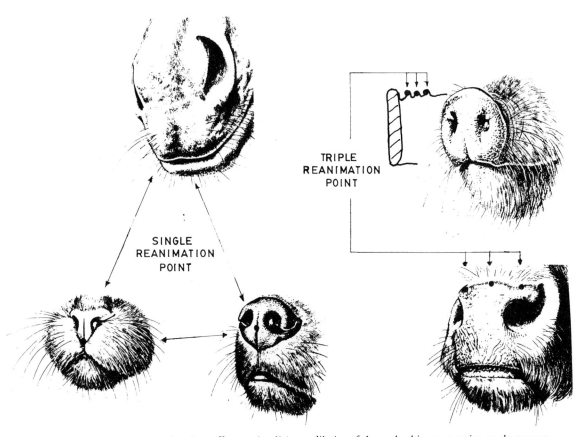

TRIPLE REANIMATION POINT

SINGLE REANIMATION POINT

Figure 10–7 For emergency reanimation, afferent stimuli (e.g., dilation of the anal sphincter, traction on the tongue, pressure on the hard palate, and light pressure on the thoracic wall over the maximal cardiac impulse point) tend to produce reflex inspiration. The philtrum points of acupuncture located on the nose serve the same purpose. Stimulation is with a hypodermic needle at the single or multiple sites indicated.

muscles. In the later part of inspiration, a gradually smaller overdistention volume is necessary to terminate inspiration. In unanesthetized animals, inputs from pulmonary stretch receptors are less important and are abolished by visual or auditory stimulation.

Termination of inflation by activation of the pulmonary stretch receptors tends to prevent overinflation of the lungs. When a demand for increased ventilation (hyperpnea) is required to eliminate an excessive concentration of alveolar carbon dioxide (e.g., during exercise and during breathing of carbon dioxide–enriched gases), a faster respiratory frequency (tachypnea) is easily obtained. This is different from dyspnea (a need for a ventilation beyond the response that the animal can provide). When pulmonary inflation is delayed by increased resistance to air flow, inspiration is lengthened to allow more time for a normal tidal volume of gas to enter the lung. In contrast, a greater pulmonary volume or an obstruction to air flow during expiration reflexly increases the time of lung emptying by forestalling the onset of the next inspiration.

In anesthetized animals, when the vagus nerves are cut to eliminate the Hering-Breuer reflexes, breathing is slower and the inspiratory muscles are more active. Records of the impulses discharged by the neurons of the phrenic nerves indicate that deepening of inspiration results from prolongation of the inspiratory discharge. After a vagotomy, lung inflation does not shorten the duration of inspiration (TI). Without inhibitory impulses from distended lungs, the amplitude of inspiration is increased and the frequency of breathing is decreased (Fig. 10–8).

Pulmonary irritant receptors, situated between epithelial cells of the airways, are inactive in eupnea (i.e., resting breathing). When activated mechanically or chemically, they send impulses in small vagal fibers toward the inspiratory cell group. Irritant receptors adapt rapidly to a sustained stimulus. Effective mechanical stimuli are lung inflation, accelerated air flow, and solid particles changing bronchial smooth muscle tone. Inhalation of cold air, cigarette smoke, inhaled dusts, and noxious agents such as sulfur dioxide, ammonia, nitrogen dioxide, or antigens also stimulates lung irritant receptors. Similarly, endogenous chemical mediators released during allergic reactions (e.g., histamine, bradykinin, slow-reacting substance of anaphylaxis or leukotriene D_4) activate irritant receptors.

When stimulated, irritant receptors reflexly constrict the airways and augment inspiratory neuron activity (i.e., frequency of inspiration and pulmonary ventilation). The rapid and shallow breathing may limit penetration of dangerous agents into the lungs and may prevent damage to the gas-exchanging surfaces. During eupnea, the irritant receptors stabilize lung compliance by initiating sporadic sighs (unrelated to the phases of inspiration or expiration), which serve to reexpand collapsed areas of the lungs. Vagotomy abolishes the reflex action of pulmonary irritant receptors.

Juxtacapillary receptors, or J receptors, in the lung interstitium near alveolar capillaries are served by small nonmyelinated (slow) vagal fibers ending near the inspiratory cell group. Adapting rapidly, they are excited mainly by lung interstitial edema and also by substances such as hista-

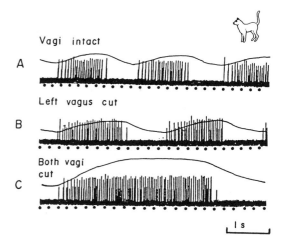

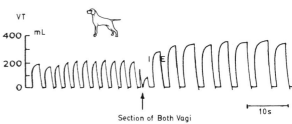

Figure 10–8 Top, Recording of inspiratory electrical impulses from two phrenic motor neurons in a decerebrate cat. Time: 0.20 second. **A,** Vagi intact, inspiration (upstroke signal) is of normal duration. **B,** Left vagus nerve cut, some prolongation of inspiration and slowing of the inspiratory cycles. **C,** Both vagi cut, slowing and deepening by prolongation of the inspiratory discharge. **Bottom,** Recording of respiration cycles before and after section of both vagi in an anesthetized dog. Vagotomy decreases the breathing rate by increasing the amplitude of the inspirations.

mine, halothane, and phenylguanide. Activation of these receptors causes laryngeal closure and apnea, followed by rapid, shallow breathing. Together with irritant receptors, J receptors may be responsible for the tachypnea (which is not dyspnea, even if very similar) seen in animals with pulmonary edema (heart failure), pneumonia, and microembolism.

Experimental injection of phenylguanide produces bradycardia with hypotension and respiratory inhibition in cats (respiratory excitation in rabbits). Inhibition of somatic muscles of the limb (even in anesthetized cats) is associated with muscular exercise, which increases cardiac output, pulmonary arterial pressure, and interstitial volume. The last-named stimulates the J receptors, which inhibit the somatic muscles, to force termination of the exercise.

Proprioceptors in the Rib Cage

Proprioceptors are nerve endings, primarily located within muscles and tendons, that receive stimuli pertaining to movements and position of the body. Three types of proprioceptors send signals to the respiratory neurons about changes in the force exerted by the respiratory muscles and the movement of the rib cage: joint, tendon, and muscle spindle receptors.

The activity of *joint receptors* (Ruffini's, pacinian, and Golgi's corpuscles) varies with the degree and rate of change of rib and limb movement. These proprioceptors sense the rate of movement, even from passive movements of the limbs. The neurogenic stimulation linked to their activity occurs even if blood circulation is cut off by a pressure cuff, which prevents muscular metabolic products from reaching the respiratory center.

The early effect of exercise on respiration is most marked as impulses from moving limbs immediately increase ventilation, which happens too rapidly to be explained by blood-borne chemical stimuli. This abrupt increase in ventilatory drive may be a learned response rather than the result of a feedback control system, with a set of impulses being sent from the brain to the inspiratory center.

Tendon organs in the external intercostals and (mostly) in the diaphragm, when stimulated by small changes in the contraction force of these muscles, inhibit inspiration. When the diaphragm is stretched, the tendon organs inhibit its contraction and inspiration. They influence muscle contraction in a manner opposite to that of muscle spindles.

Muscle spindles are numerous in the external intercostals and important for intercostal reflexes. Stretching external intercostal muscles increases their force (facilitation) of contraction. Muscle spindles help coordinate breathing during changes in posture and stabilize the rib cage when breathing is impeded by an increase in airway resistance or a decrease in lung compliance.

Pain and Temperature Effects on Breathing

Local nociception (pain) to the skin (by heat, pin prick) results in temporary apnea followed by hyperventilation. Impairment or damage to the afferent (ascending) spinal pathways may cause simple respiratory dysfunction (such as apnea during sleep) or a general depression of respiration.

In several animal species whose sudation is inadequate for evaporative heat loss, the respiratory system helps regulate body temperature. When placed in a hot environment, these animals hyperventilate to increase heat loss through the respiratory passages. Hypothalamic thermoreceptors accelerate the frequency of breathing during hyperthermia. In goats, an increase in rectal temperature of only 1° C causes thermal polypnea (breathing frequency goes from about 40 per minute to 270 per minute, and lowers $PaCO_2$ from 39 to 25 torr. Dogs, cats, and birds depend to a large extent on respiratory heat elimination for control of their body temperature. When the rectal temperature of ducks and chickens goes from 41.5° to 42° C, the respiratory frequency may increase 10-fold (from about 25 to nearly 250 per minute).

Arterial Baroreceptors in Respiratory Reflexes

A sharp rise in arterial blood pressure produces apnea, whereas sudden hypotension results in hyperpnea. The apnea is mainly from stimulation of the baroreceptors of the carotid sinus and aortic arch. Impulses from these receptors reflexly inhibit the inspiratory center.

Hyperpnea due to a fall in arterial pressure is caused mainly by withdrawal of inhibitory impulses, which are normally discharged at low frequency when blood pressure is normal. Baroreceptor impulses may normally exert a tonic restraining influence on the respiratory center, but their general influence on respiratory control is much less than that of the chemoreceptor reflexes. Denervation of the baroreceptors, which induces hypertension, has no permanent effect on breathing.

Control of Medullary Inspiratory Centers by Chemoreceptors

The main goal of respiration is to maintain proper concentrations of hydrogen ions, carbon dioxide, and oxygen in the body fluid. Ventilation is modified by nerve impulses from chemoreceptors (i.e., receptors sensitive to chemical changes in blood and other extracellular fluids). According to their localization and their chemical sensitivity, two types of chemoreceptors are recognized: central (medullary) chemoreceptors influenced directly by hydrogen ions and indirectly by carbon dioxide, and peripheral (arterial) chemoreceptors, which are more sensitive to anoxia (i.e., lowered fractional concentration or partial pressure of oxygen in arterial blood) than to hypercapnia.

Action of Central Chemoreceptors on Respiration

The central chemoreceptors are located in a bilateral area near the ventral surface (less than 0.3 mm) of the medulla, in the vicinity of the exit of cranial nerves IX and X. These neurons respond to acidity by increasing respiration and to alkalosis by depressing respiration. They generate nerve impulses directed to the intrinsic medullary respiratory center for inspiration. Augmentation of ventilation favors the elimination of carbon dioxide from the blood and alveoli. It also lessens the formation of hydrogen ions from dissociation of carbonic acid, which is previously formed by catalytic hydration of blood carbon dioxide (Table 10–1).

TABLE 10–1   Respiratory Stimulation in Man by Greater Content of Carbon Dioxide in Atmospheric Air

Carbon Dioxide		$PaCO_2$	$\dot{V}_T$	f	$\dot{V}_I$
Atm (%)	Alv (%)	(torr)	(mL)	(/min)	(L)
0.03	5.6	41	673	14	9.4
0.79	5.5	40	739	14	10.4
2.02	5.6	41	864	15	12.9
3.07	5.5	40	1,216	15	18.2
5.14	6.2	45	1,771	19	33.7
6.01	6.6	48	2,104	27	56.8

Hydrogen ions are the *primary stimuli,* and the only important direct stimuli, for central chemoreceptor neurons. Local application of a mock cerebrospinal fluid (CSF) having a low pH, which is the result of either a high carbon dioxide or a low bicarbonate content, provides hydrogen ions that especially excite sensor neurons in the chemosensitive area. Subsequent changes in hydrogen ion concentration have considerably less effect in stimulating the central chemoreceptor neurons than changes in carbon dioxide. As hydrogen ions do not easily cross either the blood-brain barrier or the blood–CSF barrier, much more stimulation of the central chemoreceptor neurons is caused by changes in carbon dioxide concentration than by changes in hydrogen ion concentration.

Blood carbon dioxide has a potent indirect effect on the central chemoreceptors. By reacting with water in the tissues, carbon dioxide forms carbonic acid, which dissociates into bicarbonate and hydrogen ions; the latter then have a potent direct stimulatory effect on the central chemoreceptors catalyzed by carbonic anhydrase:

$$CO_2 + HOH \underset{\text{DEHYDRATION}}{\overset{\text{HYDRATION}}{\rightleftharpoons}} HCO_3^- + H^+$$

An increase in the blood carbon dioxide concentration brings a rise in the carbon dioxide tension in the interstitial fluid of the medulla and in the CSF, and in both of these fluids the carbon dioxide immediately reacts with the water to form hydrogen ions. Paradoxically, more hydrogen ions are released into the chemosensitive area when the blood carbon dioxide concentration increases than when the blood hydrogen ion concentration is augmented. For this reason, the central chemoreceptors are affected more by changes in blood carbon dioxide concentration than by changes in blood hydrogen ion concentration, even if the latter are the primary stimuli.

CSF contains less protein than plasma and a weaker protein-buffering system, and the bicarbonate-to-carbon dioxide ratio $(HCO_3 \cdot H^+/CO_2)$ is the principal buffer.

$$pH = pK_a + \log (HCO_3^-)/(CO_2)$$
$$\text{or } pH = 6.1 + \log (\text{bicarbonate})/(0.03^* \times P_{CO_2})$$
$$7.4 = 6.1 + \log (24)/(0.03 \times 40)$$
$$7.4 = 6.1 + \log 20$$
$$7.4 = 6.1 + 1.3$$

This explains that a given increment in carbon dioxide concentration in the CSF causes far more changes in hydrogen ions than in plasma. Diffusion of hydrogen ions from the CSF into the chemosensitive neurons seems to be the major factor in the control of respiration. One of the advantages of this CSF buffer system influencing pulmonary ventilation is the rapidity with which it can function because of the proximity of CSF to the very rich blood supply of the arachnoid plexus. Within seconds after modification of the carbon

---

* Millimoles per liter per torr of P_{CO_2} dissolved in plasma.

dioxide tension of blood, the partial tension of carbon dioxide and the hydrogen ion concentration of the CSF are changed.

Pulmonary Ventilation Is Increased by Hypercapnia. An increase in blood carbon dioxide tension provokes a marked augmentation of pulmonary ventilation (Fig. 10–9). Within 10 minutes, an acute increase in partial pressure of carbon dioxide is obtained by breathing a gas mixture of oxygen with 3, 5, and 7 percent carbon dioxide.

Regulation of Alveolar Ventilation by Carbon Dioxide. The concentration of carbon dioxide, a ubiquitous end-product of metabolism, greatly affects chemical reactions of cells and tissue pH. Stimulation of the central chemoreceptors by carbon dioxide provides an important feedback mechanism for regulation of the concentration of carbon dioxide throughout the body. Tissue carbon dioxide tension is maintained within normal ranges by stimulation of the central chemoreceptors and by accelerating alveolar ventilation to remove the excess of alveolar carbon dioxide removed from plasma. In this way, through the central chemoreceptors, the intrinsic medullary inspiratory centers maintain the carbon dioxide tension of the tissue fluids at a relatively constant level.

A cross-circulation experiment with dogs can be used to demonstrate that central chemoreceptors account for all the ventilatory acceleration brought by carbon dioxide without the intervention of peripheral chemoreceptors. The recipient dog's head is perfused exclusively by arterial blood from the donor dog through anastomoses of the common carotid arteries of the donor to the vertebral arteries of the recipient. Ventilation and arterial carbon dioxide tension are determined before, during, and after the donor inhales carbon dioxide at 3 and 5 percent (with 20 percent oxygen and adjusted to 100 percent with nitrogen) for 20 minutes. The sensitivity of the respiratory centers of both dogs to carbon dioxide tension is similar, as indicated by the regression lines relating ventilation in both dogs as a function of arterial carbon dioxide tension of the donor dog only (see Fig. 10–9).

Effects of Peripheral Chemoreceptors on Ventilation

Peripheral chemoreceptors located outside the central nervous system are responsive to hypoxemia as well as to increased carbon dioxide and hydrogen ion concentrations. They also transmit signals to the intrinsic medullary inspiratory centers to help regulate respiratory activity in emergency and pathophysiological states.

These arterial chemoreceptors, known as glomera because of their extensive capillary network, are situated near the walls of arteries in the carotid and aortic bodies (Fig. 10–10) and have efferent nerve connections. A glomus is organized in compact or disseminated lobules, islands, or "glomoids" around highly convoluted capillaries. Histologically, a glomus consists of many glomus (epithelioid, main, receptor, or type I) cells covered by a few sustentacular

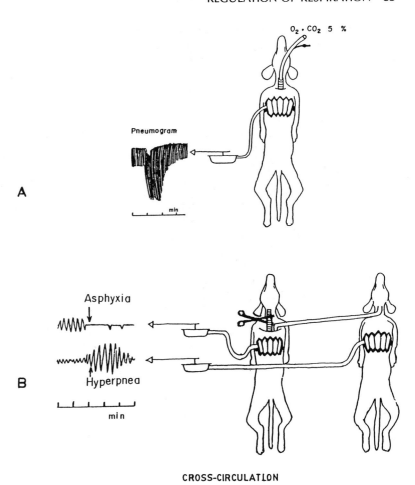

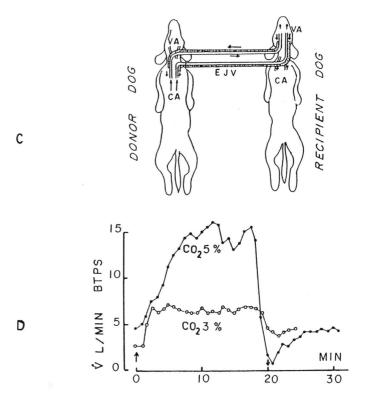

Figure 10–9 Control of ventilation by central chemoreceptors. **A,** As the carbon dioxide content of a gas mixture is raised from 0.03 to 5 percent, the alveolar content increases from 5.6 to 6.2 percent, and the blood carbon dioxide tension from 40 to 45 torr. To compensate for this higher carbon dioxide level in blood, pulmonary ventilation is doubled. **B,** When carbon dioxide-rich blood (asphyxiated and anoxic *dog A*) is infused experimentally into the head breathing air (*dog B*), the central chemoreceptors of dog B perceive the excess carbon dioxide, higher pH, and lack of oxygen in the blood of dog A, and pulmonary ventilation is increased. **C,** In experimental cross-circulation, the donor's carotid arterial blood is perfused into the recipient's head through the vertebral arteries. Return from the recipient to the donor is by a different circuit depriving the donor's head of blood. **D,** Time course of ventilatory response in the recipient dog when the donor dog was given 5 percent and 3 percent carbon dioxide to breathe and its arterial blood was perfused into the recipient dog's head through the vertebral arteries.

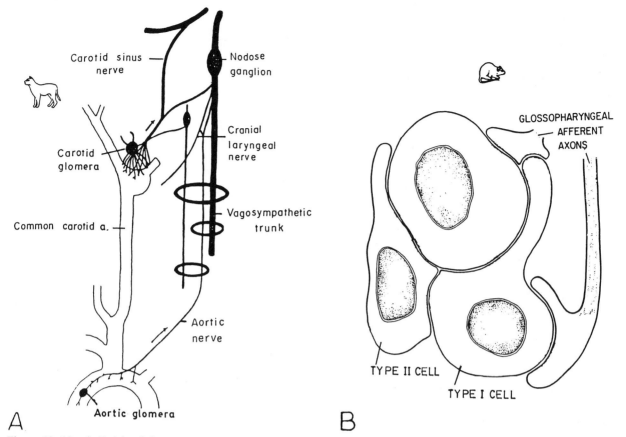

Figure 10–10 **A,** Peripheral chemoreceptors in the carotid and aortic glomera (bodies). Impulses to the medullary inspiratory centers follow the carotid sinus nerve from the carotid body and the aortic nerve from the aortic bodies. **B,** The transduction of the chemosensory discharges into the carotid or sinus is by either type I (glomus) or type II (sustentacular) cells.

(capsule, interstitial, satellite, or type II) cells. A few ganglion cells (sympathetic or parasympathetic) occur near the carotid body. In the rat, the proportions of glomus, sustentacular, and ganglion cells are about 350, 90, and 1, respectively.

The carotid bodies are located bilaterally next to the carotid sinuses at the junction of the external and common carotid arteries. They are innervated by fibers (10 to 20 glomus cells per fiber = a sensory unit) passing through the carotid nerve (sinus, Hering's nerve), a branch of cranial nerve IX (glossopharyngeal). The aortic bodies, formed by a number of glomus cell clusters, are located along the arch of the aorta and other great intrathoracic arteries. Their afferent innervations pass into the aortic (depressor, Cyon's) nerve, a branch of cranial nerve X (vagus). In the cat, the vagi also supply innervation to miniglomera around the common carotid arteries. The carotid and aortic nerves, also known as buffer nerves, carry barosensory and chemosensory fibers.

In the early 1930s, a systematic study of the carotid and aortic reflexes involved perfusion of the carotid glomera with Ringer's solution altered by a decrease in oxygen or a rise in carbon dioxide tensions. From the results new concepts of respiratory (and circulatory) control were established, and the 1938 Nobel Prize in physiology was awarded to Heymans.

Activation of Arterial Chemoreceptors by Anoxia. A decrease of the arterial oxygen tension (PO_2) below the normal level, or hypoxemia, activates the peripheral chemoreceptors (Fig. 10–11). Lack of oxygen does not affect the central chemoreceptors but acts on peripheral chemoreceptors located in the carotid and aortic bodies, which transmit signals to the medullary inspiratory centers to increase pulmonary ventilation.

The ventilation of a normal dog is immediately doubled when nitrogen is inhaled for only 30 seconds. After denervation of the arterial chemoreceptors, ventilation is not increased by 60 seconds of nitrogen inhalation. Instead, ventilation is reduced because anoxia depresses the medullary inspiratory centers. In contrast, ventilation is increased just as much by inhalation of 5 percent carbon dioxide when the peripheral chemoreceptors are denervated as when they are intact. It is evident that the peripheral chemoreceptor reflexes contribute little (20 percent in the dog) to the stimulation of breathing when arterial carbon dioxide is increased.

With progressively higher altitudes, alveolar oxygen tension decreases and ventilation increases. At an altitude of 1,200 m, alveolar oxygen pressure is lowered from a normal value of 103 torr to 84, whereas the alveolar carbon dioxide tension falls from 39.7 torr to 37.0, and ventilation is increased only from 7.6 L per minute to 8.0 (Table 10–2).

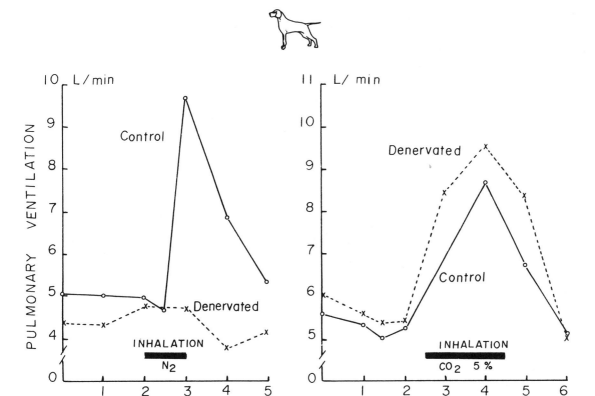

Figure 10–11   Peripheral chemoreceptors are activated by anoxia and are almost indifferent to hypercapnia. **Left panel,** Sudden anoxia (inhalation of nitrogen) causes a hyperventilatory response within 30 seconds in a normal dog but not in a dog with denervated arterial chemoreceptors. **Right panel,** Inhalation of carbon dioxide produces the same effect in a normal dog and in a dog with denervated peripheral chemoreceptors.

However, even at an altitude of 6,000 m, when alveolar oxygen tension is reduced to about one-third of normal, respiration is stimulated only moderately, since the reduction in carbon dioxide tension to 30 torr obviously limits the response for increased ventilation.

Limited Quantitative Effect of Hypoxemia. The quantitative effect of lowered arterial oxygen tension (severe hypoxemia) is to increase alveolar ventilation only about 1.5- to 1.7-fold, whereas lowering blood pH to 7.0 has a fourfold effect, and a 10-fold increase is caused by increasing the carbon dioxide tension by 50 percent. It is clear that the normal effect of hypoxemia on respiratory activity is very slight, especially when compared with the effect of carbon dioxide tension (Fig. 10–12). The cause of the poor effect of oxygen tension changes on respiratory control is an inhibi-

tory (limiting or "braking") effect caused by both carbon dioxide and hydrogen on the central chemoreceptors. The increase in ventilation is very modest, even when alveolar oxygen tension is decreased below 50 torr, because higher ventilation blows off carbon dioxide from the blood and thus reduces blood carbon dioxide tension and hydrogen ion concentration. The powerful central chemoreceptor inhibitory effect exerted by low carbon dioxide and hydrogen ion concentrations is similar to a braking action, which counteracts the stimulation of the arterial chemoreceptors by the diminished oxygen tension. Thus, hypocapnia and alkalosis keep the hypoxemia from provoking a marked increase in ventilation until the oxygen tension falls to values that are incompatible with life for more than a few minutes.

Index of Sensitivity to Hypoxemia. Oxygen deficiency plays only a small role in the normal regulation of respiration, for three major reasons. First, the respiratory system ordinarily maintains an alveolar oxygen tension higher than the level needed to saturate completely the hemoglobin of arterial blood. It does not matter whether alveolar ventilation is normal or excessive; blood can be no more than fully saturated. Second, blood flow through the carotid and aortic bodies is the highest of any tissue in the body. The glomic arteriovenous oxygen difference is less than

TABLE 10–2   Stimulation of Respiration by Altitude

Altitude (m)	0	1,200	2,400	3,600	4,800	6,000
PBatm (torr)	760	656	560	480	410	352
PAO$_2$ (torr)	103.0	84.0	66.0	53.3	42.6	34.8
PACO$_2$ (torr)	39.7	37.0	36.2	33.6	31.3	30.0
V̇I (L/min)	7.6	8.0	9.7	10.5	11.6	

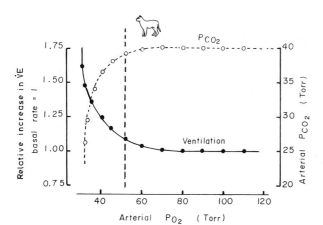

Figure 10–12 Limited hyperventilating effect of low arterial oxygen tension (<50 torr). The maximal relative increase in expiratory minute volume ($\dot{V}E$) is limited to 1.75 times the normal pulmonary ventilation; because of carbon dioxide blow-off, carbon dioxide tension is less than 25 torr. This low carbon dioxide tension inhibits the central chemoreceptors and counteracts the influence of hypoxemia.

1 percent (i.e., venous blood leaving the glomera still has an oxygen tension nearly equal to that of the arterial blood) so at all times the oxygen tension of the tissues in these glomera remains almost equal to that of arterial blood. Third, hypoxemia has an overall effect of reducing pulmonary ventilation by removing carbon dioxide and creating alkalosis, both of which depress the central chemoreceptors. However, if these two parameters (P_{CO_2} and pH) are maintained at normal values, sudden hypoxemia causes ventilation to increase by as much as do hypercapnia and acidosis (Fig. 10–13).

Situations in Which Hypoxemia Overcomes the Limiting Action of Hypocapnia and Alkalosis. In normal animals, the role of hypoxemia on arterial chemoreceptors and pulmonary ventilation is secondary to the role of hypercapnia and acidosis on the central chemoreceptors. The importance of hypoxemia to the arterial chemoreceptors becomes major in cases of arterial hypotension, dysfunction at the respiratory membrane, or chronic hypoxia. In arterial hypotension, the peripheral chemoreceptors stimulate pulmonary ventilation, even if oxygen tension is normal.

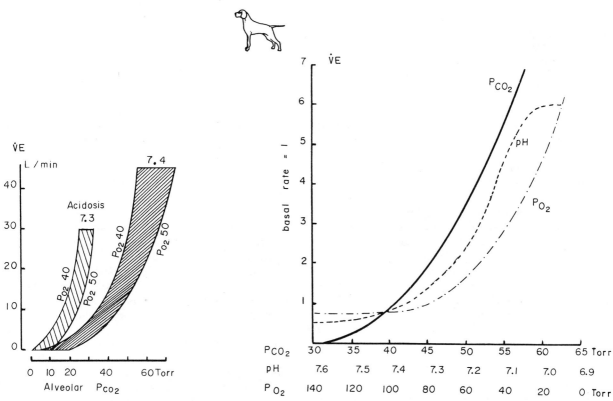

Figure 10–13 **Left panel,** A comparison of the increase in $\dot{V}E$ (pulmonary minute ventilation) as a result of hypoxemia (oxygen tension of 40 to 50 mm Hg during acidosis (pH, 7.3) and normal (pH, 7.4) conditions, and during hypo- and hypercapnia. When excess hydrogen ions and hypocapnia are present, hypoxemia is relatively inefficient to stimulate pulmonary ventilation. However, when pH and carbon dioxide tension are about normal, hypoxemia is more efficient as a stimulus of pulmonary ventilation. **Right panel,** The relative effect of the variation of one blood factor when the two others remain constant is presented. Higher carbon dioxide tension, lower pH, or lower oxygen tension produces a similar relative increase in $\dot{V}E$ (i.e., pulmonary hyperventilation) under this experimental protocol.

In lung ailments such as pneumonia and emphysema, carbon dioxide and hydrogen ion exchanges are mostly impaired, and hyperventilation resulting from hypoxemia is not followed by reduced arterial carbon dioxide tension and hydrogen ion concentration. Instead, those parameters either remain constant in the blood or increase. Thus the braking effect of these other two control systems on the hypoxemia system is not present and the system develops its full power and can increase alveolar ventilation by as much as five to seven times.

Chronic hypoxia due to high altitude first leads to a blunting of the hyperventilation response to hypoxemia, and it is only after acclimatization that hypoxemia causes hyperventilation. At high altitude, frequency of breathing first increases slightly to improve ventilation to a maximum, which is only about 66 percent above normal. This minor improvement of ventilation is due to the braking effect of the carbon dioxide and hydrogen ion system on the potential hyperventilating action of hypoxemia. After about a week, the central chemoreceptors become adapted, or less responsive, to the inhibition of hypocapnia and alkalosis. The inhibitory effect on the hypoxemia system is gradually lost, and alveolar ventilation can rise about five to seven times.

Action of Hypercapnia and Acidosis on Peripheral Chemoreceptors.   In the dog, in response to hypercapnia, the receptor cells of the carotid and aortic glomera discharge to produce one-fifth of the hyperventilation of central chemoreceptors. In the cat, the carotid glomera also respond to a decrease in arterial pH, but the aortic bodies do not.

VARIATIONS IN THE MEDULLARY INSPIRATORY CONTROL

The activity of the respiratory center may be depressed by acute brain edema resulting from brain concussion or from salt intoxication (in the pig). Occasionally, respiratory depression resulting from brain edema can be relieved temporarily by intravenous injection of hypertonic glucose. This solution osmotically removes some of the ICF in the brain, thus relieving intracranial pressure.

Overdose of anesthetic is perhaps the most prevalent cause of respiratory depression and arrest. The best volatile agent for anesthesia is one that depresses the medullary respiratory center least while depressing the cerebral cortex most. Ether is among the best of the anesthetics by these criteria; halothane, cyclopropane, ethylene, and nitrous oxide are almost as good.

Periodic Breathing

An abnormality of respiration called periodic breathing occurs in a number of disease conditions after overventilation and subsequent apnea (Fig. 10–14). Two usual types of periodic breathing are Cheyne-Stokes breathing and Biot's breathing. *Cheyne-Stokes breathing* is characterized by periodic waxing and waning of the amplitude of respiration (see Fig. 10–14). Periods of apnea or merely of reduced respiratory amplitude alternate with periods of hyperpnea. The transition from one to the other is typically gradual. In contrast, *Biot's breathing* is characterized by abrupt alternation of periods of apnea and hyperpnea. The Cheyne-Stokes type of rhythm is more common and is seen during barbiturate anesthesia and in decompensated heart disease, elevated intracranial pressure, narcotic poisoning, high altitude, and overbreathing. The cause of periodic breathing is not the same in all instances, but it seems that there is either a delay of blood from the lung to the brain or changes in the central chemoreceptors' sensitivity to carbon dioxide.

Partial Airway Occlusion

In dogs in different states of sleep, partial airway occlusion, induced by reducing the diameter of a tracheotomy

Figure 10–14 Types of periodic breathing. Biot's breathing presents abrupt alternation of apnea and hyperpnea. Cheyne-Stokes breathing shows periodic waxing and waning of the respiratory movement between periods of apnea.

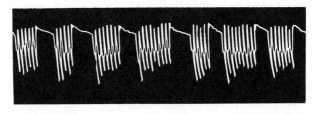

BIOT

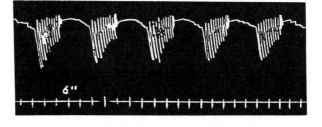

6"

CHEYNE-STOKES

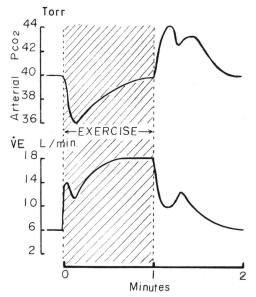

Figure 10–15 Comparison of arterial carbon dioxide tension and pulmonary minute ventilation ($\dot{V}E$) during exercise and recovery. The sudden initial hyperventilation (neural component) is not related to hypercapnia, whereas it is associated with an excess of carbon dioxide (humoral component) in the remaining part of the physical exercise. At the onset of rest, a paradoxical neural pulmonary hypoventilation coincides with hypercarbia. Then the humoral control takes over to cause a more intense pulmonary ventilation that gradually returns the carbon dioxide tension to normal.

tube by 58 percent, decreases the respiratory rate and the minute volume but increases the alveolar carbon dioxide tension by 5 torr. In the waking state, this partial airway occlusion does not alter these respiratory parameters to a significant degree.

Ventilatory Response to Exercise

From the onset of exercise, ventilation increases immediately and remains about constant during the following 20 to 30 seconds. After this lag, it increases progressively and, if the exercise is not too intense, reaches a steady state. The initial, fast ventilatory increase is termed the *neural component,* and the second, slower increase, the *humoral component.*

The changes in expired volume ($\dot{V}E$) and in arterial carbon dioxide tension during a 1-minute period of exercise and during the minute immediately following differ (Fig. 10–15). The ventilatory responses to exercise provide an interesting picture of the various mechanisms by which respiration is regulated. At the start, pulmonary ventilation increases without an initial elevation in arterial carbon dioxide, while the brain excites the skeletal muscles. The increase in pulmonary ventilation may be great enough to actually lower arterial carbon dioxide tension below the normal value, although the exercising muscles are beginning to produce large amounts of carbon dioxide. An explanation is that the ventilation forges ahead of the increase in carbon dioxide

formation. The brain provides anticipatory, or feedforward, stimulation of ventilation even before it is needed. After a short delay, the decrease in arterial carbon dioxide tension finally acts on the central chemoreceptors to reduce the pulmonary ventilation back toward normal for a fraction of a minute. Soon after, the large amount of carbon dioxide formed by the muscles gradually raises the carbon dioxide tension toward the normal level, and the pulmonary ventilation increases once again.

The opposite effects occur when exercise is over. The shutting off of the brain stimulus instantly returns the pulmonary ventilation toward normal. This gets ahead of the decrease in muscle carbon dioxide formation, and a sequence of chemical-directed feedback readjustments occurs before the pulmonary ventilation finally becomes stabilized.

In ponies, during the hyperpnea at the onset of exercise, proprioceptive input from muscles limits rather than stimulates pulmonary carbon dioxide delivery. After chronic carotid glomera denervation, tidal volume is still increased during the first 15 seconds of exercise (Fig. 10–16).

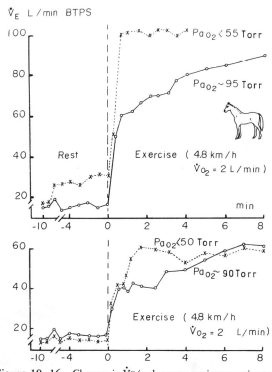

Figure 10–16 Changes in $\dot{V}E$ (pulmonary expiratory minute volume) in ponies with carotid body denervation, at rest and during a treadmill exercise at 4.8 km per hour (oxygen consumption 2 L per minute) under low (< about 50 torr) and normal (about 90 torr) arterial oxygen tension. During the first minute of exercise, pulmonary ventilation is higher at the hypoxemic tension trials than at the normal oxygen tension trials. The hyperventilating effect of carbon dioxide occurs (on the central chemoreceptors) earlier in the hypoxemic tension trials than in the normal oxygen tension trials. Possible explanations are the synergic effect on the central chemoreceptors of hypoxemia and a modest increase in carbon dioxide tension or of earlier accumulation or release of carbon dioxide during hypoxemia. After a few minutes, both sets of pulmonary ventilation results are about equal.

GLOSSARY OF TERMS RELATED TO RESPIRATION

Acapnia: See hypocapnia.

Acidemia: See acidosis.

Acidosis: A condition of increased hydrogen ion concentration in body fluids, which, if uncompensated, lowers pH of body fluids; acidemia.

Alkalemia: See alkalosis.

Alkalosis: A condition of decreased hydrogen ion concentration in body fluids, which, if uncompensated, leads to increase in pH of body fluids; alkalemia.

Anoxemia: A reduced fractional concentration (FaO_2) or partial pressure (PaO_2) of oxygen in arterial blood; hypoxemia.

Anoxia: An abnormal reduction of oxygen in body tissues; hypoxia or oxygen deficiency.

Apnea: Cessation of breathing.

Apneusis: A condition marked by long (10 to 20 seconds) inspiration unrelieved by expiration. Each inspiration is long and gasping. It follows experimental transection of the lower portion of the pons (apneustic center).

Asphyxia: Suspended animation from suffocation, with anoxia and hypercapnia in blood and tissues; suffocation.

Bradypnea: Abnormally slow rate of breathing, without great modification of tidal volume but with a lower minute volume.

Dyspnea: Difficult or labored breathing, usually associated with exercise or pulmonary or cardiac problems (i.e., with a demand for oxygen and production or accumulation of lactic acid).

Eupnea: Normal, easy breathing; minor variations in frequency and rhythm, with occasional changes in tidal volume, are within the definition.

Hypercapnia: The presence of an abnormally high fractional concentration ($FbCO_2$) or partial pressure ($PbCO_2$) of carbon dioxide in blood; hypercarbia.

Hypercarbia: See hypercapnia.

Hyperoxemia: Excessive acidity of the blood.

Hyperpnea: Abnormally deep breathing, with a considerable increase in tidal volume and, to a lesser degree, in frequency. This term should not be applied if breathing is difficult.

Hyperventilation: An increase in the minute volume leading to a blow off of carbon dioxide; polypnea.

Hypocapnia: A diminution in the fractional concentration ($FbCO_2$) or in the partial pressure ($PbCO_2$) of carbon dioxide in blood; acapnia.

Hypopnea: Abnormally shallow breathing (i.e., reduced in depth, with little change in frequency).

Hypoventilation: See oligopnea.

Hypoxemia: A deficiency of oxygen in the blood; deficiency of oxygenation.

Hypoxia: Low oxygen content or tension; deficiency of oxygen in inspired air.

Oligopnea: A decrease in minute volume; hypoventilation.

Panting: Swift and labored breathing.

Polypnea: A striking increase in respiration causing an increase in minute volume, due to either higher frequency or increased tidal volume; hyperventilation.

Suffocation: A state of asphyxia in which consciousness is lost, without known appreciation of pain or distress; struggling or choking asphyxia associated with obstruction of the upper airway; asphyxia.

Tachypnea: Rapid breathing, when the depth of breathing is not modified significantly, producing a higher minute volume.

REFERENCES

Bainton CR. Effect of speed versus grade and shivering on ventilation in dogs during active exercise. J Appl Physiol 1972;33:778.

Berger AJ, Mitchell RA, Severinghaus JW. Regulation of respiration. N Engl J Med 1977;297:92–97, 138–143.

De Mesquita S, Aserinsky E. Partial airway occlusion during sleep and waking in the dog. Respir Physiol 1981;43:77.

Diamond J, Howe A. Chemoreceptor activity in aortic bodies of the cat. J Physiol (Lond) 1956;134:319.

Eyzaguirre C, Fitzgerald RS, Lahiri S, Zapata P. Arterial chemoreceptors. In: Shepherd JT, Abboud FM, eds. Handbook of physiology. Section 2. The cardiovascular system. Vol III. Peripheral circulation and organ blood flow. Part 2. Bethesda, MD: American Physiological Society, 1983.

Houk JC. Control strategies in physiological systems. FASEB J 1988;2:97.

Kao FF, Suntay RG, Li WK. Respiratory sensitivity to carbon dioxide in cross-circulated dogs. Am J Physiol 1962;202:1024.

Long S, Duffin J. The neuronal determinants of respiratory rhythm. Prog Neurobiol 1986;27:101.

McRitchie RJ, White SW. Role of trigeminal, olfactory, carotid sinus and aortic nerves in the respiratory and circulatory response to nasal inhalation of cigarette smoke and other irritants in the rabbit. Aust J Exp Biol Med Sci 1974;52:127.

Pan LG, Forster HV, Bisgard GE, Kaminski RP, Dorsey SM, Busch MA. Hyperventilation in ponies at the onset of and during steady-state exercise. J Appl Physiol 1983;54:1394.

CHAPTER 11

RESPIRATORY REGULATION OF ACID-BASE BALANCE

Cellular metabolism produces a continuous influx of volatile and nonvolatile (fixed) acid, or hydrogen ion, residues in the extracellular fluid (ECF). Defense against this acidification of the normally alkaline ECF (i.e., regulation of the number of hydrogen ions or pH) is important for homeostasis. In fact, the importance of a nearly constant extracellular pH (about 7.4 ± 0.05) is second only to the control of the supply of oxygen. The process of pH regulation requires the coordinated functions of the blood buffers and of two of the major organs, the lungs and the kidneys. The blood buffers immediately prevent any change in the concentration of free hydrogen ions by binding any excess into undissociated substances. Then within minutes, the respiratory system eliminates volatile acidity. At a much slower rate (over hours), the urinary system removes the nonvolatile acid radicals such as bicarbonate, sulfate, and phosphate.

The contribution of the respiratory system is of major importance, since it deals with the ubiquitous, abundant, and volatile carbon dioxide (i.e., dehydrated carbonic acid). Daily, the lungs process about 100 times more milliequivalents of acid than does the urinary system.

This chapter presents the elements of ECF pH regulation by the respiratory system. It includes an overview of the perturbations of carbon dioxide elimination that lead to respiratory acidosis and respiratory alkalosis and of the evaluation of acid-base status in animals.

pH AS AN INDICATOR OF ACID-BASE BALANCE

The pH of blood (the negative logarithm of the hydrogen ion concentration) is used as an indicator of the acid-base status of ECF. In the normal range of blood pH (7.35–7.45), the ratio of fixed acids to volatile acids is about 20 to 1.

Abnormal states of hydrogen ion concentration affect blood pH: a lower pH (acidemia) follows hypercapnia (hypoventilation), and pH is increased (alkalemia) following hypocapnia (hyperventilation). Blood pH below 7.35 also denotes a state of *acidosis*—the nonvolatile-to-volatile acids ratio is below 20 to 1. Blood pH above 7.45 points to a state of *alkalosis*—the nonvolatile-to-volatile acids ratio is above 20 to 1.

In absolute terms of pH, alkalemia accompanies alkalosis, and acidemia parallels acidosis; however, acidosis can occur without acidemia if compensatory mechanisms have operated adequately. Acidosis may be initiated either by an increase in the volatile acids (denominator; i.e., of respiratory origin) or by a decrease in the nonvolatile acids (numera-tor; i.e., of nonrespiratory, or metabolic, origin). In compensated acidosis, the nonvolatile-to-volatile acids ratio is returned to nearly 20 to 1 and the pH to 7.4, even if there is still acidosis. The compensation process is established over a period of hours by renal retention of nonvolatile acids (numerator) if the acidosis is of respiratory origin. If the acidosis is nonrespiratory in origin, the compensation is effected by the lungs, which hyperventilate to reduce the absolute level of volatile acids (denominator).

Several control processes may be mobilized to prevent acidosis or alkalosis or to readjust the pH of body fluids. These are the acid-base buffer systems of the body fluids that damp pH changes; the pulmonary ventilation, which reduces or increases the removal of volatile acids; and the adjustment of urinary excretion or retention of nonvolatile acids. Acid-base readjustments operate at different rates. The response of acid-base buffers occurs within seconds, that of pulmonary ventilation takes 1 to 15 minutes, and that of the kidney mechanism requires several hours or days.

Acid-Base Buffer System for Control of Body Fluid pH

An acid-base buffer system (i.e., a poorly dissociated [weak] acid or base with one of its salts) prevents important changes in pH when either a stronger acid or a base is added to it. The animal body relies on three major acid-base buffer systems: plasma carbonic acid–bicarbonate, inorganic phosphate, and organic acids (plasma proteins, and hemoglobin of erythrocytes). In vitro, the acid-neutralizing power of the various buffers of the blood is distributed as follows: 53 percent bicarbonate, 35 percent hemoglobin, 7 percent plasma protein, and 5 percent phosphate.

In vivo, the inorganic *phosphate* (HPO_4/H_2PO_4) buffer is important only in *intracellular* fluids (ICF) and in renal tubular fluids. In *ECF*, the organic acids of the *protein* buffer systems (in cells, plasma, and hemoglobin) exert the most powerful quantitative effect (75 percent) in a sluggish manner. The *carbonic acid–bicarbonate* pair represents 23 percent of the chemical buffering capacity of ECF, which is about 12 times the intracellular buffering potential of inorganic phosphate.

In spite of different buffering capacities, all the buffer systems exist in equilibrium. A change in the buffering capacity of the entire system is reflected by a change in the capacity of one component. It is sufficient to examine one element to gain an understanding of the response capacity of the entire buffering system. The bicarbonate buffer system is used to evaluate the status of the acid-base system of the body, mostly because its components are readily regulated, the carbonic acid (actually the dissolved carbon dioxide) by the lungs, and the bicarbonate by the kidney.

BICARBONATE BUFFER SYSTEM

The bicarbonate buffer system, the principal buffer of blood and of ECF, consists of a mixture of carbonic acid and bicarbonate ions. Carbonic acid, a very weak acid (low degree of dissociation into hydrogen ions and bicarbonate ions), is transformed almost entirely (999/1,000) into carbon dioxide and water by the erythrocytic carbonic anhydrase. As a net result, a solution of carbonic acid has a high concentration of dissolved carbon dioxide and a weak concentration of hydrogen ions, or acid.

$$CO_2 + H_2O \rightleftarrows H_2CO_3 \rightleftarrows HCO_3^- + H^+$$

The relation of the pH, the bicarbonate, and the carbonic acid of the principal buffer of the extracellular fluid is expressed in the Henderson-Hasselbalch equation, in which pKa is the negative logarithm of the acid ionization constant.

$$pH = pKA + \log (base/acid)$$
$$pH = pKA = \log (HCO_3/H_2CO_3)^*$$
$$pH = pKA = \log (HCO_3/alpha \times PCO_2)$$

With pKA = 6.1, HCO_3 = 24 mmol per liter, and H_2CO_3 = alpha × PCO_2 = 0.03 × 40 torr = 1.2 mmol per liter
(CO_2 coefficient of solubility = 0.03 mmol per liter per torr)

$$pH = 6.1 + \log (24/1.2)$$
$$6.1 + \log 20$$
$$6.1 + 1.3$$

hence pH = 7.4 as long as $HCO_3/(0.03 \times PCO_2)$ is 20.

EFFECTS OF RESPIRATION ON ACID-BASE BALANCE

During normal respiration, the oxygen requirements of the body are satisfied, and carbon dioxide is transferred from blood to expired air. These functions are accomplished without much variation in blood pH because of the efficient service of the two major buffer systems (i.e., the organic acids [reduced hemoglobin-oxyhemoglobin] and carbonic acid–bicarbonate). Important variations in the pH of venous and arterial blood are damped by binding of some hydrogen ions (of carbon dioxide origin) to oxylabile groups (–NH) of reduced hemoglobin and by erythrocytic formation of bicarbonate, which is temporarily shifted into plasma.

---

* In practice, the concentration of dissolved carbon dioxide is used as the concentration of carbonic acid in the equation (i.e., H_2CO_3 = alpha × PCO_2).

Role of Reduced Hemoglobin-Oxyhemoglobin Buffer during Respiration

From its source in the mitochondrial cristae of tissue cells, carbon dioxide diffuses out of cells into interstitial fluids and across the vascular endothelium into the intravascular fluid (plasma). From the plasma, most of the carbon dioxide readily diffuses into the erythrocytes; however, the plasma retains some carbon dioxide in solution (carbon dioxide is 20 times more water-soluble than oxygen). Also, a small fraction of plasma carbon dioxide is slowly hydrated to carbonic acid, which immediately dissociates to yield two plasmatic ions, a bicarbonate anion and an hydrogen cation. Therefore, the carbonic acid level is always negligible in plasma.

Because of the catalytic action of carbonic anhydrase C (a zinc-requiring enzyme), the carbon dioxide diffused inside the erythrocytes is rapidly hydrated into carbonic acid, which rapidly dissociates into intracellular bicarbonate and hydrogen ions. Since some of the intracellular hydrogen cations bind with anions of weak acids (e.g., hemoglobin not saturated with oxygen) to form un-ionized acids in the cytoplasm of the erythrocyte, an excess of intracellular bicarbonate anions occurs. As anions easily migrate across the erythrocyte plasma membrane, bicarbonate diffuses out and is added to the bicarbonate of plasmatic origin, if and when it is replaced or exchanged for another anion (chloride), which then moves from plasma into the erythrocyte. Chloride, the most abundant plasma anion (100 mmol per liter), is usually involved in this necessary replacement, which permits removal of intraerythrocyte bicarbonate, hence the term *chloride shift* (Hamberger shift) given to the process. Evidently, the bicarbonate is formed in the erythrocyte, and its removal from the erythrocyte into plasma is related to (1) the capacity of hemoglobin to hold the corresponding hydrogen ion, (2) the obligatory replacement of bicarbonate by another anion (chloride) inside the red blood cell, and (3) the additional diffusion of carbon dioxide from plasma into the erythrocyte.

A protein such as reduced hemoglobin, with basic (hydrogen cation–accepting, e.g., –NH₂) as well as acidic (hydrogen cation–donor, e.g., –COOH) groups, can buffer hydrogen ion changes induced by acids or by bases. Histidine, a component of hemoglobin (35 residues per hemoglobin molecule), has imidazole groups (–NH) with important buffering capacity in the physiological range of hydrogen ions in red blood cells.

Oxyhemoglobin is a stronger acid (more easily dissociated) and a poorer hydrogen ion acceptor than reduced hemoglobin. Oxygenation of blood causes the transformation of reduced hemoglobin into oxyhemoglobin and the release of hydrogen ions from this stronger organic acid.

In the pulmonary blood, the arrival of oxygen in the erythrocytes weakens the intraerythrocyte reduced hemoglobin–hydrogen cation bond, liberates hydrogen ions in the cytoplasm of erythrocytes, and initiates a series of events. Plasma bicarbonate is recalled into the red blood cells to bind to these free hydrogen ions. Carbonic anhydrase in the erythrocytes immediately dehydrates the just-formed carbonic acid into carbon dioxide, which is forced to diffuse out of the erythrocyte into the plasma and thence into the alveolar air.

Role of the Carbonic Acid–Bicarbonate Buffer during Respiration

It is evident from the Henderson-Hasselbalch equation that modification of the arterial carbon dioxide tension influences the pH of blood. An increase in carbon dioxide, without a concomitant rise in bicarbonate, disturbs the bicarbonate:carbon dioxide ratio, decreasing it below 20, and lowers the blood pH below 7.35 (acidosis). There is an excess of hydrogen ions or a deficiency of base (Fig. 11–1). During respiration, an increase in free hydrogen ions is avoided because of the production of bicarbonate by the red blood cells.

In contrast, a decrease in arterial carbon dioxide tension causes the bicarbonate:carbon dioxide ratio to exceed 20 and the pH to rise above 7.45 (i.e., reflecting a state of loss of hydrogen ions or addition of base called alkalosis; see Fig. 11–1).

The Henderson-Hasselbalch relationship between blood pH, total aggregated base or nonvolatile acids (metabolic component), and weak volatile acids (respiratory component) can also be paraphrased as follows: pH is proportional to the ratio of metabolic component to respiratory component.

DISTURBANCES IN THE RESPIRATORY COMPONENT OF BLOOD pH

Changes in the respiratory component, or volatile acids (the weak acids represented by carbonic acid and by the

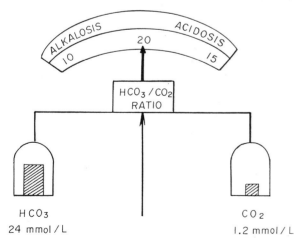

Figure 11–1 Acid-base balance is influenced by the bicarbonate:carbon dioxide ratio. In alkalosis, the ratio is increased because of loss of carbon dioxide (respiratory acid) or gain in bicarbonate (metabolic base). The situation is reversed in acidosis, in which the ratio is reduced by a gain of acid or a loss of base.

organic-acids form of oxygenated and nonoxygenated hemoglobin), can be monitored by measuring carbonic acid (expressed as dissolved carbon dioxide, alpha · Pco_2, S · Pco_2, or simply Pco_2 [S, soluble]). Primary defects in ventilation of the alveoli with increased and decreased carbon dioxide tension are processes, called, respectively, respiratory acidosis and respiratory alkalosis.

The total amount of buffer base (BB, nonvolatile acids, or anions) in whole blood is approximately 48 mmol per liter. About half of this is usually bicarbonate ions (25 mmol per liter) in plasma, and the other half is hemoglobin. Whenever the bicarbonate portion of the buffer base, or metabolic component, is greater than normal, there is metabolic alkalosis, and there is metabolic acidosis when it is less than normal.

Primary disturbances in the metabolic component tend to be compensated for by rapid changes in the respiratory component to readjust the bicarbonate:carbon dioxide ratio to 20. Conversely, primary disturbances in the respiratory component result in metabolic adjustments that are established less rapidly by the urinary system.

Respiratory Acidosis

Retention of carbon dioxide in pulmonary hypoventilation is a cause of acute respiratory acidosis, as it increases the denominator without changing the numerator of the Henderson-Hasselbalch equation. The pH falls rapidly as the carbon dioxide increases. A rise in carbon dioxide tension, from 40 to 60 torr, has the result of lowering the pH from 7.4 to 7.29; for example:

pH in respiratory acidosis:
$$6.1 + \log 28°C/(0.03 \times 60)*$$
$$\text{or } 6.1 + \log 15.6$$
$$6.1 + 1.19 = 7.29.$$

Respiratory acidosis due to an increase in blood carbon dioxide tension may occur because of inadequate ventilation in obstructive lung disease and during general anesthesia. A chronic hypercarbia or hypercapnia, from pneumonia, pulmonary emphysema or pulmonary congestion, initiates a metabolic response by the kidney that damps the effect on the reduction of blood pH. By retaining bicarbonate (and increasing the numerator), the kidney partially compensates for the respiratory acidosis. Renal compensation is rarely complete and cannot bring the pH entirely back to normal, for example:

pH in compensated respiratory acidosis:
$$6.1 + \log 33°C/(0.03 \times 60)*$$
$$\text{or } 6.1 + \log 18.3$$
$$6.1 + 1.26 = 7.36$$

The intensity of the renal compensation can be evaluated by measurement of plasma standard bicarbonate and plasma total carbon dioxide.

Plasma standard bicarbonate is the bicarbonate concentration in plasma separated anaerobically from whole blood and saturated with normal tensions of carbon dioxide (40 torr) and oxygen (100 torr). Heparinized venous blood samples, kept on ice for 2 hours or less, are reliable indicators of acid-base status of animals in most cases. Arterial blood gas evaluation is preferable for animals with respiratory problems, since the important parameters are the tensions of oxygen and of carbon dioxide.

Plasma total carbon dioxide estimation is done by the Harleco carbon dioxide analyzer. Approximately 95 percent of the total carbon dioxide content is bicarbonate, which is increased during compensated respiratory acidosis.

Respiratory Alkalosis

Hypocarbia, or hypopnea with increased blood pH, is associated with hyperventilation or excessive elimination of carbon dioxide from the alveolar air. The interest in the process is not purely physiological, since hyperventilation is associated with hypoxemia in vascular disease, pulmonary disease, and high altitude; with increased metabolism in hyperthyroidism; with excessive stimulation of the inspiratory centers in central nervous system disease; and with lack of sufficient negative pleural pressure in partial pneumothorax. It may also be induced during general anesthesia by excessive use of the respirator to assist pulmonary ventilation.

Respiratory Compensation in Metabolic Acid-Base Disturbances

Metabolic acid-base alterations, more common in animals than are respiratory disturbances, are reflected by changes in bicarbonate concentration (i.e., a base deficit [− BE] or a base excess [+ BE]). The respiratory component

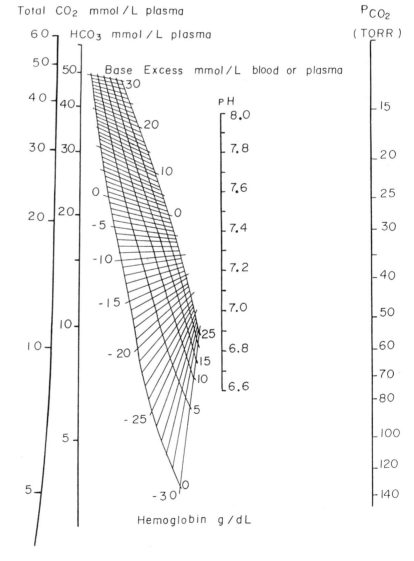

Figure 11–2 Siggard-Anderson alignment nomogram. To determine the deviation of BB, the carbon dioxide tension, pH, and hemoglobin of a particular blood sample are determined. A line is drawn from the point on the carbon dioxide tension scale through the corresponding point on the pH scale. Plasma bicarbonate can be read directly. The BB status, related to hemoglobin concentration, is read on the intersection of this line with the appropriate (actual or extrapolated) hemoglobin concentration line. The deviation of BB is considered as an excess of base when the value is + BE and as a deficit of base when the value is − BE. Total bicarbonate and total carbon dioxide concentrations also may be read on the line.

of acid-base balance is frequently required to intervene and bring rapid but incomplete readjustment of the blood pH.

In *metabolic acidosis,* the classic type of acidosis, a base deficit in bicarbonate coexists without modification of carbonic acid (expressed as SCO_2) concentration. Typical disease conditions that cause metabolic acidosis include ketosis, diabetes (acetoacetic, beta-hydroxy butyric), colonic diarrhea (loss of bicarbonate), and renal diseases (loss of bicarbonate or retention of sulfate and phosphate radicals). Also, a decrease of blood bicarbonate occurs after administration of some diuretics (inhibitors of carbonic anhydrase) or of parenteral solutions containing little or no bicarbonate, which expand the extracellular volume. Respiratory compensation soon begins to eliminate some carbon dioxide from blood by alveolar hyperventilation. The primary metabolic disturbance, or the base deficit, may remain, but a reduction in denominator in relation to the numerator raises the pH to a nearly normal level.

By using a mean acid-base alignment nomogram, also called the Siggard-Anderson acid-base alignment nomogram, it is possible to estimate the base deficit (in millimoles per liter of blood or plasma; Fig. 11–2). A straight line joining any two known points (total carbon dioxide, buffer base excess at a known hemoglobin, pH, carbon dioxide tension) may be used to compute the other variables at its intersection with their lines. This interpolation method also permits calculation of concentration of bicarbonate and of standard bicarbonate. A less complete (without the concentrations of total carbon dioxide and total bicarbonate) mean acid-base alignment nomogram has been constructed for swine (Fig. 11–3). In dogs and cows, the nomogram for humans may be used with minimal error. The base deficit

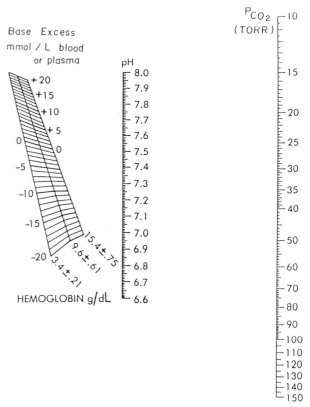

Figure 11–3   Mean acid-base alignment nomogram designed for swine blood. Determination of carbon dioxide tension, pH, and hemoglobin is required. A line drawn from the carbon dioxide tension and pH values intersects with the hemoglobin line to give the base excess status (i.e., +BE or −BE).

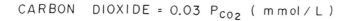

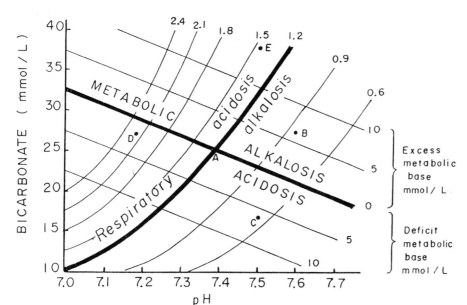

Figure 11–4   The pH-bicarbonate (Davenport) diagram, a tool for teaching (not used clinically) the concepts of acid-base, is an in vitro system containing only the bicarbonate buffer (bicarbonate–carbonic acid) and pH. The carbonic acid is expressed as dissolved carbon dioxide (i.e., 0.03 mmol per liter L × $PaCO_2$). The diagram is divided in areas, or sectors, of metabolic and respiratory disturbances (acidosis, alkalosis) of acid-base balance. The diagram is entered by plotting pH and bicarbonate on the abscissa and ordinate. Normal pH and bicarbonate intercept at point A, on the 1.2 mmol per liter line of the carbon dioxide curve (ratio = 20). Hypothetical points B, C, D, and E represent examples of acid-base dysfunctions (see text).

obtained from the nomogram can be used to estimate the bicarbonate required to restore blood pH to 7.4, using the formula:

$$\text{Bicarbonate (mmol/L)} = 0.4 \text{ M} \times \text{base deficit}$$
$$\text{or } -\text{BE, where M} = \text{mass in kilograms.}$$

Metabolic alkalosis is a relatively less common acid-base disturbance than metabolic acidosis. Its principal characteristics are base excess, loss of acid, and rise in blood pH. In ruminants, metabolic alkalosis may result from grain overload (sudden excessive ingestion), causing ruminal stasis, and from excessive feeding of urea, leading to increased ammonia formation. In all animals, metabolic alkalosis is associated with administration of alkaline drugs and of diuretics (not carbonic anhydrase inhibitors), causing excessive urinary excretion of chloride and hydrogen ions, with vomiting (accumulation of bicarbonate and deficit of chloride and hydrogen ions), and with dehydration (excessive sweating, potassium depletion).

Respiratory compensation by hypoventilation that produces hypercarbia is usually not efficient. The numerator (bicarbonate) of the Henderson-Hasselbalch equation remains elevated, but since the denominator is also increased, the bicarbonate:carbon dioxide ratio tends to return to a nearly normal level. Eventually, the kidney increases its excretion of bicarbonate to correct the primary metabolic disturbance (base excess).

A rapid evaluation of the relative degrees of metabolic and respiratory disturbances can be obtained with the pH-bicarbonate diagram (Fig. 11–4). To use the diagram, the pH and the bicarbonate concentration are found and plotted on the grid. In a normal situation (point A), the coordinates are 7.4 for pH and 25 mmol per liter for bicarbonate. Point B (7.63, 27) is an example of metabolic alkalosis (excess base of 7 mmol per liter) combined with respiratory alkalosis, or a deficit of carbon dioxide (0.8 instead of 1.2 mmol per liter). Point C (7.5, 18) represents metabolic acidosis (base deficit of 6 mmol per liter) with respiratory alkalosis (0.7 instead of 1.2 mmol per liter carbon dioxide). Point D (7.2, 28) is metabolic acidosis (base deficit of 2 mmol per liter) associated with respiratory acidosis (2.2 instead of 1.2 mmol per liter carbon dioxide). Point E (7.51, 38) describes metabolic alkalosis (base excess of 15 + mmol per liter bicarbonate) linked to a respiratory acidosis (1.4 instead of 1.2 mmol per liter carbon dioxide).

REFERENCES

Christensen HN. Body fluids and the acid-base balance. 2nd ed. Philadelphia: WB Saunders, 1964:p. 506.

Cornelius LM, Rawlings CA. Arterial blood gas and acid-base values in dogs with various diseases and signs of disease. J Am Vet Med Assoc 1981;178:992.

Dobson A. Acid-base balance in animals. In: Phillipson AT, Hall LW, Pritchard WR, eds. Scientific foundations of veterinary medicine. London: W. Heinemann Medical Books, 1980:pp. 112–125.

Feldman BF, Rosenberg DP. Clinical use of anion and osmolal gap in veterinary medicine. J Am Vet Med Assoc 1981;178:396.

Jones NL. Blood gases and acid-base physiology. Toronto: BC Decker, 1980.

Masoro EJ, Siegel PD. Acid-base regulation: its physiology and pathophysiology. Philadelphia: WB Saunders, 1971.

Raffe MR. Acid-base balance. In: Stetter DH, ed. Textbook of small animal surgery. Philadelphia: WB Saunders, 1985.

Scott Emuakpor D, Maas AHJ, Ruigrok TJC, Zimmerman ANE. Acid-base curve nomogram for dog blood. Pfugers Arch 1976;363:141.

Severinghaus JW. Blood gas concentrations. In: Fenn WO, Rahn H, eds. Handbook of physiology. Section 3. Respiration. Vol II. Washington, DC: American Physiological Society, 1965:pp. 1425–1487.

Weikopf RB, Townsley MI, Riordan KK, Harris D, Chadwick K. Acid-base curve and alignment nomograms for swine blood. J Appl Physiol 1983;54:978.

CHAPTER 12

THE CARDIOVASCULAR SYSTEM

HISTORICAL BACKGROUND

William HARVEY, a pioneer without previous models, really began modern physiology and medicine with publication (1628) of the measurement of blood volume by drainage in sheep. He measured the amount of blood put out by the heart in a single beat, and calculated that the amount forced out of the heart in a few minutes would be much more than could be in the body at any one time. Harvey, a great thinker, created new physiological concepts and understood the need for quantification. His conception of one-way flow of blood in a continuous circulatory system had to await the demonstration of capillary anastomoses between arteries and veins, which were found by MALPIGHI (1661) while studying the lungs of frogs and by VAN LEEUWENHOEK, who first described workable microscopes. One of the staunch supporters of Harvey's work was PECQUET, who described the thoracic duct, the *receptaculum chyli,* and its connection to the venous system for return of lymph, the fluid leaked out of the system. VIEUSSENS (1641–1715) described the course of the coronary vessels in relation to the structure of the heart and noted the valve in the large coronary vein as well as in the coronary sinus. Harvey had elegantly shown the presence and role of valves in the veins.

A century later, in 1733, Stephen HALES, an unconventional vicar, reported his direct measurement of blood pressures in a variety of animals, including horses (femoral artery). He used the trachea of a goose to convey blood from the artery to a vertical tube.

Two centuries after Harvey, the early French physiologist MAGENDIE showed the importance of the blood transport of nutrients, and his famous pupil Claude BERNARD discovered vascular nerves and the functions of vasoconstriction and vasodilation in regulating blood supply to the various parts of the body. Precise biophysical studies on the cardiovascular system began with Ernst WEBER and his brother Eduard, who measured the pulse wave, and Carl LUDWIG, who contributed to progress by inventing the kymograph (a smoked-paper drum recorder with adjustable speed) and the mercury manometer (a floating pen above a column of mercury) for recording blood pressure changes under varying conditions. The Webers discovered the cardioinhibitory function of the vagus nerve, and MAREY showed a relationship between blood pressure and cardiac action. In Lyon, at the oldest veterinary school of the modern era, CHAUVEAU, using air transmission (Fig. 12–1), described the pressure changes in the heart cavities and, with a special device, proved that the second heart sound was due to closure of the aortic valve. He is quoted as saying, "The atrium of the heart is writing his history."

Early efforts to describe the flow of blood in an artery were made by Chauveau and his pupils. They developed an ingenious apparatus to record the pulsatile changes in the velocity of arterial blood. The fundamental principle was to arrange that the force of the stream moved an obstructing vane, the movement of which was proportional to the force or velocity of the stream.

In the 20th century, EINTHOVEN (1880–1927) devised the string galvanometer, recorded the electrical cardiac potentials, and established the fundamental concepts of electrocardiography for bipolar limb leads.

It is amazing that the baroreceptor reflex function of the carotid sinus was elucidated only in 1924, by HERING. It is curious to note that the word "carotid" is derived from a Greek word meaning "deep sleep." Many efforts had been contributed toward this phenomenon by HEYMANS and his pupils. The basic principle for estimating the cardiac output was described by FICK (1829–1901), and the basic respiratory function of the circulating blood was enunciated by BARCROFT (1872–1947). The latter results had consequences for aviation, mountaineering, diving, and space physiology, a field opened by Paul BERT (1833–1886).

The field of cardiac catheterization can be traced to a veterinary practitioner, DESLIENS (1923), who measured heart pressures with rubber catheters used in urology. FORSSMANN (1929) is credited with opening this field with historical observations of pressures in his own right ventricle.

The needs of body cells are met by the *blood,* which serves as a transport medium, the *vessels* through which the blood flows, and the *heart,* which acts as a pump. The flow of blood through the cardiovascular system is governed by the dynamics of the pumping action of the heart, the characteristics of the blood as a fluid, and the attributes of the blood vessels.

Bleeding a horse from the jugular vein is one way of gaining access to the circulation of blood from the periphery to the heart. Since venous pressure is minimal, to maintain the flow of blood proper technique requires occlusion (tourniquet) of the jugular vein between the peripheral side of venipuncture and the heart. Conversely, an artery leads blood under considerable pressure away from the heart, and puncture of the carotid shows a pulsating flow of blood. The arterial flow of blood is further increased by occlusion of the carotid at a point craniad to the puncture, and it is stopped by compression between the heart and the puncture site.

The mammalian heart is a muscular pump that provides the force to move fluid through the vessels. Catheters introduced in the left and right sides of the heart through the carotid artery and jugular vein may be used to measure pressure and output from each ventricle. A five- to sixfold pressure difference is found between the left and right ventricles, but equal volumes of blood are pumped out of each side of the heart because they are connected in series.

The objective of this chapter is to present the essential elements of blood volume, blood constituents, blood coagulation, and blood viscosity in small and large animals.

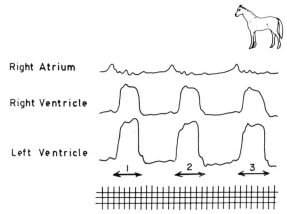

Figure 12–1 Historical tracing (Chauveau and Marey, 1859) of endocardial pressures in the right atrium, the right ventricle, and the left ventricle during three cardiac cycles in a standing horse.

BLOOD VOLUME

Total blood volume can be determined accurately only by simultaneously measuring both plasma and erythrocyte (red blood cell, RBCs) volume using dilution methods. Total blood volume can also be approximated indirectly by estimating the volume of plasma and determining the peripheral venous value of the erythrocyte packed cell volume (PCV), or hematocrit. Upon centrifugation, a blood sample prevented from coagulating separates into columns according to specific gravities—the plasma on top is separated from the erythrocytes on the bottom by a thin layer of leukocytes. The high-speed microhematocrit centrifuge allows rapid and accurate measurement in a capillary tube. Specific gravity of plasma is about 1.025, and that of RBCs around 1.080, whereas 1 mL of whole blood has nearly 1.050 times the mass of water. Except in the dog, the cell:plasma ratio at the periphery (large veins and arteries) is higher than the PCV in small vessels; consequently, the concentration of erythrocytes is not identical in all parts of the adult circulatory system (Fig. 12–2). In association with dilution techniques using Evans blue dye (T-1824) or ^{51}Cr-labeled erythrocytes, with appropriate corrections to body PCV (i.e., the mean PCV in large and small vessels), the venous PCV can be used to estimate accurately blood volume.

In cattle, blood volume obtained by summation of direct measurements of both RBC and plasma volumes is 51.2 mL per kilogram, whereas it is 53.7 mL per kilogram when calculated with the body hematocrit correction (0.904) (Table 12–1).

The blood volume varies indirectly with body mass and directly with the metabolically active body mass (i.e., it is greater in muscles than in adipose tissue). At equal body masses, adipose or untrained animals (working horses) have lower blood volume than trained animals (racehorses). The larger blood volume of physically active animals is not accompanied by a higher basal metabolic rate because of the temporary adjustment of the vascular system.

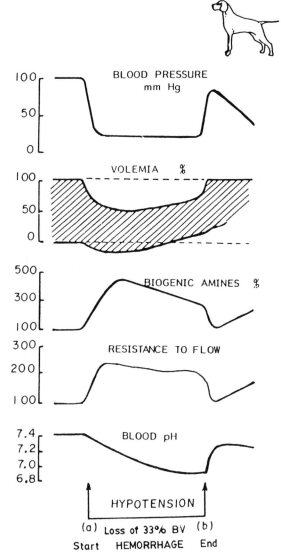

Figure 12–2 Experimental hemorrhage (*a*): loss of 33 percent of the blood has the almost immediate effect of reducing blood pressure and blood volume and causes a gradual decrease in blood pH. It also brings a rapid production of biogenic amines and vasoconstriction, which raises the resistance to blood flow. When the intravascular volume is returned by massive infusion of either the hemorrhaged blood or a crystalloid solution (*b*), blood pressure, intravascular blood volume, and blood pH immediately rise to their normal values, whereas production of biogenic amines and vasoconstriction recede only temporarily.

TABLE 12–1 Volumes for Body and PCV, Erythrocytes, Plasma, and Blood in Young Female and Male Cattle

Parameter	Direct Methods	Body PCV Method
Body PCV (L/L)		0.3023
Venous PCV (L/L)	0.3338	
Body/venous PCV ratio		0.904
Erythrocyte volume (L/100 kg)	1.53	1.62
Plasma volume (L/100 kg)	3.59	3.74
Total blood volume (L/100 kg)	5.12	5.37

Endotoxins are toxic lipopolysaccharide constituents of gram-negative bacteria. During endotoxic shock, an immediate decline in blood pressure accompanies a considerable redistribution of blood volume. Central (thoracic) blood volume is reduced, whereas hepatic and splanchnic blood volumes are increased.

Regulation of Blood Volume

If blood volume is reduced to less than a third, the ensuing shock soon becomes irreversible (Table 12–2). Lesser levels of blood loss are life threatening. The major forms of shock—*hypovolemic* by hemorrhage or loss of plasma, *septic* by bacterial toxins, and *cardiogenic* by improper cardiac pumping—are not clearly separate entities, as hypovolemia is a common factor. Fluid therapy represents a way of restoring blood volume and of reducing the local acidosis that develops because of inadequate oxygen supply (Fig. 12–3).

The replacement therapeutic fluid should be a colloid solution retained in the vascular space or a crystalloid solution distributed over the entire extracellular fluid space. Each milliliter of lost plasma should be replaced by 3 mL of balanced electrolyte solution.

Colloid versus Crystalloid Infusion

In shock, or reduction of blood volume, resulting from obstruction of the small intestine, the gut then secretes an excess of fluid and electrolytes that are not reabsorbed. Colloid solutions are superior to electrolyte solutions for resuscitation of animals with this condition. In dogs, intravenous 0.9 percent saline increases systemic arterial pressure only transiently, whereas the rise is sustained when colloids are used. Both fluids improve intestinal blood flow and reduce vascular resistance, but these effects last longer with colloids. Saline fails to raise the oncotic pressure (osmotic pressure of plasma proteins) of plasma, secretive filtration exceeds absorptive intestinal flux, and the crystalloids with water are soon lost in the intestinal lumen (Table 12–3).

Regulation of Blood versus Body Fluid Volume

The low pressure cavities of the heart, the atria, are the main contributors to the control of blood volume. Several other factors, such as aldosterone and antidiuretic hormone (ADH, or vasopressin), also play a role in the regulation of blood volume.

TABLE 12–2 Blood Volumes in Mature Animals

Species	Blood Volume (mL/kg)
Cat	66.7
Chicken	74
Cow	57.4
Dog	92.5
Goat	70
Guinea pig	72
Horse (racing)	109.6
Horse (working)	71.7
Pig	57
Rabbit	56.4
Rat	54.3
Sheep	58

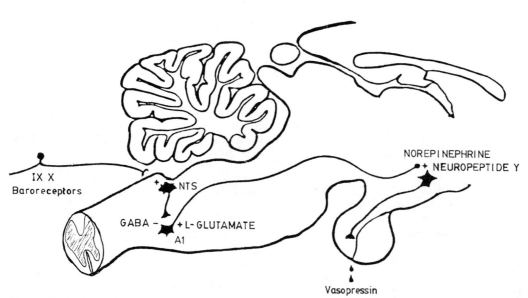

Figure 12–3 Lowered central venous pressure initiates baroreceptor stimulation reaching the nucleus tractus solitarii (NTS) through fibers in cranial nerves IX and X. Neurotransmitters in the interneurons can inhibit (GABA) or facilitate (L-glutamate) the baroceptor signals. Hypothalamic vasopressin secretion in the hypothalamic supraoptic and paraventricular nuclei (SON-PVH) is mediated by norepinephrine or neuropeptide Y.

TABLE 12-3 Arterial Pressure, Jejunal Blood Flow,
Vascular Resistance, and Capillary Hydrostatic
and Oncotic Pressures in Dogs Infused with Colloid
and Crystalloid Fluids

Parameter and Fluid	Control	20 min	60 min
Arterial pressure (mm Hg)			
Colloids	131.7	156.5	150.0
Crystalloids	118.3	136.7	122.5
Blood flow (mL/min/100 g)			
Colloids	22.1	54.9	45.9
Crystalloids	28.0	80.1	35.4
Vascular resistance (mm Hg)			
Colloids	5.9	3.4	3.1
Crystalloids	5.2	2.2	3.9
Capillary hydrostatic pressure (mm Hg)			
Colloids	12.8	16.8	15.8
Crystalloids	13.4	15.8	13.0
Capillary oncotic pressure (mm Hg)			
Colloids	21.7	25.7	24.2
Crystalloids	21.3	10.5	13.5

Many cells in the atria contain secretory granules that release substances, *atrial natriuretic factors* (ANFs), in response to stretch caused by increased perfusion pressure or expanded blood volume. Polypeptides (21 amino acids) with a cysteine-disulfide bridge essential for their activity, these ANFs bind specifically and intensely on the glomeruli and only slightly on the distal tubules and collecting ducts. Even in low concentrations, ANFs induce significant diuresis and natriuresis (excretion of Na) without any change in glomerular filtration rate. The production of ADH, usually stimulated by hemorrhage, is decreased by ANFs.

The onset of ANF action occurs within 2 to 3 minutes, in contrast to that of aldosterone (sodium-retaining mineralocorticoid hormone). The concentration of ANFs in coronary sinus blood is two to seven times higher than that in the systemic blood. It is probable that ANFs are true circulating hormones (humoral messengers) establishing the major endocrine connection between the heart and the kidneys.

Release of Vasopressin

Cells in the hypothalamus (supraoptic and paraventricular nuclei) that secrete vasopressin (ADH) receive signals directly from nerve cells in the medulla oblongata. These alpha$_1$-noradrenergic neurons receive input from the nucleus tractus solitarii (NTS) in the medulla oblongata, the terminal of primary afferent cardiovascular baroreceptors and chemoreceptors. Lowered central venous pressure initiates a signal that increases the production of vasopressin in the hypothalamus and causes its release from the neurohypophysis. Facilitating neurotransmitters are L-glutamate for the alpha$_1$-neurons in the medullary region and norepinephrine as well as neuropeptide Y (NPY) in the hypothalamus. Inhibition is induced by gamma-aminobutyric acid (GABA) in the NTS of the medulla oblongata (see Fig. 12-3).

BLOOD CONSTITUENTS

Plasma

Plasma, the suspension fluid for blood cells, may account for 55 to 70 percent of the uncoagulated blood, depending on the animal species. It is obtained from blood treated with an anticoagulant. It is unpigmented in small animals (cats and dogs) and in small ruminants (goats and sheep). Pigments from bile (bilirubin) or feeds (carotene) impart yellow tinges to the blood plasma of cows and horses.

Many anticoagulants can be used to get clot-free blood samples for transfusion or for centrifugation to separate plasma from cell constituents.

Heparin, a polysaccharide conjugated with sulfate, is a natural anticoagulant produced by basophils (a kind of leukocyte) in the blood and by mast cells throughout the body. Mast cells are part of the connective tissue surrounding capillaries in the lungs and other organs. From these tissues, heparin is released into the capillaries. A concentration of 0.2 mg per milliliter of blood is effective as an anticoagulant. One unit of heparin represents about 0.01 mg of heparin sodium. Temperature influences the anticoagulant activity of heparin (e.g., at 0°C, 1 mg heparin prevents coagulation of 100 to 500 mL of blood, but of only 10 to 20 mL of blood at room temperature).

Removal of calcium ions by *sodium citrate* and similar salts may also be used to prevent coagulation. Potassium salts should not be used to prepare blood for transfusion because of the possibility of producing heart block. Other anticoagulants acting on calcium ions are *oxalates* (sodium, potassium, and ammonium salts) and the chelating agent, the sodium salt of *ethylenediaminetetraacetic acid* (EDTA).

Fluoride salts act as anticoagulants by poisoning the enzymes involved in the coagulation process.

Chemical and physical analyses reveal that the composition of blood plasma is extremely complex and reflects the many functions of blood. Proteins (albumin, fibrinogen, and globulins) have been identified in the plasma. Albumin values exceed those of the globulins in humans, sheep, goats, rabbits, dogs, guinea pigs, and rats. The relative proportions of albumin to globulins are nearly equal, but the globulins tend to predominate in horses, cows, and pigs.

The plasma proteins, which are colloidal and nondiffusible, help maintain a colloid osmotic (oncotic) pressure of 25 to 30 mm Hg. Nearly 75 percent of this oncotic pressure is due to the smaller and more numerous albumin molecules, the balance is due mostly to globulins. This oncotic pressure opposes the hydrostatic blood pressure in the capillaries and thus prevents edema due to excessive passage of fluid into the tissues. The water-holding capacity of the blood depends on the concentration of plasma proteins.

These plasma proteins, albumin, fibrinogen, and most of the globulins (alpha, beta, and gamma) originate in the liver. Severe liver damage or prolonged dietary protein deficiency markedly reduces the syntheses of plasma proteins. The reduction of plasma fibrinogen prolongs the prothrombin time and blood coagulation time.

The globulins of the complement system, and the immunoglobulins, which are responsible for most of the plasma antibody activity, are of extrahepatic origin. They are formed in the lymph nodes and other tissue cells of the macrophage (formerly known as the reticuloendothelial) system of the spleen and bone marrow.

Blood serum, also simply called serum, is similar to plasma without fibrinogen, some calcium ions, and other coagulating factors. During the clotting process, these components of plasma are removed, and the watery fluid remaining after clot retraction is referred to as serum.

Globulins

The globulin group of plasma proteins includes kininogen, plasminogen, complement system, and the immunoglobulins.

Kininogen. An alpha₂-globulin, called *kininogen,* is the source of certain polypeptides, the *kinins* (kallidin or lysylbradykinin, a decapeptide, and bradykinin, a nonapeptide), that cause powerful arteriolar vasodilation and also increased capillary permeability. These small polypeptides result from the breakdown of kininogen by transformation of *kallikreinogen,* a normally inactive proteolytic blood enzyme, into *kallikrein,* the active enzyme. The process occurs in a cascade fashion, somewhat like the blood clotting mechanism. The activated Hageman factor (factor XIIa) of blood clotting and plasmin contribute to the activation of kallikreinogen (Fig. 12–4).

Plasminogen. A beta-globulin of blood plasma, *plasminogen,* or *profibrinolysin,* is the inactive form of *plasmin,* or *fibrinolysin,* a proteolytic enzyme causing the lysis of fibrin in clotted blood. The activation of plasminogen to plasmin occurs through thrombin, activated factor XII, lysosomal enzymes from damaged tissues, factors from the vascular endothelium, and streptokinase (a substance from streptococci). Normal small amounts of plasmin, formed all the time in the blood, are inactivated by an alpha₂-globulin of blood plasma called alpha₂-macroglobulin, or alpha₂-antiplasmin. Plasmin plays an important role in removing obstructions from the vascular system after damaged vessels are plugged by the coagulation system and repaired.

Complement System. About 10 percent of the plasma globulins circulate as proenzymes of the *complement system,* which is involved in direct lysis of invading microorganisms (bacteria, protozoa). They represent a group of nine proteins (C1 to C9) activated by a cascade of reactions reminiscent of blood coagulation, and the formation of kinins and of plasmin. These proteins can be grouped in

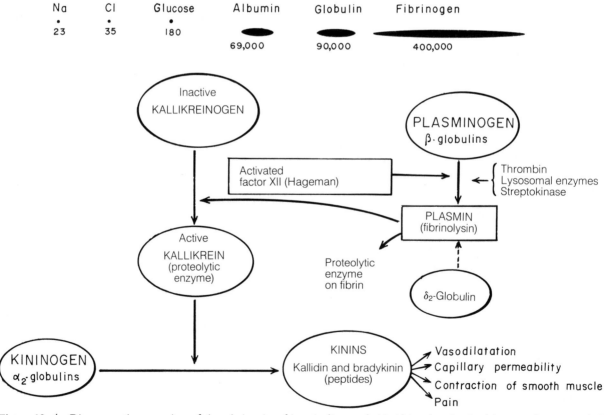

Figure 12–4 Diagrammatic comparison of the relative size of ions (sodium and chloride) and molecules (glucose, plasma proteins). **Bottom,** Cascade of events leading to the production of biogenic amines (kinins) from plasma globulins (alpha and beta).

three functional units (1) for recognition of antigen-antibody complexes, C1; (2) for activation, C2, C3, and C4; and (3) for attacking the membrane of target cells, C5, C6, C7, C8, and C9. The activation process of these normally inactive enzyme precursors is either through the *classic pathway* or the *alternative pathway*. The classic pathway is started by an immune response (antigen-antibody reaction), while the alternative pathway is initiated by a nonimmune factor, such as toxins (Fig. 12–5).

The recognition unit of the classic pathway (C1) is a macromolecular complex that consists of peripheral subunits (C1q, C1r, and C1s) connected by fibrillar strands to a central core, which gives it the appearance of a "pot of flowers." The heads of the "flowers" (C1q) bind to the stem piece (Fc) of immunoglobulins (IgG, IgM); this activates C1 into an active enzyme (C$\overline{1}$) able to act on C4 and C2 to form C3. It does this by cleaving C4 and C2 into fragments (C4a, C4b, C2a, C2b) that recombine as an active enzyme (C$\overline{4b2a}$), a C3 convertase, cleaving C3 into C3a and C3b. Convertase C5, C$\overline{3b4b2a}$, is then formed by combination of C3b, C4b, and C2a, to split C5 into C5a and C5b. Finally, C5b unites with C6, C7, C8, and C9 to form the lytic membrane-bound complex (Fig. 12–6).

The alternative pathway is identical to the classical pathway from C3 onward. It is initiated without C$\overline{1q}$, but requires the action of factor D (a serine protease) on factor B (another serine protease) combined to activated C$\overline{3b}$. The result is formation of a C3 convertase, C$\overline{3b8b}$, which differs from the classic pathway's C3 convertase (i.e., C$\overline{4b2a}$).

Immunoglobulins. Immunoglobulins (Igs) originate in lymphoid cells (B lymphocytes and plasmocytes), molecular weights of 150,000 to 900,000 daltons, and may represent about 20 percent of all blood plasma proteins.

They share a basal molecular structure: two heavy (H) and two light (L) polypeptide chains arranged in a Y fashion with interchain and intrachain disulfide bonds. The intrachain disulfide bonds may be visualized in the "stick model" or better in the "domain model," where the foldings in the H and L chains are represented as loops (Fig. 12–7). Each H chain is paired to an L chain by an interchain disulfide bond, and both H-L pairs are linked by one or two interchain disulfide bonds in the hinge region.

The Ig molecule has two major functional regions: the *hypervariable*, or variable, region, which combines with antigen, and the *constant* region, which includes the Fc piece able to combine with receptors on cell membranes and to attach to the complement complex (see Fig. 12–6). The terms variable and constant refers to the consistency of the amino acid sequences. The constant region determines much of the physical and chemical properties of the Ig (diffusivity and adherence). Upon proteolytic digestion of the Ig, the variable regions carry the fragment antigen–binding, or Fab fragment, and the constant region includes the fragment-crystallized, or Fc fragment, or simply the Fc piece.

Four classes of immunoglobulins are recognized in most animals: IgG, IgA, IgM, and IgE (Fig. 12–8). A fifth class, IgD, is found in humans but has yet to be isolated from the lymphocytes of domestic animals.

IgG accounts for 70 percent of Ig in the blood plasma of humans, although most of the IgG is outside the blood vessels. In ruminants, subclasses IgG_1 and IgG_2 reflect functional differences in the Fc piece. IgG_1 is selectively taken up by the epithelial cells of the ruminant mammary gland, and the IgG_1 content is higher in colostrum (first milk) of ruminants than during lactation. In contrast, IgG_2 is taken up by the phagocytes of sheep and cattle, although the plasma concentration of IgG_1 is higher than that of IgG_2. A

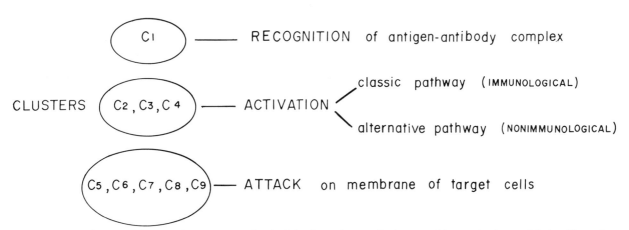

Figure 12–5 Clusters of the complement system involved in the antigen-antibody recognition, activation, and lysis of bacteria or protozoa.

A

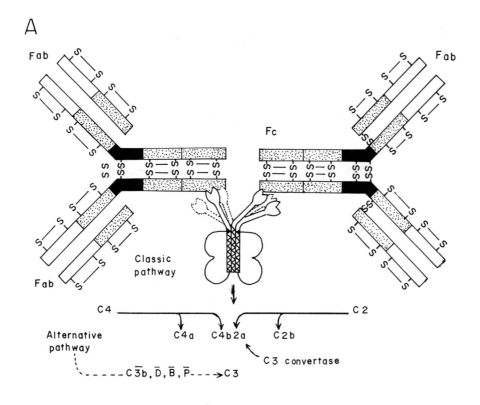

B

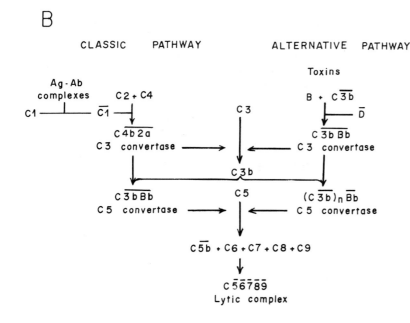

Figure 12–6 The complement system. **A,** The recognition unit of the macromolecular complex (inactive plasminogen consisting of subunits connected by fibrillar strands to a central core) binds to immunoglobulins by the fibrillar strands ("flowers"). **B,** Activation of the proenzymes, through the classic pathway or through the alternative pathway, results in the formation of the lytic membrane-bound complex.

special immunoglobulin, the so-called T globulin, is found at mucous epithelial surfaces in the horse. The amino acid sequence of T globulin is similar to that of IgG, but its high carbohydrate content makes it somewhat similar to IgA, which is also found in mucous membranes. In foals, a hemolytic syndrome (neonatal erythrolysis) is produced when the ingested colostrum contains Igs, of a yet undetermined class,

against their erythrocytes. In young ruminants, anti-erythrocyte Igs in colostrum, which are not IgG₁, are neutralized in some way during their passage through the gut, but this does not operate in the foal.

IgA, in its dimer form, is the predominant class localized in intestinal secretions because of its resistance to digestion by the proteolytic enzymes of the gut. Two IgA

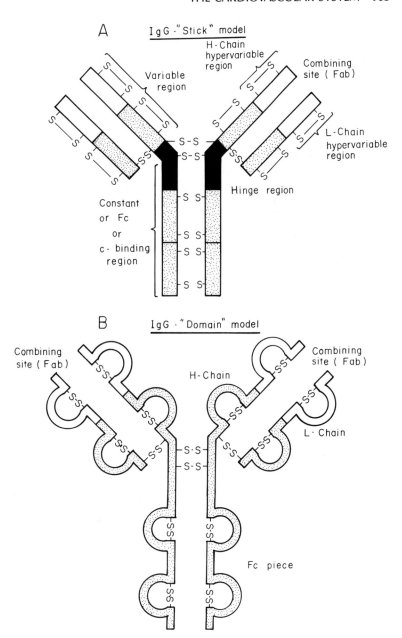

Figure 12–7 **A,** "Stick" model of a monomer immunoglobulin (IgG) with the regions (variable, hypervariable, hinge, and constant or binding) of the heavy chains, and the hypervariable regions of the light chain. **B,** Domain model indicating the combining sites and the foldings of heavy and light chains.

molecules are united at their Fc piece by a J, or joining, chain. Secreted IgA (SIgA) also has an additional glycoprotein, called a secretory piece, attached to the J chain region of the molecule. This secretory piece is thought to protect SIgA from disruption by proteolytic digestive enzymes. SIgA functions to eliminate circulating antigens via the bile, salivary glands, and lacrimal glands and thus excludes antigens that would otherwise enter the body from the gut. Other forms of IgA are a monomer resembling IgG and a tetramer. The half-life of IgA is short, about 48 hours.

The *IgM* macromolecule (a pentamer) has functions that can be taken over by IgG. It can localize in the milk and in the pulmonary and intestinal secretions of sheep and cattle, where it supports the role played by IgA. The IgM molecule

has five sets of L and H chains united at the opposite end of their variable regions or combining sites by a J chain, just like the dimer IgA.

IgE would have a larger Fc piece, which would bind on the plasma membranes of mast cells or basophils and stimulate them to degranulate. The released histamine sets off a hypersensitivity reaction, which is important in the various skin allergies of dogs. In the intestinal wall of the sheep, these degranulated mast cells (globule leukocytes) appear to be associated with the self-cure phenomenon in helminthiasis. The immediate hypersensitivity reaction at the site of contact or attachment of parasites plays a role in rejection not only of intestinal parasites but also of blood-sucking ectoparasites.

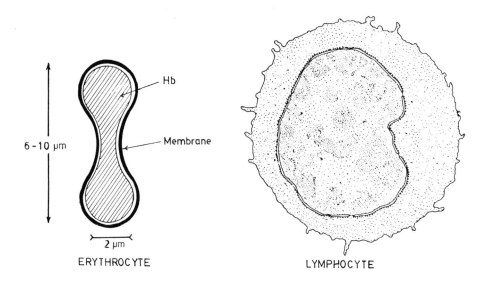

ERYTHROCYTE

LYMPHOCYTE

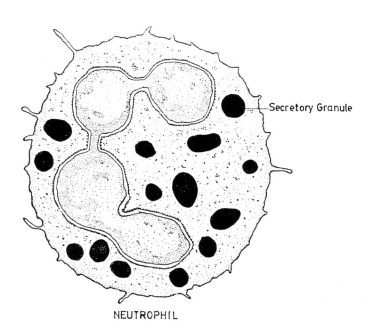

NEUTROPHIL

Figure 12–8 Diagrammatic view of an erythrocyte (lateral view), a lymphocyte, and a neutrophil, with their relative dimensions, to show the large surface of the erythrocyte relative to its volume, the large single nucleus of the lymphocyte, and the segmented nucleus and secretory granules of the neutrophil.

Blood Cells

Three classes of blood cells (corpuscles) are recognized: RBCs, leukocytes (white blood cells, WBCs), and thrombocytes (platelets). The red color of blood is due to hemoglobin (Hb), an iron-containing protein, in the erythrocytes.

Red Blood Cells

The RBC, nucleated in birds but anucleated in mammals, is actually a "flattened bag" of Hb that can be deformed into almost any shape without rupturing. The shapes of the anucleated RBCs change remarkably as they pass through capillaries. The thickness of the RBC is about 2 μm, but the diameter ranges from 4.5 to 12 μm in various species (Table 12–4). Total RBC surface area can be estimated from blood volume and erythrocyte number, diameter, and thickness. The amazingly large total surface area of RBCs plays a great role in the respiratory, or gas-transport, function of the blood. In mammals, the ratio of erythrocyte surface area to body weight is relatively constant (about 60 m^2 per kilogram).

The major function of RBCs is to transport Hb, an intracellular protein, which in turn carries oxygen from the lungs to the tissues. Free Hb dissolves in the plasma, and about 3 percent of it leaks through the glomerular membrane of the kidney. Therefore, to remain in the bloodstream, Hb

TABLE 12–4 Diameter, Surface Area, and Number of Erythrocytes in Mature Animals

Species	Diameter (μm)	Surface Area (m^2/kg)	Number ($10^{12}/L$)
Cat	6	63	7
Cattle	6	62	7
Chicken	11 × 7	44	3
Dog	7	68	7
Goat	4	56	14
Horse	6	67	11
Pig	6	63	7
Sheep	5	58	11

must be bound inside RBCs. As an organic acid, the Hb in the anucleated RBCs also acts as an excellent acid-base buffer (as do most proteins) that accounts for as much as 50 percent of all the buffering power of whole blood.

In adult animals, RBCs are composed of 62 to 72 percent water and about 35 percent solids. Hemoglobin represents some 95 percent of the solids and as much as 34 g per deciliter of RBCs, or 12 to 14 g per deciliter of whole blood. The other 5 percent of solids is made up of *proteins* (in the stroma and cell membrane); *lipids,* such as phospholipids (lecithin, cephalin, and sphingomyelin), free cholesterol esters, and neutral fats; *vitamins* (operating as coenzymes); *glucose* (energy); *enzymes* (cholinesterase, phosphatases, carbonic anhydrase, peptidases, and those concerned with glycolysis); and *minerals* (phosphorus, sulfur, chloride, magnesium, potassium, and sodium). Marked inter- and intraspecies differences exist in the electrolyte composition of RBCs. General values for the major cations of RBCs, sodium and potassium, may be reversed in some species (Table 12–5).

The average number of RBCs in blood is 5 to 7 × 10^{12} per liter. The number varies greatly among species (Table 12–4), within species (because of breeds), and within individuals of a species (because of age or disease). Another cause of variation in erythrocyte counts is their nonuniform distribution within the vascular system. Since plasma fluids are constantly shifting across capillary walls, RBC counts vary as well between arterial and venous blood samples. The difference between total and circulating cell volume amounts to more than half the available RBC mass. About a third of this noncirculating part of the RBC volume, or erythrocyte store, accumulates in the spleen. This difference disappears after splenectomy. The spleen can be regarded as a reserve that is

TABLE 12–5 Levels of Sodium and Potassium in the Erythrocytes of Different Animal Species

Species	Sodium (mmol/L)	Potassium (mmol/L)
Cat and dog	105	7.5
Cattle and sheep*	80	15
Pig	10	105

* Sheep RBCs are of two genetic types with regard to potassium content: one with >25 mmol per liter, and another with <25 mmol per liter.

called up when there is increased demand on oxygen transport capacity in stress situations (asphyxia and physical exercise) or production of epinephrine (an adrenal medullary hormone). In the horse, total mobilization of the RBCs stored in the spleen can be demonstrated during vigorous exercise or after administration of epinephrine (2 µg per kilogram), when the venous PCV rises from 0.29 L per liter to 0.45 L per liter.

Compared with that of other species, the *erythrocyte sedimentation rate* (ESR) is relatively rapid in the blood of horses and of swine (in a tube at 45° C, horse ESR is 15 mm per 20 minutes; that of swine, 15 mm per 60 minutes). Consequently, proper counting or PCV techniques require prevention of blood settling. The usual method is to affix the blood container (tube) on a slanted, slowly rotating disk, which gently inverts the tube at each cycle. Sedimentation of erythrocytes apparently proceeds in three stages: formation of rouleaux, rapid settling, and final packing. The larger the rouleaux, the more rapid the ESR, which is also nonspecifically increased during states of inflammation and of cell or tissue destruction.

An isotonic sodium chloride solution known as *physiological saline* is equivalent to an aqueous solution of 0.85 to 0.9 percent sodium chloride. This concentration is satisfactory for practical use with mammalian blood cells. *Fragility of erythrocytes* (i.e., the extent to which the total osmotic pressure of plasma can be lowered without causing hemolysis of RBCs) varies between species. The concentration of sodium chloride initiating hemolysis indicates the osmotic resistance of the weakest RBC (*minimum resistance*). The concentration at which hemolysis is total corresponds to the resistance of the strongest RBC (*maximum resistance*). RBCs of most species undergo hemolysis at sodium chloride concentrations that range from about 0.65 percent for the weakest to 0.45 percent for the strongest. The RBCs of chickens and dogs are exceptional (0.45 to 0.35 percent), and so is the maximum resistance to hemolysis in horses, which have some strong erythrocytes that resist until 0.35 percent sodium chloride.

In animals, the life span of RBCs ranges from 90 to 140 days (mean, 120 days) (Table 12–6). The life span of RBCs seems longer by at least 1 week in growing animals (e.g., 127 days in lambs and 110 days in sheep; 72 days in gilts and 65 days in pigs). For several small laboratory animals, the life span of RBCs is much shorter: 45 to 50 days in rabbits and rats, and 20 to 30 days in mice. RBCs originate continuously in the bone marrow at a daily rate sufficient to replace about 1 percent. Erythropoiesis (formation of RBCs) can be accelerated by hypoxia due to an insufficient number of RBCs or to a decreased concentration of functional hemoglobin, which causes the release of erythropoietin (a humoral agent) by the kidney. Destruction of exhausted erythrocytes, also a continuous process, occurs in the macrophage system (liver, spleen, red bone marrow, and lymph nodes). The iron and protein parts of Hb are recovered and recycled into new Hb. The pigmentary moiety of Hb is transformed into bile pigments (bilirubin, biliverdin), which are excreted in feces and urine.

The normal oxygen-carrying potential of erythrocytes can be expressed by indices: mean corpuscular volume (MCV), mean corpuscular Hb (MCH), and mean corpuscular

TABLE 12–6   Average Life Span of Erythrocytes in Domestic Animals

Species	Days
Cat	70
Chicken	28
Cow	160
Dog	120
Goat	125
Horse	145
Pig	65
Sheep	110

TABLE 12–7   Ranges and Mean Values of Corpuscular Indices of Oxygen-Carrying Potential in Animal Species

Species	MCV (fL)	MCH (pg)	MCHC (g/L)
Cat	39–55 (45)	13–17 (15)	310–340 (330)
Cattle	40–60 (52)	11–17 (14)	260–340 (310)
Dog	60–77 (70)	19–25 (23)	310–340 (330)
Goat	19–37 (27)	5–7 (6)	300–350 (320)
Horse	34–58 (46)	12–18 (15)	310–370 (350)
Pig	50–67 (63)	17–23 (20)	300–340 (320)
Sheep	23–40 (33)	9–12 (11)	290–350 (320)

Hb concentration (MCHC) (Table 12–7). The mean volume of each erythrocyte (MCV), expressed in femtoliters (fL, or 1×10^{-15}L), is calculated from the PCV (liters per liter) and the erythrocyte count (L/L ÷ no. of RBCs × 10^{-12}/L). MCH is reported in picograms (pg, 10^{-12}g) from a computation of Hb level (grams per liter) divided by the erythrocyte count. MCHC, expressed in grams per liter, is the expression of Hb level (grams per liter) divided by the PCV liters per liter.

Leukocytes

The leukocytes, or WBCs, the mobile units of the body's defense system, are much less numerous than the RBCs (i.e., 1 WBC per 400 to 1,300 RBCs in mammals, and 1 WBC per 100 RBCs in birds). These nucleated cells are at least two to three times larger than the erythrocytes because of their more spherical shape and larger diameter (Fig. 12–8).

A part of the protective system of the body, WBCs fight constantly against different infectious and toxic agents that gain entry via the skin, and the respiratory, intestinal, urinary, and reproductive systems, and even the membranes of the eyes. Without WBCs, the body could not live in symbiosis with these agents. The defense system, composed of circulating WBCs, the macrophage system, and lymphoid tissue, protects by seeking and destroying invading agents via phagocytosis and by forming antibodies for humoral and cellular immunity. Another facet of the complex responses of these cells to aggression is the release of potent chemicals that damage the sources of foreign antigens.

The WBCs are grouped in granulocytic and mononuclear series (Table 12–8). The granulocytic series refers to neutrophils (heterophils in birds), eosinophils, and basophils. These cells have a granular appearance and in clinical terminology are called simply "polys" (short for polymorphonuclear), because their nuclei become polymorphic as they mature. The mononuclear series includes monocytes and lymphocytes. These cells are transients in blood: lymphocytes recirculate from lymph tissues to blood, monocytes migrate to tissues and may swell as much as fivefold to become macrophages (i.e., large cells mobile between blood and tissues).

The number of WBCs increases (leukocytosis) during inflammation. Conversely, it is decreased (leukopenia) in viral diseases such as feline panleukopenia.

Neutrophils

Most numerous of the granulocytes, neutrophils function within the blood or tissues primarily to perform phagocytosis and to supply enzymes, mostly lysosomal, to lyse bacteria and viruses. Mature cells are capable of diapedesis: they have ameboid activity, can crawl on fibrils, and respond to chemotaxis and antigen-antibody reactions. Chemotaxis and diapedesis are interrelated. Chemotaxis occurs when neutrophils and macrophages move either toward or away from a source of chemical substances, such as bacterial toxins and degenerative debris. These products dilate the pores between the endothelial cells, render the capillary wall sticky for neutrophils and monocytes, and allow these WBCs to squeeze through (diapedesis) in response to the chemotaxis (Fig. 12–9).

Phagocytosis is the process of engulfment, involving adhesion, ingestion, and digestion of particles by leukocytes. An important function of neutrophils and monocytes, phagocytosis is selective, avoiding ingestion and digestion of normal cells and structures. Immune factors (opsonization), rough and strongly negative electrical surfaces without protein coating, all are factors that enhance the susceptibility of foreign structures or substances to phagocytosis.

TABLE 12–8   Relative Percentages of Different Types of Leukocytes in Adult Animals

WBC	Cat	Chicken	Cow	Dog	Goat	Horse	Pig	Rabbit	Sheep
Basophils	<1	3	<1	<1	<1	<1	1	0	<1
Eosinophils	4	7	4	9	4	4	5	1	4
Lymphocytes	30	55	60	25	55	35	50	55	60
Monocytes	5	10	5	5	5	5	4	14	5
Neutrophils	60	25	30	60	35	55	40	30	30

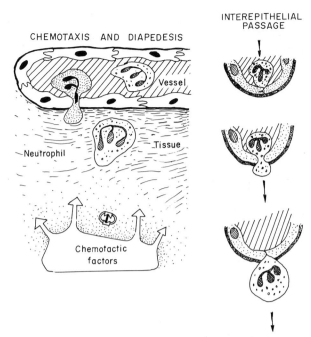

CHEMOTAXIS AND DIAPEDESIS

Vessel

Neutrophil

Tissue

Chemotactic factors

INTEREPITHELIAL PASSAGE

Figure 12–9 Diapedesis of neutrophils between cells of the vascular endothelium in response to stimulation by chemotactic factors.

Opsonization refers to the presence of components of serum, such as antibodies or complement, that attach to particles and promote their phagocytosis by WBCs.

Antibodies are immunoglobulins that have functional regions: the *hypervariable* regions are able to combine with antigens, and the *constant* regions react with receptors on cell membranes and with serum complement.

Complement is a collective term for a group of globulins (proenzymes and enzymes) in serum that join with antibodies in antigen-antibody reactions. They activate a cascade of effects that attract and stimulate neutrophils and monocytes to destroy invading microorganisms (bacteria, protozoa).

The WBC first attaches to the particle (adhesion) to be phagocytosed then projects pseudopodia in all directions around the particle. The pseudopodia meet on the opposite side and fuse to create an enclosed chamber containing the phagocytosed particle (ingestion). The chamber invaginates into the cytoplasm and breaks away from the plasma membrane. This free vesicle (phagosome) inside the cytoplasm soon unites with a lysosome to become a phagolysosome. Many lysosomal digestive enzymes (proteolytic) are thus added to lethal lysozyme and oxidizing agents (superoxide, hydroxyl ions, and hydrogen peroxide) formed in the membrane of the phagolysosome (Fig. 12–10). The amount of superoxide released during the phagocytosis of bacteria is measurable in a scintillation counter, which counts minute flashes of light (chemiluminescence) from the WBCs (neutrophils: 10 times more luminescent than macrophages). The results reflect the phagocytic index (i.e., the degree of phagocytic response of WBCs obtained from individual animals).

Neutrophils cannot phagocytose particles larger than bacteria. After phagocytosis of 5 to 25 bacteria, toxic substances and enzymes released inside the neutrophil inactivate and kill the granulocyte. The half-life of neutrophils in circulating blood is about 6 hours, and the entire pool (blood and reserve adhering to capillary endothelium) is replaced twice every day. They leave the blood to go into tissues without returning, and most are lost on the mucosal surfaces of the urinary, digestive, and respiratory tracts.

Neutrophils have a generation time of about 7 days in the bone marrow. Generation of neutrophils by myeloid marrow cells is controlled by *chalones,* or *colony-stimulating factors* (polypeptides and glycoproteins) controlling mitosis by negative feedback. The capacity for generation of lymphocytes is interpreted by analysis of the total and differential WBC count. A regenerative shift in the differential count indicates that more neutrophils are being made, as indicated by the numbers of cells circulating and by the immature forms present. A degenerative shift, where there is a low or normal total number of cells and a higher percentage of monolobed (band) than of multilobed (segmented) neu-

Figure 12–10 Phases of phagocytosis in a neutrophil: adhesion, ingestion, digestion, and elimination.

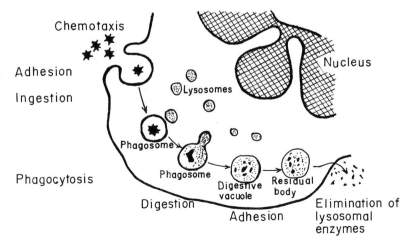

Chemotaxis

Adhesion

Ingestion

Phagocytosis

Nucleus

Lysosomes

Phagosome

Phagosome

Digestion

Digestive vacuole

Residual body

Adhesion

Elimination of lysosomal enzymes

trophils, implies that the marrow is not producing cells quickly enough. Anoxia (tissue damage, muscle exercise) induces neutrophilia.

Eosinophils

Eosinophils are much less numerous than neutrophils (2 to 3 percent of total WBCs). Although eosinophils exhibit chemotaxis and operate as weak phagocytes, their presence is related to certain stages of the reaction to parasitic migration rather than to the defense against usual bacterial agents. They become prominent in tissues where allergic reactions have occurred. The source, generation time, and life span of eosinophils are similar to those of neutrophils.

Basophils

Basophils, the least numerous, least mobile, and least phagocytic of the granulocytes (0.5 percent of total blood WBCs), seem to be the circulating form of mast cells and to have essentially a secretory function. Both types of cells liberate large amounts of heparin (a natural anticoagulant) and histamine (a vasodilator), as well as smaller quantities of bradykinin and serotonin. IgE antibodies, with large Fc pieces, have a propensity to become attached to the plasma membrane (homocytotropic antibodies) of basophils and mast cells. When specific antigen reacts with the antibody on the plasma membrane of these cells, massive release (basophilic degranulation) of heparin, histamine, bradykinin, serotonin, and lysosomal enzymes occurs. The immediate allergic (hypersensitivity) reactions are vasodilation, increased capillary permeability, and an influx of eosinophils attracted by an "eosinophilic chemotactic factor" liberated from the basophils and mast cells. Degranulated basophilic cells known as "globule leukocytes" are seen in the intestinal wall of sheep and are associated with the self-cure phenomenon in helminthiasis. During the flush of pasture growth in the spring, some antigens react with the antibodies on the basophilic cells to bring degranulation and release of vasoactive amines. This hypersensitivity reaction causes adult worms in the abomasum to be rapidly rejected and expelled.

Generated in the bone marrow, basophils have a life span of 10 to 12 days. They disappear from blood after administration of corticosteroids, adrenocorticotrophin (ACTH), and thyroid hormones.

Monocytes

The monocyte, a cell generated in the bone marrow, is reminiscent of a neutrophil with a larger monolobed nucleus. In blood, it is a temporary (half-life 10 hours), mobile, and immature cell that has very little ability to fight infectious agents. Monocytes account for only 3 to 5 percent of blood leukocytes, but the pool of monocytes is much greater, as 3 to 4 times more monocytes are standing in reserve within capillaries, simply adhering to the walls.

Monocytes show diapedesis, ameboid activity, and chemotaxis. Once outside the blood vessels, monocytes are activated: they increase their diameters as much as fivefold, and their cytoplasms fill with granules of lysosomes and mitochondria. They have then matured and are called *macrophages*.

Macrophages

More powerful phagocytes than neutrophils, macrophages can engulf particles much larger than bacteria (e.g., necrotic tissue, dead neutrophils) and five times more particles than neutrophils. Their lysosomes contain, in addition to proteolytic enzymes, large amounts of lipases, which can digest lipid membranes of certain microorganisms. Macrophages can extrude the residual breakdown products, such as the antigenic material contained in the phagocytosed particles, which may activate lymphocytes to produce antibodies; therefore, unlike neutrophils, macrophages are able to function for extremely long periods of time (months) without being killed by the toxic substances and enzymes released during phagocytosis.

Tissue Macrophage System. A large portion of the macrophages become attached to tissues and remain there as a first line of defense unless they are called to other functions. When macrophages are appropriately stimulated, they may break away from tissues, becoming mobile macrophages responding to chemotaxis, and may be able to perform all their defensive functions. This combination of mobile and fixed macrophages is now collectively known as the tissue macrophage system (formerly, the reticuloendothelial system). Macrophages in tissues differ in appearance and have different names: in the *alveoli of the lung* they are alveolar macrophages; in the *brain*, microglia; in the *liver*, Kupffer cells; in *lymph nodes, spleen*, and *bone marrow*, tissue macrophages; and in *subcutaneous tissue*, histiocytes, clasmatocytes, or fixed macrophages.

Lymphocytes

Lymphocytes, smaller and less mobile than macrophages, respond to chemotaxis. Not phagocytic, they are associated primarily with immune responses. Over 99 percent of the lymphocytes are found in tissues, and the few in the blood are in transit, since lymphocytes constantly recirculate between tissues and blood by crossing the interepithelial passage in capillaries. It is not possible to determine by microscopic observation where lymphocytes have come from or what their function may be.

Lymphocytes are made in the lymph nodes, bone marrow, spleen, thymus, tonsils, and the lymph follicles on many mucous membranes (e.g., Peyer's patches of the intestine). They circulate from, between, and among these locations, in and out of blood and lymph, and from lymph nodes and nodules. In calves, 200×10^6 lymphocytes enter the blood every minute by the thoracic lymph duct; 10 percent of them are new, and the remainder are recirculating. On the basis of their life span, two populations of lymphocytes exist, one at 2 to 4 days, and another at 100 to 200 days.

Two functional groups of look-alike lymphocytes are recognized—B *lymphocytes*, for production of circulating antibodies capable of attacking invading agents (*humoral immunity*), and *T lymphocytes,* activated lymphocytes designed to destroy foreign agents (*cell-mediated, or cellular, immunity*). Both of these functional types of lymphocytes are derived originally from stem cells in the bone marrow. During late fetal or early neonatal life, before they end up entrapped in the lymphoid tissue, the lymphocytes are "preprocessed." Genes cause the formation of large RNA molecules with many small functional segments, each of which codes for only an individual portion of an antibody (never the complete antibody) or of a specific protein on the cell surface of activated lymphocytes. For the *T lymphocytes* this occurs in the *thymus,* and for the *B lymphocytes* it happens in the *bone marrow* in man, in the Peyer's patches of sheep and swine, and in the *bursa of Fabricius* in birds. These preprocessed lymphocytes are transported through the blood to the lymphoid tissues and are entrapped there.

In the lymphoid tissue, millions of B and T lymphocytes exist as dormant *preformed* cells capable of duplicating (cloning) with specificity toward a foreign antigen (e.g., toxin, protein, protein-hapten [a low-molecular-weight compound—<8,000 daltons—not antigenic alone]). A great quantity of antibodies (Igs) may be produced by the progeny of a B lymphocyte, and they eventually circulate throughout the body. The progeny of sensitized T cells reach lymph, blood, and tissues and recirculate for months.

To produce antibodies, some B lymphocytes are activated (primary response by antigens from macrophages, helper T cells), swell and change into *plasma cells,* which then divide every 10 hours. A mature plasma cell has a potential to produce each second, about 2,000 molecules of immunoglobulin antibodies, over a period of weeks. Other activated B lymphocytes are not formed into plasma cells but replicate themselves to enhance the number of preformed dormant B lymphocytes. Subsequent exposure to the same activating antigens (secondary response) causes a greater and longer production of immunoglobulins from these numerous *memory cells.* This is the rationale for vaccinating animals (injecting antigens) several times over a period of time (multiple-dose vaccination) to improve the protection through greater antibody production.

Activated T lymphocytes produce other activated T cells instead of antibodies and T lymphocyte memory cells in a way similar to the formation of B lymphocyte memory cells. The progeny of activated T lymphocytes are made up of different functional types of T cells: cytotoxic, helper, and suppressor.

Cytotoxic T Cells (Tc) are direct attack cells able to kill microorganisms and the animal's own cells. Also called *killer cells,* they are attracted to the surface of the victim cells (usually invaded by viruses), attach to these cells, swell, and release cytotoxic lysosomal enzymes, without themselves being harmed.

Helper T cells (Th) are the most numerous T cells. They help by secreting (1) "lymphokines," which increase the activation of B cells, cytotoxic T cells, and suppressor T cells by antigens; (2) soluble interleukin 2 (IL2; one of the lymphokines) to stimulate the activity of other T cells; and (3) macrophage migration factor (another lymphokine), which activates the macrophage system.

Suppressor T cells (Ts), or *regulatory T cells* (Tr), can suppress the functions of both cytotoxic and helper T cells by negative feedback.

Owing to unusual lymphocyte recirculation, the number of lymphocytes is high in the peripheral blood of pigs, chickens, and ducks. T lymphocytes can be differentiated immunologically from B lymphocytes. T lymphocytes' membrane receptors can bind nonspecifically to sheep erythrocytes (E rosette formation) and to phytohemagglutinins (PHAs) in cows, goats, pigs, and sheep. In man, with commercial fluorescent monoclonal antibodies directed toward lymphocyte membrane glycoproteins, it is possible to sort the T cells in peripheral blood. In piglets and growing ruminants, a subclass of T lymphocytes, called null cells, are unresponsive to spontaneous erythrocyte rosette formation and PHA. In calves, the number of null cells decreases with age and the rise in T cells, and in mature cattle null cells are practically absent in blood. In adult pigs and sheep, about 40 percent of the peripheral blood lymphocytes would be null cells.

Thrombocytes

Thrombocytes (platelets) are small (3-μm), colorless, round or rod-shaped, anucleated bodies found in the circulating blood of mammals. Thrombocyte counts are about 300,000 to 450,000 per microliter of blood in mammals, and less than one-tenth that amount in chickens. They develop in about 5 days from buds on megakaryocytes in the bone marrow, which are pinched off and released into the blood. The half-life of platelets is relatively short (8 to 11 days) in the circulating blood, where they are eliminated mostly by macrophages in the spleen. Platelets have numerous functions in the animal body, but their principal role is to prevent hemorrhage when blood vessels are injured. Within seconds after disruption of the endothelial lining, platelets adhere to the subendothelial structures and form a sphere because of contractions of their microfibrils. The platelet-plugging mechanism is important for closure of minute ruptures that happen in very small vessels, including those through the endothelial cells themselves, and of more serious bleeding situations.

The ultrastructure of platelets reflects their specialized functions. The thick glycocalyx plasma membrane retains various plasma factors of clotting such as fibrinogen, and factors V, VIIc, and XI. The plasma membrane contains phospholipids that are precursors of prostaglandins and several platelet factors. Invaginations of the plasma membrane permit endocytosis and exocytosis. The cytoplasm contains calcium ions, enzymes, and as many contractile protein fibrils (actin and myosin: 20 percent) as those in smooth muscle cells. Besides organelles such as glycogen and mitochondria, granules containing adenosine diphosphate (ADP), adenosine triphosphate (ATP), serotonin, various factors of clotting, and lysosomes are also found in the cytoplasm of platelets.

Thrombocytopenia (too few platelets) is usually associated with small punctate hemorrhages in body tissues and purplish blotches (purpura) on unpigmented skin. Without making specific counts of platelets in the blood, thrombocytopenia is detected by noting whether or not a clot of blood retracts. Clot retraction depends on the presence of large number of platelets entrapped in the fibrin mesh of the clot.

An impetus to the quantitative study of platelets is related to the use of aggregometers, which precisely measure the primary and secondary stages of platelet aggregation.

The optical aggregometer is used with platelet-rich plasma (PRP) prepared by centrifugation of citrated blood. A small aliquot is pipetted into a heated (37°C) glass cuvette. A light beam is driven through the cuvette, and any transmitted light (most of it is scattered by the stirred platelets) is detected with a photoelectric cell. When the platelets tend to clump together, the concomitant increase in transmitted light is proportional to the aggregation response.

The electronic aggregometer measures the increase in the electrical resistance of the PRP during the aggregation of platelets induced by collagen. The higher electrical impedance is due to the accretion of platelets on the electrodes.

Platelets produce the most potent agent for their aggregation, thromboxane A_2 (TXA$_2$). A derivative of arachidonic acid, TXA$_2$ also causes contraction of smooth muscle fibers in the platelets (retraction) and in the walls of blood vessels (vasoconstriction). Another derivative of arachidonic acid, prostacyclin (PGI$_2$), which originates from vascular endothelial cells, has opposite effects: it inhibits platelet aggregation and relaxes smooth muscle fibers.

Atrial thrombi, composed primarily of platelets and fibrin strands, can be averted by administering acetylsalicylic acid (aspirin), which prevents production of both TXA$_2$ and PGI$_2$. Aspirin does not cause lysis of formed thrombi but limits their growth and prevents recurrences by inhibiting the synthesis of TXA$_2$.

Blood clots in pulmonary vessels (pulmonary thromboemboli, PTE) and disseminated intravascular coagulation (DIC) are often secondary to hypercoagulation states (e.g., feline cardiomyopathy, canine heartworm infection, hyperadrenocorticism, and renal dysfunctions).

COAGULATION OF BLOOD

The existence of a cardiovascular system and of a blood circulation in animals carries a considerable hazard, that of bleeding to death as the result of any break in the vascular wall. Thus, means for reducing leakage are essential for survival. Constriction of the damaged vessel is the most obvious mechanism besides hemostasis or coagulation of blood. Hemostasis involves adhesion and aggregation of blood platelets to create a plug in the wall of the damaged blood vessel.

Over 40 different substances that affect blood coagulation have been found as inactive proenzymes in the blood and tissues. Some substances in plasma promote coagulation, the *procoagulants* (e.g., TXA$_2$). Others regulate or inhibit coagulation, the *anticoagulants* (e.g., heparin, PGI$_2$, alpha$_2$-mac-

roglobulin, and C protein). Whether blood coagulates or not is determined by the balance between these two groups of substances.

Procoagulant Substances in Blood

When a vessel is ruptured, the general concept is that the procoagulants in the area are activated to transform soluble fibrinogen (Factor I) into insoluble fibrin by an enzyme called thrombin. The production of fibrin to enmesh platelets and blood cells to form a clot takes place in three stages: *prothrombin activator* formation; *cleavage of prothrombin* (globulin) into thrombin; and *transformation of fibrinogen* into fibrin threads.

The prothrombin activators (i.e., the thromboplastins, Factor III) are derived from the damaged tissues and the action of calcium ions. Prothrombin (Factor II) is a globulin formed in the liver only if adequate absorption of vitamin K from the gut occurs. The blood clotting factors have an international nomenclature but are known by many other names as well (Table 12–9).

Blood clot formation involves a complex sequence of protein interactions. Most of the plasma proteins taking part in the coagulation or hemostatic process circulate as inactive proenzymes. The sequential activation of these proenzyme proteins into their active enzyme protein forms occurs through intrinsic and extrinsic reaction mechanisms.

Intrinsic Mechanism of Blood Coagulation

The intrinsic mechanism of blood coagulation refers to the enzyme reactions, which activate specific proenzymes when blood is brought in contact with a "foreign surface" (collagen fibers, a negatively charged surface, kinins, glass, or long-chain saturated fatty acids). Any surface other than

TABLE 12–9 Blood Clotting Factors: International Nomenclature and Synonyms

International Classification	Synonyms
Factor I	*Fibrinogen*
Factor II	*Prothrombin*
Factor III	*Tissue thromboplastin*
Factor IV	*Calcium*
Factor V	*Proaccelerin,* labile factor, accelerator globulin (AcG)
Factor VII	*Proconvertin,* autoprothrombin I, stable factor, serum prothrombin conversion accelerator (SPCA)
Factor VIII	*Antihemophilic factor* (AHF), platelet cofactor I, antihemophilic globulin (AHG), plasma thromboplastic factor A, von Willebrand factor
Factor IX	*Christmas factor,* platelet cofactor II, autoprothrombin II, plasma thromboplastic factor B, plasma thromboplastin component (PTC)
Factor X	*Stuart factor,* Stuart-Prower factor
Factor XI	*Plasma thromboplastin antecedent* (PTA)
Factor XII	*Hageman factor*
Factor XIII	*Fibrin-stabilizing factor* (FSF), fibrinase, Laki-Lorand factor

the intact endothelial lining of the blood vessel wall is considered foreign to both the plasma coagulation proteins and the blood cells. Damage to a vessel wall or exposure to air thus initiates the clotting process. Once started, the chain of reactions of blood clotting culminates in the generation of thrombin and the formation of an insoluble fibrin mesh.

Chronologically, the factors associated specifically with the intrinsic mechanism of blood coagulation are Hageman factor (Factor XII), plasma thromboplastin antecedent (Factor XI), plasma thromboplastin component (Factor IX), and Stuart factor (Factor X).

Disseminated intravascular coagulation, the development of microclots or thrombi in minute vessels, is a prelude to more intense deterioration of the circulation of blood in capillaries.

Extrinsic Mechanism of Blood Coagulation

The extrinsic mechanism of blood coagulation relates to the activation reactions, which are initiated sequentially in the damaged blood vessel. They occur because of trauma to the surrounding tissues and release of tissue juices.

Formation of a prothrombin activator with the help of Factors V, VII, and X is an essential part of the extrinsic mechanism of blood coagulation. Tissues contain a specific lipoprotein, tissue thromboplastin, that causes rapid fibrin formation when it enters the bloodstream. In essence, the extrinsic clotting mechanism activates Factor X directly and bypasses the initial stages of the intrinsic mechanism to induce a faster rate of fibrin formation. This benefits the animal when tissues surrounding a damaged blood vessel are also injured and requires an extremely efficient clotting mechanism.

The intrinsic and the extrinsic mechanisms of blood coagulation are complementary systems designed to cope with the trauma to which the blood vessels are exposed. The two mechanisms are not competing with each other and are not, in fact, very distinctive in nature.

The factors consumed during clotting of blood that are not found in serum are fibrinogen (Factor I), prothrombin (Factor II), proaccelerin (Factor V), antihemophilic factor (Factor VIII), and fibrin-stabilizing factor (Factor XIII).

Anticoagulant Substances Added to Blood

Heparin, a substance synthesized in mast cells of the lung, liver, and intestinal mucosa, is not a normal constituent of blood. A polysaccharide containing many sulfate groups, heparin inhibits blood coagulation in vitro and in vivo for 3 to 4 hours when administered at a dose of 0.5 mg per kilogram. It acts mainly by neutralizing the action of thrombin. Heparin owes its action to its ability to potentiate the activity of antithrombin III and its strong electronegative charges (sulfate groups). Antithrombin III is a physiological inhibitor of several enzymes, notably Factor Xa and thrombin. Heparin also accelerates the activity of another antithrombin, heparin cofactor II. The negative charges of heparin can be completely neutralized, and its anticoagulant action antagonized by electropositive substances such as toluidine blue and protamine. During anaphylactic shock, degranulation of mast cells releases histamine and heparin, which respectively cause a fall in blood pressure and a reduction in the clotting of blood. In addition to its antithrombotic effects, heparin causes an increase in the physiological plasminogen activator, which may result in fibrinolytic activity (i.e., may help lyse thrombi).

Substances that decrease the concentration of calcium ions can prevent blood coagulation outside the body. Soluble oxalate compounds precipitate calcium ions from the plasma by forming insoluble calcium oxalate. Since oxalate is toxic to the body, citrate salts (ammonium, potassium, or sodium) are preferred as anticoagulants for blood destined for reinfusion (transfusion). They form un-ionized calcium compounds and lower the ionic calcium available for blood clotting. Other anticoagulants, such as the salts of tetraethylammonium acid, are used mostly in vitro to prevent blood clotting by chelating the calcium ions in a manner similar to that of citrate.

VISCOSITY OF BLOOD

Viscosity of a fluid is defined in terms of physics as the ratio of the shearing stress to the rate of shear. Units of viscosity are expressed in centipoises (cP), for absolute viscosity, or in relation to the viscosity of water, which has a *relative viscosity* of 1. The *absolute viscosity* of whole blood in vivo is about 2.7 cP in man. Heparin reduces blood viscosity. The viscosities of blood, plasma, and serum are usually expressed in units of relative viscosity. The characteristics of the proteins in serum and plasma as well as the number of erythrocytes in the blood affect the viscosities of these fluids.

The viscosity of a fluid containing proteins is influenced by the concentration and the size of these large molecules. The relative viscosity of plasma is between 1.9 and 2.3. Since serum has a lower concentration of large proteins (fibrinogen, globulins), its relative viscosity is slightly less (1.7 to 2.0) than that of plasma. Viscosity is also diminished in anemia and hemodilution (excess infusion of electrolytes).

The relative viscosity of blood increases when the number of erythrocytes becomes greater (e.g., in dehydration, polycythemia), which is reflected by a higher PCV (i.e., relative volume of erythrocytes in a liter of blood). Higher viscosities accompany higher PCVs (Fig. 12–11); for this reason, blood viscosity is usually higher in male animals than in females. Within the usual range of PCVs seen in animals (0.40 to 0.55 L per liter), the absolute viscosity of blood is 2.0 to 3.3 cP, which corresponds to relative viscosity values between 3 and 5 (see Fig. 12–11).

The flow of blood is maximal when PCV and viscosity are at normal values. In large vessels, erythrocytes move at random and contribute some viscous resistance to blood flow. In small vessels (<0.3 to 0.5 mm in diameter), the values for PCV and viscosity decrease to facilitate the flow of blood. In such capillaries, the viscosity of blood is 50 percent less than in large vessels, since erythrocytes line up in the

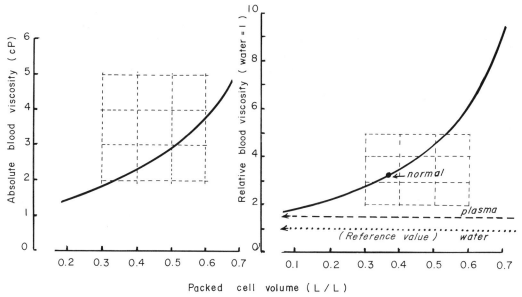

Figure 12–11 Relationship of PCV to absolute blood viscosity. The relative blood viscosity, which is related to the erythrocyte content, is normally much higher than that of plasma. Compared with water (1), plasma or serum has a relative viscosity of about 1.8.

axial part of the bloodstream to create a cell-free zone close to the endothelial wall. The phenomenon is known as *plasma skimming* because of the low PCV.

However, some counteracting effects in capillaries render blood viscosity about equivalent in small and in large vessels. The slow progression (1mm per second) of blood in capillaries, with erythrocytes adhering to each other (agglutination or rouleau formation) and to the endothelium, may increase viscosity as much as 10 times. Such an increase in the viscosity of blood in capillaries is likely to occur in horses and pigs, whose erythrocytes normally have a higher tendency to agglutinate and show a higher sedimentation rate. By momentarily slowing or blocking the progression of blood, structural obstructions or constrictions in the walls of capillaries also contribute to increasing the apparent viscosity of blood.

The term *sludged blood* refers to the slower progression of blood in the microvasculature resulting from agglutination of erythrocytes or microthromboses. Blood acidity then increases as a result of continued production and accumulation of carbonic or lactic acid. A greater content of volatile acid metabolites (mostly carbonic acid) in addition to a higher PCV makes venous blood more viscous than arterial blood.

The viscosity of blood is one of the factors that determine the arterial blood pressure. The other agents involved in regulating arterial blood pressure are the force of the heart pump, the quantity of blood in the arteries, the flexibility or elasticity of arterial walls, and the vasomotor changes (vasodilation or vasoconstriction of small vessels) in the peripheral resistance.

REFERENCES

Allen D, Jr, Kvietys PR, Granger DN. Crystalloids versus colloids: implications in fluid therapy of dogs with intestinal obstruction. Am J Vet Res 1986;47:1751.

Cardinal DC, Flower RJ. The electronic aggregometer: a novel device for assessing platelet behavior in blood. J Pharmacol Meth 1980; 3:135.

Didisheim P, Hattory K, Lewis JH. Hematologic and coagulation studies in various animal species. J Lab Clin Med 1959;53:866.

Greenwood B. A simple double-centrifugation technique for the separation of sheep leukocytes. Vox Sang 1968;15:315.

Gregersen MI, Rawson RA. Blood volume. Physiol Rev 1959;39:307.

Jain NC. Schalm's veterinary hematology. 4th ed. Philadelphia: Lea & Febiger, 1986.

Kaneko JJ. Clinical biochemistry of domestic animals. 4th ed. NY: Academic Press, 1989.

Korner PI, Smith ID. Cardiac output in normal unanaesthetised and anaesthetised rabbits. Aust J Exp Biol 1954;32:499.

Marcilese NA, Figueiras HD, Valsecchi RM, Camberos HR. Blood volumes and body:venous hematocrit ratio in cattle. Cornell Vet 1966; 56:142.

Persson SGB, Ekman L, Lydin G, Tufvesson G. Circulatory effects of splenectomy in the horse. Zbl Vet Med A 1973;20:456.

Pond WG, Hoput KA. The biology of the pig. Ithaca: Comstock Publishing Associates, 1978.

Rackear DG. Drugs that alter the hemostatic mechanism. Vet Clin North Am (Small Anim Pract) 1988;15:67.

Smith LL, Foster RL, Muller W. Intrinsic cardiac output variability in the anesthetized normal and splenectomized dog. Am J Physiol 1962; 202:1155.

Teule GJJ, den Hollander W, Bronsveld W, van Lambalagen AA, Heidendal GAK, Thijs LG. Noninvasive detection of blood volume redistribution in canine endotoxin shock. Circ Shock 1981;8:627.

White L, Saines H, Adams T. Cardiac output related to body weight in small animals. Comp Biochem Physiol 1968;27:559.

CHAPTER 13

THE HEART PUMP

The almost simultaneous contractions of the cardiac ventricles pump blood at a rate of about 1 beat per second in large animals and several beats per second in small animals. Equal volumes of blood are ejected by the ventricles into the pulmonary and aortic arteries. The right ventricle propels into the pulmonary artery a partially oxygenated (venous) blood toward the lungs, and the left ventricle sends into the aortic artery a fully oxygenated blood toward the tissues (Fig. 13–1).

In the fetus, gas exchanges occur at the placenta instead of at the lungs. The oxygen saturation is about 80 percent in the blood of the umbilical vein and about 60 percent in that returning by the umbilical artery. The ductus venosus (DV) diverts some of the oxygenated (67 percent saturation) umbilical blood into the vena cava, the remainder mixing with the portal blood (about 25 percent saturation). The vena cava directs oxygenated blood to the right ventricle, which communicates with the left ventricle through the foramen ovale (FO). Some blood also passes from the right ventricle to the descending aorta via the ductus arteriosus (DA). Blood ejected from the right ventricle bypasses the pulmonary circuit (Fig. 13–2). Both ventricles *pump in parallel* with identical arterial pressures and almost similar masculature thickness (the right ventricle is slightly thicker).

At birth, the "placental branch" of the fetal circulation is terminated, the umbilical vessels and sinus venosus (SV) constrict, and their blood is infused into the neonate. The loss of maternal oxygenation causes asphyxia, which triggers respiratory gasping and inflation of the lungs and lowers the resistance in the pulmonary blood circuit. Functional closure of the FO and DA occurs after 1 to 2 days, but permanent closure requires a few weeks. The DA obliterates because of the highly oxygenated pulmonary blood and because of production of bradykinin (lungs), catecholamines (adrenal medulla), and prostaglandins. With initiation of higher peripheral resistance in the aortic blood circuit, and closure of the FO and DA, the two sides of the heart begin to *pump in series,* with great differences in arterial pressures.

The left ventricular musculature hypertrophies to create an arterial pressure several times higher than that of the right ventricle. Because of bronchial shunts, a small fraction of blood from the left heart bypasses the right heart and pulmonary alveoli and is allowed to return to the left atrium without being fully oxygenated.

This chapter presents a succinct account of (1) the events during the pumping action of the heart, (2) the volumes of blood ejected at each heart cycle and during a given period of time, (3) the factors and structures that control heart rate, (4) the sounds that occur during the

cardiac cycle, and (5) the electrical activity associated with cardiac contraction.

MECHANICAL EVENTS DURING A CARDIAC CYCLE

To relentlessly propel oxygen and nutrient-laden blood to the cells and clean the extracellular environment of metabolic residues, the dynamics of the heart must constantly change. Some of the major mechanical events of the cardiac cycle concern the pumping action, the alternating contraction and relaxation phases, the opening and closing of the atrioventricular and arterial cardiac valves, and the changes in pressure and volume generated in the systemic circulation.

Pumping Action of the Heart

The thin-walled atria contribute very little to the pumping action of the heart, which is a function shared by the left and right ventricles. Even if both sides of the heart simultaneously deliver the same quantity of blood, the left heart pump is morphologically and mechanically very different. This is understandable, considering that blood from the right heart exits into a short and straight circuit of relatively large vessels, whereas the left heart must move blood into a longer, more diverse, and narrower network of vessels. In other words, the left heart pumps against high resistance in the systemic circulation, and the right heart pumps against low resistance in the pulmonary circulation. Conditions that increase the resistance to blood flow in the pulmonary circuit cause right ventricular hypertrophy, as the heart increases its muscle mass to assume adequately the function of a higher force pump.

Operation of the left pump (i.e., contraction of the left ventricle) simply involves a reduction in the transverse axis with very little shortening of the longitudinal axis. At the same moment, the pumping action in the less powerful right ventricle results from the summation of three activities, one from the left ventricle itself and two that are related to the contraction of the other ventricle, the left one. The right ventricle contracts by shortening its longitudinal axis (i.e., by moving the base of the right heart toward the apex). The right ventricle is also helped by the concomitant contraction of the left ventricle. As it reduces its transverse diameter, the contracting thick-walled left ventricle moves the lateral thin wall of the right ventricle toward the convex interventricular septum. Although slight, this movement is very effective in ejecting blood from the right ventricle because of a "bellows

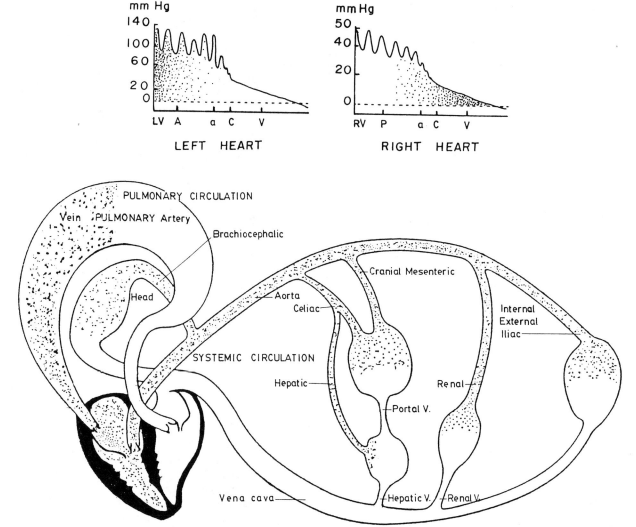

Figure 13–1 Adult blood circulation in the pulmonary and systemic circuits. **Top,** Similar relative blood pressure patterns occur in the pulmonary and the peripheral circulation. The systolic and diastolic pressures gradually decline from the ventricles (*RV, LV*) and arteries (*a*) and subside into a nonpulsatile pressure, which dwindles from the capillaries (*C*) to the veins (*V*). The actual pressures are much higher in the systemic (left heart) than in the pulmonary (right heart) circulation. **Bottom,** The simpler and shorter right heart circulation pumps blood to the lungs for oxygenation (stippling). Distribution of oxygenated blood from the more powerful (thicker muscle mass) left heart is more complex. Blood is pumped craniad to the head and forelimbs as well as caudad to the viscera and rear limbs.

effect".* In addition, as the left ventricle shortens and increases the convexity of the septum, it pulls the free right ventricular wall toward the septum and causes a passive reduction in the volume of the right ventricular chamber. This third component of the right heart pumping action is described as the *left ventricular aid.* Because of this left

ventricular aid, some blood can flow out of the uncontracting right ventricle during cardiac cycles when only the left ventricle is contracting.

Intracardiac Pressure Events during a Cardiac Cycle

During a cardiac cycle, the period of ventricular contraction is called *systole,* and the period of ventricular relaxation is called *diastole* (Fig. 13–3). Even if similar volumes of blood are expelled, the pressure changes are much higher (five- to sevenfold) in the left heart than in the right heart.

The pressure events of the cardiac cycle begin midway through diastole as blood is passively entering each ventricle

---

* A bellows is a closed boxlike device with sides that can be spread apart or pressed together to draw or to expel a fluid. A slight movement of the sides displaces a large volume of fluid without much change in the pressure.

Since the right ventricle may be looked upon as a pocket hanging from the heavy-walled left ventricle, contraction of the left ventricle moves the free wall of the right ventricle toward the interventricular septum, thus simulating the action of a bellows.

THE HEART PUMP **117**

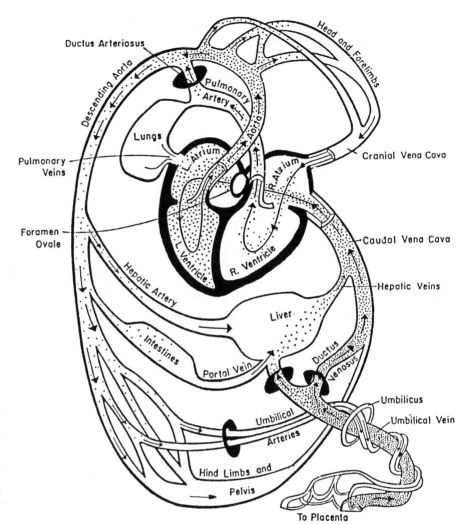

Figure 13–2 Fetal circulation with communications between the atria through the foramen ovale and between the pulmonary artery and the aorta by means of the ductus arteriosus. Almost identical force (same muscle thickness) is developed in both sides of the heart. Oxygenation of blood occurs at the placenta. Oxygenated blood (stippling) is brought to the right ventricle through the umbilical vein, ductus venous, caudal vena cava, and right atrium. From the right ventricle, some oxygenated blood flows into the pulmonary artery and ductus arteriosus to reach the aorta, but most enters the left ventricle through the foramen ovale and is ejected into the aorta. Structures circled in black (ductus venosus, umbilical arteries and vein, ductus arteriosus, and foramen ovale) become nonfunctional at birth.

at low pressure from the respective atrium. Atrial pumping is not necessary for ventricular filling in resting animals. Toward the end of diastole, the atria contract to increase slightly the ventricular volumes and pressures.

During early systole, the ventricular pressure rises drastically in the left heart. After a short time, the left ventricular pressure is sufficient to force the aortic valves to open, to reduce the ventricular blood volume, and to raise the aortic pressure. The parallel pressure events in the right ventricle are much lower but sufficient to open the pulmonary valves. In early diastole, the relaxation and expansion of each ventricular cavity lower the pressure in both ventricles and cause blood to pour in from the atria at a rapid rate.

Propulsive Force in Each Ventricle

Blood flows from the heart into the arteries when adequate pressures are generated in the ventricles. The circumferential tension (T, or force per centimeter) needed to produce these ventricular pressures (P, or force per square centimeter) is related to the geometry of the heart chambers.

The force increases in proportion to the diameter (D = 2R) of the left and right heart ventricles (Laplace's law, T = P × D). The diameter of a ventricle can be characterized by the two principal radii of curvature, R_1 and R_2 (Fig. 13–4). By transforming the formula of Laplace's law, the pressure equals the *tension* developed in the ventricle wall from contraction of the cardiac muscle, divided by the *sum of the two radii of curvature* (in centimeters):

$$P = T \div (R_1 + R_2).$$

The sum of R_1 and R_2, or the dimension of the diameter of the heart, reflects the demands for developing particular pressure values. The importance of this dimension can be illustrated by examining the results of changing the radii of the heart. For a given tension (force) developed during contraction, as the dimension of the diameter (R_1 and R_2) decreases, the pressure (P) increases. On the other hand, if the radii of curvature of a ventricle are lengthened by a factor of 2 (doubling the chamber size), tension is augmented by a factor of 4 to produce the same pressure.

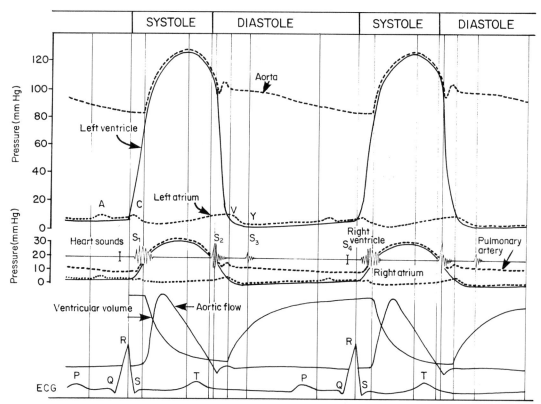

Figure 13–3 Coincident events during the cardiac cycle. **Top,** Pressure changes in the aorta and the left ventricle. In the left atrium: *A*, atrial contraction; *C*, atrial pressure artifact caused by the ventricular contraction; *V*, peak of the atrial pressure rise due to venous blood pouring into the atrium; *V*, decline of atrial pressure ("y" descent) associated with rapid ventricular filling in early diastole. **Middle,** Small pressure changes in the pulmonary artery, the right ventricle, and the right atrium. Heart sounds: S_1, AV valve closure; S_2, arterial valve closure and AV valve opening; S_3, end of rapid ventricular filling; S_4, atrial contraction; S_3 and S_4 are usually inaudible. **Bottom,** Left ventricular volume decreases during systole and increases during diastole; aortic blood flow peaks during midsystole and is reversed temporarily in early diastole; waves of the ECG: *P*, atrial activation, and atrial recovery in the last portion; *QRS*, ventricular activation; *T*, ventricular recovery.

The energy and oxygen demands of the heart (i.e., the work requirements) depend on the tension created during the ventricular contraction to produce an efficient pressure for blood flow. Myocardial oxygen consumption, which is about 9 mL per minute per 100 g of heart under basal conditions, can increase several-fold with exercise and can decrease with hypothermia.

Action of the Cardiac Valves during a Cycle

The heart pumps blood unidirectionally from the venous side to the arterial side. This one-way flow of blood is due to the operations of four cardiac valves: two arterial valves and two atrioventricular valves. Each side of the heart pump has an atrioventricular valve and an arterial valve.

The *arterial* (aortic and pulmonary) *valves* of the heart, or the *semilunar valves*, are located at the exits of the left and right ventricles. They prevent retrogression of blood from the arteries to the ventricles. Both valves consist of *three* tough but flexible *flaps, or cusps,* attached symmetrically around the

valve rings. When the arterial valves open during ventricular systole, they form a triangular orifice.

The two *atrioventricular valves* of the heart (the tricuspid on the right side, and the mitral on the left side) prevent the return of blood from the ventricles into the atria. Each atrioventricular valve contains *two large primary cusps* attached completely around the valve ring. The *tricuspid* valve has an additional prominent *secondary cusp*. The total area of the cusps, much greater than that of the orifice they guard, ensures a snug and leak-proof fit upon closure of the valves. Chordae tendineae connect the lower side of the cusps to the papillary muscles on the ventricular walls. The mode of attachment of the *chordae tendineae* to the papillary muscles is such that contraction of the latter prevents eversion of the flexible cusps of the atrioventricular valves into the atrium and tends to hold the cusps together rather than pull them apart.

Because the flow of blood must be venoarterial, the atrioventricular valves open passively whenever the pressure on the venous side exceeds the pressure on the arterial side of the cusps. Closure of the atrioventricular valves possibly

RIGHT VENTRICULAR EJECTION

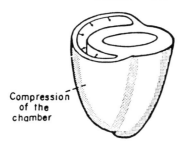 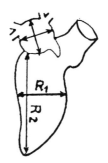 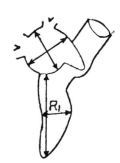

LEFT VENTRICULAR EJECTION

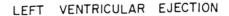

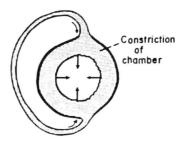 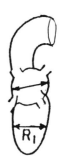 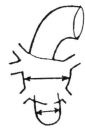

Figure 13–4 Ventricular pumping in the dog. **Top,** Right ventricular ejection results from compression of the chamber by shortening of the free wall; right and left projections of the contour of the contrast silhouettes, at the start and at the end of systole, to show the reduction in R_1 and R_2. **Bottom,** Left ventricular ejection is by constriction of the chamber, mostly from a reduction in the transverse axis and a minor contribution by a slight shortening of the longitudinal axis; contour of the contrast silhouettes during early and late systole to show the reduction mainly of R_1.

occurs through two mechanisms. The obvious mechanism is the backflow of blood (e.g., the mitral valve closes as the left ventricle begins to contract when some blood is regurgitated in the countercurrent direction). The other mechanism is present and readily seen in pathological conditions in which there is a lag, or delay, in the conduction of excitation between atrium and ventricle. Under these circumstances, the atrioventricular valves close immediately after atrial systole, reopen during the delay time, and reclose during ventricular systole. The first closure, at the end of atrial systole, is caused by the force of eddy currents behind the open cusps. The second closure results from the normal backflow of blood during ventricular contraction.

Pressure and Volume Changes in the Systemic Circulation

In the systemic circulation, blood pressure and blood ejection changes are due to specific physical events during the cardiac contraction cycle and to the closing or the opening of the atrioventricular (mitral) and arterial (aortic) valves in the left side of the heart. The *left atrium* reaches its minimal volume during atrial systole and refills during ventricular ejection.

The *intraventricular pressure* rises rapidly at the onset of the contraction of the thick-walled left ventricle. As soon as the intraventricular pressure exceeds the pressure in the left atrium, it forces the left atrioventricular valve (*mitral*) to close. Since the aortic valve is also closed, the left intraventricular pressure builds up rapidly to exceed the pressure in the aorta. Then the *aortic valve* opens, and ejection of blood proceeds from the left ventricle into the aorta. This *ventricular ejection* of blood changes with the volume of the ventricle. It is *rapid* during the isovolumetric contraction phase, then is *reduced* during the hypovolumetric contraction phase, and is finally *minimal* during the isovolumetric relaxation phase.

Ventricular pressure exceeds *aortic pressure* only during the phase of ventricular systole, which coincides with the highest aortic flow and the phase of rapid ventricular ejection of blood. The *inflow* of blood into the aorta then *exceeds runoff* into the peripheral arteries. As inflow and runoff of blood reach *equilibrium,* the pressure levels off, but it reaches a summit that signals the onset of reduced ventricular ejection. During reduced ventricular ejection, aortic flow decelerates, ventricular pressure falls below aortic pressure, but forward flow of blood continues.

Toward the end of systole, when the ventricle starts to relax and runoff from the aorta still exceeds the output of the heart, the *ventriculoaortic pressure difference* is negative (about − 15 mm Hg). This "reversed gradient" induces a *brief retrograde flow* of blood, which helps bring the cusps of the aortic valve into apposition.

The *closure of the aortic valve* is preceded by a sharp dip in aortic pressure, the *incisura,* which is followed by a secondary rise. The incisura conveniently indicates the *end of ventricular systole* and the beginning of ventricular diastole.

When the aortic valve is closed, the flow of blood from the left ventricle into the aorta is null, but blood continues to flow into the peripheral arterial bed during ventricular diastole. The *diastolic flow of blood* is due mainly to the *momentum* applied during systole and to the *elastic recoil* of the distal aorta and large arteries.

CARDIAC OUTPUT

Cardiac output represents the volume of blood that flows from either the right or left ventricle of an animal during a given period of time. It is usually symbolized as $\dot{Q}$ and is expressed in liters per minute. It can also be considered as the product of the volume of blood pumped per heart beat (*stroke volume*) and the number of heart beats per minute. The cardiac output level can be modified by changes in the rate of cardiac contraction, the stroke volume, or both. In normal animals, moderate exercise increases the cardiac output by accelerating the heart rate, as the stroke volume is relatively unchanged. *Total cardiac output* refers to the sum of the volumes of blood ejected from *both ventricles* over a period of time. It is calculated by doubling the cardiac output of one of the ventricles.

Stroke Volume

The stroke volume (SV) is the quantity of blood pumped, or ejected, from a ventricle at each systole. It is the difference between the volume of blood found in the ventricle at the *end of diastole* and the *residual volume* of blood remaining at the *end of systole.* In the resting heart, this residual volume is almost equal to the stroke volume. Besides serving as a small adjustable blood reservoir, the *residual volume* permits transient disparities between the output of the two ventricles.

The stroke volume increases either because of higher end-diastolic volume (larger filling of the ventricle with blood) for a given force of contraction, or greater force of contraction resulting in a lower end-systolic residual volume.

During diastole, stretching of ventricular muscles from increased filling causes more forceful contraction and a larger stroke volume. This regulation of the stroke volume is called the *intrinsic control,* or *heterometric autoregulation,* of the heart, because it depends on the inherent properties of cardiac muscle. It also provides a simple way of regulating cardiac output according to changes in demands.

The importance of end-diastolic volume is pointed out in the *Frank-Starling law of the heart,* or the relationship of initial myocardial fiber length (initial volume) to tension (pressure) development in the ventricle. The greater the filling, the greater the stroke volume (Fig. 13–5).

The stroke volume can be calculated by dividing cardiac output by heart rate:

$$SV \ (mL) = \dot{Q} \div HR$$

In greyhounds, denervation of the heart increases the stroke volume three to four-fold though a *homeometric autoregulation* mechanism (intrinsic, but without stretching of muscle fibers) related to myocardial catecholamines. This increased stroke volume associated with sympathetic influences is abolished by propranolol blocking of beta-adrenergic receptors.

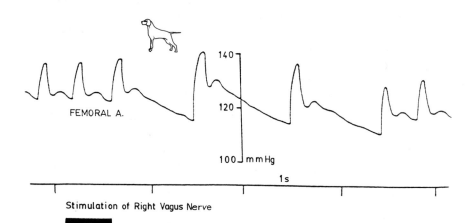

Figure 13–5 Frank-Starling law of the heart: the greater the filling the higher the stroke volume. Peripheral electrical stimulation of the right vagus nerve slows the heart (from about 180 to 60 beats per minute), permits dilation of the heart with more blood, and increases the stroke volume. This is evidenced by a higher femoral arterial pressure (about 140 mm Hg systolic pressure and 115 mm Hg diastolic pressure, compared with 136/122).

FEMORAL A.

140

120

100 mm Hg

1 s

Stimulation of Right Vagus Nerve

Measurements of Cardiac Output

Historically, measurement of cardiac output is associated with the use of flow meters. Commonly, accurate estimation of cardiac output is made with techniques based on oxygen consumption and arteriovenous oxygen concentrations (Fick principle), and the indicator dilution principle.

A variety of *flow meters* exist. Most require surgical insertion into the stream of flowing blood, or placement on the surface of the artery through which the flow of blood is to be measured.

One of the earliest apparatuses for measuring vascular blood flow was devised by MAREY and CHAUVEAU. Their flow meter, then known as a *hemodromometer,* used the kinetic energy of blood to move a small vane placed in the bloodstream. The vane moved a small air-filled, tambour-like device that recorded changes in the flow rate of blood.

The latest surface electromagnetic flow meters detect a potential difference generated when an electroconductor fluid (saline, blood, digestive contents) moves through a perpendicular magnetic field. The induced voltage is proportional to the rate of fluid flow.

A noninvasive cardiac output method uses an ultrasonic flow meter attached to the surface of a blood vessel. It is based on the Doppler effect produced by the flow of erythrocytes in a blood vessel exposed to ultrasonic waves (3,000,000 Hz). Ultrasonic vibrations are generated by a piezoelectric crystal of barium titanate excited with high-frequency electrical pulses. When ultrasonic waves are applied to the bloodstream, the flow of red blood cells causes responses of lower frequencies upstream than downstream. With higher blood flow, a greater difference exists between upstream and downstream frequencies.

The Fick Principle

According to the Fick principle, the cardiac output can be calculated by measuring the oxygen consumption per minute and the arteriovenous oxygen difference (Fig. 13–6):

$$\dot{Q} = \dot{V}O_2 \ / \ (CaO_2 \ - \ CvO_2).$$

The amount of substance (oxygen) taken up by the circulation per unit of time is equal to the difference between arterial and venous levels of the substance, multiplied by the blood flow (cardiac output). The volume of oxygen consumed in a minute is determined by spirometry. The arterial blood may be sampled from any artery, and mixed venous oxygen blood, by catheterization of the pulmonary artery. The levels of oxygen in the blood samples are measured by electronic methods. In normal mammals, the ratio of cardiac output to oxygen consumption is about 20 to 1 (e.g., in a 10-kg dog with an oxygen uptake of about 5 mL per kilogram per minute [i.e., 50 mL per minute], the cardiac output can be estimated at $50 \times 20 = 1,000$ mL per minute.

Initially, the necessary oxygen data were measured by the Van Slyke mercury manometric method for blood gas analysis, which used an ingenious apparatus recognized as tedious to operate.

Indicator Dilution Methods for Cardiac Output. A dilution method uses a known quantity of indicator (dye, radio-

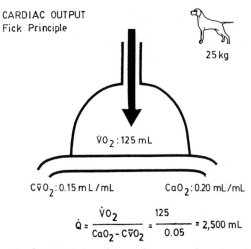

CARDIAC OUTPUT
Fick Principle

25 kg

$\dot{V}O_2 : 125$ mL

$C\bar{v}O_2 : 0.15$ mL /mL $CaO_2 : 0.20$ mL /mL

$$\dot{Q} = \frac{\dot{V}O_2}{CaO_2 - C\bar{v}O_2} = \frac{125}{0.05} = 2,500 \text{ mL}$$

Figure 13–6 Calculation of the cardiac output from the minute volume of oxygen consumption ($\dot{V}O_2$) and the arteriovenous difference in blood oxygen concentrations ($CaO_2 - C\bar{v}O_2$). The example calculates the cardiac output in a 25-kg dog when oxygen consumed is 125 mL per minute and arterial blood contains 0.20 mL of oxygen per milliliter, whereas the mixed venous blood has only 0.15 mL per minute. According to the Fick principle, the volume of blood pumped by the heart in a minute is $Q = \dot{V}O_2/(CaO_2 - C\bar{v}O_2)$ or $125/(0.20 - 0.15) = 2,500$ mL.

active isotope, or chilled physiological saline) added to the blood at one site and quantitatively measured at another site. From the exact amount of indicator or of thermal dilution in the blood, the volume of blood can be calculated. The method involves a series of measurements made at precise intervals after the infusion. The logarithm of each measurement is plotted against postinjection time to construct a straight-line curve.

Echocardiography is also used to evaluate cardiac output.

Expression of Cardiac Output

In animals, cardiac output correlates better with body weight (linearly) than with body surface (curvilinearly); thus, it is preferable to relate cardiac output to body weight.

In most animals, cardiac output in liters per minute represents about 10 percent of body weight in kilograms:

$$\dot{Q} = 0.1 \times kg^*$$

e.g., in a normal 5-kg cat, the cardiac output is about $0.1 \times 5 = 0.5$ L per minute $= 500$ mL per minute, and the approximate oxygen consumption should be near $500/20 = 25$ mL oxygen per minute.

Because of the relationship between metabolism and body size, cardiac output in homeotherms should be directly

---

* The exact equation to estimate the cardiac output is $\dot{Q} = 0.1017 \times kg^{0.9988} = x$ L/min.

proportional to body mass$^{0.75}$ or kg$^{0.75}$. Since blood is the medium to carry oxygen, the blood flow should also be proportional to body mass$^{0.75}$ or kg$^{0.75}$. Several species have cardiac outputs that are proportional to body mass$^{0.75}$, but each species has a particular cardiac output–body mass relation.

In birds, the relation between $\dot{Q}$ and body mass is represented by a different equation: $\dot{Q} = 0.2907 \times kg^{0.69} = x$ L per minute, and this larger cardiac output is paralleled by higher blood pressures and heart rates.

In spite of the limited correlation between the cardiac output and the body surface, the *cardiac index* (in liters per minute per square meter) is the commonly used clinical index. Body surface is calculated from the body mass according to the formula: $m^2 = 0.11 \times kg^{0.73}$, and cardiac index = cardiac output ÷ body surface.

Experimental Modification of Cardiac Output

Light anesthesia does not affect cardiac output but does reduce oxygen consumption. Anesthetized animals used as controls are not comparable to unanesthetized animals but are in a different steady state. For rabbits anesthetized with urethane, using the Fick principle, the mean cardiac output is 130 mL per minute per kilogram, and the mean oxygen consumption is about 7 mL per minute per kilogram (nearly the 20 to 1 ratio).

In dogs, splenectomy increases the mean variation (expressed as a percentage) from the mean value of the cardiac output. The average variation is 10.5 percent in normal dogs and 15 percent in splenectomized dogs when cardiac output is measured with radioiodinated serum albumin as the indicator substance. Apparently, the spleen stabilizes the blood volume and prevents variations of venous return to the heart and of cardiac output.

REGULATION OF HEART RATE

Together with stroke volume, heart rate establishes the value of the cardiac output. Within and between species, the *resting heart rate* seems to be inversely related to body mass. Large animals have a *slower* heart rate than smaller ones. Athletic animals (e.g., hare) and animals trained for exercise (e.g., greyhound) also have slower heart rates than sedentary (e.g., rabbit) and untrained animals (e.g., mongrel dog) of the same species. The heart also beats at a slower rate in male and adult animals than in female or young animals (Table 13–1).

Physical exercise causes the heart to accelerate (*tachycardia*) to three to eight times the resting rate to increase cardiac output. More oxygenated blood is then supplied to the skeletal muscles and skin, whereas less blood is directed to the splanchnic region. Athletic and trained animals show the highest exercise-to-rest ratios, whereas the lowest are seen in sedentary and untrained animals (Table 13–2).

TABLE 13–1 Representative Heart Rates in Resting Animals

Animal	Beats per Minute
Bull	50
Calf	150
Cat	130
Chicken	300
Cow	60
Dog	95
Goat	75
Guinea pig	250
Hare	65
Horse	35
Kitten	235
Monkey (rhesus)	240
Mouse	600
Pig	95
Pigeon	200
Piglet	225
Puppy	200
Rabbit	275
Rat	350
Sheep	75

Extrinsic Control

In resting animals, the heart rate is under the constant control of the cardioinhibitory and cardioacceleratory centers located in the medulla oblongata. These centers, continuously receiving afferent impulses from all over the body, send signals to the sinoatrial (SA) node, controlling the *chronotropic action*, or rate, of the heart. Inhibitory signals are dispatched in the left and right vagus nerves, whereas acceleratory signals travel in sympathetic nerves.

Experimental stimulation of the right vagus nerve usually has a greater negative chronotropic effect than similar stimulation of the left vagus. The right vagus nerve is distributed to the SA node predominantly, and its stimulation produces bradycardia or even complete cardiac arrest for a few seconds. An extranodal pacemaker takes over to produce extrasystoles and "escape" from the inhibition caused by the right vagal stimulation. The left vagus nerve exerts its action mostly on the atrioventricular (AV) conduction tissue, and its stimulation produces various degree of AV block. Experimental stimulation of the sympathetic fibers on the left side increases myocardial contractility (augmentor) more than heart rate (accelerator). Right side sympathetic nerve stimulation results in a greater cardiac acceleration of a much

TABLE 13–2 Representative Resting and Exercise Heart Rates in Athletic Horse and in Trained and Untrained Dogs

	Rest	Exercise	Exercise : Rest Ratio
Dog—greyhound	40	320	8
Dog—mongrel	90	270	3
Horse	30	210	7

less intense contractile force than does similar stimulation of the left sympathetic nerve.

Adjustment of the heart rate, by balancing the braking (inhibitory) effect of vagal discharges against the accelerating (facilitating) effects of sympathetic stimuli, is a form of *reciprocal innervation* at the SA node. Reciprocal innervation also exists in the medullary centers where neural activation of the cardioinhibitory center simultaneously suppresses the cardioacceleratory center.

Evidence that these centers continuously control heart rate is obtained by surgical or pharmacological transection of either vagus or sympathetic nerves. At rest, immediate changes follow the disconnection of the chronotropic medullary centers from the SA node. Vagotomy or administration of a bolus of atropine (parasympatholytic drug) causes the heart rate to accelerate (tachycardia). This effect is remarkable in the hare and the horse, *species with a naturally intense vagal tone.* Conversely, sympathotomy (excision of the stellate ganglia) or administration of propranolol (beta-noradrenolytic) slows the heart rate slightly by removing the normally

weak sympathetic tone. Propranolol has a most pronounced effect during exercise, when the sympathetic nervous system is dominant.

The medullary cardioregulatory centers are influenced considerably by impulses originating in stretch receptors (baroreceptors) in carotid sinus and aortic arch arteries (Fig. 13–7), or in venoatrial junctions (pulmonary and venae cavae) and from the cerebral cortex.

Variations in arterial blood pressure modify the impulses issued from the carotid and aortic baroreceptors, which in turn influence the medullary cardiac centers to alter the heart rate. A drop in arterial pressure induces acceleration of the heart, whereas a rise in arterial pressure causes bradycardia. This regulation of the heart rate is often referred to as Marey's law of the heart.

Distention of the atria (venoatrial junctions) by elevation of the central venous pressure (e.g., by administration of fluids) accelerates the heart rate (Bainbridge reflex). Since an increase in blood volume also stimulates the arterial baroreceptors to produce an antagonistic (decelerating) effect, the

Figure 13–7 Baroreceptors in the aortic arch and sinus of the internal carotid in the dog. The afferent impulses from the carotid sinus travel to the medulla oblongata in the sinus nerve, which merges into the glossopharyngeal nerve (cranial nerve IX), and those from the aortic arch converge into the aortic nerve, which integrates with the vagus nerve (cranial nerve X).

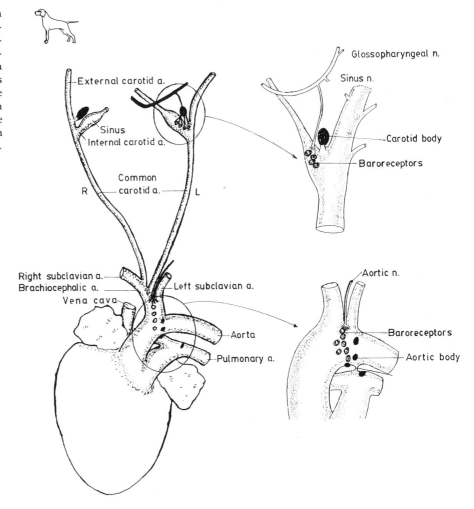

response becomes inversely related to the rate of infusion or loading. Slow infusion provokes an acceleration of the heart, whereas rapid infusion slows the heart.

Excitement, anxiety, and fear signals from the cerebral cortex also exert considerable effects on the medullary cardio-inhibitory and cardioacceleratory centers. Cardioacceleration during physical activity is marked by an intense sympathetic tone of central origin. The heart rate even accelerates ahead of physical exertion, before the actual increase in metabolism occurs.

HEART SOUNDS

The relationship of the heart sounds to the cardiac cycle events is examined by using a microphone on the chest or a phonocardiograph for recording a tracing of the amplified heart sounds. The first two heart sounds are present, but the less distinct third and fourth heart sounds are not always detected (Fig. 13–8). Usually, the phonocardiogram is recorded concomitantly with an electrocardiogram (ECG) to

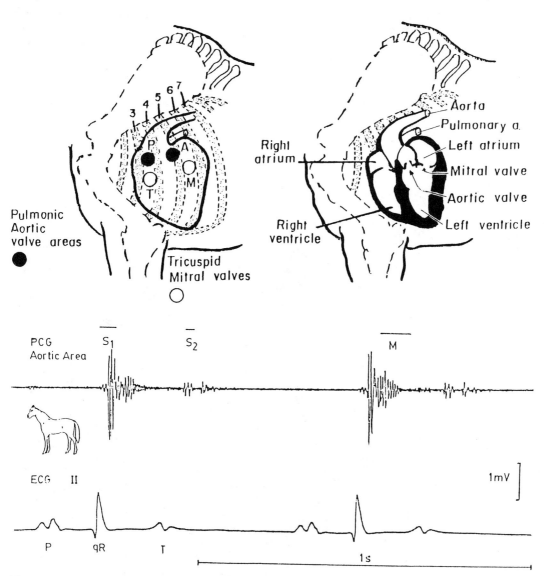

Figure 13–8 Heart sounds. **Top left,** Specific areas of the left thoracic wall of the horse for auscultation of the atrioventricular valves (M, mitral valve area, left sixth intercostal space; T, tricuspid valve area, left third intercostal space, ventral) and of the arterial valves. (P, Pulmonic valve area, left third intercostal space, dorsal; A, aortic valve area, left fifth intercostal space). **Top right,** Schematic representation of the aortic and mitral valves of the left heart. **Bottom,** First (S_1) and second (S_2) heart sounds over the aortic area in the horse with coincident electrocardiogram (ECG, lead II). A notched P wave and a negative T wave highlight the ECG. During the second heart cycle, an innocent murmur (M) is added to S_2 (i.e., an innocent diastolic murmur). Innocent systolic or diastolic murmurs occur in 60 percent of thoroughbred horses without cardiovascular problems.

help delineate the precise timing of the heart sounds relative to the other events of the cardiac cycle. Briefly, at the beginning of ventricular systole, closure of the atrioventricular valves produces the first heart sound. In late systole, in the aorta and pulmonary artery, closure of the arterial (semilunar) valves causes the second heart sound. The rapid ventricular filling phase of the heart cycle explains the third heart sound, and atrial systole accounts for the fourth heart sound.

Abnormal heart sounds known as *murmurs* occur when valve abnormalities (stenosis or reduced opening, incompetence, regurgitation, backflow, or leakage) are present. However, about 60 percent of thoroughbred horses present "functional murmurs" (innocent murmurs) at auscultation of the base of the heart, over the aortic and pulmonic areas, without having any pathological abnormality in the valves or the chambers of the heart. It may represent a slight asynchrony in the systoles of left and right heart.

The normal range of human audition lies between 20 and 16,000 Hz, but the maximal sensitivity is found within the speech frequencies (1,000 to 2,000 Hz). The audible components of the heart sounds and murmurs occupy the 30- to 250-Hz interval. The normal first and second heart sounds are within 60 and 100 Hz, whereas the third and fourth heart sounds are below 40 Hz.

Compared with the second sound ("dub"), the *first heart sound* ("lub") is lower in pitch, louder, and of longer duration. This is because the larger atrioventricular valves (mitral and tricuspid) close at lower pressures than the arterial valves (aortic and pulmonary). A muscular component has been suggested for the first sound, but the intensity of the vibrations recorded from contracting cardiac fibers is probably not sufficient to be heard on direct auscultation. More probably, the sudden closure of the atrioventricular valves produces oscillations of blood in the ventricular chambers and in the walls of these cardiac structures. These mixed and unrelated low frequencies, usually with a crescendo-decrescendo quality, are transmitted through body tissues and picked up by the stethoscope.

The *second heart sound* complex, more snapping than the first sound, results from closure of the arterial valves and accompanying vibrations of the heart and chest wall. The momentum of the blood rushing back toward the ventricle overstretches the valve cusps, and the recoil creates oscillations in both the arterial and the ventricular cavities. A normal splitting of the second heart sound may be perceived, especially during inspiration, when the aortic valve closes before the pulmonic valve. The functional valvular delay can then be explained by the different blood pressure and blood flow in the aortic and pulmonary arteries. During inspiration, the effective pulmonary venous filling pressure remains unchanged, since the intrathoracic pressure is identical for the pulmonary veins, the left atrium, and the left ventricle. On the right side of the heart, inspiration lowers the intrathoracic pressure and causes an accelerated flow of blood with a more rapid filling of the thin-walled ventricle. As a consequence, the ejection of blood from the right ventricle is delayed, and there is an interval between closure of the aortic and pulmonary arterial valves.

The *third heart sound,* a few low-intensity and low-frequency vibrations, is occasionally heard in early diastole. In the horse, it may be split into two separate sounds. A logical, but yet unproven, explanation is the back-and-forth oscillation of blood and of the ventricular walls as the atrioventricular valves open and blood rushes in from the atria.

The *fourth heart sound* consists of a few low-frequency vibrations attributed to oscillation of blood and cardiac chambers during the atrial contractions.

Auscultation of the Heart

The different valve sounds can best be distinguished by auscultation over specific areas of the chest wall (see Fig. 13–8). When the stethoscope is placed on any one of the "special" valve areas, even if the sounds from all the other valves can also be heard, the sound from the special valve is louder than the other sounds.

Continuous murmurs are heard in animals with patent ductus arteriosus and with arteriovenous fistulas. The murmur of patent ductus arteriosus is most intense during systole, when the pressure difference in the aorta and the pulmonary artery is greatest and flow through the shunt is most rapid.

Low-Frequency Microphone

A microphone specially designed to detect low-frequency sound waves can amplify the heart sounds. Permanent recordings of these heart sounds for archival purposes and for direct analysis are possible with a high-speed polygraph.

Evaluation of the Cardiac Valves with Echocardiography

Echocardiography, a noninvasive technique, consists of sending short pulses of high-frequency sound waves (ultrasound) through the chest tissues and heart and visualizing the echoes reflected from the various structures. The timing and the pattern of the reflected waves provide information on the diameter of the heart, thickness of the ventricular walls, and direction and magnitude of the movements of the valves and other components of the heart. On a screen monitor, it produces clear, well-defined echocardiograms, which are helpful in evaluating normal and pathological features in the cardiac walls and valves.

To identify the mitral valves (Fig. 13–9) in the horse, the echo beam penetrates the right thoracic wall in the vicinity of the fifth intercostal space, 25 cm from the right sternal border. The transducer, covered with sonic coupling gel, scans the right thoracic window. With the apparatus in the A (amplitude) mode, the transducer is slowly moved caudad and ventrad until the whipping motion of the mitral valve is observed between the septum and left ventricular wall. Scanning is performed from the apices of the ventricles,

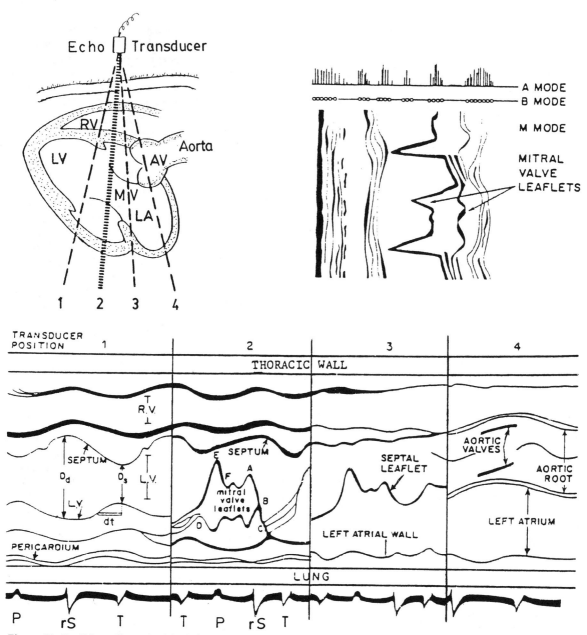

Figure 13–9 Echocardiography. **Top left,** Diagram of the path of an echocardiographic beam (*position 2*) passing through the chest wall, the outer right ventricular wall, the interventricular septum, the leaflets of the mitral valve, and the left outer ventricular wall. By varying the position of the echo transducer (positions 1 to 4), additional structures (aortic valve, left atrium) can be scanned. **Top right,** The amount of reflection is portrayed: in A (amplitude) mode, as amplitude versus tissue depth; in B (brightness) mode, as intensity versus tissue depth; and TM (time) mode, where the scan lasts 5 seconds in the B mode. In each mode, the beam is illustrated as penetrating through the heart at the level of the mitral valve and capturing both septal and lateral leaflets of the mitral valve. **Below,** Returning images when the echo transducer is changed from position 1 to 4. In position 2, *DC* represents ventricular diastole (mitral leaflets apart); *DE,* rapid filling, *EF,* reduced filling; and *FA,* atrial contraction. The mitral valve closes at C and opens at D.

dorsad to the basilar positions of the atrioventricular valves, and finally to atria and aortic root.

During the cardiac cycle, to make permanent recordings of the movements of the valves and of the walls, the setting must be changed to the TM (time) mode.

The end-diastolic dimension (Dd) and the end-systolic dimension (Ds) can be measured and used to estimate the ejection fraction by computing from the equation: percent difference in dimensions (percent D) = (Dd − Ds) ÷ Dd. The echocardiogram can also detect fluttering of the mitral valves, which is associated with pathological valve lesions.

CARDIAC ELECTRICAL ACTIVITY

Experimental stimulation of a resting single cardiac cell evokes a depolarization, either monophasic (when one of the recording electrodes is within the cell) or diphasic (when both electrodes are outside the cell). As in other glandular or muscular cells, an activity (contractility) of equivalent duration immediately follows depolarization.

The sudden monophasic depolarization, or reversal of potential, is followed by a typically long plateau and by a repolarization to resting level. The depolarization may be slow or fast, depending on the localization of the cells in the heart. The resting potential is -60 mV in the slow response and -90 mV in the fast response. In cells from the conducting tissue (sinoatrial, or SA, node; atrioventricular, or AV, node), the slow response is a more rounded and of slower spike potential than the fast response seen in the other atrial and ventricular cardiac cells.

The automaticity of the heart is based on the SA node cells, which discharge (slowly and spontaneously) once the firing threshold is reached. The rate of depolarization (rhythm) is faster with sympathetic activity and slower with activation of the parasympathetic system. The fast-responding cells have a sharp spike of higher amplitude, a longer plateau, and a shorter refractory period (Fig. 13–10).

The SA node cells, which impose a rhythm (rhythmicity) to the rest of the cells of the heart, are the *natural pacemaker*. In their absence (excision, destruction), an *ectopic pacemaker* develops in the remaining conducting system, with AV node cells having priority over Purkinje cells, which are located in the more peripheral part of the conducting system.

The depolarization of slow-response cells is not related to the usual intracellular transfer of sodium ions through fast channels in the plasma membrane. Tetrodotoxin, which blocks the channels, does not alter the action potentials of these cells. In contrast, calcium ions increase the amplitude of the depolarization, and blockage of the slow calcium channels (by verapamil) reduces the amplitude and automaticity of the slow-response cells.

The depolarization initiated at the SA node spreads radially to the atria and to the rest of the heart via the conduction system (AV node, bundle of His, right and left [thicker] bundle branches, and ramifying Purkinje fibers). The atrial pathways involve mostly ordinary atrial muscle fibers (conductivity) but also an interatrial tract from the SA node to the left atrium, and three internodal tracts of mixed fibers that connect the SA node to the AV node. In some animals (e.g., cow), the Purkinje fibers are grouped and encapsulated in small bundles.

Electrocardiography

The global resting or depolarization potentials of the myriad of myocardial cells associated with the heart beat are propagated in the body fluids, which act as good conductors. In electrocardiography, after electronic amplification, the algebraic sum of these electrograms is recorded at the periphery of the body, usually from electrodes affixed to the limbs and from specific points on the thoracic wall (indirect leads). Experimental ECGs can also be obtained after surgically opening the thoracic cavity and placing electrodes on the surface of the heart (direct leads).

The first peripheral recording (ECG) of the electrical changes accompanying the beating of the heart in man and in dog was made in 1887 by WALLER with the capillary electrometer. The terms used to identify the recorded components of these electrical changes were coined by EINTHOVEN, who introduced an instrument that was much easier to use, the string galvanometer, to quantify these electrical events. Einthoven won the Nobel prize in 1924.

In a dipole (a positive and a negative electrode in a volume conductor), a positive wave is obtained when the activation forces are directed toward the positive electrode,

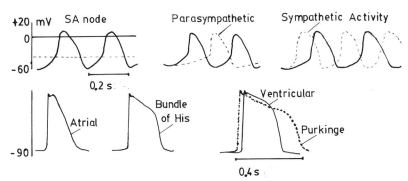

Figure 13–10 Monophasic responses of slow and fast types of cardiac cells. Spontaneously, once a threshold is reached, the slow-type cells depolarize (from -60 mV) at a rate faster in the sinoatrial (SA) node (cardiac pacemaker) than in the atrioventricular (AV) node. Parasympathetic activity slows the rate of the pacemaker, whereas sympathetic stimulation accelerates its automaticity. The depolarization (from -90 mV) of atrial, bundle of His, ventricular, and Purkinje fiber cells is of the fast type. The slow rate of repolarization of these cells (Purkinje < ventricular < bundle of His) helps protect the ventricles from the high atrial rates.

whereas a negative wave occurs when the depolarization forces move away from the positive electrode. By placing a positive electrode over the left ventricle, and a negative electrode over the skin, the changes in the electrical events produced during the cardiac cycle may be recorded (Fig. 13–11).

Wave Pattern of the Electrical Potentials of the Cardiac Cycle

The first visible wave (*P wave*) begins with the depolarization of the right atrium and ends with the depolarization of the left atrium. The left atrial depolarization (activation force) may be directed slightly away (negative wave) from the positive electrode, causing a dip in the P wave. In the horse, because of the time required for excitation to reach the left atrium, the P wave is notched (bifid). The last portion of the P wave includes the repolarization of the atria.

As the wave of excitation passes down the conduction system, the depolarization in the bundle tissue produces only small potentials, not sufficient to produce a deflection. Transmission of the impulse into the ventricles is also prevented by a nonresponsive fibrous ring supporting the valves and great arteries. The normal impulse is thus delayed and

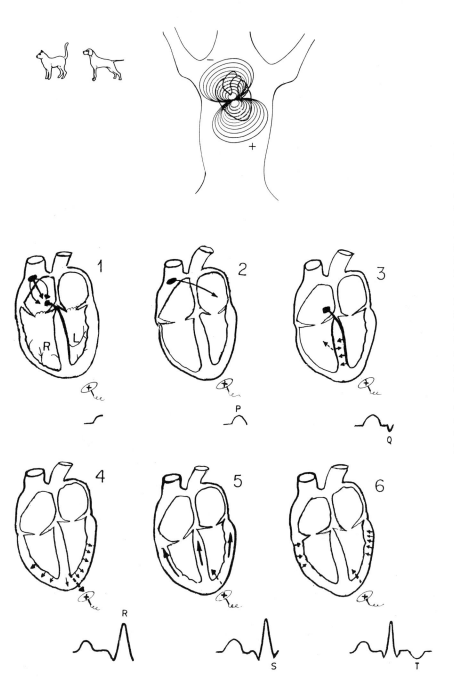

Figure 13–11 Top panel, Genesis of the ECG. In small animals (e.g., dog and cat), the total electrical activity of the myocardial cells can be determined at an external point and oversimplified in a concept known as the dipolar hypothesis. The heart is considered as the center of a dipole (i.e., an electronegative field and an electropositive field). **Lower panel,** Detection of conduction pattern of activation forces as detected from a positive electrode facing the apex of the left ventricle. The depolarization is positive when it is directed toward the positive electrode and negative when it is moving away from it. The activation starts in the SA node and reaches the atrioventricular node directly (*1*) through internodal tracts (ventral, middle, and dorsal) and ordinary atrial myocardial fibers, and the left atrium (*2*) through a ventral interatrial myocardial band as well as ordinary atrial myocardial fibers. Bundle branches there produce a negative Q wave (*3*). The activation then proceeds to the apex of the ventricular masses (*4*) and then to the base of the ventricles with the septum (*5*), ending in the repolarization of the ventricles (*6*).

directed to the ventricles by a unique route, the bundle of His. This delay, which allows the ventricles to fill with blood before their contraction, is reflected in an *isoelectric segment*. During this interval, the atria repolarize, whereas the activation impulses are conducted through the AV node, the bundle of His, and the Purkinje system at a velocity evaluated at 1 to 4 m per second.

The second electrical complex (QRS) is associated with the ventricles. It appears when a significant area of ventricular myocardium is invaded by a wave of excitation. The very variable configuration of this QRS complex depends on the sequence of ventricular excitation and the direction taken by the excitatory waves (see Fig. 13–11).

The conduction system (bundle of His) of the ventricles divides subendocardially into a left branch and a right branch, causing the apex and the walls of both ventricles to depolarize from the endocardium to the epicardium. The wave of excitation from endocardium to pericardium spreads at a velocity of about 0.3 to 0.4 m per second, which is considerably slower than that in the Purkinje conduction system.

Species may be classified into two categories according to the degree of endocardial and epicardial penetration. In the first category (cats, dogs, primates, rodents), the fibers extend 25 to 50 percent of the way from endocardium to epicardium. In the other category (birds, horses, ruminants, swine), as the fibers penetrate the entire distance in the free walls and base, the impulse spreads away from the positive electrode, and the deflection is downward (negative) (Fig. 13–12).

Actually, three phases of ventricular electrical activity concur to produce the Q, R, and S deflections of the QRS complex of the ECG. The *Q wave* (q wave, when small) is a negative deflection (transmitted away from the positive electrode) because the depolarization moves first toward the right bundle branch and then to the left bundle branch. It represents the first phase of ventricular depolarization (see Fig. 13–3) involving the interventricular septum (except the basal portion) and the papillary muscles.

The second phase of ventricular depolarization is a positive deflection, called the *R wave* (r wave, when small). Because the mass of the left ventricle exceeds that of the

Figure 13–12   Top panel, Possible types of P waves. **Middle,** Classification of animal species according to their type of ventricular depolarization (in black) and direction of depolarization. In large animals the progress of depolarization is unidirectional. In carnivores, depolarization moves from the apex toward both the septum and the epicardium. **Bottom,** Types of possible simpler QRS complexes.

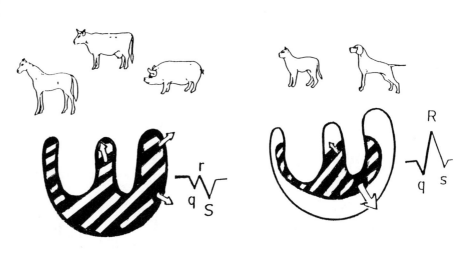

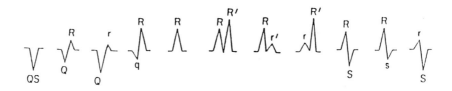

right, leftward electrical forces predominate over rightward ones. The spread of depolarization through the left ventricular mass is toward the positive electrode (i.e., it is recorded as a positive deflection (see Fig. 13–3).

The third phase of ventricular depolarization produces the *S wave* (s wave, when small). The last part of the ventricles to be activated are the basal regions of the free walls and of the septum. Since the depolarization moves away from the positive electrode, a downward, or negative, S wave is recorded. Wave forms of some QRS complexes may be abridged to only QS, QR, Qr, qR, R, Rr', RS, Rs, or rS.

After the depolarizations producing the *QRS complex*, the electrical activity returns to baseline, producing an isoelectric segment called the *ST segment*. The last wave of the electrocardiogram, the *T wave*, indicates repolarization from the epicardial surface toward the endocardium. During exercise, well-trained horses have a monophasic positive T wave, whereas untrained horses show a diphasic T wave. When depolarization and repolarization occur in the same direction, the T wave is inverted with respect to the QRS complex. Conversely, when these processes occur in opposite directions, the T wave and the QRS are on the same side of the isoelectric line.

Uses of Electrocardiography in Animals

Measurement of the cardiac electrical activity is now used as a noninvasive method to evaluate the physiology and

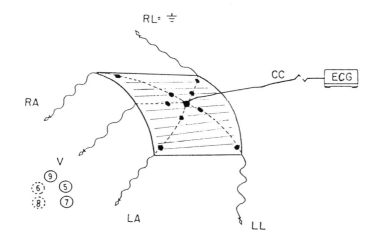

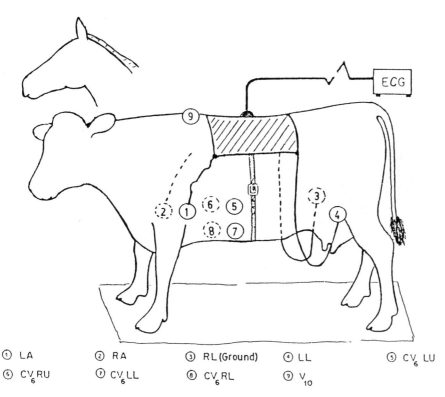

Figure 13–13 Electrode saddle for electrocardiography in large animals. Supported on the back of the animal subject, the wires are easier to manipulate and easier to position quickly. Artifacts in limb leads (bipolar and unipolar, or augmented) and in cardiac or chest leads are minimized by avoiding any discomfort to the animal.

① LA ② RA ③ RL (Ground) ④ LL ⑤ CV_6LU
⑥ CV_6RU ⑦ CV_6LL ⑧ CV_6RL ⑨ V_{10}

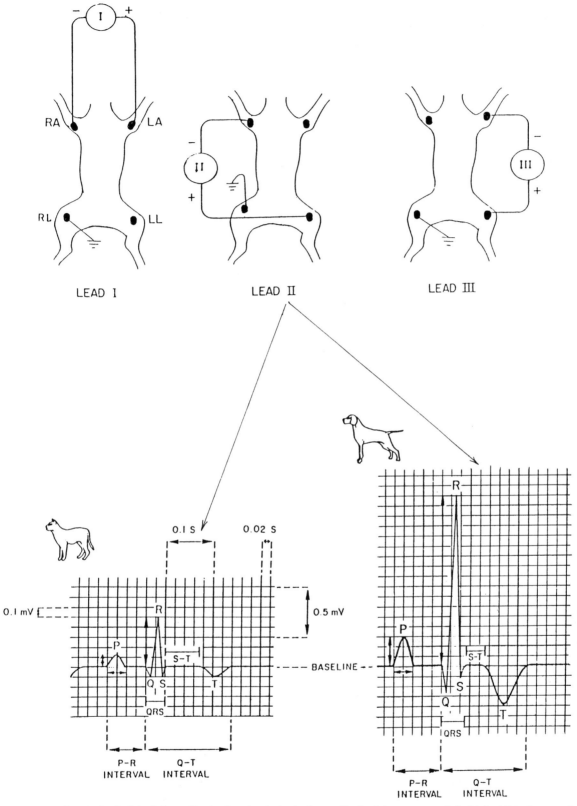

Figure 13–14   Bipolar limb leads in small animals and variation in the amplitude of the waves recorded with lead II in the cat and the dog. The recording in the dog has higher P, Q, R, and T waves than those in the cat, as well as longer PR, ST, and T parameters.

pathology of animals' hearts. Progress in electrography, improvement of portable electrocardiographs, and methods for analysis of traces have made electrocardiography an everyday working tool in small- and large-animal medicine. Electrocardiography is used during examination to evaluate the position of the heart, the relative sizes of its chambers, the

integrity of the conduction system, and the cardiac effects of treatments (electrolytes and drugs).

Even though they are inadequate in some species (e.g., horse), the standard bipolar limb leads (I, II, III) and base-apex lead (cow and horse), augmented unipolar leads (aVR, aVL, aVF), and unipolar chest leads (CV6RU, CV6LU,

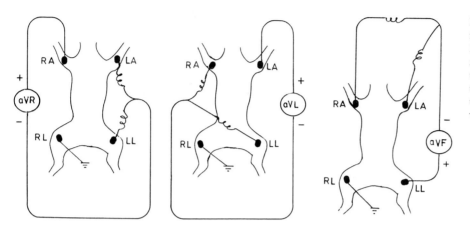

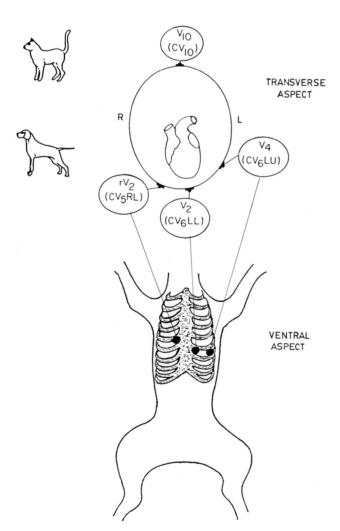

Figure 13–15 In small animals, functional arrangements of the limb leads in the unipolar augmented system (upper panel) and of the successive positions for placing the exploring electropositive electrode on the chest (transverse and ventral aspects).

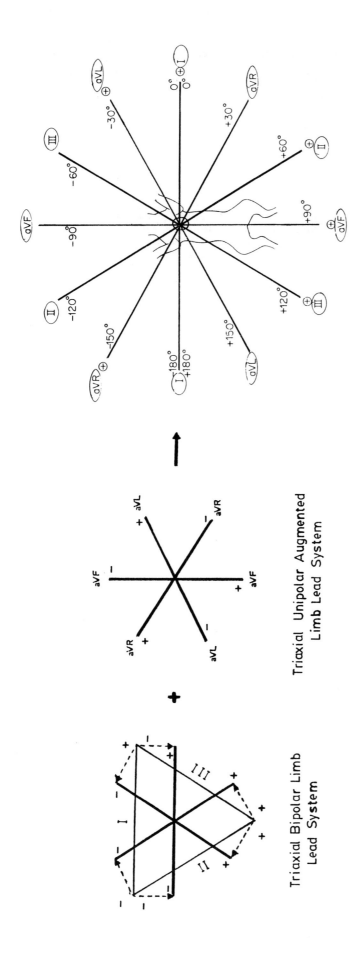

Triaxial Bipolar Limb Lead System

Triaxial Unipolar Augmented Limb Lead System

Hexaxial Lead System

Figure 13–16   By transposing each bipolar limb lead to establish a central (zero potential) midpoint, a triaxial limb lead system is formed. The unipolar limb lead system also corresponds to an analogous triaxial system. A hexaxial lead system is formed by superposing the two triaxial systems. This hexaxial system is useful in calculating the instantaneous mean electrical axis from the parameters from all the leads during depolarization of the heart.

CV6LL, CV6RL, V10) are widely used and documented. For large animals, an electrode saddle conveniently keeps wires untangled, provides them with support, and allows the use of very lightweight alligator clip electrodes. This effort to cause a minimum of discomfort to the animal is rewarded by elimination of most movement artifacts and maintenance of the required parallel alignment of the limbs (Fig. 13–13).

The standard bipolar limb leads are the counterparts of the human leads: RA (−, right foreleg) and LA (+, left foreleg) = I; RA (−) and LL (+, left rear leg) = II; and LA (−) and LL (+) = III. The bipolar base-apex lead for cows and horses: LA (+) over cardiac apex and RA (−) at the base of the neck on the right side, using the RA electrode as a ground and recording on lead I of the ECG (Fig. 13–14).

In the augmented unipolar leads (1.15 × the bipolar limb leads), a switch compares two of the bipolar limb leads with a third limb lead. The aVR lead compares RA with the two others, the aVL does the same with LA, and the aVF pairs LL against RA-LA (Fig. 13–15).

The unipolar chest leads use the limb electrodes as a central indifferent electrode (−) paired with a chest electrode (+), which is positioned on specific points on the thorax. CV6LL (left lower) is over the costochondral junction of the left sixth rib, CV6LU (left upper) is on the left sixth rib on a line going through the point of the left shoulder, V10 is over the dorsal spinous process of the seventh thoracic vertebra, CV6RL (right lower) is over the costochondral junction of the right sixth rib, CV6RU (right upper) is over the right sixth rib on a line crossing the point of the shoulder. This lead is not used in small animals such as cats and dogs (see Fig. 13–15).

In small animals, the mean electrical axis and the position of the heart in the thorax can be determined from the ECG records of the standard bipolar limb leads and of the augmented unipolar limb leads (Fig. 13–16). A hexaxial lead system is obtained by superposing the two triaxial limb lead systems (bipolar and unipolar).

REFERENCES

Bonagura JD, Herring DS, Welker F. Echocardiography. Vet Clin North Am (Equine Pract) 1985;1:311.

Deroth L. Electrocardiographic parameters in the normal lactating Holstein cow. Can Vet J 1980;21:271.

Fregin GF. The cardiovascular system. In: Mansmann RA, McAllister ES, Pratt PW, ed. Equine medicine and surgery. 3rd ed. vol. 1. Santa Barbara, CA: American Veterinary Publications, 1982.

Grubb BR. Allometric relations of cardiovascular function in birds. Am J Physiol 1983;245:H567.

Korner PI, Smith ID. Cardiac output in normal unanaesthetised and anaesthetised rabbits. Aust J Exp Biol 1954;32:499.

Parmley WW, Talbot L. Heart as a pump. In: Berne RM, ed. Handbook of physiology. Section 2. The cardiovascular system—the heart. Vol 1. Bethesda, MD: American Physiological Society, 1979.

Rudolph AM, Hegmann MA. Fetal and neonatal circulation and respiration. Annu Rev Physiol 1974;36:187.

Rushmer RF. Organ physiology. Structure and function of the cardiovascular system. Philadelphia: WB Saunders, 1972.

Scher AM, Spach MS. Cardiac depolarization and repolarization and the electrocardiogram. In: Berne RM, ed. Handbook of physiology. Section 2. The cardiovascular system. Vol. 1. Bethesda, MD: American Physiological Society, 1979.

Smith LL, Foster RL, Muller W. Intrinsic cardiac output variability in the anesthetized normal and splenectomized dog. Am J Physiol 1962;202:1155.

Sperelakis N. Origin of the cardiac resting potential. In: Berne RM, ed. Handbook of physiology. Section 2. Vol. 1. Bethesda, MD: American Physiological Society, 1979.

Tilley LP. Essentials of canine and feline electrocardiography: interpretation and treatment. 2nd ed. Philadelphia: Lea & Febiger, 1985.

White L, Saines H, Adams T. Cardiac output related to body weight in small animals. Comp Biochem Physiol 1968;27:559.

CHAPTER 14

BLOOD PRESSURES

The distribution of blood flow through the various vascular beds is controlled by changes in the caliber of the vessels leading to the capillary networks, a form of flow control that at all times requires an adequate pressure head within the arterial system. The high pressure within the systemic arteries supplies the force to propel blood through the network of narrow channels (microcirculation). Because of a tradition linked to the historical importance of the mercury manometer in cardiovascular physiology, blood pressure is always expressed in millimeters of mercury (mm Hg) and presented as a fraction whose numerator is systolic pressure and whose denominator is diastolic pressure.

In most animals, the hydrostatic head of pressure normally oscillates in the range of 80 to 140 mm Hg, the *capillary refill time* in the oral mucous membranes (lip) is then less than 2 seconds. When the arterial pressure falls below the critical level of 45 to 50 mm Hg (hypotension), not enough blood reaches the brain and tissues, producing unconsciousness and impaired function of the heart and kidneys. A state of hypertension is recognized when the arterial pressure reaches excessive values (180/95 mm Hg in dogs and 200/145 mm Hg in cats). Measurements of arterial blood pressure may be used to evaluate the cardiovascular system, somewhat as other vital signs monitored clinically: temperature (T), heart rate (H), and respiratory rate (R).

MEASUREMENT OF ARTERIAL PRESSURES

The hydrostatic pressures in arteries are obtained experimentally through direct (invasive) methods and clinically by indirect (noninvasive) ones.

Direct Blood Pressure Measurement

Direct blood pressure measurement involves cannulation or transcutaneous puncture of an artery, which is then connected to a manometer or a transducer and finally to a recording system.

The classic method of recording blood pressure directly with a mercury manometer is not very different from that used by Stephen HALES, except that a column of mercury replaces the column of blood. Since the specific gravity of mercury is 13.6 times that of water (sp. gr. 1.000) and nearly 13 times that of blood (sp. gr. 1.050), the column is shortened by that much. A noncoagulating fluid (manometric fluid) is placed between the blood and the mercury to avoid any reduction in the blood volume and to prevent coagulation of blood in the tubing. Ideally the interface of manometric fluid and blood should be just outside the cannulated vessel. By bending the glass tube into a U and

obturating one end, the displacement of mercury is over a shorter length. Blood (or a manometric fluid) acting on the mercury pushes the column down in the proximal arm of the U tube and up in the distal arm. The difference between the levels of mercury in each arm of the U tube represents the blood pressure in millimeters of mercury. The historical kymographic recording system of Karl LUDWIG included a light vertical lever floating on the mercury of the distal arm and supporting a crosspiece (lever or pen) in contact with a moving surface (sooted paper) driven by a kymograph.

The mercury manometer, which cannot follow the rapid changes in pressure, is inadequate for recording rapidly and widely fluctuating pressures. Because of its inertia (weight) and its resistance to flow into the manometer, the column of mercury oscillates only slightly above and below the mean arterial blood pressure.

Accurate direct measurements of carotid or femoral arterial pressure are obtained with pressure transducers that can convert fluid displacements into recordable high-speed electrical signals (Fig. 14–1).

Clinically, the direct methods are not used because of the increase in pressure associated with restraint, pain, necessity for tranquilization, and the hazards of femoral arterial puncture. Accurate noninvasive techniques and instrumentation have been developed and adopted to measure arterial systemic pressure in dogs and horses.

Measurement of Indirect Arterial Pressures

In animals, the usual noninvasive indirect method to measure blood pressure is based on occlusion of arterial blood flow by an inflatable cuff placed around the limb. Compression of a leg artery (brachial in a horse; cranial tibial or femoral in a dog) with an occlusive cuff of appropriate size results in an auscultatory silence at a point distal to the occlusion. Upon slow and gradual decompression of the artery, the pressure when a first sound is heard indicates the systolic pressure. Upon further decompression, the sound changes and finally disappears at a value that corresponds to the diastolic pressure (Fig. 14–2).

More sophisticated noninvasive indirect methods utilize the occlusive cuff with Doppler or oscillometric techniques in a fashion similar to the simpler and less expensive auscultatory indirect method (Fig. 14–3).

Systolic, Diastolic, Pulse, and Mean Arterial Pressures

Values of the systolic and diastolic arterial blood pressures (Table 14–1) can be used to calculate the pulse pressure and the mean arterial pressure. *Systolic pressure* (P_S) is the highest pressure in the systemic arteries while blood is being

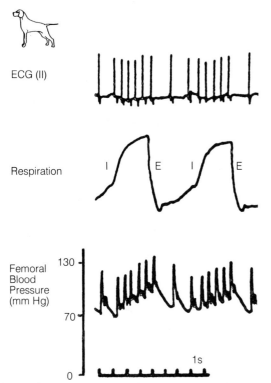

ECG (II)

Respiration

I   E   I   E

Femoral
Blood
Pressure
(mm Hg)

130

70

1s

0

Figure 14-1 Measurement of arterial pressure by the direct method. Heart rate (EKG), inspiratory (I) and expiratory (E) phases of respiration, and femoral artery blood pressure in a dog. Femoral blood pressure is recorded by the percutaneous direct method. A (special) Seldinger needle is introduced into the femoral artery, a spring guide wire is passed through the needle and advanced beyond its tip. After the needle is withdrawn from the artery and removed from the guide wire, the catheter is slipped over it and into the blood vessel, and finally the spring is withdrawn for pressure measurement. Each inspiration increases the heart rate (sinus arrhythmia) and boosts the femoral blood pressure by 15 to 20 mm Hg.

ejected from the left ventricle into the aorta (see Fig. 14-1). *Diastolic pressure* (P_d) is the lowest pressure measured during the resting phase of the heart, or diastole. The difference between systolic and diastolic pressures ($P_s - P_d$) determines the *pulse pressure* (P_p). The *mean blood pressure* ($\overline{P}_a$) is equivalent to an average arterial pressure in the system during the cardiac cycle. It is slightly lower than the arithmetic mean of the systolic and diastolic pressures. An estimate of the mean arterial blood pressure is obtained by adding 33 percent of the pulse pressure to the diastolic pressure, that is,

$$\overline{P}_a = P_d + \tfrac{1}{3}(P_s - P_d), \text{ or } P_d + \tfrac{1}{3}P_p.$$

The peak systolic pressure depends largely on the left ventricular stroke volume, the peak rate of ejection, and the distensibility of the aortic walls. During the inspiratory phase of respiration, systolic pressure may rise by about 15 mm Hg because of greater ventricular blood ejection associated with passive dilation of the intrathoracic blood cham-

bers and vessels. Inspiration, besides adding oscillations to the arterial pressure recording, also accelerates the heart rate (respiratory arrhythmia).

After ventricular systole is complete, the aortic valves are closed by a retrograde surge of blood, causing the dicrotic notch on the pressure pulse recording. After the aortic valves close, the arterial pressure gradually falls as blood flows out through the network of vessels. The rate of diastolic pressure diminution is determined by the pressure at the end of the systole, the rate of outflow throughout the vessels, and the diastolic interval. The minimal diastolic pressure depends primarily on the total peripheral resistance and on the heart rate.

Pulse pressure varies with the diastolic filling time. The pulse pressure is less when the heart rate is fast. The strength, or volume, of the pulse pressure depends on the difference between systolic and diastolic pressures. The pulse pressure widens (bigger pulse) in animals with arteriovenous fistulas (decreased peripheral resistance) and to some degree in animals with slow heart rates. A higher systolic pressure, with an increase in both pulse pressure and mean pressure, occurs without changes in peripheral resistance because of three factors: larger stroke volume, bigger ejection rate, and less arterial distensibility. These factors are exaggerated by the distortion of the pressure pulse during its transmission to the site of measurement. A higher degree of distortion may occur with valve or heart insufficiency (Fig. 14-4).

Pressures in Central and Peripheral Arteries

The systolic pressure measured at a peripheral artery is higher than that measured closer to the heart. In the femoral or brachial arteries, the systolic pressure peak is 10 to 20 mm Hg higher than that in the aorta. In beagles tranquilized with acepromazine (1 mg per kilogram), transcutaneous punctures of the femoral and aortic arteries, both coupled to a high-fidelity recording system, reveal differences in blood pressure in these arteries (Table 14-2).

The femoral systolic pressure is higher than the aortic, but the diastolic pressure is greater in the aorta than in the femoral artery of the dog. Consequently, the pulse pressure is higher in the femoral artery than in the aorta, but the mean arterial pressure in the femoral artery (90 mm Hg, or 70 + 60/3) is slightly lower than that in the aorta (95 mm Hg, or 80 + 45/3).

Arterial Pulse

The arterial pulse corresponds to a pressure wave produced by the sudden entrance of blood into a distensible tube. The tube bulges, the pressure rises at that point and is propagated at high speed along the vessel. The velocity of the pulse wave is about ten times that of the blood.

The ejection of blood from the left ventricle into the great arteries at a rate faster than its passage into the circulation is at the origin of the arterial pulse. It causes the vessel to distend at the next point while it begins to shrink at the first point because of elastic recoil. At that first point, the pressure continues to rise because of the momentum given to the

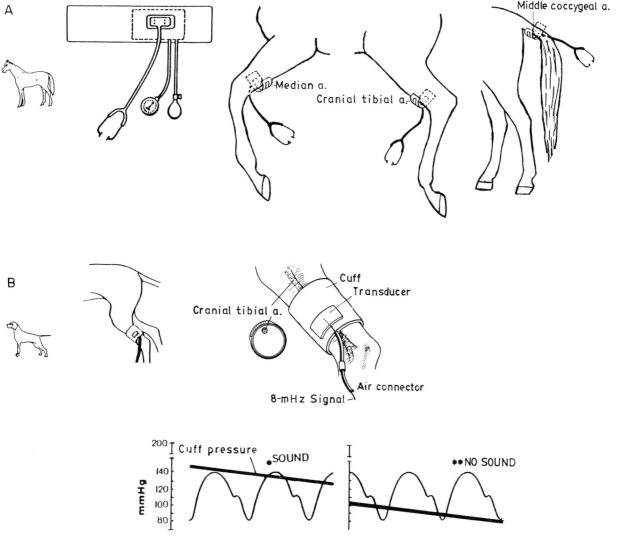

Figure 14–2   Measurement of arterial pressure by the indirect method with an occluding cuff, a pressure manometer, and auscultation. In the *horse,* the occluding cuff is usually placed over the forelimb (median artery) or over the base of the tail (middle coccygeal artery), and sometimes on the hind leg over the cranial tibial artery. The cuff is inflated to 20 to 30 mm Hg above the point of auscultatory silence. By slowly reducing the occlusion, the systolic pressure is found when the first sound is produced. Diastolic pressure is recorded when, upon further decreasing the occlusion, the auscultatory (Korotkoff) sounds disappear. **B,** In the *dog,* an apparatus combines a cuff with a transducer and a polygraph. The cuff is placed on the rear leg, over the cranial tibial artery, and the arterial pressure waves, occlusion (cuff) pressures, and signs of sound (*) and no sound (**) are recorded. The first sound (*) appears during the second arterial pulse wave, when the cuff's pressure falls below systolic pressure; the sounds disappear (**) when the occlusion pressure drops below the diastolic pressure.

blood and then falls progressively; so it goes, on down the vessel.

The contour of the arterial pulse is determined by cardiac output (stroke volume multiplied by heart rate) and peripheral vascular resistance (tone of arteries and arterioles). The form of the recorded arterial pulse changes as it passes down the arterial tree from the central (aorta) to the peripheral (carotid, radial, and femoral artery) circulation. The peripheral systolic wave is higher and more sharply peaked, whereas the peripheral diastolic wave declines and carries additional oscillations.

In animals, the arterial pulse is palpated to evaluate the number of pulsations of an artery per minute. In animals, it is felt on arteries that are most accessible: in *cats and dogs* the femoral or cranial tibial artery; in *cows,* the external maxillary, middle coccygeal, axillary (brachial), or saphenous artery; in *horses* the submaxillary, coccygeal, or transverse facial artery; and in *pigs,* the radial artery.

During palpation of the relatively slow arterial pulse of the horse, the normal dicrotic pulse (two summits) has a lower second summit, which may be relatively higher in arterial hypotension, equal (pulsus bisferiens) in aortic regur-

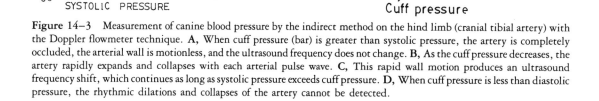

Figure 14–3 Measurement of canine blood pressure by the indirect method on the hind limb (cranial tibial artery) with the Doppler flowmeter technique. **A,** When cuff pressure (bar) is greater than systolic pressure, the artery is completely occluded, the arterial wall is motionless, and the ultrasound frequency does not change. **B,** As the cuff pressure decreases, the artery rapidly expands and collapses with each arterial pulse wave. **C,** This rapid wall motion produces an ultrasound frequency shift, which continues as long as systolic pressure exceeds cuff pressure. **D,** When cuff pressure is less than diastolic pressure, the rhythmic dilations and collapses of the artery cannot be detected.

gitation, or leaping (sharp rise and fall—"B-B shot," "water-hammer," or Corrigan's pulse) in patent ductus arteriosus. A succession of strong and weak pulses (alternating pulse) is felt in myocardial deficiencies (see Fig. 14–4). Transrectal palpation of the abdominal aorta and of its branches (cranial mesenteric, internal iliac, external iliac, and circumflex iliac artery) is useful in detecting thrombosis affecting colonic digestion and rear-leg irrigation.

VENOUS PRESSURE

The veins are dilatable channels that return blood from the capillaries to the heart. They also function as a local muscle pump when they are compressed by surrounding muscles and as a blood reservoir of varying capacity.

TABLE 14-1   Representative Values of Systemic Arterial Pressures in Adult Animals

Species	Systolic (mm Hg)	Diastolic (mm Hg)	Pulse (mm Hg)	Mean Arterial (mm Hg)
Canary	225	150	75	175
Cat	140	90	50	107
Chicken	175	145	30	155
Cow	140	95	45	110
Dog	120	70	40	87
Guinea pig	100	60	40	73
Horse	130	95	35	107
Mouse	110	80	30	90
Pig	140	80	60	100
Rabbit	120	80	40	93
Rat	100	70	30	83
Sheep	140	90	50	107
Turkey	250	170	80	197

TABLE 14-2   Simulataneous Aortic and Femoral Arterial Blood Pressure Measurements in Tranquilized Adult Beagles—Direct Method

Artery	Systolic (mm Hg)	Diastolic (mm Hg)	Pulse (mm Hg)	Mean Arterial (mm Hg)
Aortic	125	80	45	95
Femoral	130	70	60	90

Circulation of Blood in Veins

Venous pressure, which decreases from the periphery (venules) to the right atrium, usually varies from 15 mm Hg to nearly zero. The latter is the normal pressure in the right atrium. The resistance to blood flow and to venous return, negligible in the large veins (except in the neck of the giraffe), is of some importance in the venules. The pressure in the venous system is preferably expressed in millimeters of mercury above atmospheric pressure. The central venous pressure (in the right atrium and thoracic vena cava) is measured in centimeters of water (1.36 cm H_2O = 1 mm Hg).

Genesis of Venous Pressure

The forces creating the venous pressure are contraction of the left ventricle, the vacuum caused by contraction of the right ventricular and by inspiration, and the squeezing of the veins by contraction of perivenous striated muscles. The postcapillary hydrostatic pressure in the venules is a remnant of the force generated by the *left ventricle*. Each contraction of the *right ventricle* helps venous return by lowering the pressure in the right atrium at the beginning of systole and during the period of rapid filling. During *inspiration*, as the intra-thoracic pressure is lowered, the large veins dilate and fill with more blood, which increases venous blood flow toward the right atrium.

Veins in the *legs* and in some of the *abdominal viscera* have *valves* to ensure unidirectional flow of blood (*venous pump*) when the vessels are compressed from the outside (muscle pump). In the valved veins of the legs, the hydrostatic pressure may be considerable because of the weight of the blood (about 1 mm Hg for each 13 mm of the column of blood). Without muscle contractions to compress the valved veins and propel blood toward the heart, this extensive hydrostatic pressure can diminish blood volume dramatically by causing fluid to rapidly leak out of the vessels. In the *hoof* of the *horse*, with the assistance of the *valved veins* and somatic *muscles* of the legs, the *compressible corium* makes a very effective muscular pump.

Postural hypotension can occur in animals that are forced to stand erect. In a *rabbit* held vertically in a trough, postural hypotension is marked by loss of consciousness caused by inadequate cardiac output, inadequate peripheral resistance, and inadequate effective blood volume resulting from dilation of the regional blood reservoir in the abdominal veins.

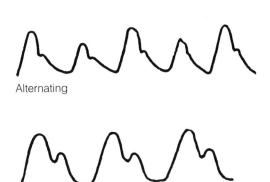

Alternating

Dicrotic

Two-Beat   (Pulsus bisferiens)

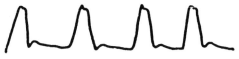

Water-Hammer

Figure 14-4   Types of arterial pulses. The slow beating of the horse heart permits identification of the normal dicrotic equine arterial pulse (two summits) where the second summit is lower than the first. It is exaggerated in arterial hypotension. An alternating pulse (i.e., a strong beat followed by a weaker beat) is abnormal and is associated with myocardial disease. The presence of two nearly equal summits of the pulse (pulsus bisferiens, or two-beat pulse) indicates aortic valve regurgitation or leakage. Arterial wall deficiencies or persistent ductus arteriosus produces a pulse with a fast rise and fall (water-hammer pulse).

These factors do not appear when the abdominal wall of the rabbit is wrapped before the animal is held vertically.

Jugular Pulse

Several waves (a, c, x, v, y) of atrial origin, transmitted to the jugular vein (*jugular pulse*), reflect the pressure changes in the right atrium associated with each cardiac cycle (Fig. 14–5).

The first positive wave (*a wave*) is associated with contraction of the right atrium. The second positive wave (*c wave*) is due to the bulging of the atrioventricular valves during contraction of the right ventricle. The third wave (*x wave*) is profoundly negative and is caused by enlargement of the right atrium when the right atrioventricular valves move away from the atrial cavity, as the base of the heart goes ventrad. The fourth wave (*v wave*) is positive and is related to arrival of some blood into the atrium and the veins during ventricular systole. The last wave (*y wave*) is negative and corresponds with opening of the right atrioventricular valve that lets atrial blood flow rapidly into the right ventricle. Insufficiency of the atrioventricular (tricuspid) valve, with marked regurgitation into the right atrium, produces a strong systolic pulsation in the jugular veins.

Central Venous Pressure

Central venous pressure (CVP) is used as an indicator of the ability of the right heart to pump the venous blood with which it is presented. The CVP is affected not only by right myocardial function but also by the venous blood volume and the venous vascular tone. It yields no information on the physiological status of the right heart.

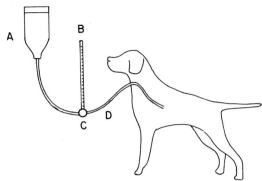

Figure 14–6 Central venous pressure measurement: *A*, infusion setup; *B*, water manometer; *C*, three-way stopcock; and *D*, intravenous catheter reaching into the right atrium. During the procedure for determining central venous pressure, the three-way stopcock is successively turned: A to B for filling B, and B to D to indicate the central venous pressure in centimeters of water.

Central venous pressure is measured by inserting a catheter into the jugular vein and connecting it through a three-way stopcock to a water manometer. The usual setup includes an intravenous infusion system (Fig. 14–6).

After sedation, local anesthesia, or short-acting anesthesia, a catheter is inserted into the jugular vein and directed into the right atrium (area of the third intercostal space). The catheter, secured in place with adhesive tape, is then connected to a three-way stopcock, two other ports of which are attached to a water manometer and to an intravenous fluid setup. The zero level of the water manometer is aligned with the right atrium (midpoint of trachea at thoracic inlet). The manometer is filled with fluid, the stopcock is turned to the jugular vein, and the fluid in the manometer is allowed to stabilize at the CVP. The operation is repeated

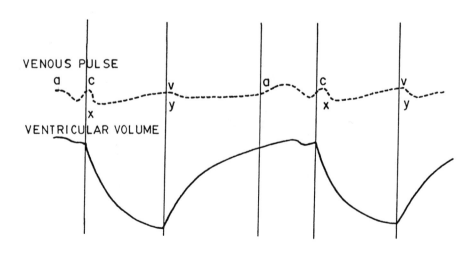

Figure 14–5 Relationship of the venous pulse, ventricular volume, and heart sounds. The *a* wave corresponds to the atrial systole and fourth sound (S_4). The *c* wave is associated with closure of the atrioventricular valves in early systole, the initial decrease of the ventricular volume, and the first sound (S_1). The *v* wave is related to closure of the arterial valves or second sound (S_2) at the beginning of diastole. The negative *x* wave is due to passive enlargement of the atrium, and the *y* wave coincides with the opening of the atrioventricular valves.

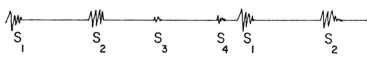

three times, and the mean is considered as the CVP, which is between -4 and 4 cm H_2O in a healthy dog.

The Veins as a Reservoir for Blood

Relatively large quantities of blood are present in the veins of the lungs, the spleen, the liver, the large abdominal veins, and the subcutaneous plexus. The veins usually contain from 65 to 75 percent of the total blood volume and, through dilation or constriction, are able to accommodate greater or lesser volumes of blood.

The walls of the larger veins (>5 mm) possess *constrictor* muscle fibers with noradrenergic sympathetic innervation. By raising the tension in the walls of the large veins, venoconstriction reduces the volume of blood in the venous circulation of viscera, thus makes more blood available to the right ventricle (increases cardiac output). During *exercise* and *hyperventilation,* as a result of a marked production of epinephrine and isoprenaline, venoconstriction and capillary vasodilation occur. The venoconstriction increases venous pressure, whereas vasodilation lowers total peripheral resistance. In the giraffe, the large veins draining the head have a heavy coat of noradrenergic smooth muscle fibers. When the head is raised, these veins constrict in order to diminish the flow of blood toward the cranial vena cava and prevent the development of an excessive hydrostatic pressure effect (about 13.6 mm blood $=$ 1 mm Hg).

By accommodating more blood in the venous reservoir, venodilation (from suppression of the venous tone) reduces the circulating blood volume and increases the venous pressure level. The elevated pressure in the veins results in production of more interstitial fluid or transudation of edema fluid and augments the pumping action in the right heart.

REGULATION OF ARTERIAL PRESSURE

Arterial blood pressure is maintained near a mean effective value by short-term and long-term regulating mechanisms.

The *short-term* controls counter acute changes in arterial pressure over seconds, minutes, or hours by modifying the heart pump and the vascular muscle tone. These short-term regulatory mechanisms include (1) the baroreceptor regulatory system, (2) the central nervous system ischemic reflex system, (3) the stress relaxation mechanism adapting the vascular dimensions to the blood volume, and (4) the capillary fluid shift mechanism.

The *long-term* regulation of mean arterial pressure, made by progressive variations in blood volume, is realized by the kidneys, which control the blood volume and the electrolyte constituents of the body fluids. The renal system operates by simple hemodynamic changes that affect arterial blood pressure, by increasing and decreasing the renal outflow of fluid and salts in response to circulatory nervous reflexes, and by providing higher or lower renal electrolyte outputs in response to aldosterone, a hormone from the adrenal cortex.

Baroreceptor Reflex System

The baroreceptors (pressoreceptors, stretch receptors), located in the walls of the arch of the aorta and above the bifurcation of the internal carotid arteries, immediately detect and react to changes in arterial pressure by negative feedback responses. The baroreceptor impulses are conducted to the medulla from the aortic arch by the aortic depressor nerve and from the carotid sinus by the carotid sinus nerve. In summary, in response to an increase in arterial pressure, the baroreceptors send nerve signals to the medullary cardioinhibitory center, which produces parasympathetic effects that counteract the arterial hypertension. Conversely, when the baroreceptors detect a low mean arterial pressure, their signals to the medullary sympathetic cardioaccelerator center bring an immediate corrective increase in arterial pressure.

Hypertension

In response to *hypertension,* the pressoreceptors send a barrage of impulses to the medulla oblongata to inhibit the sympathetic, and excite the parasympathetic, nervous systems (Fig. 14–7). Inhibition of the sympathetic nuclei results in dilation of the peripheral arterioles and reduction of peripheral resistance and arterial tension. At the same time, excitation through the vagi of the parasympathetic nuclei sending fibers to the heart further depresses both cardiac activity and arterial pressure (Fig. 14–8).

In anesthetized cats, bradycardia is produced after less than 2 minutes of experimental baroreceptor stimulation (a sudden application of 200 mm Hg to the isolated carotid sinus). Analysis of the response reveals, first, a high vagal tone and, after 45 seconds, a less pronounced inhibition of sympathetic nerves. In dogs and rabbits, aortic nerves are more effective afferent pathways than carotid sinus nerves to produce bradycardia. In rabbits, because aortic nerves run separately from the vagi, they can be easily removed, leaving the less efficient carotid sinus nerves as the afferent pathway for baroreflex cardiac slowing.

It should be reiterated that the pressoreceptor system is a short-term, not a long-term, regulator of arterial pressure. In conscious rabbits, the reflex bradycardia in response to a sudden higher arterial pressure does not persist for longer than 30 minutes, and the heart rate is eventually restored to normal during continuous arterial baroreceptor stimulation. If, because of some circulatory abnormality, the arterial pressure remains elevated for several weeks, the pressoreceptor system gradually adapts itself to this pressure level and then functions to oppose any change of pressure from the new level.

Hypotension

When the *arterial pressure falls,* the pressoreceptors emit fewer signals to the medulla oblongata. The sympathetic system is excited, and the parasympathetic system is inhibited. The arterial blood pressure then rises as a result of both the higher pumping action of the heart (inotropic action) and

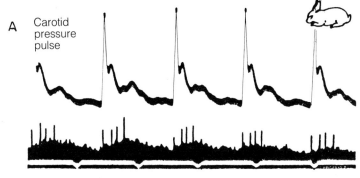

A   Carotid
    pressure
    pulse

Afferent Impulses from Carotid Sinus

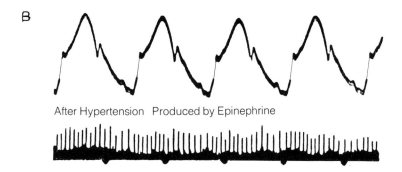

B

After Hypertension   Produced by Epinephrine

Figure 14–7 In rabbits, in response to experimental hypertension (epinephrine injection), a single carotid sinus baroreceptor produces bradycardia. The injection of a bolus of epinephrine changes the curves of the arterial pressure pulse, and the number of afferent impulses changes from pattern A (control) to pattern B (time = 1.5 seconds). In A, the heart rate is about 300 beats per minute, and the frequency of afferent discharge is near 20 per second. In B, the heart rate is lowered to 240 beats per minute, and the afferent impulses have tripled to 60 per minute.

the constriction of the peripheral vessels that elevates the peripheral resistance.

The importance of the baroreceptor mechanism in the regulation of arterial pressure is shown by occlusion of the carotid arteries of a dog, without and with reduction of cerebral blood perfusion. When the carotid sources of blood to the brain are restricted, the considerable reserve capacity of the basilar-vertebral artery supply system becomes available to prevent cerebral anoxia. Without cerebral anoxia, occlusion (partial or total) of the carotids produces only small changes in the systemic blood pressure. Unilateral occlusion of a common carotid artery decreases the perfusion of the carotid sinus region and doubles the normal basilar blood flow to the brain (9.5 ml per minute per 100 mg of brain), but systemic arterial pressure rises by only 8 percent. Occlusion of both common carotids triples the basilar arterial blood flow, whereas systemic arterial pressure is only 27 percent higher than normal. When the basilar blood flow is reduced to produce cerebral anoxia, partial or total occlusion of the common carotid artery greatly increases systemic arterial pressure.

Central Nervous System Ischemic Reflex Mechanism

The other short-term reflex regulation of arterial pressure is far more powerful than the baroreceptor reflex. The central nervous system ischemic mechanism is of particular

value when the arterial pressure approaches lethal levels (<45 mm Hg), and cerebral blood flow is inadequate. The ischemic response becomes activated at the lowest arterial pressure at which an animal can survive for 1 to 3 hours. This pressure-regulating mechanism, which can be considered a last resort, activates the sympathetic system to induce severe vasoconstriction and to facilitate myocardial contractility in an attempt to prevent the arterial pressure from falling to lethal levels. This powerful nervous ischemic response operates successfully in animals that recover from severe shock.

Stress Relaxation Mechanism in Veins

This short-term mechanism, which operates through the venous reservoirs, prevents rapid changes in systemic arterial pressure. When the blood volume increases rapidly, the veins of the circulatory system simply stretch over a period of a few minutes to accommodate the increased quantity of blood. The stress relaxation mechanism occurs without excessive elevation of the arterial pressure, since it is mainly the venous reservoir that increases its volume.

Conversely, during hemorrhage, the blood vessels (mainly the veins) begin to contract around the remaining blood volume. The force exerted by the vascular walls against the blood returns almost to normal within a few minutes. As a result, cardiac output and arterial pressure often rise back to normal, even with reduced blood volume. However, this is

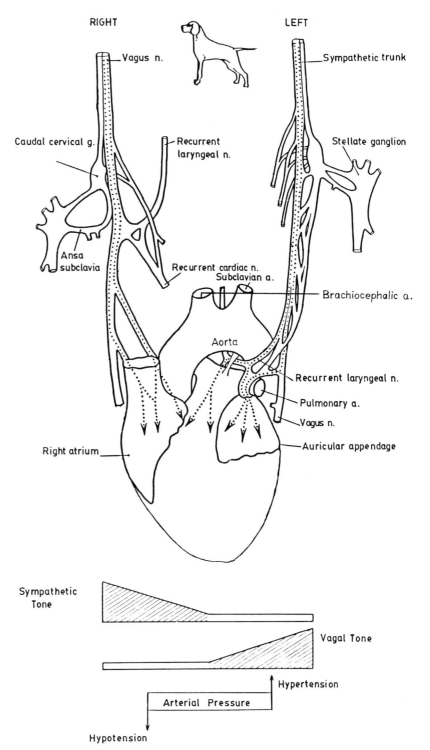

RIGHT

LEFT

Vagus n.

Sympathetic trunk

Caudal cervical g.

Recurrent
laryngeal n.

Stellate ganglion

Ansa
subclavia

Recurrent cardiac n.
Subclavian a.

Brachiocephalic a.

Aorta

Recurrent laryngeal n.

Pulmonary a.

Vagus n.

Right atrium

Auricular appendage

Sympathetic
Tone

Vagal Tone

Hypertension

Arterial Pressure

Hypotension

Figure 14–8 In dogs, excitation of the sinus or the aortic nerves or hypertension detected in the arterial baroreceptors stimulates the medullary cardioinhibitory center (increases vagal tone) and inhibits the vasoconstrictor center (decreases sympathetic tone). Conversely, hypotension stimulates the cardioaccelerator and vasoconstrictor centers (increases sympathetic tone) and inhibits the cardioinhibitory center (lowers vagal tone).

a much more slowly reacting mechanism than the 5- to 30-second pressoreceptor reflex mechanism.

Rapid loss of 15 percent of the blood volume is almost lethal to an animal whose circulatory reflexes have been blocked and are unable to protect the arterial pressure. If the animal survives this loss of blood, the arterial pressure gradually rises back to normal values over a period of 30 to 60 minutes. The pressure returns about half-way to normal every 10 minutes (e.g., 0 minute: 40 mm Hg; 10 minutes: 70 mm Hg; 20 minutes: 85 mm Hg; 30 minutes: 93 mm Hg).

Capillary Fluid Shift Mechanism

This last short-term regulatory mechanism helps temper changes in arterial pressure, particularly when the blood volume becomes too small or too great. During a rapid and voluminous transfusion to an animal, arterial pressure rises in a few seconds to as much as twice the normal values. During the ensuing 10 to 60 minutes, the arterial pressure gradually returns to normal, partly because of the reflex and stress relaxation mechanisms and of leakage of fluid out of the circulation into the interstitial spaces. Indeed, if the circulation is greatly overloaded with blood, the pores in some capillary beds are greatly stretched, which leads to even more rapid loss of fluid and protein from the circulation.

Long-Term Regulation of Arterial Pressure by the Kidneys

The long-term hemodynamic response of the kidneys to arterial hypotension is to conserve fluid and salts to augment the blood volume in the systemic circulation. Conversely, in hypertension, as a negative feedback mechanism to reduce the arterial pressure, the kidneys eliminate more fluid and salts from the circulation and reduce the blood volume. The renal control of blood volume is quantitatively the most important of all the kidney mechanisms for arterial pressure regulation.

Many different humoral mechanisms operate in conjunction with the kidneys. Some hormones are particularly important for regulation of mean arterial pressure (e.g., aldosterone and renin-angiotensin system).

SPECIAL CIRCULATIONS

The arterial perfusion of some specific organs (lungs, brain, and ruminant stomach) occurs under conditions that differ greatly from those in the systemic circulation.

Lungs

To form a closed-loop system, the pulmonary circulation is connected in series with the systemic circulation. Blood flow is equivalent in both circulations. The pressure in the pulmonary artery is only one-seventh that in the large systemic arteries (aorta) because of the shortness of its vessels and the low peripheral resistance they offer to blood flow.

Chronic lung diseases, which impair the flow of blood and increase the peripheral resistance, induce pulmonary hypertension with subsequent hypertrophy and dilation of the right ventricle. A similar experimental hypertension in the pulmonary circulation is induced by ligating one of the pulmonary arteries (Fig. 14–9). Local hypoxia also results in pulmonary hypertension by sympathetic constriction of the small arterioles, which raises the resistance to flow and the pressure inside the vessels (see Fig. 14–9).

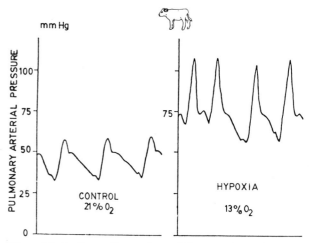

Figure 14–9 In a calf, experimental ligation of one of the two pulmonary arteries (left panel) produces hypertension in the pulmonary circulation (mean arterial pressure, 38 mm Hg). This hypertension is enhanced (mean arterial pressure, 84 mm Hg) with hypoxia (air with only 13 percent oxygen instead of the normal 21 percent).

Brain

The brains of ruminants and rabbits, like those of primates, are perfused mostly by way of the internal carotid arteries. In these species, ligation of the carotid arteries results in unconsciousness within 5 seconds, and irreversible brain damage in 4 to 5 minutes.

In contrast, the dog's internal carotid artery is poorly developed and is not the principal supplier of blood to the brain. The vertebral arteries of the dog contribute substantially to brain perfusion, as ligation of both carotids is well tolerated.

The brain, ten times more active than other tissues, produces more heat and needs to be cooled constantly. The circulation to the brain is characterized by a considerable degree of independence from the blood flow to other regions. A cooling system renders the brain independent from hyperthermia in the rest of the body.

In several animal species, a flow- and temperature-regulating mechanism is the ramification of a vessel into a plexus of smaller vessels that then reunite into a single draining vessel. Such a mechanism, termed *the rete mirabile*, is found in several species of animals and may act as a heat exchanger between arterial and venous blood.

In resting animals, the brain is cooled by venous blood coming from the the nasal cavity, which is finally drained into the jugular vein (Fig. 14–10). During hyperthermia, an additional countercurrent heat exchange seemingly occurs between the warmer carotid blood (37°C or higher) and the cooler jugular blood. In man, during hyperthermia blood is cooled in the vasodilated skin of the head and is drained into three big emissary veins located at three widely separated sites on the head.

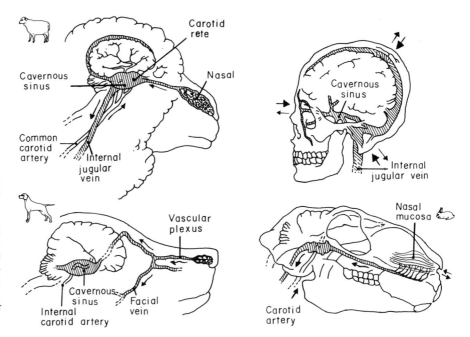

Figure 14–10 Vascular arrangement for selective brain cooling in animals. The nasal mucosa provides the normal cooling mechanism for cerebral blood of domestic animals. In addition, a system exchanges heat between the warmer carotid blood and the cooler jugular blood. In man, the heat in cerebral blood is dissipated mostly by vasodilation of subcutaneous vessels of the head.

Ruminant Stomach

The aim of the blood supply to the ruminant stomach is similar to that in other tissues (Fig. 14–11). Reticulorumen (RR) blood flow is influenced by the production of volatile fatty acids inside the RR vat, and the cyclical contractions of the forestomachs. During feeding, the RR blood flow is more voluminous. In addition, more blood perfuses the forestomach 2 to 4 hours after feeding because of chemical stimulation resulting from fermentation in the forestomachs. The increase in portal blood flow results from the richer blood flow in the RR epithelium, which is the only region where blood flow increases after feeding.

Omasal blood flow decreases during ingestion of food or feeding. This is a paradox, because the omasal epithelium is adjacent to the RR epithelium, and both have similar histology. The lower omasal blood flow may serve to reduce absorption of nutrients and delay the establishment of satiety, which would occur too early during feeding.

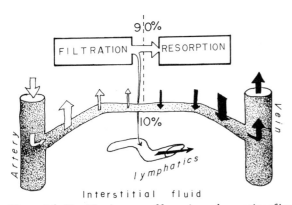

Figure 14–11 Usual pattern of formation and resorption of interstitial fluid in tissues. Filtration from blood occurs under a gradient of hydrostatic pressure. Venous (90 percent) and lymphatic (10 percent) resorption of interstitial fluid into the circulating blood is driven by osmotic gradients. The interstitial fluid contains substances from the cytoplasm of cells or added to the interstitial compartment by epithelial transfers.

REFERENCES

Alexander N, de Cuir M. Role of aortic and vagus nerves in arterial baroreflex bradycardia in rabbits. Am J Physiol 1963;205:775.

Brown AM, Duke HN, Joels N. The part played by cerebral anaemia in the response to occlusion of the common carotid arteries in the cat. J Physiol 1963;165:266.

Dobrin PB. Vascular mechanics. In: Shepherd JT, Abboud FM, eds. Handbook of physiology. Section 2: The cardiovascular system—peripheral circulation and organ blood flow. Vol III, Part 1. Bethesda, MD: American Physiological Society, 1983.

Franke FE. Sympathetic control of the dog's nasal blood vessels. Proc Soc Exp Biol Med 1966;123:544.

Hall LW, Nigam JM. Measurement of central venous pressure in horses. Vet Rec 1975;97:66.

CHAPTER 15

THE URINARY SYSTEM

Among the vital organs, such as the lungs, heart, and liver, the kidneys play a dominant role in the regulation of homeostasis. They produce urine and control (1) conservation of essential body constituents and useful nutrients, (2) elimination of waste products, (3) water and electrolyte balance, (4) acid-base balance (metabolic component), and (5) some metabolic functions of detoxification, oxidation, deamination, and enzyme activities. To accomplish these functions, the kidneys are provided with an abundant blood supply and a parenchyma with structures to purify plasma by filtration, absorption, and secretion or excretion. Renal neurohumoral secretions permit liaison with the rest of the organism, and sensor cells permit detection of some of the variants to be modulated.

The purpose of this chapter is to present the general architecture of the renal parenchyma, vessels, nerves, and functional units; the osmotic differences in the renal parenchyma; and renal dynamics.

GENERAL ARCHITECTURE OF THE KIDNEY

An understanding of the operation of the kidney requires a working knowledge of the basic morphological and functional unit, the nephron. Without overlapping into histology, some of the essential structural aspects of the kidney are presented here.

Renal Parenchyma

Examination of a longitudinal section of the kidney through the hilus gives the best illustration of the organization of the renal parenchyma. The pale cortex is seen to be sprinkled with barely visible red dots, the glomeruli, and the darker central medulla has distinct radial striations (Fig. 15–1A). The arrangement in lobes is not readily apparent, as the cortex and medulla are fused, except in the bovine kidney, which is lobate. The major components of the medulla are the loops of the nephron, the medullary collecting ducts, and particular types of blood capillaries.

Renal Vessels

The branching of the renal blood vessels is complex. The *renal artery* (division of the aorta) enters at the hilus and divides into branches radiating as *interlobar arteries* between adjacent lobes toward the cortex. From these, at the corticomedullary level, arise the *arcuate arteries*. The latter give nearly straight *interlobular arteries,* which enter the cortex and burgeon into short, straight *afferent arterioles* ending in the glomeruli (i.e., the initial part of the nephrons [Fig. 15–1B]).

A *first network* of as many as 50 parallel *capillaries* begins in each glomerulus (glomerular capillaries) as ramifications *from* the *afferent arteriole,* which merge *into* the *efferent arteriole.* The glomerular vessels are, in fact, the only capillaries in the body that drain into another arteriole (Fig. 15–1C). The diameter of the efferent arteriole is narrower than that of the afferent arteriole, fluid being lost by filtration through the walls of the glomerular capillaries.

In turn, the efferent arteriole of upper (cortical) glomeruli then breaks up into a *second network* of capillaries, the *peritubular capillaries,* which run parallel to the tubules before draining into the renal cortical vein. Some glomeruli, mostly in the juxtamedullary zone, may have a *third network* of straight (hairpin) capillaries called *vasa recta.* These straight capillaries extend into the inner medulla before looping back upward to empty into the arcuate veins in the juxtamedullary zone (Fig. 15–2).

Some interlobular arteries avoid the arcuate artery and originate directly from the interlobar artery. Straight arterioles, similar to vasa recta, originate directly from the interlobar and arcuate arteries.

On the basis of the pattern formed by their efferent vessels and according to their position in the renal cortex, glomeruli have been classified as superficial, midcortical, and juxtamedullary (Fig. 15–3). Superficial glomeruli have long efferent vessels that course to the kidney surface as *stellate venules* of the interlobular vein, often visible as star shapes on the kidney. Efferent vessels from midcortical glomeruli either divide abruptly to form peritubular plexuses near the glomeruli or form a long meshed capillary network in the medulla. Juxtamedullary efferent arterioles most often course downward to form vascular bundles, though a few divide near the glomerulus. Vasa recta capillaries drain into venules, which converge into the arcuate vein, the interlobar vein, and the renal vein.

The lymphatic circulation is prominent in the renal cortex where lymphatics follow the course of the interlobular vessels and drain into the arcuate veins. The medullary lymphatics, when they occur, drain the vasa recta system of excess protein and join the arcuate vein. After converging at the hilus of the kidney, the lymphatic vessels course as perivascular channels to the cisterna chyli and the thoracic duct. Renal lymphatics are very small and are best seen after experimental ligation of the ureter, which causes interstitial edema and marked dilation of the lymph vessels. About ten lymph channels drain each kidney of a volume of lymph nearly equivalent to the volume of urine (0.1 mL per minute). They form an essential safety net to prevent accumulation of fluid and build up of hydrostatic pressure.

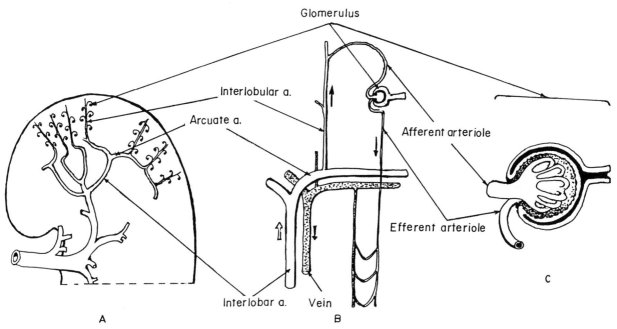

Figure 15–1 **A,** Vascular structures of the cortex and medulla of the kidney: distribution in the parenchyma of renal (hilus), interlobar (between lobes), arcuate (corticomedullary junction), interlobular (cortex) arteries. **B,** Ramification from the interlobar artery of the arcuate and interlobular arteries; origin of afferent arterioles from the interlobular arteries and of the efferent arteriole from the glomerulus. **C,** Glomerular capillaries between afferent and efferent arterioles. Glomerular space leading into the lumen of the proximal tubule (Bowman's capsule).

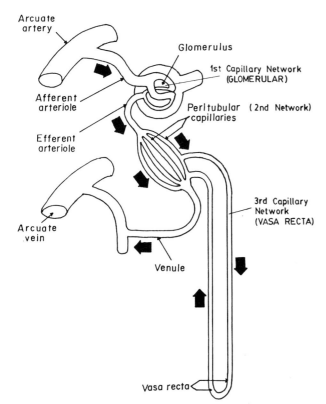

Figure 15–2 Diagram of the drainage of the efferent arteriole into peritubular and vasa recta capillaries, which then empty into the arcuate vein.

Renal Innervation

Nerve fibers enter the kidney with renal blood vessels. They are mostly efferent sympathetic fibers responsible for vasoconstriction of afferent and efferent arterioles, renal tubular cells, and juxtaglomerular cells. Other components are afferent sympathetic fibers and some cholinergic fibers, both of unknown function. Pain fibers in the visceral sheet of peritoneum adhering to the renal capsule are stimulated by acute swelling of the parenchyma (hydronephrosis, acute nephritis, acute nephrosis) and consequent stretching of the renal capsule. In hydronephrosis, a collection of urine in the pelvis of the kidney forms a cyst by producing distention and atrophy of the organ. Acute nephritis is suppurative inflammation of the kidney with a short and severe course. Acute nephrosis is any disease of the kidney characterized by degenerative lesions of the renal tubules and marked by scanty urine, with little edema (noninflammatory) or albuminuria.

Renal Functional Units

Each individual glomerulus and its efferent tubule form a nephron, the renal functional unit. Nephrons are classified as short-looped or long-looped, depending on whether their loops of Henle (loop of the nephron, nephronic loop) turn in the outer or inner medulla. Most animal species have both types of nephrons: superficial glomeruli are short-looped nephrons, juxtamedullary glomeruli are long looped, and midcortical glomeruli are of both types. Some species have only short-looped nephrons (beaver, muskrat) or long-looped nephrons (cat, dog).

Zonation into an outer and inner medulla is based on tubular criteria. The inner medulla, with a broad basis tapering to a thin papilla, contains the thin segments of the long-looped tubules of Henle (see Fig. 15–3). Within the outer medulla are two zones, the outer and inner stripes. The inner stripe is defined as the region in which thin descending limbs overlap thick ascending limbs. The inside border of the outer medulla, defined by the beginning of the thick ascending limbs of Henle's loops, contains thin limbs and collecting ducts (see Fig. 15–3). The corticomedullary margin of the outer medulla is usually taken arbitrarily as the level of arcuate arteries or the level of the lowest glomeruli.

The tubules of the nephron are divided into proximal convoluted tubule, loop of Henle, and distal convoluted tubule. The tubular surface approximates that of the blood capillaries, 12 square meters. A loop of Henle consists of four segments: a thick descending limb (*pars recta* of the proximal tubule), thin descending limb, thin ascending limb, and thick ascending limb (*pars recta* of the distal tubule). The terminal portion of the thick ascending limb contains the *macula densa,* which interacts with glomerular vascular ele-

ments (juxtaglomerular cells?) in a tubuloglomerular feedback mechanism for local adjustment of vascular resistance.

The traditional divisions of the distal tubule are ascending thick limb (*pars recta*) of the loop of Henle, the macula densa region, and the distal convoluted tubule. New knowledge (morphological and physiological) makes it more suitable to divide the distal tubule into a medullary ascending thick limb of the loop of Henle (MAT), a cortical ascending thick limb of the loop of Henle (CAT), and the distal convoluted tubule (DCT). The *macula densa* would now be incorporated into the CAT (Fig. 15–4).

The collecting duct, which can be divided into cortical, medullary, and papillary portions, drains the tubules of several nephrons. It plays a vital role in the control of acid-base balance and potassium homeostasis, and it is the primary site of action of antidiuretic hormone (ADH).

OSMOLAL ANATOMY OF THE RENAL PARENCHYMA

In all species, the osmolality of the cortical kidney tissue is the same as that of plasma, approximately 300

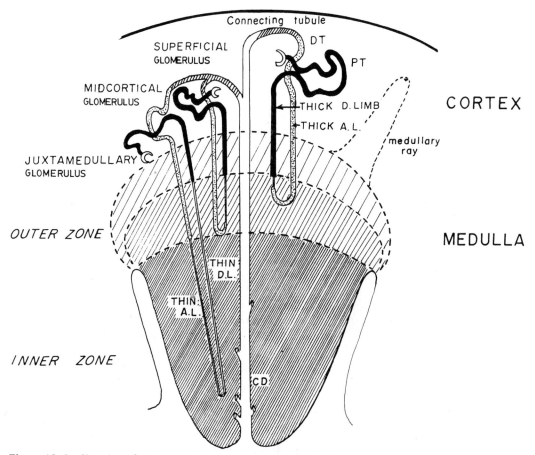

Figure 15–3 Short-looped nephrons originate from superficial and midcortical glomeruli. Long-looped nephrons have glomeruli in the midcortex and the juxtamedullary cortex. The inner medulla (only thin segments) and the outer medulla with its outer (thick descending and ascending) and inner (thin descending overlap thick descending) stripes are delimited.

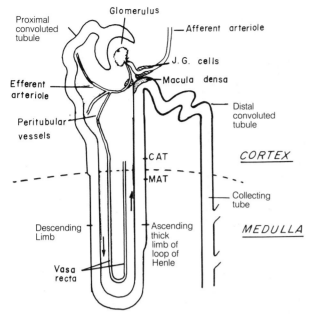

Proximal convoluted tubule

Glomerulus

Afferent arteriole

J.G. cells

Macula densa

Efferent arteriole

Peritubular vessels

Distal convoluted tubule

CAT

MAT

CORTEX

Collecting tube

Descending Limb

Ascending thick limb of loop of Henle

MEDULLA

Vasa recta

Figure 15–4 Simplified diagram of a nephron with its glomerulus continued by traditional divisions of the S-shaped tubule, and of a collecting duct shared by several nephrons. Also shown are the location of the juxtaglomerular cells and the macula densa. The terminology of the new divisions of the distal tubule and collecting duct is also indicated: MAT, medullary ascending thick limb of the loop of Henle; CAT, cortical ascending thick limb of the loop of Henle; DCT, distal convoluted tubule.

mOsm per liter. Within the medulla, osmolality increases progressively from the corticomedullary junction to the papilla; in some species, it can be as high as 5,600 mOsm per liter.

To achieve hyperosmolality in the medullary interstitium, several mechanisms cooperate. Collectively they are called the countercurrent multiplier mechanism of the loops of Henle (Fig. 15–5), because some of them require countercurrent fluid flows in the loops of the nephron and collecting duct. In the thin segment of the loop of Henle, sodium and chloride are passively transported into the interstitium; from the thick segment of the ascending limb of the loop of Henle, ions (sodium, chloride, potassium, calcium, magnesium) actively cross into the interstitium; from the inner medulla collecting duct, urea diffuses passively while ions are also transported actively into the interstitium. These can occur because of special characteristics of blood flow that prevent removal of excess solutes from the interstitium: very sluggish flow of blood in the medulla, and a countercurrent exchange of solutes and fluid between the two arms of the vasa recta. As blood progresses down the loops, it gradually gains particles of solutes to be isoosmolal to the interstitium. As it goes up the other arm of the vasa recta, the process is reversed: blood osmolality gradually decreases to the renal cortex level (see Fig. 15–5). These conditions maintain high concentrations of solutes at the tip of the loop with negligible washout of solutes.

The ratio of the maximal medullary osmolality to cortical osmolality is an index of the concentration potential between animal species (Table 15–1). These values can serve as a basis to explain that the beaver cannot have a urine with more than twice the osmotic concentration of plasma. They can be used to understand why the urine of the cat may be more concentrated than that of the dog. The concept is useful to compare and predict the potential for concentration of urine in different species. The relative depth of the medulla (corticopapillary) is also related to the ability of the kidney of an animal species to concentrate urine (Fig. 15–6).

RENAL HEMODYNAMICS

The kidneys represent less than 0.5 percent of the body mass, but 15 to 20 percent of the cardiac output circulates in their rapidly dividing system of vessels. Most blood is directed to the cortical area (74 percent), and the rest goes to the outer medulla (21 percent), inner medulla (2.5 percent), and hilar and perirenal fat (2.5 percent). In the cortex, blood passes in greater quantity, and its velocity is also greater than that in the medulla. Flow of blood is sluggish in the vessels of the medulla and slowest in the inner medulla. Oxygen consumption, which is slight (total: about 6 mL per 100 g per minute) compared with that in other tissues, follows the same pattern as blood flow and blood velocity: highest at the cortex (9 mL per 100 g per minute) and lowest at the inner medulla (0.4 mL per 100 g per minute).

In the renal cortex and the outer medulla, blood flow is autoregulated; it remains relatively stable despite large changes in arteriolar blood pressure (80 to 200 mm Hg). Two hypotheses, myogenic and metabolic, compete to explain, in part, this intrinsic capacity to compensate for changes in perfusion pressure by changing vascular resistance so that blood flow remains relatively steady. The *myogenic theory* is based on the intrinsic contractile response of smooth muscle to stretch. As the pressure rises, the blood vessels are distended, and the vascular smooth muscles in their walls contract. Conversely, if the pressure falls, vasodilation occurs. According to the *metabolic theory,* when blood flow is lowered, metabolites accumulate and dilate the vessels. As blood flow increases, these metabolites tend to be washed away.

Renal Vasoconstriction

By renal oncography (or renal plethysmography), evident changes in renal volumes occur upon stimulation of renal nerves. The predominant adrenergic fibers exert vasoconstrictive effects and lower renal blood flow to reduce the volume of the kidney encased in the oncometer. Severe hypoxia also produces vasoconstriction through a chemoreceptor–vasomotor center–sympathetic nerve reflex. Exercise reduces blood flow by vasoconstriction. As a result of vasoconstriction, renal blood flow is redistributed: it is decreased from its 90 percent value in the renal cortex (ischemia) and is

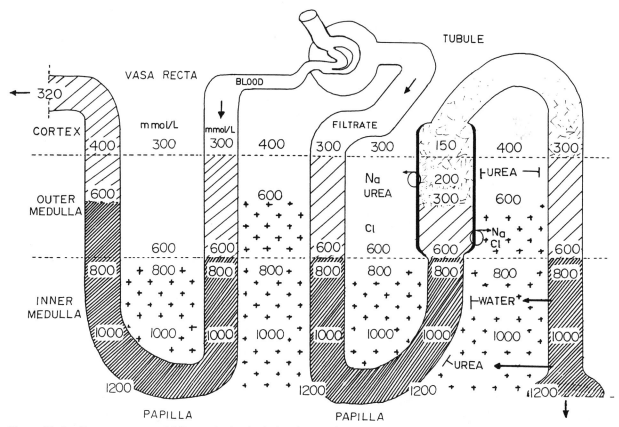

Figure 15-5 Countercurrent multiplier mechanism in the long loops and the vasa recta. Because of a continuous input of solutes (urea and sodium chloride mostly) in the interstitium, the descending vasa recta carries blood that is several times hyperosmolal to plasma at the tip, then gradually returns to near isoosmolality in the ascending vasa recta. In the process, the interstitium does not lose solute, but tubular fluid loses water from the collecting duct to the interstitium.

TABLE 15-1 Osmolality of Renal Medulla and Cortex and Their Ratio in Animal Species

Species	Medulla (mOsm/L)	Cortex (mOsm/L)	Medulla-Cortex Ratio
Beaver	600	300	2
Camel	3,180	300	10.6
Cat	3,300	300	11
Cattle	2,600	300	8.7
Dik-dik (antelope)	4,060	300	13.5
Dog	2,400	300	8
Donkey	1,600	300	5.3
Goat	2,900	300	9.7
Impala (antelope)	2,500	300	8.3
Kangaroo rat	5,600	300	18.7
Man	1,500	300	5
Oryx (antelope)	3,000	300	10
Pig	1,100*	300	3.6
Rabbit	1,800	300	6
Rat	2,400	300	8
Sheep	3,500	300	11.7
Zebu cattle	1,400	300	4.7

* Identical with sea water (1,100 mOsm/L)

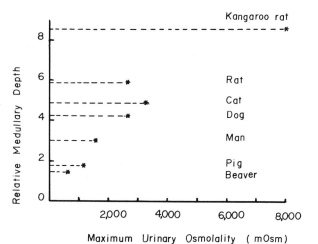

Figure 15-6 Relation of the relative thickness of the renal medulla in several species of animals and the maximal urinary osmolality or the renal water recuperation potential.

increased from its 10 percent value (hyperemia) in the medulla. This reversal of flow causes a washout of sodium chloride from the interstitium and reduces the ability to produce concentrated urine. Catecholamines (epinephrine, norepinephrine) in small doses cause greater constriction in the efferent than in the afferent arterioles, so that the glomerular filtration rate (GFR) is maintained, but renal blood flow (RBF) is decreased. However, a large dose depresses the GFR. In addition, the action of epinephrine includes constriction of renal veins, which results in swelling of the kidneys. Ether, barbiturates, and other anesthetics also have renal vasoconstrictive effects.

Epinephrine and norepinephrine are hormones from the adrenal medulla. They are postganglionic mediators of nerve transmission in sympathetic fibers. Norepinephrine does not have the effects of epinephrine on cardiac output and on glycemia.

Oncography is the recording of volume changes detected by an instrument (oncometer) that consists of a capsule enclosing an organ such as the kidney or the spleen.

Renal Vasodilation

Vasodilation may result from a high-protein diet. Sympatholytics lower arterial pressure and blood flow. Hydralazine directly relaxes arterial smooth muscle to lower arterial pressure and hyperdynamizes the heart (increases heart rate, stroke volume, and cardiac output) to improve blood flow.

Renal blood pressure gradually decreases from the renal artery to the renal vein. Graphically, the decline in pressure is represented by two sloping stages, at each end of the arteriovenous circuit, separated by an abrupt pressure drop between the capillaries of the efferent arteriole and the venous peritubular capillaries (Fig. 15–7).

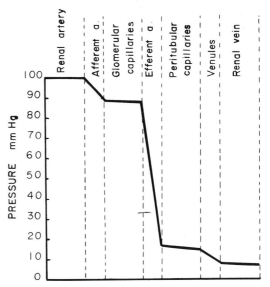

Figure 15–7 Hydrostatic pressure of blood in the renal arteriovenous compartments.

REFERENCES

Beeuwkes R. The vascular organization of the kidney. Annu Rev Physiol 1980;42:531.

Bulger RE, Dobyan DC. Recent advances in renal morphology. Annu Rev Physiol 1982;44:147.

Kriz W. Structural organization of the renal medullary counterflow system. Fed Proc 1983;42:2379.

Mayerson HS. The physiologic importance of lymph. In: Hamilton WF, Dow P, eds. Handbook of physiology. Section 2. Circulation. Vol II. Washington, DC: American Physiological Society, 1963:pp.1035–1073.

Stephenson JL. Renal concentrating mechanism. Fed Proc 1983;42:2377.

CHAPTER 16

FORMATION OF URINE

Formation of urine is the renal mechanism that regulates the composition of plasma and the excretion of nitrogenous waste. The simplistic working principle is to put a portion of the extracellular fluid outside the organism, then recover from it what is useful and add to it, if necessary, what must be eliminated rapidly. The process requires formation of a primitive urine by a filtration apparatus, the glomerulus, and its circulation in microscopic vessels (tubules and collecting ducts) composed of specialized cells. Substances are transferred from this filtrate to cells (reabsorption) or from cells to the filtrate (secretion or excretion). The basic functional unit responsible for urine formation is the nephron. This chapter describes the glomerular structures of the nephron involved in the mechanisms of filtration, the tubules and collecting duct operating reabsorption and secretion or excretion, and the concept of clearance.

GLOMERULAR FILTRATION

Structure of the Glomerulus

The glomerulus represents an extensive capillary network embedded in a capsule forming a collection space that opens into the tubular lumen of the nephron (Fig. 16–1). The capsule (Bowman's capsule, or glomerular capsule) is a double-walled, hollow structure with a space (urinary chamber, capsular space, or Bowman's space) between the two layers, continuous with the lumen of the proximal tubule.

The outer, or parietal, layer of the capsule is made up of squamous epithelial cells and their basement membrane. The cells, bound closely by junctional complexes, and their basement membrane are continuous with the epithelium and basement membrane of the proximal tubule.

The inner, or visceral, wall of the capsular space is formed of cells called podocytes (visceral epithelial cells) with numerous large arms extending out of the cell body. These large arms, in turn, give rise to pedicels that interdigitate with adjacent pedicels and adhere to the glomerular basement membrane (Fig. 16–2). These pedicels are bridged by a thin structure called the filtration slit membrane. The glomerular basement membrane separates the podocytes from the capillary endothelial cells.

Glomerular capillary walls, made up of extremely thin endothelial cells, are fenestrated by a multitude of endothelial pores (see Fig. 16–2). The capillary endothelium is on the glomerular basement membrane, on the side opposite the podocytes.

A third type of glomerular cell, the mesangial cell, situated between the capillaries (see Fig. 16–2), forms the supporting stalk of the glomerulus and physically stabilizes the capillary loop. It contains an abundance of myofilaments and is able to contract in response to a variety of stimuli (e.g., angiotensin II, antidiuretic hormone [ADH]). Contraction of the mesangial cells may decrease the caliber of all the attached vessels and reduce the glomerular surface area for ultrafiltration (i.e., may lower the glomerular ultrafiltration coefficient [K_f]). The glomerulus also contains numerous *receptors* for hormones (parathormone, PTH) or vasodilator substances (PGEs, or prostaglandins E_1 and E_2; prostacyclin, or PGI_2; acetylcholine; bradykinin; and histamine), and *enzymes* for the synthesis of several hormones (renin, PGI_2, PGE_2, and thromboxane A_2, or TXA_2).

Filtration Barrier

The glomerulus acts as an ultrafilter that passes electrolytes and small molecules (e.g., glucose) but retains large molecules (e.g., proteins) and cellular elements (red and white blood cells). Since a small quantity of plasma albumin can appear in the glomerular filtrate, it is inferred that the size of the filtration barrier is near 70,000 daltons (i.e., the molecular mass of plasma albumin). Hemoglobin released from hemolyzed erythrocytes and dissolved in plasma can cross the glomerular barrier and appear in the urine, as its molecular mass is less than 70,000 daltons. The filtration barrier is 100 times more permeable than the capillaries of skeletal muscle.

The filtration barrier is made up of three layers (Fig. 16–3): the *porous capillary endothelium* (see Fig. 16–2), which stops substances of more than 450,000 daltons; the *basement membrane,* with a collagen-like structure sufficiently loose to let substances of 160,000 daltons pass freely; and the *filtration slit membrane,* which bridges the pedicels and is the main impediment to substances of 40,000 to 70,000 daltons of molecular mass.

Effective Filtration Pressure

The formation of the glomerular filtrate (primitive urine) results from the interaction of force or pressure vectors creating the filtration gradient, the effective filtration pressure (EFP). The *driving force* is the hydrostatic pressure inside the glomerular capillaries (glomerular arterial pressure), which is about 90 mm Hg. The glomerular arterial pressure (P_c) value is nearly that of the mean arterial pressure (diastolic pressure plus one-third of pulse pressure). It is higher than in other capillaries because the glomeruli are relatively close to the aorta and are at the end of short, straight afferent arterioles.

The *opposing forces* are (1) the oncotic pressure (π_{pl}) of the

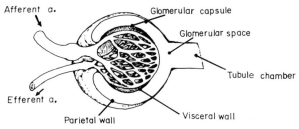

Figure 16–1 Glomerulus embedded in the glomerular capsule and creating the parietal and visceral walls of the glomerular space, which opens into the tubular lumen.

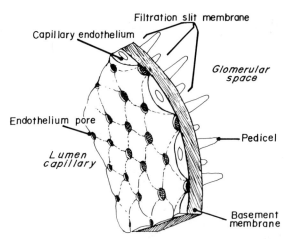

Figure 16–3 Layers of the filtration barrier of the glomerulus: capillary endothelium (with endothelial pores), basement membrane of loose conjunctive *fibrillae*, and pedicels separated by the filtration slit pores of filtration slit membrane.

plasma proteins in the blood processed in the glomerular capillaries (about 30 mm Hg), and (2) the hydrostatic pressure in the glomerular space (P_t) (Fig. 16–4).

The effective filtration pressure is influenced by changes (1) in the hydrostatic pressures in the glomerular capillaries (P_c) by a pressure beyond the autoregulated interval of 75 to 150 mm Hg or in the glomerular space (P_t) by ureteral obstruction or by edema of the kidney inside the tight renal capsule; and (2) in oncotic pressure (π_{pl}) by a decrease in plasma protein (hypoproteinemia).

Juxtaglomerular Complex

Near the glomerulus, the walls of the afferent and efferent arterioles present a covering of specialized granular cells, the juxtaglomerular cells. These cells are in contact with special cells (*macula densa*) in the wall of the distal convoluted tubule of the same nephron (see Fig. 16–4). This juxtaglomerular complex regulates the glomerular filtration through a *tubuloglomerular neuroendocrine feedback*. A lack of chloride in the tubular fluid detected by the macula densa is signaled causing afferent arteriolar dilation and efferent arteriolar constriction to increase the filtration and blood flow in the glomerulus.

Filtration Fraction

The fraction of the renal plasma flowing in both kidneys that becomes glomerular filtrate is called the filtration fraction. The average filtration fraction is nearly 20 percent of the total plasma going through the kidneys.

Glomerular Filtration Rate

The glomerular filtration rate (GFR) is the quantity of glomerular filtrate formed in all the nephrons of both kidneys. It is directly related to the effective filtration pressure (EFP) and the ultrafiltration coefficient (K_f), which is a function of the surface area. Over 99 percent of this filtrate is recovered in the tubules, the remainder being urine.

The GFR can be represented by the *clearance* of a substance that is only filtered and is not transported (reabsorbed, secreted, or excreted) by the tubular cells. The clearance concept is theoretical, since it represents the volume of plasma that is completely cleared of a substance per unit of time (milliliters per minute). Obviously, no single milliliter of blood has all of that substance removed in one transit through the kidneys. At each passage, a little portion of substance is removed from each of the milliliters of blood perfusing the kidneys.

GFR varies with changes in hydrostatic and oncotic pressures that affect the effective filtration pressure; with changes in permeability and surface area of the filtration barrier (ultrafiltration coefficient) by renal disease; and with changes in the number of functional nephrons owing to

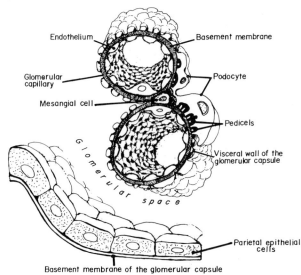

Figure 16–2 **A,** Arrangement of cells in the afferent and efferent arterioles, the capillary endothelium, and the visceral and parietal walls of the glomerular capsule. **B,** Fenestrations in the capillary endothelium; relations of mesangial cells with the basement membrane, the capillary endothelial cells, and the pedicels of the podocytes (visceral epithelial cells of the glomerular capsule).

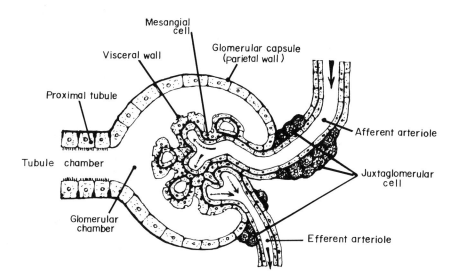

Figure 16–4 Interaction of the pressure vectors in the glomerulus to provide the effective filtration pressure.

glomeruli-destroying disease or loss of renal tissue through trauma or surgery.

An increased GFR results in loss of water and solutes from the organism. A deficit in GFR has opposite effects, causing insufficient elimination of unwanted products. Variation of ± 5 percent is sufficient to bring excessive deprivation or retention of water and solutes.

TUBULE AND COLLECTING DUCT TRANSPORTS

Glomerular filtrate must continuously evacuate the initial, or glomerular, part of the nephron to enter the second part of the nephron, the tubule. Along this course, the tubule cells selectively reabsorb and excrete or secrete substances.

Since 99 percent of the water (with dissolved substances) in the glomerular filtrate is reabsorbed in the tubules and the collecting ducts, reabsorption is quantitatively more important than secretion or excretion. Some substances, such as glucose and amino acids, are reabsorbed entirely and are not found in urine. Tubule cells excrete substances already in the plasma or synthesize substances from components present in plasma and secrete them in the fluid circulating in the tubule lumen.

A substance is excreted by the tubule cells when it is present in the plasma. Substances secreted by the tubule cells are not present in the plasma but are synthesized from chemical units found in it. Practically, this distinction is ignored, and it is common usage to refer only to the secretion of the tubules.

Structures of the Tubules

Proximal Tubule

The proximal tubule is the longest part of the tubule portion of the nephron. Its structure is well-suited for reab-

sorption and secretion. In kidneys perfused with a tissue fixative, the lumen is open, whereas in renal tissues fixed without perfusion or from biopsies, the tubules are collapsed.

Cells of the proximal tubules have an acidophilic cytoplasm, and their nuclei lie basally. The luminal margin is lined by a brush border layer of microvilli that increase the surface in contact with the tubule fluid (primitive urine) by a factor of 20. These microvilli, similar to those of the small intestine, participate in glucose and amino acid absorption. The cells are tightly attached to each other by *zona occludens* (tight junctions), which leave considerable lateral intercellular space (Fig. 16–5). Numerous basal channels, made by folds in the basal membrane, multiply the surface area adjacent to the basement membrane. Mitochondria, found mostly near the lateral surface and also near the basal mem-

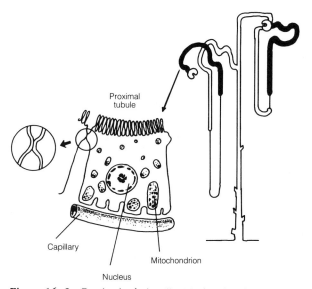

Figure 16–5 Proximal tubule cell with abundant brush border, elongated mitochondria, and basal channels.

brane, supply energy for active transport—*active reabsorption* of sodium, calcium, potassium, chloride, phosphate, and urate and *active secretion* of hydrogen, organic acids, and bases. It should be recalled that glucose and amino acids are absorbed by sodium cotransport; once inside the cell, they diffuse out while sodium is actively expelled at the basolateral membrane.

The bulk of the glomerular filtrate is reabsorbed in the proximal tubule. About 80 percent of the water and electrolytes and essentially all filtered glucose, amino acids, and proteins are removed in this segment, which also secretes many organic acids and bases.

Loop of Henle

The cells of the thick descending part (*pars recta*) of the loop of Henle differ slightly from those of the proximal tubule: they are more cuboidal, with brush borders still well-developed.

In the thin segment, the cells are flattened and do not have a brush border (Fig. 16–6). The few small mitochondria indicate the limited metabolic activity of these cells. The descending portion, highly permeable to water and moderately to urea and most other ions, is primarily for simple diffusion of substances in either direction between the filtrate and the medullary interstitium. Comparatively, the descending portion is less permeable to water and solutes such as urea and ions.

In the thick ascending limb of the loop of Henle, the cells are not identical with those of the distal tubule. Brush border is absent on the apical surface, which has only a few microvilli; the nucleus is near the apex; the cytoplasm is excessively rich in mitochondria; and the basal channels are numerous. Sodium, potassium, and chloride are cotransported in the thick ascending limb, and the tubule fluid becomes hypotonic to plasma when it reaches the distal tubule.

Distal Tubule

The distal tubule originates at the junction of the inner and outer medulla as the medullary ascending thick (MAT) limb of the loop of Henle. It has cells connected by relatively shallow tight junctions, which are provided with elaborate basolateral interdigitations and long mitochondria (Fig. 16–7), and are stimulated by aldosterone to reabsorb sodium chloride. The thinnest part of the distal tubule, known as the cortical ascending thick (CAT) limb of the loop of Henle, has a few stubby mitochondria that are not orderly arranged and respond to parathyroid hormone (PTH) for reabsorption of calcium.

The distal tubule courses between the afferent and efferent arterioles of its glomerulus and ends with a small segment of specialized cells known as the *macula densa*. In these cells, the nuclei are closely grouped into what looks like a dense spot, and the polarity is reversed, with the active

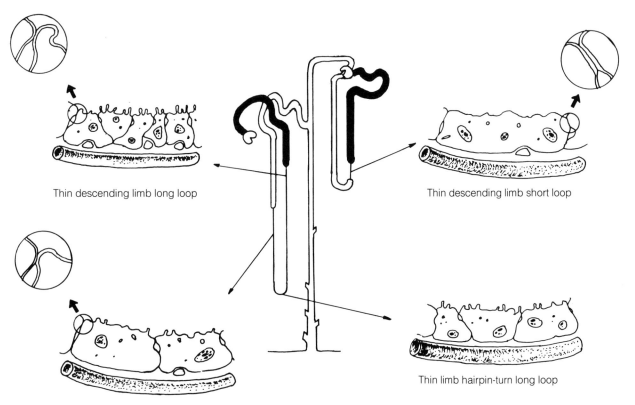

Thin descending limb long loop

Thin descending limb short loop

Thin ascending limb long loop

Thin limb hairpin-turn long loop

Figure 16–6 Flattened cells of the thin limbs of the loop of Henle, with one or two small mitochondria and without brush borders.

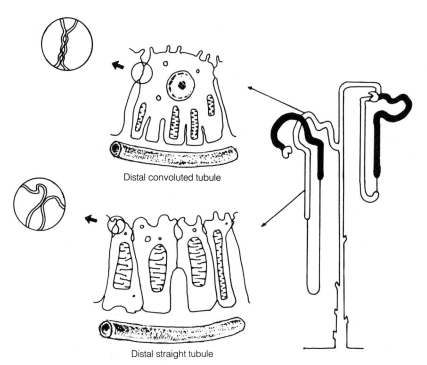

Distal convoluted tubule

Distal straight tubule

Figure 16–7 Changes in the morphology of cells in the distal tubule: **A,** straight, **B,** convoluted.

surface toward the base instead of the apex, as in other tubule cells. The cells of the macula densa are the detector in the tubuloglomerular negative-feedback mechanism leading to glomerular production of renin.

The last tubule segment of the nephron, the *distal convoluted tubule* (DCT), arises abruptly from the post–*macula densa* segment cortical ascending limb of the loop of Henle. The cells are taller and excessively interdigitated and contain long mitochondria (Fig. 16–7). The DCT ends in the connecting tubule, which connects the nephron with the collecting duct. In its terminal portions, the DCT may have (rat, not rabbit) intercalated cells as in the connecting segment. The role of the DCT is mainly to reabsorb sodium, potassium, chloride, and divalent ions.

Connecting Tubule

It is still debated whether the connecting tubule is part of the nephron or of the collecting tube. The cells of the connecting tubules are of two types: principal (light cells) and intercalated (dark cells). The principal cell has a clear cytoplasm, a central nucleus, and several small mitochondria. The less common intercalated cell (absent in the inner medulla) has a more intensely staining cytoplasm and carries more and larger mitochondria.

Collecting Duct

The collecting duct courses from the cortex, through the medulla and empties into the pelvis. It can be divided into cortical (CCD), medullary (MCD), and papillary (PCD) portions. The epithelial cells that line the collecting duct are of two main types: the common principal cell, found along the entire collecting duct tree, and the intercalated cell, identical with those of the connecting tubule, which appears to be localized in the cortex and outer medulla (Fig. 16–8).

The collecting duct is more than a passive conduit collecting fluid from several nephrons. Mostly through the intercalated cells, it acts as the final mediator of normal fluid and electrolyte balance. It plays a vital role in the control of acid-base balance and potassium homeostasis in addition to being the primary site of action of antidiuretic hormone (ADH).

THE CONCEPT OF RENAL CLEARANCE

The concept of clearance can be used to assess renal function. Renal clearance represents the virtual volume of plasma totally cleared of a substance per unit of time (C_x), usually milliliters per minute. Its determination requires a timed collection of urine to measure the urine flow, or minute volume ($\dot{V}$), and the concentration of the substance (in milligrams per milliliter) in plasma (P_x) and in urine (U_x). Calculations are figured according to the following formula:

$$C_x = (U_x \times \dot{V})/P_x$$

The renal clearance of any substance that is not protein bound and is freely filterable may be determined. By comparison with the clearance of inulin and of creatinine, which are only filtered and reflect GFR, the extent of any tubule and collecting duct reabsorption or secretion can be evaluated (Table 16–1). A substance that has a clearance *less* than that

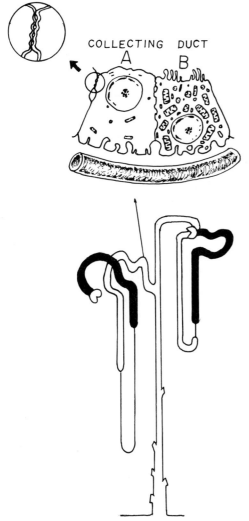

COLLECTING DUCT
A B

Figure 16–8 Principal cell (**A**) and intercalated cell (**B**) of the collecting duct.

TABLE 16–1 Renal Clearance of Various Substances

Substances	Clearance (mL/min/kg)
Filtered only	
Creatinine	2
Inulin	1.8
Filtered and reabsorbed	
Bicarbonate	0.007
Calcium	0.017
Chloride	0.02
Glucose	0
Magnesium	0.07
Phosphate	0.36
Potassium	0.17
Sodium	0.013
Sulfate	0.67
Urea	1
Uric acid	0.24
Filtered and secreted	
Diodrast	8
PAH	8.36

cantly excreted nor absorbed by the tubules. Changes in the C_x to C_{cr} ratio result from changes in C_x. The advantage of a ratio relationship is derived from the *mathematical elimination* of volumetric and timed urine measurement. The remaining requirements are the chemical determination of the substance and of the creatinine in a sample of plasma and of urine.

The mathematical transformation is as follows:

$$C_x/C_{cr} = \frac{(U_x \times V)/P_x}{(U_{cr} \times V)/P_{cr}}.$$

By simplifying the volumes (V), the relation becomes

$$C_x/C_{cr} = \frac{U_x/P_x}{U_{cr}/P_{cr}}$$

which can be transposed as

$$C_x/C_{cr} = (U_x/P_x) \times (P_{cr}/U_{cr})$$

and expressed as a percentage ratio

$$\% \ C_x/C_{cr} = (U_x/P_x) \times (P_{cr}/U_{cr}) \times 100.$$

In the horse, the percentage clearance ratio is 0.2 to 1 percent for sodium and phosphate, and 16 to 65 percent for potassium. In tubule failure, these values are elevated.

Further simplification for computing the urinary clearance ratio of phosphorus to creatinine has been reported. The concentration of phosphorus and creatinine in a single urine sample has been measured and the percentage calculated: $U_P/U_{cr} \times 100$. The rationale behind this test is that a relatively constant amount of creatinine is generally excreted by the kidney. The ratio is reduced in phosphorus deficiency, owing to decreased urinary excretion. The ratio is increased in calcium deficiency or phosphorus excess, owing to increased renal excretion of phosphorus.

of inulin or creatinine has undergone net reabsorption, whereas a substance with a clearance *greater* than that of inulin or creatinine has obviously been secreted by cells of the tubules or the collecting duct.

In practice, the clearance of endogenous creatinine is preferred to that of inulin (a polysaccharide derivative of fructose), which is cumbersome. Creatinine, an end-product of creatinine phosphate catabolism, has plasma and renal concentrations that are reasonably constant and can be measured colorimetrically.

Creatinine Clearance Ratio

The ratio of the clearance of a substance (C_x) to the clearance of creatinine (C_{cr}) indicates the extent to which that substance is being excreted or conserved by the tubules. This is so because the relationship of creatinine clearance to GFR is a constant; once creatinine is filtered, it is neither signifi-

Sodium Sulfanilate Clearance Test

This clearance test has been used in the horse and the dog to assess GFR and to detect renal disease before azotemia (increased blood urea nitrogen, BUN) develops. Sodium sulfanilate (20 percent solution) is given intravenously (10 mg per kilogram), then heparinized blood is sampled at 30, 60, and 90 minutes. The concentrations of sodium sulfanilate, measured colorimetrically, are plotted on semilogarithmic graph paper, and the clearance half-time is calculated. The average sodium sulfanilate clearance is 40 ± 4 minutes for a normal horse and 55 to 80 minutes (mean 65) for a normal dog. The clearance rate of sodium sulfanilate from blood measures glomerular function in a way similar to that of inulin and creatinine clearance. The kidney of the horse clears sodium sulfanilate more rapidly than the kidney of the dog, and glomerular filtration rate is greater in the horse than in the dog.

Clearance of Paraaminohippuric Acid

Besides being filtered, 90 percent of paraaminohippuric acid (PAH) passing through the glomerulus and remaining in the plasma is secreted by the tubule cells into the glomerular filtrate. On a single pass through the nephron, PAH is cleared from plasma. The clearance rate of PAH is used for estimating the flow of plasma through the kidney. The quantity of plasma cleared of PAH each minute corresponds to the volume of plasma that must have passed through the kidney during that period of time. With a correction for the amount of PAH not cleared or still in the blood when it leaves the kidney (10 percent), the amount of plasma flowing through the kidney (renal plasma flow, RPF) can be calculated by the formula

$$RPF = (Clearance\ PAH/90) \times 100.$$

With the value from Table 16–1 (i.e., 585 mL),

$$RPF = (585/90) \times 100 = 650\ mL.$$

USE OF DIALYSIS TO SUPPLEMENT INEFFICIENT RENAL FUNCTION

When the kidneys fail, it is possible to use the peritoneum or an artificial membrane as an alternative way of eliminating the waste products of metabolism and regulating the volume and composition of body fluids. The concepts of dialysis (i.e., the passive transmembrane diffusion of particles from one medium to another) are applied during peritoneal dialysis and hemodialysis.

Peritoneal Dialysis

Peritoneal dialysis is the process of mildly filling the peritoneal cavity with a dialysate fluid, allowing it to remain there about 45 minutes, and then removing it. The peritoneum acts as a semipermeable membrane with a large surface, and substances or fluid is exchanged between the blood and the fluid in the peritoneal cavity.

Introduction of a hypotonic solution causes fluid to move from the dialysate into the blood. When the introduced fluid is isotonic (1.5 percent glucose with electrolytes), urea, potassium, and xenobiotic substances (e.g., antibiotics, ethylene glycol, arsenic, barbiturates) are removed from the blood into the dialysate. Conversely, intraperitoneal introduction of hypertonic fluid (4.5 or 7 percent glucose with electrolytes) results in the transfer of extracellular fluid into the dialysate, thus reducing blood pressure or edema in tissues.

Hemodialysis

Conceptually, hemodialysis is identical with peritoneal dialysis except that, since it involves an extracorporeal circulation process, it is less practical in veterinary medicine. Hemodialysis is currently utilized in humans; because of its labor intensity and technical requirements, in animals its use is limited to research.

The objective of the hemodialysis process is to transfer blood metabolic waste substances across an artificial semipermeable membrane into a circulating dialysate. Blood from the femoral artery is returned into the femoral vein without some highly diffusible products of protein catabolism (urea, creatinine, phosphate, and potassium). The hemodialysis apparatus (artificial kidney) consists of a thin membrane (0.015 mm, surface of 1 m^2) that separates noncoagulable circulating blood from an isotonic solution. The membrane can be multiple parallel sheets of cellulose, cellulose tubes, or thousands of hollow tubes in which blood circulates countercurrent to the dialysing fluid.

REFERENCES

Brost DF, Bramwell K, Kramer JW. Sodium sulfanilate clearance as a method of determining renal function in the horse. J Equine Med Surg 1978;2:500.

Brown CM. Examination of the urinary system. In: Robinson NE, ed. Current therapy in equine medicine. Philadelphia: WB Saunders, 1983.

Bulger RE, Dobyan DC. Recent advances in renal morphology. Annu Rev Physiol 1982;44:147.

Chapman WH, Bulger RE, Cutler RE, Striker GE. The urinary system—an integrated approach. Philadelphia: WB Saunders, 1973.

Cowgill L, Bovee KC. Current status of hemodialysis and renal transplantation. In: Kirk RW, ed. Current veterinary therapy, small animal practice VI. Philadelphia: WB Saunders, 1977.

Gourley IM, Parker HR. Peritoneal dialysis. In: Kirk RW, ed. Current veterinary therapy, small animal practice VI. Philadelphia: WB Saunders, 1977.

Guyton AC. Textbook of medical physiology. Philadelphia: WB Saunders, 1980.

Schryver HF, Hintz HF. Minerals. In: Robinson NE, ed. Current therapy in equine medicine. Philadelphia: WB Saunders, 1983.

Traver DS, Salem C, Coffman JR, Garner HE, Moore JN, Johnson JH, Tritschler LG, Amend JF. Renal metabolism of endogenous substances in the horse: volumetric vs. clearance ratio methods. J Equine Med Surg 1977;1:378.

CHAPTER 17

RENAL ELECTROLYTE BALANCE

As an organ that regulates electrolyte balance, the kidney works in concert with the nervous system and some endocrine glands. Secretions of the parathyroid gland (parathormone, PTH), the adrenal cortex (aldosterone), and the neurohypophysis (antidiuretic hormone, ADH) are related to the transfer of electrolytes and water in the tubule of the nephron and in the collecting duct. The objective of this chapter is to present the absorption and secretion of solutes in the glomerular filtrate by cells in specific postglomerular areas.

ABSORPTION FROM THE TUBULE AND COLLECTING DUCT

Proximal Tubule

About 65 percent of all reabsorption processes takes place in the proximal tubule, and yet the osmotic concentration of the remaining glomerular filtrate is not changed and remains isotonic with that of plasma. This is because of the *obligatory reabsorption of water* in the proximal tubule (65 percent of the 99 percent of the water in the ultrafiltrate), which is driven by osmotic diffusion. The active and passive absorption of some solute lowers its concentration in the tubule fluid and raises it in the proximal peritubule fluid, causing osmosis of water. The reabsorption of the remaining 34 percent of water (i.e., the *facultative reabsorption of water*) may occur in the loop of Henle (15 percent), the distal tubule (10 percent), and the collecting duct (9 percent). Normally, only about 1 percent of the water in the glomerular ultrafiltrate escapes reabsorption and finds its way into the urine.

The proximal tubule is the site of active reabsorption of sodium, phosphate, sulfate, vitamins, acetoacetate, lactate, citrate, ketoglutarate, amino acids, glucose, urate, and proteins (see Fig. 17–7). Chloride (60 percent) is actively reabsorbed only in the latter part of the tubule. The basolateral membrane of proximal tubule cells actively absorbs potassium from the intercellular space. Besides water, chloride (40 percent in the upper proximal tubule), bicarbonate, luminal potassium, magnesium, calcium, and urea are passively absorbed by diffusion, possibly in the wake of actively absorbed solutes. The morphology of the proximal tubule is well-adapted to its extensive role in absorption. It is the longest segment of the nephron, its luminal surface has a dense brush border, and it presents a myriad of intercellular and basal channels.

Proximal tubule cells are well-equipped to accomplish their major functions, the reabsorption of sodium, which energizes numerous coupled or cotransport transfer of other substances. Sodium-potassium-ATPase is present in the basolateral cell membrane but is absent from the brush border (Fig. 17–1). Sodium cotransport proteins are found in the apical and basolateral membrane for absorption of glucose, galactose, amino acids, inorganic acids (phosphate, sulfate), organic acid metabolites (lactate, citrate, ketoglutarate), protons, and hydroxyl ions. The junctional complexes between adjacent tubular cells are permeable to small molecules of solutes and provide a paracellular shunt pathway, which is an additional route for passive movements (coupled to active sodium transfer) of ions. Carbonic anhydrase enzyme is found in the brush border, the cytoplasm, and the basolateral membrane. The brush border carbonic anhydrase facilitates bicarbonate absorption by catalyzing the breakdown of luminal carbonic acid. The cytosolic carbonic anhydrase provides an intracellular supply of protons (H^+) for the secretory process associated with bicarbonate absorption. The basolateral-bound carbonic anhydrase helps bicarbonate to exit from the cell.

Absorption of Cations

Sodium is the major cation absorbed from the proximal tubule. The others are potassium, calcium, and magnesium.

Sodium. The volume of extracellular fluid (ECF) is maintained by the osmotic action of sodium. A fall in plasma (ECF) sodium concentration causes water to move rapidly into cells and brings a rise in the hematocrit, or packed cell volume. A rise in plasma sodium concentration is accompanied by shrinkage of cells, which lose water to the ECF, and also lowers the hematocrit value. When a change in plasma volume occurs, the kidney responds by handling sodium differently in the proximal tubule, the loop of Henle, and the distal tubules.

After entering the cytoplasm of proximal cells by *diffusion,* sodium is *actively removed at the basolateral membrane.* Once sodium is in the intercellular space and basal channels, it may move into the peritubular capillary or *diffuse back* (backleak) into the lumen through the junctional complexes (Fig. 17–2). *The tubule load* of sodium (i.e., the total amount that filters through the membrane into the tubules each minute) is about 15 to 20 mmol. Sodium ions do not have a *tubule transport maximum* (Tm; i.e., a maximum rate at which they can be absorbed).

Potassium. Potassium ions *diffuse* through the junctional complexes of the proximal tubule cells, from the glomerular filtrate into the interstitium and the peritubular capillary (Fig. 17–3). They can also be reabsorbed *actively into the proximal tubule cells*, at the *basolateral membrane*, where a sodium-potassium-ATPase can admit K^+ in exchange for removal of Na^+. At the end of the proximal tubule, total

A

B

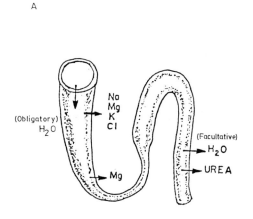

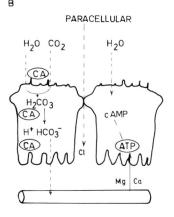

Figure 17–1 *A,* Sites of the obligatory and of the facultative reabsorption of water in the renal tubule. *B,* Proteins (enzymes) of the proximal tubular cells used for sodium cotransport, sodium-potassium-ATPase (ATP), and for the active processes of absorption and secretion (carbonic anhydrase, or CA). The paracellular shunt pathway is for passive movement of small ions (e.g., Cl).

reabsorption of potassium is 65 percent of the tubular load. PTH decreases the reabsorption of potassium and sodium in the proximal tubule.

Calcium. The cells of the proximal tubule reabsorb 65 percent of the calcium in the glomerular filtrate, the remainder being absorbed in the loop of Henle (20 percent), the distal tubule (10 percent), and the collecting duct (5 percent). The mechanisms for calcium reabsorption are still unknown; *passive* (diffusion) *and active* processes are believed to participate.

Vitamin D₃ (1,25-dihydroxycholecalciferol) secreted by the proximal tubule facilitates calcium reabsorption and the synthesis in the distal tubule and the collecting duct of a soluble calcium-binding protein (CaBP) that is larger (28,000 daltons) than the one found in the intestine (12,000 daltons). PTH activates alpha-hydroxylase in the cells of the proximal tubule to transform 25-hydroxycholecalciferol, of hepatic origin, into 1,25-dihydroxycholecalciferol, or 1,25-dihydroxyvitamin D₃. Calcitonin inhibits this alpha₁-hydroxylase and also decreases the tubular reabsorption of calcium.

PTH, a small protein of 9,500 daltons, originates mostly from the chief cells. Its secretion is related to the concentration of calcium ions perfusing the parathyroid gland. A reduction in the normal calcemia causes a release of the hormone. PTH increases calcium reabsorption *only in the distal tubule and collecting duct, not in the proximal tubule.*

Calcitonin, a peptide hormone of 3,000 daltons, is secreted by parafollicular cells of the thyroid to lower calcemia when it is above normal (hypercalcemia). Its effect on the kidney is not opposed to that of PTH; it also causes *phosphaturia and natriuria.* It increases calciuria but does not influence excretion of hydrogen and acid-base balance.

Magnesium. The proximal tubule reabsorbs only 25 percent of the tubule load of magnesium by a specific transporter located at the antiluminal, or contraluminal, membrane. The reabsorptive mechanism is directly dependent on tubule load and on luminal magnesium concentration. More magnesium ions (about 50 percent of the tubule load) are reabsorbed in the ascending limb of the loop of Henle. A tubule maximum transport (Tm) for magnesium does not exist in either the proximal tubule or Henle's loop. PTH increases the reabsorption of magnesium.

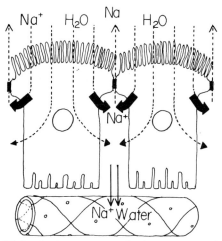

Figure 17–2 Passive transport of sodium into the cell of the proximal tubule and active transport of sodium into the intercellular space and the basal channels. Water follows passively.

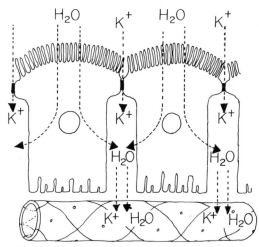

Figure 17–3 Passive absorption of potassium by the paracellular shunt pathway and by the peritubular capillary.

Absorption of Inorganic Anions

Bicarbonate.   Passive reabsorption of bicarbonate in the proximal and distal tubules is facilitated by carbonic anhydrase, an enzyme found at the brush border, cytoplasm, and basolateral membrane of the tubule cell. The enzyme catalyzes both the synthesis of carbonic acid from water and carbon dioxide and the dissociation of carbonic acid into hydrogen and bicarbonate ions.

Acidification of the filtrate in the proximal tubule is the primary phase in the mechanism of bicarbonate reabsorption. The process of hydrogen secretion involves a sodium-hydrogen antiporter in which cellular hydrogen ion is secreted in exchange for luminal sodium (Fig. 17–4). This luminal hydrogen reacts with luminal bicarbonate to form carbonic acid, which is decomposed in the brush border by carbonic anhydrase into carbon dioxide and water, both of which can diffuse into the tubular cytoplasm. For each proton secreted into the lumen a bicarbonate is generated in the cell and must exit across the basolateral membrane by a mechanism probably related to carbonic anhydrase, though this is still unclear.

Acetazolamide, a diuretic agent, inhibits carbonic anhydrase and tubule reabsorption of bicarbonate. As more bicarbonate is excreted, an excess of very alkaline urine is produced.

Chloride.   Passive diffusion of chloride (40 percent) occurs in the paracellular spaces (Fig. 17–5) because of a progressive increase in the chloride concentration along the proximal tubule. About 60 percent of chloride is actively

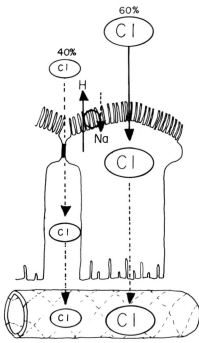

Figure 17–5   Reabsorption of chloride in the proximal tubule is by active mechanisms (60 percent) and by diffusion (40 percent).

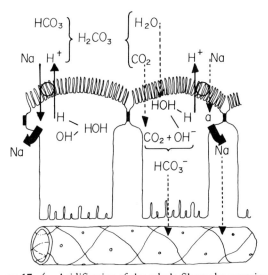

Figure 17–4   Acidification of the tubule filtrate by secretion of H^+ is the primary step in bicarbonate absorption by the cells of the proximal tubule. Tubule carbonic acid is decomposed into water and CO_2, both are absorbed passively and utilized to form a new bicarbonate molecule ($CO_2 + OH^- = HCO_3$), which is transported into the peritubular capillary, and new hydrogen to be actively secreted in exchange for sodium by a Na-H antiporter, or exchanger.

reabsorbed in the latter part of the proximal tubule. This active reabsorption of chloride involves several mechanisms; for example, coupling to sodium transport depolarizes the brush border (luminal, apical) membrane and increases its permeability to chloride, acidification of the proximal tubule (secretion of hydrogen) and high luminal chloride content stimulate chloride uptake in the brush border.

Phosphate, sulfate, nitrate, and *urate* are actively reabsorbed by transport mechanisms, which are saturable for phosphate, sulfate, and urate. The Tm values for these anions are set at a normal tubule load (about 0.1 mmol per minute, 0.05 mmol per minute, and 15 mg per minute). With an increase in plasma concentration of phosphate, sulfate, or urate, the tubule loads exceed the Tm, and phosphate, sulfate, or urate is not absorbed but is excreted in the urine. Conversely, when the plasma level of phosphate, sulfate, or urate drops, the tubule load is below the Tm, and phosphate, sulfate, or urate is reabsorbed.

PTH, calcitonin (from parafollicular cells of the thyroid), and 1,25-dihydroxyvitamin D_3 reduce the Tm for phosphate and favor phosphaturia. In the dog, pentobarbital anesthesia also perturbs the tubule transport of phosphorus and causes hyperphosphaturia.

Endogenous Organic Acids

Small amounts of naturally occurring organic anions (*citrate, malate, beta-hydroxybutyrate, ascorbic acid*) are found in the urine in small amounts. Their reabsorption takes place by mechanisms obscured by multiple factors: secretion and reabsorption, high passive permeabilities, transport by other segments of the nephron, transport rate (which is dependent on acid-base balance), or all of these.

Nutritional Substances

In the glomerular filtrate, substances of particular importance to body nutrition (*glucose, amino acids, vitamins, acetoacetate, lactate, ketoglutarate, and proteins*) are completely reabsorbed by cells of the proximal tubule through active processes linked to sodium absorption. Most of these substances have tubular transport maximums (e.g., glucose 325 mg per minute, lactate 75 mg per minute, amino acids 1.5 mmol per minute, proteins and acetoacetate 30 mg per minute), almost none of these substances enter the loop of Henle.

Proteins are reabsorbed through the brush border of the proximal tubule by an active mechanism known as pinocytosis. The proteins attach themselves to the membrane, and this portion of the membrane then invaginates into a vesicle, which eventually becomes a part of the cytoplasm.

Urea

Urea, the primary waste product of protein catabolism measured as BUN, is reabsorbed passively from the glomerular filtrate. Mathematically, 50 percent of the tubule's load is taken up in the proximal tubule, then 30 to 40 percent is absorbed in the distal tubule and in the collecting duct. However, this is without considering the amount of urea that is recirculated.

Urea reabsorbed in the collecting duct is recirculated through the interstitium, into the descending limb of the loop of Henle. ADH facilitates this recirculation of urea by increasing the epithelial permeability of the collecting duct to urea and of the distal tubule to water. This recirculation of urea occurs several times, permitting urea to remain with sodium chloride in the renal medullary interstitium, where both create an osmotic concentration that is characteristic for each animal species. Thus, a waste product is used outside the ECF to create an osmotic gradient that may be used to recover water and to produce a urine several times more concentrated than plasma.

Loop of Henle

The descending limb of the loop is concerned mostly with water, which is passively displaced from the tubule lumen to the hyperosmotic interstitium. This loss of water causes the tubule fluid to reach its maximal osmolality at the tip of the hairpin loop, where it is isoosmotic to the interstitium. The ascending limb is impermeable to water.

The cells of the epithelium of the thin ascending limb of the loop of Henle actively reabsorb some sodium and chloride; however, most of the chloride, sodium, potassium, calcium, and magnesium is actively reabsorbed in the thick ascending portion of the loop. The major driving force would be the active reabsorption of chloride ions, with positive ions following. Osmolality of the tubule fluid decreases pro-

gressively as these electrolytes are extracted from the lumen, without water, into the renal medullary peritubular interstitium. Tubule fluid leaving the thick ascending limb has an osmolality lower than that of plasma; that is, it is very dilute.

Distal Tubule

The reabsorption of *sodium* from the filtrate in the distal tubule is under the control of the adrenal mineralocorticoid hormone aldosterone. This sodium reabsorption is of great importance, even if it is quantitatively smaller (25 percent) than sodium reabsorption in the proximal tubule (65 percent). The sodium remaining in the tubule fluid is almost entirely reabsorbed without any accompanying water. Potassium and hydrogen ions, added to the tubule fluid by secretion in exchange for retained sodium, are eliminated in the urine.

Aldosterone production, triggered by an increase in the concentration of plasma potassium and by angiotensin II, is sustained by a minimal production of adrenocorticotropin (ACTH) from the adenohypophysis. Its mode of action is as follows: the steroid enters the tubule cells, combines with a receptor protein, and diffuses into the nucleus. Stimulation of the intranuclear DNA molecules and formation of RNA molecules result in an increased cellular production of the proteins (carriers or enzymes) required for the transfer of sodium and potassium.

The distal tubule is a final arbiter of sodium elimination. Under normal conditions, the distal nephron transport is set to nearly match the fraction of the tubule load that is not reabsorbed in the proximal tubule. The excreted amount, which maintains the sodium balance, is approximately equal to that ingested in food. Similarly, during sodium loading or sodium deprivation, appropriate amounts of sodium are either eliminated or reabsorbed to maintain balance. With sodium loading, less sodium is reabsorbed by the proximal tubule, and a larger load is delivered to the distal tubule. The increment in glomerular filtrate presented to the distal tubule is not completely reabsorbed and passes into the urine. The lack of complete absorption is associated with a decrease in or a lack of aldosterone.

The distal tubule reabsorption of *potassium* occurs in a fashion parallel to that of sodium: a maximum of 25 percent can be absorbed in the distal tubule (which begins with the thick portion of the descending limb of the loop of Henle), and 65 percent in the proximal tubule. Accordingly, a concentration as low as only 10 percent of the tubule load of potassium may be presented to the collecting duct.

Reabsorption of *calcium* in the distal tubule is increased by PTH, probably through the CaBP secreted in the proximal tubule. Urea is absorbed passively in the distal tubule.

Collecting Duct

The dilute tubule fluid delivered in the collecting duct can become concentrated or not, depending on the presence or absence of ADH. Without ADH, the epithelium of the collecting duct is practically impermeable to water, and little if any water is osmotically attracted to the medullary interstitium.

Hyposthenuria (production of urine of low specific gravity) is associated with inhibition of ADH by an excess of kinin-generated prostaglandin E_2 (PGE$_2$) in the distal tubule and collecting duct. This is associated with failure to transform PGE$_2$ into PGF$_{2\alpha}$ by PGE-9-ketoreductase, a process that favors reabsorption of water. PGE$_2$ synthesis is increased by hypokalemia. Conversely, increased intake of salt enhances the activity of PGE-9-ketoreductase, formation of PGF$_{2\alpha}$, antinatriuresis, and water retention by the collecting duct.

ADH is a peptide hormone of hypothalamic origin (supraoptic and paraventricular nuclei) that migrates and is stored bound to a protein (neurophysin) in the neurohypophysis. Liberation of ADH from the neurohypophysis and neurophysin is triggered by an increase in the osmolality of plasma (osmosodium receptors in the supraoptic nucleus), by a decrease in plasma volume (voloreceptors in the left atrium), and by lowered arterial pressure (baroreceptors in the carotid artery and aorta). Trauma, anxiety, morphine, nicotine, tranquilizers, and anesthetics also release ADH; alcohol inhibits the action of ADH.

ADH increases the epithelial permeability of the collecting duct. It binds to the basolateral membrane of the cell, stimulates adenylcyclase to increase the intracellular level of cyclic adenosine monophosphate (cAMP), which then activates a kinase (protein) that dephosphorylates some proteins of the membrane to modify the cell permeability to water, urea, and possibly sodium (Fig. 17–6). Under the action of ADH the cell morphology changes: the cell enlarges, the apical microvilli disappear, and the intercellular space increases. The tight junctions near the apical poles of adjacent cells remain intact. Water seems to enter the cell at the apical membrane and exit into the hypertonic intercellular spaces.

In vitro, with batrachian epithelium, ADH would be associated with three types of cell membrane receptors for water, urea, and sodium. Specific selective blockers exist for water (lanthanum) and for urea (PGE$_2$ and PGF$_{2\alpha}$).

As a result of the reabsorption of water caused by ADH, together with the higher concentration of urea in collecting duct fluid, the permeability of the collecting duct to urea increases. Urea reabsorbed in the collecting duct is recirculated in the thin limbs of the loop of Henle. This reabsorption is probably passive, since there is no Tm (associated with a saturable active transport mechanism) for urea. The proximal tubule reabsorption exceeds 50 percent. This is explained with urea secretion, in the next section.

Final control of renal reabsorption or excretion of *magnesium* is exercised by the collecting duct (Fig. 17–7). Urinary magnesium depends on the plasma magnesium concentration. Secretion occurs with hypermagnesemia and when there is excessive aldosterone, but reabsorption is associated with hypomagnesemia.

SECRETION BY THE TUBULE NEPHRON AND COLLECTING DUCT

Passive Secretion

Transepithelial renal transport of a substance is the outcome of two unidirectional fluxes, reabsorption and secretion. For *urea,* the net flux is considered to be a loss of 10 to 20 percent of the tubule load. On a mathematical basis, since 50 percent of urea is reabsorbed in the proximal tubule, the distal tubule and collecting duct would reabsorb less urea (i.e., only 30 to 40 percent of the tubular load). However, the absolute quantity of urea *reabsorbed* in the distal nephron and collecting duct, *equivalent* to the quantity *passively secreted in the thin limbs of the loop of Henle,* is more than 50 percent.

To explain and visualize the importance of reabsorption and secretion, it may be considered that of 100 parts of urea filtered in the the glomerular space, only 50 remain at the end of the proximal tubule (Fig. 17–8). Gradually, in the thin limbs of the loop of Henle, urea is added to the tubule fluid, which eventually contains 110 parts of urea as it enters the distal tubule (i.e., the secretion is 60 parts urea). As urine carries only 15 parts urea, reabsorption in the end-tubes of the kidney (under the control of ADH) represents $110 - 15$, or 95, parts urea, which is close to the tubule load of 100 parts.

Active Secretion

Potassium is secreted predominantly by cells of the distal tubule and, to a lesser extent, by those of the collecting duct. By an active mechanism involving aldosterone, potassium enters the cytoplasm in exchange for sodium. From the cytoplasm, by simple diffusion, potassium is then trans-

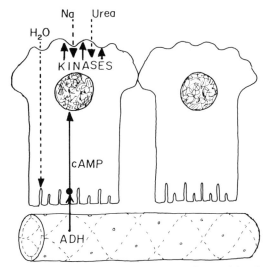

Figure 17–6 Acting on the basolateral membrane of distal tubule cells, ADH stimulates the synthesis of kinases to modify permeability of the apical membrane to water, sodium, and urea.

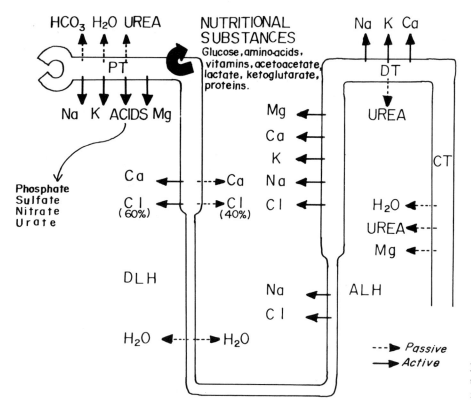

Figure 17–7 Synopsis of absorption in the tubule and the collecting duct.

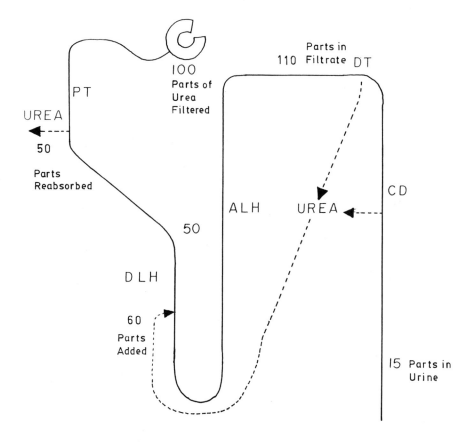

Figure 17–8 Diagram of the recirculation of urea involving absorption, in the proximal and distal tubules and the collecting duct, and secretion, from the interstitium into the thin limbs of the loop of Henle.

ported across the apical membrane into the tubule fluid (Fig. 17–9). Renal secretion of potassium, regulated by aldosterone, is far more important in maintaining the ECF potassium concentration than in controlling the sodium concentration.

Aldosterone is a steroid hormone, a mineralocorticoid (affects electrolytes of the ECF) secreted by *zona glomerulosa* cells of the adrenal cortex. Its renal effect is to increase tubular secretion of potassium and tubular reabsorption of sodium. Factors that increase the secretion of potassium are alkalosis (respiratory and metabolic), sodium loading, potassium loading, drugs (acetazolamide, thiazide, mannitol or urea diuresis). A lack of aldosterone results in an excessive loss of sodium in the urine and hyperkalemia from inhibition of secretion of potassium.

The renal control of extracellular bicarbonate is provided by secretion of *hydrogen ions* in the tubules and collecting duct. Secreted hydrogen is found in urine as (1) ammonium (chloride, usually) (i.e., $H^+ + NH_3 = NH_4$) 60 percent; (2) titrable acid (i.e., hydrogen combined with a weak acid anion [urate]), 40 percent; and (3) free hydrogen, in negligible quantity, but most effective in lowering the urinary pH to the limit of 4.5.

Renal hydrogen is actively secreted by epithelial cells in the proximal tubule, distal tubule, and collecting duct in response to an increase in carbon dioxide concentration in ECF (e.g., increased metabolic rate, decreased respiration). The major production of hydrogen (80 percent) is in the proximal tubule, but the production of hydrogen in the collecting duct has the greatest influence on lowering the urinary pH to its limit of about 4.5. The process begins with diffusion of carbon dioxide into the tubule epithelial cells. Under the influence of carbonic anhydrase, carbon dioxide

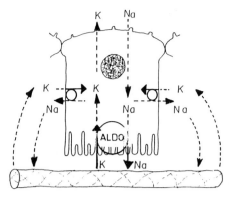

Figure 17–9 Potassium diffuses out of the cytoplasm of a distal tubule cell into the tubule fluid. It is brought into the cell by an active mechanism involving aldosterone (ALDO) in exchange for sodium at the basolateral membrane.

combines with water to form carbonic acid. The latter dissociates into bicarbonate ions and hydrogen ions, which are secreted by active transport through the apical membrane.

Organic acids (e.g., paraaminohippuric acid, PAH) and organic bases (e.g., tetraethylammonium, TEA) are *secreted only in the proximal tubule*. The processes are saturable (Tm substances) and rapid. Competition for secretion has been observed between acids and between bases, but not between acids and bases.

Ammonia is produced in the tubule epithelial cells by deamination of amino acids: glutamine (60 percent) and glycine and alanine (40 percent). It is continuously secreted from the cytoplasm by diffusion through the apical membrane of the tubule cells. In the tubule fluid, ammonia

Figure 17–10 Synopsis of the secretion processes in the nephron and collecting duct.

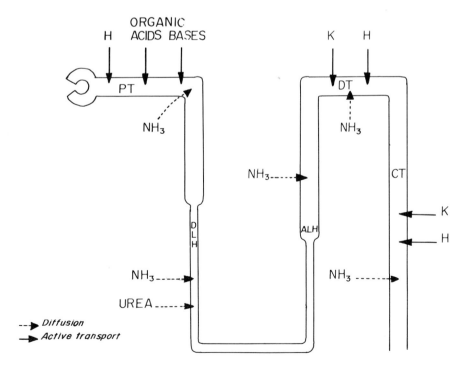

(NH₃) combines with hydrogen to form ammonium (NH₄), which then combines with the most abundant anion, chloride, in ammonium chloride (Fig. 17–10).

REFERENCES

Jamison RL, Work J, Schafer JA. New pathways for potassium transport in the kidney. Am J Physiol 1982;242:F297.

McGiff JC, Wong PYK. Compartmentalization of prostaglandins and prostacyclin within the kidney: implication for renal function. Fed Proc 1979;38:89.

Rector FC. Sodium, bicarbonate, and chloride absorption by the proximal tubule. Am J Physiol 1983;244:F78.

Suki WN. Calcium transport in the nephron. Am J Physiol 1979; 237:F1.

Ullrich KJ, Rumrich G. Intraluminal transport system in the proximal renal tubule involved in secretion of organic anions. Am J Physiol 1988;254:F453.

Warnock DG, Eveloff J. NaCl entry mechanisms in the luminal membrane of the renal tubule. Am J Physiol 1982;242:F561.

Welling DJ, Welling LW. Cell shape as an indicator of volume reabsorption in proximal nephron. Fed Proc 1979;38:121.

Wong NLM, Dirks JH, Quamme GA. Tubular reabsorptive capacity for magnesium in the dog kidney. Am J Physiol 1983;244:F78.

CHAPTER 18

RENAL ACID-BASE BALANCE

One of the important homeostatic roles of the kidneys is to regulate the composition of body fluids. With the lungs, they constitute a physiological buffer system able to give up or bind hydrogen ions. The lungs briskly excrete weak acids (molecules or ions giving up hydrogen ions) as carbon dioxide. The kidneys, at a comparatively sluggish pace, regulate the net rates of base (molecules or ions that bind hydrogen) excretion and selective reabsorption of cations and ions.

The relationship between total bases (metabolic component) and weak acids (respiratory component) is represented by the blood pH, an index of the status of the acid-base balance. Another indicator of the state of the acid-base balance is the plasma bicarbonate concentration, also called the *alkali reserve*. The role of the kidney in maintaining the acid-base balance is to avoid major changes in the pH by adjusting the bicarbonate concentration of the extracellular fluids.

The relationship between pH and the bicarbonate−carbonic acid buffer is summarized in the Henderson-Hasselbalch equation:

$$pH = pK + \log [HCO_3^-]/[H_2CO_3] + [\text{dissolved } CO_2]$$
$$\downarrow \qquad \uparrow$$
$$CO_2 + H_2O$$

$$= 6.1 + \log \frac{24 \text{ mmol/L}}{1.2 \text{ mmol/L}}$$
$$7.4 = 6.1 + 1.3$$

Disturbance in the bicarbonate−carbonic acid ratio, which is usually about 20 to 1, would cause the pH to increase (alkalosis) or decrease (acidosis) (Fig. 18−1). Because of the physiological buffers, lungs and kidneys, the ratio remains nearly stable, even though the absolute concentrations of bicarbonate and carbonic acid change because of nutrition, metabolism, and muscle activity.

Acids from proteins (phosphoric, sulfuric), lipids (phosphate, ketoacids), or bases from plants (bicarbonate, potassium) are added to the extracellular fluids during normal metabolism. The acids (A^-H^+) react with extracellular sodium bicarbonate of the bicarbonate−carbonic acid buffer to produce a salt (Na^+A^-) and carbonic acid. The carbonic acid is immediately dissociated into water and carbon dioxide, which is excreted by the lungs. The remaining acid radical A^- is eventually excreted in the urine. Digestion of plant material leads to formation of acids (acetic, propionic, butyric) and adds an excess of bicarbonate and potassium, which must be removed from the body in urine.

This chapter describes the renal mechanisms for regulation of the bicarbonate content of the bicarbonate−carbonic acid buffer of extracellular fluids: (1) reabsorption of the filtered bicarbonate; (2) replenishment of plasma bicarbonate as a result of bicarbonate synthesis in an exchange for secreted hydrogen ions, which are excreted mostly as ammonium (from amino acids) and to a lesser extent as *titrable acidity* (amount of base required to titrate urine back to the pH of blood); and (3) excretion of excess organic acids and bases. Formation of acid urine in carnivores and of alkaline urine in herbivores and metabolic acid-base disturbances are also discussed.

REABSORPTION OF FILTERED BICARBONATE

In normal animals, the concentration of bicarbonate in the glomerular filtrate as it enters the proximal tubule is about 24 mmol per liter (range 17 to 30). It reflects a normal *anion gap,* that is, the residual or unmeasured anions in the plasma, which includes phosphates, sulfates, organic acids, and protein anions. The value of the anion gap is calculated as follows:

$$\text{Anion gap} = (Na^+ + K^+) - (HCO_3^- + Cl^-)$$
$$= (145 + 5) - (110 + 24)$$
$$= 16 \text{ mmol/L (range 10 to 25)}.$$

As potassium is often omitted from the calculation, the value of the anion gap is then about 11 mmol per liter. A larger anion gap indicates the presence of unidentified anions, which may correspond to an acid (lactic acid, ketone bodies: acetoacetate, beta-hydroxy butyrate) causing acidosis.

Most of this filtered bicarbonate is passively reabsorbed in the proximal tubule by a roundabout process involving also absorption of sodium ions and secretion of hydrogen ions (Fig. 18−2). Stated in other words, recovery of sodium bicarbonate from the tubular filtrate is coupled to a furtive acidification that does not change the tubule pH.

Sodium bicarbonate in the ultrafiltrate dissociates into sodium ions (passively introduced into the tubule cells) and bicarbonate anions. A bicarbonate anion unites with a hydrogen ion actively secreted into the tubule lumen to form the unstable carbonic acid, which immediately reverts to water and carbon dioxide. The carbon dioxide passively penetrates the luminal cell membrane and is reunited with water as carbonic acid, which dissociates into bicarbonate and hydrogen ions (by cellular carbonic anhydrase catalysis). This newly formed bicarbonate ion diffuses into the peritubular fluid, and the hydrogen ion is pumped out of the cell to initiate a new cycle of bicarbonate recovery.

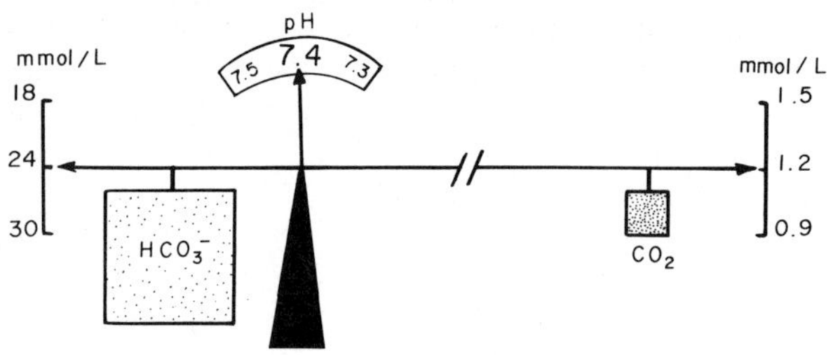

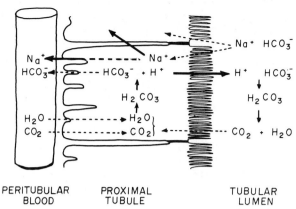

Figure 18–1 The pH of extracellular fluid remains at 7.4 as long as the concentration ratio of bicarbonate to carbonic acid is 20 to 1. Disturbances in the ratio cause immediate alkalosis or acidosis, which may be compensated for by changes to reestablish the ratio (e.g., 30 to 1.5 in alkalosis, or 18 to 0.9 in acidosis).

Figure 18–3 Active secretion of hydrogen ion in exchange for sodium, which is reabsorbed passively, in the distal tubule. Acidification of tubule fluid occurs.

REPLENISHMENT OF PLASMA BICARBONATE

Acidification of Tubule Fluid Buffers

After all the sodium bicarbonate in the tubule fluid is removed, the mechanism of Na^+ and H^+ exchange can still be pursued. Then, hydrogen ion is added to the tubule buffer systems (phosphate primarily as Na_2HPO_4/NaH_2PO_4) with the conversion of disodium phosphate into monosodium phosphate (Fig. 18–3).

At the initiation of this process, intracellular carbon dioxide is hydrated to carbonic acid, which dissociates as bicarbonate and hydrogen ions. The hydrogen ion is then actively transported across the apical membrane into the tubular lumen where it replaces a sodium ion on the tubular buffer. As a result of this sodium and hydrogen ion exchange, bicarbonate disappears from the urine, titratable acidity rises,

and pH decreases (possibly to its lower limit) because of acidification of the tubule buffer systems (the Na_2HPO_4 to NaH_2PO_4 ratio may then reach 1 to 200), and more sodium bicarbonate is returned to the extracellular fluid than was filtered at the glomerulus. A greater excretion of calcium occurs at the lower urine pH, and production of parathormone (PTH) is stepped up to diminish reabsorption and to increase loss of phosphate.

Formation of Tubular Ammonium

The tubular cell can also generate ammonia to regain sodium from neutral salt in addition to recovery of HCO_3^-

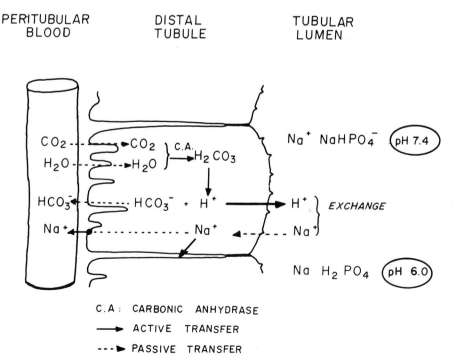

PERITUBULAR BLOOD   DISTAL TUBULE   TUBULAR LUMEN

Figure 18–2 Mechanism for passive reabsorption of bicarbonate in the proximal tubule. The process requires a concomitant absorption of sodium and active secretion of hydrogen.

C.A: CARBONIC ANHYDRASE

→ ACTIVE TRANSFER

---▸ PASSIVE TRANSFER

and acidification of the tubular buffer to a much lower pH than that of the plasma. Ammonia formation, from deamination of amino acids (mostly glutamine, but also lysine and alanine), is stimulated by the fall in pH within the tubule fluid. After ammonia has diffused into the tubule fluid, it forms ammonium (NH_4^+) by uniting with hydrogen ions previously secreted into the tubular fluid. As in the two previous mechanisms, H^+ hydrogen ion is generated intracellularly and secreted actively in the tubule lumen in exchange for sodium ion. The sodium ion is reclaimed into peritubular vessels together with the bicarbonate anion resulting from the intracellular hydration of carbon dioxide, which is immediately ionized into carbonic acid ($H_2CO_3 = HCO_3^- + H^+$) (Fig. 18–4).

This renal mechanism permits removal of anions of neutral salts (chloride, sulfate, urate, phosphate), additional sodium and hydrogen ion exchange without further reducing the urinary pH, and regeneration of HCO_3^- for the major extracellular fluid buffer (HCO_3^-/H_2CO_3). The urinary chloride concentration is inversely correlated with the excretion of bicarbonate. Chloride is the principal urinary anion when bicarbonate excretion is low. Conversely, when bicarbonate excretion is high, urinary chloride content is reduced.

URINARY EXCRETION OF ORGANIC ACIDS AND BASES

Organic acids (R—COOH) and bases (R—NH$^+$) of endogenous or exogenous origin that undergo active proximal tubule secretion and are actively and passively reabsorbed from the tubule fluid may not necessarily be excreted in large amounts in voided urine. The excreted quantity of these substances depends on the difference between the amounts added by filtration and by secretion and the amount removed by reabsorption.

The rate of active secretion of organic acids or bases is influenced by the concentration of the substances in the plasma. Different secretion systems exist for organic acids and for organic bases (Fig. 18–5).

Passive reabsorption is more extensive than active reabsorption, which is limited to the proximal tubule and is dependent on the maximal tubular excretory capacity (Tm). Excretion of these organic substances occurs only after saturation of the carrier mechanisms (e.g., citrate, malate, ascorbic acid, beta-hydroxybutyric, urate).

The magnitude of passive tubular reabsorption is determined by the membrane permeability or lipid solubility of the nonionic moiety of the substance and the concentration gradient of the nonionic form, which is influenced by the pH of the tubular fluid. A rapid urine flow rate also affects reabsorption by shortening the time in which a substance can diffuse out of the urine and by decreasing the concentration gradient because the urine is dilute.

As a general rule, dissociation of organic acids and bases is governed by tubular pH. When the filtrate is acid, organic weak acids are nonionized, and their transport across the cell membrane is accelerated, since they are more lipid soluble. Also, when filtrate is acid, the reabsorption of weak acids is increased; thus, acidification of the tubular filtrate reduces the excretion of weak acids. Conversely, when the filtrate is basic, organic weak acids are ionized, and transport across the cell membrane is reduced, since they are less lipid-soluble or their particles are larger than the membrane channels. Their reabsorption is also reduced, and their excretion thus increased. Therefore, alkalinization of the tubular filtrate favors the excretion of organic weak acids.

The opposite is true for organic weak bases, which are nonionized in an alkaline ultrafiltrate, hence their reabsorption is favored and their excretion reduced. To cause maximal excretion of organic weak bases, the filtrate must be acidified to transform the nonionic base into the ionic, or nonpermeating, form and diminish reabsorption.

Figure 18–4 In the distal tubule, sodium is passively recovered in exchange for ammonium, which is the result of active secretion of hydrogen and passive secretion of ammonia in the lumen of the tubule.

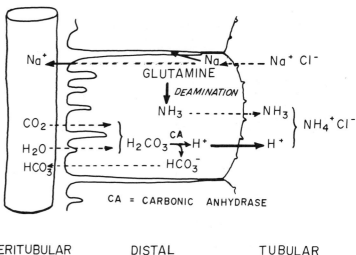

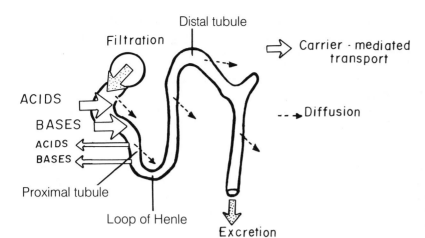

Figure 18–5 Both active absorption and secretion of organic acids take place in the proximal tubule, but the net result is secretion.

The primary function of the renal organic secretory system seems to be elimination of compounds (other than drugs) (Table 18–1) arising from the ordinary diet, from the metabolism of intestinal bacteria, or from endogenous compounds. Examples are degradation products of steroid hormones, bile salts, vitamins, prostaglandins, dyes, and urate.

Special Case of Urate

In mammals, uric acid derives from purine metabolism. It represents a minor excretory product in dogs and rats, since of the quantity filtered and secreted, over 50 percent is reabsorbed, leaving at most 40 percent of the tubule load in the urine.

Some species (Dalmatian dog, calf, pig, goat, rabbit, guinea pig) have a strong secretory component with or without simultaneous reabsorption of urate. Dalmatians excrete more uric acid (140 percent of the tubule load, three times more than other breed of dog) because the secretion rate is

much greater than the reabsorption rate of uric acid. The rabbit also shows a net secretion of uric acid (160 percent of the tubule load). In the pig, either no uric acid or very little is reabsorbed, as in birds and reptiles. In the cat, net reabsorption of urate occurs, but published evidence for secretion is lacking.

RELATION OF COMPOSITION OF FOOD TO RENAL ACID-BASE BALANCE

The pH of plasma remains within narrow limits in spite of challenges by acidic components from tissue metabolism, muscle activity, and foods; however, the pH of urine is influenced by the composition of foods. Starvation or a high-protein intake lowers urinary pH in all animal species. Carnivores void acid urine because of sulfate and phosphate in the meat, but eating a diet with a high plant content alkalinizes urine. Herbivores' urine is alkaline because of the high-potassium content of plants.

Acid Urine in Carnivores

The pH of carnivores' urine fluctuates during the prandial digestive phase. During gastric digestion and intense secretion of hydrochloric acid, the plasma alkaline tide brings a urinary excretion of base (potassium bicarbonate) from the bicarbonate–carbonic acid extracellular fluid buffer. The urine is alkaline during this period.

As the meal reaches the duodenum, a plasma acid tide accompanies the outpouring of bicarbonate-rich pancreatic juice into the small intestine. The kidney responds to this by acidifying the urine (to less than pH 6) to regain bicarbonate and eliminate the excess of hydrogen ions and by augmenting the excretion of ammonium chloride, sulfate, urate, and phosphate salts. Also, as urea synthesis by the liver is greater, less urea and water are reabsorbed in the distal tubule and the collecting duct, and the volume of urine increases during this period.

TABLE 18–1 Renal Tubular Transport of Organic Acids or Bases

Weak Acids	Weak Bases
Acetazolamide	Amphetamines
Acetylsalicylic acid	Atropine
Ampicillin	Dopamine
Chlorpropamide	Erythromycin
Diodrast (iodopyracet)	Histamine
Ethacrynic acid	Isoproterenol
Furosemide	Meperidine
Indomethacin	Morphine
Nitrofurantoin	Procaine
Penicillin	Quinidine
Phenobarbital	Thiamine
Phenylbutazone	Trimethoprim
Probenecid	
Salicylic acid	
Sulfonamides	
Thiazide diuretics	

Alkaline Urine in Herbivores

In ruminants, mastication of plant material causes a substantial quantity of bicarbonate to be extracted from the extracellular fluid into the saliva. The resulting slight acidosis stimulates the kidney to acidify urine for regeneration of bicarbonate and to excrete acid. Plasma alkaline and gastric tides are not seen in ruminants because abomasal and pancreatic secretions are continuous.

Plants eaten by herbivores have a high-potassium content. Because of higher concentration of potassium in fresh grass, herbs, and alfalfa, grazing animals produce more urine of a higher osmolality than animals fed grass hay. This potassium is secreted with bicarbonate and carbonate anions in the distal tubule (Fig. 18–6). The urinary excretion of potassium exceeds the tubular load (i.e., the quantity of potassium filtered at the glomerulus). The urine is much more alkaline (pH > 9) than plasma (pH 7.4), since it is without recovery of bicarbonate, titrable acidity, and production of ammonia. Because of the excess of base in the buffer system, much dibasic potassium phosphate (K_2HPO_4) and little monobasic potassium phosphate (KH_2PO_4) is excreted; also, chloride is reabsorbed instead of bicarbonate anions.

Ewes at pasture during spring, summer, and fall produce an alkaline urine containing as much as 128 mmol of potassium per liter. During winter stabulation, the poorer potassium content of feeds is reflected by an acid urine that carries three times less potassium (38 mmol per liter).

METABOLIC ACID-BASE DISTURBANCES

Acid-base balance can be disturbed by physiological (Table 18–2) and nonphysiological factors. Veterinary interest in acid-base disturbances has long been limited because of the difficulty in measuring blood pH and carbon dioxide tension. The easiest measurement, alkaline reserve, is inadequate to detect acidosis or alkalosis (metabolic or respiratory). An increase in plasma bicarbonate can occur in respiratory acidosis as well as in metabolic alkalosis. A decrease in the alkaline reserve may result from metabolic acidosis as well as from compensation of respiratory alkalosis (Fig. 18–7).

The metabolic component (bicarbonate anion) of the bicarbonate–carbonic acid buffer system is primarily affected in metabolic alkalosis (increased) and in metabolic acidosis (decreased). It is secondarily modified in conditions that involve primarily the respiratory component, carbonic acid (or $S \cdot PCO_2$ + dissolved carbon dioxide [S, soluble]). Then, in compensatory attempts to reinstate the 20-to-1 ratio of the buffer system, the metabolic component is increased in respiratory acidosis and, conversely, is lowered in respiratory alkalosis (Fig. 18–8).

TABLE 18–2 Physiological Factors Affecting Acid-Base Balance

Acidosis	Alkalosis
Catabolism	Adenohypophyseal hormones
Glucagon	Aldosterone
Neurohypophyseal hormones	Anabolism
Progesterone	Estrogens
Protein diet	Insulin
Sympathetic stimulation	Parathormone
Testosterone	Vagal stimulation
Thyroxine	Vegetable diet

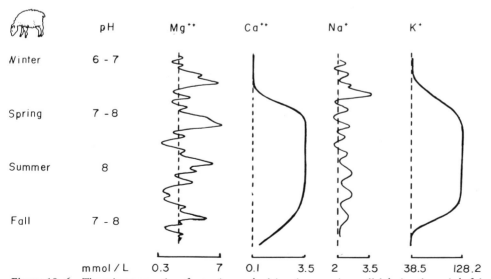

Figure 18–6 The urinary excretion of potassium and calcium increases in parallel during the period of the year when sheep are at pasture.

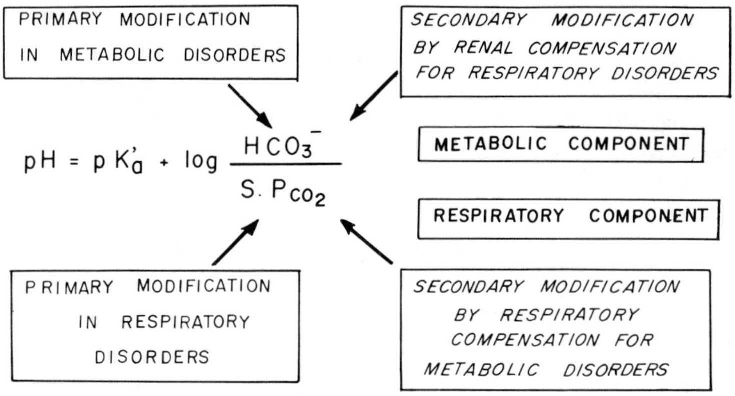

$$pH = pK'_a + \log \frac{HCO_3^-}{S \cdot P_{CO_2}}$$

PRIMARY MODIFICATION IN METABOLIC DISORDERS

SECONDARY MODIFICATION BY RENAL COMPENSATION FOR RESPIRATORY DISORDERS

METABOLIC COMPONENT

RESPIRATORY COMPONENT

PRIMARY MODIFICATION IN RESPIRATORY DISORDERS

SECONDARY MODIFICATION BY RESPIRATORY COMPENSATION FOR METABOLIC DISORDERS

Figure 18-7 Primary modifications of metabolic or respiratory components produce alkalosis or acidosis. Secondary renal modifications of bicarbonate happen in respiratory alkalosis. Secondary respiratory modifications occur in metabolic alkalosis.

Metabolic Acidosis

Metabolic acidosis may result from excess addition of acids, loss of bases, or retention of fixed acids.

Acid Production in Excess of Renal Excretion Capacity. In cows, lactic acid intoxication may occur from rumen fermentation of feeds that lack roughage (insufficient buffering by saliva), contain too much cereal or sucrose-rich plant material (apples, sugar beets), or cause a sudden change in the rumen ecology (sudden change of feeds). In horses, lactic acid intoxication is also seen in horses after prolonged intensive muscle activity. Oxalic acidosis is caused by ingestion of ethylene glycol, which is very palatable to small animals.

Loss of Bases. Subtraction of bases from the intestinal secretions accompanies diarrhea in young animals (puppy, colt, calf).

Retention of Fixed Acids. In acute renal failure, excretion of chloride, sulfate, and phosphate is perturbed because of a smaller quantity of functional nephrons. The number of nephrons per kidney is 190,000 in the cat, 430,000 in the dog, and 4 million in the cow.

In metabolic acidosis, the anion gap is usually increased (Fig. 18-9). An exception is when metabolic acidosis is caused by loss of bicarbonate anions (diarrhea); then, chloride (hyperchloremia associated with sodium reabsorption) replaces the bicarbonate, and the anion gap does not change.

Metabolic Alkalosis

Metabolic alkalosis is associated with a rise in plasma pH and bicarbonate. It may result from digestive tract disorders in ruminants (high intestinal obstruction; atony, torsion, or displacement of the abomasum) when gastric juice is prevented from moving into the intestinal tract. In small animals, loss of hydrochloric acid through vomiting causes metabolic alkalosis by a similar mechanism. The sequestration of hydrochloric acid, or loss of hydrogen cations, is matched by an equivalent gain of plasma bicarbonate anions. For each millimole of hydrochloric acid secreted into the stomach by the parietal cells, another millimole of bicarbonate is formed and released into the blood draining the stomach. Under normal circumstances, hydrochloric acid is eventually neutralized by pancreatic bicarbonate, and hydrogen balance is maintained. When hydrochloric acid is lost, an

PARAMETERS IN ACID-BASE IMBALANCE

| PARAMETER | METABOLIC | | RESPIRATORY | |
	ACIDOSIS	ALKALOSIS	ACIDOSIS	ALKALOSIS
pH	↓	↑	↓	↑
HCO_3^-	⬇	⬆	↑ (dashed)	↓ (dashed)
P_{CO_2}	↓ (dashed)	↑ (dashed)	↑	↓

---- Secondary effect

Figure 18-8 Primary modifications of bicarbonate characterize metabolic disturbances. Primary modifications of carbonic acid are limited to respiratory disturbances. Conversely, secondary changes in bicarbonate are associated with respiratory disturbances and in carbonic acid with metabolic disturbances.

ANION GAP IN METABOLIC ACIDOSIS

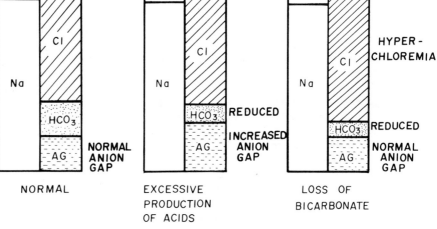

Figure 18–9 In metabolic acidosis, the plasma anion gap is usually increased because of poor excretion of organic acid anions. However, it remains normal if the metabolic acidosis is caused by excessive loss of bicarbonate in intestinal secretions (diarrhea), as hyperchloremia compensates for the loss of bicarbonate anion.

equivalent amount of bicarbonate remains unneutralized, causing elevation of the plasma bicarbonate concentration. Loss of plasma potassium can lead to metabolic alkalosis, since hydrogen cations move into the cells to replace the extruded potassium, and the excess hydrogen cations in the tubular cells promote secretion of hydrogen ions in the ultrafiltrate and a gain of bicarbonate in the peritubular blood of the proximal tubule.

REFERENCES

Bristol DG. The anion gap as a prognostic indicator in horses with abdominal pain. J Am Vet Med Assoc 1982;181:63.

Cowan TKJ, Phillips GDK. Potassium and sodium balance during dietary potasssium restriction in sheep. Can J Anim Sci 1973;53:653.

Gossett KA, French DD. Effect of age on anion gap in clinically normal quarter horses. Am J Vet Res 1983;44:1744.

Moller JV, Sheikh MI. Renal organic anion transport system: pharmacological, physiological and biochemical aspects. Pharmacol Rev 1983;34:315.

Ogilvie TH, Butler DG, Gartllley CJ, Dohoo JR. Magnesium oxide–induced metabolic alkalosis in cattle. Can J Comp Med 1983;47:108.

Quintanilla AP. Acute acid-base disorders. 1. Laboratory characterization. Postgrad Med 1976;60:68.

Roch-Ramel F. Renal excretion of uric acid in mammals. Clin Nephrol 1979;12:1.

Roch-Ramel F, Wong NLM, Dirks JH. Renal excretion of urate in mongrel and Dalmatian dogs: a micropuncture study. Am J Physiol 1976;231:326.

Weiner IM. Urate transport in the nephron. Am J Physiol 1979;237:F85.

CHAPTER 19

RENAL WATER BALANCE

On a daily basis, an animal consumes a volume of water and loses an equal amount, mostly as urine, but some fractions through breathing (sensible and insensible loss), sweating (except in dogs, cats, and swine), and stool moisture (Fig. 19–1).

The regulation of body water is equivalent to the regulation of body osmolarity, osmolarity being the number of active particles (electrolytes, molecules) per unit of plasma (i.e., about 270 to 300 mOsm per liter in large animals, and 280 to 310 mOsm per liter in small animals). Although freezing-point depression offers a direct measure of plasma osmolarity, it is more convenient to use plasma sodium as an index of body osmolality. Plasma sodium concentration measures approximately 50 percent of the total osmolality (the other half being the total number of anions) because it is 90 percent of the total cations in plasma.

The hormones that influence body osmolarity through the kidneys are antidiuretic hormone (ADH, which modulates renal water excretion), aldosterone (which modulates sodium balance), cortisol, and, to a lesser extent, parathormone (PTH). The vasoactive hormones, angiotensin, epinephrine, and norepinephrine, which reduce renal blood flow and glomerular filtration rate (GFR), affect body osmolarity by modifying urine production. Diuretics (agents that promote production of urine) can also influence body osmolarity. Atrial natriuretic factor (ANF) also causes natriuresis and diuresis. This chapter deals with body osmolarity under the influence of hormones that act on the kidneys, hormones produced by the kidney, and antidiuresis and diuresis.

HORMONES THAT ACT ON THE KIDNEYS

Antidiuretic Hormone

Antidiuretic hormone (ADH) is a polypeptide (nine amino acids) synthesized in the supraoptic, and possibly the paraventricular, centers of the hypothalamus. Production of ADH by these nerve cells is mediated by changes in intracellular fluid volume. When plasma osmolarity is high, water moves out of the cells, intracellular volume is decreased, intracellular osmolarity is increased, and ADH is produced. The reverse occurs when osmolarity is reduced. The initial product passes down the axon bound to a carrier protein, neurophysin, and is stored in axonal bulbs close to the basement membrane of the capillaries of the neurohypophysis (Fig. 19–2). The stored material (neurophysin and ADH) is liberated by the process of exocytosis by various stimuli: alterations in blood volume and in plasma osmolarity, decreased arterial pressure, increased blood temperature perfusing the hypothalamus, pain and emotions, and drugs (acetylcholine, nicotine, morphine, barbiturates).

ADH acts on the hypothalamus, the kidneys, and the pancreas. It inhibits the thirst center in the hypothalamus. The action on the kidney occurs in the glomeruli, the tubules, and the collecting ducts. ADH increases the GFR by bringing more glomeruli into operation. ADH attaches to the basolateral membrane of the tubular and collecting duct cells. The attachment activates adenylate cyclase, which converts adenosine triphosphate (ATP) into cyclic adenosine monophosphate (cAMP). The intracellular messenger is necessary to facilitate transports (by increasing the size of the aqueous channels) from lumen to the interstitium. The intracellular levels or action of cAMP is influenced by prostaglandin E, calcium, magnesium, and adrenal steroids. ADH alters the permeability of cells in the pancreas as in the kidneys; it favors the output of water from the canaliculi and decreases the volume of secretion.

About 91 percent of the water filtered at the glomerulus has already been reabsorbed when the tubular fluid reaches the collecting duct. Modulation of the remaining 9 percent is normally effected in the collecting duct under the influence of ADH. Concentrated urine is produced only as an event secondary to the presence of a hyperosmolar renal medullary interstitium. Maintenance of interstitial hyperosmolality depends on both factors of the renal countercurrent multiplier system: selective permeability of tubule segments and active transport of solutes.

Countercurrent exchange refers to the exchange of solute, water, or heat between fluids flowing in opposite directions along closely opposed limbs in a folded loop. A *countercurrent multiplier system* exists when such a folded loop also possesses an intrinsic mechanism for active transfer between the limbs (e.g., chloride transfer by the epithelium of the thick ascending loop of Henle).

Theoretical explanations of the countercurrent multiplier system are still being debated. The following principles are the latest proposed to explain the concentration of urine in the medullary loop of the doubly folded S-shaped configuration of the nephron and vasa recta (Fig. 19–3):

1. Solute is supplied by ascending Henle's limb (AHL, *the countercurrent multiplier*) to the interstitium, which extracts water from the tubular fluid in descending Henle's limb (DHL) and collecting duct (CD).

2. The cortical loop allows diluted tubule fluid in the AHL to return to isotonicity with cortical plasma before it reenters the medulla.

3. The folded vasa recta (*countercurrent exchanger*) and surrounding interstitium (the central core) provide an expansion chamber for the performance of osmotic work and a mixing chamber for salt and urea. This mixing induces passive salt transport out of the AHL.

4. The system acts as a solute-cycling multiplier from the AHL to the vascular core and the osmotically equilibrated DHL and CD.

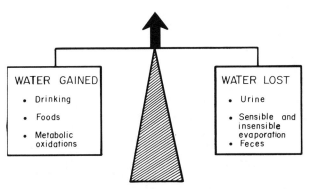

Figure 19–1 Major sources of water gain and loss during the water balance process.

5. The short-looped nephrons provide urea to drive salt transport out of AHL of long nephrons in the inner medulla.

Production of Hypertonic Urine (Baruria, Hypersthenuria)

In the presence of a high ADH titer, the cells of the distal tubule and collecting duct become highly permeable to water. Hypotonic fluid (100 mOsm per liter) entering the

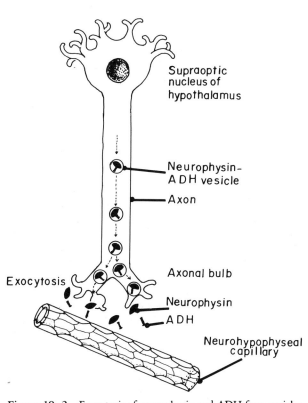

Figure 19–2 Exocytosis of neurophysin and ADH from vesicles formed in the supraoptic nucleus of the hypothalamus and held in the axonal bulbs near the neurohypophyseal capillaries.

distal tubule then rapidly loses water until it becomes isotonic with the surrounding cortical interstitium (300 mOsm per liter). As this fluid continues through the medullary collecting duct, it loses additional water to the hypertonic medullary interstitium and emerges from the collecting duct hypertonic to cortical or arterial plasma (see Fig. 19–3).

By increasing the cell permeability of the collecting duct and allowing water from the lumen to transfer into the hyperosmolal medullary interstitium, ADH reduces the water loss. ADH also reduces the urinary excretion of ions other than sodium by increasing the reabsorption of magnesium in the loop of Henle and of magnesium, calcium, potassium, and chloride in the thick ascending limb. ADH, metabolized in both the liver and the kidneys, is excreted in bile and urine; its half-life is 20 minutes.

Production of Hypotonic Urine (Hyposthenuria)

When ADH secretion is low, cells of the distal nephron are almost impermeable to water. Hypotonic tubular fluid (100 mOsm per liter) passing through the distal tubule and collecting duct loses very little water, and a urine hypotonic to renal cortex or arterial plasma is produced (Fig. 19–4).

Aldosterone

Biosynthesis of aldosterone, a mineralocorticoid and the most potent of all adrenal steroids, occurs in the outer layer, the *zona glomerulosa,* of the adrenal cortex. It may originate from pregnenolone or corticosterone. Its secretion is responsive to a rise in plasma potassium, to low plasma sodium, and to the humoral factors angiotensin II (A II) and adrenocorticotropin (ACTH).

Angiotensin II is related to the production of a renal hormone, renin, itself resulting from a fall in extracellular fluid volume and sodium depletion. In hypovolemia, the decreased renal perfusion stimulates the juxtaglomerular apparatus to produce renin (Fig. 19–5). The hormone activates a precursor (angiotensinogen) that liberates angiotensin I (A I), which is then converted to angiotensin II in the lung. Angiotensin II is a potent vasoconstrictor and stimulator of the adrenal cortex to produce aldosterone. Though ACTH is able to sustain the secretion of aldosterone, it is not its main stimulus.

Aldosterone traverses the cell membrane and combines with an intracellular receptor protein of the tubule target cell. The steroid-receptor complex reaches the cell nucleus and directs the genetic apparatus to accelerate the production of specific enzymes to either enhance or reduce the reabsorptive activity of the distal tubule cell.

Aldosterone is involved in the fine control of sodium balance. It controls the renal tubular reabsorption of a small, although important, fraction of the sodium tubule load. As a result of this regulation of the body sodium by the kidneys, renal water conservation and extracellular fluid volume are increased. The general function of aldosterone is to promote renal retention of sodium (also effective on the intestine)

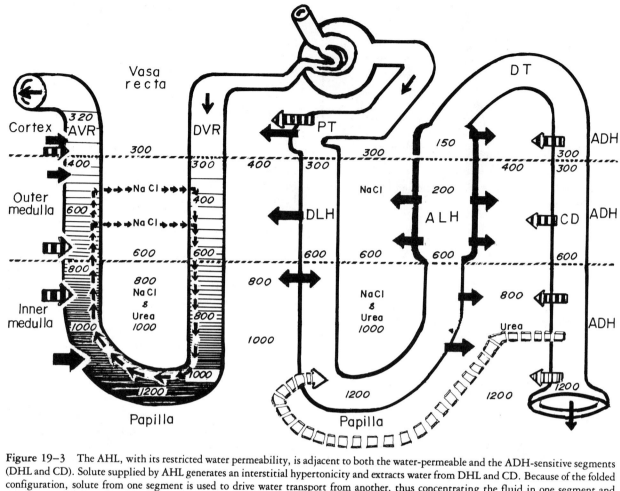

Figure 19–3 The AHL, with its restricted water permeability, is adjacent to both the water-permeable and the ADH-sensitive segments (DHL and CD). Solute supplied by AHL generates an interstitial hypertonicity and extracts water from DHL and CD. Because of the folded configuration, solute from one segment is used to drive water transport from another, thus concentrating the fluid in one segment and diluting the fluid in the other. The solute deposited in the medullary interstitium can escape in two ways: by concentration difference between AVR and DVR (dissipative loss of solute) and by difference in volume flow between AVR and DVR (useful osmotic work of concentration). When concentrations are equal in AVR and DVR, solute from AHL takes from DHL and CD its isotonic equivalent of water.

while enhancing potassium loss. The sodium reabsorption by the distal tubule is accomplished independent of potassium secretion. Aldosterone also stimulates the excretion of hydrogen, ammonium, and magnesium ions by the distal tubule.

Metabolism and excretion of aldosterone are performed by the liver and kidneys. Conjugated to glucuronic or sulfuric acid, aldosterone is secreted in bile and in the proximal tubule. There is an enterohepatic recirculation of aldosterone, which is excreted in bile.

Cortisol

Cortisol, a glucocorticoid with the highest secretion rate, originates from cells in the middle layer of the adrenal cortex, the *zona fasciculata*. ACTH regulates the production of cortisol. The increased plasma concentration of cortisol at the hypothalamus and the adenohypophysis induces a feedback mechanism that decreases the secretion of corticotropin-releasing factor (CRF) and ACTH.

ACTH secretion is increased by emotions and stress. The plasma concentration of cortisol, highest in the morning (>10 μg per deciliter) and lowest (<5 μg per deciliter) in midafternoon, is at least 1000 times more than that of aldosterone (5 to 10 ng per deciliter).

Cortisol increases GFR and tubule secretory activity. The slight mineralocorticoid action induces sodium retention and potassium excretion in the distal nephron, but much less effectively than does aldosterone.

Urinary excretion of calcium is also enhanced. It favors mild diuresis (high urine flow) and permits maximal excretion of excess body water because of an action opposite to that of ADH. Cortisol also promotes reabsorption of bicarbonate and the occurrence of metabolic alkalosis (alkalemia).

Less than 5 to 10 percent of the plasma cortisol is free and active. The remainder, bound to cortisol-binding globulin (CBG, >75 percent) and to albumin (15 percent) is inactive and unavailable to the organism. In contrast, 50 percent of plasma aldosterone is free and available. Cortisol is metabolized in the liver, and its numerous metabolites are

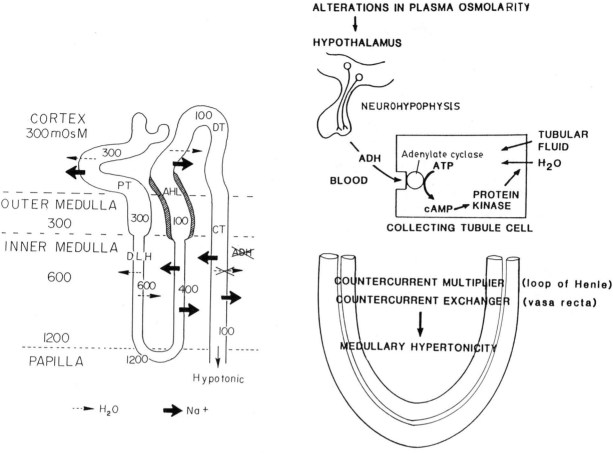

Figure 19–4 Production of dilute urine by insufficient water reabsorption in the distal tubule and the collecting ducts because of a lack of ADH. The water permeability at the apical surface of the cells of the distal tubule is not increased. ADH is needed to activate adenylate cyclase for production of cAMP, which activates protein kinases that facilitate permeability of distal tubule cells to water. Water cannot move from the lumen of the distal tubule into the peritubular capillaries, even if it is attracted by the normal medullary interstitial hypertonicity, which is maintained by the countercurrent multiplier (loops of Henle) and countercurrent exchanger (vasa recta) systems.

excreted in bile and urine as glucuronides and sulfates. The half-life of cortisol is about 90 minutes.

Parathormone

Renal excretion and reabsorption of calcium and phosphorus are modulated by PTH secreted by chief cells (agranular) of the parathyroid glands. PTH is a linear polypeptide (84 amino acids). Its secretion is responsive to hypocalcemia, hypomagnesemia, and low concentration of vitamin D_3 and to hyperphosphatemia in the blood perfusing the parathyroid.

PTH decreases the GFR, but its most important function is the regulation of urinary phosphorus excretion and, consequently, of plasma phosphorus concentration. It adjusts the rate of phosphorus excretion to conserve or eliminate phosphorus from the body. Excretion of phosphorus occurs in the gut (30 percent) and the kidney (70 percent). Administration of PTH—and, similarly, hypercalcemia—decreases the reabsorption of phosphorus in the proximal tubule, the loop of Henle, and the distal tubule. As a result, phosphorus

excretion is increased and plasma phosphorus concentration is lowered.

Conversely, PTH increases reabsorption of calcium (increases Tm) and raises the plasma calcium concentration. This hypercalcemia causes the tubule load to exceed the Tm for calcium, and in spite of an enhanced tubular reabsorption of calcium, urinary excretion of calcium is increased.

PTH also increases excretion of sodium, potassium, and bicarbonate. Conversely, it improves reabsorption of magnesium and ammonium and causes the titratable acidity of urine to be lowered. Another important effect of PTH is to favor the renal hydroxylation of 25,hydroxycholecalciferol into 1,25,dihydroxycholecalciferol (vitamin D_3). PTH is excreted in urine. Reported values for its half-life in a cow are 20, 30, and 50 minutes.

Other Hormones

The osmolarity and volume of body fluids are also influenced by other hormones that have some effect on the kidneys.

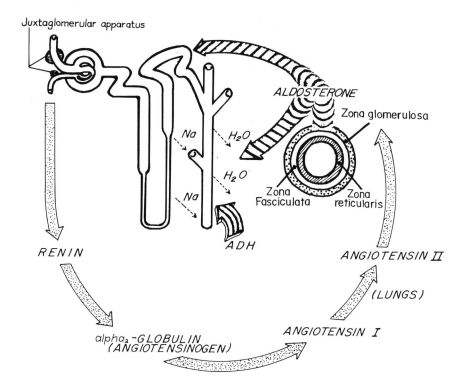

Juxtaglomerular apparatus

Figure 19-5 Regulation of volume and osmolarity of the extracellular fluid by the ADH and the renin-angiotensin-aldosterone systems.

Thyroid Hormones

Triiodothyronine (T_3) and *thyroxine* (T_4) modulate transports in tubule cells by stimulating general cellular activities. The urinary excretion of calcium is higher, whereas that of phosphorus is lower. *Thyrocalcitonin* (calcitonin) regulates tubule transport of calcium and phosphorus during states of hypercalcemia. It increases urinary output of phosphorus, calcium, magnesium, sodium, and chloride in cows, goats, rabbits, and rats but is without effect in dogs. In rabbits, the effects occur in the medullary portion of the thick ascending limb of Henle and the distal tubule.

The ovarian steroid hormones, progesterone and estrogens, have diverging renal effects. *Progesterone* decreases water and sodium retention by distal tubule cells and is considered an endogenous antagonist to aldosterone. *Estrogens* augment excretion of phosphorus but lower sodium, water, and calcium output.

Somatotropin (growth hormone), a polypeptide from the adenohypophysis, decreases the excretion of phosphorus, calcium, and magnesium in dogs.

Pancreatic Hormones

Insulin causes calciuria but favors retention of phosphorus and sodium. *Glucagon* increases the urinary excretion of phosphorus, calcium, magnesium, and sodium.

Vasoactive hormones (*epinephrine* and *norepinephrine*) constrict renal blood vessels. At moderate doses, when constriction is equal in both afferent and efferent arterioles, the quantity of blood perfused may be reduced by as much as 50 percent without significant change in GFR. At higher intra-

venous doses, a more intense constriction of the afferent arteriole results in reductions of both renal blood flow and GFR. In addition to these actions, the slower peritubular blood flow reduces sodium but increases phosphorus excretion in urine.

Atrial natriuretic factor (ANF, natriuretic factor), a small polypeptide of atrial origin released in response to expansion of plasma volume (atrial distention) and to sodium loading, has renal vasodilatory and vasorelaxant (anti-angiotensin II) effects. By inhibiting adenylate cyclase in tubule cells, it prevents reabsorption of water and sodium and increases their urinary excretion. It also accelerates blood flow in the renal interstitium and reduces the interstitial hyperosmolality.

HORMONES PRODUCED BY THE KIDNEYS

Renin-Angiotensin-Aldosterone System

Renin, a glycoprotein (36,000 daltons) formed principally in the epithelial cells of the juxtaglomerular apparatus, is enzymatically active in various organs and is dedicated to the formation of angiotensin I. For this reason, it is part of the renin-angiotensin system.

Renin is produced by activation of an enzymatically inactive prorenin and liberated in the renal afferent arteriole or lymph. Plasma prorenin concentration is increased during sodium depletion, pregnancy, and diuretic therapy but is lowered with sodium loading. In vivo, renal kallikrein may be the activator of prorenin into renin; in vitro, acidification and low temperature activate prorenin.

The concentration of renin is regulated by several mechanisms: beta-adrenergic agonists (sympathetic system), prostaglandins (PGs and arachidonic acid), and kinins. Systemic hypotension (decrease in blood volume and renal perfusion pressure) and sodium deprivation (hyponatremia, diuretics, low sodium in tubular fluid perceived at the *macula densa*) trigger the baroreceptor reflex that stimulates the beta-adrenergic receptors of the juxtaglomerular apparatus to release renin. Renal hypotension also brings about release of renin by a mechanism mediated by prostaglandin, probably PGI_2, which is independent of the adrenergic nervous system.

The substrate of renin, angiotensinogen, is a plasma glycoprotein (55,000 daltons) of hepatic origin. Renin cleaves one peptide bond in angiotensinogen to release the biologically inactive decapeptide Ang I. Angiotensin-converting enzyme (mostly in the lungs, the juxtaglomerular apparatus, and the glomerulus) then cleaves a dipeptide from Ang I to produce the biologically active peptide Ang II (Fig. 19–6). The continuous hepatic production of angiotensinogen is increased by synthetic estrogens or glucocorticoids, by thyroid hormones, and by Ang II. Pharmacological inhibition of this enzyme is used to treat essential hypertension, a problem of clinical interest in humans but of limited (academic) interest in animals.

The half-life of Ang II is about 1 minute, nearly a third of circulating Ang II is transformed into angiotensin III (Ang III) by aminopeptidase of plasma and adrenal tissue. As active as Ang II in stimulating secretion of aldosterone, Ang III has only 30 percent of the pressor effect of Ang II. The effects of angiotensins are listed in Table 19–1.

1.25-Dihydroxycholecalciferol

The kidneys are responsible for the final step in the transformation of vitamin D_3 (cholecalciferol) into a biolog-

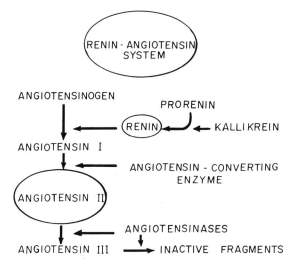

Figure 19–6 Relationship between the units of the renin-angiotensin-aldosterone system. Activation of renin is associated with plasma kallikrein, and catabolism of A II and A III is performed by various enzymes (angiotensinases).

TABLE 19–1 Actions of Angiotensins

Production of aldosterone, ADH, and glucocorticoids
Contraction of vascular and extravascular smooth muscle
Negative feedback on renin production
Thirst
Central pressor (hypertensive) effect
Sodium transfer in colon and kidneys

ically active form. They hydroxylate 25-hydroxycholecalciferol into 1,25-dihydroxycholecalciferol under the stimulation of PTH.

After vitamin D_3 is absorbed from the ingesta or is produced in the skin in response to ultraviolet radiation, it is biologically inactive and is stored in the liver. The liver performs hydroxylation of cholecalciferol into 25-hydroxycholecalciferol and precisely regulates its concentration in the plasma.

Under the stimulation of PTH, cells of the proximal tubule hydroxylate 25-hydroxycholecalciferol into 1.25-dihydroxyvitamin D_3. The most important function of dihydroxyvitamin D_3 is to cause formation of calcium-binding proteins (CaBP) in the cytoplasm of renal distal tubules and collecting ducts and of intestinal epithelial cells. CaBP facilitates diffusion of calcium ions into the cytoplasm of these cells and contributes to the regulation of calcemia and, indirectly, of phosphatemia and phosphaturia.

Calcitonin (thyrocalcitonin) inhibits the activation of 25-hydroxyvitamin D_3 to 1,25-dihydroxyvitamin D_3 in the proximal tubule.

Erythropoietin

Erythropoietin (EP), a glycoprotein (45,000 daltons) originating in the glomerulus, controls the proliferative sequence of erythrocytes in the bone marrow. This effect is seen after a lag of 2 to 3 days and extends over a period of nearly 10 days.

EP derives from a profactor (beta$_2$-globulin), synthesized in the liver and transported to the kidney. In the glomerular tuft, the profactor is converted to active EP by a renal enzyme, renal erythropoietic factor (REF). A slight extrarenal production of EP probably occurs in the liver.

Secretion of EP is stimulated by altitude (decrease of P_B and of P_{O_2}), androgens, cobalt salts, renal hypoxia, and hemorrhage (Table 19–2). Estrogens inhibit production of erythropoietin. The half-life of erythropoietin is about 5 hours. The liver inactivates EP, which is also found in urine.

TABLE 19–2 Factors Influencing Production of Erythropoietin

Increased secretion of EP because of lack of oxygen in tissues
    Large needs: ACTH, glucocorticoids, thyroid hormones
    Small supply: anemia, angiotensin (decreased RBF), cobalt (cellular anoxia), hypoxia, ischemia
Decrease in secretion because of excess oxygen in tissues
    Small needs: fasting, hypothyroidism
    Large supply: hyperoxia, polyglobulia

Prostaglandins

Cells of the interstitium, the collecting ducts, and the arterial wall of the kidney can synthesize prostaglandins (PGs). The PGs (20-C, unsaturated bonds) are not hormones in the strictest sense and are called "parahormones," or "local hormones." These arachidonic acid derivatives are synthesized mostly to serve a defensive function, locally, and on demand by the cyclooxygenase pathway.

The major active compounds are PGE_2, prostacyclin (PGI_2, or epoprostenol), thromboxane A_2 (TXA_2), and $PGF_{2\alpha}$. PGD_2, endoperoxides (PGG_2, PGH_2), and products of the lipoxygenase pathway for oxidation of arachidonic acid (leukotriene D_4, LTD_4) are also produced, but their role in the kidneys is not clear. The PG most likely responsible for the majority of the physiological effects is PGE_2, which originates in medullary and collecting duct cells. $PGF_{2\alpha}$, formed in the glomerulus, is derived from PGE_2 (Fig. 19–7). PGI_2, synthesized in the vascular walls (interlobar and afferent arteries) in the cortex, has a systemic action like that of a hormone, since it is the only active PG not degraded in the lung. Other PGs are not stored, and their transport between cortex and medulla is improbable, as, after synthesis, their extremely short half-life allows only an immediate local action.

Prostaglandins contribute to the regulation of renal blood flow, water and sodium transport, and glomerular filtration; directly to renin and ADH release; and indirectly to A II, aldosterone, and kallikrein release. Medullary and inner cortical circulations are improved by PGs. This vasodilation would protect against vasoconstrictive agents such as A II and norepinephrine. Secretion of renal PGs is stimulated by triamterene, a potassium-sparing substance.

To control water and electrolyte excretion, PGE_2 and PGI_2 influence three fundamental renal mechanisms: ADH-dependent osmotic water permeability of the collecting tubule, blood flow, and sodium chloride transfers (natriuresis and chloruresis). Excessive PG production can oppose the effect of ADH, increase the medullary blood flow, and reduce the transport of sodium chloride and urea out of the tubular fluid into the interstitium (Fig. 19–8). These actions enhance the excretion of water and formation of a more dilute urine by weakening the combined actions of ADH and the renal countercurrent system.

Prostacyclin and PGE_2 stimulate the juxtaglomerular apparatus for renin release (Fig. 19–9) during renal arterial hypotension in the dog. This PG pathway for release of renin would be parallel to the activation of the baroreceptor system via beta-adrenergic receptors during systemic hypotension. Most of the PGs generated intramurally do not enter the bloodstream and are destroyed locally in vascular walls near the site of generation. In the dog, PGI_2 causes vasodilation, diuresis, and natriuresis.

The effect of ADH is inhibited by PGs, even though ADH stimulates the production of PGs. By causing a decrease in the interstitial osmolal gradient, the medullary PGs also favor the production of dilute urine.

The *kallikrein-kinin system* stimulates the production of PGs in the cortex.

Thromboxane A_2 (TXA_2) and LTD_4, which are synthesized under abnormal conditions, constrict vessels. TXA_2 also causes aggregation of thrombocytes and thus has biological effects opposite those of PGI_2, which is a vasodilator that inhibits aggregation of thrombocytes. Production of PGE_2 results in arteriolar vasodilation, but $PGF_{2\alpha}$ causes venoconstriction.

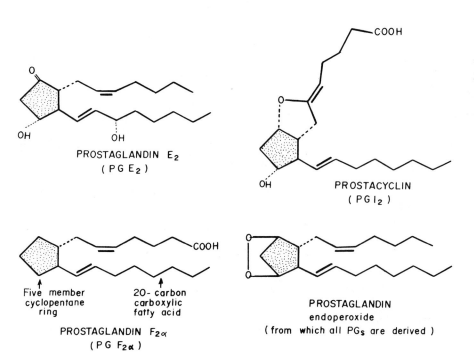

PROSTAGLANDIN E_2
($PG\ E_2$)

PROSTACYCLIN
($PG\ I_2$)

Five member cyclopentane ring

20- carbon carboxylic fatty acid

PROSTAGLANDIN $F_{2\alpha}$
($PG\ F_{2\alpha}$)

PROSTAGLANDIN
endoperoxide
(from which all PGs are derived)

Figure 19–7 Structures of the major renal prostaglandins (E_2, I_2, and $F_{2\alpha}$) and of their endoperoxide precursor.

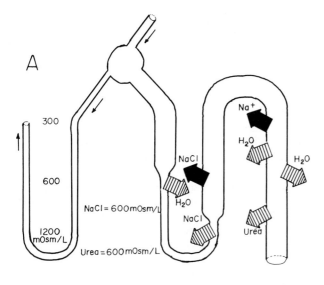

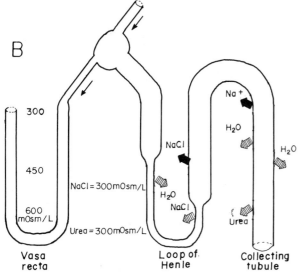

Figure 19–8 Renal countercurrent system (rabbit). **A,** Under normal conditions, when interstitial osmolality is maintained at a peak of 1,200 mOsm per liter by reabsorption of sodium chloride and urea and vasa recta blood flow is low. **B,** With higher medullary PG production, the vasa recta blood flow increases, the interstitial osmolal concentration decreases (300 mOsm per liter each of sodium chloride and urea), and reabsorption of sodium chloride, urea, and water is lower.

ANTIDIURESIS AND DIURESIS

Urine production is modified by homeostatic mechanisms that lead to antidiuresis or diuresis to maintain body osmolality within narrow limits.

Antidiuresis

Antidiuresis refers to conditions in which urine flow is low and osmolality high. The conservation of water but loss

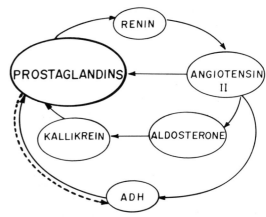

Figure 19–9 Relationships among renal prostaglandins and ADH, renin-angiotensinogen-aldosterone system, and kallikrein.

of solutes (sodium) in the urine causes dilution and corrects an initially excessively concentrated extracellular fluid. From a physiological standpoint, the most important stimuli for the release of ADH stored in the neurohypophysis are a rise in body fluid osmolality (osmotic stimulus) and volume depletion of extracellular fluid (nonosmotic stimulus such as hemorrhage).

ADH or A II (after renin release) liberated by volume depletion also induces a vasoconstriction that decreases renal blood supply and results in antidiuresis. ADH, a more potent renal vasoconstrictor than A II, reduces GFR and water losses by an effect other than increased distal tubule permeability to water. Antidiuresis by A II lowers the output of water and sodium by two mechanisms—a direct effect on the nephron and stimulation of the adrenal cortex to liberate aldosterone.

Relative situations of antidiuresis are described in animals:

Nocturnal Antidiuresis. In temperate climates, animals produce less urine by night than by day.

Diurnal Antidiuresis. In tropical climates, water losses by respiration or sweating cause less urine to be voided by day than by night.

Seasonal Antidiuresis. The urine output is less in summer than in winter.

Postural and Exercise Antidiuresis. A smaller volume of urine is produced when animals stand up than when they lie down. Exercise causes less urine to be discharged than in a resting state.

Dietary Antidiuresis. Eating dry foods causes carnivores to produce less urine than they do when they eat meat. Feeding on hay or dry pastures decreases the output of herbivores' urine in comparison with the volume of urine when they feed on fresh green plants.

Diuresis

The term *diuresis* means an increase in the rate of urine production. By measuring the concentration of solute in the abundant urine, a distinction can be made between water diuresis and osmotic diuresis.

Water Diuresis

Water diuresis, excretion of a dilute urine, raises extracellular fluid sodium concentration. The urine is dilute because it contains more water than needed to carry the solutes at their plasma concentrations, that is, it contains "free water," or "solute-free water." Excretion of copious dilute urine is associated with absence or inhibition of ADH.

Inadequate synthesis of ADH by the hypothalamoneurohypophyseal system (i.e., central or pituitary *diabetes insipidus*) is a rare syndrome that occurs genetically in Brattleboro rats. The term *diabetes* means excessive urine production, and the attribute *insipidus* qualifies the urine as being tasteless (in comparison to *diabetes mellitus,* in which urine is sweet). In diabetes mellitus, caused by lack of pancreatic insulin, an excess of urine containing sugar is produced. A nephrogenic form of diabetes insipidus, in which the kidney is unable to respond to ADH, is associated with drugs (tetracycline, methoxyflurane), hypokalemia, and hypercalcemia.

A decrease in plasma osmolarity by water loading (excessive water intake or extracellular fluid volume) causes water diuresis. It suppresses release of ADH and decreases the secretion of renin by the kidney and of aldosterone by the adrenal cortex. Renal adjustment begins after a lag of 15 minutes and is completed within 1 to 2 hours in ruminants and in about 3 hours in carnivores. Nonosmotic factors also inhibit the release of ADH. The most important are hypothermia, expansion of plasma or blood volume, and drugs (alcohol, diphenylhydantoin, thyroid hormones, cortisol, epinephrine, and atropine).

Osmotic Diuresis

Osmotic diuresis is the excretion of urine that contains large amounts of solutes (i.e., excretion of both water [pressure diuresis] and solutes [pressure natriuresis] is increased). It is generally produced when a solute that cannot be reabsorbed from the tubular filtrate is present in the plasma and is filtered at the glomerulus. The greater the quantity of unabsorbed osmolal substance, the greater the quantity of water that is not reabsorbed.

The process of osmotic diuresis can occur with metabolically inert organic molecules such as *mannitol,* sucrose, and urea. After intravenous injection, these molecules, which easily pass the filtration barrier, remain in the tubular ultrafiltrate, exert osmolal activity to retain water, and initiate profuse urine production. Osmotic diuresis is also seen with glucose, when insulin production is insufficient to prevent hyperglycemia. The tubule load of glucose is beyond the proximal tubule transport maximum capacity, and excessive water and glucose are carried in the urine (diabetes mellitus).

Intravenous injection of hypertonic mannitol or of sucrose is used not only to induce osmotic diuresis but also to exert an osmotic decrease in the extracellular water content of brain tissue. Mannitol is useful in reducing meningeal edema, whereas sucrose is of practical use in shrinking the cerebral cortex prior to surgery on the cranium.

Electrolytes can also be at the origin of osmotic diuresis when activity of tubule cells is either normal or impaired by diuretic drugs.

Within an hour after feeding on pasture plants rich in water (75 percent) and potassium, herbivores eliminate the excess potassium in their alkaline urine. The phosphorus, chloride, urea (from the proteins), and water (70 percent) of meat eaten by carnivores are found in the acid urine produced during the postprandial hour. By osmotic diuresis, animals eliminate the excess sodium chloride resulting from parenteral (intraperitoneal, subcutaneous, or intravenous injection) administration of isotonic saline, also in less than an hour. Almost immediate diuretic osmosis is produced by injecting sodium sulfate intravenously and suddenly increasing the tubular load of sulfate, a nonabsorbed solute, which is eliminated with calcium ions.

Most diuretic drugs affect the tubular epithelium to impair sodium, chloride, and potassium reabsorption (natriuresis, chloruresis, kaliuresis) and thereby reduce water reabsorption (diuresis) by osmolal entrapment (i.e., osmotic diuresis).

Xanthine (caffeine, theophylline) decreases tubular reabsorption of sodium besides increasing the glomerular filtration rate. *Thiazides* act on the proximal tubule by inhibiting reabsorption of sodium, chloride, and potassium. *Furosemide* and *ethacrynic acid* are loop diuretics that inhibit active reabsorption of chloride by cells of the ascending limb of the loop of Henle and associated sodium reabsorption in the interstitium of the medulla. Retention of potassium is favored while sodium is excreted when certain drugs are administered: spironolactone inhibits aldosterone, triamterene and amiloride inhibit reabsorption of sodium and chloride in the proximal and distal tubules, and mercurial diuretics inhibit all the tubules. *Carbonic anhydrase inhibitors* (acetazolamide) operate on the proximal and distal tubules to produce a urine with excessively high concentration of sodium bicarbonate and potassium but very little chloride.

Atrial distention, in addition to causing production of ANF, reduces sympathetic neural tone. This lowered sympathetic activity decreases tubular reabsorption of sodium and exerts an osmosis-like diuretic effect.

REFERENCES

Ackerman U. Cardiovascular effects of ANF extract in the whole animal. Fed Proc 1986;45:2111.

de Rouffignac C, Corman B, Roinel N. Stimulation by antidiuretic hormone of electrolyte tubular reabsorption in rat kidney. Am J Physiol 1983;244:F156.

Inagami T, Chang JJ, Dykes CW, Takii Y, Kisaragi M, Misono KS. Renin: structural features of active enzyme and inactive precursor. Fed Proc 1983;42:2729.

Knepper M, Burg M. Organization of nephron function. Am J Physiol 1983;244:F579.

McGiff JC, Wong PYK. Compartmentalization of prostaglandins and prostacyclin within the kidney: implications for renal function. Fed Proc 1979;38:89.

Mitchell AR. Drugs and renal function. J Vet Pharmacol Ther 1979;2:5.

Oates JA, Whorton AR, Gerkens JF, Branch RA, Hollifield JW, Frolich JC. The participation of prostaglandins in the control of renin release. Fed Proc 1979;38:72.

Ondetti MA. Biochemistry of the renin-angiotensin system. Fed Proc 1983;42:2722.

Pastoriza-Munoz E, Mishler DR, Lechene C. Effect of phosphate deprivation on phosphate reabsorption in rat nephron: role of PTH. Am J Physiol 1983;244:F140.

Sealy JE, Atlas SA, Laragh JH. Prorenin in plasma and kidney. Fed Proc 1983;42:2681.

Stephenson JL. The renal concentrating mechanism: fundamental theoretical concepts. Fed Proc 1983;42:2386.

Stokes JB. Integrated actions of renal medullary prostaglandins in the control of water excretion. Am J Physiol 1981;9:F471.

Tewksberry DA. Angiotensinogen. Fed Proc 1983;42:2724.

CHAPTER 20

THE URINARY COLLECTING AND VOIDING SYSTEM

The formation of urine is an uninterrupted process of the nephron and collecting duct. Urine that has reached the papilla is continuously forced to progress into a conducting system made up of connected reservoirs and ducts. The apparatus of the upper excretory urinary system consists of the pelvis and the ureters. The lower excretory urinary apparatus includes the bladder and the urethra. Active unidirectional peristalsis takes the urine from the tip of the papilla down to the bladder. Urine slowly accumulates in the bladder, which accommodates to large fluctuations in urine volume by varying its surface area, and is voided outside the body by micturition. This chapter is concerned with the physiology of ureters and bladder, the process of micturition, and the principal characteristics of urine in animals.

THE URINARY COLLECTING SYSTEM

The function of the urinary collecting system is to transport sterile urine at low pressure through the upper urinary excretory apparatus. The walls of the pelvis and ureter are made up of three layers: an external connective tissue adventitia, a thin muscularis, and a transitional epithelial mucosa. The smooth muscle layer contains longitudinal (outer and inner) and circular (middle) fibers that, through peristalsis, actively propel urine issued from the renal collecting tubules to the bladder. A small active flow of ions (sodium-potassium-chloride cotransport) stimulated by antidiuretic hormone (ADH) exists across the papillary surface epithelium, which also contains sodium-potassium ATPase (Fig. 20–1). In horses, the mucous membrane of the renal pelvis and the proximal ureter carries large mucous glands.

The urinary collecting system begins at the *renal calyces*. The submucosal circular layer of smooth muscle of the calyces contracts twice as fast (12 times per minute) as the renal pelvis to propel urine from the calyceal system into the renal pelvis.

The *renal pelvis,* shaped like a funnel, empties into the upper ureter (Fig. 20–2). Pressure within the pelvis remains low (5 to 15 cm H_2O) during contractions of its circular muscles, which occur at a rate of about 6 per minute in dogs and rabbits (unicalyceal), and in pigs (multicalyceal). Once initiated, the pelvic contractions are propagated throughout the upper urinary tract; thus, the renal pelvis controls ureteral peristalsis. (The renal pelvis is absent in the ox because of the unfused renal lobes.)

Excessive pressure in the renal pelvis raises the tubular fluid pressure and may retard or stop glomerular filtration. Also, renal blood flow decreases and renal parenchyma sometimes atrophies to leave a thin shell of renal parenchyma stretched by a fluid-filled pelvis.

Ureters are small, flattened fibromuscular tubes innervated by parasympathetic (stimulation) and sympathetic (inhibition) fibers. On the basis of the orientation of its circular muscle layer, the *ureter* can be divided into three segments: proximal (upper), middle, and distal (lower, juxtavesical). An oblique orientation is found in the upper and lower segments, and true circular fibers are present only in the middle segment. Their peristalsis (1 to 5 per minute) propels urine at a rate of 2 to 3 cm per second. Between peristaltic waves, the ureter normally collapses and is closed. Stable basal electromyographic activity (about 20 per minute), without mechanical consequence, is seen on both ureters. This electrical activity is unrelated to the propulsive peristalsis.

Distention of the renal pelvis and ureters increases the frequency of contractions, the normal response to an increase in diuresis. The ureter, a tube fixed at both ends, becomes tortuous when distended because it increases not only in diameter but also in length. Excessive distention of the ureter (e.g., by calculi) is painful and reduces renal blood flow ipsilaterally.

The ureterovesical junction lacks an anatomical sphincter. Reflux of urine from the bladder into the ureter is prevented by a functional sphincter created by the passage of the ureter through the bladder wall in an oblique fashion at the lateral angle of the trigone (Fig. 20–3). When the bladder is distended, the dorsal and ventral walls of the ureter are pressed together.

The urinary *bladder* is a smooth muscle chamber divided into three zones: body (detrusor muscle), trigone (ureters and urethra), and bladder neck. Because of accommodation, the body of the bladder stretches to receive large volumes of urine with only a minimal increase in intravesical pressure, which has a baseline of 2 to 4 mm Hg. The mucosa of the collapsed bladder shows extensive macroscopic epithelial folds as well as microscopic apical membrane folding. As the bladder slowly fills, first macroscopic folds then microscopic folds are smoothed out. A further increase in surface area and in storage capacity of urine can be achieved by incorporation of cytoplasmic vesicles into at least the apical membrane. During distention, the apical membrane can support a supply of cytoplasmic vesicles, which are removed during bladder collapse.

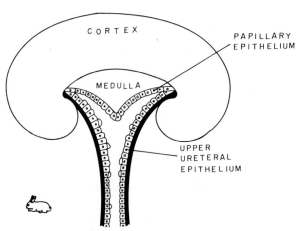

Figure 20–1 Bisection of a kidney and the initial part of the ureter to show the diagrammatic arrangement of the papillary and of the upper ureteral epithelium.

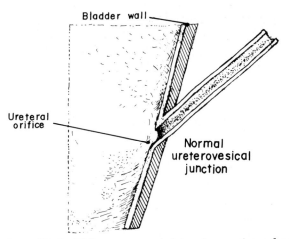

Figure 20–3 Oblique ureterovesical junction creating a functional sphincter to prevent reflux of urine in the ureter.

Continence is maintained by the internal vesical sphincter in dogs. In goats, the neck of the urethra functions as an extension of the urinary bladder and not as a sphincter; a competent internal sphincter is lacking, but the function is ensured by continuous tonicity of striated urethral muscles.

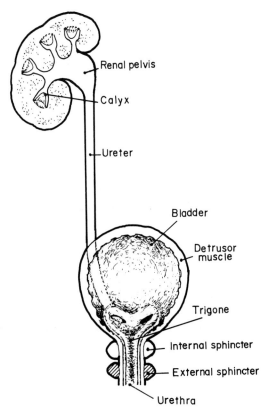

Figure 20–2 The urinary collecting (calyces, pelvis, ureter, bladder) and voiding (detrusor, trigone, internal and external sphincters, urethra) systems.

THE URINARY VOIDING SYSTEM

At a volume threshold, the detrusor muscle contracts to simultaneously widen and shorten the neck of the bladder, to raise the intravesical pressure acutely (Fig. 20–4) by 10 to 30 mm Hg and to initiate micturition reflexly. Triggering of the voiding reflex is by funnelling of the bladder neck and of the proximal urethra. In dogs, it occurs with relaxation of tone in smooth muscles and elastic fibers of the internal sphincter. In goats, urethral muscle tone decreases, and relaxation of the external sphincter follows. Dogs and swine void in short spurts, and cattle and horses in a continuous stream.

Innervation

Information on the degree of distention of the bladder and urethra passes to the spinal cord and is modulated by brainstem, spinal reflex centers, and volition. Micturition involves a sensorimotor reflex in the sacral area (S-2 to S-4) caudad to L-5. Craniad to this point, the spinal cord relays only central facilitatory control from anterior pons and posterior hypothalamus and inhibitory control from the cerebrum and midbrain. The hypogastric nerve receives sensory innervation from the fundus of the bladder. The trigone and bladder neck send sensory signals through the pelvic nerve, and the sensory innervation to the urethra is via the pudendal nerve. The pelvic nerve is motor to the bladder and provides sacral parasympathetic outflow to the detrusor muscle (Fig. 20–5). The abundant lymphatics of the bladder drain by the iliac nodes (external, internal, and common).

Atony of the bladder is a common phenomenon in all patients with spinal injuries and compressions because of nerve damage or of pain associated with contraction of the abdominal press. Prolonged urinary retention favors ammo-

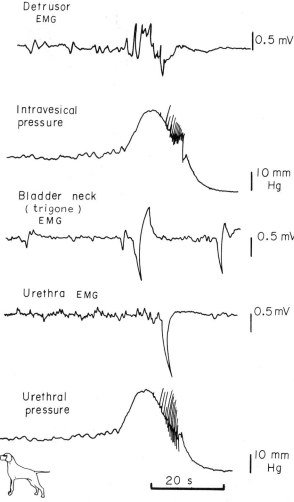

Figure 20–4 Electromyographic recordings of pressure events in the bladder and urethra leading to voiding in an anesthetized dog.

niation of urine and subsequent irritation of the bladder mucosa but also causes permanent injury to the bladder musculature. The bladder may then remain atonic and be unable to function normally in micturition.

In animals, facilitation of micturition is associated with olfaction. Investigation of previous elimination sites stimulates most animals to urinate. Emotions cause emptying of the bladder (e.g., fear or emergency in ruminants, new environment [territorial markings], playing and joy in small animals). Frequent emission of a urine containing pheromones (olfactory signals to males) is characteristic in female animals during estrus.

Sensory stimuli can facilitate micturition. In large animals, transrectal tapping on the bladder, monotone whistling, or perivulvar titillation trigger micturition. In small animals, rhythmic deep (7 to 8 per 5 seconds) suprapubic manual pressure, simple abdominal massage, and abdominal massage with a warm, damp cloth or sponge actuate urina-

tion. In adult cats and dogs, only indirect transabdominal compression of the bladder is efficient.

By cortical inhibition (e.g., house training of pets) urination can be delayed until the environment is favorable. For this retention of urine, relaxation of the detrusor and contraction of the internal sphincter are brought about through the hypogastric nerves. Puppies and female dogs void in a crouching position. Male dogs raise a hind leg while projecting a few jets of urine to mark their territory.

Modification of Bladder Function by Drugs

Drugs that affect the bladder are those that stimulate the bladder detrusor muscle (cholinergics or parasympathomimetics) and those that inhibit the bladder detrusor muscle (anticholinergics, parasympatholytics). Whether or not sympathetic fibers have motor function is controversial.

The most effective cholinergic drug, beta-methylcholine chloride, has the same action as the labile acetylcholine on the smooth muscle fibers of the bladder. This drug increases the muscle tone and the force of contraction at micturition.

The parasympatholytic drug atropine relaxes, or decreases the tone of, the bladder muscle by blocking the postganglionic actions of acetylcholine. The causes of increased bladder tone include prolonged partial, acute, or chronic irritation by calculi, and cystitis. Quaternary amines (methantheline bromide and propantheline bromide), antihistamines, and tranquilizers also have a relaxing effect on the bladder.

In the normal urethra, the turbulent flow has a scrubbing action on the urethral walls that washes off bacteria and debris. Laminar flow and lower velocities leave a thin layer of stationary fluid in which bacteria may grow.

Sheep, goats, and dogs have bladders that can be quantitatively drained by gravity when they are catheterized. In cattle, in which there is always urine below the urethral opening, complete drainage of the bladder by catheterization is difficult. In ruminants a small suburethral diverticulum lies directly ventrad to the urethral orifice and must be avoided during catheterization of the bladder.

Bladder Substitution

As a substitute for a damaged or nonfunctional bladder, a section of ileum can be surgically fashioned into a receptacle to receive the ureters (Fig. 20–6). The ileal segment then acts as a reservoir for urine, which can then be transferred to a watertight external appliance.

GENERAL CHARACTERISTICS OF URINE

Physical characteristics of urine are influenced by factors related to diet (water in beverage and feeds), water loss

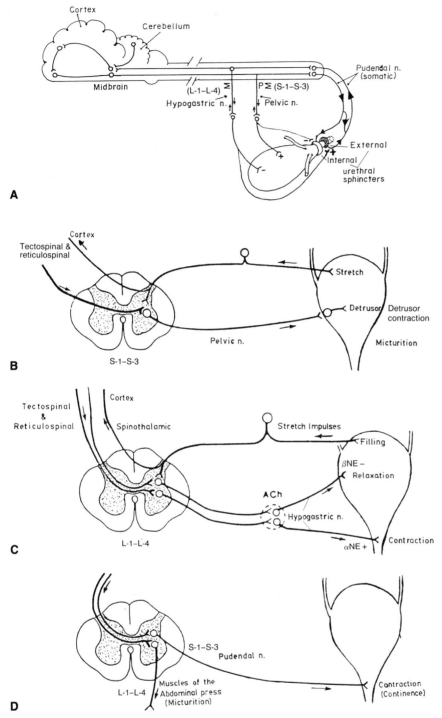

Figure 20–5   Innervation of the urinary voiding system. **A,** The sacral parasympathetic motor center controls the bladder and the internal and external sphincters. The lumbar sympathetic center, not essential for voiding, influences micturition: beta-receptor relaxation of detrusor, and alpha-receptor constriction of trigone, bladder neck, and urethra. The central centers (cortex, hypothalamus, cerebellum, and midbrain) exert mostly facilitatory, but also some inhibitory, influences on the sacral voiding center. **B,** Parasympathetic nervous system (S-1 to S-3) involved during contraction of the bladder. **C,** Sympathetic nervous system plays a role during filling of the urinary bladder. Preganglionic fibers (L-1 to L-4) travel in the hypogastric nerve to the caudal mesenteric ganglion and synapse on postganglionic neurons. Some neurons reach beta-adrenergic receptors on the body of the bladder to cause relaxation of smooth muscles and to facilitate filling. Others reach alpha-adrenergic receptors on the bladder neck to cause contraction of the smooth muscles to facilitate emptying and to force continence. **D,** Efferent neurons of the somatic nervous system travel in the pudendal nerve to striated muscles. Some neurons reach the external urethral sphincter (female: in midurethral portion; male: in membranous portion). Other neurons innervate the skeletal muscles of the abdominal press (i.e., favor emptying of the urinary bladder).

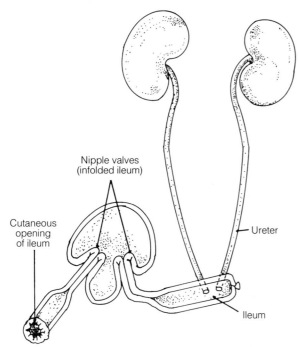

Nipple valves
(infolded ileum)

Cutaneous
opening
of ileum

Ureter

Ileum

Figure 20–6 Continent ureteroileostomy as a substitute for damaged urinary bladder. An isolated ileal segment receives the ureters and serves as a reservoir for storage of urine and as a channel to evacuate urine to the exterior. In the bladder-like part, two nipple valves are constructed to prevent reflux of urine into the prosthetic ureter and to provide continence, or prevent continuous outflow to the exterior.

(air humidity and temperature, hair coat, evaporation), and neuroendocrine factors.

Volume of urine is between 15 and 30 mL per kilogram every 24 hours. Mean daily urine production is lowest in cats, horses, and pigs (about 15 mL per kilogram per 24 hours); goats and sheep follow (about 25 mL per kilogram per 24 hours); and cows and dogs are top urine producers (30 mL per kilogram per 24 hours).

The *pH of urine* is related to what food the animal consumes. Herbivores eat plants rich in potassium and produce alkaline urine, whereas carnivores produce acid urine because of phosphate and sulfate salts from meats. Omnivores' urine can be acid or basic alkaline, depending on the major components of the feeds.

The *specific gravity* of urine in adult animals is usually between 1.020 and 1.035; it may reach 1.060 in dogs and 1.080 in cats. Pigs' urine has the lowest specific gravity (1.020), and cows and horses the highest (1.035). The specific gravity of urine of cats, dogs, goats, and sheep is 1.030. In young animals, the mean specific gravity of urine is about 1.015. The terms *baruria* and *hypersthenuria* refer to urine with osmolality and specific gravity higher than that of plasma or glomerular filtrate (>1.010); *isosthenuria* indicates osmolality and specific gravity identical with that of plasma or glomerular filtrate; and *hyposthenuria* describes urine with lower osmolality or specific gravity than that of plasma or glomerular filtrate.

Urine is usually *clear* when voided, except in horses because of mucus produced in the renal pelvis and the proximal ureter and of sedimented calcium carbonate crystals. Upon standing, calcium carbonate in the urine of cows soon precipitates to cloud the relatively fresh fluid. The color of urine, ranging from pale yellow (dilute) to dark yellow (concentrated), is caused by urochrome, a combination of urobilin and urobilinogen to a peptide.

REFERENCES

Beck RP, Daniel EE, Fimper P, King C. Electromyographic and pressure studies in the canine bladder. Am J Obstet Gynecol 1976;125:603.

Bradley WE, Timm GW. Physiology of micturition. Vet Clin North Am 1974;4:487.

Constantinou CE. Renal pelvic pacemaker control of ureteral peristaltic rate. Am J Physiol 1974;226:1413.

Constantinou CE, Djurhuus JC. Pyeloureteral dynamics in the intact and chronically obstructed multicalyceal kidney. Am J Physiol 1981;241:R398.

Hartman W, Van de Watering CC. The function of the bladder neck in female goats. Zentralbl Veterinarmed A 1974;21:430.

Hatey F, Ruckebusch Y. Etudes électromyographiques de la motricité des uretères chez le chien. Ann Rech Vet 1972;3:533.

Koushanpour E, Kriz W. Renal physiology. Principles, structure, and function. 2nd ed. New York: Springer-Verlag, 1986.

SECTION III

THE DIGESTIVE SYSTEM

CHAPTER 21

INTRODUCTION TO THE DIGESTIVE TRACT

Initiated at the time of gastrulation, the digestive tract is basically a tube within the body. In direct communication with the outside world, the lumen of the gastrointestinal tube is a part of the external environment. In the initial part of the tube, solid foods are ingested, diluted with saliva and mucus, chewed, and directed into the first dilation (the stomach). Ingested fluids reach the stomach almost directly without much alteration. The rest of the gastrointestinal tract can be considered as a long continuous tube of variable diameter. In this hollow structure, food is mixed with secretions poured from cellular glands lining the lumen and from glands with excretory canals (liver, pancreas).

The gastrointestinal tract is a frontier between the outside world and the extracellular fluid (ECF) of the body. To gain access to the internal environment, nutriments and simple molecules must be extracted from food by digestion processes. Only then can these substances enter the body by selectively passing through the lining of the gastrointestinal tract. The absorption process occurs mostly in the coiled small intestinal segment, which has an extensive blood perfusion and a large surface area for optimal selective absorption. Therefore, the mucosa of the digestive system serves as a protective barrier that prevents many swallowed substances from gaining access into the circulating ECF of the body. For instance, many bacteria contained in food cannot cross the gastrointestinal mucosa with the nutrients.

The gastrointestinal organs also contribute to production of immunological factors that defend the animal organism against toxic and infectious substances and supply some of the energy to maintain body temperature at about 38°C in mammals and near 40°C in birds.

DIGESTION

Digestion is the chemical transformation of solid food into simpler molecular forms that can be taken up from the lumen of the small intestine. It also includes the mechanical propulsion of the fluid mixture (food and secretions) within the gastrointestinal tract. The chemical and mechanical actions of digestion take place successively in the mouth, pharynx, esophagus, stomach, and upper small intestine. These functions are under neurohumoral control.

In adult herbivores (ruminants, horses, rabbits), a comparative approach to the different types of digestive functions must be considered. The digestive reservoirs, the digestive processes of transport and fermentation, and the digestive fluid balance are adapted for efficient use of plant materials, which are high in cellulose and low in nutritive value.

Neurohumoral Control of the Gastrointestinal Tract

Functions of the digestive tract are regulated by the extrinsic nervous system and by the gastrointestinal hormones, secreted in one area of the tube to act locally or on different target organs. The extrinsic nervous system consists of both efferent and afferent fibers in the vagal, sacral, and splanchnic nerves. Parasympathetic fibers, in the vagal and the sacral nerves, are the most important regulators of normal events (Fig. 21–1). Transection of the parasympathetic nerves results in significant stasis of ingesta in the stomach. The splanchnic nerves contain sympathetic fibers that are less important, as sympathectomy does not produce visible signs of digestive dysfunction.

The intrinsic nervous system, represented by the myenteric plexuses, is essential to gastrointestinal function. However, without the assistance of the extrinsic nervous system, the intrinsic nervous system cannot maintain functions at a level adequate for homeostasis. Removal of the control exerted by the extrinsic nervous system significantly modifies normal gut function. The effect of vagotomy is variable, changing motility in the small intestine only slightly but greatly decreasing gastric motility and gastric secretion.

The dynamic picture of gastrointestinal physiology is currently dominated by the neuroendocrine concept of regulation. It displaces the concept of the nervous control of digestive secretions demonstrated by Pavlov. In 1902, Bayliss and Starling discovered secretin, and digestive endocrinology was born. In the past three decades, discoveries on gut hormones have made such great strides that, except for the obvious vagal effect on the stomach, gut hormones overshadow the nervous system as controllers of digestion.

With progress in biochemical methods of extracting and synthesizing peptides, the structure and amino acid sequences of peptide molecules from the digestive tract have been determined. Besides the recognized gastrointestinal hormones (gastrin, secretin, cholecystokinin [CCK], and gastric inhibitory peptide [GIP]), a host of short peptide molecules have been found in the gut, and their amino acids have been sequenced. Some examples are vasoactive intestinal peptide (VIP), motilin, pancreatic polypeptide (PP), enkephalin (ENK), and enteroglucagon. Since all the known gastrointestinal hormones are peptides, it is postulated that each peptide isolated from the digestive tissues is also a hormone.

With the radioimmunoassay technique, some gastrointestinal peptides present in the gut endocrine cells are also found in nerve cells. Some gastrointestinal peptides are even present in both the digestive tract and the central nervous

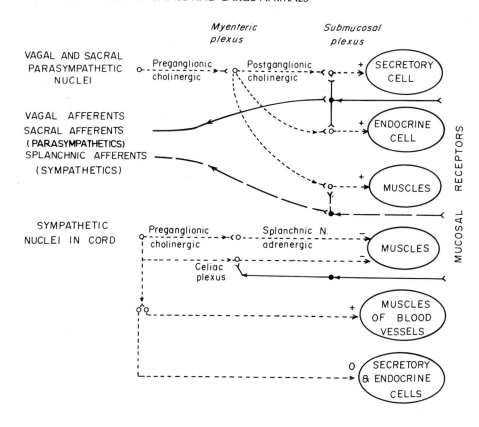

Figure 21–1 *Afferent signals* from mucosal receptors travel in vagal, sacral, and splanchnic nerve fibers. Through synapses within the submucosal plexus, the vagal and sacral stimulatory messages are dispersed locally to cholinergic secretory and endocrine cells. The submucosal plexus also serves to radiate splanchnic cholinergic effector signals to stimulate smooth muscle cells in the proximity of mucosal receptors. Submucosal receptor signals, traveling in the splanchnic fibers, form synapses in the celiac plexus to bring adrenergic relaxation of smooth muscle cells. Parasympathetic *efferent signals* in the vagal and sacral pre- and postganglionic fibers stimulate gastrointestinal secretory, endocrine, and muscle cells. Sympathetic efferent signals cause relaxation of gastrointestinal smooth muscles and constriction of the smooth muscle of blood vessels and are without effects on gastrointestinal secretory and endocrine cells.

system (Fig. 21–2). Peptides common to both the central nervous system and the digestive tract may be classified into several families. One of these includes substance P and neurotensin; both have been isolated from the brain and the gut and their amino acid sequences are known.

Digestive Reservoirs

In carnivores, the relatively large stomach acts as a reservoir for large amounts of animal tissues hastily ingested within the span of a few minutes. In contrast, the stomach of

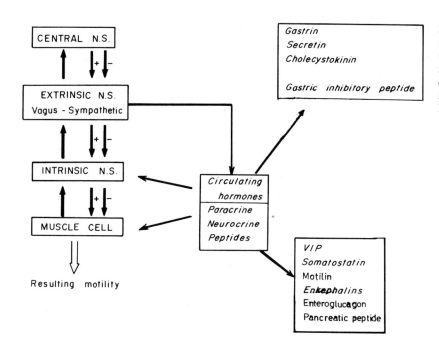

Figure 21–2 Relationships between the nervous system (central, extrinsic, and intrinsic) and gastrointestinal peptides (hormones: gastrin, secretin, CCK, GIP; and candidate hormones: VIP, somatostatin, motilin, enkephalins, enteroglucagon, and PP).

horses is filled and emptied several times during the period required (about 2 hours) to eat a typical meal of 2 to 3 kg of oats (Fig. 21–3).

The function of the pylorus corresponds to its etymological meaning, "gate of the stomach." The ileocecal sphincter, separating the small and the large intestine, also has the connotation of an intestinal gate. In fact, it has been termed "the apothecaries' gate or barrier" because drugs delivered by apothecaries (ancient name for pharmacists) were supposed to correct the constipation induced by persistent closure of this sphincter.

Mechanical propulsion of the nutrients through the stomach is a more important motor function (Fig. 21–4) in herbivores (ruminants, horses, rabbits) than in carnivores (cats, dogs). Omnivorous animals, such as pigs, feed on both animal and vegetable substances.

Transport Processes

In the upper small intestine mostly, several well-defined transport processes are involved in moving molecules of nutrients from the intestinal lumen across the apical membrane into the epithelial cells of the mucosa and subsequently through the basolateral membrane of these cells into the blood. These absorptive processes depend on activities of mucosal structures and surfaces (Fig. 21–5), metabolism, and circulation. Besides absorbing materials from the lumen, the mucosal lining also secretes fluids into the lumen. Luminal materials not absorbed from the gut are propelled along to the colon and are eliminated as feces.

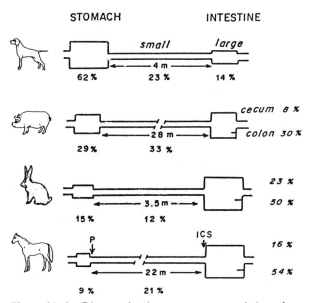

Figure 21–3 Diagram showing among monogastric (monolocular stomach) species the large capacity of the canine stomach (62 percent of the volume of the entire digestive tract), which under natural conditions corresponds to the volume of a meal. In contrast, the volume of the equine stomach is less than 9 percent of the volume of the whole digestive tract. *P*, Pylorus; *ICS*, ileocecal sphincter.

Fermentation Processes

The large intestine, or hindgut, is a viscus with specific digestive functions related to its distal location and to its volume and length. The volume of the large intestine tends to increase from carnivores (cats, dogs) to herbivores (horses, rabbits); the pig represents an intermediate species. The bulkier large intestine of horses and rabbits reflects its nutritional significance as a fermentative vat.

Chemically complex substances from the small intestine reach the large intestine. These unabsorbed residues of food are mixed with some digestive secretions and some microorganisms. Such very moist (almost fluid) contents, rich in components (nitrogen, energy, and minerals), are highly favorable to intense development of an active microflora (1 to 3 $\times$ 10^{10} bacteria per gram of fresh content). The large intestine is indeed the habitat of the greatest number of microbial species. Microbial enzymes help complete the breakdown of the substrates that have resisted the action of the mucosal enzymes of the small intestine. In addition, the large intestine has absorptive functions, since the proportion of water in the feces (60 percent) is much lower than in the ileum (90 percent).

Obviously, the extent of these processes depends on the retention time of digesta in the large intestine, which accounts for 85 percent of total retention time in pigs (about 24 to 36 hours) and in dogs. Even in dogs, a prolonged increase in the protein content of the meal induces the development of an ammonia-producing flora (Fig. 21–6).

Fluid and Electrolyte Balance

In a 20-kg dog, of a total volume of less than 3 L (2,700 mL) of fluid presented to the intestine, about 20 percent (600 mL) comes from the diet, and 2,100 mL comes from endogenous digestive secretions (salivary glands, stomach, liver, pancreas, small intestine). Each day, the volume of fluid crossing the gut wall greatly exceeds the volume of ECF, and only a fraction of the fluid (about 35 mL) normally ingested actually appears, or is lost, in the feces (Fig. 21–7).

The proximal small intestine (duodenum and jejunum) is the major site of water absorption. About 50 percent of the 2.7 L is absorbed in the jejunum, and about 1 L, or 37 percent, of the total volume of fluid presented to the ileum is absorbed. Another 12 percent of the total volume of fluid is absorbed in the colon, leaving less than 1 percent to be excreted, or lost, in the feces. The efficiency of absorption, or fractional water extraction, increases distally. The colon extracts about 90 percent of the water presented to it and is the final determinant of fecal consistency. Disruption of this complex exchange, caused either by more secretion or by less absorption, increases fecal water output and results in diarrhea. Damage to the distal part of the bowel (e.g., colitis) provokes small-volume diarrhea, with tenesmus and mucus in the feces.

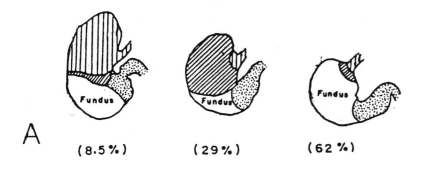

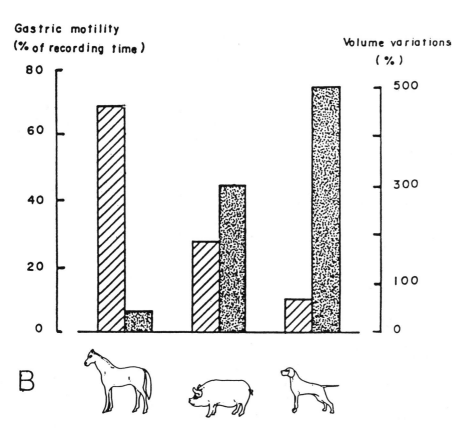

Figure 21–4 **A,** Distribution of nonglandular (vertical hatched area) regions of the stomach and relative surface of the fundus as the hydrogen ion secretory area; relative capacity of the stomach as a percentage of the volume of the entire digestive tract is shown in parentheses. **B,** Relative motor, or contractile, activity of the stomach and its variations in volume.

DIGESTION IN ADULT RUMINANT SPECIES

In ruminant herbivores, the true glandular stomach is preceded by multichambered dilations associated with specialized mixing motor functions and fermentative processes. Before weaning, the esophageal groove directs suckled colostrum and milk from the cardia toward the true glandular stomach, or abomasum, through the as-yet undeveloped omasum. At maturity, the well-developed reticulum and rumen form a fermentation vat corresponding to more than 70 percent of the volume of the digestive tract (Fig. 21–8).

The major end-products of anaerobic breakdown of dietary fiber are primarily short-chain fatty acids (SCFAs: acetic, propionic, and butyric). Considerable amounts of SCFAs are produced in the reticulum as well as in the hindgut of monogastric herbivores such as horses; these animals derive as much as 80 percent of their maintenance energy from SCFAs. The major sources for anaerobic fermentation are plant polysaccharides (cellulose, pectins, and hemicelluloses).

Certain peculiarities are related to the presence of a reticulorumen: (1) mixing of the contents by *specific movements* (at a rate of about 1,440 per day) that are controlled in the brainstem and occur as a vagovagal reflex; (2) *eructation,* a mechanism whereby the ruminant animal controls the large quantities of gas produced as a result of microbial fermentation (12 to 25 L per minute in cattle fed green alfafa); (3) *rumination* as a way of obtaining a correct degree of grinding of the roughage; and (4) *copious voluntary intake* to fill the rumen, or, more exactly, to replace the food materials digested in the reticulorumen, and the undigested part, which

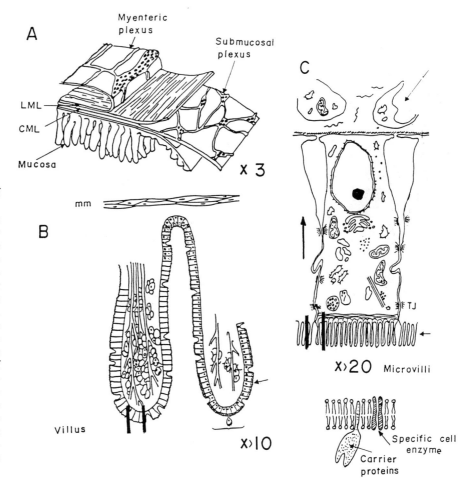

Figure 21–5 Amplification of the surface of the small intestine. **A,** Folds of the mucosa increase the surface area of the intestinal wall by a factor of 3. **B,** Villi increase the mucosal surface area by a factor of at least 10. **C,** Microvilli (brush border) increase the surface by a factor of at least 20. The total surface is about 100 m^2 for a 4-m long small intestine of a dog. Villus movements occur from the muscularis mucosae, whereas propulsion of the contents is related to contractions of the circular and longitudinal muscle layers (*CML* and *LML*) coordinated by a neural network made up of the myenteric plexus and the submucosal plexus. The greater the number of tight junctions (*TJ*) between cells, the more efficient is water absorption.

passes out of the reticulorumen. In cows, if gut-fill is correct and physical breakdown of feed is normal, the time spent in alimentary behavior reaches nearly 12 hours per day (Fig. 21–9).

Rumen digestion has received much attention. Microbial attack and digestion of food components in the rumen have been observed with scanning electron microscopy. Limits to digesta progression through the digestive tract have been explored with digesta flow markers and particle-sizing devices. Analyses of diet composition have been simplified, and specific nutrients are produced by genetically altered microbes. A search for the site of digestion in vivo is done with new cannula designs, digesta flow markers, and constitutive microbial markers. Ruminants are maintained on intragastric or intravenous infusions of purified nutrients in order to quantitate their nutrient requirements.

The purpose of this section is to present a clear and comprehensive view of the digestive tracts of animal species that consume different diets. In spite of rapid advances in basic knowledge, little is known about the integration of various gastrointestinal functions, which are very different in carnivores and in herbivores. Among herbivores, animals with pregastric (preacid) fermentation (ruminants, and some pig-like animals such as the peccary and babirusa) have

gastrointestinal functions quite different from those of herbivores with postgastric (postacid) fermentation (e.g., lagomorphs, rodents, and perissodactyls).

For these reasons, the first chapters, on microbial ecosystems and immunology of the gut, and the last ones, on

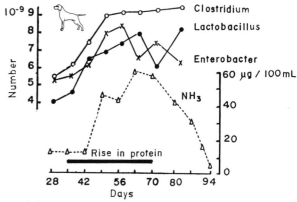

Figure 21–6 Long-term increase in fermentation rate of colonic contents caused by raising by 20 percent the amount of crude protein in a dog's food.

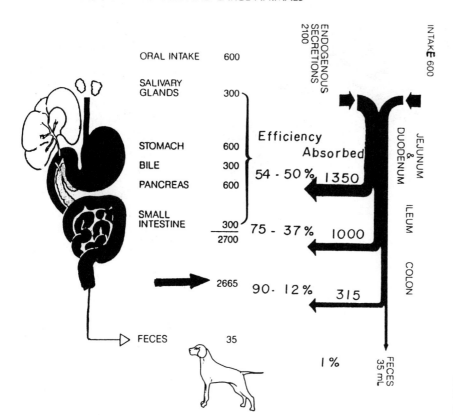

Figure 21–7 An account of electrolyte and water secretion and absorption in the canine gastrointestinal tract.

secretory and absorptive functions under neuroendocrine control, are presented generally with special notation of species' differences. In contrast, alimentary behavior and gastrointestinal motility are analyzed separately for species that rely on fermentation in the reticulorumen and those whose fermentation occurs in the large intestine (folded or replicated colon in the horse, helicoid colon in pigs, and cecal

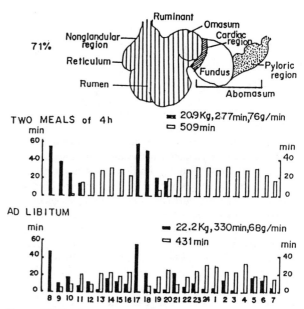

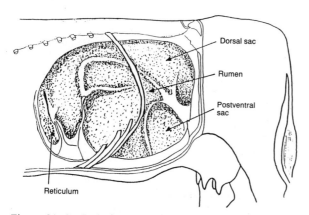

Figure 21–8 Reticulorumen. The reticulum lies against the costal part of the diaphragm. Its ventral relations are the sternal part of the diaphragm, the caudad end of the sternum, and the xiphoid cartilage close to the abomasum. The rumen is divided into dorsal and ventral sacs.

Figure 21–9 Arrangement of the ruminant stomach and 24-hour alimentary behavior of an adult (700-kg) cow fed an excess (25 kg) of roughage, either in two 4-hour meals (8:00 and 17:00) or ad libitum. The rate of ingestion is about 68 to 76 g per minute, and the time spent eating (*black columns*) is between 277 and 330 minutes per day. The time spent ruminating (rechewing the cud) is 430 to 509 minutes per day (*white columns*).

enlargement in rabbits). The references have been selected to illuminate other aspects of digestive function, to assess information perhaps more relevant to pathophysiology, and to satisfy those who feel that the grass might be greener on the other side of the fence.

REFERENCES

Burroughs CF. Diarrhea and constipation. In: Ettinger SJ, ed. Textbook of veterinary internal medicine. 2nd ed. Philadelphia: WB Saunders, 1983.

Campling RC, Balch CC. Factors affecting the voluntary intake of food by cows. Br J Nutr 1961;15:523; 531.

Church DC. The ruminant animal. Englewood Cliffs, NJ: Simon & Schuster, 1988.

Dobson A, Dobson MJ. Aspects of digestive physiology in ruminants. Ithaca, NY: Comstock Publishing Associates, 1988.

Dulphy JP, Faverdin P. L'ingestion alimentaire chez les ruminants: Modalités et phénomènes associés. Reprod Nutr Dev 1987;2:129.

Hart NL. The behavior of domestic animals. New York: WH Freeman, 1986.

Johnson LR. Physiology of the digestive tract. Vol. 2. New York: Raven Press, 1986.

Owens FN. New techniques for studying digestion and absorption of nutrients by ruminants. Fed Proc 1987;46:283.

Rerat A. Digestion and absorption of carbohydrates and nitrogenous matters in the hindgut of the omnivorous nonruminant animal. J Anim Sci 1978;46:1808.

Ruckebusch Y. Gastrointestinal motor functions in ruminants. In: Wood J, ed. Handbook of physiology, Vol. 4. Gastrointestinal motility and circulation. Washington, DC: Physiological Society, 1988.

Ruckebusch Y, et al. La mécanique digestive. Paris: Masson INRA, 1982.

Stevens CE. Comparative physiology of the vertebrate digestive system. NY: Cambridge University Press, 1988.

Stromberg DR. Small animal gastroenterology. Davis, CA: Stone Gate Publishing, 1979.

CHAPTER 22

MICROFLORA AND IMMUNOLOGY OF THE DIGESTIVE TRACT

Within a day or so after an animal is born, its entire digestive tract is populated by strains of microorganisms from the environment. Before birth, the gastrointestinal tract is sterile, but afterwards no sterile regions are found in the digestive system. The density of the gastrointestinal microflora is expressed in number per gram of dry mass or per milliliter of digesta. Since a single bacterium corresponds approximately to a sphere 1 μm in diameter, 10^{12} bacteria completely fill the volume of 1 mL, or 1 mm^3. By allowing at least 50 percent for water content and for a multitude of undigested organic particles, the maximum number of bacteria is about 5.10^9 to 5.10^{10} per gram of digesta. Values above 10^{11} are uncommon. Microorganisms in the aboral parts of the gut are essentially anaerobes. Facultative anaerobes are found only in the proximal parts. Gut bacteria contribute to the digestion or transformation of food by transforming the ingested components of foods and by modifying the morphology and metabolic activity of the intestinal mucosa. The gastrointestinal immune system and the mechanical barrier formed by epithelial cells, glycocalyx, and the mucous coat protect the host from substances introduced into the lumen of the gut.

This chapter discusses the factors that affect the composition, maintenance, and functions of this digestive microflora in monogastric animals in terms of (1) environment and age, (2) composition of diet and of ingested food, and (3) morphology, secretions, and motility of the gastrointestinal tract. The rumen microflora, with its anaerobic cellulolytic bacteria for digestion of cellulose, is discussed in another chapter with ruminant digestion.

This chapter also briefly reviews the cells of the gastrointestinal immune system, the role of Peyer's patches, which can absorb antigens and respond by firing off effector cells into the intestinal lymph, and the synthesis of secretory IgA and its passage into the intestinal lumen.

MICROFLORA OF THE DIGESTIVE SYSTEM

Influence of Environment and Age

Environment and Digestive Flora

The composition of the gastrointestinal microflora has been studied in animals reared from birth in unprotected and protected environments.

Animals Reared Conventionally. Under usual farm conditions the microflora of an animal constitutes a complex, uncontrolled, and dynamic open ecosystem. Microorganisms in food, water, and the surroundings enter at one end of the tract, and waste products and microbes exit at the other end. The microorganisms in the system are either indigenous or transient. Indigenous (autochthonous) species are inhabitants of microbial communities established on or in the body and do not damage the host animal. The indigenous microbial communities of the gastrointestinal tract are regulated by allogenic (host animal) and autogenic (microbial interaction) processes. The allogenic processes involve the environment and the diet. Transient (allochthonous) species only pass through a region or temporarily colonize a habitat vacated by the indigenous inhabitants for one reason or another.

Animals Protected from the Conventional Environment. These are obtained initially under aseptic conditions. Mammals are delivered by hysterotomy (cesarian section) or are immediately dipped after birth in an antiseptic solution. For avians, dipping the incubated egg in an antiseptic a day before hatching sterilizes the shell without killing the embryo.

Germ-free animals and gnotobiotic animals are kept in sterilized plastic isolators (Fig. 22—1B and C) and are provided with aseptic air, water, and food. Air is sterilized by filtering; sterile food, water, and equipment are transferred from a container to the isolator through a double-door air lock, which is kept sterile by spraying with peracetic acid, an oxygen-liberating compound that kills spores in less than 20 minutes and leaves a nontoxic acetic acid residue. These animals are not without viruses, mycoplasmas, chlamydiae, toxoplasmas, and parasites transmitted during fetal life. Calves, cats, dogs, hamsters, kids, lambs, mice, piglets, chickens, guinea hens, turkeys, rabbits, and rats have been raised as germ-free animals. A gnotobiotic or gnotophoric animal carries one known strain of bacteria that was implanted experimentally.

Specific pathogen—free animals (SPF) are initially germ-free animals that are kept in surroundings free of and protected from specific microorganisms (Fig. 22—1D).

Age and Digestive Flora

The gastrointestinal tract can be considered as a series of distinct habitats—mouth, stomach, small intestine, and large intestine. Each habitat possesses a characteristic microflora that is in equilibrium and forms a part of the open ecosystem with the host. The establishment of a stable gastrointestinal microflora occurs in successive steps during the preweaning and postweaning periods.

Preweaning Period. In conventional animals, the dam is the major contributor to the microbial flora of the

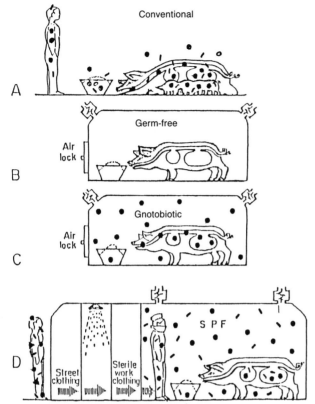

Figure 22–1 **A,** A conventionally reared animal exposed to microorganisms in the environment and its food. Its digestive tract may have a microflora of hundreds of different species of bacteria. **B,** A germ-free animal does not have a digestive microflora and is kept in the sterilized environment of an isolator. Air goes in through a filtered inlet and out through a filtered outlet. Sterilized food, water and utensils are introduced through an air lock. **C,** In a gnotobiotic animal, the gastrointestinal tract is colonized by a known flora. Such an animal is kept in an isolator just as a germ-free animal is. **D,** A specific pathogen–free (SPF) animal is protected from conventional congeners and specific microorganisms. The microflora of the gut is very different from that of conventionally reared animals of the same species.

neonate. With a germ-free neonate, implantation of microbes may require 24 to 48 hours to stabilize at 5.10^9 to 5.10^{10} per gram of digesta.

In suckling animals raised conventionally (Fig. 22–1A), the high gastric pH of food in the stomach permits rapid multiplication of ingested bacteria. Some pass unharmed into the small intestine and continue multiplying there.

In artificially reared conventional piglets, the pH of the stomach content may remain high, multiplication of bacteria from the environment may increase until up to 5 weeks of age, and scouring may result. Such a gastric flora can convert fermentable carbohydrates to lactic acid and small amounts of volatile fatty acids. An inverse relationship exists between microbial lactic acid production and hydrochloric acid secretion. The acidity produced by lactic acid seems to suppress hydrochloric acid secretion, so the gastric pH remains high

enough for proliferation of some microorganisms. In a protected environment (Fig. 22–1D), piglets develop fewer gastric bacteria, and secretion of hydrochloric acid is established sooner than in conventional farm conditions.

The digestive tract of preweaned animals (calf, kitten, piglet, and puppy) harbors several kinds of microorganisms: *Bacteroides, Clostridium perfringens, Escherichia coli, Lactobacillus,* and *Streptococcus.* Also, *Staphylococcus aureus* is found in puppies and yeasts (*Candida species*) occasionally in kittens.

Postweaning Period. After weaning, when *gastric* secretion is well established and an animal is fasting, the number of bacteria is only 10^1 to 10^2. Growth is limited to (mostly) acid-resistant organisms such as *Clostridium, Streptococcus, Lactobacillus, E. coli;* some fungi; and some facultative anaerobic bacteria. Only microorganisms such as *Lactobacillus* and *Bifidobacterium* can colonize the gastric mucosa (Fig. 22–2).

In the *small intestine,* the microflora is qualitatively similar to that of the stomach. The number of organisms in the empty proximal small intestine is about 10^1 to 10^2 per gram, and gram-positive species (e.g., *Streptococcus, Clostridium, Lactobacillus,* and *Staphylococcus*) outnumber gram-negative species. In the distal part, the predominant gram-negative species (coliforms, enterococci) begin to approach the composition of the flora of the large intestine and number 10^3 to 10^4. Some bacteria present at birth disappear at weaning; others appear at weaning and persist in the digestive tract. They may act as a defensive barrier by making enterocytes unavailable to pathogens or by creating an environment that is detrimental to pathogens. Acting as antigens, live or dead microorganisms stimulate secretion of immunoglobulins (sIgA) by both plasma cells in the lamina propria and enterocytes.

In the *large intestine* of herbivores, the microflora is a very complex ecosystem that acts as a cellulose digester in much the same way as the rumen does, but on a lesser scale. A fairly constant number of organisms (10^{10} to 10^{11} per gram—over 400 species from 40 genera) populate the colon. *Bacteroides* and *Bifidobacterium* are predominant, followed by *Eubacterium, Enterobacter,* gram-positive cocci, and *Lactobacillus.* Bacteria constitute a third of the fecal mass, and anaerobes outnumber facultative anaerobes by a factor of 10^2 to 10^4.

Changes in the Microflora Associated with Food and Diet

The diet of the host animal exerts direct and indirect effects on the gastrointestinal flora. The direct action is by changing the nutrients available to indigenous bacteria; the indirect effect is to modify the physiological and the immunological responses of the host animal.

Influence of Food on Digestive Flora

Conventionally reared piglets fed twice daily ad libitum maintain a high *gastric* pH, permitting bacteria and lactic

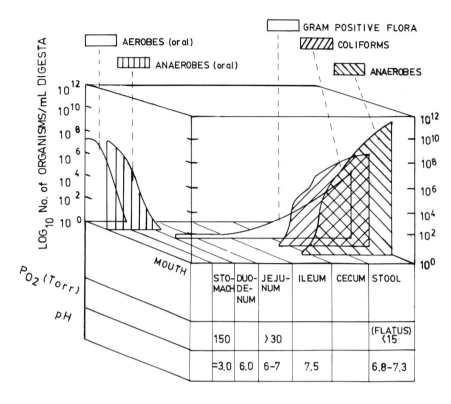

Figure 22–2 General outlook of the digestive flora. Anaerobes and coliforms predominate in the distal small intestine (ileum) and the large intestine. More oral aerobes and anaerobes cohabit in the mouth than in the stomach. Coliforms are absent from the gastric mucosa and the proximal small intestine (duodenum, jejunum), but the minimal amount of gram-positive microbes and yeast increases progressively along the distal intestinal tract.

acid to develop more rapidly than if they were fed restricted but frequent meals. When such piglets are restricted to small meals at hourly intervals, the rise in gastric pH is minimal and gastric juice can exert its maximal bactericidal and proteolytic effects. In pigs, starvation lowers the number of lactobacilli fixed on the gastric epithelial surface. A similar effect is noted in rodents given a high-protein diet.

The number of microorganisms in the stomach and small intestine is usually low but can increase when nutrients are present. Following a meal, oral organisms (*Bacteroides, Streptococcus, Lactobacillus, Neisseria*) are washed away with saliva and can be found as transient residents of the stomach contents (10^4 to 10^5 per gram) before most of them are destroyed by gastric acid. Food increases the number of organisms in the small intestine by 10^2 to 10^3 in the cranial and caudal segments.

Influence of Diet on Digestive Flora

By ingestion of *colostrum* (the first perinatal mammary secretion) perinatally, postnatal antibodies are passed from the dam to the calf, colt, lamb, kid, kitten, piglet, and puppy. Enterocytes can absorb only the immunoglobulins (IgG, IgA, and IgM) of colostrum by pinocytosis during the first 24 hours, before "closure" of the epithelial cells of the small intestine. These maternal antibodies give the neonate passive immunity against specific pathogenic microorganisms until it can initiate its own active immunity.

Colostrum. A fluid accumulates in the mammary gland during the last month of pregnancy or after injections of 17 beta-estradiol and progesterone. This lacteal secretion has a

higher content of Na^+, Cl^-, and protein, but a lower content of K^+ and lactose, than milk.

Immunoglobulins represent the most important class of proteins in colostrum. In bovines, the levels of IgG_1 decrease in maternal plasma 2 weeks before calving but increase in the colostrum, as a result of a selective transfer (Table 22–1). This transfer is maximal 1 to 3 days before calving, so that at parturition the concentration of Igs in colostrum is five times that in the plasma. The same plasma-to-colostrum transfer phenomenon, coinciding with the high levels of total estrogens, occurs in sows 1 week before farrowing (Fig. 22–3).

In sows, cows, and mares, IgGs are the major constituents of colostrum, which is more a transudate from plasma than a true secretion; however, the concentration of Igs falls

TABLE 22–1 Immunoglobulin Concentrations in Colostrum and Plasma of Some Domestic Animals

	IgA (mg/dL)	IgE (mg/dL)	IgG (mg/dL)	IgM (mg/dL)
Colostrum				
Bitch	5–22	—	1–3	0.1–0.6
Cow	1–7	—	34–39	3–13
Ewe	1–7	—	8–13	7–12
Mare	5–15	—	15–50	1–3.5
Sow	9–11	—	30–70	3–32
Plasma				
Bitch	0.2–1.2	0.2–0.4	5–17	0.7–2.7
Cow	0.1–0.5	—	17–27	2.5–4
Ewe	0.1–0.5	—	17–20	1.5–2.5
Mare	0.6–3.5	—	5–20	0.8–2
Sow	0.5–5	—	17–29	1–5

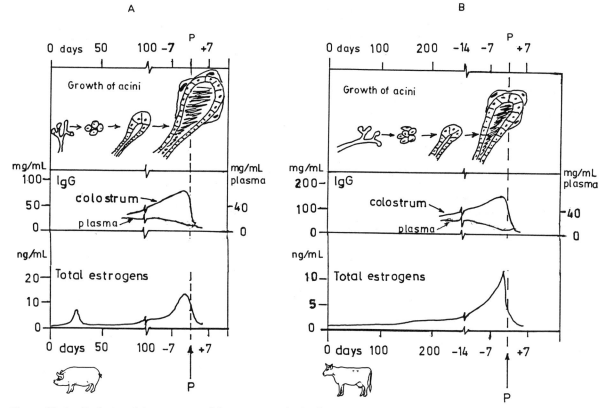

Figure 22–3 Evolution of the structures of the mammary gland, of the IgG₁ secretions in serum and lacteal fluid, and of the total production of estrogens during pregnancy and at parturition (P) in the sow (A), and the cow (B).

within a few days of lactation. The Igs in milk (mostly IgA, IgM, and IgG) are synthesized in the mammary gland (Fig. 22–4). In fact, IgA is predominant in sow's milk throughout lactation.

Pigs produce more gastric lactic acid (90 versus 50 percent) and less volatile fatty acids (propionic, butyric, and valeric acids) on a whey diet than on a cereal diet. In older pigs being fed cereals, gastric production of formic acid may

exceed that of butyric acid. In such pigs being fed whey, gastric production of formic acid may be greater than that of propionic acid. By cecotrophy (coprophagia) rabbits introduce indigenous cecocolonic bacteria in the stomach as transients.

The microflora varies in response to diet, probably more so in the small intestine than in the large intestine. Microbial effect is a major factor in digestion of nonstarch polysac-

Figure 22–4 In the sow, transfer of Igs from plasma to colostrum and to milk. During pregnancy, all (100 percent) the IgGs in the sow's colostrum are derived from plasma, whereas a great proportion of IgA and of IgM is synthesized by the mammary gland. During lactation, more IgA, IgM, and IgG are produced by the mammary cells, and less immunoglobulins are transferred from the plasma.

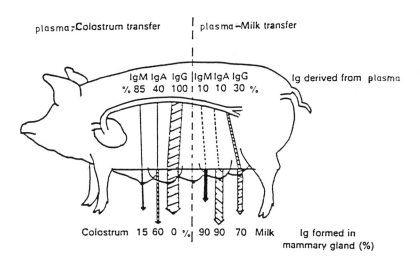

charides, the major chemical component of dietary fiber. Fibers rich in pectin but poor in lignin (e.g., cabbage, carrots) stimulate microbial growth to further increase and complete the digestion of fiber. In the small intestine this is likely to be in the ileum, where the bacterial population is higher than in the duodenum or jejunum.

Microbial enzymes involved in biochemical reactions in the small intestine are affected by diet. A high-protein diet increases the luminal concentration of anaerobic *Bacteroides* species that are principally responsible for production of beta-glucuronidase, a deconjugating enzyme. Several endogenous and xenobiotic compounds undergo enterohepatic circulation related to the microbial flora. As glucuronide or sulfate products, they are excreted in bile and deconjugated by the microbial enzymes, and most of the free compounds are reabsorbed and partially reconjugated by aborally situated mucosal cells. In the blood, they are returned to the liver for reexcretion in bile (or in urine for the fractions that escape the liver). The compounds that undergo this *bile-intestine-liver recirculation* are *bile salts, sex steroids* (estrogens, progesterone, testosterone), *urobilin, chloramphenicol, and morphine,* to prolong their biological half-life and keep their fecal level low. Oral *antibiotics* (penicillin, ampicillin, neomycin) *decrease the enterohepatic circulation* of these products and increase their fecal excretion by reducing by a factor of 5 the enzyme-producing gastrointestinal microflora. Human contraceptive failure is associated with oral antibiotic therapy.

In horses on a high-fiber diet (chaffed lucerne, meadow hay) cellulolytic anaerobic fungi with monoflagellate zoospores colonize the hindgut. They grow on fibrous plant fragments and produce large quantities of hydrogen gas during fermentation, and they are able to form stable cocultures with the methanogenic bacteria present in the gut. In rodents fed a high-carbohydrate diet, the pH of the large intestine is lower than that of rodents fed protein-rich food.

Diet seems to have a limited effect on the fecal flora. When the protein content of the diet is low, the number of fungi increases and that of staphylococci decreases, and when protein content is high, there is a rise in *Bacteroides* and proteolytic bacteria and a drop in clostridia and saccharolytic bacteria. A diet low in vitamin A reduces the fecal concentration of streptococci. Malnutrition increases the number of yeast in feces. Low-residue diets reduce the volume of feces, which then consist of desquamated cells, mucus, and microorganisms. The mucosal cells normally discarded from the intestinal epithelium then serve as a source of nutrients.

Influence of Gastrointestinal Morphology, Secretions, and Motility

The microflora is specialized to cope with the demands of life in the gastrointestinal tract, and the constant replacement of the mucosal epithelium as dead cells are extruded in the lumen of the gut. Luminal bacteria are found in the digesta, while mucosal bacteria are attached to the intestinal mucosa. Adhesion of the bacteria to the mucosa is provided

by specialized antigenic structures (pili or fimbria, glycocalyx) and secretions (agglutinins) that serve as anchors to the villus or crypt, or simply by the layer of mucus covering the mucosa, without any other means of fixation. The intimate association of host and mucosal bacteria leads to closer interaction than that between host and luminal bacteria. Mucosal bacteria are probably the external factors that have the greatest influence on the animal host. The association of microorganisms and the epithelial surfaces is also important to sustain a bacterial strain during a radical change in diet or during starvation.

Gastrointestinal Morphology and Digestive Flora

In areas of sudden dilation of the gut, stagnation of digesta may occur, and with it, an increase in the bacterial count and in the concentration of bacterial enzymes. The fundus of the stomach can be considered as the first area of stagnation where bacterial proliferation occurs in monogastric animals. The cecum and colon, the major stagnation areas in the monogastric digestive system, have the highest concentrations of bacteria.

Gastrointestinal Secretions and Digestive Flora

Coliform bacteria can divide every 20 minutes (this occurs after death of the host) and, if they are unchecked, would rapidly overwhelm the host. Host and microbial factors slow the multiplication of intestinal bacteria and limit it to one to four times per day. *Gastric acid* is important in reducing the bacterial population in the proximal small intestine and in fighting pathogenic bacteria. The absence of hydrochloric acid is accompanied by a rise in intraluminal pH, a proliferation of coliform and anaerobic gram-negative bacteria, and an increase in the number of streptococci, lactobacilli, and fungi in the small intestine. *Bile* also contributes to the inhibition of many microorganisms in the small intestine.

Gastrointestinal Motility and Digestive Flora

Peristalsis is the major host defense against bacterial overgrowth in the digestive system. When peristalsis diminishes, bacterial growth is accelerated.

In the stomach, mucosal cells retain some bacteria, but luminal microbes are propelled out of the stomach with the contents by gastric peristalsis. Duodenal peristalsis moves luminal content at a rate more rapid than that at which microorganisms can multiply. Agglutination by antibodies creates bacterial aggregates that are more easily eliminated by peristalsis. In the distal ileum, the content moves sluggishly, and microbes of the large intestine are occasionally found in high concentrations. The cause of this contamination is contents of the large intestine crossing the ileocecal valve into the ileum (antiperistalsis). Few microbes associate with epithelial surfaces of the cecum and colon (e.g., strains of *E. coli* [K88, K99, and K987P]). Bacteria in the lumen of the large intestine, eliminated passively in the feces by intestinal transit, are dead and are not detectable in the feces.

Interaction between Normal and Invading Digestive Flora

In comparison with animals reared conventionally, germ-free animals have a thinner and less cellular gut wall; smaller Peyer's patches with fewer germinal centers; longer, thin, and pointed villi; shallower crypts; a predominance of mature cuboidal, instead of columnar, enterocytes; greatly reduced mucosal surface; and lower rates of cellular turnover (desquamation and renewal of cells). The lamina propria, without plasma cells, possesses only a few lymphocytes and macrophages. The cecum in germ-free rats is ten times more voluminous. Besides these morphological changes, the following physiological gastrointestinal alterations have been noted in germ-free animals: slower gastric emptying, more alkaline intraluminal pH, and decreased motility and transit. Absorption of glucose, xylose, and calcium increases, an effect similar to that of adding antibiotics to animal feed. Cecal and colonic water absorption is reduced. Any allochthonous strain can colonize the gastrointestinal tract, since there is a "biological" vacuum space. Exposure of a germ-free animal to bacteria increases the numbers of plasma cells, lymphocytes, and macrophages in the lamina propria (i.e., it stimulates the immune system of the gut). Acceleration of the turnover rate of enterocytes, blunting of villi, and hypertrophy of crypts also follow bacterial colonization of a germ-free animal.

A primary function of the normal, or indigenous, flora is to oppose invasion by pathogens. Microbial interactions, direct and indirect autogenic processes, are important in the large intestine, where several populations interact to promote or limit growth of other bacteria.

The *direct autogenic factors* are nutritional competition, and production of toxic bacterial by-products (bacteriocins, fatty acids, hydrogen sulfide, and bacterial antibiotics). By using the available oxygen, facultative anaerobes help produce an anaerobic medium for survival of anaerobes. *Bacteriocins* are proteins secreted by bacteria that kill closely related bacteria. Examples include *colicins* (bactericidal chemicals produced by strains of *E. coli*). Fatty acids (acetic, butyric) are powerful stabilizers of the flora (especially Enterobacteriaceae) in the large intestine. *Bacillus subtilis* and *Pseudomonas aeruginosa* produce gastrointestinal antibiotic substances.

Indirect autogenic factors include bacterial deconjugation of compounds, microbial immunological responses, and stimulation of peristalsis.

THE GASTROINTESTINAL IMMUNE SYSTEM

The intestinal wall is the most voluminous immunological organ in an animal, since at least 25 percent of the intestinal mucosa and submucosa is lymphoid tissue. The lymphoid tissues in the intestine, called *gut-associated lymphoid tissue (GALT)*, are part of the mucosal immune system, which also includes bronchial tissue, the mammary gland, and the female genital system.

Gut-Associated Lymphoid Tissue

The cell population of GALT is found in the connective tissue of the lamina propria (as lymphocytes and plasma cells), between the epithelial cells lining the intestinal villi (as intraepithelial lymphocytes), in organized lymphoid nodules (e.g., Peyer's patches), and in scattered isolated lymphoid follicles.

Lamina Propria Lymphoid Cells

B lymphocytes, plasma cells, T cells, macrophages, eosinophils, and mast cells are interspersed in the vascular and lymphatic connective tissue of the intestinal lamina propria. B lymphocytes migrate from Peyer's patches to the lamina propria to complete their maturation into plasma cells. Most intestinal plasma cells (70 to 90 percent) produce IgA antibodies, about one-fifth produce IgM, and a few generate IgE. IgG-producing cells are oddities in the lamina propria but are prevalent in peripheral lymph nodes and spleen. Some T lymphocytes participate in cell-mediated immunity by their effect on other types of cells, such as macrophages and monocytes. Both B cells and T cells, after stimulation by antigens, become the memory bank for future antigenic encounters. Three to four days are required for cells to migrate from Peyer's patches to the lamina propria (Fig. 22–5).

Intraepithelial Lymphocytes

Large intraepithelial lymphocytes (IEL) are situated between the enterocytes lining the villous surface, near the basement membrane in the basal part of the epithelium. They constitute about one-sixth of the intestinal surface, and a large portion of them are T cells that have migrated from Peyer's patches. The functional role and ultimate fate of IEL are not known.

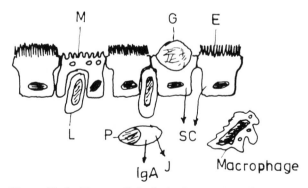

Figure 22–5 Plasma cells in the lamina propria produce mostly the monomer IgA (75 percent), some pentamer IgM (20 percent), and little IgE (5 percent). They also produce J chains for the dimer sIgA and for IgM. The secretory components (SC), found in sIgA and IgM, come from the basolateral membrane of enterocytes and goblet cells (G). (L, Lymphocyte; M, M cell.)

Peyer's Patches

Peyer's patches, also known as patches of aggregate nodules, are organized aggregates of peripheral lymphoid tissue on the antimesenteric wall of the gut that play a key role in the initiation of the mucosal IgA response and in the expression of local mucosal immunity. They are located in the lamina propria, extending as deeply as the submucosa, and are separated from the intestinal lumen by a specialized follicle-associated epithelium (FAE), which can be permeated by lymphocytes. Each Peyer's patch may have as many as six lymphatic follicles (oval, 800 μm in length) separated by thymus-dependent interfollicular areas (Fig. 22–6).

The FAE, similar to that found in the tonsils, contains 81 percent enterocytes, 9 percent cells with microfolds instead of microvilli (hence the name "M cells") interspersed among the more cuboidal enterocytes, mucus-producing goblet cells (8 percent), and Paneth cells (2 percent). The proportions of preeffector lymphocytes are about 25 percent T lymphocytes, 55 percent B lymphocytes, and the remainder non–B- or non–T lymphocytes, which are not K, or natural killer, cells. The FAE is distinguished by its sunken appearance within the epithelium.

M cells contain, besides stunted microvilli and a luminal membrane with many small folds, numerous antigen-accessible vesicles within their apical cytoplasm (see Fig. 22–6). In close association with underlying lymphocytes, their function is to transport antigen across the intestinal epithelium by pinocytosis.

The *dome area,* immediately below the specialized epithelium, allows transport of antigens to the preeffector cells (Fig. 22–7). Antigens can enter Peyer's patches only from the intestinal lumen, but the B and T cells are derived from the recirculating lymph pool. In the dome and interfollicular areas, T lymphocytes predominate.

Follicles contain a *germinal center* consisting largely of B lymphocytes producing IgA, IgE, IgG, and IgM, and few

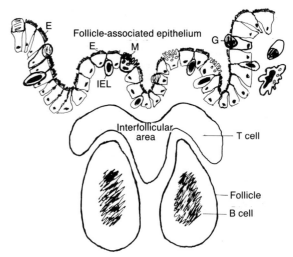

Figure 22–6   Areas of Peyer's patches: follicles, FAE (containing enterocytes; M cells; goblet cells; Paneth cells; and preeffector lymphocytes: T, 25 percent; B, 55 percent), dome area for transfer of antigens and rich in T lymphocytes, central core of B-preeffector cells, and thymus-dependent interfollicular area (rich in T lymphocytes).

plasma cells. The rim of the follicle presents lymphocytes without B- or T-cell markers.

Primary Cells of the Gastrointestinal Immune System

Foreign antigenic materials (microbes, viruses, parasites, food products, drugs, chemicals) may penetrate the mechanical barrier of the normal or abnormal (diseased) intestinal mucosa and stimulate preeffector cells of the

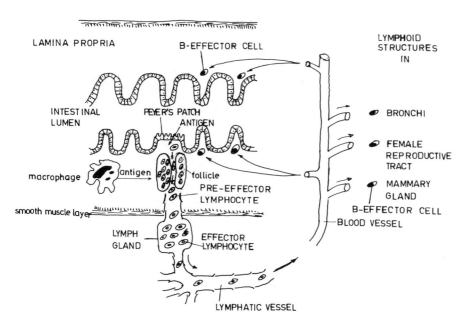

Figure 22–7 Upon antigen stimulation, preeffector cells fired off from Peyer's patches migrate into the lymphatic and blood circulations. They finally populate the lamina propria of the intestine and of other mucosal lymphoid organs (respiratory, reproductive, mammary gland) to complete their maturation.

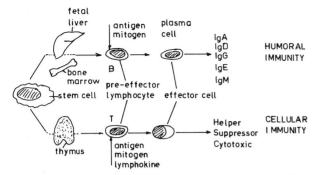

Figure 22–8 Lymphocytes of the immune system. B lymphocytes are formed in the bone marrow in mammals or the bursa of Fabricius in birds. They are activated by antigens or mitogens and then mature into cells that produce antibodies such as IgA, IgD, IgE, IgG, and IgM or humoral immunity. Likewise, when thymus-derived lymphocytes are stimulated by antigens or mitogens, they proliferate and mature into T effector cells to produce cell-mediated or cellular immunity.

GALT to become effector cells (Fig 22–8). The cells involved in these immune responses are primarily B and T lymphocytes, and secondarily macrophages, mast cells, eosinophils, and basophils.

B Lymphocytes

B lymphocytes (derived from bursa of Fabricius in avians and from bone marrow in mammals) differentiate into plasma cells that synthesize and secrete antibodies (immunoglobulins) (Table 22–2). IgA is predominant in intestinal secretions.

T Lymphocytes

T lymphocytes may differentiate into one of several subclasses of a heterogenous population of T cells, variously known as cytotoxic T cells, T helper cells, and T suppressor cells (Fig. 22–9). On antigenic stimulation, cytotoxic T cells release chemicals to damage target cells. T-helper cells cooperate in the induction of B-effector cells to humoral antibody synthesis and in the induction of other T cells. Suppressor T cells inhibit the induction of B cells and of other T cells. T cells can produce other products, such as lymphokines, and are responsible for cell-mediated immunity. Mitogens for T lymphocytes are plant lectins (plant proteins) such as phytohemagglutinins (PHA) and concanavalin A (Con A), thymic hormones (thymus humoral factor,

TABLE 22–2 Molecular Weight of Immunoglobulins

Immunoglobulin	Daltons
IgA	160,000
IgD	190,000
IgE	200,000
IgG	150,000
IgM	1,000,000

or THF, thymopoietin, and thymosin), amphotericin B (a polyene antibiotic), and a host of immunomodulating drugs.

Macrophages, Eosinophils, Mast Cells, and Basophils

Macrophages prepare antigens for induction of B-effector cells into plasma cells and T cells into cytotoxic cells. By phagocytosis, they also play an important role in clearing foreign material coated with antibody.

Eosinophils are found in the blood of the intestine and of other tissues that communicate with the outside environment (e.g., skin, lungs, genitourinary tract). Antigens at the surface of the intestine, including parasites, allergy-causing foods, and drugs, react with mastocytes to attract eosinophils. A chemotactic factor liberated from mast cells and basophils also attracts eosinophils. Eosinophils produce a chemical that inhibits discharge of histamine from basophils and a lysozymal enzyme that inactivates the slow-reacting substances of anaphylaxis.

Mucosal *mast cells* are stimulated into activity by T lymphocyte–derived lymphokines. The function of mast cells depends on their degranulation (Fig. 22–10), that is, the extracellular discharge of vasoactive amines (histamine, serotonin). Mast cells are involved in the classic immediate anaphylactic reaction and in the genesis of "delayed in time" late-phase reactions to a variety of antigens.

Migration of Intestinal Lymphoid Cells

Intestinal lymphoid cells are interrelated through migrations from one site to another. T and B lymphocytes from Peyer's patches populate the lamina propria and the intraepithelial sites, where they mature into T-effector or plasma cells. After initial antigenic stimulation, B and T cells migrate from Peyer's patches by way of the lymphatic and blood circulations, to the intestine (lamina propria and intraepithelial) and other extraintestinal organs of immunity—mammary gland, genital tract, and respiratory tract (see Fig. 22–7).

Intestinal Mucosal Immunity

Immunoglobulins A, E, and M are proteins produced by cells in the intestinal lymphoid organs. The mucosal immunity operates independent of the humoral system of the body. The IgG found in the lamina propria is derived from serum and is not a local intestinal product.

IgA

IgA is the major immunoglobulin to originate from antibody-producing cells in the intestinal lamina propria. The IgA in intestinal secretions is termed secretory IgA, or sIgA.

Secretory IgA is a dimer consisting of two monomers, a secretory component (SC), and a J chain (Fig. 22–11). The

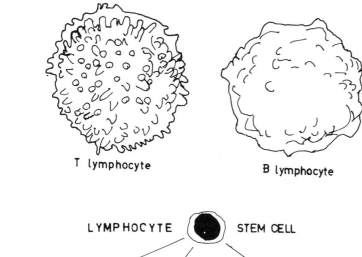

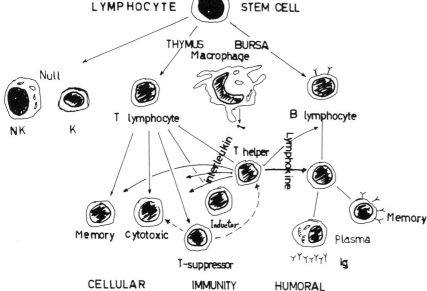

Figure 22–9 **A,** Scanning electron microscopy of T lymphocyte (rough surface) and B lymphocyte (smoother surface). **B,** The lymphocyte stem cells give rise to nonkiller (null) cells, killer cells, T lymphocytes, and B lymphocytes; upon antigenic stimulation T and B lymphocytes further mature into cells that produce cellular immunity (T cells: helper, inductor, suppressor, cytotoxic, memory) or humoral immunity (immunoglobulins from plasma cells, memory B lymphocyte).

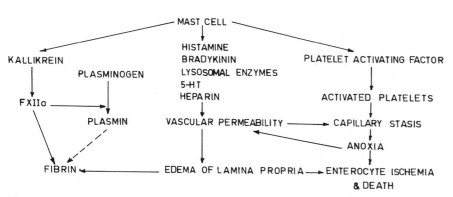

Figure 22–10 Probable events after T-lymphocyte lymphokine-induced degranulation of mucosal mast cells with discharge of kallikrein, histamine, and platelet-activating factor (PAF). These nonspecific pathways may be common to several forms of immunologic or inflammatory damages to intestinal mucosa. For example, some of these substances attract eosinophils and undergo phagocytosis. Kallikrein enzymatically activates Factor XII of blood coagulation and the plasmin-complement cascade of events. The histamine-related changes in vascular permeability eventually alter the functions and structures of the intestinal wall.

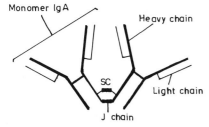

Figure 22–11 Secretory IgA, a dimer of IgA, with the SC and J chain.

secretory component, a glycoprotein believed to be produced by the goblet (mucus) cells, is incorporated onto dimeric IgA when the latter crosses the membrane of enterocytes into the intestinal lumen. SC increases the resistance of sIgA to digestion by proteolytic enzymes and serves to anchor IgA to the mucosal surface. The J chain, like IgA, is produced by plasma cells and connects the two monomers of IgA.

From the lamina propria, IgA-J-IgA is transported through the enterocytes, to acquire SC, into the intestinal secretions (Fig. 22–12). Secretory IgA prevents absorption of antigens by the intestinal mucosa, resists proteolytic degradation by either bacteria or digestive enzymes, acts against dietary antigens to prevent food allergies, and functions as a regulator of the intestinal flora.

Figure 22–12 Dissemination of IgA into the lymphatics and blood and of IgA-J-IgA through the lymph and blood circulation pathways and through the intestinal epithelium into the lumen as IgA-J-SC-IgA, or sIgA.

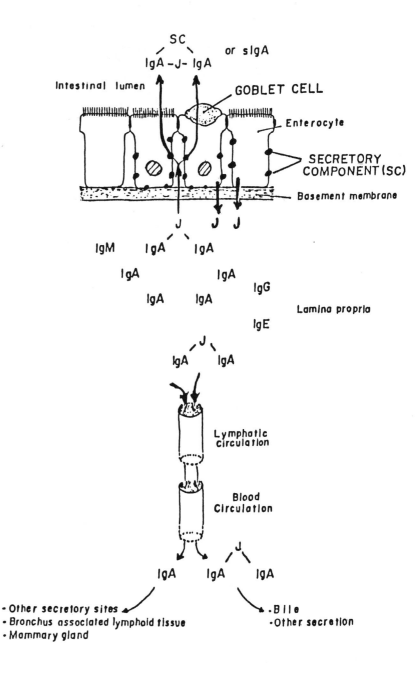

IgE

IgE is involved in allergic disorders: antigen-antibody-receptor reactions cause release of histamine and slow-reacting substance of anaphylaxis by mastocytes. The intestinal level of IgE is increased by intestinal parasites. IgE does not bind SC and does not adhere to cell membranes.

IgG

IgG is rapidly degraded after entering the lumen of the gut. It can mediate cell lysis and stimulate phagocytosis.

IgM

IgM, produced locally in the lamina propria, may also be derived from serum. It is a pentamer possessing a J chain. It is transported across the intestinal epithelium by a processus similar to IgA. The concentration of IgM in intestinal secretions is one-twentieth that of IgA.

REFERENCES

Bauchop T. The gut anaerobic fungi: Colonisers of dietary fibre. In: Wallace G, Bell L, eds. Fibre in human and animal nutrition. Wellington: The Royal Society of New Zealand, 1983.

Brandtzaeg P, Baklien K. Intestinal secretion of IgA and IgM: a hypothetical model. In: Immunology of the gut. Ciba Foundation Symposium 46 (new series). New York: Elsevier, 1977.

Clarke RTJ. The gut and its micro-organisms. In: Clarke RTJ, Bauchop T, eds. Microbial ecology of the gut. New York: Academic Press, 1977.

Coates ME, Fuller R. The gnotobiotic animal in the study of gut microbiology. In: Clarke RTJ, Bauchop T, eds. Microbial ecology of the gut. New York: Academic Press, 1977.

Drochner W. Aspects of digestion in the large intestine of the pig. Adv Anim Physiol Anim Nutr 1987;(suppl 17).

Ducluzeau R, Raibaud P. Ecologie microbienne du tube digestif. New York: Masson, 1979.

Hartiala K. Metabolism of foreign substances in the gastro-intestinal tract. In: Lee DHK, ed. Handbook of physiology. Bethesda, MD: American Physiological Society, 1977.

Hirsh DC. Microflora, mucosa, and immunity. In: Anderson NV, ed. Veterinary gastroenterology. Philadelphia: Lea & Febiger, 1980.

Kagnoff MF. Immunology of the digestive system. In: Johnson LR, ed. Physiology of the gastrointestinal tract. New York: Raven Press, 1981.

Kidder BE, Manners MJ. Digestion in the pig. Bristol: Scientecnica, 1978.

Masek K. Current status of drugs which modulate the immune response. Trends Pharmacol Sci 1983;4:318.

Pfeiffer CJ, Hanninen O. Alimentary excretion of environmental agents and unnatural compound. In: Lee DHK, ed. Handbook of physiology. Bethesda, MD: American Physiological Society, 1977.

Prins RA. Biochemical activities of gut micro-organisms. In: Clarke RTJ, Bauchop T, eds. Microbial ecology of the gut. New York: Academic Press, 1977.

Savage DC. Effects of food and fibre on the intestinal luminal environment. In: Wallace G, Bell L, eds. Fibre in human and animal nutrition. Wellington: The Royal Society of New Zealand, 1983.

Simon GL, Gorbach SL. Intestinal flora in health and disease. In: Johnson LR, ed. Physiology of the gastrointestinal tract. New York: Raven Press, 1981.

Smith MW, Peacock MA. Lymphocyte-induced formation of antigen transporting "M" cells from fully differentiated mouse enterocytes. In: Robinson JWL, Dowling RH, Riecken EO, eds. Mechanisms of intestinal adaptation. Lancaster: MTP Press Ltd, 1982.

Strombeck DR. Small animal gastroenterology. Davis, CA: Stonegate Publishing, 1979.

CHAPTER 23

FEEDING BEHAVIOR

Feeding behavior may be defined as the overall actions of an animal that lead to ingestion of suitable edible food to satisfy organic needs. Animals reject most inedible substances because of innate reflexes and lack of appetite for them. Feeding behavior implicates two antagonistic processes: initiation of a need to eat (hunger) and cessation of this need when the animal is satiated. The stimulus of hunger initiates the search for and intake of food, and satiety stops it. Most of the research on food intake has not been centered on induction of eating, by stimulation of the *feeding center in the lateral hypothalamus,* because it is difficult to quantify hunger or the need of an animal to eat. In contrast, satiety is easier to observe at the end of a meal. Uncontrolled hyperphagia, or bulimia, can be noted after destruction of the *satiety center* in the *ventromedial hypothalamic nuclei.*

In animals, maintenance, growth, and production activities require the expenditure of energy derived from oxidation of the components of food that can be utilized by the cells. Digestion involves the processes of physical, chemical, and microbial breakdown of foods that cannot be absorbed directly.

The physical grinding of plant material by mastication is an important process of digestion in herbivores. Plant and animal tissues used as foods contain similar types of chemical substances (proteins, lipids, carbohydrates, minerals, and vitamins) but contain vastly different proportions of each. Animal tissues have a remarkably low carbohydrate content compared with plant tissues (Table 23–1). The principal chemical action during digestion is brought about by enzymes issued in the digestive secretions or by enzymes from bacteria and protozoa. In ruminants, horses, and rabbits, the cooperative rather than competitive relationship of animals with gastrointestinal microorganisms is of major importance for digestion of plant material.

FOOD PREHENSION IN CARNIVORES

Dogs, like their wild ancestors, tend to eat rapidly and may consume enormous meals. For instance, a male Labrador retriever may consume 10 percent of its body weight in canned food at once. Cats, as solitary hunters, tend to feed frequently and on smaller meals. A mouse represents the size of a meal for a house cat.

Dogs and cats may use their forelimbs to hold food, which is passed into the mouth largely by head and jaw movements without much grinding. Although mastication is basically a voluntary act under the control of higher nervous centers, it usually takes place involuntarily. Rhythmic movements of the mandible (lower jaw) constitute the *chewing reflex,* and lowering of the mandible in response to the extension of the tongue represents the *linguomandibular reflex.*

Cats and dogs convey fluids into the mouth by rapid extension and retraction of the tongue, which has a free mobile end formed into a ladle. The cat also bears numerous dorsal lingual spicules, which help retain fluids and bring them into the mouth with each retraction of the tongue.

In contrast, other animals draw liquid into the mouth by suction. The mouth is held closed and submerged beneath the fluid while the tongue exerts a pump-like effect to create sufficient negative pressure to draw the fluid into the mouth. Likewise, sucking involves the creation of negative pressure in the mouth by means of the tongue and cheeks; that is how rodents ingest liquids.

Salivation

The serous secretion of the parotid glands, the mucous secretion of the sublingual glands, and the mixed secretion of the submandibular glands are stimulated reflexly by food, mastication, and temperature. Through the roots of cranial nerves VII, IX, and X, the afferent nerves from the taste receptors proceed into the brainstem and connect with the upper and lower salivary nuclei in the region of the tractus solitarius (Fig. 23–1).

The secretion of the salivary glands is at the origin of several discoveries. More than a century ago, Claude BERNARD (1852) showed that some days or weeks after section of the chorda tympani, the cannulated submandibular duct of dogs was still delivering saliva. This phenomenon was termed *paralytic secretion.*

The same year, COLIN published his technique on parotid gland fistulation in horses and oxen. He reported that the bovine parotid was different from other salivary glands in that it secreted *continuously,* even between meals.

In 1927, the Russian physiologist Ivan PAVLOV (1849–1936) published his work on *conditioned* (salivary) *reflexes* in dogs. Pavlov attributed the flow of saliva (and gastric juice) to the presence of food in the mouth as an unlearned response (a reflex, innate response), or, as he called it, an unconditioned response. Classical conditioning is defined as the formation (or strengthening) of an association between a conditioned stimulus (CS) and a response to an unconditioned stimulus (US). With repeated presentation of a conditioned stimulus in a controlled relationship with an unconditioned stimulus, the response is eventually elicited by the CS alone. The original response to the US is called an *unconditioned response,* and the learned response to the CS is termed a *conditioned response.*

TABLE 23–1 Percentage Composition of Some Plant and Animal Products

Products	Water	Carbohydrate	Lipid	Protein	Ash
Muscle	72	0.6	4.3	21.4	1.5
Wheat grain	13	71.2	1.9	12.2	1.7
Pasture grass	80	10.0	1.0	3.2	2.4

Conditioned Salivary Secretion

Conditioned salivary secretion (e.g., in response to light) can be established in a dog. Usually, when a light is turned on (CS), the dog makes some exploratory movements in his feed dish but does not salivate. If after a few seconds, meat (US) is delivered to the feed dish, the dog eats, and a recording device (Fig. 23–2) registers copious salivation. After several trials in which the light stimulus always precedes the meat stimulus, which results in salivation (the reinforcement response), the dog salivates when the light stimulus is turned on even though the meat stimulus does not follow.

In the usual order of events, the conditioned reflex can best be remembered by the animal if the CS is not always applied alone but is occasionally followed by the uncondi-

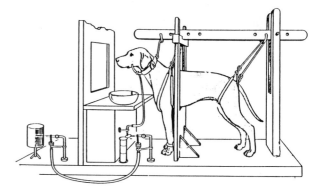

Figure 23–2 Recording and experimental arrangements used by Pavlov in classical salivary conditioning. Mechanical devices (not shown) permit the light (conditioned stimulus) to appear in the window and the meat powder (unconditioned stimulus) to appear in the food bowl.

tioned stimulus. This conditioned response may be regarded as a simple habit, because a learned association is demonstrated to exist between the CS and the conditioned response.

Food Preferences and Aversions

Food preferences develop in puppies and kittens as a result of experience. Dogs in a group that is initially fed soybeans may refuse to touch any new food or to eat meat. Animals deficient in sodium show a strong preference for sodium, but this is not usual for other mineral deficiencies.

Conditioned aversion in nature protects animals from repeated ingestion of food that produces gastrointestinal illness or food allergy. Animals that ingest a sublethal amount of a toxic pest control bait subsequently will avoid it. Aversion to cannibalism is widespread among carnivores.

In cats, aversion to meat is conditioned by stuffing meat with lithium chloride (Fig. 23–3). Aversion to sheep meat is conditioned to coyotes to control sheep predation. After a couple of experiences with lithium-poisoned lamb meat, coyotes no longer chase sheep, or if they attack and kill the prey they do not eat it.

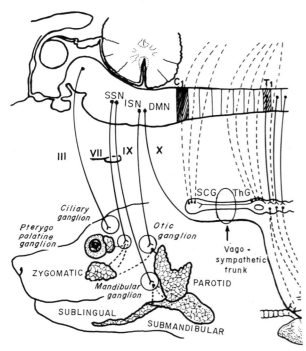

Figure 23–1 Neural regulation of salivary secretion in the dog. The submandibular and sublingual glands are supplied by parasympathetic secretory nerves originating in the superior salivary nucleus (*SSN*). Preganglionic fibers proceed through the facial nerve (cranial nerve VII) and the chorda tympani. The parotid gland obtains its parasympathetic nerve supply from the inferior salivary nucleus (*ISN*), the efferent fibers travel through the glossopharyngeal nerve (*IX*). Sympathetic fibers come from the superior cervical ganglion (*SCG*). (ThG, Thoracic ganglion; DMN, dorsomedial nucleus of ventral column of spinal cord.)

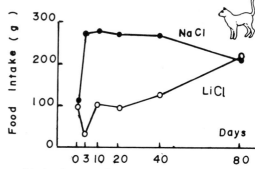

Figure 23–3 Aversion of the cat (measured as food intake) to food containing lithium chloride compared with food containing salt.

Swallowing

Swallowing, or deglutition, is a motor activity involving the whole esophagus. In dogs, swallowing is more a somatomotor than a visceromotor process, because the canine esophagus consists of striated muscles innervated by somatic motor nerves. In pigs, the distal part of the esophagus is made of smooth muscle fibers, and both the striated cranial part and the distal smooth part exhibit an autonomous peristaltic activity that is influenced by the autonomic nervous system.

The complex action of transferring food and liquid from the oral cavity to the stomach starts with a movement of the tongue that positions the food bolus centrally, between the tongue and hard palate, in a position suitable for swallowing (Fig. 23–4).

The swallowing center is located in the rhombencephalon (metencephalon, hindbrain). An animal rendered decerebrate by transection of the midbrain can still swallow food placed in its throat. The various phases of the act of swallowing are coordinated partly in this center, and by various subservient motor nuclei. Stimulation of the afferent fibers of the glossopharyngeal and vagus nerves, between their entry into the medulla and the nucleus solitarius, simultaneously causes deglutition and salivation. Through the glossopharyngeal nerve, the swallowing center receives impulses from receptors in the mouth and the epiglottis. The presence of the food bolus elicits a series of reflexes, which divide swallowing into pharyngeal and esophageal stages.

During the *pharyngeal stage* of swallowing, peristaltic contractions of the pharynx propel the bolus from the base of the tongue into the laryngopharynx and the relaxed pharyngoesophageal sphincter. The pharyngoesophageal, or upper esophageal, sphincter (UES) is formed by the cricopharyngeal muscle and subjacent esophageal circular muscles. Following the passage of the bolus into the cranial esophagus, the UES contracts to return to its naturally closed state and to initiate the esophageal phase of swallowing (Fig. 23–5).

The *esophageal stage* of swallowing includes the peristaltic propulsion of the bolus from the cranial esophagus to the gastroesophageal junction. This is called *primary peristalsis*, a reflex contraction of the muscles of the esophagus that progresses uninterrupted to the gastroesophageal, or lower esophageal, sphincter (LES). Primary peristalsis is linked to the integrity of the vagal nerves. When a bolus temporarily pauses or several boluses accumulate in the proximal esophagus, the local stimulus results in a secondary peristaltic

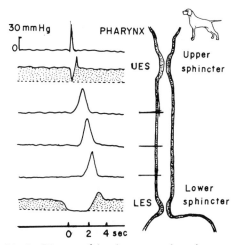

Figure 23–5 Diagram of the pharyngoesophageal, upper esophageal, sphincter (*UES*), the esophagus, and the lower esophageal sphincter (*LES*) intraluminal pressures after a swallow in a dog. Pressure scales are approximate. Velocity of the bolus is 5 cm per second: the bolus goes from UES to LES in 4 seconds.

wave (*secondary peristalsis*) that pushes the food to the gastroesophageal junction.

The LES is a physiological high-pressure zone that separates the esophagus from the stomach. The opening of the LES is a passive mechanical event stimulated by the force of an oncoming bolus. The relaxation of the sphincter is an active reflex process mediated neurologically, as the LES begins to relax before esophageal pressure peaks in the distal esophagus (see Fig. 23–5). Synchronization of LES relaxation with the oncoming esophageal wave is required for normal passage of a bolus. Vagotomy abolishes peristalsis in the body of the esophagus and decreases the synchronous relaxation of the LES with deglutition. These alterations are attributed to the absence of afferent innervation of the mucosa rather than to the section of the efferent fibers.

FOOD PREHENSION IN HERBIVORES

Prehension of food differs among herbivorous animals. In some species, the main prehensile structure is the lips (upper or lower). Others use mainly their tongues, and some rely mostly on their incisor teeth.

In the *horse*, the sensitive, mobile upper and lower lips are the main prehensile structures used during feeding.

Figure 23–4 Phases of progression of the bolus during the pharyngeal stage of swallowing. 1, When the bolus reaches the base of the tongue, it (2) is propulsed into the relaxed cricopharyngeal sphincter following the closure of the larynx. 3, The bolus enters the esophagus during relaxation of the cricopharyngeal sphincter.

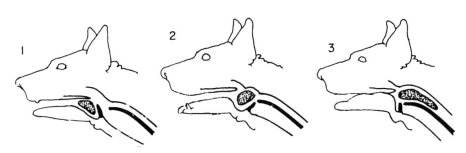

During grazing, the lips are drawn back to allow the incisor teeth to sever the grass at its base. Under natural conditions, the *pig* digs up the ground with its snout (rooting), and grass is carried into the mouth largely by the action of the pointed lower lip. In other common grazing herbivores, the lips possess only limited movements.

In *ruminants,* lips, tongue, lower incisor teeth, and the dental pad at the rostral end of the hard palate act as organs for prehension of food. *Grass and roughage eaters,* the traditional *grazers* (GR) (cattle, sheep), have a small mouth opening and short lips with a relatively long tongue. They curve their tongue around mainly monocotyledonous forage (grass, hay), which is then drawn between the lower incisor teeth and the upper dental pad and severed by a movement of the head. In sheep, a cleft in the upper lip permits very close grazing. *Concentrate selectors* (CS), the traditional *browser ruminants* (deer, moose, giraffe), have a large mouth opening, which permits them to use their lower incisor teeth to strip twigs or to gnaw on fruits and flowers of dicotyledonous plants. Intermediary opportunistic mixed (IM) feeder ruminants (goat) can adapt to either feeding type but prefer the low-fiber, dicotyledonous plants. They will even climb suitable trees to get their preferred foods.

Dietary Selection

Free-ranging horses usually prefer grasses and legumes, but a wide variety of shrubs, herbs, woody plants, and even roots may be selected. Horses and ponies selectively graze strips sown with tall fescue, white clover, dandelions, and timothy but avoid sections containing red fescue and red clover.

Sheep consistently select a diet low in protein but otherwise adequate, and ewes continue to make the same choice throughout pregnancy. Correct self-selection of diet, an example of satisfying nutritional needs by taste through either "appetite instinct" or learning, is not found in ewes.

Eating Rate

Horses and ponies confined to stalls or pens and given free access to hay exhibit the same feeding patterns observed in free-ranging animals and usually eat during 10 to 12 hours daily, in sessions lasting 30 to 180 minutes. In contrast, confined horses eat concentrate or pelleted feed rapidly and spend the remaining time in boredom (i.e., standing, lying down, searching, chewing wood) (Fig. 23–6).

Diurnal patterns of intensive eating in the early morning, late afternoon, and during the evening are the rule. After 2 or 3 weeks of continuous access to a single feed, ponies stabilize their body weights, consuming 2 to 3 percent of their total body weight in dry matter in a 24-hour period. Horses similarly limit their dry matter intake. The time spent grazing by brood mares is about 10 hours per 24 hours, and 30 minutes more from the third week after foaling than nonlactating mares (Fig. 23–7).

The number of diurnal sucks in the foal is very high 48

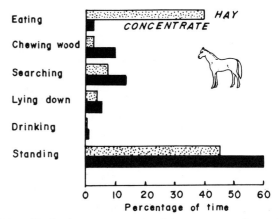

Figure 23–6 Average percentage of time spent on various activities by horses fed hay and concentrate.

hours after birth but decreases rapidly with age, whereas grazing time increases from 10 percent of the observed time in May to 67 percent in October. These changes are related to a decrease in the foal's growth rate. During the first week after foaling, the mares are disturbed in their grazing by about 20 periods of suckling.

In pigs, feeding behavior is polyphasic, and the time spent eating is less than 10 to 15 minutes, two or three times a day. In contrast, the babirusa (a pig-like animal of Indonesia) browses leaves several hours per day. Structurally, the babirusa's stomach differs from that of domestic pig by its enormous diverticulum ventriculi. When seen in longitudinal section, the stomach of the babirusa has similarities to the rumen of the domestic sheep. A diverticulum presents portions recalling the dorsal and ventral sac of the rumen (Fig. 23–8).

Taking into account the alimentary behavior and the nature of food, sheep consume pelleted grass faster than chopped grass or hay (Tables 23–2 and 23–3).

Isolated ewes restricted to an intake at two-thirds of ad libitum rate spend less time eating but ruminate more than

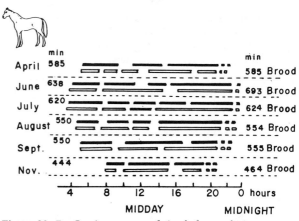

Figure 23–7 Grazing patterns of a herd of mares during summer and fall. Solid bars indicate nonlactating mares; open bars indicate brood mares.

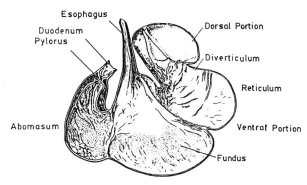

Figure 23–8 Section of the stomach of the babirusa, an Indonesian pig-like animal, showing a diverticulum, with dorsal and ventral portions for fermentation of leaves, recalling the reticulum of sheep.

those fed ad libitum. Grouped ewes in either situation spend as much time eating, but the ones restricted in their intake ruminate more.

Analyses of the ruminoreticulum fill in cattle (500 kg) show that the proportion of dry matter (DM) is similar (about 25 percent), whatever the regimen. However, the ruminoreticular DM content after alfalfa is ingested (lucerne hay) (62 kg, or 9.5 kg DM) is 9.2 kg, whereas it is 12 kg—much higher—after grass (82 kg, or 9.0 kg DM). The higher turnover rate of the ruminoreticulum contents with alfalfa than with grass explains this discrepancy, in that less DM remains in the digestion vat with alfalfa.

Masticatory Movements

In herbivores, mastication, or chewing, refers to the mechanical breakdown of food in the mouth by diduction (opening) and occlusion (closing) of both sets of upper and lower molar teeth during eating or rumination. Grinding of plant tissues in horses and in ruminants (Fig. 23–9) occurs by lateral movements of the mandible, which, along with others of pulsion (forward) and retropulsion (backward), are possible because of the flexibility of the temporomandibular joint.

TABLE 23–2 Rate of Intake of Hay and Dried Grass in Sheep Fed ad Libitum

		Dried Grass	
	Hay (86% DM)	Chopped (88% DM)	Pelleted (88% DM)
Rate of eating (g/30 min)			
0–30 min	220	182	324
30–60 min	132	125	131
60–90 min	100	125	108
Intake/kg sheep	1.5	1.6	2.6
Mean retention time (hr)	69	60	21

TABLE 23–3 Effects of Grouping and Isolation of Sheep on Feed Intake with ad Libitum and Restricted Feeding Regimens

	Ad libitum		Restricted	
	Grouped	Isolated	Grouped	Isolated
Rate of eating (g/30 min)	265	240	295	285
Time spent (hr/day)				
Eating	3.7	5.1	3.9	3.8
Ruminating	5.2	5.3	7.4	7.5
Intake (kg)	1.6	1.6	1.0	1.0

Since the upper jaw (maxilla) is wider than the lower jaw (mandible), mastication occurs only on one side of the dental table at a time. Because of this lateral movement, the teeth wear with chisel-shaped grinding surfaces, the sharp edge of the lower teeth being innermost and that of the upper teeth outermost. In horses, these sharp inner and outer edges must be filed to prevent tongue and lip injuries and inadequate chewing of hay. The teeth of herbivores wear unevenly because they are made of substances with different degrees of hardness, but this characteristic increases the grinding efficiency of the dental tables.

Most mammals masticate on one side or the other in various alternating sequences. Rodents are exceptions to this, as they shift their teeth in a forward and backward (propalineal) pattern. Movements of the tongue and lips propel the food toward the active, or working, dental side whenever the jaws are widely separated. The usual mediad motion of the mandible on the working side then drives all or part of the food across the dental table, cutting or shearing the food, while the upper and lower dental cusps slide past each other. The nonworking tooth rows remain out of direct contact for most of the orbits of a sequence. The food is in contact with both sets of cusps on the working side, and a portion of the food is transferred to the nonworking surface during the closed portion of each orbit. Unless there is a switch of the masticatory side, the food is transferred back toward the working side when the jaws open again.

Swinging in simply definable planes occurs only in carnivores. Masticatory orbits are asymmetrical in almost all mammals. The jaws move in three-dimensional space: downward rotation at the condyles is coupled with unilateral or bilateral condylar translation. All phases of the orbit are affected by the *nature and size of the food particles*. Goats and cats show different orbital patterns when the food type or the size of the food particles is changed.

The lower incisors of ruminants are very mobile, with a possible labial displacement of as much as 3.6 mm linearly, graded up to a load of 0.5 N in sheep (Fig. 23–10). Such patterns are consistent with the view that periodontal tissues are viscoelastic.

In steers with an esophageal fistula to collect grazed and masticated grass, the percentages of particles longer than 1.7 mm and shorter than 0.5 mm, respectively, are 22 and 27 percent with bermuda grass and 31 percent and 21 percent with flaccid grass. Steers housed in stanchions spend more time chewing 20-mm long particles of grass than 5-mm particles (Table 23–4).

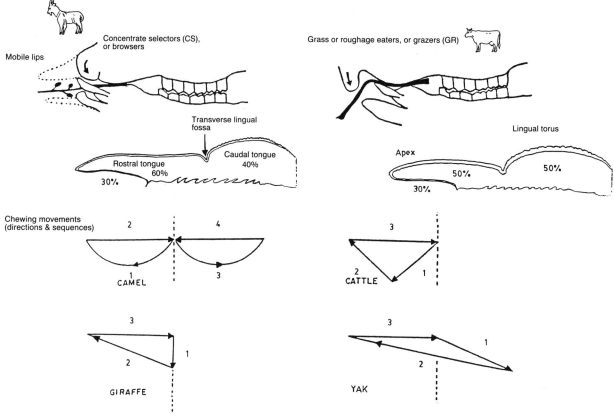

Figure 23–9 Masticating movements in herbivores. **Top Row,** Upper and lower lateral dental tables in concentrate selector and grazer ruminants (note absence of upper incisors, replaced by dental pad). **Second Row,** In concentrate selectors, the rostral part of the tongue is relatively longer than the caudal part (60 versus 40 percent). However, in grazers, the central lingual fossa separates the tongue into equal rostral and caudal portions, but the epithelium covering the tongue is thicker. The apex (free end) of the tongue is of the same relative length in both types of ruminants. **Third and Fourth Rows,** Directions and sequences of mandible movements during prehension and rumination chewing.

Salivation and Esophageal Motility in Ruminants

The pH of saliva of preruminants (young ruminants) tends to be slightly acidic, as in carnivores, but may rise to 7.5 after stimulation. In adult ruminants the salivary secretions are continuous and alkaline (pH about 8) due to the large amount of bicarbonate that is provided to neutralize the short-chain fatty acids (SCFAs) in the rumen (Fig. 23–11).

The esophagus of cattle and sheep is striated muscle throughout its entire length, whereas in pigs and horses the caudal esophagus is made up of smooth muscle. In standing, conscious sheep, esophageal motility shows fast retrograde

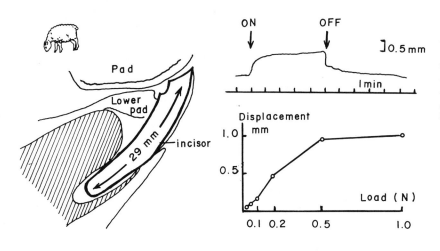

Figure 23–10 Arrangement of supporting tissues of the sheep incisors (mean length 29 mm). Displacement, in millimeters, produced by suddenly applying a load (0.1 to 1 N) for 5 minutes. The motility is force dependent for linguolabial loads placed on (*on*) or removed from (*off*) the incisors.

TABLE 23–4 Effects of Particle Size of Grass on Chewing
and Rumination Time in Steers

	Median Particle Length (mm)	
	5	20
Daily intake (kg)	12	13
Chewing time		
Eating (min/kg DM)	8.4	10.3
Ruminating (min/kg DM)	17	25
Rumination		
Boli/kg DM	19	31
Time chewing (min/bolus)	0.85	0.78

(orad) peristalsis and normal aborad peristalsis (28 cm per second) during swallowing of saliva. Retrograde peristalsis (66 cm per second) is regularly triggered by esophageal distention coinciding either with the added reticular contraction of regurgitation during rumination or with eructation.

REGULATION OF FOOD INTAKE

Seeking, prehension, mastication, salivation, and swallowing of food are under the direct control of the brain. Some tumors of the hypothalamus result in excessive obesity. By studying lesions and by stimulating specific areas of the hypothalamus, an appetite center and a satiety center have been determined.

The *appetite center* is identified with both lateral hypothalamic nuclei. Lesions of the lateral hypothalamic areas result in aphagia; conversely, continuous stimulation of these areas induces voracious eating in rats and in goats (Fig. 23–12). The *satiety center* is located in both ventromedial hypothalamic (VMH) nuclei. Lesions of the VMH areas produce hyperphagia and obesity in adult rats and cats, as do microinjections of barbiturates.

The onset of feeding is brought about by a reduction in negative signals from the satiety center to the appetite center. The appetite center is then free to operate and stimulate food seeking and intake. The end of a meal would be due to an increase in plasma glucose, amino acids, or peptides, hyperthermia, dehydration, or gut fill activating the satiety center to halt the operation of the appetite center.

Theories on Appetite Regulation

Initially, the *glucostatic theory* assumed that the level of excitability to food was related to the blood concentration of glucose, since intravenous infusion of glucose reduces the subjective feeling of hunger in man. Prolonged injection of glucose into animals also reduces food intake; however, appetite has not been reported to be inhibited by parenteral administration of glucose.

The *amino acid balance theory* is supported by a lack of correlation between satiation and the arteriovenous glucosemia difference and by the fact that maximal satiety follows ingestion of protein food or amino acids, even when arteriovenous glucosemia is low. Amino acids are considered as food intake regulators in growing pigs. A homeostatic mechanism would control free amino acid levels in plasma and tissues by reducing the inflow of amino acids from food when plasma amino acid concentrations exceed requirements. When energy-yielding substrates are more available than amino acids to build proteins, as in low-protein diets, food intake is also depressed. Conversely intake of carbohydrate food is lowered when diets are too rich in proteins (Fig. 23–13).

The amino acid balance theory and the glucostatic theory run into considerable difficulties in diabetes mellitus,

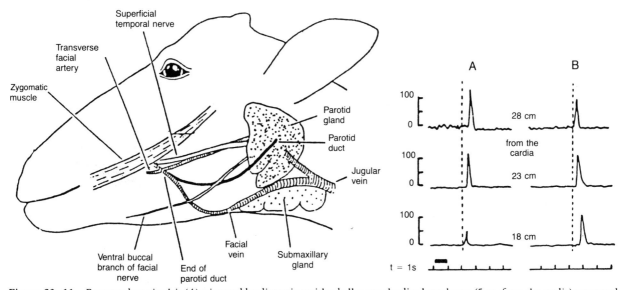

Figure 23–11 Retrograde peristalsis (*A*) triggered by distention with a balloon at the distal esophagus (5 cm from the cardia) compared with normal (aborad) esophageal peristalsis (*B*) caused by deglutition of saliva in a sheep. *Left Panel:* Diagrammatic arrangement of the facial vein, parotid salivary duct, transverse facial artery, and superficial temporal nerve on the lateral subcutaneous surface of the sheep's head.

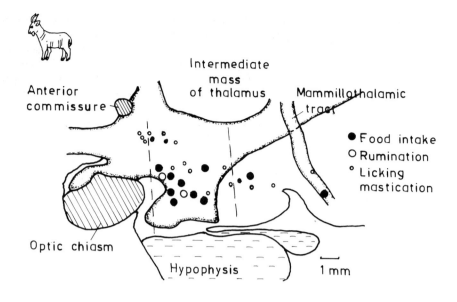

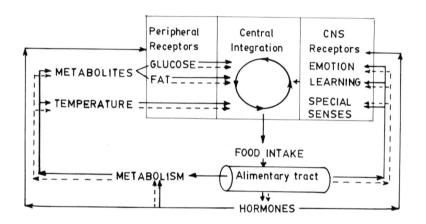

Figure 23-12 Schematic representation of the control systems regulating food intake. Central integration occurs through stimulating (→) or inhibitory (---→) neurotransmitters. Parasagittal section of the hypothalamus showing the lateral hypothalamic nuclei, or feeding center.

during which hyperphagia occurs although the blood levels of amino acids and glucose are very high. On the other hand, in liver disease, appetite and amino acidemia are suppressed.

Gut fill or *rumen fill* is considered to be a regulator of feeding behavior in ruminant species. Short (about 7 mm) indigestible polypropylene fibers placed in the rumen of sheep to increase its volume do not affect ingestive behavior. It should be noted that, because of rumination (and remastication), these particles are recovered in the feces in a more finely ground condition. When longer polypropylene fibers (about 30 mm) are given, food intake is depressed (see Fig. 23–13), but 95 percent of the particles remain unchanged in the rumen after 28 days. The faster rate of passage of particles out of the ruminoreticulum is due to their more rapid breakdown. Grinding and pelleting of a highly digestible roughage are not associated with any major change in the voluntary intake. The grinding and pelleting of straw lead to an increase of about 25 percent in voluntary intake, because of the increased rate of passage out of the ruminoreticulum.

The *thermostatic theory* suggests that food consumption has a certain dependence on the temperature of the body and of the environment. The basis of the thermostatic theory rests on an increase in the hypothalamic temperature during feeding and other activity (which is poorly correlated to cessation of feed intake in goats) and on the fact that heat stress depresses food intake in rabbits.

The *dehydration theory* is founded on the observation that satiation follows dehydration of the digestive tissues and that appetite is stimulated by hydration of the digestive tissues. Ingestion of food and secretion of digestive juices dehydrate the glandular tissues of digestion, which would signal inhibition of food intake. Earlier observations on dogs reported that, during ingestion of food, water passes gradually from the tissues into the digestive juices. Hyperosmolal chyme (digesta from the stomach or gizzard) draws water into the lumen of the small intestine to distend the duodenum and also contributes to digestive tissue dehydration in chickens.

The different theories of appetite regulation should be examined with consideration of the different types of nutrition of herbivores and carnivores. The amino acid balance

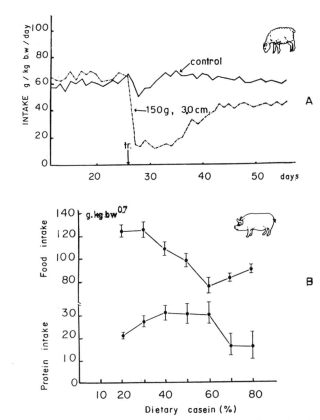

Figure 23–13 Physical and chemical regulation of appetite. **A,** Wethers consume less hay after receiving 150 g of 3-cm polypropylene fibers in the rumen. **B,** Food intake is lower in pigs when protein intake rises from 20 to 30 percent.

theory is hardly applicable to plant-eating animals, nor is the glucose balance theory relevant to predatory animals. Appetite regulation (satiety) may be controlled by certain metabolites. If this occurs, it should be assumed that the control is mediated through cellulose end-products in herbivores and through amino acid homeostasis in carnivores.

Metabolites as Satiety Factors in Ruminants

Short-chain fatty acids (SCFAs) are considered as possible components in a feedback system for the regulation of feed intake in ruminants. Intraruminal administration of acetate or propionate before or during a meal usually depresses feed intake in cattle. In cattle, intravenous infusion of acetate or propionate also reduces feed intake.

In sheep and goats, intravenous, intraduodenal, or intraabomasal infusion of acetate produces variable results. In growing lambs, the abomasal infusion of isocaloric amounts of acetic (44 g per day) and propionic (31 g per day) acids diminishes feed intake, but the abomasal infusion of equivalent amounts of the sodium salts has no effect on feed intake. Abomasal infusion of 0.5 mol acetic, propionic, or hydrochloric acid lowers feed intake with each acid. Reduction of feed intake and aciduria (acid urine) result when the

acid concentration infused into the abomasum is raised to 1.0 mol. SCFAs (acetic, propionic, or half-and-half by weight mixture) added to the feed (5.1 g per 100 g feed) do not change the feed intake. Similarly, when equal amounts of these acids are added as sodium salts, feed intake remains unchanged. It is evident that SCFAs reduce feed intake of lambs only when they are supplied in great excess and in the acid form.

Effect of Frequency of Feeding

Food intake is influenced by the frequency of feeding. In cats, food and water intake are lower when frequent small meals are fed than with a single daily meal. Over a period of 10 days, after adaptation to the schedule of frequent small meals, cats eat 52 g per day and drink 127 mL per day, much less than the 86 g per day and 179 mL per day that are consumed on the single-meal schedule.

Effects of Taste Factors in Ruminant Feed Intake

Cattle have taste receptors on the tongue that respond to the four primary flavors: salty, sweet, sour, and bitter. The strong movements of the tongue during prehension help present the flavors of sapid substances to the gustatory receptors. Ruminants have lower rejection and higher acceptance values toward bitter substances than many other animal species. They also show no satiation for sweet substances, and unlimited intake can occur (e.g., molasses in diets).

The behavioral mechanisms for sodium homeostasis are well developed in cattle. When a single parotid duct of a steer is cannulated, the steady secretion of parotid saliva causes loss of sodium from the body. During development of sodium depletion by loss of saliva, the intake of food and water gradually diminishes, with concurrent hypovolemia, hypoosmolality, and a drop in plasma pH (to 7.2). Eventually, a compensation process develops to reduce salivary flow and to reverse the sodium:potassium ratio in saliva from 145:5 to 5:130 mmol. Continuation of sodium depletion for more than 8 days brings anorexia.

Normal hungry steers trained to press a plate for food rewards find hypertonic solutions of sodium salts to be aversive. Conversely, sodium-depleted cattle will eat even powdered salt and sodium bicarbonate. Motivation for salt increases in animal in a **T** maze with the onset of the sodium deficit. Sodium-deprived steers learn immediately which arm of the **T** maze harbors a sodium reward and thereafter move first to this arm, indicating memory even after an interval of 6 weeks. When sodium-depleted steers are allowed a supplement of sodium, normal sodium metabolism is restored and abnormal salt intake behavior disappears. These results demonstrate that ruminants have a clear specific taste for sodium cations and that the anion is not important. Other metabolic ions (calcium, magnesium, potassium, ammonium) produce poor response to the operant procedure, except lithium chloride and lithium sulfate, which are also very effective.

Endogenous cues regulating long-term feeding activity are probably more complex in cattle than in any other species. The apparently simpler short-term regulating factors are more difficult to assess in ruminants because of the presence of rumination. This specialized act of ingestive behavior is needed for cellulose digestion after optimal fill of the rumen. Ruminants pay for their ability to garner energy from plant material that has a meager content of both sodium and water, which are essential to buffer acid production in the rumen. To compensate, ruminants must produce a large amount of alkaline saliva, which provides the fluid needed for fermentation, buffers the acids of fermentation, and assists in the processes of remastication and reinsalivation during rumination.

Effects of Estrogens on Food Intake

The effects of estrogens on food intake seem quite universal among animal species. Observations after ovariectomy in rats are taken as evidence that estrogens lower feed intake (Fig. 23–14), but experimental results question the notion that estrogens exert an inhibitory role on feed intake. One of the problems is that the female rat cycles continuously throughout the year, with a short estrous cycle of 4 to 5 days. The female rat is subjected to much more estrogenic influence than other species, which cycle only on a seasonal (carnivores) or a monthly (ruminants) basis.

In ruminants, when estrogen secretion increases during estrus, food intake decreases. In adult cows, the administration of estrogens lowers both food intake and body weight. These results are in opposition to the former husbandry practice of giving estrogenic chemical (diethylstilbestrol) in food to increase the growth rate and meat quality of cattle and sheep. In reality, the weight gain–promoting effect of estrogens is manifested only by growing cattle and sheep, because of greater production of adenohypophyseal growth hormone (somatotropic hormone, or STH).

TABLE 23–5 Intake, Rumination, and Retention Times of Food in Early Lactating Cows Fed Two Types of Diets

	Diet A*		Diet B†	
	Before Calving	After Calving	Before Calving	After Calving
Intake (kg DM/day)	12	15	14	19
Eating (hr)	5	8	4	5
Rumination (hr)	9	10	4	6
Mean retention time in gastro-intestinal tract (hr)	68	70	56	46

*Alfalfa hay to concentrate (2:1)
†Pellets (alfalfa, beet pulp, concentrate) + 1.5 kg long hay

Adjustment of Feed Intake with Lactation in Cows

After calving, the cow's needs for energy and protein increase rapidly in parallel with the lactation demands for lipid, protein, and lactose. The mechanisms that increase food (DM) intake to meet the requirements for milk production are poorly understood. Whatever the diet, a deficiency of nutrients (needed for milk synthesis) seems to stimulate the lateral hypothalamus to induce the drive for food seeking. There is no explanation for the delay of 1 to 2 weeks taken by a dairy cow to adjust the level of food intake to meet the needs of milk production. It is possible that the high concentration of blood estrogen near calving is a factor in this higher but still inadequate food intake. After calving, the higher blood level of free fatty acids (FFAs), which are released from adipose tissue for milk fat synthesis, is still below the 300 mEq/L threshold required to inhibit feeding.

The behavioral and digestive mechanical events recorded during the increased food intake following calving are given in Table 23–5. With pelleted food, the rate of passage

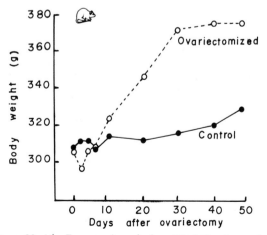

Figure 23–14 Estrogens lower body weight in female rats. Body weight increases after removal of the ovaries (ovariectomy), the main source of estrogens in rats that have unlimited access to food.

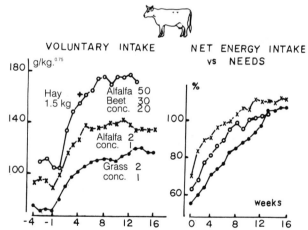

Figure 23–15 Changes in voluntary dry matter intake and percentage of net energy intake in relation to energy needs in lactating cows fed three diets: (A) hay (1.5 kg) plus a mixture of alfalfa, beet pulp, and concentrate; (B) alfalfa plus concentrate (2:1); and (C) grass plus concentrate (2:1). Intake of A is always greater than that of B, which is always greater than that of C. Energy needs match intake after 8 weeks (170 g/weight (kg)$^{0.75}$) with A, after 10 weeks (140 g/kg$^{0.75}$) with B, and after 13 weeks (120 g/kg$^{0.75}$) for C.

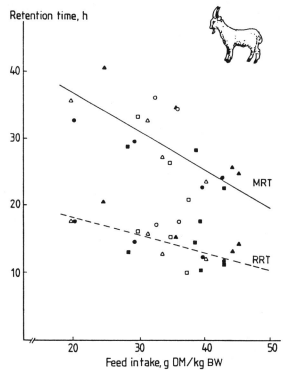

Figure 23–16 Relationship between the level of feed intake (DM/kg) in dairy goats and mean retention times in the ruminoreticulum (RRT) (12 to 18 hours) and in the entire digestive tract (MRT) (25 to 35 hours).

of digesta is faster when the intake is higher, whereas with alfalfa and concentrates, the rate of passage of digesta is slower, and less feed is eaten in a period twice as long. It is recognized that the intake of a mixture of grass hay and concentrate is lower than the same amount of concentrate with alfalfa, which is in turn less well accepted than pelleted foods offered with only 1.5 kg of long hay (Fig. 23–15).

Ruminoreticulum Retention Times

Retention time of feed particles in the ruminoreticulum is a factor of great importance for the utilization of nutrients in the feed and for limiting the level of food intake. Because of the action of rumen microorganisms and the thorough

mastication of the feed, the size of the particles of digesta gradually decreases. In sheep and goats, passage out of the rumen is related to a critical particle size (about 1 to 2 mm). In goats, sheep, and cattle, higher feed intake reduces the retention times of feed particles and of water both in the entire gastrointestinal tract and in the ruminoreticulum (Fig. 23–16). Ad libitum feed intake in ruminants appears ultimately to be controlled mostly by distention of the reticulum and of the proximal part of the rumen.

REFERENCES

Andersson B, Larsson B. Influence of local temperature changes in the preoptic area and rostral hypothalamus on the regulation of food and water intake. Acta Physiol Scand 1961;52:95.

Baile CA. Control of feed intake in ruminants. In: McDonald IW, Warner ACI, eds, Digestion and metabolism in the ruminant. Armidale: University of New England Publishing Unit, 1975.

Bell FR. Aspects of ingestive behavior in cattle. J Anim Sci 1984;59:1369.

Berkovitz KB, Moxham BJ, Newman HN. The periodontal ligament in health and disease. Oxford: Pergamon Press, 1982.

Church DC. The ruminant animal. Englewood Cliffs, NJ: Simon & Schuster 1988.

Davis DD. Notes on the anatomy of babirusa. Zoology 1940;22:363.

Finco DR, Adams DD, Crowell WA, Stattelman AJ, Brown SA, Marsanti JA. Food and water intake and urine composition in cats: influence of continuous versus periodic feeding. Am J Vet Res 1986;47:1638.

Forbes JB. The voluntary food intake of farm animals. London: Butterworths, 1986.

Gans C, Devre E, Gorniam GC. Analysis of mammalian masticatory behavior: progress and problems. Ztbl Vet Med C 1978;7:226.

Hecker JF. Experimental surgery on small ruminants. London: Butterworths, 1974.

Hofmann RR. Anatomical adaptations of the ruminant digestive system. In: Dobson A, Dobson MJ, eds. Aspects of digestive physiology in ruminants. Ithaca, NY: Comstock Publishing Assoc., 1988.

Journet M, Remond B. Physiological factors affecting the voluntary intake of feed by cows: a review. Livestock Prod Sci 1976;3:129.

Larsson S. On the hypothalamic organization of the nervous mechanism regulating food intake. Acta Physiol Scand 1954;32(Suppl. 115):1.

Lindberg JE. Retention times of small feed particles and of water in the gut of dairy goats fed at different levels of intake. J Anim Physiol Anim Nutr 1988;59:173.

Martin-Rosset W, Doreau M, Cloix J. Etude des activités d'un troupeau de poulinières de trait et leurs poulains au paturage. Ann Zootech 1978;27:33.

Papas A, Hatfield EE. The effect of oral and abomasal administration of volatile fatty acids on voluntary intake of growing lambs. J Anim Sci 1978;46:288.

Pond KR, Ellis WC, Akin DE. Ingestive mastication and fragmentation of forages. J Anim Sci 1984; 58:1567.

CHAPTER 24

GASTROINTESTINAL MOTILITY

This chapter is concerned with the motility of the stomach, pylorus, small intestine, and large intestine.

The *stomach* receives and stores food, mixes it with gastric secretions, and meters delivery of the mixture (chyme) to the duodenum. As a motor unit, the stomach has three functional areas: a proximal fundus, a central body, or corpus, and a distal antrum. The antrum contributes to mixing of the gastric contents and acts as a pump to deliver them, as chyme, to the duodenum.

The *pylorus,* a low-pressure muscular sphincter, has little or no role in regulating gastric emptying of liquids. The important function of the pylorus is to prevent the entrance into the duodenum of large food particles. Another function is to hinder gastric reflux of bile, which in dogs and pigs is delivered close to the pylorus.

The *small intestine* extends from the pylorus to the proximal end of the large intestine. In dogs, it is about 4 m long when it is fully relaxed, and its motor function is essential for the absorption of the nutrients and the simple molecules resulting from digestion of foods. Once these substances are absorbed into the blood, they are obligatorily directed to the liver.

The *large intestine* has several major functions: absorption of electrolytes and water from the luminal contents, postgastric fermentation of polysaccharides in monogastric (unilocular-stomach) herbivores, and storage and periodic expulsion of residue material (feces).

GASTROINTESTINAL MOTILITY AND THE SMOOTH MUSCLE LAYERS

The musculature of the alimentary canal consists of two layers of smooth muscle, an outer one of continuous longitudinal fibers and an inner one of circular fibers. The inner circular layer is thickened at the pylorus to form the *pyloric sphincter* and also between the small and large intestine to form the *ileocecal sphincter.* A network of interconnecting nerve fibers and ganglion cells is present between the two smooth muscle layers (*myenteric plexus*) and in the submucosa (*submucosal plexus*).

In vitro, with a 2- to 3-cm segment or strip of small intestine in a temperature-regulated water bath containing glucose, oxygen, and ions, the movements (called *pendular movements* in the rabbit) of the outer longitudinal layer can be recorded. They can also be altered by drugs (e.g., inhibition by epinephrine, enhancement by acetylcholine) (Fig. 24–1).

In vivo, when the lumen is distended by fluid, the movements of the muscular layers are coordinated by the intrinsic myenteric and submucosal plexuses. Contractions of the inner circular layer result in a stricture of the lumen, with division of its contents. These local contractions (called *segmental contractions*) occur in a series, at a frequency of about 10 to 15 per minute, to cause local mixing of the contents. The coordinated action of both layers of smooth muscle results in aboral propulsion of the digesta. This occurs because of the local contraction of the inner circular muscular layer, which moves along the intestine behind a dilation in the lumen associated with an action on the outer longitudinal muscular layer. The onward propulsion of contents is a motor activity called *peristalsis.*

Peristaltic activity is caused by an increase in pressure that stimulates sensory nerve endings, either directly by activating stretch receptors or indirectly by releasing chemical mediators. The stimulated sensory nerves reflexly excite efferent nerve fibers contained in the intrinsic plexuses. Peristalsis is abolished by removing the mucosa and is disrupted by drugs that act at various points on the reflex pathways. For example, peristalsis ceases with blockade of nerve conduction in the submucosal plexuses by local anesthetics or of ganglionic transmission at the myenteric plexuses.

MOTILITY OF THE STOMACH

The fundus of the stomach is chemically important for hydrogen cation secretion. Mechanically, the stomach relaxes at the time of eating to accommodate food without raising the intragastric pressure (Fig. 24–2), and it also prevents immediate aboral propulsion of entering food. The fundus of the stomach does not show electrical or electromyographic smooth muscle activity with either mucosal or serosal electrodes.

Electromyographical Activity

Electromyographic activity, which is present only in the mid-corpus and antrum of the stomach, consists of electrical potentials generated in the mid-corpus that spread over the body and the antrum in the direction of the pylorus. The potentials appear regularly and may or may not be associated with motor activity. The low potentials, which are not coincident with circular smooth muscle contractions, are called *slow waves* (SWs), or *electrical control activity* (ECA). The wider potentials, which coincide with motor activity of the inner circular smooth muscle fibers, are called *spike potentials* (SPs), or *electrical response activity* (ERA).

SW, or ECA, is an omnipresent gastric event occurring constantly at a frequency of 5 cycles per minute in the dog.

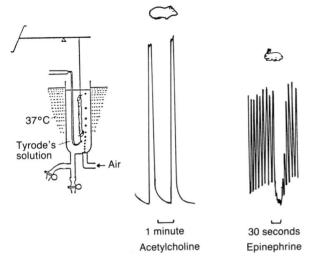

37°C

Tyrode's
solution

← Air

1 minute
Acetylcholine

30 seconds
Epinephrine

Figure 24–1 Typical record of spontaneous repeated contractions (pendular movements) in vitro of rabbit jejunum and of the extensive inhibitions produced by addition of epinephrine (1 μg) to the reactive bath. In contrast, guinea pig ileum does not show spontaneous repeated contractions, but single ones can be induced by adding acetylcholine (1 μg) or histamine, serotonin, or prostaglandins.

Whether or not the corpus and antrum contract with each wave of the cycle depends on a second electrical event, the SP, or ERA. This explains why the number of corpus and antral contractions does not always correspond to the number of SW potentials generated from the pacemaker in the middle of the corpus every 12 seconds.

Antral Pump

The *antrum* and the *pylorus* are the discriminating sieving mechanisms that separate solids from liquids and allow solids to be retained in the stomach longer than liquids. The sequence of terminal antral contractions (see Fig. 24–2) is related to the sieving and grinding actions of the antrum. Larger gastric particles remain in the stomach, suspended in a liquid peripheral to the moving central stream of smaller particles, which are propelled through the pylorus. As the pylorus closes, these larger particles are suddenly tumbled by reversal of the flow (retropulsion) of the fluid in which they are suspended. The stir developed by the sudden reversal of velocity breaks apart the larger particles.

In beagle dogs, digestible foods are broken down to particles of approximately 1 mm in diameter before they are emptied from the stomach. With nondisintegrating particles larger than 5 mm, the postfeeding gastric residence time is about 7.5 hours.

Gastric Emptying

The fluid material that leaves the stomach and enters the duodenum is called *chyme*. Gastric emptying is influenced by the volume and composition of the meal (the nutritive density) (Kcal/mL). In theory, the rate of gastric emptying is equally slowed by isocaloric amounts of fat, protein, and carbohydrate. In fact, dietary fats leave the stomach very slowly because they trigger a negative feedback mechanism that affects not only the proximal part of the intestine but also the rest of the intestine.

The inhibitory control of gastric emptying begins in the duodenum, with involvement of regulatory receptors specific for osmolality, acidity, fats, and the amino acid tryptophan. Gastric emptying of glucose can be described as a closed-loop system in which the duodenum inhibits gastric emptying. As the gastric antrum contracts, it empties into the duodenum an amount of glucose that supplies a species-specific quantity of calories, which produces a corresponding time-specific inhibition of gastric emptying. Once the inhibitory effects cease, antral contractions once more deliver into the duodenum another batch of calories, which again inhibit gastric emptying. For test meals of glucose (4 Kcal/g) containing 7, 15, and 25 g/dL, respectively, the rate of calorie delivery to the duodenum by the stomach is 1.05, 1.16, and 1.10 Kcal per minute (Fig. 24–3).

MOTILITY OF THE PYLORUS

Closure of the pyloric sphincter narrows the lumen of the gastroduodenal junction, causes less fluid to enter the duodenum, and slows gastric emptying. This contraction of the thickened inner circular layer at the pylorus is tonic in nature compared with the advancing antral contraction.

Since 1930, it has been recognized that artificially holding the pylorus open does not change the rate of gastric emptying; however, some findings question this concept, since human pyloric myotomy accelerates gastric emptying of liquids after vagal denervation of the stomach, and canine pyloric myotomy or pylorectomy also increases gastric emptying. Contraction of the pylorus occurs with splanchnic nerve stimulation, whereas alpha-adrenergic blockers relax the contracted pylorus. The pyloric sphincter is not inhibited by atropine.

The transpyloric flow of chyme represents a volume about equal to that of the meal (Fig. 24–4). The material crossing from the stomach into the duodenum is composed of small particles of food matter suspended in gastric juice. Transpyloric flow is increased by intraarterial naloxone, which suggests that vagal excitation of the pylorus could be mediated by enkephalin-containing nerves, and by vasoactive intestinal peptide (VIP), a gastrointestinal hormone that may also mediate vagal inhibition.

Vomiting

In most animals except horses, vomiting is a protective reflex to disgorge ingested contents from the stomach (and sometimes from the duodenum) through the mouth. The purpose of vomiting is to relieve gastric overdistention or to

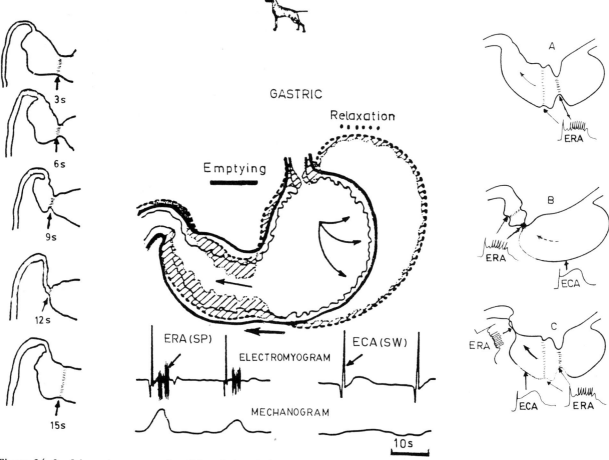

Figure 24–2 Schematic representation of the relationship between canine gastric action potentials and contractions before and during ingestion and digestion. **Right,** Before ingestion of food, slow waves (*SW*) or electromyographic control activity (*ECA*) move at 12-second intervals from mid-corpus (**A**), toward antrum (**B**), without any mechanical activity. Gastric contractions occur when spike potentials (*SP*) or electromyographic response activity (*ERA*) are superimposed on each slow wave (**C**). **Center,** Feeding is accompanied by gastric relaxation to prevent an increase in intragastric pressure. Gastric emptying is associated with SP. **Left,** Propulsion of gastric contents is visualized at 3-second intervals.

expel noxious or undesirable ingesta from the gastric reservoir.

In ruminants, the process of vomiting is rare and impractical, since rumination includes a phase of regurgitation, which brings material from the large forestomach system into the mouth. Acidic abomasal contents may be regurgitated into the forestomachs. Horses do not vomit, except *in extremis,* with rupture of the stomach, as they seem to lack the necessary mechanism to relax the lower esophageal sphincter. Pigs vomit readily, but the physiology of the process has not been studied. In dogs and cats, vomiting is a well-developed reflex that is clinically very important.

The vomiting reflex is heralded by nausea, a sensation of gastric discomfort or malaise with disgust for food, and also by salivation, tachygastria, and hypotension. It is controlled by a vomiting center located in the medulla oblongata near the tractus solitarius and the dorsal motor nucleus of the vagus nerve. The vomiting center responds to autonomic input and to input from a dorsal bilateral chemoreceptor

trigger zone (CTZ) situated in close proximity (in the area of the postrema) near the floor of the fourth ventricle of the medulla.

The afferent arm of the vomiting reflex carries signals from autonomic afferent fibers and input from the vestibular nuclei (via the cerebellum and the CTZ). Irritant substances entering the stomach, digestive disturbances such as "overeating syndrome" on concentrated diets, obstructive objects in the pharynx and upper esophagus (choke), and pain from renal calculi stimulate the medullary vomiting center. The CTZ receives signals from higher nerve centers when the animal is experiencing strong emotion; after brain trauma; and from the vestibular system (e.g., vagal inputs, motion sickness, and certain systemic diseases or intoxications). Since the CTZ appears to lack the normal blood-brain barrier, it responds to certain chemicals (e.g., apomorphine, morphine, xylazine, cytotoxic drugs, digitalis, ergot extracts, veratrum alkaloids). The CTZ is also activated by afferent signals from the gut (e.g., copper sulfate) as well as

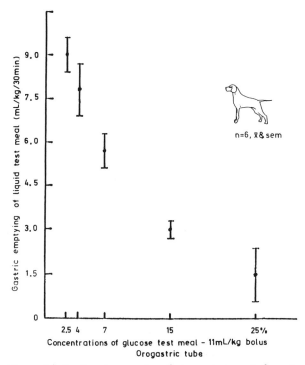

Figure 24–3 Gastric emptying of glucose test meals from the canine stomach following administration by orogastric tube of a standard fluid volume (11 mL/kg) containing hypotonic (2.5 and 4 percent) and hypertonic (7, 15, and 25 percent) glucose concentrations. The rate of gastric emptying decreases as osmolality increases.

5-hydroxytryptamine (5-HT, or serotonin) and peptides from enterochromaffin cells.

The emetic reflexes are still incompletely understood. Cells of the CTZ synapse with many gamma-aminobutyric acid (GABA) receptors, which can be partially blocked by some tranquilizing drugs. The effector neurons of the CTZ respond to dopamine, which is released from other neurons by apomorphine, whereas its release is prevented by metoclopramide.

The latency in the emetic action of some cytotoxic drugs implies that their molecules must undergo hepatic processing to gain the emetic effect. Severe emesis induced by either cytotoxic drugs or radiation is prevented by 5-HT₃–receptor antagonists. These agents are effective against a variety of anticancer therapies in the ferret. Their site of action may be the visceral afferent neurons of the gut.

The efferent arm of the vomiting reflex coordinates the complex muscular contractions and relaxations needed to produce successful retrograde evacuation of the stomach contents. It operates through several nerve pathways (cranial nerves V, VII, IX, X, and XII).

When gastric irritation or distention is the primary stimulus, an episode of unproductive retching may precede vomiting. In *retching,* gastric contents enter the esophagus but not the pharynx. Retroperistalsis initiated in the duodenum leads to increased electrical spiking activity in the duodenum and the stomach (Fig. 24–5). Simultaneously, the gastric cardiac area and the lower esophageal sphincter relax, and inspiratory movements create a more negative intrathoracic pressure, which facilitates reflux of gastric contents into the thoracic esophagus. During *vomiting,* the upper esophageal sphincter relaxes, the glottis closes to protect the lungs, the soft palate is elevated to protect the nasal cavities, and projectile expulsion of the vomitus occurs through the mouth under the pressure of the contracting abdominal muscles. Vomiting may continue for as long as the triggering stimulus persists, but it usually ends after the stomach is empty.

Chronic vomiting may lead to metabolic alkalosis due to loss of chloride and hydrogen ions, when the fluids lost are mainly of gastric origin. A more paradoxical metabolic acidosis occurs when intestinal retroperistalsis causes vomiting of alkaline fluids (bile, duodenal juice, and pancreatic juice) from the small intestine.

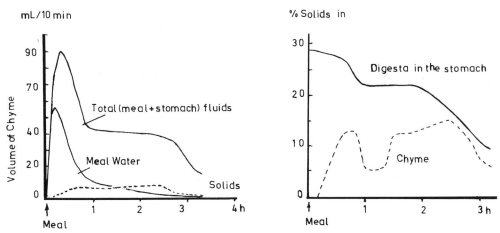

Figure 24–4 Postprandial gastric emptying within the 3 hours following ingestion of a mixed (solids and liquids) meal in the dog. The proportion of solids decreases from 30 to 10 percent because of pyloric discrimination between solids and liquids and also because of the progressive reduction of the solids to smaller particles.

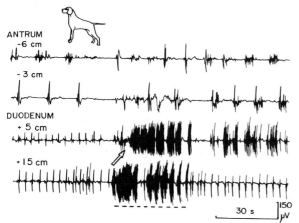

Figure 24–5 Antiperistalsis of the duodenum preceding vomiting in the dog. The arrow indicates the ejection of duodenal contents following antral inhibition and retrograde duodenal contractions, which explains the presence of bile-stained intestinal contents in the vomitus.

MOTILITY OF THE SMALL INTESTINE

The small intestine is the site of two types of motility: repeated, localized, and alternating narrowings of the lumen, called *rhythmic segmentation,* and propagation of a ring of contraction over some distance, called *peristalsis.* Rhythmic segmentation helps mix the chyme with the intestinal and other digestive (pancreatic juice, bile) secretions and in-

creases the contact of nutrients with absorptive mucosal surfaces. Peristalsis is mainly for propulsion.

Interdigestive Motility

In dogs that have fasted over 12 hours, the interdigestive small intestinal motility is organized in cycles of successive periods of inactivity and of irregular and regular motor activity. Each cycle starts at the stomach and moves distally, with a gradual reduction in the rate of electromyographical slow waves (18 per minute at the duodenum, 15 per minute at the ileum) (Fig. 24–6). The purpose of these irregular and regular contraction phases may be to cleanse the gastrointestinal tract of undigested materials, inspissated secretions, desquamated cells, and bacteria before the next meal.

Long-term analyses correlate interdigestive small intestine motility and electrical activity of the smooth muscles. From the electromyographical results, it is evident that interdigestive small intestinal motility is the result of a succession of cycles, or complexes, called *interdigestive myoelectrical complexes* (IDMCs) or *migrating myoelectrical complexes* (MMCs), that repeat every 90 to 120 minutes. These IDMCs, or MMCs, include three forms or patterns of motor activity: inactivity, a mixture of peristalsis and rhythmic segmentation, and rhythmic segmentation alone. In electromyographical parlance, the patterns, or phases, of the MMC are termed: *quiescence, or no spiking activity* (NSA), also known as phase I, or slow waves (SW); *irregular spiking activity* (ISA), a mixture of quiescence and spiking activity also known as

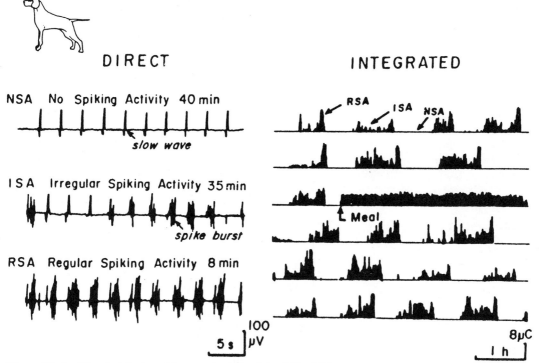

Figure 24–6 Electrical rhythm without mechanical activity (*SW* or *NSA*) in the canine duodenum and electrical rhythm where spike bursts are superimposed irregularly (*ISA*) or regularly (*RSA*) to coincide with mechanical activity of the duodenum. ISBs occur almost continuously during the 3 to 6 hours after a meal.

TABLE 24–1 Terms and Synonyms Used in Smooth Muscle Electromyography of the Stomach and Small Intestine

Electrical activity without motor activity (electrical control activity [ECA])
  Nonspiking activity (NSA): Slow wave (SW); quiescence; phase I
Electrical activity with motor activity (electrical response activity [ERA])
  Irregular spiking activity (ISA): phase II
  Regular spiking activity (RSA): phase III

phase II; and *regular spiking activity* (RSA), pure spiking activity also known as phase III (Table 24–1). The relative duration of each phase of an MMC is usually as follows: NSA, 20 percent; ISA, 75 percent; and RSA, 5 percent.

Effect of Feeding

In dogs, a meal abolishes the NSA and RSA phases of the MMC, so the motor activity becomes continuous ISA. This is interpreted as a disruption of the appearance of the phases of the MMCs at the level of the gastroduodenal junction.

In pigs, when the meal is divided into several very small portions (snacks), eating does not disrupt the appearance of the phases of the MMCs but only alters the duration of the initial ISA phase, which is prolonged and postpones the subsequent NSA phase (Fig. 24–7). In contrast to the situation in monogastric animals, it is noteworthy that in adult ruminants, the phases of the MMCs are always present and are not disturbed by feeding or delivery of abomasal contents into the duodenum.

Propulsion of Chyme

During the RSA phase of the small intestinal motility cycle, segmentation-like contractions propagate slowly along the gut at a velocity proportional to the length of the small intestine (Fig. 24–8). This motility pattern causes mixing within the intestinal lumen and greater contact and renewal of chyme with the brush border enzymes of the small intestinal mucosa. It also retards the passage of chyme and acts as a barrier against retrograde flow of chyme during the peristaltic contractions that characterize ISA activity. The peristaltic movements of the ISA phase are more efficient (and do not cause retrograde flow of chyme) when they begin aborad to a place on the gut previously narrowed by a phase of RSA activity.

Comparative Aspects of Small Intestinal Propulsion of Chyme

In mammals, the entire spiking activity is regulated by slow waves, whose frequency decreases as they move aborally from the upper to the lower small intestine. The decreasing frequency of slow waves and superimposed spike bursts are responsible for the aborad propulsion of chyme.

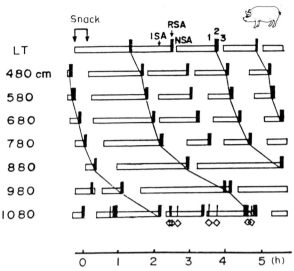

Figure 24–7 Aborad propagation of migrating myoelectrical complexes (MMCs, integrated analyses) along the distal small intestine of a pig. The eight sets of electrodes are placed on the serosa from the union of the duodenum and jejunum (ligament of Treitz, *LT*). The phases of the MMC are represented diagrammatically: ISA, or phase II (*1*); RSA, or phase III (*2*), and NSA, or phase I (*3*). Note that a snack fails to disrupt the MMC.

In birds, no comparable regulatory factor for propulsion of chyme exists in the upper part of the small intestine. Retroperistalsis, or aborad-orad motor patterns, are similar to those of emesis (Fig. 24–9).

The digestive transit of food ingested by birds is the result of two opposite forces: the stomach (gizzard) motility acts against the small intestinal retroperistalsis. When retroperistalsis ceases, aborad progression of digesta can occur. Compared with turkeys, chickens have a lower frequency of gastric contractions and a higher frequency of duodenal slow waves. The two species are similar in that intestinal slow waves do not have a characteristic wave form, and spike bursts occur at random at any point in the slow wave. This may mean that there is no true peristalsis toward the ileum.

The motor activity of the gizzard against the duodenum is strongly enhanced by vagal activity. At night, as a consequence of lower vagal tone, there is less gastric activity but more retroperistalsis. After vagotomy (Fig. 24–10), gizzard activity is lower, the intense duodenal activity is almost continuous, and the diurnal variations disappear.

Pathophysiology

The MMC pattern appears to be a complex and fragile organization. Like a sudden increase in the volume of intestinal contents, different pathological situations lead step by step to disruption of the daily MMC pattern.

The postprandial MMC pattern in dogs (the duodenal inflow of chyme in dogs increases threefold after feeding) resembles the MMC disruption elicited by experimentally doubling (500 mL per hour instead of 250 mL per hour, administered through a duodenal cannula) the duodenal

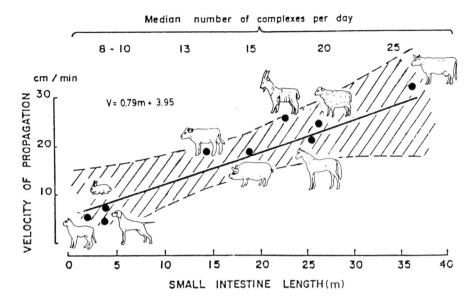

Figure 24–8 Relationship between the velocity of propagation of the RSA phases of the MMC and the length of the small intestine. The median daily number of jejunal complexes is higher in ruminants than in carnivores because of the MMC-disrupting effect of feeding in carnivores. The hatched area refers to 95 percent confidence limits.

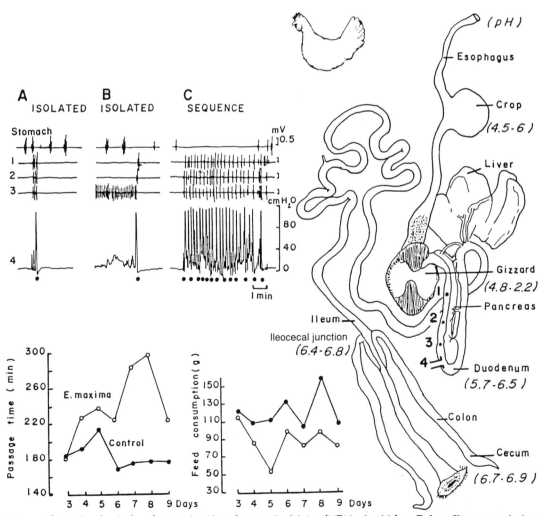

Figure 24–9 Duodenal (aborad) peristalsis (**A**) and retroperistalsis (orad) (**B**) in the chicken. **Below,** Shorter transit time at the level of the gizzard and lower feed consumption in a chicken infected by *Eimeria maxima*. **Right,** Note the range of pH values in the gizzard.

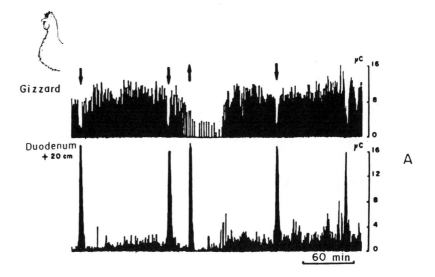

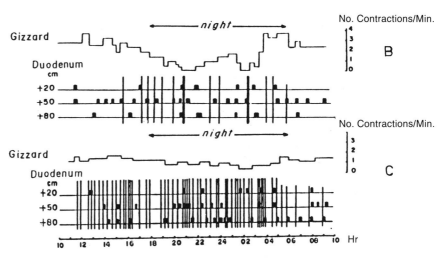

Figure 24–10 **A,** Low-speed recording of the motility of the gizzard and duodenum in the chicken. The gizzard is inhibited at the onset of a period of strong duodenal contractions (μC), and the activity of the gizzard is stopped at the occurrence of retroperistalsis on the duodenum (μC). **B,** Reduced gizzard and increased duodenal motor activities at night. **C,** After vagotomy, the activity of the gizzard is reduced and without diurnal variations, whereas the duodenal motor activity is strongly enhanced. In **B** and **C,** vertical bars represent peristalsis or retroperistalsis (*thicker bar*); squares represent local activity.

content of chyme in sheep. When food intake is increased thus, all MMCs reach the ileum, and supernumerary MMCs start in the jejunum, causing an increase in the total number of MMCs. Nevertheless, beyond an upper limit of MMCs, disorganization occurs and repetitive groups of spikes invade the entire small intestine. Such events occur in species as different as dogs, pigs, and sheep (experimentally).

Pathological disorders associated with an excessive flow of chyme into the lumen of the small intestine induce disorganization of the MMC pattern. Examples include gastric ulcer in rats and dogs, nutritional diarrhea secondary to eating heated soybean flour, helminthiases, infectious diseases, and electrolyte disorders. In man and animals, the integrity of the MMC pattern may be considered an indicator of good health.

Ileus is a persistent lack of tone and motor activity (contractions) of the smooth muscle, usually of the small intestine. It is probably triggered by noxious stimuli impinging on the neurons of the enteric nervous system. Precipitating factors may include allergy or chemical toxicity, bowel infection or peritonitis, extreme pain or trauma, and

surgery. Ileus is often accompanied by the hazardous sequela of gaseous distention.

THE ILEOCECAL SPHINCTER

The ileocecal, or ileocolic, sphincter is thought to control transit of contents between the small and large intestine. It regulates the flow of digesta from ileum to cecum and prevents retrograde flow. Ileal stimulation reflexly relaxes the ileocecal sphincter. Isoprenaline, a beta-adrenergic receptor agonist, also causes its relaxation and indicates the presence of inhibitory beta-adrenergic receptors.

Colonic stimulation contracts the ileocecal sphincter. Stimulation of the distal end of the splanchnic nerves causes sphincter contraction and relaxes the surrounding intestine. In the cat these responses are mimicked by phenylephrine, both in vivo and in vitro, which suggests an alpha-adrenergic stimulatory mechanism (Fig. 24–11).

The comparison of the ileocecal sphincter with the pyloric sphincter suggests that an excitatory alpha-adrenergic receptor would be present at both sphincters. In

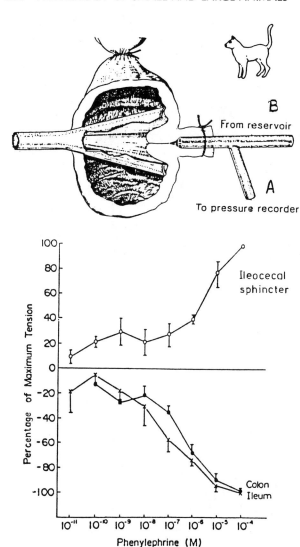

Figure 24–11 Schematic illustration of the ileocecal sphincter in the cat, with recording of transsphincteric flow. The pressure necessary to induce flow through the closed ileocecal sphincter is measured from a small side branch to the perfusion tube (A). The pressure is recorded continuously as the reservoir (B) is raised to find the column height at which the saline just starts to flow through the ileocecal sphincter (i.e., the opening pressure).

contrast to the pylorus, the ileocecal sphincter does not respond to the gastrointestinal hormones (secretin, gastrin, cholecystokinin) or to glucagon, but it is minimally affected by the calcium chelator ethylenediaminetetraacetic acid (EDTA).

MOTILITY OF THE LARGE INTESTINE

The mixing and storage functions of the colon are linked to specific patterns of motility, especially in animals that are hind-gut (postgastric) fermenters (horses, rabbits, pigs).

The simplest form of colon is a uniform tube—2 cm

long in ferrets, 15 cm in rats, 30 cm in dogs (Fig. 24–12). Sacculations of the cecum and the colon are developed in horses, rabbits, and pigs. Functional particularities responsible for pellet formation operate in small ruminants, rabbits, and rats.

Motility of Canine Colon

Displacement of the contents in the canine colon is related to the propagation of powerful contractions. Electromyographically, these contractions correspond to *isolated spike bursts* (ISPs) and *grouped spike bursts* (GSB). The ISBs, of long duration (lasting longer than 5 seconds), are propagated either orad or aborad for a short distance. GSBs, of short duration (lasting less than 5 seconds), occur during periods of activity lasting about 5 minutes and are repeated at 20- to 30-minute intervals. These GSBs occupy 6 to 25 percent of the recording time, migrate slowly from the proximal to the distal colon, and are termed *migrating spike bursts* (MSBs) (Fig. 24–13). They are probably equivalent to the "rhythmic pulsations and tone changes" described 5 decades ago.

Motility of Pig Sacculated Colon

In 1 day the cecum and ascending (spiral) colon of the pig exhibit about 1,400 ISBs of long duration, which are propagated in either direction and occupy 16 percent of the recording time. A similar percentage of GSBs of short duration occur as MSBs.

The role of ISBs of long duration is demonstrated by feeding a high-residue diet (e.g., dried food rich in cereals for dogs, or rich in cellulose for pigs), which causes the number of ISBs of long duration to decrease though the volume of the stool may be doubled. In fact, the faster propulsion of the high-residue digesta by the ISBs of long duration is due to the absence or disappearance of retrograde peristalsis, or orad ISBs. The decrease in colonic motility observed after addition of fiber supports the use of bulking agents for the treatment of constipation and of irritable colon syndrome, a disease associated with an increase in colonic contractile activity.

Motility of Rabbit Cecocolon

For the formation of either soft or hard feces, the rabbit is provided with special large intestinal motility, which is controlled by a mid-colonic pacemaker area. This site, at the origin of antiperistaltic waves of contractions directed toward the cecum, is also involved in the physical separation of liquid and solid digesta delivered by the cecum.

When pellets or hard feces are formed, the role of the thick-walled spindle-shaped fusus coli, located between the proximal haustrated and distal undifferentiated colon, is regulated by endogenous prostaglandins (Fig. 24–14).

Soft feces, usually produced in the morning, are immediately consumed by rabbits (*cecotrophy*) to replenish the

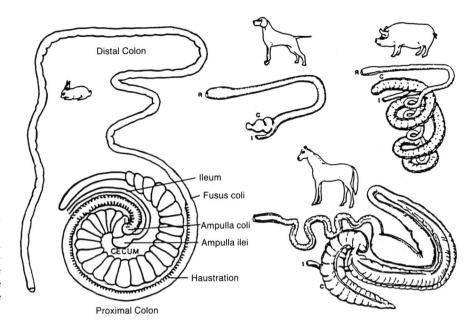

Figure 24-12 Gross morphologic variations in the mammalian colon (*I*, ileum; *C*, cecum; *R*, rectum). In most carnivores, the colon is a uniform tube without sacculations. In the other species, variable degrees of sacculations occur at the cecum and at the rostrad end of the colon.

gastrointestinal flora and provide amino acids and vitamins. These soft feces appear at the anus because of inhibition of the motility of the proximal colon and hyperactivity of the distal colon. This arrangement causes digesta from the cecum to reach the rectum rapidly.

Motility of Horse Large Intestine

In horses, the large intestine is highly responsive to changes in the volume of intraluminal contents. When the volume of cecal contents is doubled, the contractile activity of the cecum and proximal colon is increased eightfold, and the rate of passage of digesta fourfold.

In the large intestine of the horse, extensive digesta retention and fermentation occur in the cecum and in the right ventral (RVC) and left ventral (LVC) segments of the proximal colon. Infusion of short-chain volatile fatty acids

(SCVFAs) into the cecum or colon increases the localized motor activity (ISBs). The degree of fullness is the principal factor in the development of propagated activity (GSBs).

The higher intraluminal pressure of the equine colon following the first hour of feeding is probably related to both chemical stimulation of the wall and its distention, mostly at the level of the LVC. These changes in pressure and in the basal tone of the colon may be recorded by means of strain-gauge transducers (Fig. 24-15).

Motility of Rat Cecocolon

Pellet formation occurs in the large intestine of the rat as a progressive enhancement of segmenting contractions (ISBs). It is organized as a cyclical pattern of activity, with spike bursts of short duration interrupted by a short quiescence every 8 to 12 minutes (Fig. 24-16). Three to four

Figure 24-13 Myoelectrical and contractile activities of the canine colon recorded from bipolar electrodes attached at 3-cm intervals to the serosal surface of the transverse colon. The distally moving pattern of electrical spikings on all four electrodes, the MSBs, is associated with slow aboral progression of intestinal contents.

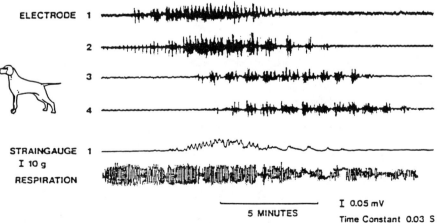

ELECTRODE 1
2
3
4

STRAINGAUGE 1
I 10 g
RESPIRATION

5 MINUTES I 0.05 mV
Time Constant 0.03 S

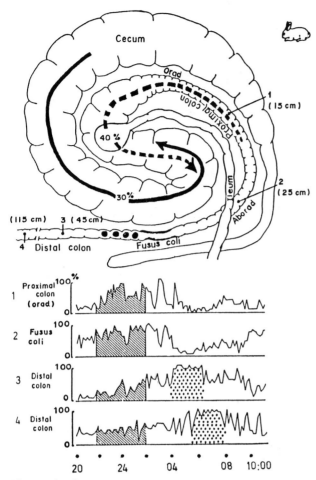

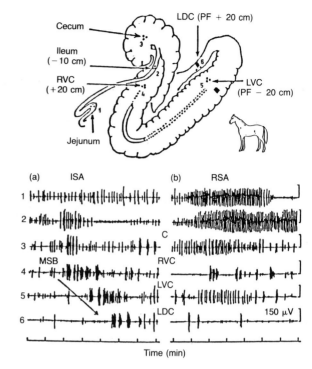

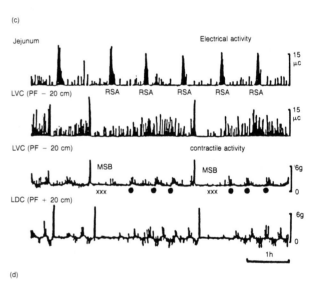

Figure 24–14 Diagram showing the emptying contractions (*arrow*) from apex to base of the rabbit cecum, which account for 30 percent of all cecal motor acitivities. On the proximal colon, about 40 percent of contractions are orad (retroperistalsis), across the ampulla (*dashed arrow*). After a meal accompanied by a period of hyperactivity (*hatched area*), the production of cecotrophs corresponds to inhibition of proximal colon motility and hyperkinesia of the distal colon (*dotted area*).

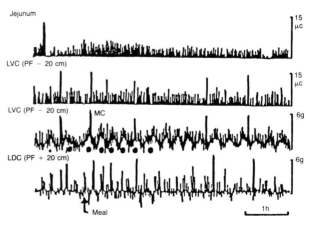

Figure 24–15 Equine large intestine showing the electrode sites (electrical activity) on the jejunum (*1*), ileum (*2*), cecum (*3*), right ventral colon (*RVC, 4*), left ventral colon (*LVC, 5*), and left dorsal colon (*LDC, 6*). Strain-gauge transducers are fixed, near sites 5 and 6, 20 cm proximal and distal to the pelvic flexure (*PF*) to record contractile activity. **A,** Electrical activity: ISA on the small intestine, and MSB passing from the cecum to the LDC. **B,** RSA on the jejunum and ileum, and ISB on the RVC, LVC, and LDC. **C,** In a fasting pony, integrated EMG activity (summed up at 20-second intervals) showing the regular occurrence of MMCs on the jejunum, and a few MSBs on the LVC coinciding with cyclical variations in muscle tone (*xxx,* absence; ●, presence). **D,** Feeding disorganizes the MMC (without NSA and RSA) on the jejunum; MSBs on the LVC coincide with more frequent changes in muscle tone.

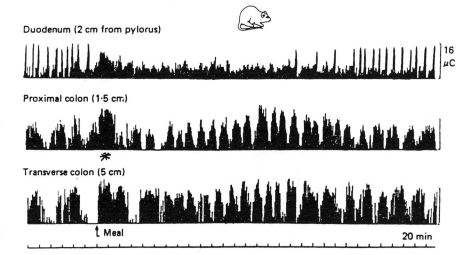

Duodenum (2 cm from pylorus)

16
μC

Proximal colon (1·5 cm)

Transverse colon (5 cm)

↑ Meal

20 min

Figure 24–16 Feeding of a rat: comparative motor response of small and large intestine spiking activity. The 5- to 7-hour disruption of the MMCs of the duodenum is preceded by a phase of hyperactivity lasting 35 to 40 minutes on the colon (*) and followed by the enhancement of the cyclical activity of the proximal and transverse colon.

hours after a meal, this pattern is increased in frequency and magnitude (GSB) as part of the gastrocolic reflex (colonic phase).

Response of Cecocolon to Eating

The term "gastrocolic reflex" is used because the chief stimulus is the entry of food into the empty stomach. Although this term has wide application, it is not appropriate to describe the increased colonic activity that occurs with eating. In neonates, sucking is usually accompanied by defecation for three reasons: the response is hormonal and is not clearly established to be neural; the stimulus originates not only in the stomach but also in the small and large intestines; and the response involves the colon and the cecum.

The cecum of the rabbit responds to eating with an increase in the frequency and the amplitude of the pressure changes or the contractions. The amplitude of the contractions may double, but the frequency increases by only 10 to 25 percent.

The colon of the rabbit is stimulated by the presentation of food. This raises the possibility of a "cephalic phase" to the gastrocolic reflex. In the dog, within 10 minutes ingestion of food causes a "gastric phase" of the reflex, which persists for longer than an hour. However, since simple gastric distention does not excite a colonic response, the stimulus is not simply gastric. This fact would suggest that there is an "intestinal phase" to the gastrocolic reflex. After the initial phase of hyperactivity, there is another one, suggesting that the entry of chyme into the colon itself is involved and that a "colonic phase" of the gastrocolic reflex exists.

The response of the colon to eating is thought to be mediated by excitatory cholinergic nerves. Adrenergic mechanisms in the perivascular nerves would also be involved. The mechanism would be stimulation of excitatory alpha-adrenergic receptors, so that the excitatory response of the colon to eating would be "deinhibition," or transient suspension of tonic neurogenic inhibition.

Flatus and Defecation

Flatus is the anal expulsion of colonic gas, which is composed mainly of nitrogen and carbon dioxide, with some methane and malodorous sulfur-containing gases. Defecation, the passage of feces through the anus, is a reflex response to distention of the rectum. A part of the reflex involves afferent and efferent somatic fibers in the pudendal nerve that control the external anal sphincter, which is also under conscious control. The other part implicates an autonomic reflex arc conveyed in the pelvic nerves. Rectal distention activates this autonomic reflex, which simultaneously causes peristaltic waves in the distal colon, contraction of the longitudinal muscles of the rectum, and relaxation of the smooth muscles of the internal anal sphincter. The external anal sphincter (striated muscle) relaxes also, and the feces are expelled, with or without assistance by abdominal straining (abdominal press), which is common in dogs and cats but does not occur in ruminants.

REFERENCES

Burrows CF, Merritt AM. Influence of alpha-cellulose on myoelectrical activity of the proximal canine colon. Am J Physiol 1983; 245:9301.

Cherbut C, Ruckebusch Y. The effect of indigestible particles on digestive transit time and colonic motility in dogs and pigs. Br J Nutr 1985;53:549.

Ferre JP, Ruckebusch Y. Myoelectrical activity and propulsion in the large intestine of fed and fasted rats. J Physiol 1985;362:93.

Leib MS, Wingfield WE, Twedt DC, Williams A. Gastric emptying of glucose in the dog. Am J Vet Res 1986;47:31.

Pahlin PE, Kewenter J. Sympathetic nervous control of cat ileal sphincter. Am J Physiol 1976;231:296.

Pairet M, Bouyssou T, Ruckebusch Y. Colonic formation of soft feces in

rabbits: a role for endogenous prostaglandins. Am J Physiol 1986;
250:G302.

Pousse A, Mendel C, Appahamian M, Kachelhoffer J, Balboni G, Plas A. A
slow-wave frequency complex of the canine small intestine during the
fasting state. Can J Physiol Pharmacol 1987;65:1132.

Roche M, Ruckebusch Y. Basic relationship between gastric and duodenal
motilities in chickens. Am J Physiol 1978;234:E670.

Ruckebusch Y. Motor functions of the intestine. Adv Vet Sci Comp Med
1981;25:345.

Sellers AF, Lowe JE, Drost CJ, Rendans VT, Georgi JR, Roberts MC.
Retropulsion-propulsion in equine large colon. Am J Vet Res
1982;43:390.

Wood JD. Physiology of the enteric nervous system. In: Johson LR,
Christensen J, Grossman MI, Jacobson ED, Schultz SG, eds. Physiology of the gastrointestinal tract, 2nd ed. New York: Raven Press, 1987.

CHAPTER 25

RUMINANT GASTROINTESTINAL MOTILITY

Embryological studies show that all four parts of the ruminant stomach (rumen, reticulum, omasum, and abomasum) are of gastric origin. The rumen and reticulum enlarge from the fundic region facing the cardia, and the omasum develops from the terminal section of the fundus of the abomasum. The volume of the abomasum is about 1.5 L at birth, or twice the volume of the nonfunctional ruminoreticulum and omasum (0.7 L). Compared with the ruminoreticulum of the adult bovine, that of the calf is vestigial (Fig. 25–1).

When the neonate sucks, milk passes from the lower esophageal sphincter to the abomasum by a closable channel, the reticular groove (Fig. 25–2). The reticular groove is closed reflexly by stimulation of pharyngeal receptors, which are activated by milk components and by the act of sucking. This very powerful reflex is necessary to allow the colostrum (first milk) and milk to pass directly into the abomasum, bypassing the then nonfunctional forestomachs of the neonate. The immunoglobulins of colostrum can then be transferred to the duodenum, where they are rapidly absorbed by a transitorily, very permeable enteric mucosa. The abomasal mucosa of the newborn ruminant is almost devoid of parietal cells, so the immunoglobulins of colostrum are not degraded by proteolytic (pepsin) enzymes. Within 12 to 24 hours after birth, trophic factors activate an explosive proliferation of parietal cells for active proteolytic digestion by pepsin. Calves that fail to ingest colostrum do not develop the passive immunity needed to withstand pathogenic forms of organisms that may gain access to the gastrointestinal tract.

The calf is born with a drive to lick and nibble, a behavior favoring the ingestion of the fauna and flora that normally colonize the ruminoreticulum. Also, by sucking three to six times a day, the calf stimulates a maternal neuroendocrine reflex for milk let-down, which is important for its survival. This maternal reflex may be impaired by adrenal catecholamines released when pain, caused by anything from sore teats to foot lesions, inhibits the contractions of the mammary myoepithelial cells.

The transition from the preruminant (milk feeder) to the ruminant state occurs early. The calf shows signs of being able to regurgitate (bring back food from the stomach to the mouth) as early as 5 days of age. At 3 weeks, calves graze about 3 hours a day. By about 7 weeks, their grazing time is about half that of adults, and their blood volatile fatty acid (VFA) levels are similar to those of adults. In the ruminoreticulum, the presence of VFAs from digestion of cellulose is a very active trophic stimulus. VFAs stimulate salivary excretion, ruminoreticular epithelium and muscle growth, and circulation and absorption in the forestomach.

CHARACTERISTICS OF THE PRERUMINANT STOMACH

Development

The development of the stomach of the lamb can be divided roughly into three stages: birth to 3 weeks of age, when the ruminoreticulum is nonfunctional; 3 to 8 weeks, when the ruminoreticulum is beginning to develop; and 8 weeks and beyond, when the ruminoreticulum is fully functional.

During the first 3 weeks of life, the lamb depends entirely on its mother's milk and is considered a nonruminant animal. The intake of milk reaches a maximum during this period, glucose absorption from the gut is very rapid, and plasma glucose concentration rises to its highest level. Enzymes in the gut and liver metabolize absorbed glucose, and carbohydrate metabolism then has a typical nonruminant pattern.

At the early ruminant stage (between 3 and 8 weeks), glycemia is lowered and blood volatile fatty acid concentrations are raised until they reach normal adult values. There is an increase in the content of plasma stearic acid and of trans- or of branched-chain acids, and of adipose tissue triglycerides. The ability of extrahepatic tissues to utilize glucose and synthesize fat from it becomes very poor. If glucose is injected, secretion of insulin and glucose tolerance are low, much as in a diabetic animal.

Reflex Mechanisms in Preruminant Digestion

Closure of the reticular groove is a reflex initiated by sucking or drinking. The afferent limb comes from receptors in the posterior oral cavity (Fig. 25–3), and the effector limb leaves the medullary center of the reflex in the vagus nerves. When the pharyngeal receptors are not properly activated, milk may be transferred into the ruminoreticulum. This event occurs when cold milk is drunk from a bucket; then the milk sequestered in the ruminoreticular fluid moves slowly into the abomasum. The reticular groove reflex may be activated experimentally in *sheep* with *copper* salt (10 mL of $CuSO_4$ 10%), and in *calves* with *sodium* salts. The reticular groove reflex is inhibited either by injection of atropine or by application of a local anesthetic to the oral cavity. In the young ruminant, this inhibition is used to make sure that a drug remains in the ruminoreticulum. Of course, a drug can be delivered directly into the ruminoreticulum through an

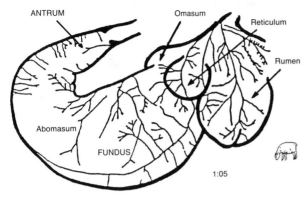

Figure 25–1 Nonfunctional ruminoreticulum and omasum of the newborn lamb. The volume of the abomasum (glandular stomach) is twice that of the forestomachs (nonglandular stomach) of ruminants at birth.

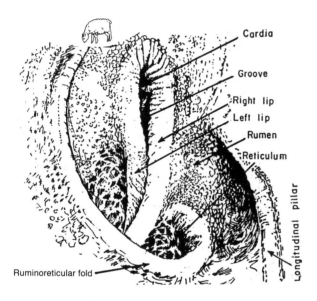

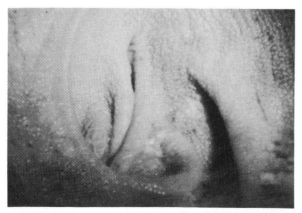

Figure 25–2 Reticular groove of the adult sheep. Diagrammatic view (**top**) and photographic view (**bottom**) from a fistula in the dorsal sac of the rumen. The reticular groove is a vertical structure with a clock-wise torsion of its lips near the reticuloomasal orifice, which is masked by the ruminoreticular fold.

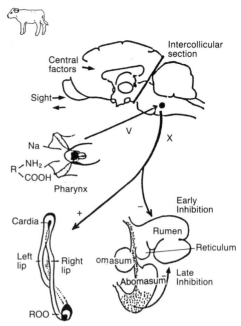

Figure 25–3 Reflex closure of the reticular groove. Diagram representing the pharyngeal receptors in the posterior mouth (afferent limb, fifth cranial nerve, *V*) converging into the center in the medulla oblongata. The efferent limb (tenth cranial nerve, *X*) carries stimulatory signals to the reticular groove, and inhibitory signals to the reticuloomasal orifice (*ROO*) and the forestomachs. A late inhibitory signal (vagovagal reflex) to the forestomachs originates from the slight distention of the abomasum by clotted milk.

esophageal (gastric) tube introduced in the nares, through the pharynx, and down the esophagus to reach into the anterior forestomachs.

An early inhibition of ruminoreticular and omasal motility accompanies the reticular groove reflex. Another important response to milk intake is abomasal fundic relaxation. Clotted milk, causing a *slight antral distention,* relaxes the fundic part of the abomasum because of a *vagovagal relaxatory reflex,* which also inhibits the ruminoreticulum. By contrast, a *considerable antral dilatation* brings an adrenergic response with *inhibition of abomasal motility.*

In the milk-fed calf, abomasal emptying is controlled by the volume of milk sucked and retained in the abomasum, and the nature of the duodenal chyme. The volume of the gushes of gastric chyme delivered into the duodenum, at a rate of 3.5 gushes per minute, depends on the volume of liquid present in the body of the abomasum. With introduction of 1 to 4 L of milk, the volume of each periodic antral gush is higher, in order to maintain constant the half-life of abomasal contents (about 30 minutes), whatever the volume of milk introduced into the abomasum.

Alkalinity in the duodenum causes *abomasal emptying* through reflex mechanisms activated by chemoreceptors and osmoreceptors in the small intestine. The empty abomasum has a pH of less than 2.0, which may rise to 6 to 6.5 on addition of digesta (Fig. 25–4).

Duodenal *acidity inhibits* abomasal emptying and gastric acid secretion via a number of gastrointestinal peptides

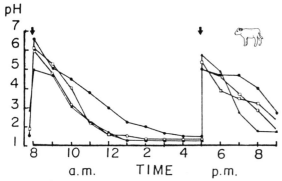

Figure 25-4 Increase of the intraabomasal pH in calves after sucking 1.5 L of milk substitute (7 percent w/v, pH 6.8) from a bottle (*arrow*). The resting or fasting pH value (1.5) returns after 4 hours.

or hormones. Somatostatin is probably the most important digestive hormone involved in this abomasal inhibition, but secretin and cholecystokinin also inhibit abomasal motility and secretion. Only in ruminants are alkaline bile and pancreatic secretions added to the duodenum at a considerable distance (20 to 35 cm) from the pylorus. This anatomical arrangement helps maintain an acid environment, which enhances the release of peptides that inhibit abomasal functions. Excessive acidification of the duodenum may lead to accumulation of a surplus of digesta in the abomasum by decreasing abomasal emptying.

Weaning Period and Abomasal Emptying

When the calf or lamb reaches the age of 24 days, a crisis may occur because of overdistention of the abomasum. At that age, in addition to milk, the preruminant is also eating concentrated solids, which tend to accumulate in the abomasum, to overdistend it, and to inhibit abomasal emptying. Results of the effect of different temperatures (4° and 40°C) of test meals on abomasal emptying and secretion indicate better abomasal performance at 4°C.

As a result of ravenous consumption of milk or milk substitute, a calf may develop hypoxia. It usually occurs with tachycardia, hypertension, and cerebral anoxia, which may lead to fatal convulsions. This situation can be avoided by preventing rapid ingestion of milk and supplying liquid food at a low (4°C) rather than a high (40°C) temperature.

PHYSICAL BREAKDOWN OF FEED IN THE RUMINANT DIGESTIVE TRACT

The physical breakdown of forages is an integral part of digestion in ruminants, its role being to increase the surface area of food presented to ruminoreticular microbes and to enhance both the rate of passage of digesta and the feed intake. These effects can be observed, together with decreased ruminoreticular digestibility, when particle size is reduced prior to feeding by chopping or grinding forage.

Particle Size of Food and Chewing

Chewing during eating and rumination is the important component in the process of reducing food to fine particles. By increasing salivation, chewing also contributes to dilution and to buffering the ruminoreticular fluid. In heifers (340 kg), the total time spent chewing (intake and rumination) alfafa hay (16.9 hours per day) is almost identical with that required to chew long hay, and for coarsely (2.1-mm particles) or finely (1.4-mm particles) chopped hay (16.6 hours). Chewing rate during rumination varies with the coarseness of the diet and the amount of feed ingested. From the total chewing time results, it is evident that less time is spent eating diets containing coarser particles, but that this is compensated by spending more time ruminating each bolus.

Diurnal analyses of the number of boluses per minute of rumination and of the chewing time of each regurgitated bolus indicate fluctuating and overlapping results throughout the day for long hay and for coarsely or finely chopped hay (Fig. 25-5).

With long hay, a dramatic decrease in the number of boluses per minute of rumination occurs near feeding time. After feeding, an abrupt rise is observed in the number of boluses processed per minute of rumination, and the return to baseline takes nearly 6 hours. The rumination of more boluses after feeding may reflect an attempt by the animal to use rumination as a means to reduce more rapidly the size of recently ingested long hay particles.

As a rule, fewer boluses are processed per minute of rumination as the size of hay particles gets smaller. This holds whether ruminants are fed long or chopped hay. The

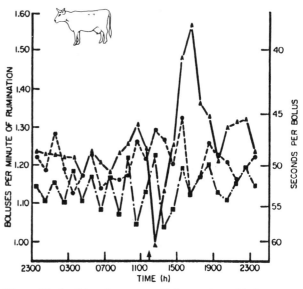

Figure 25-5 Diurnal patterns of the number of boluses per minute of rumination and the chewing time per bolus in heifers fed long alfalfa hay (▲—▲), and chopped alfalfa hay (●---●, coarse; ■---■, fine). Feeding (*arrow*) was 8, 8.4, and 8.5 kg of dry matter per day.

mean fecal particle size is greater when finely chopped hay is fed than when long or coarsely chopped hay is provided. This would suggest a less effective rumination (i.e., less ability to cause physical degradation of the digesta).

The breakdown of grass hay particles in the rumen and in the mouth can be studied with esophageal-fistulated sheep. Ingesta, intercepted either during regurgitation or during deglutition, can be analyzed for volume and particle size. Sheep muzzled during the nonfeeding period to restrict ruminating regurgitate more voluminous boluses with larger particles than congeners allowed to ruminate without hindrance. During feeding, the muzzled sheep have more chewing movements than nonmuzzled sheep, and the swallowed boluses contain smaller particles. The effectiveness of particle breakdown, which normally increases with time after feeding, is lost by muzzling, as rumen contents and feces show a higher proportion of large grass hay particles.

Pseudorumination

When the ruminating behavior cannot be expressed, a very irregular and shorter pattern of chewing occurs to mimic natural rumination (Fig. 25–6). It is due to lack of stimulation of reflexogenic areas owing to absence of solid contents. In sheep, this occurs when strands of long grass silage become matted or tangled into a mass, which remains caudad to the cranial pillar of the rumen and cannot be broken down into boluses that can be regurgitated. It is also seen experimentally when calves with the ruminoreticulum isolated are fed volatile fatty acids (VFAs) via a rumen cannula and casein via an abomasal cannula. The frequency of

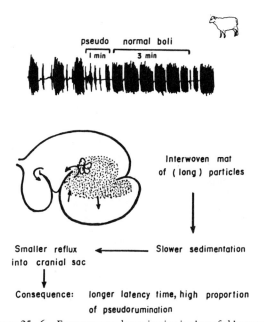

Figure 25–6 Frequent pseudorumination in sheep fed long grass silage. After the meal, the solid contents become entangled in the caudal sac of the rumen, with lack of reflux into the cranial sac. Psuedorumination is due to insufficient stimulation of the reflexogenic areas that induce rumination.

pseudorumination is reduced by increasing the amounts of VFAs in the rumen. By contrast, the addition of indigestible particles into the isolated ruminoreticulum brings more tactile stimulation on the rumen wall and enhances the frequency of pseudorumination.

Rumination and Its Components

The ruminoreticulum of artiodactyls is more than just a simple storage compartment for forage. Its main function is to perform as a fermentation chamber, and it is also an important absorption site of nutrients and simple molecules (Fig. 25–7). The remaining part of the forestomachs, the omasum, processes the food after it has been fermented in the rumen and reticulum. Perissodactyls (nonruminant herbivores such as horses, rhinoceroses, tapirs) also possess a fermentation chamber, which is located at the junction of the small and large intestine. In these animals, the cecum and the enlarged colon contiguous to the cecum also absorb the nutrients and simple molecules produced by cecocolic fermentation.

An essential feature of the ruminant forestomachs is the structure connecting the reticulum and the omasum, the reticuloomasal orifice (ROO). It acts like a sieve, causing food to be retained in the rumen and reticulum for a considerable time. The ROO restricts passage of food into the omasum and the secretory abomasum, allowing only particles that have been reduced to a certain size to pass. This fragmentation of food to the proper particle size is achieved by the combined physical and microbial processes of ruminoreticular rumination and fermentation.

Rumination, the phenomenon of "chewing the cud," or rechewing the coarse ruminoreticular contents ingested at some earlier time, is a characteristic feature of ruminant animals. The urge to ruminate is strong and leads to single or successive cycles of rumination lasting about 60 seconds, which, all together, represent as much as 8 hours per day.

The time spent ruminating by a given animal depends on the texture of the food and the amount of food ingested. Ruminants fed concentrates or pelleted hay ruminate less than those that receive hay. When the texture of food is unchanged, the rumination time is related to the quantity eaten. In stall-fed animals, there is a circadian rhythm in the periods of rumination. Cattle may ruminate from 35 to 80 minutes per kilogram of roughage consumed and do two-thirds of their ruminating at night, when rumination is favored by rest, recumbency, and drowsiness (also seen at milking time). Deep sleep frequently follows a period of rumination at night.

Rumination is centrally mediated by the "gastric centers" of the medulla oblongata and the ventral hypothalamic area. Not all the factors that stimulate or inhibit rumination have been clearly defined. Tactile stimulation of the reticular and ruminal epithelia is a powerful stimulus for rumination, especially when digesta moves over the ruminoreticular fold during contractions. The craniocaudal pillar complex harbors receptors to monitor the volume and texture of ruminoreticular digesta. The time allowed for the physical break-

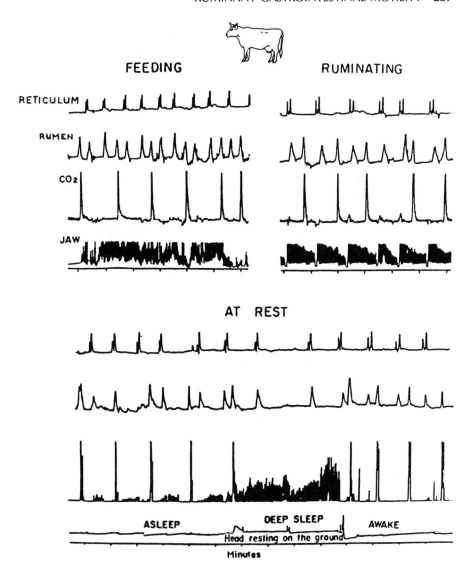

FEEDING **RUMINATING**

RETICULUM

RUMEN

CO2

JAW

AT REST

ASLEEP   **DEEP SLEEP**   AWAKE
Head resting on the ground

Minutes

Figure 25–7 Pressure changes in the reticulum and the rumen, carbon dioxide peaks in the esophagus (eructation), and jaw movements in a feeding cow (left), in a ruminating cow (right), and in a resting cow (asleep, deeply asleep, and awake) without any jaw movements.

down of food through rumination is controlled by sensory information about the digesta that is perceived at or in these pillars (Fig. 25–8). The types of sensory information are *digesta texture,* from tactile stimulation; *digesta consistency,* from the resistance opposed to the contracting pillars; and *rumen fill,* from the stretch of the pillars.

Intravenous injection of a very low dose of epinephrine (3 μg/kg) induces rumination in sheep by enhancing the afferent input from the reticular wall. Opiate antagonists (naloxone) not only stimulate rumen motility but also enhance epinephrine-rumination, even in sheep fed pellets (Fig. 25–9). In goats, conditioned-reflex rumination can be obtained by associating a series of light flashes with gentle stroking of the reticular epithelium. Rumination is inhibited in cattle and sheep by a large dose of epinephrine, and in sheep by the opioid-system pathway.

A rumination cycle includes four phases of activity: *regurgitation* of semifluid bolus from the ruminoreticulum, its simultaneous *remastication* and *reinsalivation,* and *reswallowing (or redeglutition)* of the finely rechewed bolus.

Regurgitation Phase

Rumination starts with the regurgitation phase, which is the swift movement of semiliquid digesta from the ruminoreticulum, through the cardia, up the esophagus, and into the mouth. Rapid antiperistalsis is provided by the esophageal striated muscle of ruminants. The antiperistaltic wave of regurgitation passes over the esophagus at a velocity of 0.2 m per second (i.e., two times [in cattle] to five to six times [in sheep] faster than the velocity of the normal peristalsis of deglutition). In about 2 seconds, the "retained" bolus has the fluid squeezed out of it. This fluid is immediately swallowed, and the remainder is then chewed, reinsalivated, and subsequently swallowed. The "tail" bolus (i.e., the excess fraction in the pharynx and esophagus of the slurry) is reswallowed within 1 second of regurgitation.

Regurgitation is heralded by a *long-lasting* (2 to 4 seconds in sheep, 1 to 1.5 seconds in cattle) *extra contraction of the reticulum,* which is immediately followed by the normal biphasic reticular contraction. The reticular extra contraction

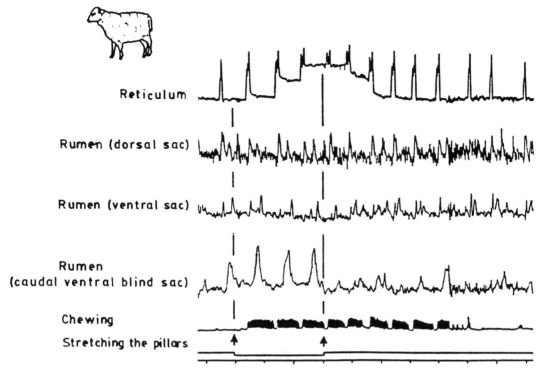

Figure 25–8 In the sheep, stimulation (for 3 minutes) of the caudad rumen pillar induces, within less than 30 seconds, a rumination period (9 cycles) that outlasts the duration of the stimulation by nearly 5 minutes.

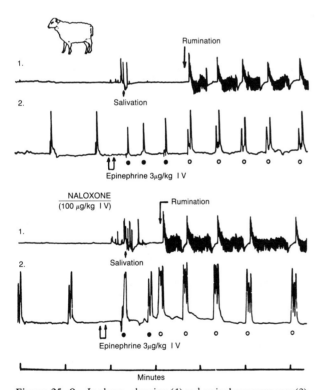

Figure 25–9 In sheep, chewing (*1*) and reticular movements (*2*) are modified after a minute dose of epinephrine (3 μg/kg IV). Salivation and reticular activity increase almost immediately, and secondary chewing (rumination) occurs within 2 minutes after injection. Naloxone pretreatment (100 μg/kg IV) enhances the intensity of the phenomenon.

floods the *open cardia* with material from the bottom of the reticulum immediately before an inspiratory effort with a closed glottis creates a brief supernegative pressure (−25 to −40 mm Hg) in the thoracic esophagus. Electromyographic and fluoroscopic evidence shows that the influx of ruminoreticular digesta into the esophagus occurs when the lower esophageal sphincter (LES) is actively opened (Fig. 25–10). Also, at this moment, the upper esophageal sphincter (UES), or cricopharyngeal muscle, is relaxed.

Simultaneous Remastication and Reinsalivation Phases

The *remastication* phase of rumination (*secondary mastication*) is characterized by chewing movements occurring at a slower and more regular rate than those associated with ingestion of food (*primary mastication*). The patterns of mandible movements are different during eating and during rumination.

During a rumination cycle that lasts about 60 seconds, most of the time (50 seconds) is taken by the chewing and salivation phases, and the remaining 10 seconds are for regurgitation and redeglutition. The rate and duration of rumination chewing are controlled by the texture (coarseness) and quantity of the food. Rumination involves a great number of remastication movements, or secondary mastications (9,000 to 25,000 daily). Feed concentrates and pelleted hay require less rumination chewing than do forages (grass, hay). When the texture of the food remains unchanged, the quantity of food is the variable that affects rumination chewing time.

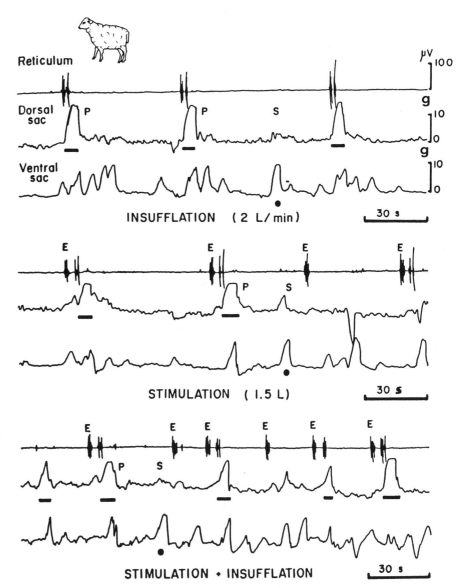

Figure 25–10 Sheep reticulum, dorsal sac, and ventral sac motility. Results of distention by gas (2 L per minute, insufflation), by polyethylene chips (1.5 L, tactile stimulation) and by a combination of both floating plastic (tactile stimulation) and gas (insufflation). Tactile stimulation alone causes less reticular extra contractions (*E*) than the combination of tactile stimulation and insufflation. Eructation (●) is provoked equally by each type of distention. Insufflation always increases the motor activity of the ventral sac.

For example, in a sheep eating 500 g of hay per 24 hours, about 350 rumination cycles occur in 368 minutes, at the chewing rate of 46 mastications per minute. A total of nearly 17,000 mastications is required during the day.

If the daily hay intake is restricted to 200 g, the average number of rumination cycles is only 225, and they occur in 210 minutes. The chewing rate is slower (40 per minute), and the total number of chewing movements required is only 8,400.

When the intake of hay increases to 800 g per day, the rumination time is doubled (451 minutes per day for the 404 cycles), and the chewing rate is higher (52 mastications per minute), so that about 23,450 mastications are needed for rumination.

The reinsalivation phase of rumination coincides with the remastication phase. The serous rumination (secondary) saliva comes mostly from the parotid gland on the side of chewing during rumination and does not contain any secretion from the mandibular glands. By contrast, ingestion (primary) saliva contains more mucous (buccal glands) and seromucous (sublingual and mandibular glands) secretions, to coat and lubricate the boluses of forage for easier swallowing.

Rumination saliva and ingestion saliva are secreted at about the same rate—and about 2.5 times the resting rate. The latter is maintained by activation of receptors of the ruminoreticular epithelium by tactile stimuli.

> In cattle fed hay, the rumination salivation rate is 2.5 times the rate of resting salivation. In sheep fed a range of dry forage diets, the rumination (parotid) salivation rate is from 0.9 to 2.6 times (mean: 1.7 times) the resting salivation rate. In *Bos indicus* cattle fed small amounts of hay, the ingestion salivation rate is 2.9 times the resting rate, and with straw, it is twice the resting rate.

Raising the percentage of dry matter (DM) or fiber in food increases saliva secretion during ingestion, resting, and rumination. When widely disparate feedstuffs are fed, parti-

TABLE 25–1 Volumes of Salivation and Deglutition in Lactating Cows Fed Hay-Crop Silage or Corn Silage, with Other Parameters Related to Salivation and Eating

Silage	Daily Intake (kg)	Eating Rate (g/min)	Swallowing Rate (bolus/min)	Swallow Volume* (mL)	Saliva mL/min	pH
Hay-crop						
Eating	34.1	96.7	2.2	89	188	8.5
Resting	—	—	—	70	152	8.5
Corn						
Eating	39.6	119.2	1.9	79	166	8.5
Resting	—	—	—	81	156	8.5

*When the animal was resting, a bolus of 139 g of the specific silage was given.

cle size seems more important in determining the rate of salivation. Less ingestion saliva is secreted when particle size decreases, and feeding diets rich in minute particles reduces production of rumination saliva. The resting and eating salivations in lactating cows fed either hay-crop silage or corn silage are different (Table 25–1). Neither silage increases ingestion salivation greatly, but hay-crop silage, which takes longer to eat (96 vs 119 g per minute), increases it more.

Saliva—of all types—is important for fermentation, as it provides 70 percent of the water present in the ruminoreticulum, and it contributes most of the phosphate and bicarbonate buffers. Saliva buffer concentration does not change with alterations of the diet. The total daily salivary buffer supply to the ruminoreticulum is related to the total amount of salivation (210 to 250 L at 4 to 8 weeks' lactation in a cow), which is itself related to the proportion of fiber in the diet.

Redeglutition Phase

A rumination cycle is concluded with the reswallowing, or redeglutition, of the now reinsalivated and rechewed portion of ruminoreticular content that was regurgitated. In sheep, the esophageal peristalsis of redeglutition propels reswallowed fluids at the rate of 35 cm per second and the remasticated bolus at 21 cm per second.

Eructation

Eructation is the physiological process of expelling ruminoreticular gases (carbon dioxide, 65 percent; methane, 25 percent; nitrogen, 7 percent; oxygen, 0.5 percent; hydrogen, 0.2 percent; hydrogen sulfide, 0.01 percent) through the cardia and the esophagus. It occurs at a rate of one to three eructations per minute but is not audible or evident at the nostrils or the mouth. Because of closure of the nasopharyngeal sphincter, a large portion of the eructated gases (carbon dioxide, methane) is inspired and recycled into the organism by absorption into the lungs. This explains how strong volatile flavors from ruminoreticular degradation of plants (garlic, onion, leek) reach the mammary glands and are incorporated into milk.

In the fluid environment of the ruminoreticulum, the chewed plant material is further macerated, softened, and disrupted by microbial enzymes to produce simpler molecules (VFAs, amino acids, and gases). These substances are beneficial to both the host and the colonizing microorganisms, which eventually are a significant source of protein for the host. A large quantity of ruminoreticular gases (0.5 to 2 L per minute in the cow) is produced by gasogenic microbes and by the reaction of salivary bicarbonate with acids. Normally, the excess gas bubbles coalesce, separate from the ruminoreticular contents to form pockets of free gas above the level of the contents, and are eliminated by eructation.

Eructation is a vagovagal reflex, with centers in the medulla oblongata. Mechanical receptors to detect distention are present in the rumen dorsal sac, in the reticular groove, around the cardia, and in the esophagus. The effector response involves clearing the submerged cardia of digesta by contraction of the cranial and caudal pillars of the rumen, simultaneously relaxing the cardia and contracting the dorsal sac, and a biphasic esophageal phase. The esophagus first experiences a *filling phase*, with an increase in esophageal pressure between the closed diaphragmatic and lower esophageal sphincters. The second esophageal phase brings *clearing contractions* (i.e., retroperistalsis bringing up gases) from the diaphragmatic sphincter of the esophagus, and an immediate aborad peristalsis to clear the esophagus of remaining fluids.

Experimental insufflation of the ruminoreticulum stimulates the eructation reflex, which is accompanied by motility of the ventral sac of the rumen to displace the gases dorsally into the rumen and cranially toward the relaxed cardia (see Fig. 25–10). This ruminal motility is an example of the secondary type of contraction of the rumen, which starts caudally (dorsal blind sac) and spreads orad. The primary type of rumen contraction always follows the biphasic reticular contraction and spreads caudally. In cattle, 66 percent of eructations coincide with the secondary type of rumen contraction, and 20 percent with the primary type. In sheep, eructation may occur independently of the rumen (4 percent), concurrently with secondary-type rumen contractions (37 percent), and most of the time with the primary type (60 percent).

CYCLICAL CONTRACTIONS OF THE RUMINORETICULUM

Periodic displacement of the left abdominal wall and of the left lumbar fossa is readily seen or palpated once or twice per minute in small and large ruminants. On auscultation over the left flank, a crescendo and decrescendo are heard that coincide with each volume change in the left flank. These alterations of the shape of the left abdominal wall are due to incessant mechanical activity in the rumen that mixes and propels the contents (food, saliva, drinking water, microorganisms) of this huge fermentation vat.

Research—by direct inspection through a large dorsal rumen sac fistula, by radiography of the ruminoreticulum after feeding radio-opaque meals, by recording pressure changes in the reticulum and rumen, by electromyography of ruminal and reticular smooth muscle, and by detection of deformation of the walls of the forestomachs—has shown the basic mechanical activity of the rumen to be of two types. The first (primary) type of motor activity, which spreads cephalocaudally over the rumen, is related to and driven by the basic motor activity of the reticulum. The second (secondary) type of rumen contraction, which moves caudocephalad, is not subordinated to the motor activity of the reticulum.

Rumination and eructation have already been mentioned as other mechanical events added to, and related to, the basic pattern of motor activity of the rumen and reticulum. Rumination events (additional reticular contraction, regurgitation, remastication, reinsalivation, and redeglutition) result from mechanical distention of the ruminoreticulum by coarse food, whereas eructation follows gaseous distention of the ruminoreticulum.

Basic Motor Activity

A basic motor activity cycle of the ruminoreticulum starts in the reticulum as a rapid biphasic contraction and ends in the rumen as a slower contraction of the primary type, which may be either uniphasic (dorsal sac) or biphasic (dorsal and ventral sacs).

The reticulum also synchronizes or activates other forestomachs' motor events, such as relaxation of the reticuloomasal orifice in cattle and sheep and relaxation of the omasum followed by contraction of the omasal canal in sheep.

The biphasic reticular contraction is of shorter duration (5 to 7 seconds) in sheep than in cattle (5 to 12 seconds), where it also causes contraction of the atrium of the rumen. The partial relaxation, or notch, in the biphasic reticular contraction is very evident in cattle and much less marked in sheep. The first phase of the biphasic reticular activity is termed the mixing contraction, and the second one the evacuation contraction of the reticulum.

Pressures obtained from transducers experimentally placed at different locations in the reticulum and rumen reflect the contractions and relaxations of these compartments (Fig. 25–11). Recordings from the ruminoreticulum show that the ratio of basic reticular-reticular (biphasic) to cephalocaudad rumen contractions may be 1:1 or 1:2. In the former situation, the reticular events are followed by a contraction of the dorsal sac of the rumen, whereas in the latter, a reticular cycle gives rise to a first contraction of the dorsal sac immediately followed by a contraction of the ventral sac.

This ruminoreticular activity propels some reticular digesta distally over the ruminoreticular fold into the dorsal sac of the rumen at intervals of 35 to 45 seconds during ingestion and rumination of food, or as long as 75 seconds in a resting ruminant. The ruminoreticular fold actually drops to facilitate caudad movement of digesta out of the reticulum. Then, the reticular groove is stretched open simultaneously, as the reticuloomasal orifice relaxes. The finer particles of digesta suspended in fluid are propelled and spiralled into the dilated funnellike reticular groove and reticuloomasal orifice by the contraction of the cranial and

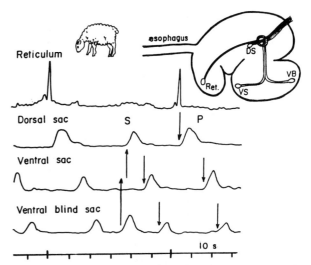

Figure 25–11 Diagram of the ovine ruminoreticulum with the positions of balloons to record motility (pressure changes) in the reticulum (*Ret*), dorsal sac (*DS*), ventral sac (*VS*), and ventral blind sac (*VB*). The reticular contraction spreads cephalocaudally (i.e., as a primary contraction, *P*) to the dorsal, to the ventral, and to the blind ventral sacs. A secondary contraction (*S, caudo-cephalad*) originates in the blind ventral sac and moves retrograde, to the dorsal sac, where it reverses direction to return aborally to the ventral sac and ventral blind sac.

ventral sacs of the rumen. Immediately upon completion of this sequence, the reticular groove and reticuloomasal orifice remain closed until the next ruminoreticular cycle begins at the reticulum.

The displacement of liquid by these cyclical ruminoreticular contractions (1 per minute, 1,440 per day) is strong enough to modify the electrical resistance between electrodes on the limbs. The changes in electrical activity of the heart measured between a pair of electrodes (right foreleg and left hindleg) are visible on an electrogastrogram (Fig. 25–12).

Development and Control of Forestomach Motility

Electrophysiological methods have revealed the existence of two evolutionary developments in the ruminant forestomachs. These are the intrinsic activity within the intramural plexuses of the forestomach and the extrinsic activity related to the gastric centers in the brain stem with their nerve pathways.

The intrinsic system forms a local nervous system, which is established at 6 weeks in the bovine embryo and is represented by the myenteric (between the muscle coats) and submucosal plexuses of the forestomachs. These plexuses are connected by nerve strands to form a mesh, which is much denser in the reticulum and rumen dorsal sac than in the rumen ventral sac or the abomasum. The intramural reflex activity (e.g., more intense muscle tone in response to distention) is related to the enteric nervous system (ENS). It is

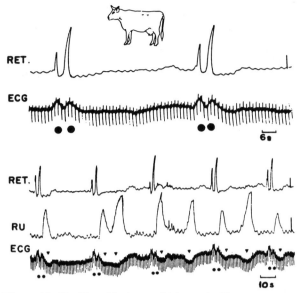

Figure 25–12 **Top,** Tracings at high speed of bovine reticular motor activity (*Ret*) and electrocardiogram (limb derivation RA-LL [right arm–left leg]) to show the interval between the biphasic reticular contractions (●), which are detected by the cardiac electrodes. **Bottom,** Slower tracings of ruminoreticular motor activity (*Ret, Ru*) and ECG to reveal the additional effect of primary and secondary ruminal contractions (▼) on the ECG.

influenced only by extrinsic nerves and is modulated by gut hormones and neurotransmitters.

The primary roles of extrinsic contractions are mixing and aboral propulsion of the contents of the forestomachs. The extrinsic system allows cyclical motor activity of the ruminoreticulum as vagovagal reflexes and coordinates this cyclical activity with the processes of regurgitation and eructation. The outflow from the gastric centers by the vagal motor neurons is strictly related to the afferent neural input. Two additional interconnected neuronal networks act as vagal relays to and from the gastric centers. One network of interneurons controls the frequency of the cyclical ruminoreticular movements; the other regulates the amplitude of the forestomach contractions through vagal discharges, first on the reticulum and later on the rumen. They are evoked by an activity of the central nervous system (CNS), which is reflexly modified by sensory inputs coming largely from the alimentary tract itself. The frequency and amplitude of extrinsic contractions are inhibited by abomasal distention (Fig. 25–13). The magnitude of the extrinsic contractions and their form (i.e., primary or secondary rumen motility, regurgitation, or eructation) are related to coarse particles or gas, which distends the reticulum or stretches the rumen pillars.

Any husbandry practice or clinical condition that affects this vagovagal reflex will modify the pattern of these extrinsic contractions and lead to digestive dysfunction. They do so by acting either on the general level of the CNS or on the volume, texture, and composition of the gut contents. As an example, the presence of a dog (sniffing, growling, barking) influences the general level of CNS activity of a cow.

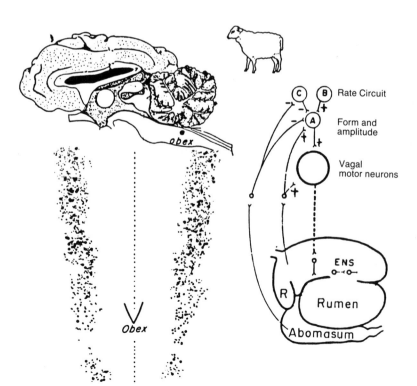

Figure 25–13 **Left panel,** The bilateral gastric centers are the located in the brain stem, near the caudal angle of the roof of the fourth ventricle, under the cerebellum. By reference to the obex, the centers extend laterally and mostly rostrally, as shown by the retrograde cellular degeneration (black dots) 16 days after rumenectomy. **Right panel,** The functional organization of the gastric centers includes the vagal motor neurons, the neurons (*A*) concerned with the form and amplitude of contractions, the neurons (*B, C*) that control the frequency of contractions. Distention of the abomasum inhibits both A and CB neurons, but tactile distention of the reticulum and stretching of the pillars evoke the vagovagal primary or secondary types of rumen contractions (modify form and shape).

It induces a state of psychological stress, which accelerates ruminoreticular motor events.

Extrinsic versus Intrinsic Forestomach Activity

The transection of one of the two vagi does not greatly inhibit the extrinsic contractions of the forestomachs, so long as the contralateral circuit continues to function. General anesthesia, which is similar to temporary severance of both vagi, reversibly abolishes the extrinsic ruminoreticular contractions.

Totally vagotomized sheep can survive when they are nourished with an intraruminoreticular infusion of VFAs, electrolytes, and vitamins together with intraduodenal administration of a solution of casein. Within 2 or 3 weeks, changes occur in the electromyographic and strain-gauge recordings. Intrinsic activity is manifested as large electrical group discharges and phasic contractions in the ruminoreticulum (Fig. 25–14). Between phasic contractions, the intrinsic activity (group discharges) is denser in the reticulum than in the rumen. The frequency of the discharges is six or seven every 10 minutes, depending on the ruminal volume.

The consistent relationship between the frequency (number, series) of discharges and the ruminal volume suggests a neurally integrated activity at the level of the myenteric plexus (i.e., enteric nervous system [ENS]). The intrinsic activity of the ruminoreticulum is blocked by atropine (0.1 mg per kg), hexamethonium (2 mg per kg), ambient cold (30°C versus 37°C), and VFAs (0.1-M acetic, propionic, or butyric acids buffered to pH 4.0). The coordinated extrinsic and phasic activities of the ruminoreticulum may be impaired at four sites of interaction between the CNS and the ENS (Fig. 25–15). Parallel pathways probably exist at the level of the ENS for intrinsic tonic activity.

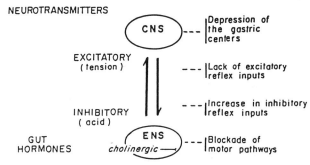

Figure 25–15 Schematic relationship between the CNS and the ENS for the control of ruminoreticular motility. Possible causes of ruminal stasis by depression of the gastric centers are anesthesia, lack of sensory tactile stimulation from a pelleted diet, vagovagal (reflex) inhibition from the distended abomasum, and blockade of cholinergic motor synapses (e.g., hypoglycemia).

OMASOABOMASAL ACTIVITY

In sheep and cattle, the reticuloomasal orifice (ostium reticuloomasicum) may be considered as the bottleneck for the outflow of digesta from the ruminoreticulum. By restricting food passage, it also limits new food intake.

The structure of the reticuloomasal orifice seems to differ in ruminants according to the texture of their food. Some ruminants regulate the size of the orifice, opening it at times for rapid passage of very large fibrous particles that cannot be broken down to a smaller size. In concentrate-selector species, the longitudinal folds (short papillae), which are larger in the reticuloomasal orifice than on the floor of the reticular groove, form a dam or sievelike mechanism. In grass and roughage eaters, these longitudinal folds are shorter and fewer and are not major obstacles to aborad progression of food particles. In all types of ruminants, these longitudinal folds mark the beginning of the primary omasal leaves (laminae), which diverge from this opening. The omasal canal is the space limited by the omasal pillar and the free edges of the laminae and represents a wide omasal entrance portion, continuing the reticuloomasal orifice.

Omasal Motility

Omasal contractions are slow and progressive. In cattle, they are independent of those of the reticulum. In sheep, the proximal and middle parts of the omasum contract about 15 to 30 seconds after the biphasic reticular contraction. The omasal contraction ends at the onset of the reticular contraction (Fig. 25–16). The rapid downward biphasic deflections that open the reticuloomasal orifice look somewhat like the mirror image of the upward deflections of the biphasic reticular contractions.

Abomasal Motility

The abomasum lies in the lower right region of the abdominal cavity. It is partly covered by the edge of the rib

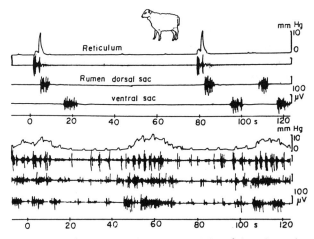

Figure 25–14 Top, *Extrinsic* motor activity of the ovine reticulum (pressure and electrical activity) and electrical activity of the rumen (dorsal and ventral sacs) before vagotomy. **Bottom,** *Intrinsic* activity of the same structures 12 days after complete truncal vagotomy.

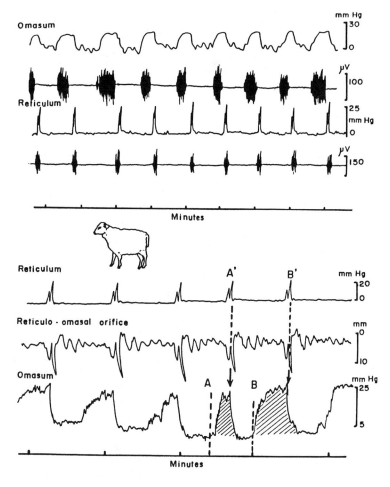

Figure 25–16 Top, Cyclical pressure and electrical changes in the omasum and the reticulum of the sheep. The omasal activity, which follows reticular activity, ceases at the onset of reticular activity. Bottom, The end of the second phase of reticular motility (*A', B'*) coincides with the relaxation of the reticuloomasal orifice (*dotted line*) and of the sustained omasal contraction (*arrow*), which begins 15 to 30 seconds (*A, B*) after the onset of the reticular contraction.

cage and extends backward under the right costal arch, where it can be cannulated.

The abomasum is the only part of the ruminant stomach that secretes digestive juices. Large folds (rugae), corresponding to 85 percent of the area of the fundic mucosa, make the construction of fundic pouches difficult. In the calf, fundic pouches have been used to collect rennin (rennet), an enzyme that coagulates milk.

The gastric secretion of the fundic area is similar to that of dogs—a watery fluid containing pepsin and hydrochloric acid, with two other major constituents that can replace each other (sodium and hydrogen ions). The pH of gastric juice in sheep fed ad libitum varies between 1.05 and 1.32. After an overnight fast, the sight of food, as well as abomasal distention, increases the abomasal acid output from 10 to 60 mEq per L. In contrast, gastric fluid collected from innervated antral pouches is slightly alkaline and contains visible strands of mucus and clumps of epithelial cells.

The motor activity of the fundus of the abomasum is restricted to shallow contractions. The more powerful antral motor activity is inhibited at the onset of a period of regular contractions on the antroduodenal junction (Fig. 25–17). These periods of regular antroduodenal contractions occur 18 to 20 times per day. Although the supply of digesta from the ruminoreticulum to the abomasum is continuous, these cyclical periods correspond to abomasal emptying.

The gastric or abomasal emptying of a fully fed ruminant is not a continuous process. This has been proved by measuring the abomasal outflow of chyme and relating it to the cyclical changes in the amplitude and frequency of the contractions of the pyloric antrum in sheep. These periods of high pressure at the abomasoduodenal junction are followed by periods of quiescence without any passage of chyme.

Transpyloric Flow of Digesta or Chyme

The flow of chyme into the duodenum usually occurs in gushes of as much as 2 to 10 mL. A cycle of abomasal emptying consists of a series of gushes during 10 to 15 minutes, followed by a period of rest when nothing or only an insignificant amount of chyme trickles into the duodenum. The summation of successive cycles gives a pyloric outflow of about 400 mL per hour in a 40-kg sheep (Fig. 25–18). During enteral perfusion of casein in a vagotomized sheep, the outflow of chyme is continuous and the cycles are less apparent owing to shorter periods of antroduodenal quiescence.

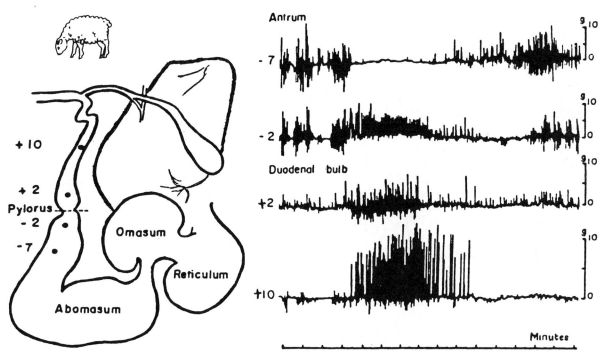

Figure 25–17 In sheep, mechanical activity of the antroduodenal junction, recorded from strain-gauge force transducers placed proximal (−2 and −7 cm) and distal (+2 and +10 cm) to the pylorus. Almost synchronized series of contractions occur on the duodenal bulb (+2 and +10) and the pyloric antrum (−2), while the more distal part of the antrum (−7) then relaxes. These contractions progress aborally at a rate of 8 to 10 cm per minute. They represent the phases of the migrating motor complex (MMC), which periodically sweeps along the small intestine in ruminants.

Measurement of abomasal emptying in the ruminant is difficult because the ruminoreticulum acts like a mixing pool system. The amount of time stained particles stay in the ruminoreticulum increases with the volume of this vat. The turnover of stained particles depends on the level of feeding and on the physical form of the food. The volume of digesta allowed to flow out of the ruminoreticulum toward the pylorus is also related to the rate of transfer through the omasum and to the rapidity of the chemical and motor processes in the abomasum.

In normal sheep given food marked with fuchsin, the marker first appears at the pylorus after 22 hours and disappears after 19 days. In sheep whose rumen is surgically removed, similar marked food is seen at the pylorus after only 6 hours and is passed out after 6 days. The rumen delays appearance of the marker at the pylorus by about 16 hours and final disappearance by 13 days. The ratio of abomasal to ruminoreticular flow is highest with a high level of feeding and when grass harvested at early maturity is fed. In sheep fed straw, a ruminoreticular digesta outflow of 5, 7, or 10 L per day corresponds to an abomasal chyme outflow of 6, 8, or 13 L per day.

In adult ruminants, the abomasal outflow is controlled by a local nerve network. The development, during 3 to 4 minutes, of regular spiking activity (RSA) on the duodenal bulb coincides with the inhibition of antral evacuation. Antral inhibition can be reproduced experimentally by moderately distending the duodenum.

INTESTINAL MOTILITY

Motility of the Small Intestine of Ruminants

The entire pattern of small intestine motor activity, the migrating myoelectric complex (MMC) of electromyographical parlance, is always present in ruminants (Fig. 25–19). In contrast, and disregarding some variations, monogastric species show MMCs only during the interdigestive, or fasting, state. In these fasting species, the migration of the components of the MMCs—no spiking activity (NSA) and intermittent (ISA) and regular spiking activity (RSA)—is associated with the propulsion of scant amounts of small intestine contents (intestinal and pancreatic secretions, bile, and desquamated cells). In these monogastric animals, the appearance of chyme in the small intestine disrupts the MMCs. The NSA and RSA phases disappear, leaving only the dominantly propulsive ISA. The situation is different in ruminants, where the small intestine constantly carries about 400 mL of chyme per hour, without altering the NSA, ISA, and RSA phases of the MMCs.

When the ruminant duodenum empties, propulsive waves appear on both antrum and duodenal bulb as long as the volume of the abomasum remains constant. Propagated aborally at a high velocity, the duodenal propulsive waves of the ISA phase (Fig. 25–20) transfer chyme beyond the duodenal flexure, to relieve the distention at the duodenal

A.

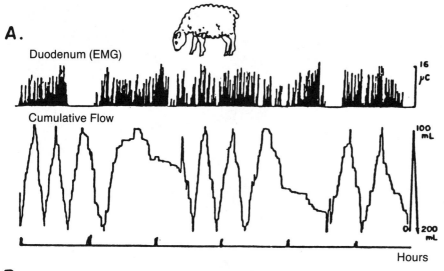

B.

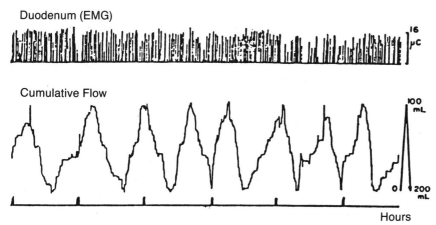

Figure 25-18 In the sheep, electrical activity of the duodenal bulb and cumulative delivery of chyme through the pylorus. **A,** In control animals, the outflow is rhythmic and is related to the initiation of well-patterned MMCs on the duodenum. **B,** In animals subjected to enteral perfusion (casein 20 g per L, 160 mL per hour) abolishes the periods of quiescence (NSA) and causes a continuous flow of chyme into the duodenum.

bulb. A constant gravimetric volume distention is present in the duodenal bulb because of its vertical position in the abdomen. The role of the short phase of regular activity, marked by RSA, is to act as a barrier to prevent backflow of chyme in the nearly vertical duodenal bulb.

Neural Control

The extrinsic nerves (splanchnic, vagus) have a regulatory function on the MMCs, since neurotomy affects only the frequency or the velocity of propagation and not the pattern of the MMCs. The daily number of MMCs decreases from 18 to 13 after splanchnectomy but rises from 18 to 25 after total extrinsic denervation (splanchnectomy and vagotomy). Vagotomy slows the velocity of propagation of the duodenal MMCs, which continue to migrate, but at only 16.7 cm per minute (about 40 percent as fast as normal). Vagotomy also abolishes the duodenal response to acid (chemical) stimulation.

In normal sheep, duodenal infusion of 0.1-M hydro-chloric acid during an NSA phase (i.e., 20 minutes after a natural RSA phase) usually induces premature phases of RSA (i.e., the chemical stimulation increases the frequency of MMCs).

The appearance of MMCs is also more frequent after administration of 5-hydroxytryptamine (5-HT), or serotonin, which plays a major role as a neurotransmitter locally, via the ENS, or on the smooth muscle cells. The effect is more pronounced near the pylorus than elsewhere, giving credence to the antroduodenal origin of MMCs in the ovine species and explaining the high concentrations of neurotransmitters at this level of the gut. Methysergide, an agonist of serotonin, also increases the frequency of the MMCs.

Motility of the Large Intestine

Variation in the anatomy of the large bowel does not explain the formation of pellets in sheep and goats or soft feces in cattle. The role of the spiral colon in the formation of pellets is indicated by the retention time of digesta, which is

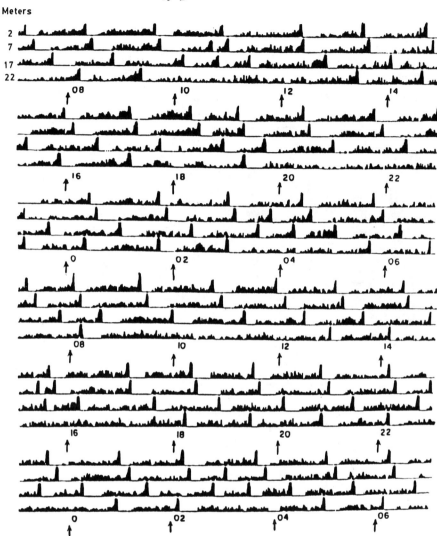

Figure 25–19 Integrated record of the MMCs initiated on the small intestine of a hay-fed sheep in a period of 48 hours. The pairs of serosal electrodes are at 2, 7, 17, and 22 m from the pylorus. The progression of each MMC along the small intestine is clearly seen, and it is evident that about 30 percent of the MMCs that start on the duodenum do not reach the ileum, 22 m from the pylorus.

20 hours in sheep (cf. 8 hours in cattle). Electromyographic studies indicate that the dominant motor activity of the ovine spiral colon is segmentation (Fig. 25–21). The isolated spike bursts (ISBs) form narrow rings to divide the content of the lumen into fairly uniform segments and to propel feces over very short distances in both directions (orad and aborad). In contrast, the major pattern of activity seen through the whole colon of cattle is grouped spike bursts (GSBs), which have a mean frequency corresponding to those of defecations.

The cecocolic segment of the large intestine represents 15 percent of the entire digestive tract in ruminants. The other segments of the large intestine (cecum, proximal colon, centripetal and centrifugal coils of the spiral colon, distal colon, and rectum) also participate in other homeostatic functions (e.g., fermentation, electrolyte and fluid balance, and evacuation of residues).

METABOLIC ROLE OF FORESTOMACHS' MICROBIAL ECOLOGY

The ruminoreticulum and omasum complexes are characterized by an anaerobic environment. The constant temperature of about 40°C, the buffering system that keeps pH near neutral, and the microenvironment are ideal for the development of anaerobic bacteria, fungi, and protozoa. Despite ingestion of food mixed with oxygen-containing air and materials, the redox potentials of the ruminoreticulum contents are held at a strongly reducing level (about -250 to -450 mV) by the activity of these microorganisms.

A newborn animal acquires an inoculum for its ruminoreticulum by licking its mother and other members of the herd. The various substrates for microbial growth are provided by the feed. The various microbial species differ in

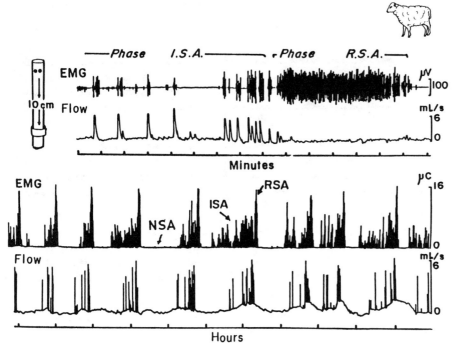

Figure 25–20 Top, Fast recordings (*minutes*) of the electrical activity and flow of chyme in the small intestine of the sheep. The flow of the contents of the small intestine occurs only during ISA and is most marked near the end of the phase. Flow of chyme is negligible during the RSA phase. Bottom, Slower recordings (*hours*) clearly show that the flow of chyme is related to the ISA phase of each cycle of electromyographic activity. Little or no flow is seen outside of the ISA phase (i.e., during RSA and NSA) of each MMC.

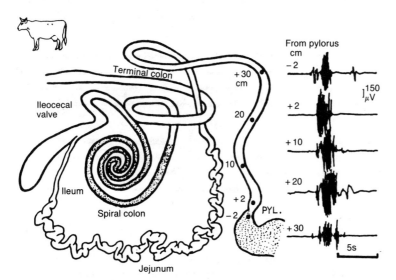

Figure 25–21 Top, Schematic representation of any ruminant gastrointestinal tract and record of a very rapid propagation of a strong peristaltic contraction (strain-gauge force transducers) from the antrum and along the duodenum of a cow (at −2, +2, +10, +20, and +30 cm from the pylorus). Bottom, In sheep, GSBs are replaced by ISBs associated with the formation of fecal pellets. In cattle, GSBs slowly migrate (2 cm/per minute) from the ileocecal valve into the spiral colon and to the terminal colon, at a mean frequency corresponding to that of defecations.

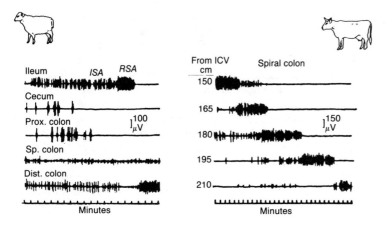

their ability to utilize these substrates and to compete for them. Special growth-promoting and growth-inhibiting factors are present in the ruminoreticulum medium. In addition, the rumination and eructation cycles influence microbial growth by macromixing and soaking ingesta, by grinding coarse particles, by removing gases (notably carbon dioxide and methane), by removing end-products (Table 25–2) through mucosal absorption, and by propelling indigestible materials onward. The gas bubbles formed during fermentation as well as the movements of the microbes themselves also contribute to important micromixing of the ingesta.

Ruminoreticulum bacteriology is a very specialized field because of the enormous diversity of species. Classification of microorganisms found in the forestomachs is based on several criteria (e.g., morphology—shape, size, ultramicrostructure—and cultural characteristics—substrate digested, end-products formed) (Table 25–3).

At least two environments for subpopulations of ruminoreticulum microorganisms are recognized: one that is free-ranging in the ruminal milieu and another that is surface adherent and can account for more than half of the total microbial population. Microbial polysaccharide glycocalyx mediates the attachment of microorganisms to ruminoreticular surfaces and provides a protective coat that makes bacterial colonies resistant to bacteriophages. Microbes can adsorb not only to the mucosal wall of the forestomachs but also to ingested plant materials (fibrous stalks, roots, leaves, grains). The adherent microbes in the digestive environment of ruminants have been studied by scanning and transmission electron microscopy. The species that adhere to the epithelia differ from those that cling to fibrous feed particles.

The surface of the tongue appears to be colonized by chain-forming microorganisms. In the rumen of young calves fed milk, the initial microbial populations include *Micrococcus, Staphylococcus, Lactobacillus, Corynebacterium, Streptococcus, Flavobacterium,* and *Escherichia. coli.* As they enter the ruminant stage, typically anaerobic bacteria appear

TABLE 25–3 Ruminoreticulum Microorganisms and Their Fermentation Substrate

Microorganisms	Substrates								
	Acids	Amylose	Cellulose	Hemicellulose	Lipids	Pectin	Protein	Sugars	Urea
Anaerovibrio					X				
Bacteroides		X	X	X		X			X
Butyrivibrio			X	X	X	X			X
Eubacterium					X				
Fusocillus					X				
Lactobacillus								X	
Lactospira						X			
Megasphaera	X								
Micrococcus					X				
Ruminococcus			X	X					X
Selemonas	X	X							X
Streptococcus		X				X			
Succinimonas									
Succinivibrio					X	X			X
Treponema						X		X	X

in the rumen (e.g., *Bifidobacterium, Eubacterium, Flavobacterium, Fusobacterium necrophorum* [*Sphaerophorus necrophorus,* a pathogen commonly recovered from liver abcesses], *Peptostreptococcus, Propionibacterium,* and *Selemonas*). About 50 percent of the bacteria adherent to the ruminoreticular mucosa are facultative anaerobes, which would use oxygen that diffuses through the epithelium. Some (about 10 percent) of the adherent gram-positive bacteria carry urease, proteases, and deaminases to degrade urea from food and saliva, urea diffused from blood into the rumen, and proteins from sloughed cells and from feed materials. In sheep nourished by liquid perfusions of short-chain fatty acids (SCFAs) with buffer into the ruminoreticulum, and of casein into the abomasum, the redox potentials of the ruminoreticulum contents rise from about -400 mV to the range of -14 to -50 mV.

The population of adherent microorganisms on fibrous feed particles includes *Butyrivibrio, Bacteroides, Ruminococcus, and Lactospira* species. These bacteria and fungi account for a large proportion of the ATP in the ruminoreticular contents. They digest cellulose, pectins, hemicelluloses, and amyloses.

The digestion of structural carbohydrates, a vital feature of ruminoreticular metabolism, is necessary to nourish the free-living microbial species that complete the ruminoreticular digestive process. Digesting fibrous carbohydrates such as cellulose, which are not digestible by the enzymes secreted by the ruminant animal, is the primary contribution of the ruminoreticular microbiota. In exchange for this benefit to the host, the microbes utilize feed nutrients that the host animal could readily digest, and they absorb some of their end-products (e.g., hexoses and amino acids). In compensation, the host digests the microbes themselves for their protein, lipid, and starch content. The ruminant animal must also adapt its metabolic pathways to contend with the biological value of the protein, which is not as high as that of some of the feed proteins. To compensate for

TABLE 25–2 Sites and End-Products of Digestion of Food in Ruminants

Sites	Nutrients Digested	End-Products
Ingested food		
Rumen	Structural carbohydrates	SCFAs, CH₄,* CO₂
	Nonstructural carbohydrates	SCFAs, CH₄,* CO₂
	Protein	SCFAs, NH₃*
Undigested food, microbial cells, endogenous materials		
Abomasum, small intestine	Nonstructural carbohydrates	Monosaccharides
	Protein	Amino acids
	Lipids	Fatty acids
Undigested residues from small intestine		
Cecum, colon	Structural carbohydrates	SCFAs, CH₄,* CO₂
	Nonstructural carbohydrates	SCFAs, CH₄,* CO₂
	Protein	SCFAs, NH₃*
Feces		

* Energy or nitrogen losses for the host ruminant.

the lack of glucose derived from the digesta that passes to the abomasum, the end-products of microbial carbohydrate metabolism (SCFAs) and of proteins (amino acids) are used to accomplish net gluconeogenesis. Propionate and glucogenic amino acids are the key to this marvelous achievement by the ruminant liver.

> The monogastric hind-gut fermenter (horse, rabbit) can catch the readily digestible ingredients but cannot benefit as much from fermentation. In the colon, the microbes cannot be digested, and many of the microbial end-products cannot be absorbed. The rabbit compensates somewhat for this deficit by means of cecotrophy.

Importance of Microbial Protein in Ruminants

Increased output of microbial protein from the ruminoreticulum is desired to increase efficiency of animal production and to reduce the need for intact protein in the feed. Several factors influence microbial growth (Fig. 25–22). The synthesis of protein and lipid from the ruminoreticulum is related to the efficiency of microbial growth. The output of microbes is the result of the amount of organic matter digested in the ruminoreticulum (adenosine triphosphate [ATP] yield) and of the efficiency with which the microbes use this ATP for growth.

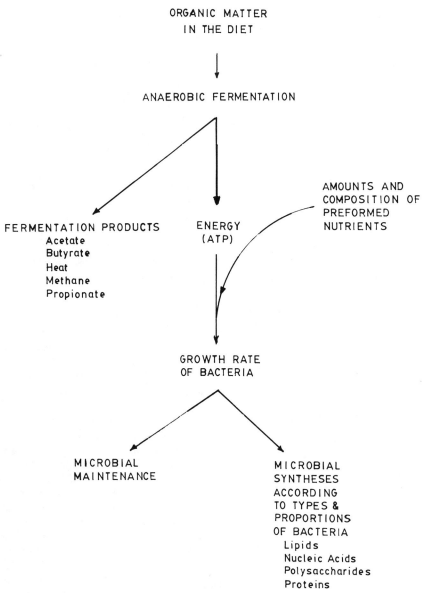

Figure 25–22 Factors influencing ruminoreticulum microbial growth or microbial protein synthesis.

Efficiency of microbial growth can be expressed in terms of yield of dry cells (or of microbial protein) per mole of ATP or per unit of organic matter fermented in the ruminoreticulum. Total microbial yield from the ruminoreticulum usually rises as the amount of organic matter fermented in the forestomachs increases. Independent of yield, microbial efficiency is often greater with less extensive digestion in the ruminoreticulum and with a lower total microbial yield. For example, despite lower total microbial yield, microbial efficiency is higher with whole-corn than with processed-corn diets.

Initially, the size of the ruminoreticular population, or biomass, had served as an index of efficiency of fermentation, with larger numbers being desirable. Studies in chemostats have discredited this index of efficiency. The ruminoreticulum microbial biomass may decline at faster passage rates, even though identical or increasing amounts of microbial protein are supplied to the duodenum. A large microbial biomass is undesirable for maximal microbial efficiency.

The overall growth rate for bacteria in the ruminoreticulum is about 6 to 7 percent per hour. This means that microorganisms must replicate at least 1.5 times each day. At this rate, a large proportion of energy is used for maintenance. Besides energy, shortages of nutrients, such as nitrogen or sulfur, are additional factors that limit microbial growth.

Specific Actions of Ruminoreticulum Microorganisms

To attack successfully specific substrates, ruminoreticulum microorganisms must have key enzymes, such as alpha-amylase, cellulase, disaccharidases, deaminases, exopep-tidases, lipases, phosphorylases, proteases, and urease. The most important outcome of the metabolic process of ruminoreticular fermentation is the formation of vast amounts of SCFAs (formerly VFAs), especially acetate, propionate, and butyrate. Some longer-chain forms of fatty acids are also produced (e.g., isobutyrate, valerate, and caproate). These short and long fatty acids are the end-products of metabolism for many ruminoreticulum bacteria and are also the principal source of energy for the host ruminant. The majority of the SCFAs are absorbed from the forestomachs (Fig. 25–23). The host's metabolism also benefits from the ruminoreticular microbes forming a microbial biomass that passes on for digestion in the abomasum and intestine. This biomass constitutes a major source of protein for the ruminant animal and includes some microbial starch and lipids as well.

Several cellulolytic microorganisms effectively deaminate amino acids to produce branched fatty acids (isobutyrate, valerate, isovalerate, and 2-methylbutyrate), which are essential growth factors for synthesis of long-chain membrane lipids. They also release ammonia, along with ureolytic microbes; ammonia is used as a primary nitrogen source by many ruminoreticulum bacteria. Often, carbon dioxide and some growth factors (phenylacetic and phenylpropanoic acids) are formed at the same time.

Complex plant lipids can be degraded by ruminoreticulum microbes; however, the highly reducing environment promotes the hydrogenation of unsaturated fatty acids, and less of the essential unsaturated fatty acids remain in the ruminoreticulum. Absorption of these hydrogenated fatty acids leads to the formation of more saturated ("harder," i.e., higher melting point) body and milk fats of ruminants and to the presence of unusual fatty acids. Hydrogen gas is removed from the ruminoreticulum by methanogenic bacteria (*Methanobacterium, Methanobrevibacter,* and *Methanomicro-*

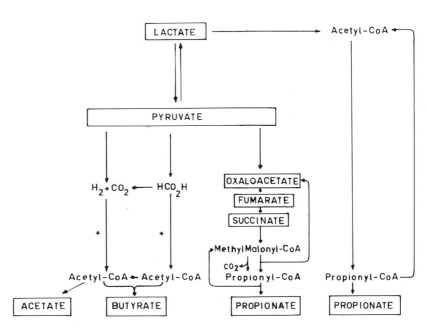

Figure 25–23 Pathways for SCFA production from pyruvate.

bium), which reduce carbon dioxide (via formic acid) to methane. *Methanosarcina* can also form methane from acetate on diets high in molasses.

Many ruminoreticulum bacteria require B vitamins for growth. It is fortunate that some microbial production of B vitamins is provided for them and for the ruminant host. However, with low-fiber diets, *Bacillus thiaminolyticus* produces an extracellular thiaminase, a transferase enzyme that destroys thiamine in the presence of appropriate substrates. This can lead to the important neurological disease known as polioencephalomalacia.

Sudden introduction of diets high in readily fermentable carbohydrate (e.g., sugars and starches) causes rapid proliferation of *Streptococcus* and *Lactobacillus,* which promote accumulation of D- and L-lactic acids in the ruminoreticulum ingesta. The ensuing excessive acidification of the contents, to pH values as low as 4.0, destroys many bacterial species and protozoa of the ruminoreticulum. Systemic acidosis results, and an irreversible breakdown of homeostasis is marked by dehydration, endotoxemia, and gastrointestinal dysfunction. Some lactate-using microbes, such as *Selemonas* and *Veillonella,* are acid sensitive. However, more acid-resistant lactate-using species (e.g., *Megasphaera*) multiply too slowly to maintain a balance, and adaptation occurs only if concentrates are increased slowly.

Bloating is another dysfunction of ruminoreticulum fermentation. It is due to trapping of evolving gases in foams, which prevent successful eructation. The foams are particularly likely to occur on legume pastures carrying alfafa and clovers. In feedlots, foams also result from slimes formed on certain concentrate diets.

Certain antibiotics that are ionophores (e.g., such as monensin and lasalocid) have come into widespread use as feed additives for cattle. They improve efficiency of feed utilization by inhibiting proteolysis and deamination and possibly by selecting for microbial species that use the succinate metabolic pathway. Thus, the molar concentrations of the SCFAs are changed in favor of propionic acid (a glucogenic fatty acid). As gram-positive bacteria are selectively inhibited, these ionophores provide a margin of safety against lactic fermentation. At the same time, they also arrest the energy-wasting process (greater than 10 percent) of methanogenesis by inhibiting the microbial species that form the precursors of methane, namely, hydrogen and formic acid. In general terms, broad-spectrum therapeutic antibiotics have a detrimental effect on ruminoreticulum microbial function.

Fungi and Protozoa of the Ruminoreticulum

Anaerobic cellulolytic fungi of the ruminoreticulum are also highly proteolytic. Ruminoreticulum protozoa are a major feature of the microbiota, normally having a population density in excess of 10^5 per milliliter of rumen fluid. The most prevalent forms are the ciliated protozoa. Their proportions vary considerably with the diet; the following genera typically are present: *Dasytricha, Diplodinium, Entodinium, Eoidinium, Isotricha,* and *Ophryoscolex.* Some flagellated species of protozoa are also present in the reticulorumen.

Most types of ciliated protozoa digest starch, and several are cellulolytic, producing SCFAs, lactic acid, and hydrogen. They are also proteolytic, and can store a form of glycogen as body starch. On high-starch diets, the *Entodinium* forms of protozoa tend to multiply.

The contribution of protozoa to the performance of the ruminant host is an extremely elusive parameter to measure. The use of chemicals that selectively kill protozoa has given equivocal results. Other avenues of research are required to unmask the impact of protozoa on the productivity of their host animals (domestic and wild ruminants) and their interaction with other microorganisms. Protozoa compete with bacteria for substrates, and since predation of bacteria is common, they play a role in the degradation of bacterial protein and appear to have a stabilizing effect in the ruminoreticulum. They seem to resist passage through the reticuloomasal orifice by segregating in the dorsal part of the ruminoreticulum ingesta.

Attempts to Control Ruminoreticulum Fermentation

Over the last 2 decades, studies have been undertaken to control ruminoreticulum fermentations. The objective of the first attempts was to protect nutrients from microbial degradation (e.g., protein in feed, by heat or chemicals) to preserve them for the ruminant host. Another avenue of research was aimed at avoiding intrarumen saturation of fats by preventing hydrogenation of unsaturated fatty acids. These efforts have not lived up to their early promises, but research continues for improvements.

Another course of research is the biotechnical manipulation of bacterial species genomes, which will bring a better understanding of ruminoreticulum microbes. It is hoped that the addition of specific functions to microorganisms would give them the edge under specified dietary conditions and would lead to productive advantages for the ruminants.

It seems more probable that fermentation will be made more efficient by pretreating feeds under controlled conditions than by manipulating the extraordinarily diverse and competitive biological environment of the ruminoreticulum. One example of a valuable goal is the development of a method of pretreatment for feeds that permits the degradation of lignin-containing plant materials.

REFERENCES

Bell FR. The mechanisms controlling abomasal emptying and secretion. In: Ruckebusch Y, Thivend P, eds. Digestive physiology and metabolism in ruminants. Lancaster: MTP Press, 1980.

Black JL, Sharkey JM. Reticular groove (*Sulcus reticuli*): An obligatory adaptation in ruminant-like herbivores. Mammalia 1970;34:294.

Bryant MP. Rumen mechanogenic bacteria. In: Dougherty RW, Allen RS, Burroughs W, Jacobson NL, McGilliard AD, eds. Physiology of digestion in the ruminant. Washington, Butterworths, 1965.

Cassida KA, Stokes MR. Eating and resting salivation in early-lactation dairy cows. J Dairy Sci 1986;69:1282.

Chai K, Milligan LP, Mathison GW. Effect of muzzling on rumination in sheep. Can J Anim Sci 1988;68:387.

Cheng KJ, Costerton JW. Adherent rumen bacteria and their role in the digestion of plant material, urea and epithelial cells. In: Ruckebusch Y, Thivend P, eds. Digestive physiology and metabolism in ruminants. Lancaster (England): MTP Press Ltd., 1980.

Church DC. The ruminant animal. Its digestive physiology and nutrient metabolism. Englewood Cliffs, NJ: Prentice-Hall, 1988.

Dunlop RH, Hammond PB. D-Lacticacidosis in ruminants. Ann NY Acad Sci 1965;119:1109.

Godfrey NW. Development of rumen function in the calf. J Agric Sci 1961;57:177.

Hungate RE. The rumen and its microbes. New York: Academic Press, 1966.

Janis C. The evolutionary strategy of the *Equidae* and the origins of rumen and cecal digestion. Evolution 1976;30:757.

Jaster EH, Murphy MR. Effects of varying particle size of forage on digestion and chewing behavior of dairy heifers. J Dairy Sci 1983; 66:802.

Kaufmann W, Hagemeister H, Dirksen G. Adaptation to changes in dietary composition, level and frequency of feeding. In Ruckebusch Y, Thivend P, eds. Digestive physiology and metabolism in ruminants. Lancaster (England): MTP Press Ltd., 1980.

Moir RJ. The comparative physiology of ruminant-like animals. In Dougherty RW, Allen RS, Burroughs W, Jacobson NL, McGilliard AD, eds. Physiology of digestion in the ruminant. Washington: Butterworths, 1965.

Prins RA, Clarke RTJ. Microbial ecology in the rumen. In: Ruckebusch Y, Thivend P, eds. Digestive physiology and metabolism in ruminants. Lancaster (England): MTP Press Ltd., 1980.

Reid CSW. Digestive physiology: The challenges today and tomorrow. In: Milligan LP, Grovum WL, Dobson A, eds. Control of digestion and metabolism in ruminants. Englewood Cliffs, NJ: Prentice-Hall, 1986.

Ruckebusch Y. Motility of the gastrointestinal tract. In: Church DC, ed. The ruminant animal. Englewood Cliffs, NJ: Simon & Schuster, 1987.

Ruckebusch Y, Malbert CH. Physiologic characteristics of ovine pyloric sphincter. Am J Physiol 1986;251:G804.

Ruckebusch Y. Gastrointestinal motor functions in ruminants. In: Schultz SG, Woods JD, eds. Handbook of Physiology, section 6. The gastrointestinal system, vol. I: Motility and Circulation, part 2. Bethesda, Md: American Physiological Society, 1989.

Webber DE, Nouri M, Bell FR. A study of the effects of meal temperature on gastric function. Pflügers Arch 1980;384:65.

Yokoyama MT, Johnson KA. Microbiology of the rumen and intestine. In: Church DC, ed. The ruminant animal: digestive physiology and nutrition. Englewood Cliffs, NJ: Prentice-Hall, 1988.

CHAPTER 26

EXOCRINE DIGESTIVE SECRETIONS

The exocrine secretions of the digestive tract are necessary for proper mastication, for deglutition, and for luminal transformation (digestion) of food into simpler constituents. Inside the lumen of the gastrointestinal tube, digestion involves a series of mechanical, chemical, and microbial processes. The main chemical action is brought about by enzymes, water, acid, and electrolytes secreted by animals in their various digestive juices. Salivary glands, stomach, pancreas, liver, and intestine can induce net transfer of large volumes of fluids from blood by active, energy-dependent mechanisms that are controlled by the neuroendocrine system.

The objective of this chapter is to describe the general characteristics of the process of active secretion (i.e., the biochemical and circulatory events). For each exocrine digestive secretion in monogastric and ruminant animals, the essentials of its origin, composition, control, and functions are reviewed.

BIOCHEMICAL EVENTS

In most stimulated secretory tissues, the secretion response is elicited by release of neurotransmitters and peptides or gut hormones. These gut hormones modulate circulatory and secretory levels in both the peripheral and the central nervous system. Dense-core vesicles of epinephrine, serotonin, or acetylcholine contain companion peptides (Fig. 26–1).

As a result, the action of the chemical transmitter of the postsynaptic cell is enhanced by co-release of the peptide. Functional interaction may exist between dopamine and cholecystokinin (CCK) and between serotonin and substance P.

In the cat mandibular salivary gland, each part of the autonomic nervous system is related to a neuropeptide (e.g., neuropeptide Y (NPY) with the sympathetic, and vasoactive intestinal peptide (VIP) with the parasympathetic (see Fig. 26–1).

By binding to specific receptors on the cell membrane, these extracellular agents activate one of two secretory response processes (Fig. 26–2). Each process involves intracellular production of one of two cyclic nucleotides (cyclic adenosine monophosphate, or cAMP, and cyclic guanosine monophosphate, or cGMP). The action of both cAMP and cGMP is to increase the amount of free intracellular calcium, which then combines with the calcium-dependent protein calmodulin to form a calcium-calmodulin complex. The complex activates a system of protein kinases responsible for the specific secretion of the cell (enzymes, electrolytes).

In the first activation mechanism of secretion, calcium is liberated from intracellular reserves by cAMP, which derives from the action of adenylate cyclase on adenosine triphosphate (see Fig. 26–2). The activation process is induced by the binding of various substances to specific receptors on the plasma membrane of secretory cells. VIP and heat-labile enterotoxins (LT) of *Escherichia coli* are examples of cAMP secretagogues (see Fig. 26–2A).

In the other secretory activation mechanism, cGMP is produced to cause transcellular entrance of extracellular calcium into the secretory cell. The formation of cGMP from guanosine triphosphate (GTP) occurs through the activation of the enzyme guanosine cyclase. It is activated by stimulation of membrane receptors' reacting to acetylcholine and parasympathomimetic substances, calcium ionophores, heat-stable enterotoxin (ST) of *E. coli*, serotonin, calcitonin, and gut hormones (gastrin; glucagon; secretin; gastric inhibitory peptide, or GIP) (see Fig. 26–2B).

The action of the intracellular complex calcium-calmodulin ions operates for the following secretions: *salivary glands* (cholinergic and adrenergic stimulation), *gastric* (cholinergic, histamine, and gastrin stimulation), *pancreatic* (cholinergic, secretin, cholecystokinin, and prostaglandin stimulation), and *intestinal* (cholinergic, VIP, and prostaglandin stimulation).

CIRCULATORY EVENTS

The circulatory system intervenes to influence the digestive mechanisms of secretion, absorption, and motility. During some situations (fasting, exercise, and stress) blood can be diverted to organs where optimal blood flow has a higher priority. The flow of blood in the vascular bed of digestive glands is then depressed and of low priority. Following feeding (Table 26–1), blood flow in the digestive glands increases dramatically, doubling or even tripling during the functional hyperemia.

As a general rule, blood flow in digestive glands is stimulated primarily by humoral agents (mostly VIP) and is inhibited by neural means. The veins of digestive glands are more richly endowed with smooth muscle than are other systemic veins. Norepinephrine raises the muscle tone of veins and arteries of digestive glands (see Fig. 26–1) and can reduce the quantity of blood in the digestive vascular bed by as much as 40 percent. Conversely, acetylcholine decreases the muscle tone of arteries and leads to a more abundant blood volume in the digestive glands. By localized tonic changes, the quantity of blood in either arterial or venous vessels of the digestive glands can be modified.

Autoregulation is a phenomenon for the maintenance of normal blood flow through capillary beds despite wide varia-

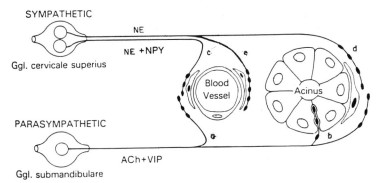

Figure 26–1 Autonomic motor innervation of the blood vessels and acini of the salivary gland. (ACh, Acetylcholine; Ggl., ganglion; NE, norepinephrine; NPY, neuropeptide Y; VIP, vasoactive intestinal peptide.)

tions in arterial inflow pressure. The responses in the resistance vessels are vasoconstriction when the arterial pressure increases and vasodilation when the pressure decreases. Autoregulation is partially controlled by locally produced metabolites (e.g., elevation in local blood carbon dioxide causes vasodilation, and depression causes vasoconstriction). The metabolites increase when flow decreases, and their activity brings about a return to normal flow.

Neural regulation by stimulation of the sympathetic segment of the autonomic nervous system brings vasoconstriction in both venous and arterial vessels of the secre-

tory glands. Vasodilation and higher blood flow from parasympathetic stimulation are indirect effects not associated with cholinergic and adrenergic mechanisms. These indirect effects may possibly be caused by serotonin, which may be involved in a local reflex or may act as a neurotransmitter.

Gut hormones (gastrin; cholecystokinin, or CCK; VIP; and glucagon), acetylcholine, crude (but not purified) secretin, NPY, and histamine increase blood flow and oxygen consumption in secretory glands. Atropine, an anticholinergic, blocks the vasodilating effect of acetylcholine, gastrin, and CCK. Prostaglandins and serotonin have very

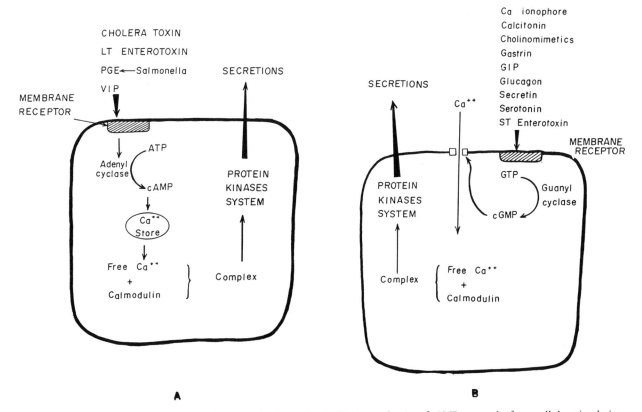

Figure 26–2 Active secretory process in digestive glands associated with the production of cAMP as a result of extracellular stimulations. **A,** Calmodulin-calcium ion complex reacts with protein kinase system to cause secretions specific to each gland. **B,** The complex, formed by calmodulin and calcium ions entered by transcellular route, acts on protein kinases to produce the secretions specific to each digestive gland. (GIP, Gastric inhibitory peptides; LT, heat-labile; ST, heat-stable.)

TABLE 26–1   Factors That Affect Blood Flow of Digestive Glands

Vasodilatory	Vasoconstricting
	Exercise
Feeding	Fasting
Glucagon	
Histamine	
Increased CO_2	Decreased CO_2
Isoproterenol	
Parasympathetic stimulation	Sympathetic stimulation
Acetylcholine	Epinephrine
CCK	Stress
Gastrin	Vasopressin
Prostaglandins	
VIP	

potent vasodilating effects on the digestive tract. Isoproterenol binds to beta$_2$-adrenergic receptors to stimulate vasodilation and improve blood flow. Epinephrine acts on alpha-adrenergic receptors to cause vasoconstriction. The acute stress seen in hemorrhagic shock may cause the neurohypophysis to produce sufficient vasopressin to explain the marked vasoconstriction.

ROLE OF THE SALIVARY GLANDS

Saliva is the fluid mixture produced by the serous and mucous salivary glands. The principal salivary glands (parotid; mandibular, or submaxillary; and sublingual) are paired and drain into the oral cavity; the others (palatine, buccal, and pharyngeal) line the mucous membranes of the mouth.

In most animals, immediate preprandial and feeding stimuli excite a seromucous salivary secretion, mostly to facilitate mastication and deglutition. The saliva of some animal species also contributes some pregastric enzymes for splitting of carbohydrates (amylase in pigs, rats, rabbits) or lipids (lipase in calves, lambs). Unlike monogastric animals, ruminants produce saliva continuously.

The salivary glands of ruminants function as the secretory tissue of the nonsecretory ruminoreticulum. The ruminant saliva keeps the ingesta fermenting in the ruminoreticulum in a proper fluid suspension and provides it with bicarbonate and phosphate buffers. The volume of saliva production in sheep and goats is about 10 to 15 L per day, and in cattle five to 10 times more. The cycle of fluid secretion and reabsorption, due to the development of an active rumen fermentation, further increases the mass of ovine parotid glands. Lambs raised conventionally (with multiple microbial strains in their gut) have twice as much parotid tissue as gnotobiotic lambs (with one or a few kinds of gut microbes). In cattle, the nasolabial glands, which are considered to be salivary in nature, constantly maintain moisture on the muzzle. The secretion of the nasolabial and salivary glands is extremely reduced during the short para-doxical sleep periods of ruminants and during hyperthermia (fever).

Origin of Saliva

Even if their specific structures are different, the salivary glands are essentially secretory cells grouped into a blind sac, an acinus, which is extended by epithelial cells that form an excretory capillary duct. Ducts from clusters of acini converge into a system of gradually larger pathways to form eventually a single main excretory duct for each salivary gland.

Somewhat like the nephron, the salivary gland has mechanisms for filtration, reabsorption, and excretion or secretion. The functional salivary unit, termed the *salivon* on account of this analogy, is represented by a capillary network that surrounds first the epithelium of the excretory capillary duct and then the cells of a single acinus (Fig. 26–3).

The capillary arterial blood flows countercurrent to the primary secretion of the acinus circulating in the excretory capillary duct. Arterial blood thus interacts initially with the duct cells and later with the secretory or acinar cells of the salivon. Interaction between blood and the duct cells causes transepithelial transfers of ions and modifies the composition of the primary, or acinar, saliva.

Filtration of water and potassium occurs from blood and from the acinar cells, which actively secrete chloride, sodium, and bicarbonate ions. Mucous salivary glands have salivons with acinar cells able to produce mucoproteins (mucin) by exocytosis. In some animal species, enzymes (amylase in pigs, rats, rabbits; lipase in calves, lambs), epidermal growth factor, or EGF (in mice), lysozymes, or higher contents of phosphate and bicarbonate (in ruminants) are added by the acinar cells. Ductal or acinar cells can also excrete substances from blood and then concentrate them in saliva (e.g., the salivary iodine level can be 10 times that of plasma iodine). Viruses (e.g., feline leukemia, rabies) are also found in the saliva of infected or carrier animals.

The primary saliva produced by diffusion and by secretion of the acinar cells is isotonic to the plasma. *In ruminants, whatever the secretion rate, saliva is always isotonic* to blood. In nonruminants, changes in salivary composition are due to modification of the fluid along the excretory capillary duct of the salivon: sodium cations and chloride anions are partially reabsorbed and potassium cations and bicarbonate anions are secreted. Net reabsorption of ions without net fluid absorption explains the hypotonicity of saliva at normal secretory rates. At high flow rates, the composition of saliva approaches that of the isotonic primary secretion, as less time is available for blood-ductule transfer of ions.

Composition of Saliva

Saliva collected from the mouth is a colorless, slightly opalescent fluid consisting mostly of water and small amounts of electrolytes. Selectively excreted in the saliva by the epithelial cells of the capillary excretory ducts, iodine

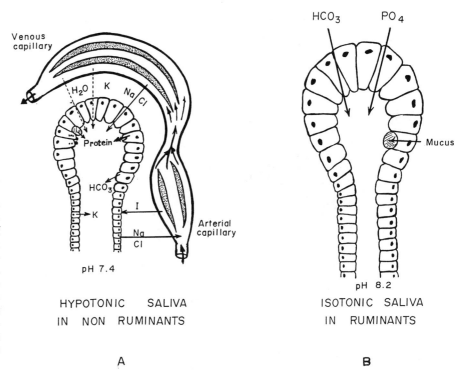

Figure 26–3 The transepithelial transfer of ions during the production of the primary saliva. The ions come from the arterial capillaries and from active acinar secretion of chloride, protein, bicarbonate, and sodium. **A,** Hypotonic saliva production in nonruminants. **B,** In a ruminant, addition of bicarbonate and of phosphate by acinar cells produces an isotonic and alkaline saliva. Feeding and ruminating saliva is bicarbonate rich, whereas continual (basal or unstimulated) saliva is phosphate rich.

may reach a concentration in saliva that is 10 times that in blood.

In nonruminants, saliva secreted at the basal rate is *hypotonic* to plasma (Na^+, Cl^-, and K^+ each 10 mEq per L; HCO_3^- 5, PO_4^{--} trace) but has the same pH as blood (7.4). When the secretion rate is faster, saliva becomes isotonic to plasma, K^+ concentration changes but little, and the concentrations of Na^+, Cl^-, and HCO_3^- increase.

Ruminant saliva is always isotonic, but its pH is alkaline (8.2). The composition of electrolytes is nearly constant for K^+ (5 mEq per L), Cl^- (15 mEq per L), and Na^+ (170 mEq per L) and shows variations for phosphate and for bicarbonate with changes in saliva flow rate (see Fig. 26–3). Significant alteration of the buffering capacity does not occur. During feeding, seromucous saliva production is mostly from mandibular glands, since *parotid secretion is profuse* only at the initiation of feeding and is scanty as eating continues. Feeding saliva of ruminants, produced at about four times the basal rate, is the richest in bicarbonate (140 mEq per L) and the poorest in phosphate (10 mEq per L). Phosphate-rich (70 mEq per L) serous saliva is produced by parotid and buccal glands during the basal (unstimulated) rate of secretion, whereas output of HCO_3^- is at its lowest (90 mEq per L).

A sheep with a unilateral permanent parotid fistula loses 1 to 4 L of saliva per day. It also develops a large sodium deficit, increased urinary chloride excretion, and an avid appetite for salt.

By substituting potassium for sodium, sheep with a parotid fistula may live for weeks with large residual sodium deficits. The sodium in food just compensates for the saliva loss. This indicates how ruminants may adapt to the salt deficit in a geographic area by eating potassium-rich grass.

The highest protein content and sulfate content are found in mucoid saliva (mucin and immunoglobulins). In ruminants, mucin is produced mostly by the mandibular glands during eating. Some salivary proteins also exist as enzymes (amylase, lipase). Amylase is present in the saliva of a number of species (pig, rat, rabbit) but is absent or present only in very low concentrations in others (cat, dog, horse, cow, goat, sheep). A lipase (pregastric esterase) active against milk fat triglycerides with short-chain fatty acids (SCFAs), mostly butyric acid, is secreted by buccal glands in a number of young ruminants, particularly the calf. Urea is secreted in ruminant saliva. A metabolite of protein or amino acid catabolism, it is produced in the liver from ammonia absorbed from the rumen, is extracted from blood, and undergoes salivary gland–rumen–blood recycling.

Control of Salivary Secretion

The nervous system controls the volume and the character of reflex salivary secretion. Knowledge of the influence of hormones on the production and composition of saliva is still rudimentary.

Neural Control of Spontaneous Salivary Secretion

Shortly after the discovery of the secretory nerves of the salivary glands, Claude BERNARD (1862) made the puz-

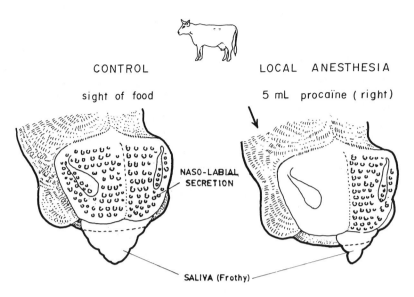

CONTROL
sight of food

LOCAL ANESTHESIA
5 mL procaïne (right)

NASO-LABIAL
SECRETION

SALIVA (Frothy)

Figure 26–4 Continuous bovine nasolabial secretion is analogous to that of parotid glands. It is reduced during sleep and may be blocked by local anesthesia.

zling discovery of *"paralytic secretion."* He observed that the mandibular (submaxillary) gland of the dog continues to secrete for long periods after neurotomy.

ECKHARD (1867) found *"spontaneous secretion"* when he noticed that the sheep's parotid gland continues to discharge saliva even if it is connected to the animal only by its blood vessels.

Using the cat mandibular gland, EMMELIN (1957) obtained pharmacological denervation and supersensitivity with gradually increasing doses of nicotine and atropine-like drugs (1 to 8 mg per kg) over a period of 10 days. This is termed *"paroxysmal secretion"* and *"degeneration secretion."*

A continuous minimal salivary secretion by the buccal glands maintains a degree of oropharyngeal humidity (Fig. 26–4). Like the nasolabial secretion, this spontaneous secretion of saliva decreases during sleep. In paradoxical sleep of adult animals, the nasolabial secretion apparently ceases, since the muzzle of the cow and the nose of the cat change from cool and humid to warm and dry. Some reflexly controlled salivary glands have what appears to be a spontaneous secretion because of constant inapparent activation of the afferent pathways of the reflex. Continuous secretion of this type occurs in the parotid and the ventral buccal glands of ruminants, the sublingual glands of cats and dogs, and the mandibular glands of rabbits.

Reflex Control of Salivary Secretion

Reflex salivation occurs by activation of the medullary salivary center, by central stimuli, or by mechanical and chemical stimuli in the mouth, esophagus, and stomach (Fig. 26–5). Salivary glands receive cholinergic (parasympathetic) and adrenergic (sympathetic) efferent fibers. The parasympathetic fibers, carried in the glossopharyngeal and facial nerves, synapse, respectively, in otic and submaxillary ganglia. Postganglionic otic fibers go to the parotid glands, and those of the submaxillary ganglia ramify to the mandibular and to the sublingual glands. Reflex salivation can be classified according to the origin of the stimuli: oral, extraoral, and experimental.

In the mouth, mechanoreceptors for texture (smooth, rough, dry, moist) and for palatability or taste (straw, grass, cereal, meat) and chemoreceptors (acid, alkaline) are stimulated to increase the volume of saliva and to determine its serous or mucous character. In ruminants, saliva associated with chewing is added to the continuous parotid and ventral buccal (inferior molar) secretions during mastication of feeding. Mastication of rumination does not induce salivation from the same salivary glands. During feeding, a profuse, predominantly mucous saliva is produced by the mandibular and sublingual glands, whereas rumination increases the

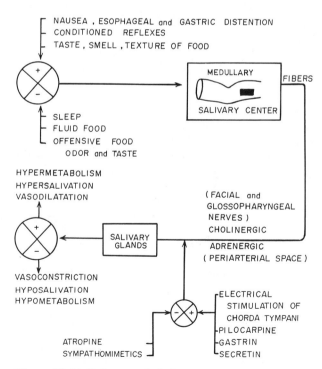

NAUSEA, ESOPHAGEAL and GASTRIC DISTENTION
CONDITIONED REFLEXES
TASTE, SMELL, TEXTURE OF FOOD

SLEEP
FLUID FOOD
OFFENSIVE FOOD
ODOR and TASTE

MEDULLARY
SALIVARY CENTER

FIBERS

HYPERMETABOLISM
HYPERSALIVATION
VASODILATATION

(FACIAL and
GLOSSOPHARYNGEAL
NERVES)
CHOLINERGIC

SALIVARY
GLANDS

ADRENERGIC
(PERIARTERIAL SPACE)

VASOCONSTRICTION
HYPOSALIVATION
HYPOMETABOLISM

ELECTRICAL
STIMULATION OF
CHORDA TYMPANI
PILOCARPINE
GASTRIN
SECRETIN

ATROPINE
SYMPATHOMIMETICS

Figure 26–5 Reflex control of salivary secretion with some pharmacological effects.

quantity of viscous saliva secreted by buccal and palatine glands.

An animal may or may not be aware of extrabuccal stimuli that activate reflex salivation. Repetitive application of neutral or noneffective stimuli, such as olfactory, visual, auditory, and nociceptive sensations, before presentation of a normal salivary stimulus can lead to development of a conditioned reflex. After an adequate learning period, the neutral stimuli alone induce salivation. Facilitating or inhibiting signals to the salivary center can originate from the hypothalamus' reticular area. Hunger, taste, and olfactory areas send facilitating signals. Inhibitory messages to the salivary center accompany emotions such as anger and anxiety or stress. Salivary reflexes are produced from unconscious stimulation of some viscera. An *esophagosalivary* reflex associates esophageal distention or irritation with salivation. *Gastrosalivary* or ruminoreticulosalivary reflexes occur after aerophagia or distention of the stomach by gas or after mechanical stimulation of the cardia, of the reticulo-omasal orifice, of the lips of the esophageal groove, of the wall of the reticulum, or of the ruminoreticular fold. Nociceptive stimuli or gastric irritation initiates nausea, which precedes vomiting. A *uterosalivary* reflex follows uterine dilation during pregnancy.

Experimentally, saliva is increased by electrical stimulation of efferent pathways, by drugs acting on the autonomic nervous system, and by denervation of glands. In dogs, electrical stimulation of the *chorda tympani* causes vasodilation and profuse secretion from the mandibular and sublingual glands. The glandular vasodilation is due to bradykinin, an octapeptide produced by the action of kallikrein (a proteolytic enzyme) on plasma alpha$_2$ globulin (kininogen). Cholinolytic agents, such as atropine (a mixture of *l*- and *d*-hyoscine) and scopolamine (*l*-hyoscine) stop the hypersalivation that follows administration of cholinomimetics (pilocarpine) or electrical stimulation of the *chorda tympani.* Sympathomimetic drugs decrease production of serous and seromucous saliva, induce vasoconstriction of the salivary glands, and cause them to expel a small quantity of thick mucoid saliva. In *the cat,* abundant serous salivation follows administration of sympathomimetics. Denervation inhibits salivary secretion in all glands, but a paralytic salivary secretion appears in the mandibular glands 24 hours after section of the *chorda tympani,* and in the parotid glands 24 hours after vagotomy. This response is associated with greater susceptibility of the denervated glands to the action of endogenous epinephrine and norepinephrine.

Hormones and Salivary Secretion

From clinical studies, it is perceived that hormones influence salivary secretion. Hypersalivation is associated with enhanced secretion of gastric hydrochloric acid, which results from excessive production of gastrin. High concentrations of secretin increase secretion of seromucous saliva and of pharyngeal fluid.

In ruminants fed a sodium-depleting diet (fresh grass), the lower sodium and the higher potassium levels of parotid saliva follow a rise in the blood concentration of aldosterone.

In man, administration of secretin or of a secretin-CCK mixture increases the salivary amylase content.

Functions of Saliva

The universal functions of saliva are (1) to keep the buccal mucosa moist, (2) to physically (fluid) and chemically (lysozyme, bicarbonate, and mucin) prevent excessive growth of resident microorganisms that produce lactic acid and neutralize the bacterial acids that would dissolve away tooth enamel and be detrimental to dental hygiene, (3) to facilitate the initial digestive motor events, mastication and deglutition, with mucin that adheres to food and to mouth, forming a thin film that reduces friction, and (4) to solubilize substances that are able to stimulate gustatory and olfactory receptors.

In some animal species, salivary enzymes (amylase in swine, chickens, rats, rabbits; lipase in young ruminants) added to foods are operative in the stomach until they are inhibited by acid in gastric juice. Generally, saliva can selectively excrete particles such as chlorate, lead and antimony salts, bromides, and iodides. Additional salivary excretion of peptides such as glucagon, somatostatin, and renin also occurs.

The alkaline saliva of ruminants also serves many special purposes (Fig. 26–6). It supplies fluid and buffers to the ruminoreticulum to make it a medium for proper and efficient growth of microbial fauna and flora for digestion of proteins and fibrous carbohydrates in ingested foods. The quantity of liquid added daily may be twice that of the extracellular fluid (ECF). The salivary bicarbonate and phosphate can buffer the acids produced during fermentation and can maintain the pH of the ruminoreticulum within the normal range (5.8 to 7.0). A salivary gland–ruminoreticulum urea cycle, related to the ammonia cycle, is supported by salivary excretion of urea, which is reabsorbed

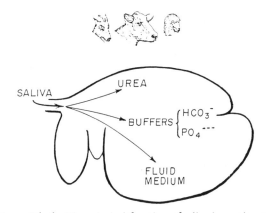

Figure 26–6 The principal functions of saliva in ruminants are to return urea to the rumen to maintain the salivary-ruminoreticulum urea cycle; to add fluid for proper microbial actions in the large ruminoreticulum fermentation vat; and to supply bicarbonate and phosphate buffers to keep the pH of the ruminoreticulum within normal limits (5.8 to 7.0).

through the ruminoreticulum wall. Salivary lysozyme has a bacteriostatic action.

Saliva contributes to the nondigestive thermoregulating function of evaporative cooling. This occurs in conjunction with panting (open-mouth polypnea) in the dog and the cat usually with the tongue protruding, or with panting and "gular flutter" (rapid oscillations of the gullet or floor of the mouth and upper throat) in birds.

DIGESTIVE SECRETION OF THE STOMACH

The mucosa lining the stomach produces several exocrine secretions: hydrochloric acid, pepsinogen (precursor of pepsin), soluble and insoluble mucus, bicarbonate-rich fluid, intrinsic factor, and basal alkaline fluid. In milk-fed preruminants, the abomasum juice also contains additional enzymes: rennin, or chymosin (milk-clotting enzyme), gastric lipase, and gelatinase. Gastric juice, a mixture of these secretions, can thus have quite a variable composition.

In nonruminants, the gastric secretion produced during the digestive (feeding or prandial) state is different from the one evolved during the interdigestive (fasting) period. The output of gastric juice during the digestive period is higher, and its composition is more complex. In pigs, in which food is stored in the cardiac glandular zone and slowly evacuated into the rest of the stomach, the secretion of gastric juice tends to be continuous, even if it is higher at feeding. In the dog, ingestion of 1 kg of food results in the production of a considerable volume of gastric secretion, about 1.3 L, compared with the slight salivary secretion (about 0.3 L).

In ruminants, the abomasal secretion is continuous and of uniform composition, except in preruminant animals, in which the flow of ingesta into the abomasum varies.

Mucosal barriers physically and chemically protect the gastric mucosa against digestion by its own major secretions, hydrochloric acid and pepsin. The gastric mucosal barrier is provided by mucus adherent to epithelial cells, by tight junctions between these epithelial cells, and by active transfer of H^+ and Cl^- ions out of the mucosa and of Na^+ ions into the plasma. This transfer of H^+ from within the crypts to the lumen occurs with a decreasing gradient: the pH is lower in the lumen than at the apical membrane.

The contribution of a surgeon of the United States Army, William BEAUMONT, stands unique in the annals of gastroenterology. His experiments and observations on the gastric juice and the physiology of digestion over nearly a decade (1825–1833) on his subject, Alexis ST. MARTIN, revolutionized scientific thought on gastric juice.

St. Martin survived an accidental shotgun discharge from a distance of a meter that hit him just under the left breast. A large portion of his side was blown off and openings were made into his lungs and stomach. Beaumont received, kept, nursed, medically and surgically treated, and sustained St. Martin, who recovered and lived with a 6-cm gastric fistula for over half a century.

The most important results of Beaumont's observations on gastric juice are his description of pure gastric juice, his analyses of its essential elements and its mucus, and the influence of emotions as well as of different foods and beverages on gastric mucosal appearance and secretion.

Origin of Gastric Secretions

The gastric mucosa is divided into nonsecretory, or nonglandular, and secretory, or glandular, zones of varying importance among species (Fig. 26–7). The *nonglandular zone* of the gastric mucosa is covered by a stratified squamous epithelium. This area occupies much of the stomach in rats and horses and all of the forestomachs of ruminants. In dogs and pigs, it is near the esophagogastric junction and takes up very little surface.

The *glandular zone* contains surface epithelial cells and gastric glands organized in pits and tubules. The epithelial cells on the surface of the mucosa produce insoluble mucus and a basal alkaline secretion. The organized glands of the gastric mucosa are regrouped into three specialized regions: the cardiac glands area; the gastric, or oxyntic glands, area; and the pyloric area (Fig. 26–8).

The *cardiac glands area* is important only in the pig, in which it occupies the cranial half of the stomach. The cardiac glands produce only insoluble mucus and basal alkaline fluid, which is plasmalike but contains more bicarbonate.

The *oxyntic glands area,* which is under the influence of gastrin, is largest in the stomach of the dog and the abomasum of ruminants (66 percent of total surface). In the pig and the horse, this area of oxyntic, parietal, and neck

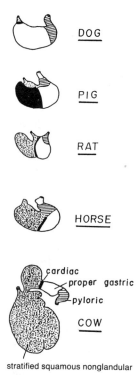

DOG

PIG

RAT

HORSE

cardiac
proper gastric
pyloric

COW

stratified squamous nonglandular

Figure 26–7 Relative importance of the nonglandular area of the stomach in the rat, the horse, and the cow. In the pig, the cardiac glandular area is almost the largest surface of the gastric mucosa.

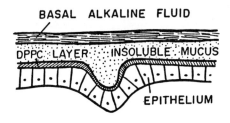

CARDIAC GLANDULAR AREA

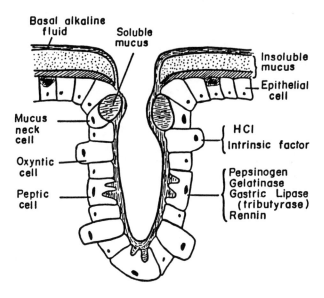

OXYNTIC GLANDULAR AREA

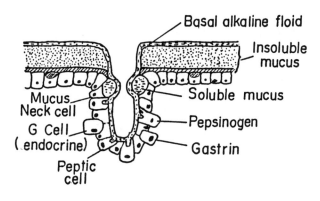

PYLORIC GLANDULAR AREA

Figure 26–8 Cellular arrangement of the specialized gastric secretory areas: cardiac, oxyntic, and pyloric. (DPPC, Dipalmitoylphosphatidyl choline.)

mucous cells has only half as much relative importance (33 percent of total surface). The secretory unit of the oxyntic glands is made of *parietal or oxyntic cells* that produce hydrochloric acid and gastric intrinsic factor; of *chief, or peptic, cells* that secrete proteins such as pepsinogen, gelatinase, gastric lipase, and rennin; and of *mucous neck cells,* which yield soluble mucus.

The *pyloric glands area,* near the gastroduodenal junction, adds soluble mucus and some pepsinogen. The G cells in the pyloric glands area are the source of gastrin, the major physiological hormonal stimulus for acid secretion.

Composition of Gastric Juice

Except in adult ruminants, which are always secreting abomasal juice, the composition of gastric juice changes with the interdigestive and digestive periods of digestion.

During the *interdigestive period of digestion,* when the stomach is void of food, the gastric glands do not secrete. Only the surface epithelial cells of the gastric mucosa produce the insoluble, or gel-forming, mucus and a constant basal alkaline fluid. The *insoluble mucus,* a mucin gel found all over the gastric mucosa, is released by exocytosis from surface mucous cells. It contains as much as 20 percent dipalmitoylphosphatidyl choline (DPPC), the substance of lung surfactant, which helps bind it to the epithelial cells. The insoluble fraction of mucus forms a layer of variable thickness (100 to 400 μm), and it imbibes the basal alkaline fluid. The *basal alkaline fluid* seems like an ultrafiltrate of plasma, which is rich in sodium, chloride, bicarbonate, and potassium but has very low concentrations of hydrogen ions and is without proteins. In the nonsecreting stomach, an active transfer of sodium and potassium occurs toward the submucosa. The luminal acid produced when the stomach is secreting totally inhibits absorption of sodium and also inhibits secretion of insoluble mucus, which precipitates as visible clumps.

The *digestive, or postprandial, period* includes the interval from the immediate prefeeding and actual feeding to the point when the stomach is empty of food. During this digestive interval, copious volumes of gastric juice are secreted. In ruminants, because of unceasing entry of digesta rich in volatile fatty acids into the abomasum, the production of abomasal juice is continuous.

Soluble mucus from the peptic and mucous neck cells of the oxyntic glands is discharged only after vagal excitation, to lubricate the digesta, and thus protect the gastric mucosa.

As the rate of digestive gastric secretion gets higher, the sodium concentration of the juice drops, the hydrogen concentration rises, and the chloride and potassium concentrations change only slightly. For every hydrogen ion actively secreted by the parietal cell, one bicarbonate ion diffuses into the blood, to create a phase of metabolic alkalosis known as the *alkaline tide.* These extra bicarbonate ions in the plasma are then excreted in the pancreatic juice or in the ileal fluid (horse and pig) to neutralize acidity (hydrochloric acid or VFAs) in the intestinal lumen.

The hydrochloric acid secreted in the stomach is isoosmotic with venous gastric blood. The concentration of hydrogen ions in gastric juice (150 mEq per L) is several million times greater than that of plasma (0.00004 mEq per L). The pH of gastric digesta during the postprandial period is between 2.5 and 6.

Pepsinogen, the inactive form of pepsin (proteolytic enzyme) is first activated by acid in the gastric lumen and then by pepsin itself in a positive-feedback process. In preruminants, the abomasal secretion of rennin decreases with age. The gastric intrinsic factor is a mucoprotein essential for the intestinal absorption of cyanocobalamin (vitamin B_{12}).

In the abomasal mucosa of ruminants and in the gastric mucosa of leaf-eating monkeys (langur), the levels of lysozyme C are many times higher than those of mammals lacking forestomachs. In ruminants and ruminant-like species, lysozyme C is a major digestive enzyme, helping make the bacteria that enter from the forestomachs available for digestion by the host's enzymes. Lysozyme C also resists digestion by pepsin.

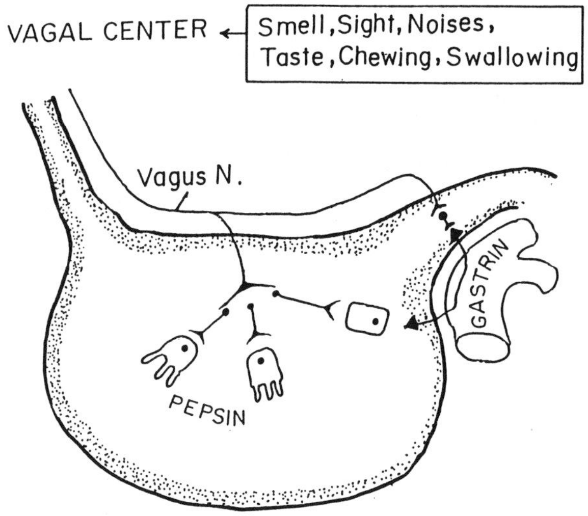

Control of Gastric Secretion

Gastric secretion is reflexly regulated by neuroendocrine mechanisms. Cholinergic and anticholinergic agents, gut hormones (gastrin, secretin, CCK), histamine, and prostaglandins influence the cellular output of substances in the gastric juice. Traditionally, in nonruminants the global secretion of gastric juice during the digestive period is considered to occur in three phases: cephalic, gastric, and intestinal. In ruminants, gastric (abomasal) secretion is continuous, as arrival of digesta from the nonglandular forestomachs into the glandular stomach is uninterrupted.

Cephalic Phase

Anticipation of food ingestion (smell, sight, preparation noises, accustomed times) and the presence of food in the mouth (taste, chewing, swallowing) activate an initial secretion of enzyme-rich gastric juice (Fig. 26–9). Acetylcholine-mediated impulses from the stimulated dorsal vagal motor centers are propagated mostly to the peptic (pepsin) cells and also to the oxyntic cells and to the gastrinogenic G cells. Secretin, from the mucosa of the small intestine, enhances secretion of the peptic cells while it inhibits the effect of gastrin on the oxyntic cells. The cephalic phase of gastric secretion is not important in nonruminants because it disappears following vagotomy and is of minimal importance in ruminants, since digesta is brought constantly into the abomasum from the omasum.

Gastric Phase

The major secretory acid response happens when food reaches the stomach and causes mechanical (distention) stimulation of the oxyntic and pyloric areas and chemical (proteins, amino acids, acidity) stimulation of the pyloric area (Fig. 26–10). In ruminants, the main stimulus to abomasal

VAGAL CENTER ← Smell, Sight, Noises, Taste, Chewing, Swallowing

Figure 26–9 Cephalic phase of gastric secretion in nonruminants. Acquired (conditioned) and natural (innate) oral stimuli acting during the vagally dependent phase.

secretion seems to be the amount of volatile fatty acids entering the abomasum. In lambs, during the first hours after birth the abomasum is deficient in parietal cells, and this lack of hydrochloric acid spares immunoglobulins from digestion. In preruminants, sucking or drinking milk causes the volume and the proteolytic contents (renin, pepsin) of abomasal juice to peak 1 to 3 hours after feeding. Cholinergic

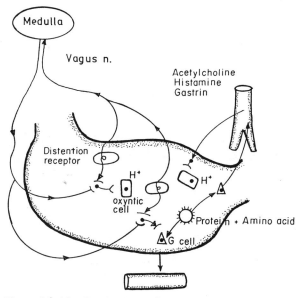

Figure 26–10 Gastric phase of gastric secretion in nonruminants. Distention of the stomach and ingesta directly stimulate cholinergic-mediated receptors in the oxyntic and pyloric areas and also induce a vagovagal reflex. These short and long reflexes increase the output of gastrin by G cells, which reinforces the stimulation of the oxyntic cells. Histamine and acetylcholine share the same effect.

reflexes, vagovagal and local, in the oxyntic and pyloric areas are responsible for the stimulation of the oxyntic cells (hydrochloric acid) and the antral G cells (gastrin). Histamine, cholinomimetics, and gastrin stimulate parietal cells by a similar mechanism, which is blocked by cholinolytics (atropine) and by histamine H_2 receptor–blocking agents (cimetidine, ranitidine). The gastric phase has more effects on oxyntic cells than on peptic cells. Gastrin, via the circulation, ultimately stimulates the oxyntic cells to secrete.

GIP antagonizes the action of gastrin on the acid-producing cells more than does CCK or secretin. Excessive acidification of the stomach (pH 2 or less) suppresses gastrin release (negative feedback) by the G cells. Some vagal fibers synapse with efferent fibers that are inhibitory to gastrin release. Prostaglandins inhibit gastric acid secretion by oxyntic cells.

Intestinal Phase

The protein products in the chyme expelled from the stomach cause release of duodenal gastrin (enterooxyntin of dog), which stimulates oxyntic cells to produce hydrochloric acid (Fig. 26–11). Other substances such as lipids and fatty acids result in liberation of duodenal CCK, secretin, and the most powerful of the inhibitors of gastrin, GIP. Hyperosmotic solutions and excessive acidity in the duodenum also inhibit gastric acid secretion.

Functions of Gastric Secretion

Some functions of hydrochloric acid are to kill microorganisms and to rupture cells to release their contents.

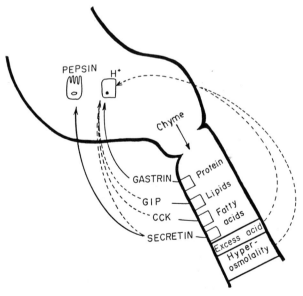

Figure 26–11 Intestinal phase of gastric secretion in nonruminants. Stimulation of oxyntic cells by gastrin and of peptic cells by secretin, both from the duodenum. Inhibition of gastrin effect is brought by other endocrines (GIP, CCK, secretin) and by excessive acidity or osmolality of the chyme emptied into the duodenum.

Hydrochloric acid lowers the gastric luminal pH for proper action of the proteolytic enzymes pepsin and rennin. Destruction of bacteria by acid chyme also prevents colonization of the proximal small intestine by undesirable microorganisms.

In neonatal preruminants, the optimal pH for milk clotting and for proteolysis is not the same. The optimal pH for coagulation of milk is 6.5 for rennin and 5.3 for pepsin, whereas for proteolysis it is 3.5 for rennin and 2.1 for pepsin. The relative activity of rennin is about half that of pepsin in the growing calf or lamb. The abomasum retains the casein curd to allow time for effective proteolysis, and the clot formed after a meal entraps most of the milk fat, and even some of the clot remaining from a previous meal. Pepsin transforms proteins into peptides.

In the pig and the horse, the fluid from the cardiac glands is rich in bicarbonate and mucus and tends to have a higher pH. This bicarbonate-mucus mixture neutralizes VFAs formed after fermentation of food in the large cardiac area in the pig or the nonglandular or squamous epithelium area in the horse.

The gastric intrinsic factor is a protein secreted by the parietal cells (cat, guinea pig, monkey, ox, rabbit) or chief cells (mouse, rat) of the gastric mucosa, and by mucous cells in the pyloric area and duodenum (hog). It unites with vitamin B_{12} to form a complex that is absorbed in the ileum. Like acid secretion, the output of intrinsic factor is stimulated by histamine, pentagastrin, and cholinergic agents but is inhibited by cimetidine (histamine H_2 receptor–blocking agent). Gelatinase liquefies gelatin.

EXOCRINE SECRETION OF THE PANCREAS

The exocrine secretion of the pancreas is an alkaline fluid, isoosmotic to blood plasma, that neutralizes the gastric acid in the duodenum. It also contains enzymes to complete the breakdown of protein, starch, and fat in the chyme. In some species (horse, pig) the pancreatic juice also contributes most of the buffering fluid needed to create a proper fermentation medium in the lumen of the large intestine. This role is similar to that of saliva in the ruminoreticulum fermentation reservoir of ruminants.

In 1824, after cannulation of the pancreatic duct of a horse, LEURET and LASSAIGNE obtained 85 mL (3 ounces) of a clear alkaline fluid. Applications of vinegar to the duodenal mucosa increased the rate of secretion.

In 1902, in a demedullated dog (with extirpated celiac and mesenteric ganglia), BAYLISS and STARLING showed that intraduodenal injection of hydrochloric acid and intravenous injection of an acid extract of the duodenal mucosa each caused pancreatic secretion to increase.

Pancreatic juice enters the duodenum through a separate duct in dogs, cats, cows, horses, pigs, and rabbits. However, in sheep, goats, and rats, the pancreatic duct joins with the bile duct to form a common biliary-pancreatic duct, which adds a mixture of bile and pancreatic juice to chyme (Fig. 26–12). Pancreatic juice is secreted in response to

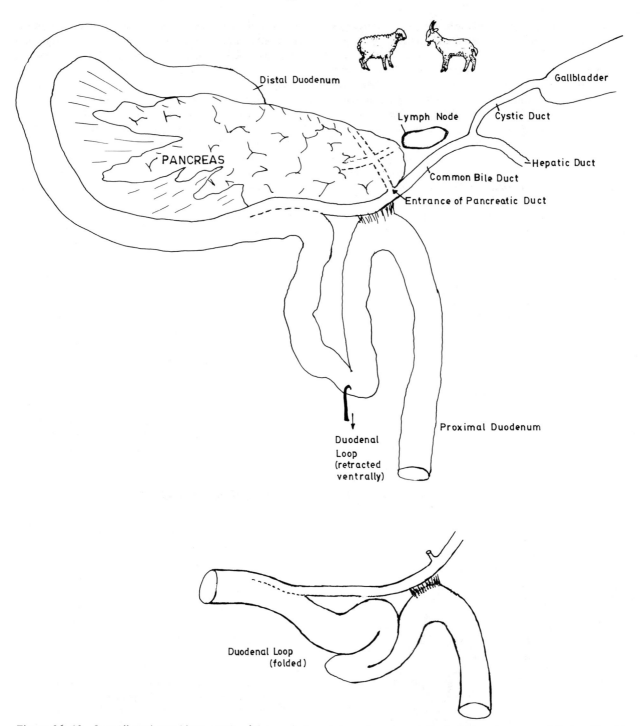

Figure 26–12   In small ruminants (sheep, goat) and the camel, the exocrine pancreatic secretion drains into the common bile duct 10 to 12 cm from its junction with the duodenum. The duodenal entrance of the common bile duct is just caudad to an inverted-S reflection of the duodenum. The proximal attachment is to the common bile duct at a point opposite the junction of the pancreatic duct, and the distal attachment is at the beginning of a semicircular union of the duodenum to the edge of the pancreas.

neuroendocrine stimuli, mostly associated with the vagus nerve and with the gut hormones secretin and CCK.

Origin of Pancreatic Juice

The exocrine pancreatic secretion originates in a system of acini and ducts, which is a secretory unit ("pancreaton") structurally and functionally similar to salivon, the basic secretory unit of the salivary glands. The acinar cells of the *pancreaton* secrete a primary pancreatic fluid into a small duct, which has walls with cells that can modify the composition of the initial secretion. Eventually, these units converge into one or more larger pancreatic ducts, which discharge the isotonic pancreatic juice into the duodenum.

The pancreatic arterial capillaries carry blood directly to the acini, and other capillaries arrive also at the acini after having irrigated the islets of Langerhans in the endocrine pancreas (Fig. 26–13). Sympathetic innervation (vasoconstriction) is limited to arterioles, while many cholinergic fibers reach acini and ducts of the pancreaton and islets of Langerhans. Pancreatic secretory activity raises basal blood flow by as much as fivefold.

The acinar cells produce a primary fluid containing electrolytes (sodium, potassium, calcium, magnesium) with enzymes (amylase, lipase) and proenzymes, or zymogens (procarboxypolypeptidase, trypsinogen, chymotrypsino-

gen). According to the prevailing theory, pancreatic enzymes are always secreted in parallel as granules in cytoplasmic vesicles extruded by exocytosis at the apical membrane of the acinar cells. In sheep, pancreatic enzymes are not always secreted in parallel. An alternative concept proposes that pancreatic enzymes are released from cytoplasmic storage pools and secreted immediately in response to specific end-products of digestion.

The cells in the walls of the ducts of the pancreatons are responsible for secretion of water and bidirectional transfer of electrolytes (sodium, potassium, bicarbonate, chloride) but keep pancreatic juice isotonic to plasma at any rate of flow (Fig. 26–14).

Bicarbonate and chloride are secreted by all the duct cells of the pancreaton, but those near the acini secrete mostly bicarbonate. If the secretion rate is low, the distal cells of the duct passively reabsorb bicarbonate in exchange for secretion of chloride. At high rates of secretion, little bicarbonate is reabsorbed by the distal cells of the ducts.

Secretion of bicarbonate is an active process involving the production of hydrogen ions, which are actively transferred out of the ductule cells into the plasma in exchange for sodium (Fig. 26–15). The active exchange of sodium for hydrogen ions is altered by drugs that inhibit epithelial transport of sodium, such as ouabain (cardiac glycoside) and ethacrynic acid (diuretic). This pancreatogenic acidification of plasma causes an *"acid tide,"* which neutralizes the gastrogenic *alkaline tide* associated with the production of hydrochloric acid. The plasma carbon dioxide resulting from this neutralization diffuses back into the ductule cells and, with the help of carbonic anhydrase, is reconverted into bicarbonate, which is actively secreted into the ductule pancreatic juice. The cellular conversion of carbon dioxide into bicarbonate may be hindered by inhibitors of carbonic anhydrase such as acetazolamide (diuretic).

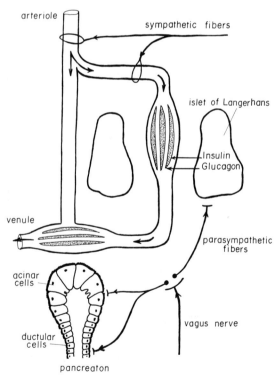

Figure 26–13 Diagrammatic arrangement of capillaries and postganglionic sympathetic and parasympathetic fibers at the functional endocrine (islet of Langerhans) and exocrine ("pancreaton") units. Sympathetic fibers are restricted to the arterioles.

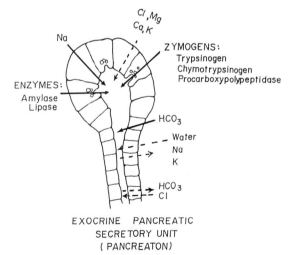

Figure 26–14 Acinar cells of the pancreaton secrete enzymes, zymogens, and electrolytes. Proximal ductule cells produce most of the bicarbonate. At low secretion rates, bicarbonate is exchanged for chloride in the distal duct cells.

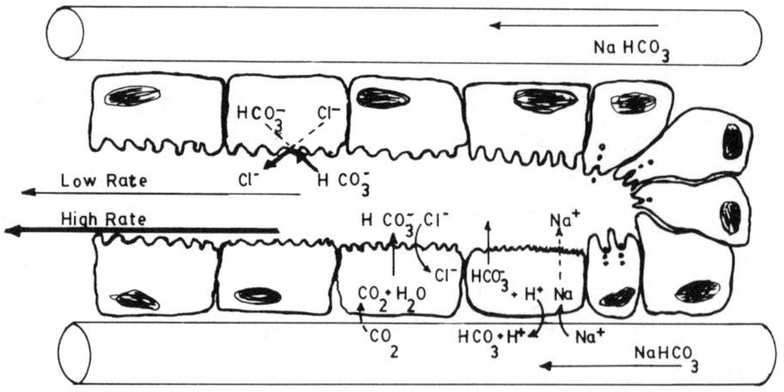

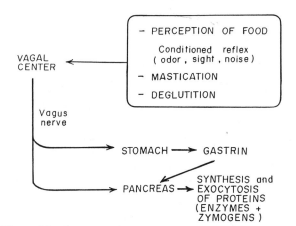

Figure 26–15 Acidification of pancreatic venous blood during secretion of alkaline fluid. H^+ is pumped into blood in exchange for Na^+, which then diffuses out of the cells into the duct fluid. Plasma carbon dioxide diffuses into the cells of the ductules, where it is converted to HCO_3^-, which is then actively excreted into the fluid produced in the proximal portion of the ductules. At high secretion rates, pancreatic juice is rich in bicarbonate. At low secretion rates, it is rich in chloride, which is exchanged for bicarbonate.

Composition of Pancreatic Juice

Concentrations of sodium and potassium in pancreatic juice are similar to those in plasma at all flow rates. So are bicarbonate and chloride levels at the basal rate of pancreatic secretion. As the production rate increases, the concentration values of these ions become reciprocal: the quantity of chloride falls, and that of bicarbonate reaches the former value of chloride. In the horse, this change is not seen; chloride and bicarbonate are equal at all flow rates. Pancreatic juice is isotonic to plasma.

The output of pancreatic juice in large animal species differs; approximate daily values are for the horse, 11 L per 100 kg; for the cow, 4 L per 100 kg; and for the sheep, 1 L per 100 kg. The profuse volume of pancreatic juice dilutes the enzymes in the pancreatic juice of the horse, and the rate of enzyme secretion appears to be extremely low in comparison with those of other species. In small animals (dog, cat), the basal (interdigestive, unstimulated) pancreatic secretory rate is negligible, but the flow during the digestive (stimulated) state is over 2 mL per minute.

The proteolytic enzymes are secreted as zymogens (i.e., inactive enzymes or proenzymes), whereas amylase and lipase are secreted as active enzymes. The activation of the proteolytic zymogens in the intestinal lumen by trypsin is an example of positive feedback. Trypsin is originally activated by an enzyme from the duodenal mucosa, enterokinase. A substance known as trypsin inhibitor prevents premature activation of trypsinogen and autolysis of pancreatic tissue. In the duodenum, the optimal pH for pancreatic enzymes (lipase, amylase, trypsin, chymotrypsin, carboxypolypeptidase) activity is near neutral.

Control of Pancreatic Secretion

Pancreatic secretion is controlled by cholinergic nerve fibers and by gut hormones (gastrin, CCK, secretin). In a manner similar to gastric secretion, regulation of pancreatic secretion is divided into three phases: cephalic, gastric, and intestinal.

Cephalic Phase

The vagal autonomic nervous system is essential for the occurrence of this initial step of pancreatic secretion. The perceptions of food (odor, sight, noise) and the contact of food with the mouth (mastication) and pharynx (deglutition) are sent to the bulbar vagal centers, from which vagal fibers convey effector signals directly to the pancreas and to the stomach (Fig. 26–16). The acetylcholine-mediated pancreatic responses are scanty secretion of an enzyme-rich juice and synthesis of new enzymes. The stomach's response is to raise the output of gastrin, which besides its oxyntic effect, stimulates apical exocytosis of proteins by acinar cells in pancreatons. Thus, in the cephalic phase of pancreatic secretion, the enzyme content is directly increased. The cephalic phase of pancreatic secretion is unimportant in ruminants.

Gastric Phase

Distention of the stomach stimulates neural and endocrine events (Fig. 26–17). One entirely neural response is a vagovagal reflex (gastropancreatic reflex). In this long pathway reflex, gastric mechanoreceptors send signals to the bulbar area through the vagus, and efferent signals are sent to the stomach and the pancreas, also via the vagus. A short pathway reflex (local) is the cholinergic release of gastrin. Both direct vagal stimuli and gastrin increase the exocytosis and the synthesis of enzymes but have little immediate action on volume and bicarbonate.

In the horse and the pig, the cephalic and the gastric phases of pancreatic secretion increase not only the enzymes but also the volume and the bicarbonate concentration of pancreatic juice. In the horse, the enzyme output is much smaller than in the pig. In ruminants, in which abomasal distention by digesta is continuous, the gastric phase is unimportant.

Figure 26–16 In nonruminants, the perception of food and conditioned reflexes induce a vagally dependent cephalic phase of exocrine pancreatic secretion. A small volume of protein-rich (enzymes, zymogens) pancreatic juice is secreted.

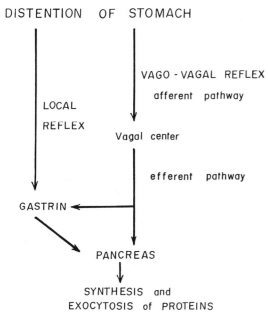

Figure 26–17   Endocrine and neural events during the gastric phase (distention of the stomach) of exocrine pancreatic secretion in nonruminants.

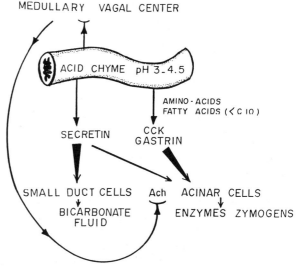

Figure 26–18   Neural and hormonal events during the intestinal phase of exocrine pancreatic secretion.

Intestinal Phase

Arrival of acid chyme (pH 3 to 4.5) into the duodenal lumen starts the principal (75 percent) secretin-mediated phase of pancreatic secretion. The small intestine mucosa contributes other gut hormones that influence pancreatic secretion, CCK, VIP, gastrin, enteroglucagon, and GIP.

Only during this limited pH window is a large amount of secretin released from a zone of the duodenal mucosa containing the inactive form of the hormone (prosecretin). Acting through cAMP mediation, secretin is the most potent stimulus for duct cell production of water and bicarbonate. Secretin exerts only a weak effect on exocytosis and synthesis of pancreatic enzymes by acinar cells (Fig. 26–18). By comparison with the basal pancreatic secretion, the effect of secretin (five to 10 times greater in the dog than in the sheep) is to raise the production of pancreatic juice as much as 150 times. In the sheep, exposure to cold increases the production of thyroxine (T_3) and the rate of gastrointestinal transit, both leading to greater output of secretin and 50 percent more pancreatic juice daily. Secretin (half-life: 3 minutes) is metabolized at the kidney. VIP, glucagon, and GIP are related to secretin (three amino acids in common) and all do increase the amount of water and bicarbonate in pancreatic juice. Since their effect is much less potent, when VIP and glucagon compete with secretin on acinar receptors they may reduce the total effect of secretin on pancreatic juice.

CCK is released mainly by L-amino acids (tryptophan, phenylalanine, valine) and fatty acids (oleic) with more than 10 carbons. Through cGMP, which mobilizes and activates intracellular calcium, CCK stimulates mostly exocytosis of acinar enzymes, but it also increases secretion of bicarbonate and greatly potentiates secretin effects on bicarbonate secretion. Gastrin and CCK share a five–amino acid sequence and belong to the same family of gut hormones. Gastrin stimulates the formation and exocytosis of pancreatic enzymes.

Chymodenin (*chymo*trypsinogen-trypsinogen *d*uodenal stimul*in*), a candidate gut hormone from the duodenum liberated by protein, causes a specific increase in the pancreatic production of chymotrypsinogen.

Acetylcholine produced locally contributes to the release of secretin and of CCK. Also, through a vagovagal or enteropancreatic (long) reflex, acetylcholine sensitizes the pancreas to the action of both secretin and CCK. Thus, acetylcholine assists the production of both ductal bicarbonate and acinar enzymes by the pancreatons. Vagotomy abolishes the cephalic phase and greatly decreases the importance of the intestinal phase of pancreatic secretion. Adrenergic stimulation is inhibitory to pancreatic bicarbonate secretion (alpha-adrenergic more so than beta-adrenergic).

Functions of Pancreatic Juice

The principal functions of pancreatic juice are to neutralize the acid chyme in the lumen of the small intestine with bicarbonate; to supply the large intestine of omnivores (pig) and of some herbivores (horse) with a large quantity of isoosmotic fluid for fermentation of food in their postgastric digestor (the cecocolic part of the large intestine); and to provide proteolytic, amylolytic, and lipolytic enzymes that operate on specific substrates at a neutral or slightly alkaline pH. Amylase hydrolyzes starch to maltose, maltotriose, and dextrins. With emulsification of fat droplets by bile salts, lipase hydrolyzes triglycerides to free fatty acids, monoglycerides, and intermediate triglyceride forms, and glycerol. The activated exopeptidase (carboxypeptidase) cleaves from the ends of the protein molecule, whereas the activated endopeptidases (trypsin and chymotrypsin) cleave peptide bonds within the protein molecule.

BILE SECRETION

In the liver, the largest gland of the body, bile formation (choleresis) is continuous. As a general rule, the delivery of this exocrine secretion into the duodenum is intermittent in monogastric species (dog, horse) and continuous in ruminants.

In animals without a gallbladder (camel, deer, dove, elephant, elk, giraffe, horse, moose, pigeon, pocket gopher, rat), the easily distended hepatic duct delivers bile directly into the lumen of the small intestine. In animals with only intermittent needs for bile, the sphincter of Oddi restricts the entrance of bile into the duodenum between digestive periods. The duodenal entrance and the morphology of this biliary sphincter are not identical in all species (Fig. 26–19). During this storage period, bile is concentrated in the gallbladder (a blind sac at the end of the cystic duct, which is a branch of the hepatic duct).

The common bile duct (i.e., terminal end of the hepatic duct [horse] or fusion of the cystic and hepatic ducts [cow,

pig]), discharges bile into the duodenum. In some animals (cat, dog, horse) the pancreatic and common bile ducts penetrate the duodenum close together (Fig. 26–20). In the sheep and the goat, the pancreatic duct empties directly into the common bile duct so that a mixture of bile and pancreatic juice enters the duodenum (see Fig. 26–12).

In the rabbit, in which the pancreatic duct and the bile duct enter the duodenum separately, Claude BERNARD showed that fat absorption occurred only after hydrolysis by lipase and emulsification by bile salts.

In the dog, DASTRE transferred the opening of the bile duct from the duodenum to the proximal jejunum and observed that fat absorption occurred only caudad to the site of delivery of bile.

Bile contains mainly bile salts (tauro- and glycobiliary acid derivatives), bile pigments (bilirubin, biliverdin), electrolytes, and phospholipids (cholesterol, lecithin). The concentrating gallbladder in some animals (e.g., dog) absorbs water, chloride, and bicarbonate from bile and secretes mucin, and increases the concentrations of some components by several-fold (Table 26–2).

Bile acids secreted by the liver are required for emulsification and digestion of lipids in chyme made slightly alkaline by the addition of hepatic and pancreatic bicarbonate. Their almost complete (95 percent) recovery in the

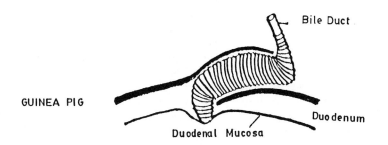

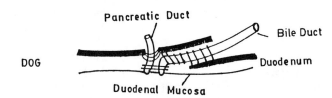

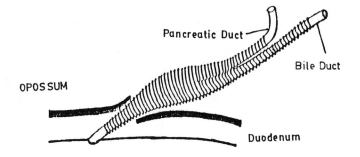

Figure 26–19 Different types of biliary sphincters in the duodenum of the guinea pig, the dog, and the opossum.

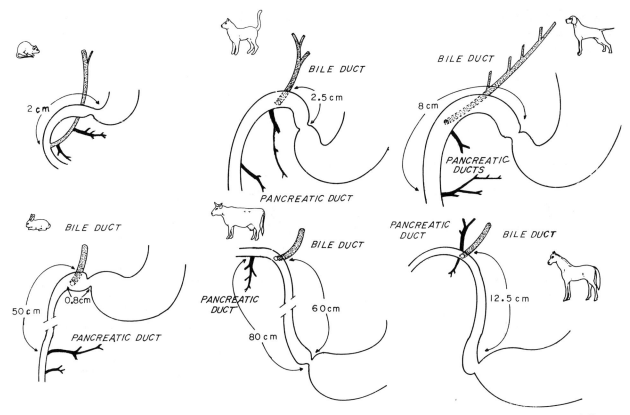

Figure 26–20 Diagrammatic arrangement and localization of the common bile duct, the pancreatic duct, and their openings in different animals.

ileum and their return to the liver by the portal circulation establishes an enterohepatic circulation of bile salts, which is important for choleresis. Bile pigments and cholesterol are excretion products from the organism. The control of bile secretion is by neurohumoral mechanisms.

Origin of Bile

Isoosmotic bile is generated continuously by a functional hepatic secretory unit, the *hepaton,* somewhat analogous to the salivon and the pancreaton. The hepatocytes drain bile into an initial bile canaliculus, which has walls with cells able to modify the composition of the primary

TABLE 26–2 Mean Content of Some Substances in Canine Hepatic and Gallbladder Biles (mmol/L), and Their GB/HEP Ratios

	Hepatic Bile	Gallbladder Bile	Ratio Gb/Hep
Bicarbonate	50	10	0.2
Bile salts	35	315	9.0
Calcium	06	30	5.0
Chloride	80	05	0.06
Potassium	07	07	1.0
Sodium	175	80	0.5

bile. In less than 9 seconds, blood is transferred via the hepatic sinusoids from the hepatic arterioles and portal venules in the portal triads to the central vein (Fig. 26–21). The structures provided to circulate blood, plasma, and bile are the hepatic sinusoids, the space of Disse, and the biliary canaliculi (Fig. 26–22).

The sinusoids carry arterial and portal blood from the portal triad to the central vein of each liver lobule. Their permeable endothelium excludes blood cells but allows plasma in the space of Disse to bathe the hepatocytes. Each of these rows of adjacent hepatocytes forms a functional secretory unit that sends bile in a microscopic bile canaliculus that is continued by an epithelial cell–lined ductule (cholangiole). The canaliculi coalesce into bile ducts carried in portal triads, and these eventually join into the large duct that leads bile into the lumen of the small intestine (Fig. 26–23).

The primary bile, actively produced by the hepatocytes, undergoes modifications as it progresses from the canaliculi into the bile ducts. Substances from plasma are rapidly taken up by the hepatocytes by active transport (e.g., bile acids), less rapidly by facilitated diffusion, and slowly by pinocytosis, or by a combination of these processes. Materials required for syntheses or excretion may bind to cell components and accumulate in hepatocytes (e.g., bile acids, free bilirubin) to be conjugated before their release from the liver cells. Passage from the hepatocytes to bile is by active processes. Water and solutes are transported through the

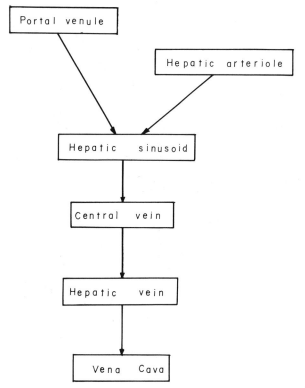

Figure 26–21 Blood flow through the hepatic lobule to the vena cava.

intercellular space according to osmotic and electrochemical gradients, rather than through the cell cytoplasm. Solutes and water may be reabsorbed or added by the epithelial cells lining the ductules (Fig. 26–24).

Composition of Bile

Bile, a fluid isotonic to plasma, is made up of water (95.5 to 97.5 percent), with secretory substances (bile salts and lecithin) and excretory substances (bile pigments, cholesterol, and xenobiotics) dissolved in an alkaline electrolyte solution (sodium, potassium, calcium, chloride, and bicarbonate) similar to pancreatic juice (Table 26–3). The composition of the diet influences the pH of bile (7.4 to 8.0); for example, meats acidify, and plants alkalinize. The composition of bile varies according to animal species and to the extent of the concentration and secretory processes in the extrahepatic biliary tract (gallbladder, common bile duct).

Biliary Acids

Bile salts account for more than 50 percent of the total solids of bile. The primary bile salts (sodium and potassium salts of cholic and chenodeoxycholic acids conjugated with glycine or taurine) are formed in the liver from cholesterol (80 percent). Characteristically, bile acids are preferentially conjugated with taurine in carnivores, with glycine in herbivores, and with both glycine and taurine in omnivorous species. In some animal species, the liver converts chenodeoxycholic acid into trihydroxycholanic acids (hyocholic acid in the pig, and alpha- and beta-muricholic acids in rat and mouse), which can be considered as primary bile acids in these animals. The primary bile salts play an important role in digestion, and their conservation by an ileal-hepatic (enterohepatic) circulation is important for the economy of the animal body. Besides bile salts, other substances are also recycled from the intestine (e.g., pancreatic enzymes, indomethacin, phenolsulphonphthalein). Because of their strong ionization, their reabsorption is limited mostly to the distal ileum. Bile salts are recirculated at least twice during a meal, several times in a day, and possibly about 20 times before elimination in the feces. Only about 5 percent of the bile salt pool is normally lost per recirculation, and it is replaced by equivalent bile salt synthesized in the liver. The presence of an excessive quantity of conjugated unreabsorbed (primary) and bacteria-deconjugated (secondary) bile salts in the large intestine may lead to diarrhea by inhibition of sodium ion transport.

Secondary unconjugated bile salts (deoxycholic, lithocholic, and hyodeoxycholic in the pig), found in the

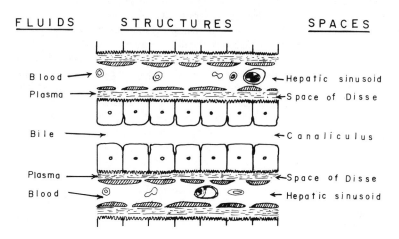

Figure 26–22 Relationship of fluids, structures and spaces involved in the secretion of bile.

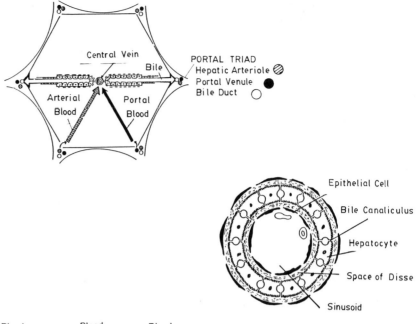

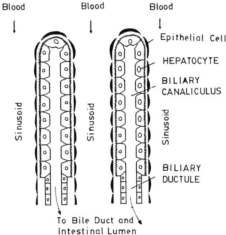

Figure 26–23 **Top,** Diagram of the paths of hepatic arterial and portal venous blood, and of bile. Blood from the portal triad (arterial and venous) flows in the sinusoids toward the central vein. Bile in the canaliculi is directed into the ductules (small ducts) and then into the bile duct in the portal triad of the hepatic lobule. **Center,** Representation of the configuration of hepatocytes around the hepatic sinusoid. **Bottom,** Schematic representation of the functional exocrine secretory unit (hepaton) of the liver.

feces as a result of bacterial action on the primary bile salts, are excretory products. Reabsorption of lithocholic acid would be harmful to the animal organism (pyrogenic, liver damage). Normally, unconjugated bile salts are not found in bile, but they may occur as a result of enterohepatic recirculation of unconjugated bile acids formed after microbial action in the lower gut. Passive reabsorption of unconjugated bile salts is possible throughout the small intestine.

Lecithin

Lecithin is converted to lysolecithin (lysophosphatidylcholine) and glycerylphosphorylcholine by phospholipases in the duodenum. Lysolecithin is reabsorbed as the major phospholipid of chylomicrons. In the sheep, lecithin (phosphatidylcholine) is the principal (95 percent) phospholipid of bile.

Bile Pigments

Metabolites of spent hemoglobin, biliverdin and its reduction product bilirubin, impart a greenish-yellow (biliverdin) to brownish-yellow (bilirubin) coloration to bile and are responsible for its bitter taste. At the end of the life span of erythrocytes (about 70 days in the cat and the pig and more than 110 days in the dog, the horse, and ruminants), hemoglobin is liberated from the ghost cells. The free hemoglobin is broken down by reticuloendothelial cells in liver, spleen, and bone marrow, which produce biliverdin and its reduction product, bilirubin.

Bilirubin binds immediately to plasma albumin for transport to the hepatocytes. The liver cells return albumin to plasma and conjugate bilirubin with glucuronide (80 percent) and sulfate (10 percent) radicals to increase its solubility in bile (Fig. 26–25). Glucuronyl transferase also

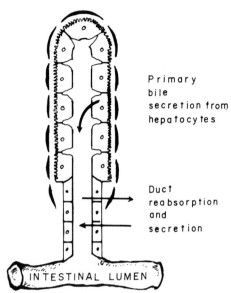

Figure 26–24 Modulation of the composition of primary bile within the secretory unit and the small ducts of the bile system.

TABLE 26–3 Composition of Ovine Bile, Pancreatic Juice, and Blood Plasma (mmol/L)

	Bile	*Pancreatic Juice*	*Plasma*
Bicarbonate	23	28	26
Bile salts	11	—	—
Chloride	118	123	114
Potassium	04.4	04.6	04.8
Sodium	150	147	146

those of the plasma and pancreatic juice (see Table 26–3). Mixed bile of the cat and rabbit has a somewhat higher bicarbonate and a somewhat lower chloride content (Table 26–4), and canine hepatic bile follows a similar trend.

Eighty percent of cholesterol is excreted in the form of biliary acids, but some is still present in bile. Bile is the major route for excretion of calcium in the feces. Some mucin is contributed by goblet cells and deep epithelial glands in the distal portion of the common bile duct.

Through bile, the liver removes many xenobiotic substances from plasma (e.g., sulfanilamides, antibiotics, cardiac glucosides, dyes, and porphyrins). The rate of removal of the dye sulfobromophthalein (bromsulphalein, or BSP) is used to evaluate the functional capacity of hepatocytes and the hepatic blood flow. In Southdown sheep and in cattle, deficient biliary excretion of porphyrin metabolites of chlorophyll is associated with a dermatosis resulting from the effect of light on the porphyrin-laden skin.

catalyzes conjugation of numerous natural (e.g., steroids) and xenobiotic substances. Drugs (e.g., phenobarbital) stimulate hepatic synthesis of glucuronyl transferase. Unconjugated bilirubin and urobilinogens formed by the action of bacteria in the intestine and reabsorbed in the portal circulation are reexcreted in bile or in urine. Antibiotics and xenobiotics are also subject to enterohepatic circulation.

Total plasma bilirubin includes conjugated and unconjugated bilirubin. Unconjugated bilirubin is measured as the indirect-reacting bilirubin (indirect van den Bergh reaction, requiring alcohol), and conjugated bilirubin as the direct-reacting bilirubin (direct van den Bergh, without alcohol) (Fig. 26–26).

Hyperbilirubinemia causes icterus (yellowness of the plasma, the sclera, and the mucous membranes). In icterus due to bile duct obstruction, the plasma level of conjugated bilirubin is elevated. Hyperbilirubinemia with an increase in the unconjugated bilirubin occurs because of excessive hemolysis and of functional problems in hepatocytes (decreased uptake, conjugation, lack of glucuronyl transferase, and secretion). A strain of rat, the Gunn rat, has an inherited glucuronyl transferase deficiency and is unable to conjugate bilirubin with glucuronic acid. Homozygous Gunn rats have chronic nonhemolytic unconjugated hyperbilirubinemia. Bile pigments in excess are systemically toxic.

Upon contact with air, bilirubin rapidly oxidizes to biliverdin. Bovine bile produced in summer is yellowish-brown (bilirubin), whereas winter bile is green (biliverdin). Upon exposure to air and light, urobilinogens and urobilins give the characteristic orange-brown color to feces.

Other Constituents of Bile

In sheep, in which bile does not remain a long time in the gallbladder, electrolytes of hepatic bile approximate

Functions of the Gallbladder

The extrahepatic biliary tract consists of the hepatic duct, the cystic duct, the gallbladder (if present), the common bile duct, and the sphincter of Oddi. The gallbladder and the sphincter of Oddi form an operative negative-feedback system. During the interdigestive period (between meals), the sphincter of Oddi is tonically active, or contracted, whereas the gallbladder is inactive and dilated. Conversely, during the digestive (prandial and immediate postprandial) period, the cystic duct and the gallbladder are actively pulsating, whereas the sphincter of Oddi relaxes and contracts phasically.

Hepatic bile flows into the gallbladder when the sphincter of Oddi is closed. In the gallbladder, the stored bile is modified. As bile accumulates, the extensive folds of the gallbladder mucosa are smoothed out, without appreciably increasing the intravesical pressure. The gallbladder is equally efficient to concentrate bile in all animal species. The extent of the concentration is directly related to the duration of storage—slight because of a short retention time in ruminants, considerable due to long storage in carnivores. In dogs, gallbladder absorption proceeds more slowly at night than during the day.

The cells of the gallbladder mucosa add mucin and hydrogen ions and actively reabsorb sodium, which leads to passive transfer of water and other electrolytes (chloride, bicarbonate). The other components of bile increase by several-fold (calcium, bile salts and pigments, lecithin, and cholesterol) but form micelles, which lower osmolal activity

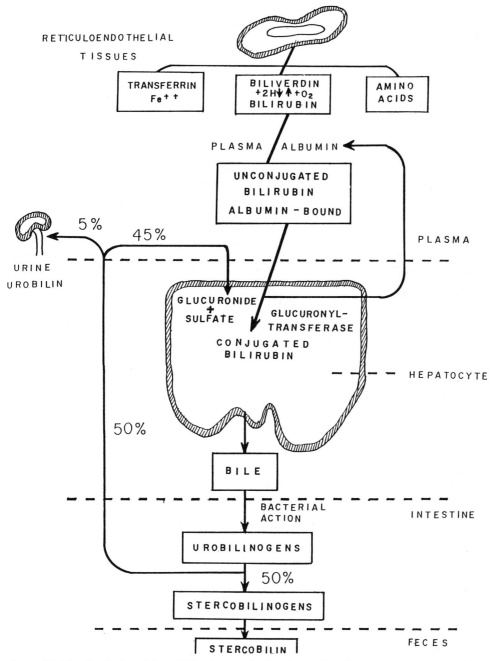

Figure 26–25 Synthesis and fate of bile pigments in the plasma, the bile, and the small intestine. An enterohepatic circulation of the bile pigments (45 percent of reabsorbed urobilinogens) occurs, in a manner similar to that for bile salts.

and tend to keep vesical bile isoosmolal to hepatic bile and plasma. When less soluble salts or substances are present in excess, the concentrating effect of the gallbladder can lead to stone formation.

Emptying of the gallbladder by contraction of its smooth muscle is brought about by a neurohumoral mechanism involving negative feedback on the sphincter of Oddi. The gallbladder is aroused by feeding and by arrival at the duodenum of chyme rich in lipids and in protein hydroly-

sates. In the dog, enhancement of gallbladder motility accompanies the presence of continuous irregular electromyographical spiking activity (ISA) on the proximal small intestine. The neural component is mostly motor vagal impulses originating with stimulation of the cephalic phase of gastric acid secretion and liberation of gastrin and thyrotropin-releasing hormone (TRH) in the dog. The humoral part is due to production of CCK by the mucosa of the proximal small intestine, which is stimulated by lipids and

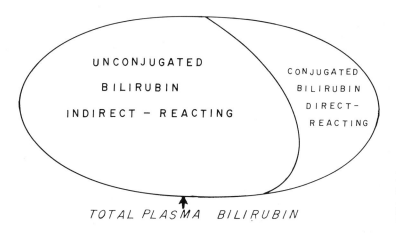

Figure 26–26 Elements of total plasma bilirubin and their van den Bergh reactions: indirect for unconjugated or free bilirubin and direct for conjugated bilirubin.

TABLE 26–4 Electrolytes in the Bile of Different Animals (mmol/L)

	Cat	Dog	Rabbit	Sheep
Bicarbonate	31	50	46	23
Calcium	—	06	04.7	—
Chloride	91	80	84	118
Magnesium	—	—	0.5	—
Potassum	03.1	07	06.9	04.4
Sodium	138	175	148	150

peptides. CCK released into the bloodstream acts to stimulate smooth muscle cells of the gallbladder and to inhibit those of the sphincter of Oddi. A neurogenic or myogenic short inhibitory reflex, which originates from the contracting gallbladder and the duodenal peristalsis, supports the relaxing effect of CCK on the sphincter of Oddi (Fig. 26–27). In the sheep, the gallbladder contracts more frequently at pasture and when feeding. Gallbladder emptying

occurs during the irregular spiking activity (IRA) phase of the migrating myoelectrical complex (MMC) on the ovine small intestine. Substances that stimulate the gallbladder to contract (CCK; a decapeptide, caerulein, isolated from frog skin) are called *cholagogues*. Gallbladder motility is inhibited by atropine.

The sphincter of Oddi contracts after administration of acetylcholine and relaxes in response to epinephrine. In the opossum, experimental oral dosing of 30 percent ethanol (10 mL) increases the electromyographical activity of the sphincter of Oddi without causing a concomitant rise in motor activity of the stomach and duodenum.

Control of the Secretion of Bile

Formation of bile by the hepatocytes, or *choleresis*, is stimulated by active reabsorption of conjugated biliary acids, by passive reabsorption of deconjugated biliary acids, and by

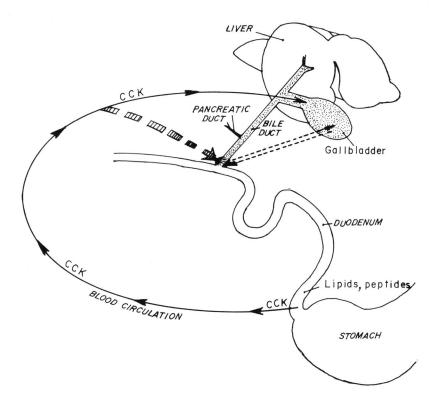

Figure 26–27 Neurohumoral control of gallbladder emptying. Nervous negative-feedback mechanisms operate between the gallbladder and the sphincter of Oddi (dashed lines). CCK also exerts positive (gallbladder) and negative (sphincter of Oddi) activations.

neurohumoral mechanisms. The hourly continuous secretion of bile is about 0.25 mL per kg in a fasting animal and reaches a peak output of about 1.0 mL per kg in a feeding animal. Substances that stimulate hepatocytes to secrete bile are called *choleretics*.

Bile acids are strong choleretics, but bile salts have little choleretic activity. Exclusion of bile acids from the intestine causes about 25 percent of the lipids ingested to appear in the feces and malabsorption of lipid-soluble vitamins. Experimental impediment to the ileal reabsorption of bile salts also causes fatty stools, because liver bile acid synthesis cannot be increased to compensate for the loss in the feces.

Secretin, a peptide hormone released from the duodenum by acid from the stomach and absorbed into the bloodstream, acts on the ductules of the hepaton to increase the alkalinity and the volume of bile. This increased secretion of water and electrolytes, mostly bicarbonate, also occurs after administration of *gastrin* and *CCK* (Fig. 26–28).

Choleresis is also observed after vagal stimulation and after administration of histamine. Conversely, choleresis is inhibited either by hepatic venous congestion or by raising the intraluminal pressure in the bile duct.

Digestive Functions of Bile

Bile is mixed with chyme (1) to add bicarbonate to neutralize the remaining gastric acid, and alkalize the digesta; (2) to act as an amphipathic (detergent, hydrotropic) agent, through its bile acids, to emulsify the lipids and to facilitate the action of the pancreatic esterases; (3) to cooperate with phospholipids (cholesterol and lysolecithin) in the alkaline digesta, to form micelles for solubilization and absorption of mono- and diglycerides; and (4) to contribute a bacteriostatic action in the upper small intestine.

REFERENCES

Blair-West JR, Bott E, Boyd GW, Coghlan JP, Denton DA, Goding JR, Weller S, Wintour M, Wright RD. General biological aspects of salivary secretion in ruminants. In: Dougherty RW, ed. Physiology of digestion in the ruminant. London: Butterworths, 1965.

Camara VM, Prieur DJ. Secretion of colonic isozyme or lysozyme in association with cecotrophy of rabbits. Am J Physiol 1984;247 (Gastrointest Liver Physiol 10):G19.

Caple IW, Heath TJ. Biliary and pancreatic secretions in sheep: Their regulation and roles. In: McDonald IW, Warner ACI, eds. Digestion and metabolism in the ruminant. Armidale: U New England Publishing Unit, 1975.

Cranwell PD, Douglas RA, Stuart SJ. Development of abomasal secretion in the milk-fed lamb. Can J Anim Sci 1984;64:95.

Denton DA. The study of sheep with unilateral parotid fistulae. Quart J Exp Physiol 1957;42:72.

Diamond JM. Transport mechanisms in the gallbladder. In: Code CF, ed. Handbook of physiology, Section 6: Alimentary canal, volume V. Washington: American Physiological Society, 1968.

Dobson DE, Prager EM, Wilson AC. Stomach lysozymes of ruminants. J Biol Chem 1984;259:11607.

Gray CH, Nicholson DC, Quincy RV. Fate of bile in the bowel. In: Code CF, ed. Handbook of physiology, Section 6: Alimentary canal, volume V. Washington: American Physiological Society, 1968.

Hoffmann AF. Functions of bile in the alimentary canal. In: Code CF, ed. Handbook of physiology, Section 6: Alimentary canal, volume V. Washington: American Physiological Society, 1968.

Kato S, Young BA. Effects of cold exposure on pancreatic exocrine secretions in sheep. Can J Anim Sci 1984;64(Suppl.):263.

Legrand-Defretin V, Juste C, Corring T, Rerat A. Enterohepatic circulation of bile acids in pigs: Diurnal pattern and effect of reentrant biliary fistula. Am J Physiol 1986;250:G295.

Lysons RJ, Alexander TJL. The gnotobiotic ruminant and in vivo studies of defined bacterial populations. In: McDonald IW, Warner ACI, eds. Digestion and metabolism in the ruminant. Armidale: U New England Publishing Unit, 1975:180.

Matsui T, Yano H, Kawashima R. Effect of calcitonin on biliary and salivary excretion of calcium and phosphorus in sheep. Can J Anim Sci 1984;64(Suppl.):225.

Roy JHB, Stobo IJF. Nutrition in the pre-ruminant calf. In: McDonald IW, Warner ACI, eds. Digestion and metabolism in the ruminant. Armidale: U New England Publishing Unit, 1975.

Ruckebusch Y. Motility of the ruminant stomach associated with states of sleep. In: McDonald IW, Warner ACI, eds. Digestion and metabolism in the ruminant. Armidale: U New England Publishing Unit, 1975.

Ruckebusch Y, Sddani G. Gallbladder motility in sheep: effects of cholecystokinin and related peptides. J Vet Pharm Ther 1985;8:263.

Schanker LS. Secretion of organic compounds in bile. In: Code CF, ed. Handbook of physiology, Section 6: Alimentary canal, volume V. Washington: American Physiological Society, 1968.

Scott D. Changes in mineral, water, and acid-base balance associated with feeding and diet. In: McDonald IW, Warner ACI, eds. Digestion and metabolism in the ruminant. Armidale: U New England Publishing Unit, 1975.

Thivend P, Debarre M, Lefaivre J, et al. Influence of sorbitol on biliary secretion in the preruminal calf. Can J Anim Sci 1984;64(Suppl.):102.

Ushijima J, Okubo M, Kato S. Composition changes in pancreatic juice in sheep caused by prevention of entry of digesta into the duodenum. Can J Anim Sci 1984;64(Suppl.):104.

Wheeler HO. Water and electrolytes in bile. In: Code CF, ed. Handbook of physiology, Section 6: Alimentary canal, volume V. Washington: American Physiological Society, 1968.

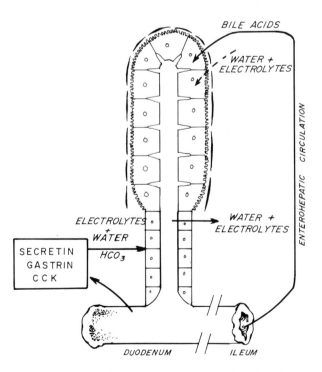

Figure 26–28 Choleresis by hepatocytes and ductules. The recirculation of bile acids stimulates hepatocytes to secretory activity. Peptide hormones activate cells of the ductules (small ducts) to add the alkaline component of bile.

CHAPTER 27

GASTROINTESTINAL ABSORPTION

The ultimate function of the gastrointestinal tract is to absorb nutrients essential to the metabolic needs of the animal body. The lumen of the digestive system is considered to be outside of the body. Most constituents must be transformed in the lumen's "outside" environment into substances that can interact with the transport systems in the intestinal mucosa. In the intestinal epithelium, processes and activities must occur at the luminal (apical) plasma membrane, within the cells, and at the basolateral plasma membrane before substances can be transferred from the lumen through the mucosal cells and into blood or lymph. Successful absorption of such substances requires that transformation of food occur first in the lumen (*luminal* or *cavital digestion*) and later in the mucosa (*mucosal digestion*).

Luminal digestion is performed by creating a special environment inside the gastrointestinal tract. The ingestion of food activates motor and secretory events to make the luminal phase of digestion possible. The *motor activities* divide the food into small particles, mix these fine particles of food with secreted liquids, propel and triturate (masticate) this mash, and activate the circulation of blood and lymph. These mechanical processes are powered by striated muscles (mastication, part of swallowing) and smooth muscles (peristalsis, retroperistalsis, rhythmic segmentation). The *secretions,* isoosmolal to plasma, dilute and lubricate the food particles, change and regulate the pH of the gastrointestinal environment, solubilize hydrosoluble substances, add enzymes for reactions of hydrolysis, and dissolve the breakdown products. Luminal digestion depends much more on the contribution of fluids by the digestive glands (salivary, gastric, intestinal, liver, pancreas) than on the ingestion of liquids by the animals. These are necessary for homeostasis of body fluids.

Mucosal digestion follows luminal digestion. Before possible absorption by the epithelial cells into the blood and lymph, the mucosal membranes, the only barrier between food particles and blood, help discriminate against potentially toxic substances ingested with food. The first step in mucosal digestion occurs near the *apical plasma membrane* and involves the selective chemical transformation of substances liberated from food during luminal digestion. Then these new products are transferred *into the enterocytes* for possible intracellular modifications, and the final step occurs when these products cross the *basolateral membrane* and pass into the circulating blood and lymph.

During mucosal digestion, most of the secretions added into the lumen of the digestive tract are ultimately recovered by reabsorption and returned to the extracellular fluid pool. Thus, the absorptive function of the gastrointestinal tract includes both reabsorption of the endogenous digestive secretions and absorption of exogenous nutrients (Fig. 27–1).

Absorption of the end-products of digestion is not known to occur in the mouth and esophagus, although some drugs are absorbed from buccal membranes. In monogastric animals, although a continuous flux of water and water-soluble substances permeates the pores of the gastric mucosa, the net rate of luminal absorption from the stomach is not important. Like the colon, the monogastric stomach has a "tight" epithelium (narrow intercellular spaces) and small pores (0.4 nm); both factors restrict the transfer of ions and water through the gastric mucosa.

This chapter discusses the process of absorption and its variation with age and with species in the different segments of the gastrointestinal tract (the polygastric or polylocular stomach and intestine, small and large).

ABSORPTION IN THE FORESTOMACHS OF RUMINANTS

In the forestomachs (ruminoreticulum, omasum) of ruminants, microbial (bacterial, protozoal, fungal) actions on the principal foodstuffs cause production of gases and various end-products of digestion. Some can be absorbed locally, whereas others pass on into the bowel for further processing.

Although it is largely stratified and squamous, the epithelium that lines the forestomach has a thin (three to four cells) layer of cornified cells and is "leaky," somewhat as the small intestine is. Absorption in the ruminant forestomachs is also facilitated by loose tight junctions (wide intercellular spaces), a discontinuous stratum granulosum, and larger pores (1 nm). Highly vascularized papillae extend the surface of the forestomachs (ruminoreticulum, 21-fold in cattle and 13-fold in sheep and goats; omasum, 25 percent) and help increase absorption.

Morphological modifications of the papillae in the ruminoreticulum occur rapidly with changes in the quality of food. Within 2 weeks, the density, shape, and mitotic activity of papillae can be increased with higher-quality food. These changes are stimulated by the presence and absorption of ammonia and volatile fatty acids (acetate, butyrate, propionate), and other organic acids such as lactate. Because of these characteristics, transport occurs from blood to ruminoreticulum and from ruminoreticulum to blood.

Methods to measure absorption of materials from the forestomachs and that are used to provide an index of absorption may be divided into two main classes: (1) those utilizing changes in the composition of the contents of the ruminoreticulum or the omasum, and (2) those based on the analysis of the blood draining the ruminoreticulum or omasum after infusion of liquid diets into the forestomachs (Fig. 27–2). Cyanide and alkaloids (pilocarpine, atropine)

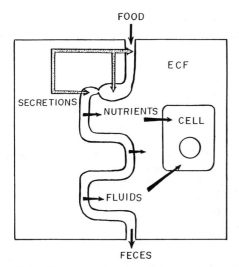

Figure 27-1 The primary function of the gastrointestinal tract is to absorb nutrients from food and to reabsorb fluids added to create the proper luminal environment for digestion in the bowel.

are some of the xenobiotic substances absorbed from the ruminoreticulum.

Gases Produced in the Rumen

In cattle, well over 60 percent of eructated gas is forced into the trachea as a result of nasopharyngeal sphincter closure. With subsequent inspiration, these gases (methane, carbon dioxide) are inhaled into the lungs and are absorbed by the blood. Onion-flavored plants cause a lactating ruminant to eructate gases carrying this flavor, which after absorption by the lungs is secreted in milk within 15 minutes, imparting to the milk "off flavors."

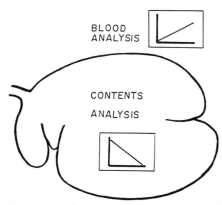

Figure 27-2 Methods for measuring forestomach absorption. Forestomach absorption is indicated either by a decrease in the composition of the contents or by an increase in the constituents of the blood draining the organs.

Volatile Fatty Acids

Absorption of the soluble products of fermentation (volatile fatty acids [VFAs] and lactic acid) occurs from the ruminoreticulum epithelial surface. In sheep and goats, allowing for differences in surface area and in concentrations, the absorption of VFA, ammonia, inorganic ions, and water resembles that of the ruminoreticulum of cattle. In the latter, the omasum is relatively larger (12 percent) in relation to the ruminoreticulum than in small ruminants (2 percent), and a higher rate of omasal absorption may be expected.

Passive ruminoreticular absorption of undissociated volatile fatty acids (i.e., acetic, propionic, and butyric) occurs with relative ease (Fig. 27-3). VFA absorption rate increases as the pH of the ruminoreticulum ingesta decreases (i.e., after feeding, when fermentable carbohydrates predominate). This process assists in maintaining the range of ruminoreticular pH between 5.8 and 7.0. The concentrations of VFAs are 10 times higher in the ruminoreticulum than in the abomasum, and most VFAs (20 mmol per hour in sheep and goat) are absorbed (85 percent in ruminoreticulum, 10 percent in omasum) before the digesta reaches the duodenum. In cattle, 76 percent of the VFAs are absorbed in the ruminoreticulum, 19 percent in the omasum and abomasum, and 5 percent in the small intestine. In the lactating goat and cow, high intraruminal absorption of propionic acid increases plasma glucose, and propionate is the major stimulant of insulin secretion by the pancreas. During fasting, the ruminoreticulum concentration of VFAs decreases, and carbon dioxide (in the form of bicarbonate) accumulates in the ruminoreticulum contents, the pH of which may rise above 7.0. In the omasum, absorption of VFAs—as well as of sodium and of ammonia—becomes greater as the flow rate of digesta increases.

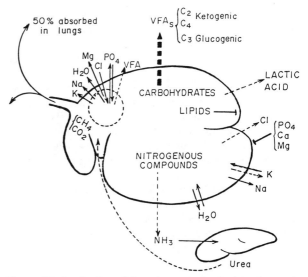

Figure 27-3 Outline of the substances absorbed in the ruminoreticulum (——, active; - - -, passive). The transfer of substances across the omasal wall is global, without specific active or passive pathways.

To be absorbed, a substance must be soluble in either the minute fat droplets or in the aqueous phase of the digesta. As the pH of the forestomach is between 5.5 and 6.5 and that of the intestinal contents is 7 to 8, the rates of absorption of the same compounds differ widely.

The difference depends on the pKa, which influences the pattern of absorption from the various compartments of the gastrointestinal tract. When pH is numerically greater than pKa (e.g., pKa of VFAs is about 4.8, and that of lactic acid is 3.7), an acidic substance becomes more ionized, whereas a basic substance becomes less ionized. Substances highly ionized in the forestomachs are trapped (i.e., poorly absorbed). VFAs are mostly absorbed in the nondissociated form. In the more alkaline small intestine, less ionized substances are readily absorbed.

Lactic Acid

The ruminoreticulum level of lactic acid is usually low. Considerable ruminoreticulum accumulation of lactic acid follows sudden ingestion of large amounts of easily digestible cereals (wheat, corn) or sugar-rich food (sugar beets). If the increase in ingestion is gradual, organisms able to convert lactate to propionate proliferate, and the ruminoreticulum may tolerate high levels of carbohydrate without lactic acid accumulation. Lactic acid diffusion through the ruminoreticulum wall is higher when the digesta is acidic than when it is neutral. The absorption rate of lactate may be from 10 to 20 times less than that of VFAs. Lactic acid is a stronger acid than the VFAs; its pKa is about 3.7 (compared with 4.8). In high concentrations, it can have a corrosive effect on epithelium.

Nitrogen End-Products (Ammonia and Amino Acids)

After a meal, the increased passive ruminoreticulum absorption of ammonia reflects a higher rate of hydrolysis of various nitrogenous materials (grass, urea). In the forestomach fluid, high ammonia concentrations are tolerated well if the pH is below 7.0, but signs of toxicity appear when the pH rises to 7.3.

The nutritional importance of normal ammonia absorption is not evident. Normally, most of the ammonia absorbed in the ruminoreticulum is converted to urea in the liver. A large part of this blood urea is returned to the forestomachs by diffusion into the ruminoreticular fluid and into saliva. This forestomach urea is reconverted to ammonia and is used by microorganisms or directed again to the liver for formation of urea, which is recirculated to the ruminoreticulum. In sheep and goats, the ruminoreticulum absorbs four times more ammonia (9 mmol per hour) than the omasum (2 mmol per hour). Amino acids are also absorbed by the ruminoreticulum.

Inorganic Ions

The epithelium of the forestomachs absorbs inorganic ions (e.g., sodium, chloride, ammonia) with water from the digesta in the ruminoreticular fermentation vat. Sodium and chloride ions are absorbed from the ruminoreticulum against a concentration gradient. The rate of active absorption of sodium increases markedly after a meal. The transfer of sodium across the ruminoreticulum wall, occurring against its electrochemical gradient, is stimulated when potassium intake is increased. With potassium-rich fresh grass, the urinary sodium content is greater and the ratio of sodium to potassium in the saliva is higher than with potassium-poor hay and meals. Chloride is absorbed passively in the ruminoreticulum but is secreted in the omasum.

The ruminoreticulum wall does not favor transfer of phosphate, calcium, and magnesium. Potassium ions are actively secreted into the ruminoreticulum, where their concentration is greater than in plasma, and this favors increased diffusion of potassium into the blood.

Absorption of both sodium (4 mmol per hour) and potassium (1 mmol per hour) from the omasum is about one-fifth that in the ruminoreticulum (sodium, 20 mmol per hour; potassium, 5 mmol per hour). Magnesium is absorbed mainly from the omasum when the dietary intake is low, but it may also be absorbed from the ruminoreticulum when dietary intake is higher. Phosphate moves in either direction across the omasal wall, but a slight net absorption is postulated.

Water

Water can move freely across the ruminoreticulum epithelium. During fasting, when the ruminoreticulum contents are hypotonic to plasma, water (about 125 mL per hour in sheep and goats) is absorbed from the ruminoreticulum. After feeding, only relatively small net movements of water occur across the ruminoreticulum epithelium, because the ruminoreticulum fluid becomes hypertonic to plasma.

The omasum of the sheep and the goat absorbs about 30 mL per hour of water (one-fourth that of the ruminoreticulum, or 10 percent of the water leaving the ruminoreticulum. A positive correlation exists between the absorption of water and the absorption of sodium, potassium, or VFAs in the omasum.

SECRETIONS OF THE SMALL INTESTINE

During luminal digestion, exocrine secretions from the small intestine perform indispensable physical and chemical functions. An enormous quantity of endogenous secretions is delivered into the intestinal tract to dilute the contents of the gut, to neutralize its acidity, and protect the mucosa during the luminal digestion.

The secretions of the small intestine contribute water, mucus, immunoglobulins, bicarbonate ions, and enzymes. Water liquefies the intraluminal content and dilutes the hyperosmolal chyme. Mucus and immunoglobulins (IgA and sIgA) adhere to the surface of the intestinal mucosa and provide protection from physical agents and bacteria. Sodium bicarbonate is added as an intestinal isoosmolal alkaline fluid to help neutralize the excessive acidity of chyme. Some active enzymes (disaccharidases, dipeptidases) come from the desquamated villous cells and participate in the luminal digestion of carbohydrates and proteins.

Normally, net intestinal secretion is not noticeable, since nearly 99 percent of the fluid produced is ultimately reabsorbed farther down the gut. The existence of a real intestinal secretion is thus challenged. Adequate evaluation of physiological intestinal secretion is difficult because of the equilibrium between the isoosmolal active secretion of sodium chloride and sodium bicarbonate by the crypt cells and the active absorptive processes in the villous cells (Fig. 27–4).

The magnitude of this transfer of fluid into and from the gut can be grasped only when diarrhea occurs. This rupture of the equilibrium between intestinal secretion and absorption may result from intestinal secretion exceeding normal reabsorption capacity or from normal secretion when reabsorption is impaired.

The functioning of the secretory mechanism of the

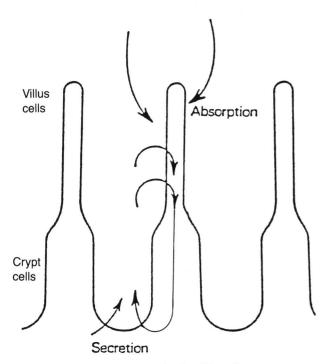

Villus cells

Absorption

Crypt cells

Secretion

Distention, Irritation, Bile salts
Vagal activity
Humoral activity (secretin, CCK, VIP, PGs, 5-HT)
Bacterial toxins

Figure 27–4 Separation of the active intestinal secretory activity (localized in the younger crypt cells) and of the active absorptive activity, which occurs in the older villous cells. Under physiological conditions, net intestinal secretion does not happen because of an equilibrium between the secretory and absorptive processes. Water and electrolytes from the crypt cells are recaptured at the tip of spatially separated villous cells. Since the venous return from the villi passes by the crypts, the absorbed water and electrolytes may be secreted back into the lumen.

immature and nonvillous crypt cells is increased by cholinergic and humoral stimuli and is exacerbated by microbial toxins. Vagal activity, enhanced by cephalic, gastric, or local intestinal stimuli (distention, irritation by bile salts, hyperosmolality), activates the secretory mechanism of the crypt cells. Gastrointestinal hormones (secretin and cholecystokin [CCK]), a candidate hormone, vasoactive intestinal polypeptide (VIP), and the omnipresent autacoids (prostaglandins E_1 and E_2, and endogenous amines: serotonin, histamine, kinins) also intensify the rate of intestinal secretion. Most bacterial diarrheas are caused by *Escherichia coli* or *Salmonella*, which produce toxins that stimulate crypt cells to produce far more than the villus cells normally can absorb. The intestinal secretion caused by these heterogeneous stimuli would involve cyclic adenosine monophosphate (cAMP). Apical transfer of chloride anions into the lumen would be mediated by cAMP, and these cavital anions would then attract sodium cations into the intestinal cavity from the sodium-rich intercellular crypt space (see Fig. 27–4).

With regard to the mature enterocytes of the villi, these stimuli impair the absorption mechanism of sodium at the apical membrane. On the villous cells, the cAMP resulting from cholinergic, humoral, and toxic factors exerts an inhibitory effect on the apical absorption of sodium chloride. Occlusion of a portion of the intestine does not alter secretion by the crypt cells but impairs absorption by the villous cells by depriving them of blood circulation. The continued secretion of the crypt cells further overdistends the intestinal segment and aggravates the normal hypoxia of the villous cells, creating a fatal positive feedback.

Submucosal (Brunner's) glands in the proximal duodenum (Table 27–1) specifically secrete mucus in response to vagal stimuli, local distention, and irritation during the digestive period. In contrast to most animal species, mucus secretion by the duodenal glands of the cat is not continuous during the interdigestive, or fasting, period. In the rest of the intestinal epithelium, mucus production results from exocytosis and apical expulsion of mucus from goblet cells and from extrusion or exfoliation of whole goblet cells.

ABSORPTION IN THE SMALL INTESTINE

The small intestine is the main site of absorption in all animal species. The duodenum absorbs largely minerals (Ca^{++} and Fe^{++}), end-products of digestion, and vitamins,

TABLE 27–1 Length of the Duodenal (Brunner's) Gland Area Distal to the Pylorus

Species	Length (cm)
Cat and dog	1–2
Cattle	400–500
Goat	20–25
Horse	500–600
Pig	300–500
Sheep	60–70

whereas the distal portion of the small intestine (jejunum and ileum) is the site of absorption of water, vitamin B_{12}, and bile salts.

In general, adrenergic stimulation and glucocorticoids enhance absorption in small and large intestine cells by favoring the basolateral transfer of sodium chloride through an increase in cAMP. Cholinergic agents, which increase the entry of Ca^{++} across the basolateral membrane and formation of cGMP on the apical membrane, stimulate digestive secretions by crypt cells and reduce intestinal absorption by the villous cells.

Structure of the Small Intestine

A cross-section of the wall of the small intestine cylinder includes microvilli, enterocytes, lamina propria, crypts, muscularis mucosa, submucosa, circular and longitudinal muscles, and serosa (Fig. 27–5). Extremely well-developed blood and lymphatic systems receive the products absorbed by the small intestine. The highly permeable blood capillaries from the mucosa and from the villi unite to form venules and veins that drain into the portal vein via mesenteric small vessels (radicles). In the resting small intestine, although only one-third of the capillaries of the villi are open, the mucosa accounts for 75 percent of the total blood flow, the remainder passing to the submucosa and the muscularis. The volume of blood flowing in the mucosa can be more than doubled during a meal. In an absorbing villus, an interstitial osmolality four times greater at the tip than at the base (1200 versus 300 mosm per L) exerts a powerful osmotic attraction to water in the lumen. The fast-flowing blood (600 times as fast as lymph) draining the small bowel carries water, inorganic salts, glycerol, short-chain fatty acids, amino acids, and monosaccharides.

The lymph capillaries of the mucosa and villi (lacteals) drain into larger lymph vessels (see Fig. 27–5). Lymph proceeds from the small intestine into the lacteal vessels of the mesentery, the cisterna chyli, the thoracic duct, and the venous system craniad to the heart. The lymphatic system carries aggregates (chylomicrons) generated in the enterocyte after absorption of end-products of lipid digestion.

Absorptive Surface

The mucosa of the small intestine possesses features that enormously increase epithelial surface area for absorption. These include foldings in the mucosa (*valvulae conniventes*), villi, and microvilli. Generally, each feature contributes to increasing the surface area by a factor of 2 or 3 for the folds, of 30 for the villi, and of 30 for the microvilli. In most species, folding of the mucosa is prominent at the proximal end of the small intestine and regresses distally. *Valvulae conniventes* are absent in the adult bovine. Each villus, approximately 1 mm long and covered by three types of cells (enterocytes, goblet cells, and enterochromaffin cells), projects freely into the intestinal lumen (Fig. 27–6). Crypts of Lieberkühn (gland-like structures) between villi show mitotic division of cells at their bases. These undifferentiated cells mature, differentiate into one of the three cell types as they move up from the crypts, and ultimately replace those that normally desquamate near the tip of each villus. Microvilli (1 μm), numerous fingerlike folds of the apical cell mem-

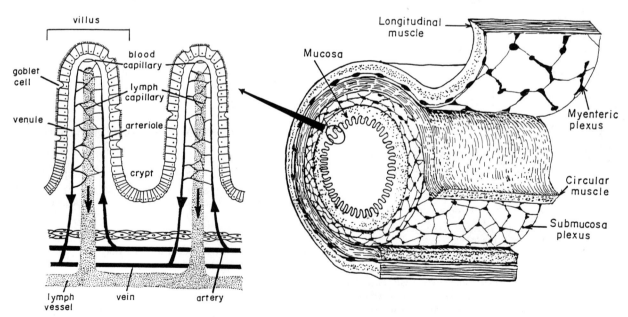

Figure 27–5 **Right,** Layers of longitudinal and circular smooth muscles (motor acitvity) cover the submucosa and mucosa (secretory and absorptive activities) of the intestine. The mucosa of the small intestine is increased by large folds, which are covered by small projections (villi) made up of enterocytes and goblet cells. In the villi, the circulation of arterial blood and lymph is countercurrent, as blood in arterioles moves in the direction opposite that of lymph in capillaries, but venous blood flows parallel to lymph.

brane, are found only on enterocytes (see Fig. 27–6). The microvilli, responsible for the greatest amplification of the surface area, also carry a glycoprotein surface coating (glycocalyx, or brush border) and an adjacent unstirred layer of water (300 μm thick). Through its enclosed digestive enzymes, the glycocalyx participates in the mucosal phase of digestion. The brush border also contains specialized transfer mechanisms to transport the end-products of digestion from the lumen of the intestine into the cytoplasm of enterocytes.

Mucosal Regeneration

The intestinal epithelium has the fastest turnover rate in the body and a high regenerative capacity. The turnover period (2 to 5 days) changes with age; it is a week in neonate pigs, 3 days in a suckling pig. A gastrointestinal hormone, gastrin, has the most important stimulant or trophic effect on intestinal cell division and renewal.

Water and Electrolytes

A critical function of the small intestine is absorption of ingested water and reabsorption of the fluid secretions delivered into the proximal part of the gastrointestinal tract. Intestinal absorptive cells absorb solute and fluid through two parallel paths: the intracellular, or transcellular (active), pathway and the extracellular, or intercellular (paracellular, passive), pathway. The intracellular pathway is through the cell, as water-soluble substances traverse the apical cell membrane and basolateral membrane (Fig. 27–7).

The extracellular pathway for many water-soluble substances is between the cells and through the tight junctions. Major barriers to water and electrolyte transepithelial transport are the "pores" in the apical membrane (smaller in the large bowel than in the small gut) for the intracellular pathway, and the tight junctions for the extracellular pathway. Resistance to flow is negligible in the basement membrane and the lamina propria.

By an active process requiring energy from ATP, Na pumps on the basolateral membranes of the enterocytes drive

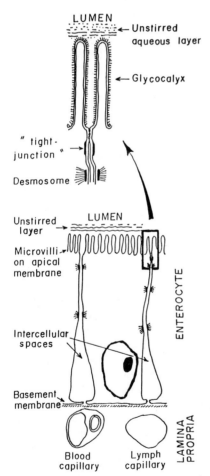

Figure 27–6 Section of the small intestine to magnify the structures for absorption (apical and basolateral parts of the plasma membrane of enterocytes). An unstirred aqueous layer and the glycocalyx (fuzzy coat) separate the lumen of the gut from the microvilli (folds) on the apical membrane of enterocytes and from the basolateral extracellular spaces between adjacent enterocytes.

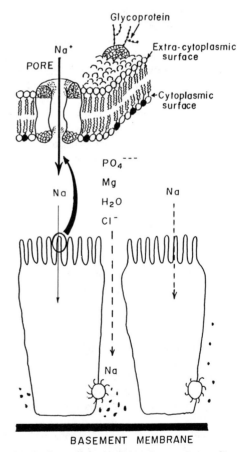

Figure 27–7 *Intracellular* (active) pathway, where sodium penetrates the apical membrane through a pore by either a passive or an active process (or both) and is actively expelled into the intercellular space at the basolateral membrane. Passive or *extracellular* pathway of absorption of water, magnesium, chloride, and phosphate, which may also be absorbed actively.

sodium into the intercellular spaces (see Fig. 27–7). The presence of this sodium initiates events that are responsible for most of the water and electrolyte absorption by the intestine: (1) it raises the osmotic pressure in the intercellular space; (2) it sets a net positive charge that attracts anions to raise further the intercellular osmotic pressure and tends to move anions in the direction of the positively charged blood; (3) as this osmotic pressure increases, water flows into the intercellular space through the cell membranes and tight junctions to raise the hydrostatic pressure between the enterocytes; and (4) this increased hydrostatic pressure pushes electrolytes and water through the basement membrane and across the capillary wall.

To drive electrolytes and water toward the capillary, the resistance between the enterocytes at the tight junction must be greater than at the basement membrane. If this is not so, electrolytes and water are directed back into the lumen. The tight junction is permeable to sodium ions, which may leak back into the lumen. In contrast, the tight junctions in the mucosa of stomach and colon are impermeable and prevent backflow from blood to the lumen in spite of large electrical potential differences and concentration gradients.

Water is absorbed by passive diffusion (extracellular pathway) and depends on sodium absorption, which participates also in absorption of amino acids, monosaccharides, and bile salts. Sodium ions can passively enter the enterocyte independently, by carrier-mediated transport, or both ways. Carrier-mediated transport of sodium is either with substrate-coupled mechanisms (hexoses, amino acids) that are specific to the small intestine or with a countertransport mechanism for luminal extrusion of hydrogen ions from the enterocyte in exchange for sodium. Availability of glucose and amino acids increases the absorption of sodium. Glucocorticoids increase small bowel and large bowel absorption of sodium by stimulating the sodium pump at the basolateral membrane. Potassium ions are absorbed by the passive mechanism.

Very little magnesium is absorbed by the extracellular pathway. Absorption of calcium, slower than that of sodium, is preferential over absorption of most other divalent cations, is carrier mediated (facilitated) by the calcium-binding protein at the apical membrane, and is active at the basolateral membrane. Strontium and barium are also bound to calcium-binding protein, whose synthesis is promoted by dihydroxy vitamin D_3 (1,25-dihydroxycholecalciferol). Parathormone catalyzes the formation of this active metabolite of vitamin D and directly enhances apical and basolateral transfer of divalent calcium. Apical membrane absorption of soluble iron (ferrous is more soluble than ferric), an active process in the duodenum and upper jejunum, is dependent on the ferritin in the enterocyte. Iron is transferred outside the enterocyte by an active mechanism. Bicarbonate absorption (intracellular) is preferential to absorption of chloride (passive), which happens by both the extracellular pathway and the intracellular pathway, in which case it is coupled to sodium (Fig. 27–8). Both passive and active processes operate for absorption of phosphate, and the active mechanism is closely related to the active transport of calcium.

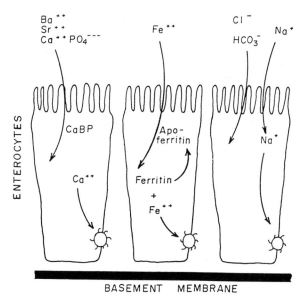

Figure 27–8 Active absorption of barium, strontium, calcium, and phosphate occurs through calcium-binding protein in the apical membrane; iron absorption is related to the endocellular presence of ferritin; chloride and bicarbonate penetrate the apical membrane by coupling with sodium.

Inorganic sulfate and trace minerals are absorbed by still undefined mechanisms.

Carbohydrates

Dietary carbohydrates are mainly starches, disaccharides, monosaccharides, and fibrous carbohydrates (hemicellulose and cellulose). The *luminal phase* of small intestine digestion results in amylase hydrolysis of starches, yielding oligosaccharides (alpha-dextrins, maltotriose, and maltose, but no free glucose), but the fibrous carbohydrates remain intact. In monogastric herbivores fed high-fiber diets, the increased bulk accelerates the transit of chyme and lowers the efficiency of luminal digestion of nonfibrous carbohydrates. During the essential *mucosal phase* of carbohydrate digestion (Fig. 27–9), specific saccharidases in the glycocalyx of enterocytes hydrolyze the oligosaccharides into monosaccharides (glucose, galactose, and fructose). These monosaccharides are then transported across the cell to gain access to the portal circulation. Glucose and galactose are absorbed mainly by the jejunal enterocytes, against a concentration gradient, by a sodium-dependent active transport mechanism. Fructose crosses the apical membrane of enterocytes of the jejunum by facilitated (mediated) diffusion. Since this transfer is not energy dependent, fructose cannot be absorbed against a concentration gradient. Enterocytes can convert fructose into glucose. Limited absorption of mannose, xylose, and arabinose seems to occur by a diffusion mechanism. Monosaccharides leave the enterocyte by diffusion at the basolateral membrane and accumulate in the

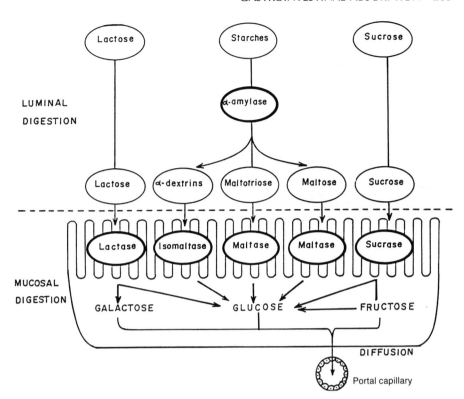

Figure 27–9 Luminal end-products of carbohydrate digestion in the small intestine, their mucosal enzymatic transformation before absorption in the enterocytes, and their passage in the portal blood capillaries.

intercellular space before entering the capillaries of the portal circulation.

Proteins

Luminal hydrolysis of endogenous (microbial, enzymatic, and desquamated) and dietary proteins begins in the stomach and is completed principally in the duodenum. The action of gastric and pancreatic proteases yields amino acids and oligopeptides. These oligopeptides are then transformed into a mixture of amino acids, dipeptides, and tripeptides by mucosal oligopeptidases in the glycocalyx (Fig. 27–10).

Enterocytes in the jejunum actively absorb unchanged di- and tripeptides more rapidly than amino acids, and intracellular peptidases then hydrolyze these peptides to amino acids. L-Amino acids resulting from luminal digestion are transferred into the enterocytes by sodium-dependent mechanisms very similar to those for hexose transport. Intracellular amino acids diffuse across the basolateral membrane to reach the intercellular space, and ultimately the portal capillaries. A much smaller volume of D-amino acids is absorbed by the intracellular pathway.

Lipids

Dietary lipids presented to the duodenum are triglycerides, cholesterol esters, and lecithins. Some tri-glycerides in chyme (e.g., those in milk) are hydrolyzed during luminal digestion to glycerol and water-soluble short-chain fatty acids, both of which are amphipathics and can enter the enterocyte rapidly by diffusion. Most triglycerides are transformed into water-insoluble monoglycerides and fatty acids, which can diffuse easily through the lipid membranes of the enterocytes. The crucial point of fatty acid and monoglyceride absorption is their solubilization in the unstirred layer, or water phase, to carry them to the glycocalyx (Fig. 27–11). Bile salts act to bring these water-insoluble end-products of lipase digestion and other fats (cholesterol, sterols, and fat-soluble vitamins) into a water-soluble negatively charged aggregate (5 nm) called a *micelle*. The micelle performs as a transport vehicle to move these lipids to the glycocalyx, where they are released to diffuse across the apical membrane into the cell. The bile salts return to the gut lumen to be almost entirely reabsorbed by an active mechanism in the ileum and to reappear in bile (the enterohepatic circulation of bile salts). Lipid-soluble vitamins, fatty acids, glycerol, monoglycerides, phospholipids, and cholesterol are re-formed into chylomicrons (2 nm). These beta-lipoprotein–covered intracellular structures can stabilize lipid products in an aqueous medium. By exocytosis or by diffusion, chylomicrons cross into the intercellular space and finally enter lymph capillaries. Glycerol and short-chain fatty acids leave the enterocyte by diffusion, gain the intercellular space, and then enter the portal capillaries.

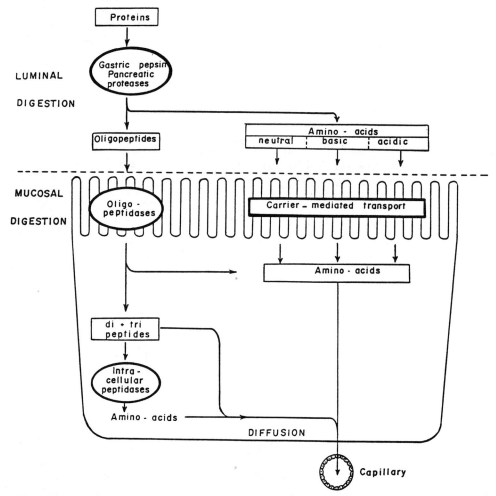

Figure 27–10   Luminal and mucosal phases of protein digestion in the small intestine, the end-products absorbed and transferred into the portal blood circulation.

Water-Soluble Vitamins

Most water-soluble vitamins are absorbed or can be absorbed by the extracellular pathway (Table 27–2). Absorption of thiamine and folicin can also occur by the intracellular pathway, and that of riboflavin by facilitated diffusion. Vitamin B_{12} requires the presence of an intrinsic factor (gastric origin) for its absorption by an active process in the ileum, but megadoses of vitamin B_{12} are absorbed passively, even without any intrinsic factor.

A specific active transport process is implicated in the ileal absorption of vitamin B_{12}. The normal ileal absorption of cobalamins depends on the presence of intrinsic factor (IF). In the absence of IF, only 1 to 2 percent of ingested vitamin B_{12} is absorbed in the small intestine (not limited to ileum).

IF joins to vitamin B_{12} as a dimer: two molecules of IF unite with two vitamin B_{12} molecules. This IF–vitamin B_{12} dimer then binds to a receptor on the brush border of the plasma membrane. The IF–vitamin B_{12} complex is split before free vitamin B_{12} actively crosses the plasma membrane and enters the enterocyte. Facilitated or active transport is probably involved for the cellular exit of vitamin B_{12}, about 6 hours after its ingestion, into portal blood, where it binds to a globulin of liver origin, transcobalamin.

TABLE 27–2   Absorption of Vitamins in the Small Intestine

Type	Water-soluble	Lipid-soluble
Passive diffusion	*Biotin, *niacin, *pantothenic acid, *pyridoxine, *thiamine, *vitamin C	Vitamin A, vitamin D, vitamin E
Facilitated passive transport	*Biotin, *folacin, *niacin, *riboflavin	Vitamin K
Active transport	*Folacin, *thiamine, *vitamin B_{12}	

*Absorbed by more than one mechanism.

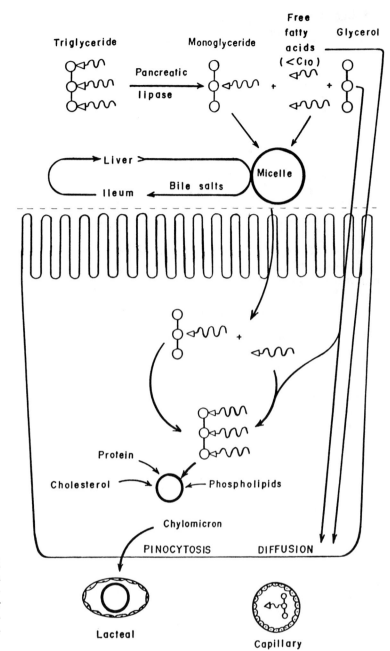

Figure 27–11 Luminal digestion of lipids, and absorption of amphipathic glycerol and short-chain fatty acids into the portal blood circulation. Lipid-soluble end-products are formed into aggregates for transport from the lumen to the enterocyte (micelle) and from the enterocyte to the lymph capillaries (chylomicrons).

ABSORPTION IN THE LARGE INTESTINE

In the large intestine of herbivores, where bacterial transformation of carbohydrates and proteins produces volatile fatty acids (acetic, propionic, and butyric) and ammonia, the mucosa is well adapted to buffer these substances and to absorb water, electrolytes, lactate, and succinate. Absorptive capacity is greatest in the proximal segment and gradually regresses caudally. Monosaccharides, amino acids, microbial proteins, and vitamins cannot be absorbed in the large intestine.

In ruminants, 90 percent of the water entering the cecum is absorbed. In the horse, the cecum is the greatest absorptive organ; the ventral colon absorbs next best, and the small colon mops up whatever is necessary to form normal fecal balls. The efficiency is such that of the 19.5 L of fluid entering the large intestine of a 100-kg pony, only about 1.5 L escapes in the feces.

The colon, a primary absorptive organ, can absorb as much as twice the usual volume it receives daily. The absorptive capacity follows a gradient, which is greatest at the proximal colon and decreases distally. In carnivores, the colon is the only absorptive organ of some importance for

TABLE 27–3 Absorptive Capacity and Fermentative Activity of the Swine Large Intestine

Substances	Absorptive Capacity (mL or mg/h/kg BW)
Glucose	500
Lactose	800
Lipids	1,000
Sodium chloride in saline	250
Starch (potato, corn)	1,500
Sucrose	500
Water	18

BW, Body weight.

reabsorption of water and electrolytes. Impairment of this reabsorptive function leads to diarrhea in all animal species and even to fatal loss of extracellular fluid (over 30 percent) in those with capacious large intestines (pig, horse).

In the pig, the absorptive capacity for water, nutrients, and minerals is very high (Table 27–3). This compensates for irregular ileocecal nutrient flux and leads to a nearly normal digestibility with minor variations in fecal consistency and concentrations of bacterial metabolites.

During the fermentative process, liberated volatile fatty acids favor water absorption and produce a dry fecal consistency. Fatty acids themselves do not induce diarrhea, which is due to impaired absorption of water in the colon. Lowering the pH of the colon contents results in lactic acid fermentation with low levels of fatty acids. Lactic acid alone can induce diarrhea. A large quantity of lactic acid must be infused intracecally to cause diarrhea, and the mechanism of the metabolic action of lactic acid in the large intestine is unclear. Conditions produced by infusions of lactic acid are quite different from those caused by fermentations that liberate lactic acid in the large intestine (Table 27–4).

As in rumen acidosis, an excess of lactic acid (due to ineffective absorption of L-, and mostly D-, lactic acid) is responsible for a higher intraluminal osmotic pressure in the colon. Lactic acid, because of its pKa value (3.7), rapidly lowers the pH, which influences the survival of the microbial population, the production of short-chain fatty acids (a source of energy), and the ionization and absorption of salts.

In sheep and cattle, the large intestine is a principal site for sodium absorption by diffusion into the epithelial cell, water is absorbed passively, but chloride is absorbed actively, whereas potassium and bicarbonate are excreted. Aldosterone, a mineralocorticoid hormone, increases colonic absorption of sodium, which is exchanged for the excretion of potassium. In the ileum and in the colon, bicarbonate is secreted in exchange for absorbed chloride (Fig. 27–12). As luminal acid may damage the mucosa, buffers are required to neutralize the organic acids resulting from bacterial action. In herbivores, much of the colonic bicarbonate is used for this purpose, while colonic phosphates from dietary sources perform this task in carnivores and omnivores.

In cattle, the amounts of ammonia or urea tolerated in the large intestine are greater than those found in the rumen. The levels of ammonia and urea in the portal blood are also striking. Nitrogen is absorbed predominantly as ammonia, and the highest tolerated level of ammonia in the portal vein is about 1,400 µg/dL. The concentration of ammonia in portal vein blood decreases during diarrhea caused by high urea and ammonia loads in the large intestine. Thus, higher fecal excretion of ammonia takes away ammonia from the large intestine and acts as a kind of regulation of "recycled" nitrogen absorbed from the colon. High concentrations of ammonia in the cecum induce severe bloody diarrhea with partial or total loss of absorptive capacity of the colon. In vivo, chronic intoxication with high levels of ammonia or urea in the large intestine is present only in situations of severe uremia. The diarrhea is caused by the interference with absorptive capacity of the colon, and the osmotic activity of urea and ammonia.

In rabbits, microbial proteins, essential amino acids, and B vitamins are also synthesized in the large intestine. By cecotrophia (i.e., coprophagia of soft feces coming directly from the cecum), these compounds are ingested at their exit from the anus. Through the normal processes of digestion, nutrients liberated from these substances are absorbed in the small bowel, as they are in ruminants.

TABLE 27–4 Comparative Effects of Infused and Fermentative Lactic Acid (LA) in the Swine Large Intestine

Parameter	Infusion	Fermentation
Cecum Level of LA	High	Moderate
Form of LA	L- = D-	L- form > D- form, but level of D- form rises as pH declines
Large intestine Level of LA	High in cecum and proximal colon Lower in distal colon and rectum	Uniform, because of continuous absorption
Bacteriostatic action	High in proximal colon	Moderate, but higher as pH declines
Fecal pH	High	Low

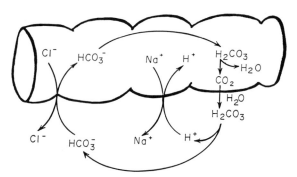

Figure 27–12 Coupling of sodium and chloride absorption in the distal ileum and the large intestine with bicarbonate excretion to neutralize organic acids of microbial origin.

INFLUENCE OF AGE ON INTESTINAL ABSORPTION

During the immediate postnatal period and at weaning, the absorptive function of the intestinal tract changes. In neonatal ruminants, dogs, pigs, and horses, all the maternal immunoglobulins are received from the colostrum during the immediate postpartum period. Absorption by the neonatal intestine is by pinocytosis or endocytosis (Fig. 27–13). This process involves (1) adsorption of macromolecules to the luminal membrane of the small intestinal adsorptive cell; (2) energy-dependent invagination of the membrane and formation of small vesicles; (3) migration of the membrane-bound vesicles inside the enterocyte and their intracellular digestion to liberate some of the macromolecules to the basolateral surface of the cell; and (4) passage by exocytosis or reverse endocytosis of the macromolecules to the intercellular space and the lymphatic system.

The neonatal duodenum can absorb only large amounts of intact protein during a period that is longer in small ruminants (4 days) than in other species (1 or 2 days). In mice and rats, small bowel absorption of intact proteins lasts until 10 to 18 days after birth. In the piglet, the basolateral membrane of the jejunum "closes" much later (2 to 3 weeks) to macromolecules, and even later in the ileum (see Fig. 27–13). This permeability of the intestinal mucosa is nonspecific to all macromolecules, mostly immunoglobulins such as IgG and viral particles, until the intestine "closes" to prevent further bulk passage of proteins. Apical membrane "closure" occurs much later than basolateral closure in each segment of the small intestine.

Structural alteration of the cell luminal membrane by pinocytosis of the macromolecules decreases the absorptive efficiency for other substances (see Fig. 27–13). Active absorption of sodium by the small intestine is reduced by about 40 percent during this period of antibody transfer. A coincident higher blood level of aldosterone acts on the colon to bring about a compensatory increase in the absorption of sodium together with excretion (secretion) of potassium. Thus, during this critical immediate postnatal period, the absorptive function of the colon is changed to offset the simultaneous impairment of sodium transfer in the small intestine.

After closure to macromolecules, the small intestine resumes efficient absorption of water and electrolytes. In the horse and the pig, which have voluminous large intestines, weaning signals a decrease in the absorption of fluid from the small intestine. Most water and electrolytes are rapidly directed to the capacious large intestine at a time when cellulolytic microbial colonies are beginning to function at this site in the gastrointestinal tracts of these species. It is the beginning of a digestive process equivalent to the one operating in the ruminant forestomachs. Absorptive function in the large intestine can, and is adjusted to, recuperate water and electrolytes to avoid excessive losses in the feces.

In cattle, zinc absorption changes with age. The apparent absorption of dietary zinc in 5- to 12-month-old calves is almost twice that of mature cows.

REFERENCES

Annison EF. Absorption from the ruminant stomach. In: Dougherty RW, ed. Physiology of digestion in the ruminant. London: Butterworths, 1965.

Banks JN, Smith RH. Exchanges of major minerals in the stomach compartments of the ruminating calf. Can J Anim Sci 1984; 65(Suppl.):215.

Bentley PJ, Smith MW. Transport of electrolytes across the helicoidal colon of the newborn pig. J Physiol 1975;249:103.

Bines JA, Hart IC. The response of plasma insulin and other hormones to intraruminal infusion of VFA mixtures in cattle. Can J Anim Sci 1984;64(Suppl.):304.

Bremmer I, Davies NT. Dietary composition and the absorption of trace elements by ruminants. In: Ruckebusch Y, Thivend P, eds. Digestive physiology and metabolism in ruminants. Lancaster: MTP Press Ltd, 1980.

Drochner W. Aspects of digestion in the large intestine of the pig. Adv Anim Physiol Anim Nutr 1987;17:1.

Emmanuel B, Kennelly JJ. Effect of intraruminal infusion of propionic acid on plasma metabolites in goats. Can J Anim Sci 1984; 64(Suppl.):295.

Engelhardt Wv, Hauffe R. Role of the omasum in absorption and secretion of water and electrolytes in sheep and goats. In: McDonald IW, Warner ACI, eds. Digestion and metabolism in the ruminant. Armidale: U New England Publishing Unit, 1975.

Ferguson DR, James PS, Paterson JYF, Saunders JC, Smith MW. Aldosterone-induced changes in colonic sodium transport occurring naturally during development in the neonatal pig. J Physiol 1979;292:495.

Giesecke D, Stangassinger M. Lactic acid metabolism. In: Ruckebusch Y, Thivend P, eds. Digestive physiology and metabolism in ruminants. Lancaster: MTP Press Ltd, 1980.

Hamilton DL, Roe WE. Electrolyte levels and net fluid electrolyte movements in the gastrointestinal tract of weanling swine. Can J Comp Med 1977;41:241.

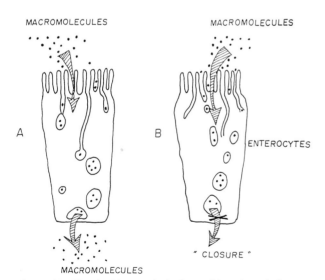

Figure 27–13 A, Pinocytosis (endocytosis) at the apical membrane for absorption of luminal macromolecules, and exocytosis (emiocytosis) at the basolateral membrane during an immediate postnatal period (2 days in duodenum, 2 to 3 weeks in jejunum, and over 3 weeks in ileum). **B**, Basolateral closure occurs at the end of these periods, but apical closure is delayed.

Hofmann RR. Comparative anatomical studies imply adaptive variations of ruminant digestive physiology. Can J Anim Sci 1984;64(Suppl.):203.

Hyden S, Sperber I. Electron microscopy of the ruminant forestomach. In: Dougherty RW, ed. Physiology of digestion in the ruminant. London: Butterworths, 1965.

Istasse L, Orskov ER. The effects of intermittent and continuous infusions of propionic acid on plasma insulin. Can J Anim Sci 1984;64(Suppl.): 148.

Langer P. Comparative anatomy of the stomach in mammalian herbivores. J Exp Physiol 1984;69:615.

McGilliard DA, Jacobson NI, Sutton JD. Physiological development of the ruminant stomach. In: Dougherty RW, ed. Physiology of digestion in the ruminant. London: Butterworths, 1965.

Ooms L, Degryse A. Pathogenesis and pharmacology of diarrhea. Vet Res Commun 1986;10:355.

Scott D. Changes in mineral, water, and acid-base balance associated with feeding and diet. In: McDonald IW, Warner ACI, eds. Digestion and metabolism in the ruminant. Armidale: U New England Publishing Unit, 1975.

Thivend P, Toullec R, Guilloteau P. Digestive adaptation in the preruminant. In: Ruckebusch Y, Thivend P, eds. Digestive physiology and metabolism in ruminants. Lancaster: MTP Press Ltd, 1980.

Vernay M. Resorption von kurzkettigen Fettsäuren in Dickdarm des Kaninchens in vivo. Dtsch tierärztl Wschr 1987;94:7.

Washabau RJ, Strombeck DR, Buffington CA, Harrold D. Evaluation of intestinal carbohydrate malabsorption in the dog by pulmonary hydrogen gas excretion. Am J Vet Res 1986;47:1402.

CHAPTER 28

NEUROENDOCRINE CONTROL OF THE DIGESTIVE TRACT

The multiple activities of the digestive system are modulated by the enteric nervous system (ENS), which is independent of the central and autonomic parts of the nervous system. Through central and local neural reflexes, the nervous system also provides specific stimuli for the release of gastrointestinal peptides, some of which are recognized as true hormones. This chapter presents two elements of the neuroendocrine control of the gastrointestinal tract, the ENS and gastrointestinal peptides.

THE ENTERIC NERVOUS SYSTEM

In addition to the components of the autonomic nervous system (parasympathetic and sympathetic fibers), a third component exists in the wall of the digestive tube. It represents a complex neuronal network, the ENS.

The term "enteric nervous system" was coined by LANGLEY (1852–1925) to describe the functional characteristics of plexuses discovered by MEISSNER (1829–1905) in the connective tissue of the submucosa of the small intestine, and by AUERBACH (1828–1897) between the longitudinal and circular smooth muscle layers.

The ENS is intrinsic to the wall of the gastrointestinal tract. With a gastric part and an intestinal part, the ENS runs uninterrupted from the lower esophagus to the anus. It consists of two nerve networks that completely envelop the gut. The first network (myenteric, or Auerbach's plexus) lies between the smooth muscle layers, and the second one (submucosal, or Meissner's plexus) lies between the inner smooth muscle (circular) layer and the submucosa. Each has groups of ganglion cells interconnected by fiber tracts (Fig. 28–1).

The ENS functions like a "brain" to coordinate and program gastrointestinal functions. Electrophysiological research on the intestinal part of the ENS has revealed sensory cells, interneurons, and motor neurons grouped in a complex arrangement that forms an independent nervous system dedicated to the regulation of digestion. The intestinal wall of the cat contains nearly 70 million nerve cells. These enteric nerve entities are not considered to be mere stations of the parasympathetic system. Similar electrophysiological studies have not been conducted on the gastric part of the ENS.

The operating model for the ENS is the same as for the central nervous system (CNS). The ENS works by means of *sensory receptors,* which may be mechanoreceptors, chemoreceptors, or thermoreceptors. Sensory information on the moment-to-moment state of the gastrointestinal wall and lumen is collected by these receptors and coded in the form of *action potentials.* Through a synaptically connected network of *interneurons,* this information is processed and is distributed to motor neurons. These *motor neurons,* which are the final common pathways to the effector systems, may initiate, sustain, or inhibit the behavior of the *effector.*

The link between the extrinsic nervous input and the enteric nervous system is complex and is still debated. It is recognized that gastroenteric reflex arcs function independent of preganglionic parasympathetic fibers. Current neurophysiological concepts suggest that the ENS contains subsets of neural circuits that are programmed for control of distinct gastrointestinal motility patterns. These preexisting programs receive command inputs that are transmitted from the CNS along vagal fibers (Fig. 28–2). This concept would explain the potent influence of a small number of vagal efferent fibers on motility in a broad region of bowel. This construct is analogous to the operation of other, better-known, neural control systems in which activation of single "command neurons" releases extensive coordinated motor responses.

Sympathetic pathways transmit command signals from the CNS that shut down gastrointestinal blood flow and motility. This is a component of the pervasive response of the sympathetic nervous system to environmental stresses. Part of the mechanism for sympathetic shutdown of the bowel is mediated by input that acts on presynaptic terminals to prevent release of excitatory transmitter substances within the ENS.

Role of the Gastroenteric Nervous System

In sheep, suppression of extrinsic parasympathetic nerves (vagal) results in abolition of the sequential and correlated ruminoreticulum contractions; however, adaptive changes occur in the ENS of the ruminoreticulum if the denervated sheep are maintained on a liquid diet. From 12 to 21 days after truncal vagotomy, wavelets are seen here and there on the reticulum and later on the rumen walls. Then, suddenly, within a 24-hour period, the ruminoreticulum presents slow and prolonged weak contractions at intervals of 120 to 180 seconds (Fig. 28–3).

Role of the Intestinal Enteric Nervous System

A simple model can be used to summarize the operation of the intestinal ENS during peristaltic motor events (Fig. 28–4). Peristalsis is activated by input from stretch receptors, which signal, via cholinergic interneurons, radial dis-

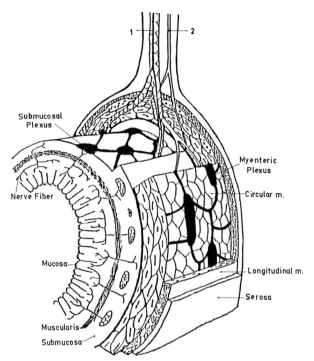

Figure 28–1 The ENS, with its intrinsic networks of neurons, interneurons, and nerve fibers that form the submucosal plexus and the myenteric plexus. The arteries link the ENS to the extrinsic nerves; the sympathetic fibers travel within the arterial wall (*1*); and the parasympathetic fibers are in proximity (*2*) to the artery.

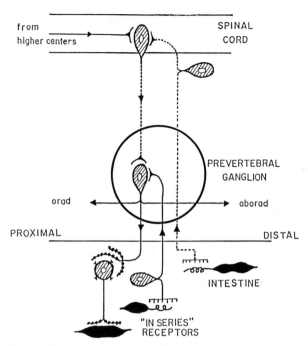

Figure 28–2 Arrangement of the components in peripheral sympathetic reflexes. By acting directly on the cells in the prevertebral ganglion, the "in series" receptors activate a local response and a more dispersed response, which spreads orad and aborad. Vagal afferent fibers may reinforce the local receptor signal through synapses with neurons in the CNS.

tention of the muscular layers. This input activates inhibitory neurons ahead of the bolus. The inhibitory neurons are depicted as being dependent on cholinergic stimulation. This hypothesis is based on (1) the predominance of fast cholinergic excitation in enteric neurons; (2) the blockade of descending inhibition by nicotinic-blocking drugs; and (3) the absence of effect of serotonin or serotonergic drugs. The cholinergic motor neurons are presented as being slowly stimulated by serotonin (AH/type 2 cells). Coordination of contraction of the circular muscle layer orad to the bolus with contraction of the longitudinal muscle layer aborad to the bolus is achieved in the model by spatial distribution of the processes of the neurons (AH/type 2).

Electromyography demonstrates that the ENS periodically elicits short periods of rhythmic depolarization (regular spiking activity, or RSA, of the myoelectrical complex) on the small intestine of sheep. This ability of the ENS is emphasized by comparing the intestinal motility pattern of a fetal lamb with that of a parasympathetically denervated segment of sheep gut. This segment of small intestine is doubly transected, then is reinstalled in continuity with the small intestine by double end-to-end anastomoses, and is denervated. The denervated segment behaves like an independent unit, with numerous (4-hour) periods of rhythmic depolarization resembling those seen before birth, when the small intestine is not developed and is not propelling chyme.

In pigs, the extrinsic innervation does not provide the pathway for initiation and propagation of myoelectrical complexes in denervated jejunal segments. In less than 10 days after autotransplantation (complete autonomic nervous system denervation), the periods of RSA reappear and recur regularly. This indicates that the pattern of reciprocal excitation and inhibition regulating the migration of the phases of RSA must be controlled by integrative networks within the ENS.

Role of Motilin

The origin of the enteric myoelectrical complexes is suggested to be at the antrum, although the frequency of the duodenal basic electrical rhythm (slow waves) is three to four times faster than in the antrum. The basis of this hypothesis is a coincident cyclical hyperactivity of the whole gastroduodenal area in fasting dogs. The release of gut hormones resulting from periodic changes in the intraduodenal pH is considered to be the factor that activates the cyclical periods of spiking activity at the gastroduodenal area. The plasma concentration of motilin increases five-fold immediately at the beginning of a cyclical period of gastric contractions and a subsequent duodenal myoelectrical complex. In the dog, duodenal alkalinization, which occurs 7 to 8 hours after feeding, stimulates release of motilin.

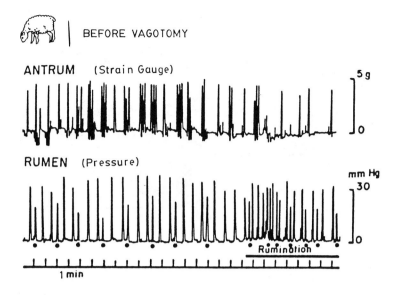

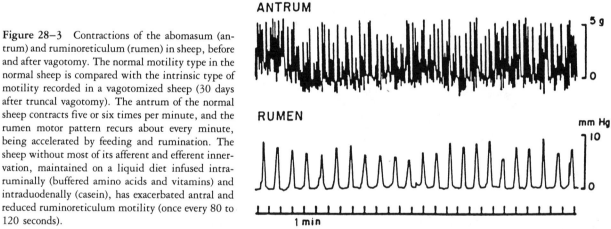

Figure 28–3 Contractions of the abomasum (antrum) and ruminoreticulum (rumen) in sheep, before and after vagotomy. The normal motility type in the normal sheep is compared with the intrinsic type of motility recorded in a vagotomized sheep (30 days after truncal vagotomy). The antrum of the normal sheep contracts five or six times per minute, and the rumen motor pattern recurs about every minute, being accelerated by feeding and rumination. The sheep without most of its afferent and efferent innervation, maintained on a liquid diet infused intraruminally (buffered amino acids and vitamins) and intraduodenally (casein), has exacerbated antral and reduced ruminoreticulum motility (once every 80 to 120 seconds).

GASTROINTESTINAL HORMONES

Gastrointestinal hormones all are peptides originating from amine precursor uptake decarboxylase (APUD) cells, which have migrated from their site of origin in the neural crest of the embryo to various digestive organs (antrum, small and large intestine, pancreas). In these structures, these cells have differentiated into specific gastroenteropancreatic (GEP) endocrine cells. Because cells that secrete gut hormones are nerve cells by origin, it is not surprising that gut hormones appear in the brain and that neurotransmitters appear in nerve cells of the intestine.

Gut endocrinology began with the discovery of the first hormones, secretin (1902) and gastrin (1905), and pro-

gressed in an unspectacular fashion until the 1960s. In contrast to glandular endocrinology, research on gut hormones was impeded by the difficulty in investigating a diffuse system of different endocrine cells scattered in a great bulk of tissue. Extirpation of cells is impossible, and tissue extracts contain a number of hormones, proteins, and peptides. Six decades elapsed before the uncertainty about the nature and specificity of these two gut hormones was resolved.

When many identified peptides isolated from the gut are injected into experimental animals, they evoke several responses and are presumed to be mediating these actions. So far, only four peptides have been confirmed as 'bona fide' gut hormones: secretin, gastrin, cholecystokinin-pancreozymin (CCK, or CCK-PZ), and gastric inhibitory peptide (GIP).

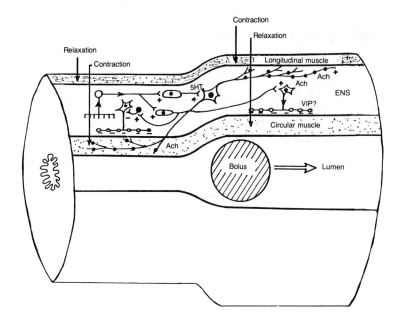

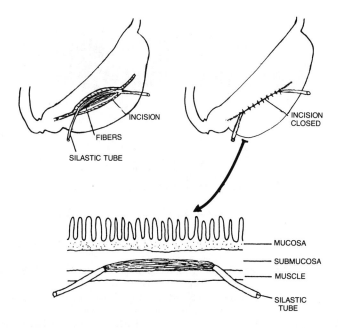

Figure 28–4 **Top,** Schematic of neural circuitry for control of the longitudinal and circular layers of smooth muscles during peristalsis. In the segment orad to the bolus, the circular muscles contract, whereas the longitudinal muscles are inhibited. Over and aborad to the bolus, the intestinal longitudinal muscles then contract, with concomitant relaxation of the circular muscles. The neurotransmitters (ACH, serotonin, VIP) may provoke a depolarization (excitation, +) or hyperpolarization (inhibition, −) at the synapses. **Bottom,** Fine hollow cellulose fibers are surgically implanted for dialysis of the gastric or intestinal submucosa. Analysis of the composition of the fluid of dialysis provides information on the neurotransmitters or neuromodulators released during the local phases (ECA or NSA, ISA, ERA or RSA) of gastrointestinal motor activity.

Most of the other gut peptides, only considered as "candidate" gut hormones, must satisfy other criteria before being recognized as "true" gut hormones.

On the basis of common amino acid sequences and their biological actions, gastrointestinal peptides have been classified into three groups. Two of these groups are represented by the secretin family and the gastrin family, and the third is a group of heterogenous peptides that fit into neither of the other families (Table 28–1).

These polypeptides, which have receptor sites in all

TABLE 28–1 Classification of Gastrointestinal Peptides

"Family," or Group	Peptides
Secretin "family," or secretin-like group	Secretin, VIP, glucagon, GIP
Gastrin "family," or CCK-like group	Gastrin, CCK, CCK-PZ
Heterogeneous group	Bombesin, or gastrin-releasing peptide; chymodenin; motilin; neurotensin; somatostatin; substance P

tissues of the gastrointestinal tract, influence motility, secretion, absorption, and growth of the digestive system. They are released in response to short or long vagovagal neural reflexes, to the presence of other hormones, and to specific stimuli that act on the gastrointestinal mucosa.

Gut Peptides Released in Response to a Meal

The gut peptides released during the digestion of a meal act on diverse targets. They affect secretion and motility of stomach and small intestine, pancreatic and biliary secretions, absorption, and epithelial growth of the gastrointestinal tract. By following the path of ingesta through the gastrointestinal tract, it is logical to consider that the gastroenteropancreatic endocrine peptides are liberated in sequence (Fig. 28–5). The first peptides liberated include somatostatin, VIP, substance P, enkephalins, and bombesin, which are present in cells located in the fundus of the stomach. Gastrin and GIP are then secreted, and subsequently secretin, CCK, motilin, and chymodenin are activated. Enteroglucagon and neurotensin are released when chyme reaches the ileum.

Somatostatin (14 amino acids) is an antitrophic peptide in all gastrointestinal tissues. It is released into the gastric venous blood and the gastric lumen by acidification of the duodenum. Considered to be a putative paracrine peptide, somatostatin can also affect adjacent cells without entering the general circulation and reduces exocrine secretions as well as the output of other endocrine peptides.

Vasoactive intestinal peptide (VIP), a 28–amino acid peptide, shares some structural similarities with secretin, glucagon, and GIP. Found in mast cells, VIP is a potent vasodilator (peripheral, splanchnic, and pulmonary) and is considered a possible nonadrenergic noncholinergic relaxant of the smooth muscles of the reticuloomasal orifice. By stimulating the intestinal mucosa to actively secrete anions and by inhibiting local neutral sodium and chloride absorptive mechanisms in the proximal colon of the dog, it causes a watery diarrhea. In cats, VIP increases the release of insulin. In birds, it is more important than secretin for stimulating pancreatic secretion.

Substance P (11 amino acids) is a vasodepressor peptide that inhibits intrinsic ruminoreticulum motor activity and acid secretion (gastrin). Substance P is a companion peptide of serotonin.

Enterochromaffin (EC) cells produce and release not only *enkephalins* but also serotonin (5HT) and substance P. Of

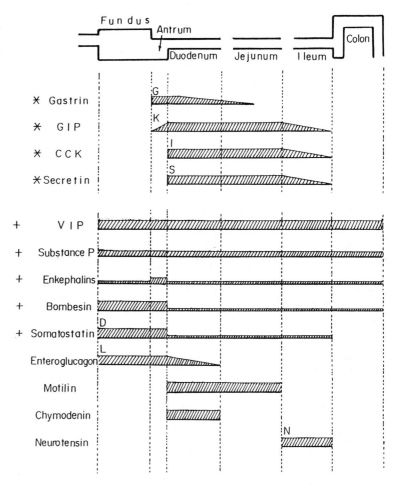

Figure 28–5 Schematic distribution of gastrointestinal peptides in the gastrointestinal tract of dogs. The concentration of each peptide is proportional to the thickness of each horizontal bar. Asterisks represent recognized hormones; pluses indicate the presence in cells of the ENS. The cells that secrete the intestinal peptides: G, K, I, S, D, L, and N.

the enkephalins (5 amino acids), methionine is two to five times more potent than leucine in producing the biological effects of morphine on smooth muscle. Enkephalins play a physiological role by increasing the amount of food eaten during a meal (sheep), by increasing gastric secretion (dog), and by suppressing pancreatic secretion and gastrointestinal motility. With VIP, somatostatin, neuropeptide Y (NPY), and gastrin-releasing peptide (GRP, or mammalian *bombesin*), enkephalins are the putative peptidergic neurotransmitters found in postganglionic nerve terminals.

The mammalian form of bombesin (14 amino acids) is termed gastrin-releasing peptide (GRP). As a putative neurotransmitter or paracrine agent it can act locally. It also functions and produces its effects in classic hormonal fashion when it is released from smooth muscle nerve terminals into the peripheral circulation. In sheep, under physiological conditions, GRP reduces food intake, elicits satiety, and controls insulin release.

Gastrin (17 amino acids) differs slightly in its composition in bovine, canine, feline, ovine, and porcine stomachs, but the pentapeptide C-terminal sequence (termed pentagastrin) is the same. More gastrin is found in the mucous membrane of the antrum than in that of the duodenum, because the former has twice as many G cells. Several factors stimulate or inhibit release of gastrin (Table 28–2).

Gastrin inhibits salivation, increases gastric secretion of acid and pepsinogen, raises the output of pancreatic enzymes (50 percent of the effects of CCK in the dog), and releases more insulin. On the oxyntic cells and the mucous cells (stomach, small intestine, pancreas, colon), gastrin increases DNA, RNA, and protein synthesis and thus augments the size and the quantity of mucosal cells. This potent gastrointestinal trophic action of gastrin is antagonized by secretin and VIP. Gastrin increases the closure of the reticuloomasal orifice, decreases the frequency of reticular contractions, and delays gastric or abomasal emptying (dog, calf, sheep).

Gastrointestinal peptide (GIP) (43 amino acids) originates from villi and upper crypt cells, most of which are in the duodenum, some in the jejunum, and a few in the ileum. GIP is released when chyme containing lipids (triglycerides), amino acids, or glucose comes in contact with these cells.

TABLE 28–2 Factors That Influence the Release of Gastrin from the G Cells in the Antrum and the Duodenum

Factors That Stimulate Release	Factors That Inhibit Release
Abomasal parasitism	Dopamine
Calcium 2.7 (sheep)	Gastric acidification: pH < 2.7–4.0
Epinephrine	GIP
Feeding	Glucagon
milk (preruminant)	Hyperglycemia
fresh food (fasted sheep)	Magnesium
Gastric pH above 4.0 (dog)	Norepinephrine
GRP	Prostaglandins
Hypoglycemia	Secretin
Isoosmolar ethanol (dog)	Somatostatin
Products of protein digestion	Vagotomy
Vagal stimulation (sham feeding)	VIP

Despite its name, the major function of GIP is to regulate the release of pancreatic insulin. During the hyperglycemia of feeding, this *incretin* action increases the production of insulin. The importance of this physiological function is the basis of the suggestion of an alternate, and probably more appropriate, name for GIP: *glucose-dependent insulinotropic peptide*. GIP also causes a higher rate of secretion (rich in chloride ions) in the jejunum and disturbs the absorption of water and electrolytes in the small intestine.

Secretin (27 amino acids), which has structural similarities to VIP, GIP, and glucagon, has no active group and requires the whole molecule to function. It is released into the circulation from duodenal and jejunal mucosal cells (3 to 1 ratio) upon their activation by acid chyme (pH 3 to 4.5) or bile salts (dog), especially sodium taurocholate in cats.

In the dog but not in the cat, in response to a meal secretin is more efficient as an inhibitor of gastric acid secretion than as a stimulant of pancreatic secretion rich in water and bicarbonate. Secretin also increases the volume and alkalinity of bile, the output of fluid from the submucosal duodenal (Brunner's) glands, and the production of pepsinogen by the gastric cells. Diuresis of a sodium- and chloride-rich urine follows the administration of secretin (or of glucagon, which shares 14 of its 27 amino acids).

Secretin reduces ruminoreticulum motility, delays gastric emptying, and decreases motility of the small intestine. It also constricts the sphincter of Oddi to shut off the flow of bile into the gut and directs it to the gallbladder. Secretin has a trophic effect on the duodenum and the pancreas, but an antitrophic action on the gastric oxyntic cells.

Cholecystokinin (CCK) (33 amino acids) is the term used to designate a single peptide that causes gallbladder contraction and pancreatic enzyme secretion. Originally, these effects were erroneously attributed to two separate substances, CCK and *pancreozymin* (PZ), which were later proved to be identical. For both actions to be optimal, a core of eight amino acids (CCK8) and sulfatation are essential. The name CCK is used because of historical precedent.

CCK is released from the duodenum and the jejunum by cold exposure, by luminal products of lipid and protein digestion, and by enteropancreatic cholinergic reflexes. The most efficient CCK releasers are fatty acids longer than nine carbons, and amino acids such as phenylalanine, tryptophan, methionine, and valine.

CCK increases gastric acid output (more in cats than in dogs), intestinal flow of lymph, acinar pancreatic production of enzymes (trypsinogen, but not lipase) and calcium, and release of hormones (insulin, somatostatin, GIP, and secretin). CCK and secretin exert a synergistic effect (effect greater than the sum of individual actions) to produce a voluminous, alkaline, and enzyme-rich pancreatic secretion. This effect is associated with activation of both cyclic guanosine monophosphate (cGMP) and cyclic adenosine monophosphate (cAMP) intracellular messenger nucleotides (cGMP is activated by CCK, gastrin, GRP, substance P, and acetylcholine; cAMP is activated by secretin, VIP, and cholera toxin).

The release of CCK stimulates the gallbladder to contract and increases motility of the small intestine and the colon. Meanwhile, the lower esophageal sphincter (LES), the ruminoreticulum, the gastric fundus, and the sphincter of Oddi all relax, and gastric emptying also ceases. Intracerebral ventricular (ICV) administration of CCK induces satiety and reduces meal size in sheep and pigs, possibly by causing generalized malaise.

Motilin (22 amino acids) is a motor-stimulating peptide present in EC cells of the duodenum and jejunum. It is released by acidification (pig) or alkalinization (dog) of the duodenum. During the canine interdigestive (fasting) phase of intestinal motor activity, the motilin plasma level is lowest during the nonspiking activity (NSA) phase (quiescent, phase I) and is highest during the regular spiking activity (RSA) phase (phase III, activity front) of the migrating myoelectrical complex (MMC). Motilin is thought to initiate the RSA phases periodically, every 90 to 120 minutes. In the fasting dog, administration of motilin causes contraction of the LES and of the stomach and increases gastric emptying of fluids (not of solids).

Chymodenin (74 to 76 amino acids) is a peptide isolated from the small intestine. It is an acronym for *chymo*tryp-sino-trypsinogen *duode*num stimulin, which causes selective secretion of chymotrypsinogen-trypsinogen without changing the output of lipase in the pancreatic juice (rabbit).

Enteroglucagon is a 37–amino acid peptide that is part of a larger peptide, *glicentin* (100 amino acids), found in the ileum and the colon. It is released as a result of local chemical and physical stimuli. Blood enteroglucagon increases after oral administration of glucose, when lipids are present in the duodenum and the ileum, and during exposure to cold. Enteroglucagon inhibits gastric acid secretion, prolongs intestinal transit time, and exerts considerable trophic actions on gastric and intestinal growth.

Neurotensin (13 amino acids) is a peptidergic transmitter found in the brain and in the mucosa of the ileum (dog). Released by lipids, the physiological action of neurotensin is still unknown but may involve inhibition of gastric acid secretion. Some of its pharmacological effects include lower gastric acid secretion and motility (dog) and higher glycemia and blood glucagon levels.

REFERENCES

Bloom SR. Gut hormones. New York: Churchill Livingstone, 1978.

Dobson A, Dobson MJ. Aspects of digestive physiology in ruminants. Ithaca: Comstock Publishing Associates, 1988.

Dockray GJ. Evolutionary relationships of the gut hormones. Fed Proc 1979;38:2295.

Milligan LP, Grovum WL, Dobson A, eds. Control of digestion and metabolism in ruminants. Englewood Cliffs, NJ: Prentice-Hall, 1986.

Pearse AGE, Polak JM, Bloom SR. The newer gut hormones. Cellular sources, physiology, pathology, and clinical aspects. Gastroenterology 1977;72:746.

Walsh JH. Gastrointestinal hormones and peptides. In: Johnson LR, ed. Physiology of the gastrointestinal tract. New York: Raven Press, 1987.

Wood JD. Enteric neurophysiology. Am J Physiol 1984; 247:G585.

SECTION IV

THE NERVOUS SYSTEM

CHAPTER 29

BASIC FUNCTIONAL ORGANIZATION OF THE NERVOUS SYSTEM

The nervous system is a tubular structure that originates from a proliferation of the fetal ectoderm known as the *neural plate*. Anatomically, it can be divided into the *central* nervous system (CNS), and the *peripheral* nervous system (PNS). The CNS consists of the brain and spinal cord, whereas the PNS comprises the nerve roots from the brain stem and from the spinal cord as well as the peripheral nerves. Whatever the arrangement proposed for the CNS (e.g., whether sensory and motor or somatic and visceral divisions), the neuron, or nerve cell, is the structural, functional, genetic, and trophic unit. This chapter describes some of the fundamental concepts of the organization of the nervous system and of the functions of axons and dendrites of nerve cells.

FUNDAMENTAL CONCEPTS

The nervous system is made up of countless cells known as *neurons* and of a certain amount of *neuroglial tissue*. The neuroglial cells are not involved in the performance of neural functions but form an interstitial, or supporting, tissue. They are involved in the nutrition of the specific neural elements by acting as intermediaries between the blood and these elements. Three types of neuroglial cells were identified at the start of the 20th century by Ramon y Cajal: *astrocytes, oligodendrocytes,* and *microglia*. The astrocytes have many arms, or projections, and contact the walls of cerebral blood vessels and of the meninges. They allow passage of electrolytes and small molecules and assist in regulating the osmotic equilibrium of the neural tissue. The oligodendrocytes appear to be the CNS's counterpart of Schwann cells, which form thin sheaths around the axons of unmyelinated nerve fibers, and of myelin layers of myelinated nerve fibers. The oligodendroglia surround nerve cells and fibers in the CNS, and defects in these fatty sheaths may lead to formation of plaques or patches of scarred nerve fibers (sclerosis). The microglia, the macrophages of the CNS, serve a janitorial role, removing debris from the brain and the spinal cord by their phagocytic activity.

Cerebrospinal Fluid

The neural tissues are protected from mechanical forces by membranes called meninges (pia mater, arachnoid, and dura mater), by bony structures, and by a special liquid, cerebrospinal fluid (CSF), which occupies about 10 percent of the cavities of the CNS. The CSF also plays an important role in maintaining hydrostatic pressure within the cavities of the nerve tissues, and it contributes dynamic exchanges of water, electrolytes, and organic molecules with blood. In addition, CSF plays a role in resistance to infection.

CSF is formed continuously from the capillaries of the choroid plexuses in specialized areas of the cerebral ventricles. By bulk flow, CSF circulates through the ventricles into the central canal of the spinal cord, and it flows into the subarachnoid spaces surrounding the nerve tissue (Fig. 29–1). In dogs, hydrocephalus is produced by blocking the aqueduct of Sylvius, a small canal connecting the third and fourth ventricles of the brain. Reabsorption of CSF into the more viscous blood occurs mainly at venous sinuses via microscopic arachnoid villi.

In most animals, the hydrostatic pressure of the CSF is variable, but usually it is between 0 and 18 cm H_2O. In the goat, pressures between 0 and 5 cm H_2O normally are measured in unanesthetized animals, but -10 to $+320$ cm H_2O is tolerated without signs of discomfort. The volume of CSF is about 20 to 25 mL, and it is produced at a rate near 0.15 mL per minute. Sampling of up to 3 mL per hour does not alter the composition of the CSF.

General Role of the Nervous System

The nervous system may be considered as a communication network, not unlike a telephone system. "Messages," or impulses, are transmitted from receiver organs to effector organs of the body, often through a central switchboard (brain and spinal cord). The receiver organs sense or respond to physical environmental stimuli, such as light, sound, odor, and pressure. The effector organs are able to produce movement and action (muscles) or secrete fluids (glands).

Unlike other cells of the body, neurons have long cytoplasmic extensions called nerve fibers, or *axons*, which are referred to as the *white matter* because of their myelin sheath. They also possess many *dendrites*, which receive information from other nerve cells or receptor organs. The *gray matter* is made up of cell bodies, the trophic units of the neuron. Any portion of the neuron separated from the cell body eventually dies from lack of nutrition; however, a sectioned nerve may regrow down the peripheral nerve path if the separated parts are in close enough proximity to permit the action of nerve growth factor.

Displacement of cytoplasm in the neuron is referred to as *axoplasmic flow*, although it occurs in both axons and dendrites. The cytoplasm flows continuously, first from the cell body toward the end of every extension and then from the far reaches to the cell body of the neuron.

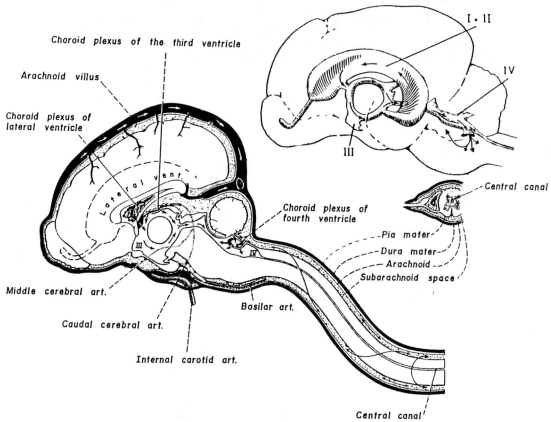

Figure 29–1 Diagram of the CNS (brain and spinal cord) surrounded by CSF produced in the choroid plexuses of the cerebral ventricles. The CNS is protected by bony structures (skull and vertebrae) and by meninges (dura mater, arachnoid, pia mater). In the brain, CSF circulates in four central cerebral ventricles and in a peripheral subarachnoid space, which extends over the spinal cord. The large insert pictures the cerebral ventricles, whereas the small insert represents the arrangement of the meninges in the spinal cord.

According to the direction of transmission of nerve signals (action potentials), the *dendrites* (peripheral processes) normally conduct an action potential *toward* the neuron cell body, whereas *axons* conduct an action potential *away* from the cell body. However, in some specialized *afferent neurons* (e.g., neurons in dorsal root ganglia) transmission is initiated in a *receptor* and travels toward the neuron and then on to a *synapse*.

In the *spinal cord*, the centrally located gray matter forms a column made of neuron cell bodies and supportive tissues. Surrounding this gray matter axis, the white matter makes up the remainder of the spinal cord, much of it as bundles of fibers running rostrad or caudad.

The spinal cord has nuclei of *motor neurons* in the *ventral horn* and in the *intermediolateral cell column* (throughout the thoracic and upper lumbar levels and the sacral levels of the spinal cord). The ventral horns contain the motor neurons that control somatic motor activity, whereas the intermediolateral cell column caters to a visceral efferent system.

Multipolar cells have numerous branching dendrites and a single axon. Those with long axons are typified by the motor nerve cells (motor neurons) in the ventral gray column of the spinal cord. The axons of these neurons emerge from the CNS to become peripheral motor nerve fibers.

Other multipolar nerve cells with short axons are designated as type II Golgi cells. Instead of leaving the gray matter, their axons break up into numerous branches in the vicinity of the cell body. By means of these cells, an afferent neuron may be placed in contact with many motor neurons. These cells are therefore known as *internuncial neurons,* or *interneurons* (Fig. 29–2).

The *dorsal roots of spinal nerves* include thick myelinated fibers and fine myelinated and nonmyelinated fibers (see Fig. 29–2). The thick fibers of the spinal cord are afferent axons, which conduct impulses originating from stretch receptors of muscles. The numerous small fibers, myelinated and nonmyelinated, are afferent axons that transmit impulses, mostly from pain, temperature, and tactile receptors.

Bipolar, pseudounipolar, and all other cells at the origin of peripheral afferent nerve fibers are located in ganglia outside the CNS. *Bipolar cells* have one axon and one dendrite. Examples of such cells are found in the retina of the eye, where light-sensitive cells have a short axon and dendrite.

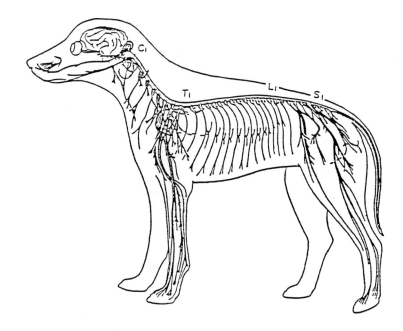

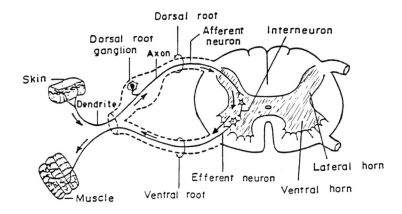

Figure 29–2 Top, Diagrammatic representation of the distribution of the peripheral somatic nervous system with its bilateral cranial (*C*), thoracic (*T*), lumbar (*L*), and sacral (*S*) nerves. **Bottom,** Representation of the gray matter with a dorsal (afferent) and a ventral (motor) root. A dendrite connects with an axon of a pseudounipolar cell in the dorsal root ganglion. In the lateral horn of the gray matter, an interneuron (multipolar cell) distributes the incoming signal to one (ipsilateral) or several (contralateral) motor cells of the ventral horn. The axon from the motor cell carries an effector signal to muscle cells.

In pseudounipolar cells, nerve impulses apparently pass from the peripheral branch to the central branch without entering the cell body. These nerve cells of the ganglia of the cranial and spinal nerves are also embryonically bipolar cells. However, the two processes have fused near the cell body into a single process, so that the neuron is *T shaped*. One branch (real dendrite) of the process functions as an axon of an afferent nerve fiber from a peripheral receptor, whereas the other branch (real axon) passes into the CNS by way of the dorsal root of a spinal or cranial nerve. *Pseudounipolar neurons,* where the peripheral branch is physiologically a dendrite, serve as axons to conduct nerve impulses centrally (Fig. 29–3).

Nerve and muscle cells have the property of *excitability*. When a suitable stimulus is applied to a nerve axon, the plasma membrane becomes excited and an electrical event (i.e., an action potential) occurs within the plasma membrane at the point of stimulation.

The action potential travels (propagates) away from this point at a fixed speed (i.e., conduction velocity) related to the diameter of the axon. The information sent along nerve axons is graded by the number (frequency per second) of identical action potentials, rather than by variations in the strength of the impulses themselves. When a skin receptor is stimulated, gently at first then vigorously, action potentials of identical strength are generated, and they travel up the afferent nerve at the same speed. However, the strong stimulation induces more signals per unit of time (i.e., more action potentials pass a given point on the nerve during a given interval) (see Fig. 29–3).

The impulses conducted along the processes of neurons (axons and dendrites) are really electrical phenomena (Fig. 29–4). An impulse modifies the electrical charge of the neuron; it changes the relationship between the positive charges on the surface of the plasma membrane and the negative charges within. This change travels along the neu-

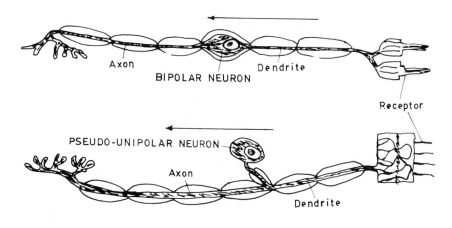

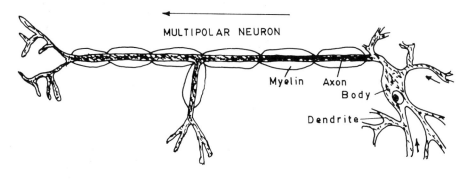

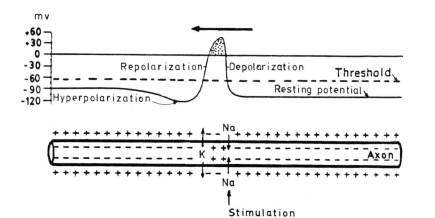

Figure 29–3 Top, Types of *afferent* neurons (bipolar, and pseudounipolar) and *efferent* neurons (multipolar internuncial or interneuron, and motor). **Bottom**, Impulse (action potential) on a nerve axon resulting from effective stimulation, which successively depolarizes, repolarizes, and hyperpolarizes the plasma membrane. The resting polarized state (−90 mV, positive charge outside, negative charge inside) is gradually reversed by an influx of sodium cations until the threshold is reached (−60 mV); then an abrupt influx of sodium cations depolarizes it to about +55 mV. Repolarization is by a sudden outflow of potassium cations, whereas hyperpolarization to nearly −120 mV (a state of inhibition or refractoriness to stimulation) is due to an excessive outflow of univalent cations (sodium and potassium).

ron by producing a breakdown of permeability of the plasma membrane in the area immediately next to the impulse. When this breakdown in permeability occurs, the charges at that new point modify their relationship, and that point then gets the impulse. In the meantime, the area that previously had the impulse begins to restore itself. This change in electrical potential is associated with an exchange of sodium and potassium ions between the exterior and the interior of the neuron. A nerve impulse travels along the neuron, either to or from the CNS, depending on whether the neuron is afferent or efferent.

The main paired nerve trunk, the ganglionated sympa-

thetic trunk on each side of the spinal column, receives *white rami communicantes* from the ventral branches of the thoracic and of the lumbar spinal nerves (Fig. 29–5). These white rami are made up of some myelinated preganglionic fibers, which extend from the ventral branch of a spinal nerve to the corresponding sympathetic vertebral ganglion. They parallel the *gray rami* (unmyelinated postganglionic fibers), which are returning from the sympathetic vertebral ganglion to their corresponding spinal nerves.

The white rami communicantes, which enter the ganglionated sympathetic trunk in the thoracic and in the lumbar regions, are the efferent connections of the sympathetic

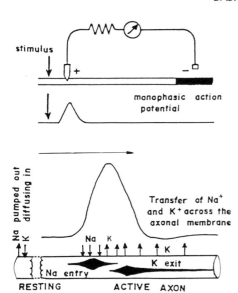

Figure 29–4   The action potential is a deviation of the resting potential. The stimulus (excitation process) causes increased permeability of the plasma membrane to sodium cations. They are transferred en masse from outside into the cytoplasm, where their positive charges progressively change the resting negative potential into a positive action potential. When the internal medium reaches maximal positivity (maximal depolarization) in relation to the external medium, a sudden reversal of potentials occurs toward the initial resting potential (repolarization). The two processes (depolarization, or change of the resting potential, and emergence of repolarization, or return to the resting potential) constitute the action potential.

system with the CNS. The rest of the sympathetic nervous system consists of nerve trunks and of ganglia associated with visceral structures of the body. For example, the greater and lesser splanchnic nerves carry sympathetic fibers to the abdominal viscera from ganglia and plexuses, such as cranial mesenteric, caudal mesenteric, and celiac. In contrast, most of the ganglia of the parasympathetic system are within the wall of the organs, and the parasympathetic nerves (pneumogastric, or vagus, and hypogastric) are represented by efferent preganglionic fibers (see Fig. 29–5).

The Blood-Brain Barrier

Brain capillaries act as stringent gatekeepers between blood and brain and control the uptake of nutrients and the release of metabolites by nerve cells. Over a century ago, it was observed (Ehrlich, 1885) that injected dyes do not cross into the CNS. The existence of a blood-brain barrier (BBB), first erroneously located in the choroid plexuses, is now accepted to be in the brain capillaries, which account for 99 percent of the BBB. The collective surface area of these brain capillaries is estimated to be over 5,000-fold that of the choroid plexuses.

The mechanism of the BBB is in part a function of lack of opportunities for pinocytosis, but it is due mostly to design features of the brain capillaries, particularly the im-

permeable tight junctions between the endothelial cells and the small number of pores or fenestrations. These tight junctions between endothelial cells of brain capillaries are permeable to small molecules and ions. Besides small molecules and ions, only lipid-permeable or carrier-transported substances can penetrate the endothelium of brain capillaries. A similar capillary barrier system is found in peripheral neural networks such as enteric ganglia.

Another obstacle to entry of substances into the CNS is the blood-CSF barrier. The capillaries of the circumventricular organs, which include the choroid plexuses, are porous and allow rapid diffusion of small molecules into the interstitial space surrounding them. However, a tight junction barrier on the ventricular side of the membrane lining the cerebral ventricles (ependyma) prevents any further penetration of larger molecules. In most species, these barriers (blood-brain and blood-CSF) are nearly fully formed in newborn animals. The neuroglial or glial cells do not contribute to the BBB effect.

Significant roles of the BBB are regulation of brain metabolism and protection of the nervous system from foreign chemicals and organisms. In addition, the BBB prevents unnecessary contact of the nervous system with large endogenous molecules that may have undesirable effects. For example, when dopamine is injected peripherally, it inhibits ruminoreticulum motility without causing central nervous effects. However, when dopamine is introduced into the CNS (e.g., intracerebroventricularly), it induces behavior changes without affecting motility of the ruminoreticulum.

FUNCTIONS OF NEURONS

This section presents the all-or-none principle and the concepts of threshold, conduction, saltatory condition, synapse, and neuromuscular junction.

All-or-None Principle

Within a *neuron,* the speed of progression of an impulse and its amplitude, or size, are relatively invariable, though they do vary from one neuron to another. A particular neuron always conducts impulses at the same velocity and amplitude, regardless of the power of the stimulus (light, sound, or pressure) that initiated the impulse. This characteristic is referred to as the all-or-none principle.

The velocity of transmission and the amplitude of an impulse are determined by differences in charges on the plasma membrane of the cell and by interchange of ions through the plasma membrane. These factors have nothing to do with the size of the stimulus. The all-or-none principle means that the energy for neural impulses resides within the neuron.

A neuron is like a fuse made of gunpowder. Such a fuse burns at the same rate and with the same amount of heat whether it is lit by a blowtorch or a match. The neuron is similar to the fuse in that the velocity and the amplitude of

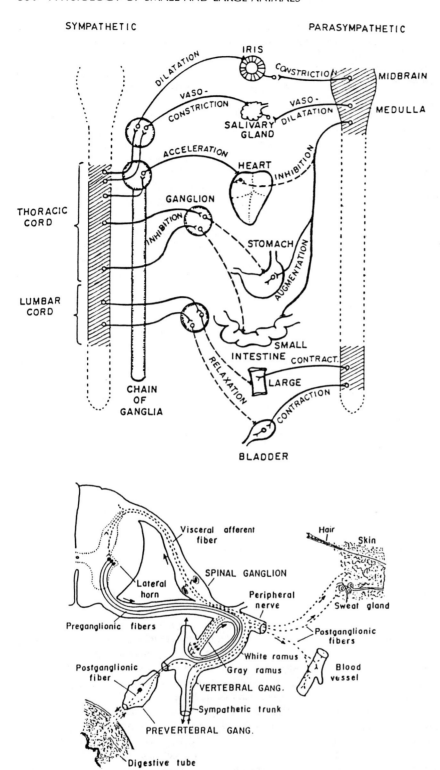

Figure 29–5 **Top,** The autonomic (efferent) innervation of some of the viscera. Each organ receives a double innervation, and the actions of the two systems (sympathetic and parasympathetic) are opposite. The sympathetic visceral efferent neurons are located in the thoracolumbar portions of the spinal cord, whereas the parasympathetic neurons are in the cranial (midbrain and medulla) and the sacral portions of the nervous system. **Bottom,** Relation of the sympathetic neurons to structures in the thoracic spinal cord, in the sympathetic trunk, and in the viscera. The direction of conduction in preganglionic fibers (solid lines) and postganglionic fibers (broken lines) is also given.

the impulse depend entirely on the state of the conductor, which should be well-nourished and not depleted of essential biochemical substances.

Differences occur in the number of impulses conducted by a neuron during a given time and in the distance between successive impulses. A strong stimulus produces a series of impulses separated by short intervals, whereas a weak stimulus causes fewer impulses to occur at greater intervals. In addition, a more intense stimulus arouses activity in more neurons.

Muscle cells of the efferent system operate on the same all-or-none principle as neurons. A muscle cell, if stimulated enough to react at all, contracts to its maximum extent. Gradations of contractions do not occur within a muscle cell. Differences in the amount of muscle pull are produced by increasing the number of muscle cells that contract. This is correlated with the number of impulses carried by a neuron and by the number of neurons that are active or firing.

Threshold for Response

A neuron does not respond at all to a stimulus below the threshold value. All stimuli above the threshold, no matter how strong, produce exactly the same effect on the neuron in terms of velocity of transmission (speed of conduction) and of amplitude of the impulse. Thus, a neuron either fires at the maximum strength permitted by its chemical structure or does not fire at all. Thresholds may be altered by repeated stimulation, and weak stimuli may *summate* to the point where they exceed the threshold.

Speed of Conduction of Impulses

Once an impulse is initiated, it propagates away from the site of excitation at a fixed speed, or *conduction velocity*. The conduction velocity is related to the diameter of the nerve axon, and to whether it is myelinated. A localized passive change in plasma membrane potential, such as one caused by subthreshold stimulation, does not spread more than a few millimeters along the nerve.

The action potential must be continuously regenerated as it propagates. An action potential at one site on an axon's surface causes local currents to flow between the active depolarized area and the adjacent inactive regions. These new active depolarized regions in turn depolarize and excite their neighboring regions, and so the impulse is propagated.

The speed of conduction of a nerve fiber is determined by the strength of the current flowing in the local circuits ahead of the impulse. One of the most important factors is the longitudinal resistance offered by the axoplasm to current flow. This, in turn, is determined by the diameter of the nerve fiber (Fig. 29–6).

Just like a wire cable, axons with the largest diameter have the lowest resistance to current flow along the axon. In large axons, the comparatively low internal resistance leads to high conduction velocity. In vertebrates, this is the only mechanism used to obtain high conduction velocity. The squid escapes from its enemies by driving itself rapidly backward through the water via gigantic (500-μm in diameter) nerve fibers, which have a conduction velocity as high as 20 m per second. In mammalian nerves, high conduction velocity is the result of myelin insulation (Table 29–1), but a large unmyelinated fiber still conducts impulses faster than a myelinated fiber of small diameter (fibers of group I are larger than those of group II). The myelin insulates the nerve between nodes, so that the local currents produced by activity at one node are forced to flow across the next nodal regions.

Saltatory Conduction of Impulses

Myelinated nerves are characterized by nodes of Ranvier, which occur at regular intervals as interruptions in the insulating myelin. The distance between nodes varies with the diameter of the nerves: it is greatest in the thickest nerves, about 0.3 to 2 mm. These nodes allow the occurrence of a phenomenon known as *saltatory conduction,* which involves jumping of nerve impulses from node to node. Only a small proportion (less than 10 percent) of the energy of saltatory conduction is lost by spread to adjacent fibers. Saltatory conduction, which is much faster and conserves more energy) permits expansion and increased efficiency of neural communication within the animal body. In higher vertebrates, it is an evolutionary advantage. In unmyelinated fibers, the nerve impulses travel only by progressive depolarization of the nerve plasma membrane.

Synapse, or Communication between Neurons

A *synapse* is the meeting site of neurons, such as the juncture of the axon of an afferent neuron with a dendrite or a cell of an interneuron (internuncial, or association, neuron). Little is known about what goes on at a synaptic connection between the presynaptic neuron and the postsynaptic neuron, but the neural impulse does not jump the synaptic cleft (or gap) like a spark. The neural impulse ceases when it reaches the end of the axon of the presynaptic neuron, and it causes biochemical substances to be secreted from vesicles in the bouton (presynaptic spherical end). The synapse works as a one-way valve, because the transmitters in the vesicles are localized in the presynaptic part of the junction.

In a cholinergic synapse, acetylcholine (ACh) is the transmitter substance. ACh is made in the mitochondria of the presynaptic terminal by acetylation of choline. The ACh formed is stored almost entirely in the many tiny vesicles found in the presynaptic nerve terminal. Each vesicle is estimated to contain about 1,000 molecules of ACh. The transmitter is released from the presynaptic endings in "packets," or "quanta," each consisting of many ACh molecules. A single quantum of transmitter probably corresponds to the contents of a single presynaptic vesicle. The postsynaptic membrane potential change is attributed to the simultaneous arrival of large numbers of quanta of ACh (Fig. 29–7).

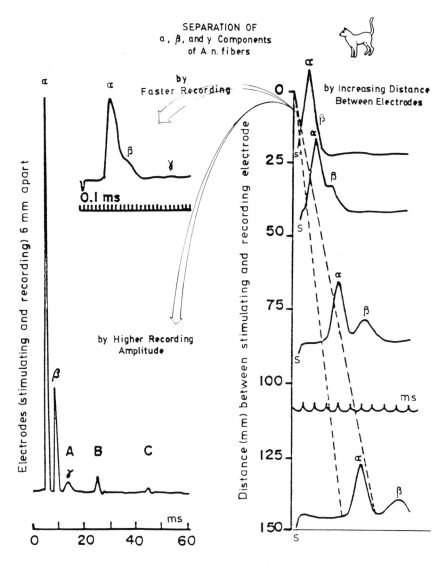

Figure 29-6 Electroneurogram (action potential) of a mixed cutaneous nerve (the saphenous nerve in the cat) recorded at a distance of 6 cm from the stimulating electrode. The peaks of the A-fiber group are indicated by α and β. At the greatest distance between stimulating and recording electrodes (143 mm), for a stimulus voltage that is just sufficient for presence of the β component, the α components become separated. The ordinate records the distance (in millimeters) between stimulating and recording electrodes. The abscissa represents time (in milliseconds). The insert corresponds to the diagrammatic representation of the α, β, and γ components of the electrical response of the A-fiber group to a single stimulus.

In sequence, the events at the origin of an *excitatory postsynaptic potential* (EPSP) are

1. Depolarization of the presynaptic terminal by an arriving action potential
2. Release of ACh from the presynaptic membrane, diffusion of ACh across the synaptic cleft, and its attachment to a receptor on the postsynaptic membrane (all of which occur within 0.5 ms)
3. Increase in permeability of the postsynaptic membrane, resulting in depolarization and in excitation of the postsynaptic membrane
4. Removal or inhibition of ACh by acetylcholinesterase

Instead of spherical endings, presynaptic inhibitory neurons have ellipsoidal endings. The origin of an *inhibitory postsynaptic potential* (IPSP) is linked to release of a transmitter, which acts on a receptor on the postsynaptic membrane to cause its hyperpolarization. Recordings with microelectrodes indicate that IPSP is virtually a mirror image of the EPSP, and that it is a hyperpolarizing potential. The

IPSP is the result of an increase in permeability of the postsynaptic plasma membrane to potassium cations and chloride anions.

Typical examples of "inhibitory neurons," present mostly in the gray matter, have short axons (e.g., Renshaw's cells, inhibitory interneurons, in the ventral horn). In the gray matter, other inhibitory interneurons of reflex arcs (path of an impulse in a reflex act) are also found. They are involved in inhibitory proprioceptive (pertaining to movements and position of the body) and in inhibitory exteroceptive (pertaining to sensations from skin and membranes) reflex arcs.

Catecholamines (e.g., epinephrine) induce hyperpolarization and increase postsynaptic membrane resistance; however, several monocarboxylic amino acids and closely related compounds decrease the postsynaptic membrane resistance during hyperpolarization. These substances have potent depressant effects on neuronal excitability in the CNS. They include gamma-aminobutyric acid (GABA), glycine, taurine, and guanidoacetic acid (Table 29–2).

GABA, uniquely located in the CNS, is released from

TABLE 29–1   Afferent Nerve Fibers Directed to the Spinal Cord

Nerve Groups	Diameter (μm)	Velocity (m/s)	Origin	Stimulus and Threshold	Connections
IA (A,α)	12–20	70–120	Spindle endings	Stretch, low	Monosynaptic agonist with motor neurons (excitatory)
	12–20	70–120	Spindle endings	Stretch, low	Disynaptic antagonist with motor neurons (inhibitory)
IB (A,α)	12–20	70–120	Golgi tendon organs	Stretch, high	Disynaptic agonist with motor neurons (inhibitory)
II (A,β,γ)	5–12	30–70	Touch-pressure	Deformation	Multisynaptic
			Flower spray ending of spindle	Stretch, low	Multisynaptic
III (A,δ)	2–5	12–30	Pain receptors	Noxious stimuli, low	Multisynaptic with autonomic connections
IV (C fibers)	0.5–1.0	0.5–2	Pain receptors	Noxious stimuli, high	Multisynaptic

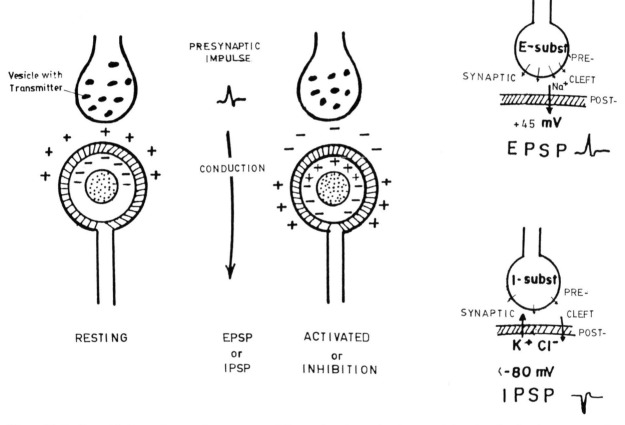

Figure 29–7   Potential changes in an excitatory synapse. When an impulse reaches the synaptic junction of an "excitatory neuron," a cathode is set up in the presynaptic membrane and in the postsynaptic membrane by the release of an E-transmitter (apparently ACh). The resulting reduced polarization allows brief inflow of sodium cations, while inducing local circuits in nearby regions. The flow of sodium cations tends to depolarize the postsynaptic membrane toward 0 mV, and an excitatory postsynaptic potential (EPSP) develops. Correspondingly, at an inhibitory synapse, an impulse releases an I-transmitter substance, which allows an outflow of potassium cations and an inflow of chloride anions through the postsynaptic membrane. As a result of this short increase in permeability to potassium and chloride ions, the whole postsynaptic membrane is hyperpolarized up to -80 mV, with the development of an inhibitory postsynaptic potential (IPSP).

the cerebral cortex. The level of GABA can be related to the electroencephalogram (EEG) pattern: more GABA emerges during sleep than during arousal. GABA is formed by decarboxylation of the dicarboxylic amino acid, L-glutamic acid.

Interestingly enough, the dicarboxylic amino acids, glutamic acid and aspartic acid, are powerful excitants of nerve cells, whereas their decarboxylation products, GABA and beta-alanine, are powerful depressants.

TABLE 29–2 Structure-Activity Relationships of Some Excitant and Depressant Amino Acids on Central Nervous System Neurons

Inhibitory Monocarboxylic and Related Amino Acids	Potency	Corresponding Excitatory Amino Acids	Potency
β-Alanine	− − −	L-Aspartic	+ + +
γ-Aminobutyric acid	− − −	L-Glutamic	+ + +
ε-Aminocaproic acid	−	D-L-Aminopimelic	+
3-Aminopropane sulfonic acid	− − − −	D-L-Homocysteinic	+ + + +
δ-Amino-*n*-valeric acid	− −	D-L-Aminoadipic	+
Glycine	− −	D-L-Aminomalonic	+
Taurine	− − −	D-L-Homocysteinic	+ + +

Neuromuscular Junction

In a Ringer's solution containing a low concentration of curare, an isolated muscle-nerve preparation does not contract when the nerve is stimulated. However, by using a glass microelectrode to record from the muscle membrane at the end-plate, a rapid and transient depolarization occurs upon stimulation of the motor nerve of the curarized muscle-nerve preparation. This is known as the *end-plate potential*, or EPP (Fig. 29–8), which normally excites striated muscle cells.

Curare, a molecule that is chemically similar to acetylcholine, can successfully compete for ACh receptors on the plasma membrane of the muscle cell. Since it is not destroyed by cholinesterase and does not cause an increase in

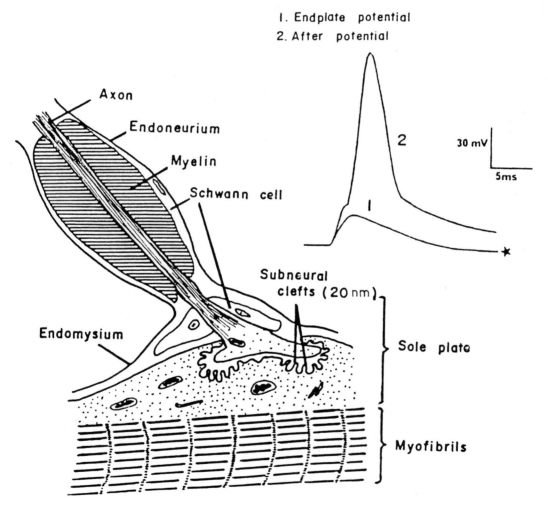

1. Endplate potential
2. After potential

Figure 29–8 At the neuromuscular junction of a motor end-plate, the endomysium covering the muscle fiber and the endoneurium covering the nerve fiber are continuous. The sarcoplasmic reticulum is extended further by invaginations to form postsynaptic membrane folds (subneural clefts). Mainly afterpotentials are recorded from intracellular electrodes in a muscle fiber close to the neuromuscular junction (*insert*) when the motor nerve is stimulated. When a blocking concentration of curare (asterisk) is added, nerve stimulation causes only a small, slow depolarization at the end-plate (EP), the end-plate potential (EPP).

plasma membrane permeability, curare prevents the post-synaptic excitation that normally follows release of ACh from the nerve terminal.

Unlike curare, two other clinically useful analogues of ACh (*succinylcholine* and *decamethonium*) cause prolonged de-polarization of the postsynaptic membrane. These drugs produce initial twitching of the striated muscles, rapidly followed by complete inhibition due to the sustained depo-larization.

A third type of peripheral motor paralysis is produced by preventing the synthesis or the release of ACh in the nerve terminal by a substance such as the *botulinum toxin*. Unlike the effects of curare or succinylcholine and decamethonium, botulinum poisoning is irreversible.

As an extension of the neurologic examination, the electromyogram (EMG) (a recording of the electrical activity of striated muscle) is used to evaluate the neuromuscular system. The equipment consists of an oscilloscope, which displays the wave forms, and an auditory amplifier, which projects a sound corresponding to each wave form. The two basic types of EMG examination are needle EMG, and nerve stimulation (Fig. 29–9). Needle EMG examination is per-formed by inserting an exploring needle electrode into a muscle to examine its intrinsic electrical activity. The elec-trical activity recorded from the muscle during needle EMG examination may be that of nerve stimulation.

Myopathy

Myopathy refers to abnormal conditions and diseases of the muscle cells and muscle tissue (the literal meaning is "muscle suffering"). In man, a group of primary myopathies is referred to by the confusing term of muscular dystrophies; they are slowly progressive diseases with hereditofamilial associations, in which regeneration is not a feature. In ani-mals, the term has been applied misleadingly to the nutri-tional myopathies of larger farm animals. Myopathies tend to be bilateral and symmetrical and to cause gait disturbances to get worse during exercise.

Paroxysmal or sudden attacks of muscle weakness and fatigue, usually precipitated by exercise, occur in *myasthenia gravis*, the classic type of episodic weakness. The characteris-tic signs of myasthenia gravis include weakness after exercise, salivation, dropped jaw, dysphagia, dysphonia, regurgita-tion, and inspiratory dyspnea. Myasthenia gravis is seen in puppies and in adult dogs and cats. Clinical improvement in response to the cholinergic drug edrophonium chloride or to the anticholinesterase drug neostigmine is diagnostic.

REFLEX, OR INVOLUNTARY, ACTIONS

A reflex is an involuntary activity in an effector organ (muscle, gland) elicited by the stimulation of a receptor organ. Most reflexes inherent to the spinal cord have five component parts that can be studied in a spinal preparation

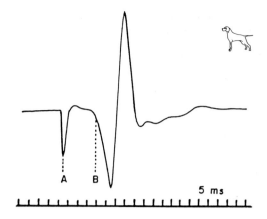

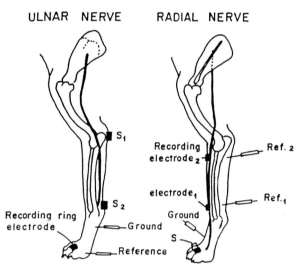

Figure 29–9 **Top,** In the dog, a biphasic response (*B*) is recorded from the muscle on the toe, following stimulation of the ulnar nerve (*A*). The interval between A and B is the latency (> 10 msec), and the conduction velocity is about 50 m per second. **Bottom,** In myasthenia gravis, repetitive stimulation of the ulnar nerve at two different sites, S_1 and S_2, results in diminution of the response. Stimulation (S) of the toe while the conduction velocity is measured between ref 1 and ref 2 along the radial nerve is used to detect sensory neuropathy. In the myopathic syndrome characterized only by generalized weakness, exercise intolerance, and a stilted, stiff gait, these reflexes and sensory perception of pain are preserved.

(Table 29–3). Through the CNS, these structures form an arc known as the *reflex arc* (Fig. 29–10). Extensor thrust reflex, flexion of withdrawal reflex, inverse myotatic (or clasp-knife) reflex, myotatic reflex, and scratch reflex are presented as examples.

Extensor Thrust Reflex

Application of pressure to the palmar or plantar surface of a dog's paw causes extension of the limb into a rigid column because of the simultaneous contraction of limb

TABLE 29–3   Component Parts of the Reflex Arc Present
in Most Reflexes Inherent to the Spinal Cord

1. The **receptor organ**, which may be located either in the muscle, in the viscera, or in the skin
2. The **afferent neuron**, which has its cell body located in the dorsal root ganglion (group I A)
3. **Internuncial neurons** of the spinal cord (for the flexion reflex)
4. **Afferent neurons**, which supply the effector organ (motor neurons for a striated muscle)
5. The **effector organ**, which may be a skeletal muscle, a smooth muscle, a cardiac muscle, or a gland

extensors and flexors. The receptors serving this response are a combination of stretch receptors in the muscles and of cutaneous pressure receptors in the paw. This reflex is the myotatic reflex modified by afferent activity from cutaneous receptors. The extensor thrust reflex is important in maintaining the posture of the animal.

Flexion, or Withdrawal, Reflex

A noxious stimulus applied to the distal part of a limb provokes a quick withdrawal of the limb from the stimulus. The motor activity elicited by this reflex is not always limb flexion, but it is always adequate to remove the body or affected part from the stimulus. When the withdrawal reflex originates from a noxious stimulus applied at the extremity of a limb, the opposite limb extends. This results from excitation of the extensor muscles and inhibition of the motor neurons to flexor muscles of the contralateral limb. This reflex is produced even in the animal whose spinal cord has been transected.

Inverse Myotatic, or Clasp-Knife, Reflex

When a limb is forcibly flexed, muscle tone increases in the extensors while it decreases in the flexors (myotatic reflex). If the flexion is continued, eventually the tone of the

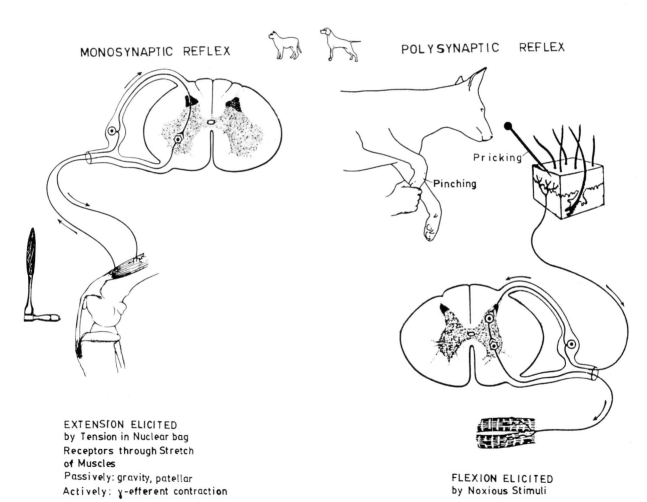

MONOSYNAPTIC REFLEX

POLYSYNAPTIC REFLEX

Pricking

Pinching

EXTENSION ELICITED
by Tension in Nuclear bag
Receptors through Stretch
of Muscles
Passively: gravity, patellar
Actively: γ-efferent contraction

FLEXION ELICITED
by Noxious Stimuli

Figure 29–10   Monosynaptic and polysynaptic reflex arcs occur, respectively, as the stretch and the flexor reflexes. The temporal characteristics of the stretch (myotatic) reflex are short latency (about 0.5 msec) and contraction limited to the muscle that has been stretched. In contrast, the flexor reflex has a longer latency, indicating involvement of an interneuron, and the protective response includes the whole of the stimulated limb (i.e., withdrawal of the limb from the noxious stimulus).

extensors is suddenly reduced, whereas that of the flexors is enhanced, causing the limb to be actively flexed. This is the inverse myotatic reflex, sometimes called the *clasp-knife reflex* (because of its characteristics in a decerebrate animal).

The receptor organ for this reflex, the Golgi tendon organ, is activated whenever the tendon is stretched by contraction of the muscle attached to the tendon. In the absence of muscle contraction, a much higher threshold for activation exists in these stretch receptors than in muscle spindles. The high threshold stretch receptors then produce a reflex (inverse myotatic), which is antagonistic to the reflex brought about by muscle spindles (myotatic).

Myotatic Reflex

Sudden stretch of a muscle or its tendon, as in tapping the patellar tendon, is an appropriate stimulus for adequate initiation of the myotatic reflex. Such a stretch applied to any tendon initiates reflex activity, which causes contraction of the stretched extrafusal fibers via the alpha-motor neurons. The gamma-motor neurons supplying the intrafusal fibers then correct their length to be ready for another response.

The myotatic reflex is a *postural reflex* because it aids in maintaining an animal in the standing position. If the stifle suddenly flexes, this action stretches the quadriceps muscle, which initiates the reflex that causes the quadriceps to con-

tract, thus extending the stifle to support the mass of the animal. These receptors are more abundant in antigravity muscles and in muscles in which control of muscle tone is of considerable importance.

The myotatic reflex is the only reflex arc with *four components instead of five*. It *does not utilize internuncial neurons* (intermediary neurons, or interneurons) because the afferent neurons synapse directly on the efferent neurons. It is also a *monosynaptic reflex arc,* as only one synapse is necessary to transmit neuronal activity from the receptor to the effector organ. In addition, it can be considered as a *proprioceptive reflex,* since it occurs within the same organ, the muscle.

Special Fibers in Striated Muscles

Special striated fibers, called *intrafusal fibers,* are more delicate, smaller, and paler than those of the rest of the skeletal muscle. Some intrafusal fibers are relatively large and long, extending the entire length of the neuromuscular spindle (muscle proprioceptor). The term *muscle spindle* comes from the overall shape of the receptor, with its bulbous swelling in the middle region. These longer intrafusal fibers tend to be *swollen in their equatorial region* (mid-region, nuclear bag region), where the fibers lose their striations and become noncontractile. The *accumulation of several nuclei* in this swollen region of the intrafusal fiber explains the term *nuclear bag fiber* (Fig. 29–11). Other, shorter and thinner,

Figure 29–11 Functions of intrafusal muscle fibers and neuromuscular spindle. The role of the gamma (γ) system is to set a new length for the intrafusal muscle fibers after contraction of the extrafusal muscle cells by the alpha (α) motor neurons. The Golgi tendon organs, which lie "in series" with the extrafusal muscle cells, have a higher threshold than the annulospiral axons and the nuclear bag region. Stimulation of the IA afferent occurs when tension is created in the intrafusal nuclear bag region, through passive stretch (gravity) and active stretch (γ efferent contraction).

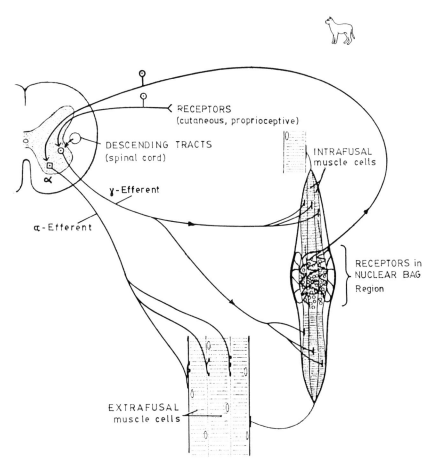

RECEPTORS
(cutaneous, proprioceptive)

DESCENDING TRACTS
(spinal cord)

γ-Efferent

α-Efferent

INTRAFUSAL
muscle cells

RECEPTORS in
NUCLEAR BAG
Region

EXTRAFUSAL
muscle cells

muscle fibers, with their nuclei arranged in a chain along much of the length of the fibers, are called *nuclear chain fibers*. The intrafusal muscle fibers are innervated at their polar ends by fine (3 to 8 μm in diameter) motor nerve fibers, the *gamma-efferent or fusimotor nerve fibers*. These fusimotor fibers constitute about *30 percent of the fibers in the ventral roots,* and they belong to the A_γ group. *Extrafusal muscle fibers* are innervated by larger nerve fibers of the A_α group (12 to 20 μm in diameter).

Scratch Reflex

The application of cutaneous stimuli to the skin over the dorsal and lateral surfaces of the thorax induces the scratch reflex in the dog. In response, the animal stands on one rear limb and scratches near the stimulated area in a manner appropriate to remove the stimulus. The scratch reflex can occur in either an intact animal or an animal whose spine has been transected, indicating that the mechanisms underlying its organization are located within the spinal cord.

REFERENCES

Bayon A, Drucker-Colin R. In vivo perfusion and release of neuroactive substances. Methods and strategies. New York: Academic Press, 1985.

De La Hunta A. Veterinary neuroanatomy and clinical neurology. 2nd ed. Philadelphia: WB Saunders, 1983.

Kelly DE, Wood RL, Enders AC. Bailey's textbook of histology. 18th ed. Baltimore: Williams & Wilkins, 1984.

Monnier M. Functions of the nervous system. Vol 1. General physiology—autonomic functions. New York: Elsevier, 1968.

Rogawski M, Barker JL. Neurotransmitter actions in the vertebrate nervous system. New York: Plenum Press, 1985.

CHAPTER 30

SENSORY RECEPTORS AND FUNCTIONS

Sensations, usually defined as feelings or impressions produced by stimulation of afferent nerves, also include "sensations" that are known to be present by analysis or experimentation but are not consciously experienced. For example, the actions of sensory nerves controlling the rate of the heartbeat and of sensory impulses from the viscera do not reach consciousness.

Sensations can be categorized according to various criteria. Sensations can be *exteroceptive* (relating to stimuli from the external world) or *interoceptive* (having to do with stimuli from within the organism). The term interoceptive, which includes sensations from viscera and from somatic structures, has been replaced by *proprioceptive,* which includes all sensations that arise within the organism. Another type of classification uses the localization of sensations. *Epicritic sensations* are sharply defined ones, such as the perception of a point of light, that can be localized with a high degree of precision. Epicritic sensation is highly developed over protruding portions of the body (nose, lips, ears, foot pads), and it can discriminate between stimulation of two closely spaced points. *Protopathic sensations,* which are poorly localized, include burning types of pain, deep muscle aches, and pain spread over a wide area.

This chapter deals with the receptor organs, the ascending spinal pathways, and the sensory functions of the cerebral cortex.

RECEPTOR ORGANS

The function of receptor organs is similar to that of transducers: they modify the form of applied energy to patterns of nerve action potentials, which can inform the central nervous system (CNS) of changing or steady states of the external and internal environments. A wide variety of receptor organs are used by the organism.

When nerve fibers are excited in any way, the sensations aroused are those that would be experienced with normal excitation of the receptors. For instance, if optic nerve fibers are electrically stimulated, the sensation of light is experienced. Likewise, mechanical stimulation (e.g., by applying pressure to the side of the eyeball) also brings about a visual sensation.

Classification of Receptors

The form of energy to which a receptor organ is most sensitive is referred to as the *adequate stimulus* for that receptor organ. The adequate stimulus for the rods and cones of the retina are light rays, the one for the hair cells of the cochlea is mechanical deformation of the hairs, and the one for pressure receptors of the skin is mechanical displacement of the skin.

Receptor organs can be classified on the basis of their adequate stimuli as *thermoreceptors, mechanoreceptors, chemoreceptors, and photoreceptors.* Some receptor organs are nonselective as to the form of energy that elicits a maximal response. Indeed, these receptor organs respond to any form of energy, which may be intense enough to be destructive to tissues. Such receptors, called *nociceptors* (noxious receptors, or pain receptors), respond to pain by eliciting a reflex activity, which causes the organism to remove itself or the body part from the painful stimulus.

Adaptation of Receptors

According to the rate of adaptation to the prolonged application of an adequate stimulus, receptor organs may be classified as *phasic* (e.g., corpuscles) or *tonic* (e.g., pacinian muscle spindles) receptors. Receptor organs found in the body exist with all gradations of rates of adaptation or accommodation. The intensity of stimulation is indicated by the frequency of discharge (i.e., the interval between impulses) (Fig. 30–1). The receptive fields of individual afferent fibers often overlap, so any natural stimulus usually excites a number of afferent fibers, and this corresponds to another means for perception of the intensity of a stimulus.

Usually, when a stimulus is applied, the frequency of discharges rises rapidly to a peak and then declines (the dynamic phase of the response). This may be followed by a longer period (static phase) during which the frequency falls slowly. An afferent unit is said to adapt rapidly if the discharge is brief. Such units are silent in the absence of a changed stimulus.

Selective Sensitivity

The receptors of afferent fibers have the important function of lowering the threshold of the axon for a particular mode or kind of stimulus. This selective sensitivity is not absolute: one class of receptor can be excited by another kind of physicochemical change, but a relatively much greater intensity of stimulation is required to reach threshold. For example, cutaneous thermoreceptors can be excited by mechanical stimuli, but the force required is about 2,000 times greater than that needed to excite the normal sensitive mechanoreceptors.

The relation between structure and function is confirmed by the combined use of electrophysiological and

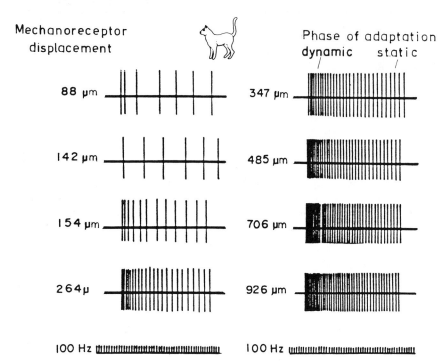

Figure 30–1 Discharge of afferent impulses in the axon of a cutaneous mechanoreceptor in the hairy skin of a cat. The mechanical stimulation is identical except in displacement (in μm). This afferent unit adapts slowly, with an initial high-frequency discharge (dynamic phase) followed by the more gradual decrease of frequency (static phase of adaptation).

histological methods. The hairy skin of monkeys, cats, and rabbits has three receptor structures with distinctive functions: Pacinian corpuscles, hair follicles, and mechanoreceptors. The Pacinian corpuscle, excited by mechanical stimuli, is very sensitive and adapts rapidly. The hair follicle, excited by hair movements, is innervated in a characteristic manner. The slowly adapting mechanoreceptors, as expanded disks (Merkel's disks) that are enclosed in nonneural structures, lie inside the basement membrane in a regular array. These three types of receptors all have distinctive responses to mechanical stimulation, which depend at least partly on the nonneural structural elements. In addition to these receptors, other afferent units, such as thermoreceptors and nociceptors, are present in the skin.

Thermoreceptors

Two main classes of thermoreceptors are recognized. *Cold receptors* are excited by a fall in skin temperature and are depressed by a rise. *Warm receptors* respond to heat in an opposite manner. The common properties shared by both classes of thermoreceptors are (1) a steady discharge at constant temperature, (2) an accelerated discharge when the temperature changes (i.e., faster for a fall in temperature for cold receptors, and faster for a rise with warm receptors), (3) a relative insensitivity to mechanical stimulation, and (4) small receptive fields.

Cutaneous Nociceptors

Cutaneous nociceptors are excited by both high and low temperatures as well as by intense mechanical stimuli. The receptive fields are small (<1 cm²), and the receptors of the afferent units do not ramify extensively in the skin. This group is classified as nociceptors because they respond only to intense stimuli. One common feature of all these nociceptors is that they become less responsive if the stimulus to the skin is repeated at frequent intervals (e.g., less than 30 seconds). The total area innervated by a cutaneous nerve is called the cutaneous area of that nerve.

The usual clinical testing procedure (i.e., gathering and grasping skin and then pinching) is applied at selected sites for the thoracic and pelvic limbs (Fig. 30–2). A withdrawal reflex or conscious response to the skin pinch indicates that the nerve and its spinal root are functional.

Abdominal and Pelvic Visceral Receptors

The abdominal and pelvic viscera are innervated by the vagal, splanchnic, and pelvic nerves. The respective ratios of afferent to efferent fibers of these nerves are 9 to 1, 3 to 1, and 1 to 1. Despite the numerical preponderance of sensory fibers, the roles of the visceral input remain rather obscure. Mucosal, epithelial, tension, and serosal receptors are recognized.

Mucosal receptors lie in or immediately below the mucosal epithelium of the stomach and small intestine. Local anesthesia of the mucosa abolishes responses to mechanical and chemical stimuli. Under experimental conditions, in anesthetized cats and rats, unstimulated gastric mucosal receptors do not discharge. Spikes are readily elicited by stroking the mucosa very lightly. Application of steady pressure or incremental distention produces "on-off" responses typical of rapidly adapting mechanoreceptors.

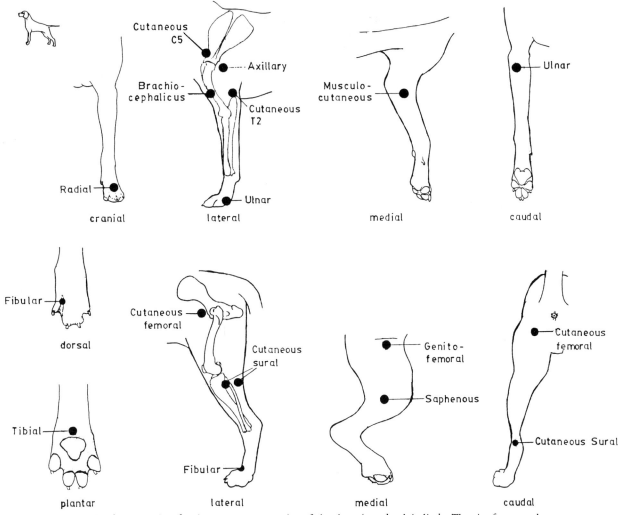

Figure 30–2 In the dog, test sites for the cutaneous sensation of the thoracic and pelvic limb. The site for musculocutaneous nerve stimulation, by grasping the skin with a hemostat, is 2 cm distal to the medial epicondyle. The radial nerve is examined at the dorsal skin of the third and fourth digits. The tibial nerve is stimulated from the skin at the proximal border of the metatarsal pad.

In addition to the rapidly adapting responses to mechanical stimuli, *epithelial receptors,* as well as mucosal receptors, may adapt slowly to certain chemical stimuli. The efficacy of the acidic solutions is related directly to their titratable acidities (regardless of their pH value) and inversely to their molecular masses. Buffered and unbuffered equimolar solutions of weak acids are equally efficacious, even if the hydrogen cation concentration may be 100 times less (i.e., 2 pH units more) in the buffered solutions.

Tension receptors are reported in the stomach and small intestine of cats and rats, the forestomach of sheep, and the bladder of cats. As slowly adapting mechanoreceptors, they give a spike discharge related to the tension prevailing in the smooth muscle layers of the viscus. They behave as if they were located in series with smooth muscle cells; an increased discharge arises actively during isometric contraction of the viscus and passively during distention of the viscus. The distention-sensitive receptors are excited also by visceral tension developed actively during spontaneous and experimentally induced contractions of the smooth muscles of the stomach, intestine, and bladder.

Tension receptors are visualized as sensors of the volume or degree of filling of the viscus. They also sense the effectiveness of a contraction in propelling (or expelling) the contents of the viscus. As sensors of the volume of gastric and intestinal contents, tension receptors are implicated in vagovagal receptive relaxation of the stomach and in postprandial satiation behavior.

Serosal receptors are slowly adapting mechanoreceptors lying either in the mesentery or under the serosa of a viscus (near its mesenteric attachment). Serosal receptor responses have been recorded from fibers dissected from uterine, mesenteric, hypogastric, and lumbar splanchnic nerves. They may indirectly monitor visceral fullness, as this is reflected in a distortion in the shape and in the position of the viscus as well as of its mesenteric attachments.

The vagueness of visceral sensations and of visceral reflexes is attributed to convergence of visceral afferent inputs in the CNS. In addition, because of an apparent economy in visceral receptor mechanisms, each receptor type is activated by a variety of visceral stimuli. A likely confusion is caused also by each form of experimental visceral stimulus, which probably excites more than one type of receptor.

ASCENDING SPINAL PATHWAYS

At each particular level of entry, the dorsal root afferent fibers send many segmental collaterals into the dorsal horn gray matter. In addition, the large afferent fibers (especially from skin and joints) emit long collaterals up the dorsal columns (dorsal fasciculi) ending in the *cuneate* and *gracilis* nuclei at the top of the spinal cord and in the medulla. The primary afferent fiber branches from the spinal cord are relayed at nuclei before ending in the cortical area (Fig. 30–3). The cortex is at the origin of three major motor segments, including the spinal cord, basal ganglia, and reticular formation.

Dorsal Columns

The dorsal columns are the principal paths for the sensations of cutaneous touch and for sensations in joints, muscles, and tendons. In animals, these sensations are disturbed by lesions in the dorsal column.

One consequence of such lesions is ataxia, inability to control voluntary movements (in the monkey, there is loss of weight discrimination). The other spinal cord pathways, such as the spinothalamic tract, carry sufficient information to allow at least partial recovery from dorsal column lesions.

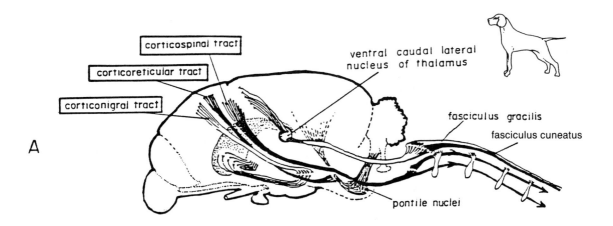

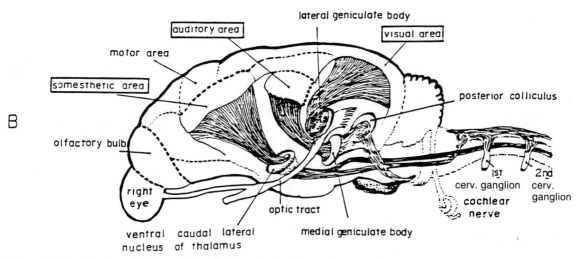

Figure 30–3 **A,** The cortical motor segments of the spinal cord, the substantia nigra, and the reticular formation are fed by the dorsal fasciculi, which is relayed at the thalamic nuclei. **B,** The afferent areas of the cortex correspond to afferent paths from the thalamus: cutaneous (and visceral), nociceptive, proprioceptive, auditory, and visual. The thalamic nuclei are shown separately for clarity, and only the auditory pathways, which are relayed at the medial geniculate body, are decussated.

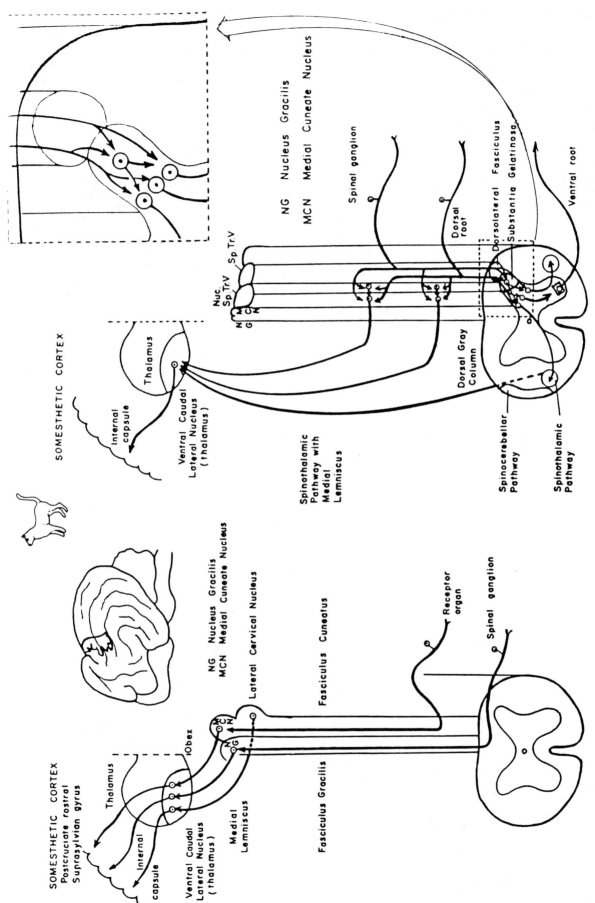

Figure 30–4 **Left,** This schematic diagram shows the general proprioceptive pathway to the somesthetic cortex for conscious perception in the cat, with projections to localized regions of the cerebral cortex, which are called primary sensory areas. The somatotopic organization of the somesthetic cerebral cortex reflects the density of receptor organs in the body. **Right,** General somatic afferent system is referred to as the pain, temperature, and touch system. In the lateral funiculus, the spinothalamic pathway is dorsal in the cat and ventral in the pig.

317

Spinothalamic Tract

This tract arises in cell bodies in the gray matter or the dorsal horns within a segment or two of the level of entry of the afferent fibers. The second-order fibers cross the midline and enter the white matter of the ventrolateral quadrant, in which they ascend to the medulla (Fig. 30–4).

A hemisection of the spinal cord causes loss of *pain and temperature* sensation on the *other side* of the body, at about two segments caudad to the lesion (*crossed spinothalamic tract*), and of sensations of *position, touch, pressure, and vibration* on the *same side* of the body as the lesion (*uncrossed dorsal column path*). This is the *Brown-Séquard syndrome*.

Surgical interruption of the spinothalamic tract is used to relieve severe or intractable pain. The operation, known as *cordotomy,* involves transection of the white matter in the ventrolateral quadrant of the spinal cord. If the surgery is successful, it results in loss of pain and temperature sensation on the opposite side of the body, at a site two segments caudal to the lesion.

In evaluating the degree of nerve tissue damage following injury and motor paralysis, interpretation of an interrupted spinothalamic pathway is based on the degree of analgesia. Animals with hypoalgesia (or depressed response to noxious stimuli caudad to the lesion) have a better prognosis than those with complete analgesia. The presence of cerebral response to noxious stimuli indicates that some pathways in the spinal cord are intact at the site of the lesion.

Specific Projection System

The cortical projections originate from nuclei in the thalamus, which send efferent fibers to restricted regions of the cerebral cortex. The sensory surfaces of skin, joints, eye, and ear project to specific sensory areas of the cerebral cortex through relay nuclei in the thalamus (Fig. 30–5). The specific cortical projections retain a high degree of point-to-point topographical precision, and electrical stimulation of part of one of these thalamic nuclei leads to excitation of only a small, restricted, and precisely defined area of the cortex.

The somatic sensory relay nuclei of the thalamus can be divided into two principal groups, the ventrobasal complex group and the posterior group. The thalamocortical radiation from the ventrobasal region of the thalamus goes to the somatosensory region of the cerebral cortex (see Fig. 30–5).

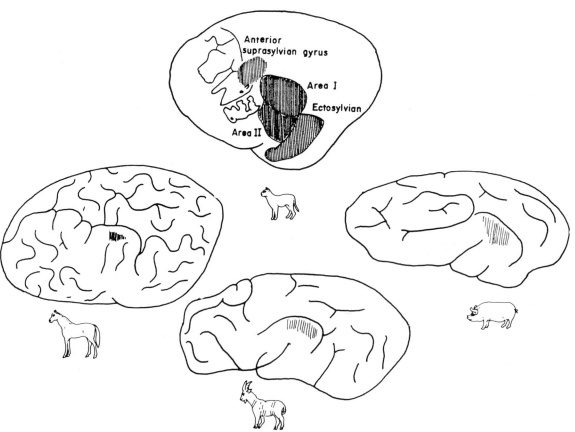

Figure 30–5 Primary (I) and secondary (II) auditory areas of the cerebral cortex of the cat are compared with the auditory receiving cortex in the goat, the pig, and the pony. In the cat, the representation of the primary somatosensory area of the body is detailed (contralateral side of the forelimb and face). The location of somatosensory area II of the cat is ventrolateral to the primary area (I).

The position and size of this region have been established by a combination of ablation techniques, evoked potential methods, and single-unit recording. It lies around, and mostly caudad to, the cruciate sulcus.

SENSORY FUNCTIONS OF THE CEREBRAL CORTEX

All sensory systems have projections from the ventrobasal complex part of the thalamus to well-localized regions of the cerebral cortex, which are referred to as *primary sensory areas*. By experimentation, four primary sensory cortical areas have been established in domestic animals: audi-

tory, visual, somesthetic, and olfactory. The vestibular and gustatory senses also have cortical representations.

The representation of the body in the ventrobasal complex of the thalamus is not linear but is related to the innervation density of the various parts. The entire body surface is represented with a distorted image (Fig. 30–6). The rabbit has a relative dominance of the trigeminal representation. The cat has a more balanced spinal and trigeminal projection. In the monkey, the hands and feet have a very rich afferent innervation and are more highly developed as tactile and prehensile organs.

By plotting the points of the skin surface that evoke primary potentials or excite specific points on the cortex, a figure of the animal's contralateral body surface is generated. For man, such a figure is referred to as *homunculus*, for cats it

Figure 30–6 **Top,** Diagrammatic illustration of the representation of the body surface in the ventrobasal complex of the thalamus, with dominant trigeminal representation in the rabbit and relative increases in the sizes of the limb and trunk areas in the cat and the monkey. **Middle,** In the cat, gyri on the neocortex, with duality (i.e., primary and secondary splanchnic, vagal, somesthetic, optic, and acoustic areas). **Bottom,** Abbreviations of Nomina Anatomica terms: *Bo,* bulbus olfactorius; *Gc,* gyrus coronalis; *Gl,* gyrus lateralis; *Go,* gyrus orbitalis; *Gp,* gyrus proreus; *GSa,* gyrus Sylvii ant.; *Gsa,* gyrus sigmoideus ant.; *GSp,* gyrum Sylvii post.; *Gsp,* gyrus sigmoideus post.; *GsSa,* gyrus suprasylvii ant.; *GsSm,* gyrus suprasylvii medius; *GsSp,* gyrus suprasylvii post.; *Lp,* lobus piriformus; *Sa,* sulcus ansatus; *Sc,* sulcus coronalis; *Scr,* sulcus cruciatus; *SeSp,* scissura ectosylvii post.; *Slp,* scissura lateralis post.; *SprS,* scissura praesylvii; *SsSp,* scissura suprasylvii post.; *To,* tractus olfactorius.

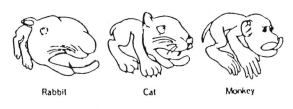

Rabbit Cat Monkey

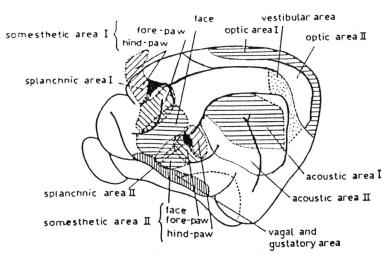

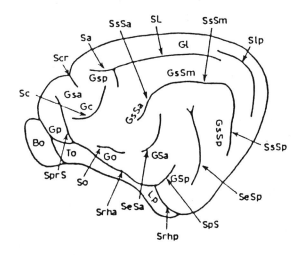

is a *felunculus*, and for dogs it is a *canunculus*, and so on, according to the genus of the animal investigated. The figure is distorted, some parts of the body being excessively represented over large areas of the cerebral cortex and other parts having very meager cortical representation. Studies on the face of ungulates indicate that only receptors in the lips and snout send impulses to the cortex. These impulses are ipsilateral in sheep and goats and contralateral in pigs and horses.

In an anesthetized animal, electrical stimulation of the cerebral cortex demonstrates somatic motor activity areas. These regions, referred to as *primary motor areas*, are closely related to the *secondary somesthetic area*, which also exhibits somatotropic organization.

In ungulates, recording of evoked electrical potential changes, which is distinct from observation of spontaneous electrical rhythms (electroencephalography) is used to study the central afferent systems. The electrical potential changes are evoked by physiological stimulation of peripheral receptors or by electrical excitation of peripheral afferent nerve fibers. Responses to stimulation of the contralateral forelimb—and sometimes of the contralateral hind limb—are observed in the anterior ectosylvian gyrus of the goat, the sheep, and the horse. In the pig, stimulation of a limb does not evoke any cerebral potential. In none of the ungulate species does stimulation of a limb produce a detectable response in the area that may be homologous with the postcentral gyrus.

Chloralose is used to facilitate transmission of afferent impulses to the cortex. In a cat anesthetized with chloralose, cortical responses are more easily evoked, as light tactile stimuli are sufficient to cause evoked responses. In contrast, administration of pentobarbital sodium to a cat anesthetized with chloralose reduces the responses evoked by stimulation of the peroneal nerve (Fig. 30–7).

Intracerebroventricular injection of small doses of tubocurarine causes some vasodilation by increasing neuronal activity. It also modifies the evoked cortical responses, which show accentuation of the positive waves, with attenuation or disappearance of the negative waves. Tubocurarine accentuates the positive waves of the evoked cortical potentials, which are elicited by contralateral stimulation of the peroneal nerve, possibly by suppression of nonspecific background activity (Fig. 30–8).

The significance of dual representation is unknown. Duality (areas I and II) appears to be a general principle of the cortical organization and also of the cerebellar organization. In addition, dual systems of fibers are present in cutaneous nerves or in perception, (e.g., area I for epicritic sensations, and area II for protopathic sensations).

Following mechanical or chemical stimulation, changes in motor activity of a viscus are due mainly to secretion of peptide hormones or to activation of the local nervous system. This affirmation is based on the fact that motility still occurs after extrinsic denervation. The importance of the role of hormones and intramural plexuses in the motility of a viscus (stomach, intestine) must not be underestimated.

In addition to conscious sensations (e.g., gustatory), sensory autonomic nervous input is permanently conveyed

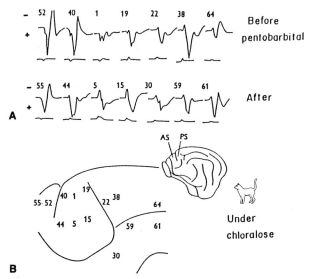

Figure 30–7 Facilitated transmission by chloralose anesthesia of the evoked cortical responses elicited by stimulation of the contralateral peroneal nerve in the cat. **A,** The evoked cortical response under chloralose, and its reduction after pentobarbital sodium injection. **B,** The numbers beside the evoked responses designate points on the anterior and posterior sigmoid gyrus (*AS, PS*) from which the records were obtained.

from the gut to the cortex. Various sensory neurons deliver to the cortex a large amount of qualitative and quantitative information concerning mechanical and chemical changes occurring within the wall of the gut. These autonomic afferent impulses reach various central nervous structures and modulate sophisticated functions, such as the control of feeding behavior (e.g., those delivered by intestinal glucoreceptors influence neurons located in the medulla).

Opioid Peptides

Discovery of opiate receptors in the brain and of opioid peptides in the CNS has triggered a new wave of research in neuroscience. Three subclasses of opiate receptors have received the greatest attention: mu (μ), delta (δ), and kappa (κ). The mu receptors, named for morphine, are activated by the classic opiate alkaloids. The delta receptors respond to the mouse vas deferens assay system, and the kappa receptors bind to the ketocyclazine class of drugs.

These receptors are widely distributed in the brain and the spinal cord, except for the cerebellum in some species. They also occur in some peripheral tissues. The mu sites, which are absent from most of the hypothalamus, may modulate pain sensation and participate in sensorimotor integration. The delta receptors, absent from the diencephalon and the brain stem, may play roles in motor integration, olfaction, and cognition. The kappa receptors are prevalent in the diencephalon, in parts of the limbic system, and in the basal ganglia. Kappa receptors are involved in regulation of water balance, food intake, neuroendocrine functions, and pain perception.

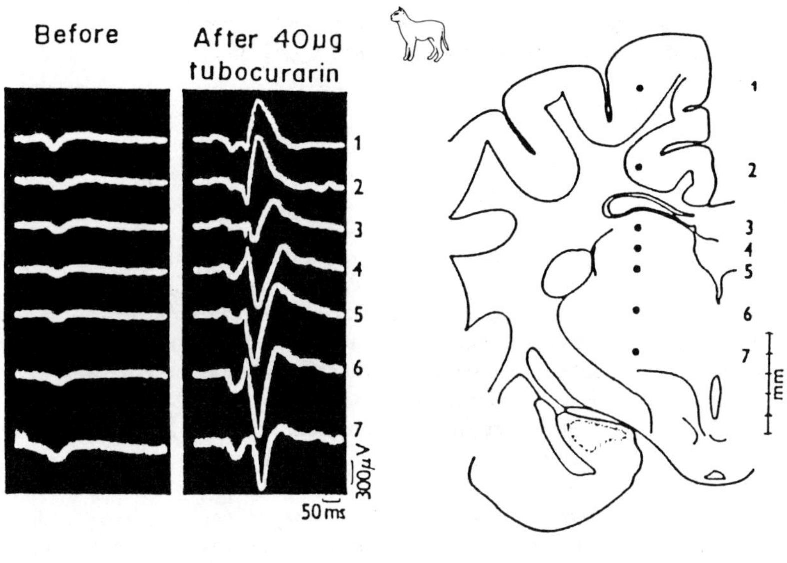

Figure 30–8   In the cat, tubocurarine facilitates transmission of the evoked thalamic responses elicited by stimulation of the contralateral peroneal nerve. The figures on the right side refer to the points shown in the diagram of the coronal section at 9 mm in front of the Horsley-Clarke tract, in the zero plane of the electrode. At the lowest point, the tip of the electrode was in the posterolateral nuclei.

Profound interspecies differences occur in the distribution and density of opioid receptors, and peptide agonists. Perhaps these diversities underlie the dramatic species variations observed in functional and behavioral responses to opiate drugs.

In animals, levels of opioid peptides are increased by exercise (jogging), skin twitching by horses, and certain acupuncture techniques to relieve pain. To provide analgesia without respiratory depression or addiction is the objective of extensive research on the opioid peptide systems. This class of substances may have broader application for animal physiology.

REFERENCES

Bailey CS, Kitchell R. Cutaneous sensory testing in the dog. J Vet Intern Med 1987;1:128.

Ewart WR, Wingate DL. Central representation of arrival of nutrient in the duodenum. Am J Physiol 1984;246:G750.

Leek BF. Abdominal and pelvic receptors. Br Med Bull 1977;33:163.

CHAPTER 31

MOTOR FUNCTIONS

Within the cerebral cortex of the different animal species, a general similarity or homology pattern is found between the cortical motor areas and the muscle control they produce. The relationship between precision of motor function and development of the underlying cellular structure is marked in the area of the brain that contains *large pyramidal cells* known as *Betz's cells*. When these cells are stimulated by electrical current, they produce responses in different limb muscles.

The *pyramidal system* is an uninterrupted, *monosynaptic corticospinal pathway* from the cerebrum to the spinal cord via the pyramids of the medulla. In contrast, the *extrapyramidal system* consists of neurons that originate in the cerebral cortex, including the motor area, and descend into the brain stem via subcortical nuclei. From specific brain stem nuclei, without going through the pyramids of the medulla, axons course to and through the spinal cord. This *multisynaptic extrapyramidal corticosinal pathway* is of great importance in domestic animals.

This chapter presents concepts regarding the pyramidal system, the extrapyramidal system, the functions of the motor system, and postural reactions and spinal disturbances and an introduction to exercise physiology.

THE PYRAMIDAL SYSTEM

The development of the pyramidal system is directly related to the capacity of an animal to perform finely skilled movements. This system is *poorly developed in domestic animals,* especially in horses, oxen, and sheep. In horses most of the pyramidal system is dedicated to the facial muscles for lip movements, which suggests that these muscles perform the most highly skilled activity of the species. In dogs, movements of the ear, of the eyelids, and of the masseter muscles are related to the pyramidal system (Fig. 31–1).

The axons of the pyramidal cells descend through the white matter of the brain (corona radiata of the motor cortex, internal capsule, crus cerebri, longitudinal fibers of the pons, and pyramids of the medulla), and 75 percent of them cross in the *pyramidal decussation.* They descend as the lateral and corticospinal tracts. In dogs, these axons terminate in the gray matter of the spinal cord, about 50 percent in the cervical part (at C6–7), about 20 percent in the thoracic part (at T1–2), and about 30 percent in the lumbosacral part (at L4–7 and S1–3). The swellings, or intumescences, at the cervical and lumbosacral levels correspond to neurons involved in spinal reflexes, which are still present after the spinal cord segments are cut off and isolated from the rest of the central nervous system (CNS) (Fig. 31–2).

THE EXTRAPYRAMIDAL SYSTEM

The extrapyramidal system includes many scattered groups of interconnected and functionally related neurons that form multisynaptic pathways from the brain to the lower motor neurons of the brain stem and spinal cord. These extrapyramidal pathways, in unison with the pyramidal system, provide tonic mechanisms to support the body against gravity and to recruit spinal reflexes during initiation of voluntary movements. These functions are performed ultimately by the influence of the extrapyramidal system on the alpha and the gamma motor neurons in motor nuclei in the brain stem, and in the ventral gray column of the spinal cord.

The *caudate nucleus,* located in the floor of the lateral cerebral ventricle mediad to the internal capsule, is a major relay. The large head, and most of the body, of the caudate nucleus are rostrad to the diencephalon. The body of the caudate nucleus extends caudad into the temporal lobe and provides a major feedback circuit with the thalamus and cortex (Fig. 31–3).

The substantia nigra, the tegmental nucleus, and the red nucleus are three structures of the midbrain (*mesencephalon*) involved in a feedback circuit through the cerebellum. The cell bodies of the *substantia nigra* are so named because they contain a melanin pigment, which accumulates with age. Located throughout the mesencephalon, this nucleus is dorsad to the crus cerebri and ventrad to the tegmentum and is bounded rostrally by the subthalamic nucleus. Neurons of the substantia nigra synthesize and secrete the neurotransmitter *dopamine,* and some of these neurons project rostrally to the caudate nucleus to form the *nigrostriatal pathway.* The *tegmental nucleus* is an ill-defined area in the reticular formation of the tegmentum of the midbrain. At the level of the rostral colliculus, the *red nucleus* is ventrolateral to the oculomotor nerve. The red nucleus receives a group of afferent axons from the ipsilateral motor area of the cerebral cortex via the internal capsule and crus cerebri (Fig. 31–4). This corticorubral system is organized somatotopically and descends through the entire spinal cord. Neurons of the thoracic limb area of the motor cortex project on the dorsal part of the red nucleus, whose neurons project on the spinal cord gray matter, which innervates the thoracic limb. Corticorubral neurons from the pelvic limb region of the motor cortex synapse in the ventral portion of the red nucleus, whose neurons descend in the rubrospinal tract (RST) to influence the pelvic limb lower motor neurons. Neurons in the rubrospinal tract are predominantly facilitatory to motor neurons of flexor muscles.

The distribution of white and gray matter is different in the brain stem (*rhombencephalon*) and in the spinal cord. The

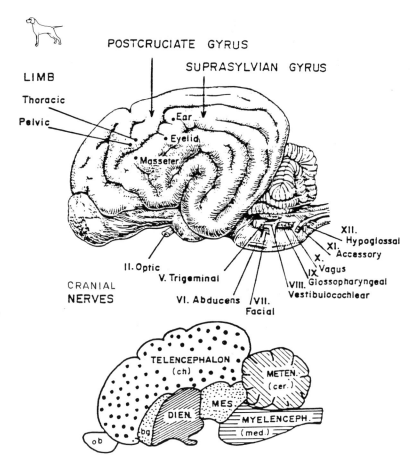

Figure 31-1 Top, Topography of the canine cerebral cortex. The pyramidal system neurons for the *right* thoracic and pelvic limbs originate in specific parts of the *left* postcruciate gyrus. The rostral part of the suprasylvian gyrus is related to the innervation of the muscles of specific areas (ear, eyelid, masseter) of the head. Bottom, Schematic median section of the canine brain with the forebrain, or telencephalon (*ob*, olfactory bulb; *ch*, cerebral hemispheres); the diencephalon (i.e., basal ganglion (*bg*), thalamus, and hypothalamus); the midbrain, or mesencephalon (*mes*); the lower brain stem with the metencephalon (*meten* or *cer*, cerebellum); and the myencephalon (*med*, medulla oblongata).

greatest portion of the *brain stem* is occupied by an ill-defined meshwork of a variety of cell types, the *reticular formation,* which extends into the tegmentum of the midbrain and into the caudal diencephalon. Defined areas within the reticular formation receive projections from the cerebellum, the spinal cord, and the extrapyramidal nuclei. In turn, the reticular formation projects to these three areas.

The *reticular formation* has many functions, including *activation of the cerebral cortex* for the awake state (ascending reticular activating system, or ARAS) and sleep mechanisms as well as several types of *control mechanisms*. These controls involve the *vital functions—respiration* and *circulation, voluntary excretion,* and *vomiting and swallowing*. A descending portion of the reticular formation influences ventral gray column internuncial activity, the alpha and gamma efferent neurons affecting muscle tone, and motor activity linked to the extrapyramidal system.

The cranial nerve nuclei of the medulla are organized into columns of cells. The *somatic motor column* contains alpha motor neurons, which are similar structurally and functionally to the neurons located in the spinal cord. These medullary cranial neurons supply the skeletal muscles of the head, which are derived from the embryonic somites—the extrinsic muscles of the eye, supplied by the oculomotor, trochlear, and abducent nerves, and the muscles of the tongue, supplied by the hypoglossal nerve (Fig. 31-5).

The *visceral motor column* contains neurons analogous to those of the intermediolateral cell column of the spinal cord and to those of the parasympathetic nucleus of the sacral spinal cord. These neurons give rise to parasympathetic innervation for muscles (cardiac and smooth) and glands (head, cervical, thoracic, and abdominal viscera). The nuclei involved in this column are indistinct (e.g., rostral and caudal salivatory, which are a part of the reticular formation) or distinct (e.g., dorsal motor nucleus of the vagus [cranial nerve X], which innervates the cervical, thoracic, and abdominal regions).

FUNCTIONS OF THE MOTOR SYSTEM

The *functions of the pyramidal system* are: (1) initiation of voluntary activity of the motor system, (2) maintenance of muscle tone to support the body against gravity and to establish the posture upon which the voluntary activity can be performed, and (3) control of muscle activity associated with visceral functions (respiratory, cardiovascular, excretory).

The *extrapyramidal system* functions by modulating muscle tone through its control over the myotatic reflex and postural reflexes. *Postural reflexes* can be divided into two

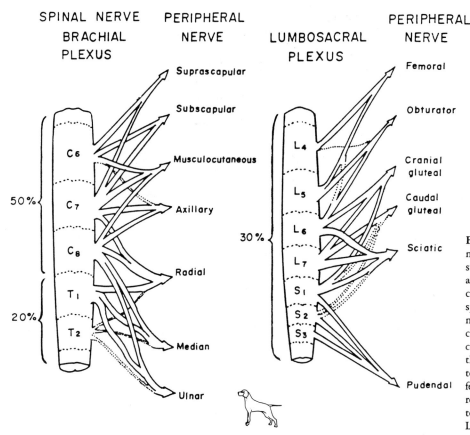

Figure 31–2 In the dog, segmental innervation from cervical swellings to thoracic limb muscles and from lumbosacral intumescences to pelvic limb muscles. The spinal nerves, from C6 to T2 segments, intertwine to form the brachial plexus (flexor, biceps, and triceps reflexes). The flexor reflex of the pelvic limb depends on the integrity of the sciatic nerve. The femoral nerve controls the patellar reflex, and the most important motor component of this reflex is the L5 ventral root.

types, *supporting reflexes* and *attitudinal reflexes*. Supporting reflexes alter skeletal muscle activity by causing the limbs to become supporting columns against the pull of gravity. Attitudinal reflexes change muscle activity to maintain the body in a position appropriate for the various movements. In other words, attitudinal reflexes control the posture of an animal so that the position of the body in space in relation to the gravitational field is adequate for various positions or movements of the head. They involve both forelimb and rear limb musculature for the production of coordinated motor activity. Two types of receptor organs, neck and labyrinthine, are operative.

Tonic neck reflexes are best illustrated by observing a cat looking up at a bird. The forelimbs extend to support the anterior portion of the body, and the rear limbs flex so that the cat assumes a "sitting" position. Conversely, if a cat is looking down into a mouse's hole, the forelimbs are flexed, and the rear limbs are extended.

Tonic labyrinthine reflexes, receptive to linear acceleration of the position of the head, maintain the creature in a normal standing position. If an animal is placed in a supine position, tonic labyrinthine reflexes cause the head to rotate on the neck. This, in turn, initiates tonic neck reflexes and brings the body into the upright position. Such a reflex response to body position is referred to as a *righting reflex.*

These responses can be observed sequentially when a cat is dropped through space from a supine position. The head is initially turned toward an upright position (as a result of tonic labyrinthine reflexes), the rest of the body quickly follows (owing to tonic neck reflexes), and the animal lands in an upright position.

In normal animals, these reflexes are assisted by the visual system, but blind animals also demonstrate them, indicating that the visual system is not essential to the righting reflex.

Paresis

Disturbance of the mechanism for initiating voluntary motor function causes *paresis* (weakness) or *paralysis,* depending on the severity and location of the lesion. The severity of the paresis increases as the location of the lesion descends in the upper motor neurons and involves more of the pathways.

Unilateral lesions of the upper motor neurons rostrad to the red nucleus cause *contralateral hemiparesis* that is so mild that it usually is not apparent in the gait. However, the response to postural reaction testing is deficient. This is exemplified by experimental removal of the motor area of the cerebrum or complete removal of the cortex of one hemisphere.

Unilateral lesions in the pons and medulla usually produce an *ipsilateral hemiparesis* of gait and a postural reaction deficiency. The gait dysfunction is more obvious if the unilateral lesion is further caudad in the medulla or the cranial cervical spinal cord. The anatomic landmark for lesions that produce an ipsilateral hemiparesis is in the region of the caudal mesencephalon and rostral pons. When the lesion occurs

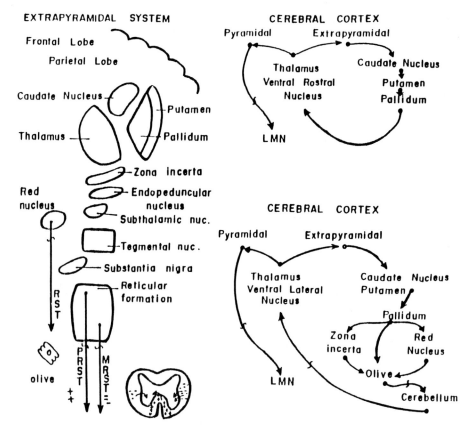

Figure 31-3 **Left,** The extrapyramidal system involves the cerebral cortex (frontal and parietal lobes) and the basal ganglia (i.e., caudate nucleus, putamen, and pallidum). Three structures are involved at the level of the diencephalon: the zona incerta, the endopeduncular nucleus, and the subthalamic nucleus. The red nucleus, the mesencephalic origin of the rubrospinal tract (RST), is connected to the tegmental nucleus, and the substantia nigra. At the level of the rhombencephalon, besides the olivary nucleus (O), the reticular formation initiates the (facilitatory) pontine reticulospinal tract (*PRST*), and the (inhibitory) medullary reticulospinal tract (*MRST*). The medullary and the pontine tracts are, respectively, inhibitory and facilitatory to contralateral extensor muscles. **Upper right,** Besides the pyramidal neurons directed to lower motor neurons (*LMN*), a feedback circuit provides a multisynaptic pathway from the extrapyramidal neurons toward the pallidum and the thalamus and cerebral cortex. **Lower right,** Another feedback circuit operates through the red nucleus and zona incerta, olive, cerebellum, toward the thalamus and cerebral cortex.

rostrad to this area, the hemiparesis is contralateral and is less marked.

Myotatic Reflexes

Derangement of the descending upper motor neuron pathways involved in the maintenance of muscle tone usually causes signs of myotatic reflexes, which are freed from the effects of the inhibitory pathways. All spinal and myotatic reflexes (patellar, biceps, triceps) may be intact or hyperactive (hyperreflexia), or clonus (alternate contraction and relaxation) may be observed. Hypertonia is manifested by increased *resistance to passive manipulation* and exaggerated contraction of muscles subjected to stretch. Flexor reflexes may show a prolonged afterdischarge, which is observed as *repetitive flexion* of the limb in the absence of repeated stimuli.

Spasticity

The loss or inhibition of myotatic reflexes results in spasticity or hypertonia and hyperactive reflexes. *Spasticity,* observed in the gait as stiffness, is particularly prominent in horses with diffuse spinal cord disease affecting the white matter. The pelvic limb stride is stiff, and the hoof often slaps the ground sharply.

Paralysis

Paralysis indicates loss of motor function to muscles. It may involve visceral structures, such as the esophagus, diaphragm, and bladder, or the muscles of the head and limbs. Motor function may be destroyed by lesions of the muscles themselves (myositis), the neuromuscular junction (botu-

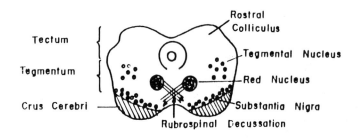

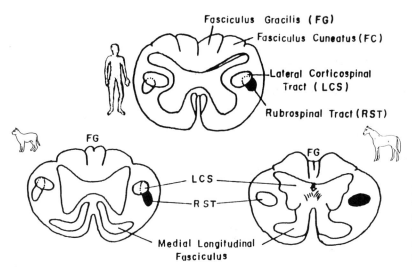

Figure 31–4 Top, Extrapyramidal nuclei of the midbrain. **Middle and bottom,** Comparison of the first cervical spinal cord segment in man, cat, and horse to indicate the relative increase in the contribution of the RST in animals.

lism, myasthenia), the peripheral nerves (trauma), the motor nerve root (polyradiculoneuritis), the gray matter of the spinal cord segment to the affected muscle (myelitis, spinal accident), the entire spinal cord (trauma), or many parts of the brain (encephalitis). Paralysis, unlike ataxia, is a sign that permits fairly easy localization of a lesion.

Paralysis can be classified clinically as *flaccid, spastic, and rigid. Flaccid paralysis,* in which affected muscles have no tone or reflexes, arises from lower motor neuron damage. It is also seen during the first 12 to 24 hours of complete upper motor neuron loss, when the affected muscles have no tone on palpation but do exhibit reflexes. *Spastic paralysis* is caused by complete loss of upper motor neuron function. This state is a dynamic one that develops from initial flaccidity, with intact reflexes in the first few hours, to a gradually increasing palpable tone and hyperreflexia. After 1 to 2 months, the animal can usually support weight on the affected limb and can make cyclical reflex leg movements (spinal walking). *Rigid paralysis* describes a state of involuntary rigidity resulting from partial loss of upper motor neuron function, direct lower motor neuron irritation (spasms), and loss of lower motor neuron inhibition loops (Renshaw's cells). Rigid paralysis is seen in strychnine toxicity or tetanus and as part of the Schiff-Sherrington sign.

The Schiff-Sherrington sign is extensor rigidity of the forelimbs that is apparent only when the animal is at rest. The animal retains full voluntary motor function in the forelimbs but has usually lost it in the hind limbs.

The sign occurs when lower motor neurons or more

craniad cord segments are released from the inhibitory tone of more caudad spinal cord segments. The Schiff-Sherrington sign is usually associated with severe thoracic cord injury caudad to T2 or more rarely with lumbar cord injury. It can develop within a few hours after the injury or may be delayed for several days.

The Schiff-Sherrington sign seen in severe thoracolumbar lesions is accompanied by paralysis of the rear legs; the forelegs are rigid when the animal stops making conscious movements with them (i.e., the front limb rigidity in this instance is not paralysis).

Involuntary Incidental Movements

In primates, dysfunctions of the extrapyramidal system in the brain result in the production of repetitive involuntary, adventitious (incidental) movements. These diseases usually affect areas of the cerebral cortex or specific extrapyramidal nuclei. Examples of adventitious movements are postural tremor, athetosis, dystonia, ballism, chorea, and myoclonus, but the presence of one of these signs is not pathognomonic for deficiency of any one nuclear area.

Postural tremor is produced by small, rapid, alternating contractions of opposed muscle groups. It is observed when the subject is at rest and often disappears with activity, especially in the hands and fingers of patients with parkinsonism. Therapy involves the replacement of a deficient neurotransmitter substance, dopamine. *Athetosis* is manifested by slow, writhing movements of the extremities;

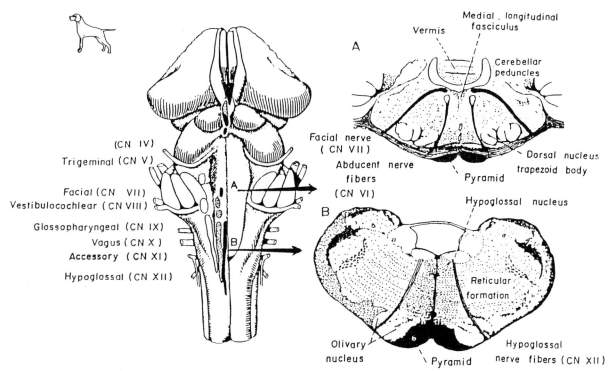

Figure 31–5 Left, Dorsal aspect of the canine brain stem shows the functional organization of cranial nerve nuclei, with their special and general *visceral* efferents (*white or dots*) and their general *somatic* efferents (*solid black*). **Right,** Transverse sections through the medulla: at the level of the facial nuclei (**A**), and at the level of the hypoglossal nuclei (**B**).

ballism by violent flailing (jerking, twitching movement) of a limb; *chorea* by continual but irregular rapid, jerky movements of different muscle groups; and *myoclonus* by repetitive, rhythmic contractions of a certain group of muscles that may persist during sleep.

Comparable diseases and signs are rare in domestic animals, except for the myoclonus of *canine distemper* (commonly referred to as chorea, flexor spasm syndrome, spasmodic twitching, or tremor). The myoclonus of canine distemper is not an expression of spinal cord hyperreflexia. Transection of dorsal roots supplying an isolated segment of the spinal cord does not abolish the myoclonus. Such a procedure abolishes the activity within muscles that are antagonistic to those exhibiting the myoclonus. This indicates that the myoclonus of canine distemper is a true flexor or extensor myoclonus (i.e., that primary activity does not occur spontaneously within the antagonist muscles). The activity within antagonist muscles that is recorded in an intact dog is reflexly elicited by stretching these muscles during the myoclonic contractions of the agonist muscles.

Canine distemper myoclonus is a disease of the spinal cord recognized by CHAUVEAU in 1862. Though it is often considered to be triggered by the brain, the rate and intensity of myoclonus in canine distemper are not altered appreciably by isolating the spinal cord from the remainder of the CNS. It appears that the rate of myoclonus depends on neurons within one, or at most two or three, spinal cord segments.

Isolating a lumbar segment from the remainder of the spinal cord does not appreciably alter the rate or intensity of myoclonic activity; however, owing to the short length of sacral spinal cord segments, considerable trauma to the spinal cord results from transection between these levels, which produces in abolition of myoclonus in muscles served by these segments.

Experimental lesions in the extrapyramidal nuclei of dogs and cats produce signs such as a tendency to circle or to turn the head to one side.

POSTURAL REACTIONS AND SPINAL TRANSECTION (SPINALIZATION)

Quiet standing is achieved through continuous fine adjustments of muscle tension in a large number of limb and trunk muscles. These adjustments express the behavior of the CNS functioning as a feedback-operated control system converting the limbs into pillars that support the body against the pull of gravity.

Reaction patterns of biceps femoris to the displacement of the floor (Fig. 31–6) are used to evaluate this coordinated activity. Detected as vertical force changes exerted in the posterior limb and as changes in electromyographical activity of muscles of the thigh, the reactions are uniform and predictable across trials and across dogs. Similar constant

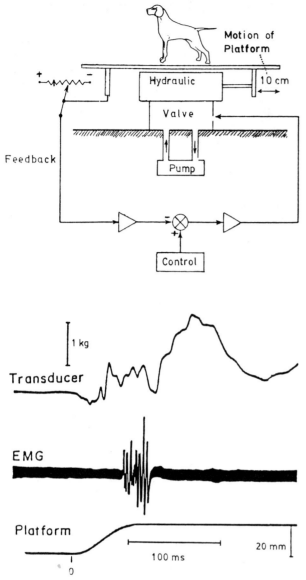

Figure 31–6 Top, Representation of an electromechanical system, with a platform running on rails, used to produce postural disturbances. Bottom, The typical reaction patterns of biceps femoris to a horizontal change in the platform (20 mm) bring a change in the force transducer record and in the EMG tracing.

patterns of reaction time are measured in the various muscles. Tests have been devised to assess proprioception and to evaluate postural reactions.

Proprioception

The common tests for conscious proprioception (muscle, tendon, and joint sense) in animals are knuckling, sway reaction, and reflex stepping (Fig. 31–7), which all are based on the tactile placing reflex. The tactile placing reflex, both a bulbospinal and a spinal reflex, is elicited only with facilitation from the cerebral motor cortex by means of the cor-

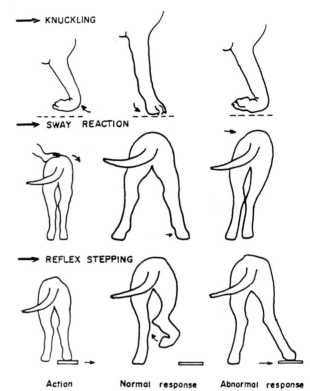

Figure 31–7 Normal and abnormal responses in a dog during examination of proprioception at the forelimb (knuckling), and at the right hind limb (sway reaction, reflex stepping).

ticospinal motor systems. Responses are diminished or absent following disturbances or transection of these descending motor pathways.

In *knuckling*, flexion and contact of the dorsal aspect of the digits with the floor or absence of tactile stimuli on the palmar aspect of the digits brings immediate extension of the digit and support of the body. In the *sway reaction*, when an animal experiences lateral and horizontal displacement, the nonsupporting limb immediately extends to support the body. *Reflex stepping*, sudden flexion of a supporting limb, follows a sudden abduction movement, or withdrawal of the surface in contact with the toes.

POSTURAL REACTIONS

Five reactions are used to test for spinal or supraspinal disturbances: extensor postural thrust reaction, flexor reflex to nociception, hopping reaction, placing reaction, and righting reaction (Fig. 31–8).

In the *extensor postural thrust reaction*, when touch and pressure receptors are activated, afferent impulses are sent to the cerebral cortex via afferent tracts in the spinal cord. From both cortical and subcortical nuclei, efferent impulses are directed to the extensor muscles to exert an antigravity effect.

Stimulation of pain receptors elicits the *flexor reflex to nociception* (i.e., withdrawal of the limb from the stimulus). Afferent pathways end in multisynaptic spinal cord reflex

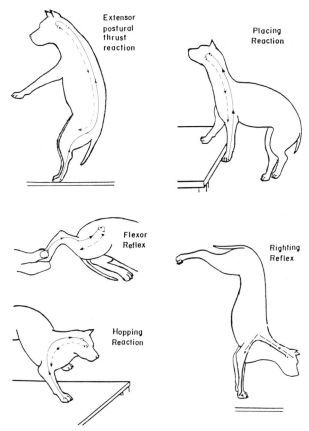

Figure 31–8 In the dog, afferent (———) and efferent (- - - -) pathways of reflexes involved in five elementary reactions: extensor postural thrust reaction, flexor reflex, hopping reaction, placing reaction, and righting reflex.

centers, from which efferent impulses are directed to the flexor muscles. Since the thalamus receives some of the pain impulses via the spinothalamic tracts, signals from the higher centers may contribute to voluntary withdrawal of the limb.

The *hopping reaction* is induced by activation of pressure and stretch receptors in the limb supporting the animal. The movements of the animal's body change the center of gravity, and afferent signals are sent to the cerebrum, the reticular formation, and the cerebellum. Efferent impulses originate from these formations toward the various muscles, which contract to realign the limb in proper position for efficient support of the animal's weight.

The *placing reaction* depends on activation of receptors on the anterior surface of the forelimb. Afferent pathways conduct impulses to the cerebrum, which monitors the tactile sensations. Cerebral and cerebellar signals are sent to initiate and coordinate the muscle contractions for placing.

The mechanism for the *righting reaction* uses the vestibular and visual systems and tactile receptors. Pathways from these receptors to the cerebrum conduct afferent signals for evaluation in the higher centers. Efferent pathways carry control signals originating in the cerebrum to the extensor muscles.

SPINAL TRANSECTION ("SPINALIZATION")

After transection of the spine at T10–12, cats show obvious loss of voluntary control and equilibrium of the hind limbs. However, after training to walk on a treadmill, these "spinalized" cats show important recovery of locomotion in the hind legs (Fig. 31–9).

After spine transection, even adult cats can recover locomotor function of the hind limbs, with weight support of the hind quarters and plantar digitigrade placement of the feet. This is apparently contrary to the observation that age at spinalization influences recovery and that adults do not regain as much locomotor function as young animals. It suggests that proper interactive training may greatly improve the recovery of such locomotor functions in adults.

ELECTROMYOGRAPHY

A small portion of each action potential passing along a muscle fiber spreads away from the muscle to the skin. When many muscle fibers contract simultaneously, the summated electrical potential at the skin is very great. When a normal muscle is stimulated, an *electromyogram* (EMG), or electrical recording of action potentials, can be made by placing two electrodes on the skin or by inserting minute needle electrodes into the muscle.

Electromyography can also be used to detect *muscle fasciculation* and *muscle fibrillation,* which occur after interruption of innervation to a muscle. A few (3 to 5) days after

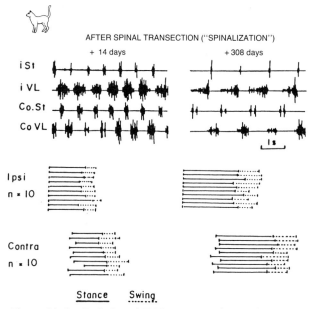

Figure 31–9 Evolution of EMG activity and gait of the hind limbs during walking at 0.2 m per second, at 14 days and 308 days after spinal transection ("spinalization") in an adult cat. The EMGs are from ipsilateral (*i*) and contralateral (*Co*) semitendinous (*St*) and vastus lateralis (*VL*) muscles. Duration of stance and of swing are expressed in seconds.

traumatic destruction of a peripheral nerve to a muscle, spontaneous impulses generated in the denervated muscle fibers cause *fasciculatory muscle movements*, which are seen as a slight ripple on the skin. Typical electromyographical records of weak periodic potentials, occurring at a rate of one every few seconds, are obtained from the skin over the muscle. After a few more days or a few weeks, the motor nerve conduction velocity is reduced from about 30 to 40 m per second to nothing, and the skeletal muscle fibers that have lost their innervation develop an intrinsic rhythmicity, with brief (1- to 2-ms), biphasic (100- to 350-μV) and rapid (3 to 10 per second) impulses, called *muscle fibrillation*. This is associated with the spread of large numbers of acetylcholine receptor proteins over the surfaces of the muscle fibers. As the muscle fibers do not fire simultaneously, the fibrillation potentials do not summate and are not strong enough to be recorded on the surface of the skin. To record an EMG of fibrillation, minute bipolar needle electrodes must be inserted into the muscle belly itself.

MUSCLE DEVELOPMENT, FATIGUE, AND METABOLISM

Skeletal muscle constitutes a major component of the carcass of meat-producing animals. Growth potential of muscle is limited postnatally to hypertrophy of its component muscle fibers. The limits of size increase are governed mainly by the maximum size at which the fibers can function efficiently.

The growth potential of muscle is determined mostly in utero. At birth, the number of muscle fibers is an indicator of the potential for postnatal growth performance. For instance, in the semitendinosus muscles of newborn pigs, there is a relationship between the relative growth potential and the number of fibers. Low–birth weight pigs exhibiting a high degree of catch-up growth have a relatively large number of fibers in these semitendinosus muscles. Piglets that show poor catch-up growth are prevented from reaching their full growth potential by environmental factors and other factors such as diseases.

In sheep, from birth to 2 years, the growth patterns of muscles of the proximal part of the pelvic limb are rapid and monophasic. This group of muscles continuously increases as a proportion of total muscle; this finding differs from earlier results indicating that the proportion of total muscle develops more slowly after weaning.

Exercise and Muscle Development

Muscle contraction is the result of a complex array of interwoven physiological events related to neurological, respiratory, and cardiovascular functions. During locomotion, the function of muscle is a collaborative achievement rather than an isolated mechanism. Muscles are the power-creating tissues of the body and are vital in determining performance.

TABLE 31–1 Factors That Influence Length and Frequency of Horse's Stride

Stride Length
  Acceleration capacity (force produced by muscles relative to body weight)
  Internal muscle architecture
  Leg length
  Range of movements of joints
Stride Frequency
  Intrinsic speed of sarcomere contraction
  Mechanical advantage of muscles
  Natural frequency of limbs
  Repetitiveness of limb movement (aerobic and anaerobic energy supply mechanisms)
  Resonant frequency between limb movement and respiratory rate

They influence both the length and the frequency of stride (Table 31–1).

The contractile properties of muscle fibers can be related to their myosin-ATPase activity. According to this criterion, a slow-twitch muscle fiber (type I) and two fast-twitch fibers (types IIA and IIB) are identified. Another classification is based on a combination of the contractile speed and the oxidative capacity of the fibers. This nomenclature recognizes slow-twitch high-oxidative, fast-twitch high-oxidative, and fast-twitch low-oxidative muscle fibers.

The oxidative potential of the type I fibers can affect their ability to contract more frequently. A high proportion of type I (slow-twitch) muscle fibers favors endurance activities by making muscles more fatigue resistant, whereas a higher proportion of type II (fast-twitch) fibers is advantageous for speed, as more frequent contractions are possible. Because power output (i.e., propulsion) is directly related to the cross-sectional area of the muscle fibers recruited, the type (size) as well as the number of fibers within a muscle is of great importance.

Normal training does not influence the proportion of type I and type II fibers or the number of fibers in a muscle, which are both genetically determined. In contrast, normal training and inactivity can greatly influence metabolic characteristics related to oxidative capacity and the diameter of muscle fibers.

Muscle Development and Anabolic Drugs

In male animals, some of the changes that occur at about the time of puberty include increased muscle development (*anabolic effect*) and thickening of bones. These effects are due to increased secretion by the testis of androgens or "male-making" hormones, which also change the secondary sexual characteristics (*androgenic action*). The increase in muscle mass is due to an increase not in the *number* of muscle fibers *but* in the *size* of individual fibers, which causes an overall gain in muscle mass. This marked effect on muscle mass has led horsemen to refer to anabolic drugs as "muscle puffers."

An increase in muscle strength of about 18 percent is purported to occur when anabolic steroids are combined with a high-protein diet and vigorous training. An increase in muscle mass may help improve the performance of sprinting racehorses and may improve stamina and endurance. A potential problem for mature horses is that muscle mass may increase without a corresponding increase in bone strength. Since the weakest point in any tendon is its point of insertion into the bone, the risk of tendon rupture is probably higher. Fillies may demonstrate overt masculinization and interference with future breeding performance because of the androgenic action remaining in most anabolic steroids.

Muscle Fatigue

Muscle fatigue is caused by at least two mechanisms: glycogen depletion and accumulation of lactic acid. Depletion of glycogen within fibers occurs during prolonged aerobic exercise. Accumulation of lactic acid, which appears during maximal exercise, causes a profound drop in pH within the fibers and perturbs the functions of actomyosin and of metabolic pathways. In both muscle fatigue mechanisms, the pool of muscle cells available for contraction is decreased, and the desired power output is reduced.

At speeds at which all the energy (ATP) is obtained via aerobic metabolism, both free fatty acids and glycogen are used as fuel sources. The state of fitness and the speed regulate the relative utilization of glycogen and of free fatty acids. The availability of glycogen is limited, whereas supplies of free fatty acids from adipose tissue are theoretically sufficient for long periods (days). In reality, the release of free fatty acids is rate limited and once the glycogen reserve is depleted, the intensity of exercise is controlled by the amount of free fatty acids available to the muscle fibers.

In horses, contrary to what occurs in man, not only does maximal exercise decrease phosphocreatine, but also stored ATP is reduced by 50 percent (Fig. 31–10). This decrease in ATP, which does not result in a concomitant increase in ADP, is a loss for the adenine nucleotide pool, as ATP is degraded to inosine monophosphate (IMP) via adenosine monophosphate (AMP). During the hour following exercise, some IMP is recycled into ATP during the recovery period, but the recovery is not complete, as a fraction of the IMP is further degraded into uric acid. The role of this decrease in ATP remains unknown in muscle fatigue, but it does not have any harmful effect on muscle, as only a small amount of the creatine phosphokinase (CPK) leaks into the plasma, and plasma aspartate transaminase (formerly called glutamic oxaloacetic transaminase, or GOT) remains unchanged.

Blood Changes During Exercise

The speed and the duration of exercise influence the intensity of changes in some blood parameters. Packed cell volume (PCV), number of erythrocytes, and hemoglobin

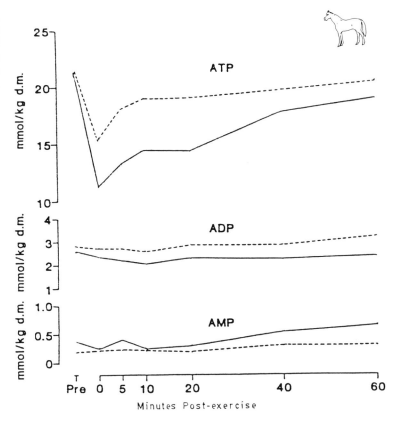

Figure 31–10 Adenosine triphosphate (ATP), adenosine diphosphate (ADP), and adenosine monophosphate (AMP) content of middle gluteal muscles of horses before exercise (*Pre*), after a single maximal exercise over 800 m (- - - -) or 2000 m (———), and during a 60-minute recovery period.

TABLE 31–2 Effect of Various Types of Physical Activity on Postexercise Packed Cell Volume and Levels of Glucose and Lactate in the Horse

Activity	PCV (L/L)	Lactate (mmol/L)	Glucose (mmol/L)
Endurance racing	0.45		4.5
3-day cross country	0.60		
Galloping	0.63	30	11
Resting	0.43		
Treadmill exercise	0.50		7
Trotting or pacing	0.58	15	

concentration increase with the speed of exercise (up to 450 to 600 m per minute). The linear correlation of PCV with exercise at moderate speeds is important, as it reflects a relative increase in the quantity of erythrocytes, which serves the body's need for oxygen transport. In horses, sustained endurance exercise at an extremely low speed (144 m per minute) has no significant effect on these parameters (Table 31–2).

The mobilization of erythrocytes is a unique hematological response to exercise in the horse. Catecholamines mobilize the erythrocytes from the splenic reservoir. When the splenic reservoir is removed by splenectomy, work capacity is reduced. During exercise, the increased PCV is positively correlated with speed, heart rate, blood viscosity, and plasma norepinephrine concentrations.

Leukocytosis is greater during endurance exercise than after galloping exercise. In addition, a large increase in neutrophils is concomitant with a lower lymphocyte count. The neutrophil-to-lymphocyte ratio (1.8 to 1 prior to exercise) is as high as 6 to 1 after 160 km of endurance exercise. The extent of the neutrophil increase correlates positively with heart rate and speed, whereas these parameters correlated negatively with the relative lymphocytopenia. An increase in plasma cortisol may explain these results, and it appears that the more stressful the exercise, the greater the change in the neutrophil-to-lymphocyte ratio.

Fitness and Performance Potential

The accumulation of lactate in the blood can be used as an indication of the degree of anaerobic metabolism required to perform muscle work. The increase in blood lactate is not linear with the increase in exercise, but it can be described as an exponential relationship.

Stride length, rather than stride frequency, is closely related to performance speed, performance velocity, and a heart rate of 200 beats per minute. It may indicate that stride length is the critical factor in energy consumption.

The oxygen consumption at a certain level of muscle exercise (e.g., at 8 m per second on the treadmill) decreases very rapidly in horses. Over a period of 5 weeks following this precipitous drop, the oxygen uptake gradually and slowly creeps up toward the baseline level. This means that the horse adapts to this work by improving the mechanical efficiency of its oxygen utilization rather than by increasing the maximum level of oxygen uptake.

REFERENCES

Barbeau H, Rossignol S. Recovery of locomotion after chronic spinalization in the adult cat. Brain Res 1987;412:84.

Breazile JE, Blauch BS, Nail N. Experimental study of canine distemper myoclonus. Am J Vet Res 1966;27:1375.

Forssberf H, Grillner S, Halbertsma J. The locomotion of the low spinal cat. I. Coordination within a hindlimb. Acta Physiol Scand 1980; 108:269.

Griffiths IR, Duncan ID. Some studies of the clinical neurophysiology of denervation in the dog. Res Vet Sci 1974;17:377.

Handel SE, Stickland NC. Catch-up growth in pigs: a relationship with muscle cellularity. Anim Prod 1988;47:291.

Iggo A. Cutaneous sensory mechanisms. In: Barlow HB, Mollon HB, eds. The senses. Cambridge: Cambridge University Press, 1982.

Lohse CL, Moss FP, Butterfield RM. Growth patterns of muscles of merino sheep from birth to 517 days. Anim Prod 1971;13:117.

Mountcastle VM. Sensory receptors and neural encoding. In: Mountcastle VM, ed. Medical physiology. 14th ed. St. Louis: CV Mosby, 1980.

Reynolds PJ, Talbott RE, Brookhart JM. Control of postural reactions in the dog: the role of the dorsal column feedback pathway. Brain Res 1972;40:159.

Rinvick E, Walberg F. Demonstration of a somatotopically arranged corticorubral projection in the cat: an experimental study with silver methods. J Comp Neurol 1963;120:393.

Snow DH. Exercise and training. In: Hickman J, ed. Horse management. London: Academic Press, 1984.

Tobin T. Drugs and the performance of horses. Springfield: Charles C Thomas, 1981.

Villablanca JR, Marcus RJ, Olmstead CE. Effects of caudate nuclei on frontal cortical ablations in cats. Exp Neurol 1976;52:389; 1977;53:31, 289.

CHAPTER 32

HIGHER NERVOUS ACTIVITY

The term "encephalization" refers to the increased power of command exerted by the more rostrad parts of the central nervous system (CNS) on the lower reflexes and their mechanisms. The higher nervous system allows the animal to maintain its motor activity under a low-voltage fast frequency (LVFF) electrical activity brought about by the reticular formation (Fig. 32–1). It is at the basis of individual behavior but also of links between individual animals and others and with the environment. The amygdala and the hippocampus (i.e., the *limbic system*) are involved in the *visual memory* and in the ability to associate an object with a *reward*. In addition, the *cerebellum* and other poorly defined structures are associated with reward-punishment mechanisms (Fig. 32–2).

Somewhat like antagonistic spinal reflexes, the go and stop mechanisms, or reward and punishment, are mutually inhibitory; however, activation of one mechanism can depress the other. Similarly, sudden deactivation of one mechanism releases the other from inhibition and by a rebound effect causes a brief period of heightened activity.

CATON (Liverpool), in 1875, first described continuous electrical activity in the exposed cerebrum of animals. Much later, in 1929, BERGER (Iena) used the string galvanometer to record that activity through the intact skull and found that it changed with sleep and wakefulness. Decades later, MORUZZI (Pisa) compared the electrical activity of the cat's brain after low, midpontine, pretrigeminal, and high transection. He found that cortical waking processes, characterized by permanent LVFF electrical activity, act independently of sensory inputs. An electroencephalogram pattern similar to that of sleep (i.e., high-voltage slow frequency [HVSF] activity and miosis) occurs when the reticular formation is depressed, as by barbiturates.

In 1954, DELGADO (New Mexico), following the early work of HESS (Zurich), reported the first experimental proof that electrical stimulation of the brain (i.e., the cerebroperiventricular system) could serve as a *punishment*. The same year, OLDS and MILNER (Canada) described the unexpected finding that electrical stimulation of the brain (i.e., the medial forebrain) could serve as a *reward*.

In 1922, SCHJELDERUP-EBBE (Norway) introduced the concept of social dominance when he observed the pecking order in domestic fowl. In 1971, WOOD-GUSCH (Scotland) reported on the dominance of high-ranking birds.

This chapter deals with higher nervous activity, taking into account the special sensory systems, the cerebellum, sleep and related states, social dominance, and biological rhythms.

SPECIAL SENSORY SYSTEMS

This section introduces the tactile and kinesthetic sensory systems, the olfactory sensory system, the gustatory sensory system, vision, the vestibular sensory system, and the auditory sensory system.

Tactile and Kinesthetic Sensory Systems

The tactile and kinesthetic sensory systems are closely interrelated with regard to peripheral receptor organs, afferent nerves, and central nerve pathways. The two sensory systems are subserved by three types of receptor organs: receptors responding to bending of hairs (peritrichal plexus), receptors activated by pressure on the skin (pacinian corpuscles, Meissner's corpuscles, and some naked nerve endings), and receptors stimulated by vibrations applied to the skin.

Hair cells located in the ampulla of the *semicircular ducts* (crista ampullaris) and hair cells associated with the *otoliths* in the maculae of the *labyrinth* are the receptors of the vestibular organ, which is involved in the righting reflex of animals (Fig. 32–3).

The *pig's snout* is a remarkable organ that is intimately related to the animal's acute sense of smell and important to its search for food and its detection of other animals. In addition, the snout is important because it is used as the pig's chief tactile and effector organ. The snout is to the pig what hands are to man. It has been observed that the pig snout is its chief executive as well as its chief tactile organ, spade as well as hand, whereas the legs are little more than props for the body (Fig. 32–4).

What can be achieved by such an apparently sensitive "chief executive organ" is astonishing. In the New York Zoo, two wild boars were put into an animal house with an outdoor concrete run having a small crack in its surface. Within 2 weeks, by rooting with their snouts, the two pigs had excavated and reduced to rubble the 3- to 4-inch thick concrete run.

Olfactory Sensory System

The receptor organs for the olfactory system are located within the nasal mucosa, in the caudodorsal portion known as the *olfactory mucosa*. The central process of the receptor cells (the axon) passes deep into the olfactory mucosa and joins

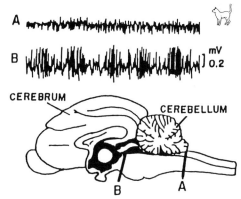

Figure 32–1 Electrical activity of the cerebrum after brain stem transections. Cut A produces an "encéphale isolé," or isolated cerebrum preparation. The EEG record has waves of low-voltage high-frequency (LVHF), which is associated with an alert animal. Cut B (postcollicular) produces a "cerveau isolé," or isolated brain preparation. The EEG pattern immediately following the transection is of the type seen in sleep, with high-voltage, low-frequency (HVLF) waves. The spontaneous recovery of the cortical desynchronization (LVHF) after 6 to 7 days suggests that strong activating processes are located rostrad to a midbrain transection.

other axons to form the olfactory nerves. The fibers of the olfactory nerves are the *smallest axons* of the mammalian nervous system, having diameters as small as 0.2 μm. Adaptation to the response does not occur (Fig. 32–5).

The *organ of Jacobson,* which is responsible for the *lip curling (flehmen) reaction* in horses and cattle, is related to the olfactory system. Special molecules called *pheromones* that are emitted by animals influence other animals via the olfactory sensory system. Recognition of species, individuals, and rhythmic status of sexuality and territorial marking by gland secretions or bodily excretions are activities based on olfaction. The olfactory sense is very important to behavior in many species of animals.

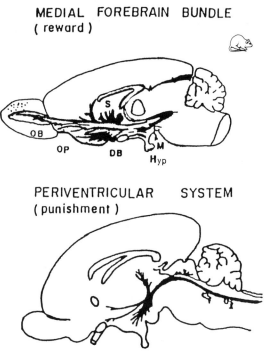

Figure 32–2 Diagram represents the presumed substrate of reward mechanism, the medial forebrain bundles, in a mammalian brain. The periventricular system of fibers is the presumed substrate of the punishment mechanism. *OB,* Olfactory bulb; *DB,* nucleus of the diagonal band; *M,* mammillary body; *S,* septum; *Hyp,* hypophysis; *OP,* optic tract.

Gustatory Sensory System

The four submodalities of human taste—sweet, salt, bitter, and sour—are not necessarily perceived by animals. The sensory perception elicited by a substance that is considered sweet by humans may be perceived as something different or may not be perceived at all by animals.

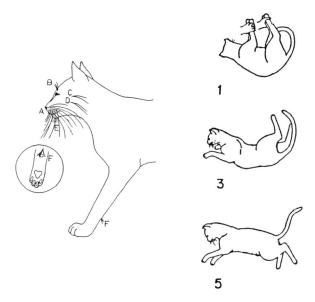

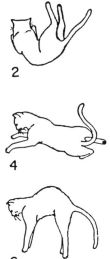

Figure 32–3 Left, Hair follicle afferent units in the cat (*A* through *F*). **Right,** In the cat, sequences of the six (*1* through *6*) postural phases of the righting reflex, which is initiated by hair cells in the ampulla of the semicircular ducts and by hair cells (with otoliths) in the macula of the labyrinth.

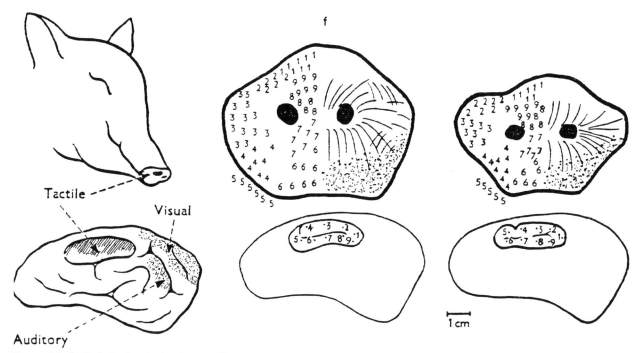

Figure 32–4 **Left,** In the pig, localization of tactile, visual, and auditory areas of the cerebral cortex. **Right,** Receptors on the snout and their location on the tactile cortical receiving area. Electrical stimulation with an electrode at points (1–9) on the brain (**lower diagram**) causes discharges at corresponding points (1–9) on the snout (**upper diagram**). Points 5 are on the lateral surface of the snout and the margin of the upper lip.

Sensory nerve responses to the application of distilled water ("water" fibers) to the taste buds have been demonstrated in some animals (cat, dog, hen, monkey, pig, pigeon) but have not been observed in other animals (calf, goat, rat, sheep) or in humans (Table 32–1).

"*Salt*" *taste fibers* in rodents (guinea pig, hamster, and rat) are excited more by sodium chloride than by potassium chloride, whereas the converse is true in carnivores (cat and dog). "*Acid*" *taste fibers* are activated by high concentrations of hydrogen ions. Sensitivity is related to pH, and threshold

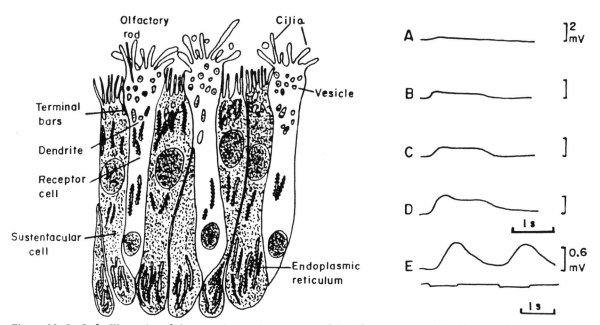

Figure 32–5 **Left,** Illustration of electron microscopic appearance of the olfactory mucosa. The olfactory rod is the part of the receptor exposed to odorants. **Right,** The intensity of depolarization of olfactory potentials (upward from the baseline) recorded from the mucosa varies according to the stimulus: *A,* purified air; *B,* butanol vapor at 0.001 M; *C,* butanol vapor at 0.01 M; *D,* butanol vapor at 0.1 M; and *E,* two butanol (0.1 M) exposures at 1-second intervals.

TABLE 32–1 Comparison of the Presence (+) or Absence (−) of Gustatory Fibers in Some Species of Animals and Birds

Stimulus	Cat	Dog or Human	Goat or Sheep	Hen	Pig or Rabbit	Pigeon	Rat
Acetic acid (0.1 M)	+	+	+	+	+	+	+
Distilled water	+	+	−	+	+	+	−
Sodium chloride (0.5 M)	+	+	+	+	+	+	+
Quinine hydrochloride (0.02 M)	+	+	+	+	+	−	+
Ringer's solution (0.15 M NaCl)	−	−	+	−	−	−	−
Sucrose (0.05 M)	−	+	+	−	+	−	+

pH is usually between 3 and 4. A solution of strong acid (e.g., hydrochloric acid) is more effective than an equimolar solution of a weak acid (e.g., acetic acid), because the latter is less dissociated. *"Bitter" taste fibers* are stimulated by bitter substances, which are usually alkaloids, such as quinine, caffeine, and strychnine.

"Sweet" taste fibers respond to solutions that contain organic compounds, such as the simpler carbohydrates, of which D-fructose (0.5 M solution) is the most effective. Other substances efficient to stimulate sweet fibers include aldehydes, ketones, amino acids, and synthetic sweetening agents such as saccharin. The more complex molecules may also excite other classes of fibers (e.g., saccharin may excite "bitter" taste fibers). *Chorda tympani* responses to sugars and saccharin are mediated by multiple receptor sites. Single cell studies suggest the existence of six different sugar receptors (for sucrose, lactose, maltose, fructose, glucose, and mannose) plus a saccharin receptor.

The statements above are based on responses to only single concentrations of stimuli, and some of the differences may actually represent concentration effects. In addition, reducing sugars mutarotate in solution, producing a mixture of stimulant molecules. Additional support to the multiple receptor theory is provided by human psychophysical studies in which the sugar taste function is found to be nonlinear and the taste responses to several sweeteners, including sugars, fail to cross-adapt. Mixtures of purely sweet and purely bitter compounds suppress the sweet taste, which may account for the nonlinearity of the taste function.

In addition to inhibition by mixtures of purely sweet and purely bitter compounds, the sweet taste response is suppressed specifically by other substances. Inhibition of response to sweet is caused by low concentrations of zinc (Zn^{++}) and copper (Cu^{++}) and by the antibiotic chloramphenicol. Zinc and copper compounds inhibit the taste responses of animals to sucrose, maltose, fructose, glucose, and sodium saccharin but hardly affect the responses to L-alanine, D-tryptophan, glycine, L-serine, L-proline, and L-valine. It seems that there is one receptor system for sugars and saccharin and another for sweet-tasting amino acids.

Vision

The eye is fashioned in two hemispheres. The small anterior hemisphere forms the transparent cornea, through which light enters the eye. The larger posterior hemisphere includes the sclera (protection), the choroid (nutrient), and the retina (receptors).

The visual receptor organs of domestic animals are very complex in comparison with the trichromacy of human color vision. The *retina* contains photopigments, which respond to adequate stimulus (electromagnetic energy) within a given range of frequencies (photoreceptors). The *rod photoreceptors* are receptive to low-frequency (380 to 600 nm) light rays, in contrast with the *cone photoreceptors,* which are receptive to high-frequency light rays (450 to 780 nm). The two types of photoreceptor cells sense light energy of two overlapping spectra.

The eye (lens, pupil, retina) of the *pig* is more like that of man than that of any other common farm animal. The vision of the pig is highly developed; its retina is rich in short, thick cones. Pigs respond to light within, and perhaps beyond, the range of wavelengths defined as visible light for humans (i.e., from below 420 up to 760 nm). Young (8-month-old) pigs fed from the same place every day *do not respond to visual stimuli for food reward.* From the time of weaning, piglets fed food scattered on the floor can learn to *discriminate between levels of brightness.* Learning experiments indicate that pigs would *distinguish between colors* or wavelengths (differences as small as 20 nm) independently of brightness.

Avian color vision is unique in its spectral range. Whereas primate color vision operates within a spectral range of 420 to 760 nm, diurnal birds have a much larger range. Pigeons are able to discriminate among wavelengths near *ultraviolet,* a part of the spectrum invisible to man. Since birds have good discrimination over a wider spectral range than man, they have better color vision.

The color vision of *mammals* is like that of humans with defective color vision. Ground squirrels, and probably cattle, dogs, and cats, have *dichromatic* color vision, similar in several respects to that of human protanopic (*red-green blindness,* confusion of red and blue-green) dichromats.

The neuroanatomical pathway for vision involves decussation of the signals from the medial aspect of the retina (Fig. 32–6).

The colliculus receives the visual projections, and additional somatic and acoustic afferents. In cats, the developmental chronology of sensory representation parallels the animal's use of modality-specific cues for tracking behavior. Somatic stimuli are effective in activating superior colliculus cells at birth, when orientation is accomplished by somatic cues. Acoustic activation and visual activation develop many days later, along with auditory and visual orientation behavior. Presumably, the organization of the superior colliculus is important for visual orientation. The visual deficits that result from destruction of the *superior colliculus* suggest that it is involved in visually guided (orienting and tracking) behavior in the cat.

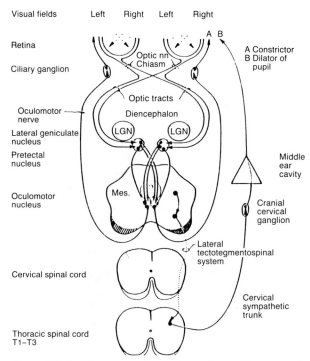

Figure 32–6 Neuroanatomical pathway for pupillary control. Miosis, the cardinal sign of an interruption in the sympathetic supply to the orbit, occurs after section of the cervical sympathetic trunk, usually following cervical trauma at the T1–T3 level.

The magnified foveal representation in the colliculus provides a zone of enhanced visual acuity, especially for binocular vision (Fig. 32–7). In addition, the forelimb of the cat is represented only by small receptive fields of neurons, whereas the facial zones have a representation with maximum tactile resolution, which can be used for exploration and for seizing and handling prey.

The field of vision in rabbits and horses is lateral, with a very narrow blind area and little binocular vision (see Fig. 32–7).

The cardinal sign of *Horner's syndrome* is miosis, usually detected by anisocoria (pupils of different diameters), which can be made obvious by placing the animal in dim light. Prolapse of the third eyelid and ptosis (drooping of the upper eyelid) are additional signs (Fig. 32–8). The diagnosis of Horner's syndrome, which occurs mostly after a lesion affecting the first thoracic segment, may be confirmed by observing the pupillary response to cocaine. Cocaine (5 percent) is instilled onto the surface of both eyes, and after 45 minutes the degree of pupillary dilatation is noted. Minimal dilatation of the affected pupil compared with full dilatation of the normal pupil confirms the diagnosis.

Vestibular Sensory System

The receptor organs of the *vestibular system* are located within the inner ear, embedded in the petrous portion of the temporal bone. The *medial longitudinal fasciculus* functions to conjugate the eye movements. Transection of the medial longitudinal fasciculus within the brain stem, either artificially or by a disease process, results in disturbance of the horizontal movement of the eyes (*nystagmus*). This is an involuntary rhythmic eyeball oscillation, either with equal movements (pendular) or a quick phase (jerk). For example, ice cold water instilled in the right ear induces a contralateral jerk nystagmus (i.e., in the eye opposite the stimulated ear) (Fig. 32–9).

Auditory Sensory System

The auditory system functions for the reception of airborne or water-borne vibratory energy. The receptor cells are contained within a highly organized structure known as the *organ of Corti*. The coiled scala media is roughly triangular in cross-section. One side of the triangle is formed by the fibrous elastic basilar membrane, which extends from the inner bony core of the cochlea to the spiral ligament lining the outer wall of the canal. The brainstem auditory evoked response (BAER) has generally been limited to testing for hearing deficit (Fig. 32–10). In veterinary medicine, it is also a tool used in the diagnosis of brain stem lesions.

CEREBELLUM

The cerebellum, much smaller than the cerebrum, lies at the back of the skull, behind the brain stem. In Latin, *cerebellum* is a diminutive of *cerebrum* (i.e., a lesser brain). As in the cerebrum, the highest functions in the cerebellum are confined to the thin layer of elaborately folded and wrinkled (to increase its area) gray matter that makes up the cortex.

The Purkinje cells of the cerebellum were among the first neurons recognized in the nervous system. They are named for J.E. PURKINJE (Czechoslovakia), who described them in 1837. The most complex of all neurons, they have a large and extensive dendritic apparatus referring impulses to a bulblike soma and a long slender axon. In humans, the dendrites of the Purkinje cells may form as many as 100,000 synapses with afferent fibers, more than any other cell in the CNS.

The histology of the cerebellum, whose macroscopic aspect resembles a tree (arbor vitae), was established by RAMON Y CAJAL (Spain) in 1888, using a staining technique developed in 1873 by GOLGI (Italy). The cerebellar tissue is impregnated with salts of silver, which colors some nerve cells deep brown or black.

The first reliable clues to the function of the cerebellum were offered by LUCIANI (Italy) and FLOURENS (France), who found disturbances of coordination and equilibrium in "decerebellate" animals. SHERRINGTON was able to demonstrate that the cerebellum coordinates the movements of the muscles but does not initiate them.

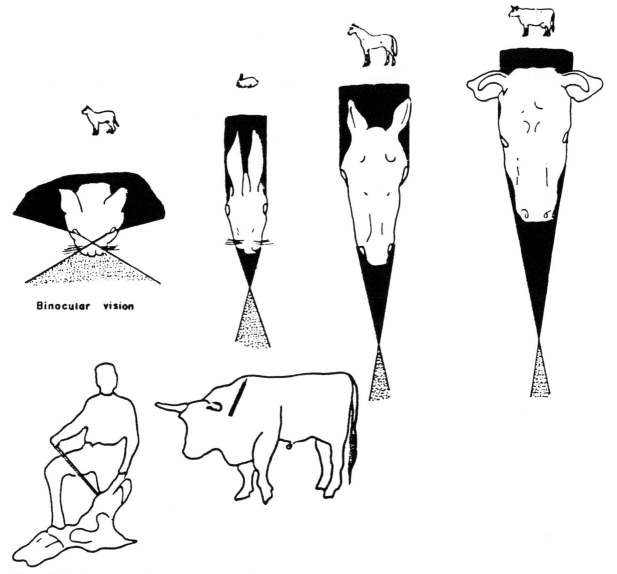

Binocular vision

Figure 32–7 In contrast to the cat, which has excellent binocular vision, some species (rabbit, horse, and cattle) with wide-set eyes have wide and excellent lateral vision but an anterior blind area that is without lateral or binocular vision. To avoid being seen by the bull, the toreador maneuvers to place himself in the blind area of the animal.

Organization of Movement

Destruction of the cerebellum is at the origin of *rigidity,* with flexion of the hindquarters (Fig. 32–11).

Microscopic examination of the cerebellar cortex of animals with neonatal cerebellar *ataxia* indicates a degeneration due to an intrinsic abnormality in the Purkinje neuron's metabolic structure that is not related to any injury (abiotrophy). Hereditary cerebellar abiotrophy and extrapyramidal nuclear abiotrophy are found in dogs (Kerry blue terriers, Gordon setters, rough-coated collies), in horses, and in cattle. Ingestion of *Solanum fastigatum* profoundly disturbs the metabolism of the Purkinje neurons, resulting in ataxia.

Somatotopy

The climbing fibers and the mossy fibers, the two afferent systems that ultimately direct impulses to the Purkinje cells, are distributed throughout the cerebellar cortex in a more or less orderly array. The two systems are present in all members of the vertebrate subphylum but are radically different in some properties and represent opposite extremes among the neurons of the CNS. The climbing fiber is virtually a private line to a Purkinje cell, whereas the mossy fibers carry sensory inputs from the spinal cord, the brain stem, and the upper motor areas of the brain (Fig. 32–12).

A single Purkinje cell may be connected to many climb-

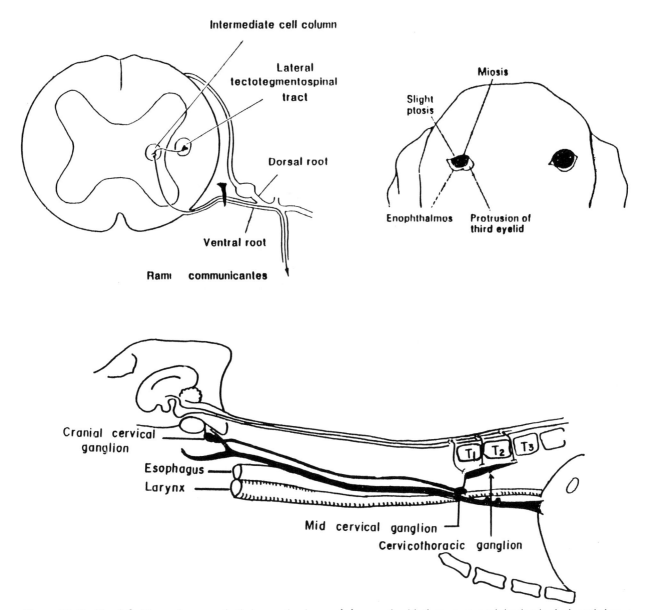

Figure 32–8 **Top left,** The ocular sympathetic innervation is regarded as a path with three neurons originating in the hypothalamus, tectum, and tegmentum. In the lateral tectotegmentospinal system, their fibers descend through the lateral pons, medulla, and cervical spinal cord. **Top right,** Anisocoria (unequal sizes of the pupils) in Horner's syndrome in the dog, resulting from paralysis or section of the cervical sympathetic fibers, which also causes miosis, enophthalmos (sinking of the eye), and protrusion of the third eyelid. **Bottom,** The neurons synapse with cell bodies of *preganglionic* neurons in the intermediate cell column of the first three thoracic segments (T1–T3). The postganglionic neurons are in the cervical sympathetic trunk. Stimulation of the part afferent to the eye results in dilation of the pupil.

ing fibers, whereas the mossy fibers, which ultimately excite many Purkinje cells, have few contacts with each of them. The cerebellum is a *central control point for the organization of movement*. Movement can be generated in the absence of the cerebellum, but the cerebellum is necessary to obtain maximum motor efficiency because it modulates, or reorganizes, the motor commands, and it coordinates the diverse input signals. As an organ of regulation, the cerebellum corrects movements before they are generated (Fig. 32–13).

Dysmetria

An animal without a cerebellum is unable to adjust the position of its limbs with respect to a goal. Overshoot or undershoot conditions, called *dysmetria,* are usually associated with disturbances corresponding to specific localization of the cerebellum. Several synapses between climbing fibers and Purkinje cell dendrites are responsible for the adjustments of movements (Fig. 32–14).

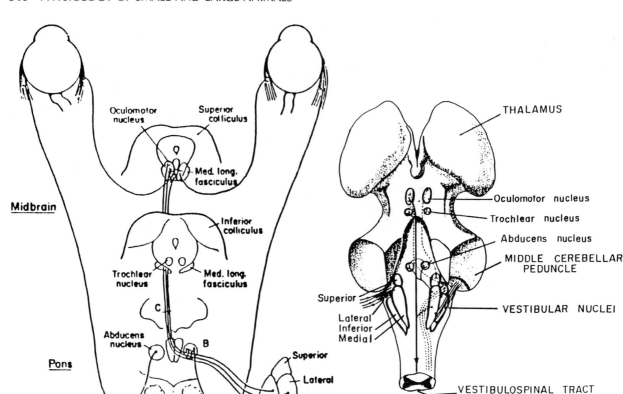

Figure 32–9 **Left,** Diagram of the relationship between the vestibular nuclei, the medial longitudinal fasciculus, and the nuclei of the extraocular muscles. **Right,** The projection fibers of the vestibular system.

SLEEP AND RELATED STATES

Sleep is a behavioral state marked by a characteristic immobile posture and a diminished but readily reversible sensitivity to external stimuli. As most definitions of behavior strongly imply action, the absence of motion may account for the omission of sleep as a behavioral function in animals.

CHABERT (Alfort) first described sleep associated with rapid eye movement (REM) in cattle in 1796. Movements of the muzzle and lowing noises occur for brief periods in lactating cows that seem to be asleep. These dreamlike phases appear more frequently a short time after calving.

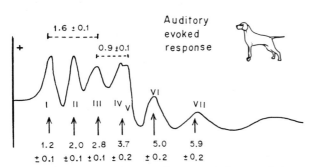

Figure 32–10 Normal BAER (brainstem auditory evoked response) in a dog, with latencies of 1.2 and 5.9 ms for the first and last responses.

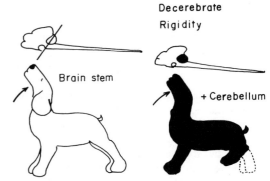

Figure 32–11 Rigidity with *extension* of the hind limbs (opisthotonos) is observed following significant damage to the brain stem. Rigidity with *flexion* of the hind limbs is observed after significant damage to the cerebellum.

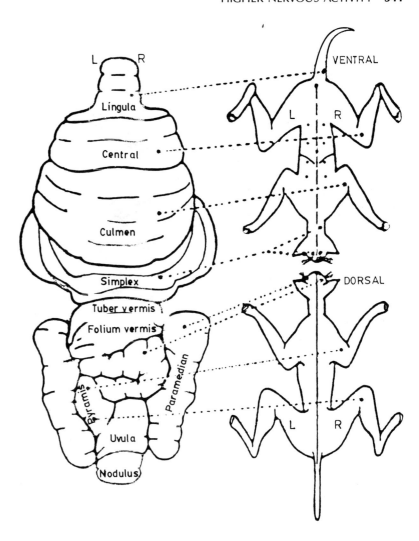

Figure 32–12 Somatotopic localization in the cerebellum of motor functions is achieved by stimulating areas over the cerebellar surface and by evoked responses following stimulation of various sensory inputs.

Nevertheless, for decades, even after the advent of electroencephalographic techniques, it was erroneously contended that adult ruminants do not sleep. It was thought that complete loss of vigilance is labile, transient, and polyphasic and that drowsiness is the most common behavior pattern observed in the recumbent ruminating animal.

The Sleep Cycle

All mammals show alternating states of rest and activity. During rest, most species indulge in both *slow-wave sleep* (SWS) and deep, or *paradoxical, sleep* (PS). In SWS, the sensory threshold is raised, and diffuse slow waves of high-amplitude electrical activity (predominantly 1 to 5 Hz, 200 μV) are recorded from the cortex. Usually of shorter duration, PS further raises sensory thresholds during periods of REM, but electroencephalographic records do not differ from those obtained during alertness (mainly 25 to 27 Hz, 50 μV); (Fig. 32–15).

During human sleep, the brain, which controls the peripheral autonomic systems, undergoes continuous oscillations (troughs and peaks) with a period length of about 90 minutes. The temporal elements of the sleep cycle, which occurs in all mammals, are remarkably constant for any species or individual. The troughs and peaks indicate sensitive and strict central control, as with other metabolic cycles and rhythms (Fig. 32–16).

During *troughs* of the cycle, subjects are difficult to arouse. Brain waves are then of high-voltage slow frequency (HVSF), whereas peripheral autonomic activities such as heart rate and blood pressure are low and regular. On the basis of the electroencephalogram (EEG), these troughs are referred to as SWS, or *synchronized* sleep.

The *peaks* of the cycle are characterized by LVFF waves, as in waking, by irregular high levels of autonomic activity, and by nystagmoid REM. Arousal threshold is variable, and reports of hallucinoid dreaming are frequent. On the basis of the EEG, the peaks are referred to as *asynchronized* sleep, or REM sleep.

Role of the Reticular Formation

Impulses are carried by fibers from the reticular formation to the cerebral cortex via a path that is yet to be

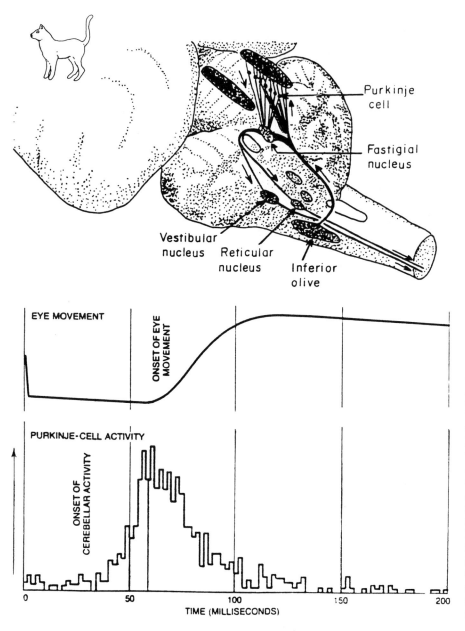

Figure 32–13 Top, Projection of climbing fibers into the cerebellar cortex. The fibers originate in the bilateral inferior olives of the brain stem and are organized in the longitudinal strips covering many cortical folds. The length and orientation of these strips suggest that the climbing fiber system participates in the regulation of movements that involve several limbs, since each strip extends across areas known to be associated with several parts of the body. Branches of the climbing fibers reach also the cerebellar nuclei (the fastigial nucleus) and are joined there by the axons of Purkinje cells from the cortex. **Bottom,** Rapid eye movements, called *saccades,* are associated with activity in the cerebellar cortex. The top graph is an average record of 100 saccades; the bottom graph is a record of the activity of a single Purkinje cell during the same 100 saccades. Purkinje cell activity begins to increase about 25 ms before the movement is initiated, which suggests that the cerebellum can coordinate or correct such movements before they are generated.

determined. The overall effect of reticular system activation on the cortex is analyzed by studying the *cortical evoked responses.* The usual surface-negative type of evoked response is nonsummating, and its decrease of amplitude, which follows reticular formation stimulation, is considered a form of occlusion. The input of the reticular formation is believed to be excitatory to the cortex.

The state of *sleep* is generally thought to be caused by diminished *corticopetal sensory influences,* and the *waking* state to be due to their increase. In the cat, sleep may be actively induced also by means of electrical stimulation of the thalamic nuclei, via permanently implanted electrodes. Upon stimulation, the animal shows diminished motor activity, seeks out a resting place, then curls up and appears to be in a natural state of sleep. The injection of acetylcholine into other regions of the brain stem through permanently implanted cannulas produces a behavior change similar to sleep.

Chemical Differentiation of Neurons and Sleep

The neurons in the brain stem can be classified into two groups by applying fluorescent dyes that bind selectively to biogenic amines. A first group of cells, which project their axons rostrad and concentrate *5-hydroxytryptamine,* or serotonin, is in the midline raphe nuclei of the pons and in the midline of the brain stem. The other group of cells, situated more laterally in the brain stem, contain catecholamines

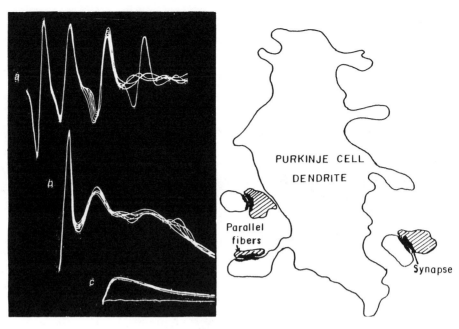

Figure 32–14 Left, Responses of a Purkinje cell to stimulation by a climbing fiber. Diphasic (*a*) action potentials are measured from outside the cell, whereas monophasic action potentials are measured from inside the cell. The response is of the all-or-nothing type. Stimulation of a climbing fiber provokes the firing of the Purkinje cell by depolarizing the cell membrane, a phenomenon that is not recorded in a damaged cell (*c*). **Right,** The diagram indicates the synapses between parallel fibers and the Purkinje cell dendrite.

(mostly *dopamine* and *norepinephrine*) and occupy most of the locus caeruleus.

This dichotomy suggests a functional duality, which is much simpler to study than the histology of the cells of the brain stem under the light microscope. In addition, a structural chemical dualism to match the troughs and the peaks of the sleep cycle is proposed. In this system, serotonin in the

raphe nuclei would produce SWS, whereas norepinephrine in the locus caeruleus would induce REM sleep.

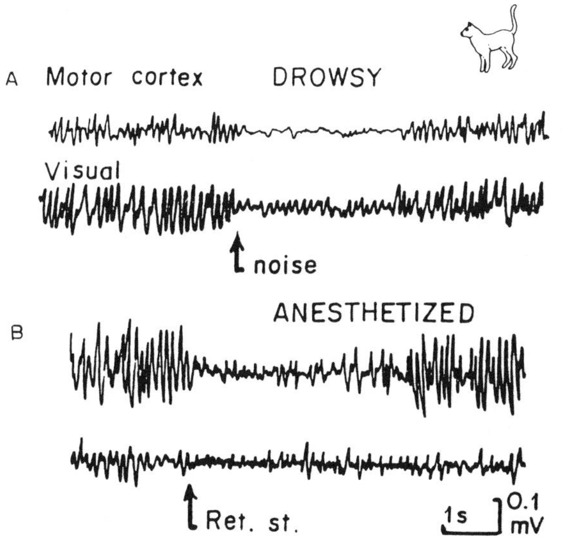

Selective Sleep Deprivation

Under stall conditions, standing cows may indulge in SWS but not REM sleep. In a recumbent position, mostly during the night, cows experience both SWS and REM sleep. In ruminants, food intake (about 8 hours per day) limits available sleep time.

Forced standing for 24 hours (day and night) causes *selective deprivation* of REM sleep. *Partial deprivation* of REM sleep results from forced standing at night, which prevents only nocturnal REM sleep but allows some during the daytime, when the animal may be recumbent.

During prolonged (8-week) absence of recumbency at night (partial sleep deprivation), the total duration of SWS increases slightly (17.0 versus 12.1 percent), and about half of it occurs during the forced nighttime standing. However, the usual 10 to 12 episodes of SWS per 24 hours are fragmented into microcycles of 2 to 5 minutes, which are separated by brief waking periods marked by stereotyped oral movements (Fig. 32–17). The amount of REM sleep is strongly reduced (0.4 versus 1.8 percent), and feeding occupies the entire free time (4 hours), which is adequate for the intake of the normal ration (8 kg of hay).

When recumbency is prevented for 20 hours per day and access to food is limited to the remaining 4 hours, hunger becomes the dominant drive. If the 4-hour free-access schedule is maintained for more than 2 to 3 weeks, the cows increase their rate of food intake, and equal free-time is divided between this fast intake behavior and REM sleep (i.e., recumbency). When the cows have adapted to these conditions, total REM sleep duration is almost equal to the

Figure 32–15 Alerting responses in the cat brain. **A,** After a sudden sensory stimulus (*arrow*), which may be a noise, a touch, or a flash of light, the EEG pattern changes to the alert type. Alerting, or desynchronization, of EEG lasts for a brief time before return of the regular alpha, or spindle, type of record characteristic of the drowsy animal. **B,** A brief electrical stimulation is delivered to the reticular formation, and it has a similar alerting effect on the EEG of the cortex.

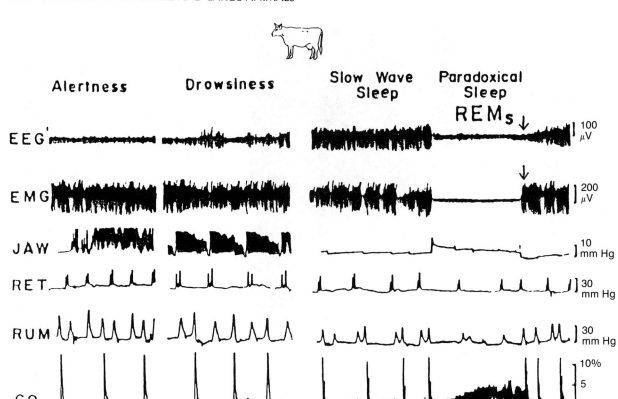

Figure 32–16 Electrographical correlates of various stages of sleep and wakefulness in cattle. As the cow becomes drowsy, the EEG deactivates, muscle tone (EMG) and chewing (JAW) decrease, and some slowing of reticular (RET) and ruminal (RUM) contractions occurs. These changes progress in slow-wave sleep. During paradoxical sleep (REMs), which ends at the right-hand arrow, the EEG becomes activated, nuchal muscle tone (EMG) is abolished, and RET and RUM rates and strength of contractions decrease further without rumination and eructation (peaks of carbon dioxide trace reflect eructation).

amount observed under field conditions. If the free time is shortened to 2 hours, which is less than the time required for intake of the usual ration, hunger is again the dominant drive (Fig. 32–18). The reduced food intake causes weight loss, which is equivalent to the emaciation seen in non–sleep-deprived subjects receiving the same quantity of food.

During the first week of recovery, after a 60-day period of partial or selective sleep deprivation, the SWS increases from 15.8 to 24.2 percent per 24 hours, but the number of episodes remains unchanged at 12 per day. During the same week of recovery, the relative duration (percentage) and the number of episodes of REM sleep per 24 hours increase: from 2.6 percent and seven, to 4.8 percent and fourteen.

Comparisons of Sleep Patterns of Domestic Animals

Natural selective forces work against the evolution of long-sleeping prey species. For example, cats sleep a great deal (more than half the time) and a preponderance of it is REM sleep (Table 32–2). In contrast, prey species (e.g., ruminants, rabbits, guinea pigs) sleep very little and have very short periods of REM sleep because a long stage of deep sleep would reduce their ability to awaken and escape capture by a predator.

The basic phylogenetic relationship is that sleep occurs in higher species only. For example, electroencephalographical signs of sleep (SW and REM) are found in birds but are absent in amphibians. Among mammalian species, even the most primitive exhibit signs of sleep.

Among animals that are able to sleep, young animals sleep more than older ones of the same species. Most of the sleep time of neonates is spent in REM sleep, which gradually decreases with maturation. For example, an 8-day-old lamb may spend about half the time sleeping, about 15 percent as REM sleep (i.e., about three times more than in adult sheep). The high proportion of REM sleep in the young probably begins in utero. About 30 days before parturition, fetal calves spend almost half of their total sleep time in REM sleep, and nonsleeping electroencephalographical signs are present only about 15 percent of the time.

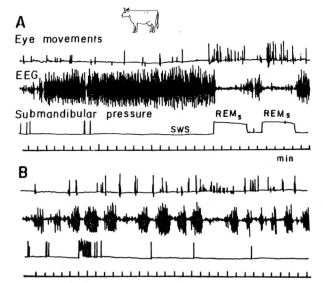

Figure 32–17 Fractioning of SWS concomitant with reduction of REM sleep toward the end of an 8-week period of nonrecumbency, which prevents REM sleep or causes REM sleep deprivation. **A,** Normal SWS followed by two REM sleep episodes. **B,** Fractioning of an SWS period by desynchronized EEG phases accompanied by action potential shifts due to eye movements. The loss of muscle tone during REM sleep is recorded as a consistent increase in submandibular pressure, which is caused by prolonged contact of the head with the floor.

The horse, the cow, and the sheep seem to sleep mostly at night, whereas the pig also sleeps a lot during the day. All these species have polyphasic REM sleep and SWS; the pig shows more episodes. The horse has the least amount of drowsiness but spends the greatest percentage of its sleep time in REM sleep.

Related States of Hypnosis, Hibernation, and Anesthesia

Hypnosis

Reflex immobility (hypnosis) is a unique state of profound immobility and relative unresponsiveness that can be triggered by several types of stimulation. The state of hypnosis is reversible; it terminates either spontaneously or upon visual, auditory, or tactile stimulation. Although the condition is usually called "animal hypnosis," the designation is somewhat anthropomorphic. The term "immobility reflex" better describes the state in terms of its physiology.

The most conspicuous feature is immobility that is probably reflexive, because it is a specific, stereotyped, involuntary, and unconditioned response to specific stimuli. The immobilization method for rabbits requires that all movements be restricted for a few seconds. Rabbits can be placed on their back while the limbs are held immobile; then careful removal of the hands is required so that sensory input does not disrupt the trance.

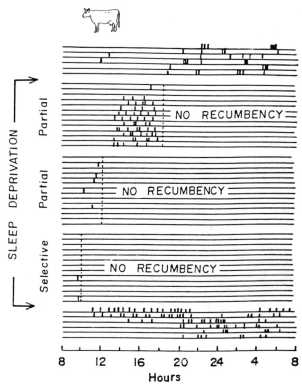

Figure 32–18 In a cow, distribution of SWS episodes 6 days before and 6 days after an 8-week period of partial REM sleep deprivation caused by nonrecumbency. Recumbency is prevented for 14, 20, or 22 hours per day, and access to food and REM sleep are permitted during, respectively, 10, 4, or 2 hours. REM sleep episodes are indicated by columns. Shift of REM sleep has a latency of nearly 1 week before it returns to about a normal level. After selective sleep deprivation, recovery takes 5 days.

Hibernation

Hibernating animals become temporary poikilotherms, with their body temperature close to that of the environment in cold weather. Unlike genuine poikilotherms, hibernating animals recover their ability to regulate high body temperatures during favorable environmental conditions and periods of activity. During periods of

TABLE 32–2 Cumulative Daily Sleep and Wakefulness in Some Animal Species over 24 Hours

Species	Alert Wakefulness (%)	Drowsiness and SWS (%)	REMs (%)
Cat	44.9	41.7	13.4
Cow	52.3	44.5	3.1
Fox	38.9	51.1	10
Guinea pig	71.6	24.5	3.9
Horse	80	16.7	3.3
Pig	46.3	46.4	7.3
Rabbit	71.3	25.5	3.1
Rat	48	45	7
Sheep	66.5	31.1	2.4

hibernation, the characteristic physiological changes include marked depression of metabolism, of heart and respiratory rates, of blood pressure, and of brain electrical activity.

> Before entering into their lethargy, animals stockpile important lipid reserves (brown fat), which are used slowly during the hibernation period. Hibernating animals of small size (marmot, hamster) that cannot accumulate important reserves awaken to feed during the winter.
>
> Pseudohibernating animals, such as the bear, can sleep during most of the winter but can be awakened rapidly, as they do not fall into profound torpor. In addition, their internal temperature is only slightly depressed.

Anesthesia

The most commonly used anesthetic agents are barbiturates (by injection) and halothane (by inhalation). These substances cross the blood-brain barrier effectively because of their marked liposolubility and lipophilia and the large amount of lipoprotein in the brain. The extensive blood supply to the brain, as opposed to the relatively poor blood supply of fat depots, permits sufficient drug to be carried to the brain for anesthesia.

Administration of thiobarbiturate in the alert sheep (20 mg per kg over a 30-second period) changes the EEG from LVFF into HVSF within 60 to 120 seconds after the injection is started. Spectral analysis reveals an EEG of slow waves with persisting synchronization of the LVFF (about 27 Hz) until awakening (i.e., about 36 minutes after injection of the thiobarbiturate) (Fig. 32–19).

The disposition kinetics of the barbiturate indicates that the drug has an apparent volume distribution of 1 L per kg, a body clearance of 3.5 mL per minute, and a half-life of 196 minutes. At the time of awakening (36 minutes), 25 percent of the administered dose is located in the central compartment, 13 percent is found in the shallow peripheral compartment (muscle), 37 percent remains in the deep peripheral compartment, and 25 percent has been eliminated. Using simulated curves, it appears that suppression of the shallow compartment (muscle) does not change the time of awakening. In contrast, when the elimination rate constant is decreased, awakening is delayed. The relatively short

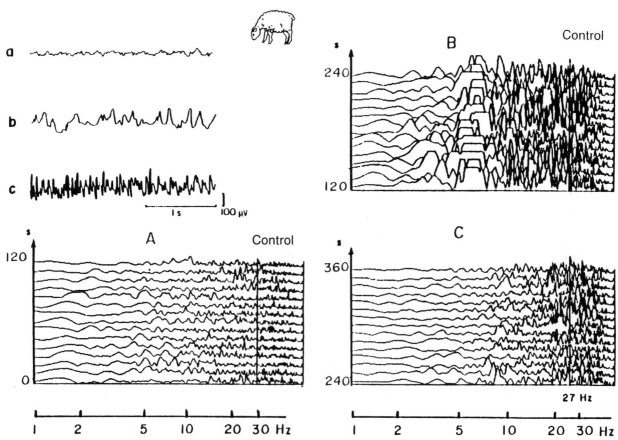

Figure 32–19 Electrocorticogram (ECoG) pattern in sleep. **A,** Desynchronized LVFF (20 μV, higher than 13 Hz) of alert wakefulness. **B,** More or less high-voltage isolated spike bursts, and more or less prolonged interval of isoelectric activity. **C,** Slow waves (i.e., synchronized HVSF [150 to 200 μV, 2 to 4 Hz]) due to thiobarbital anesthesia (20 mg per kg). The corresponding spectral analyses of the EEG recording (duration of each horizontal line is 8 seconds) show the first stage of thiobarbital anesthesia. Logarithmic scale for the x-axis, with a vertical line at 27 Hz; y-axis in millivolts squared per octave.

duration of thiopentobarbital anesthesia in sheep (36 minutes) is probably due to elimination of the drug by hepatic metabolism and uptake by body fat. This hypothesis differs from the widely accepted view that the duration of barbiturate anesthesia is independent of the rate of hepatic metabolism.

In the early 16th century, opium and alcohol were used in attempts to lessen the pain of surgery. In 1824, HICKMAN (England) gave carbon dioxide to animals to produce general anesthesia before surgery. From 1843 to 1844, COLTON, WELLS, MORTON, and RIGGS (USA) tried dental extractions after inhalation of nitrous oxide. In 1846, MORTON (USA) used ether vapor (handkerchief soaked in ether) for dental extractions. In 1884, KOLLER (Germany) initiated local anesthesia with cocaine, in searching for a pain-killing drug to put into the eye before surgery.

Episodic sleep, or narcolepsy, is characterized by excessive drowsiness in humans. However, in dogs, the principal clinical sign is cataplexy (immobility and rigidity)—sudden paroxysmal attacks of flaccid paralysis that may last from a few seconds to several minutes. Attacks may be induced also by excitement. Respiration and cardiac function are not affected. The frequency of attacks may vary from one every other day to several hundred per day.

SOCIAL DOMINANCE

Social dominance is defined as "priority of access to an approach or priority away from an avoidance situation." Hypervigilance (i.e., hyperactivity of the CNS seen only in the search for food) is related to three major functions of this social status: leadership, reduction of aggression, and sexual priority.

Both fowl and pigs, which are raised under extremely intensive management conditions, have been observed under these artificial conditions. The progressive development of aggression and of problems in social behavior related to crowding, changes in group membership, and social isolation can be easily studied in these species.

Fowl

Aggressive behavior between any two domestic fowls is usually *unidirectional,* as one bird can repeatedly peck the other without provoking reprisal. This relationship can be maintained by threat and submission rituals, which do not require direct physical attack.

A perfect *linear hierarchy* of dominance relationships is common in smaller flocks. Social status declines uniformly from the alpha bird (which can peck all others in the groups) to the omega bird (which is submissive to all its flockmates). However, *triangular hierarchy* can sometimes occur (e.g., A pecks B, B pecks C, and C pecks A). Triangular relationships exist more often in larger flocks.

Consistent social relationship between *chicks* occurs within 24 hours of hatching, and early interindividual pecks

are exploratory rather than aggressive. Aggressive behaviors resembling those of mature birds are not observed until hierarchies form at about 6 weeks. If birds are still in *heterosexual flocks* at 10 to 15 weeks, *two unisexual peck orders* appear to develop with relatively little intersex aggression (Fig. 32–20).

Certain *postures* (semi-crouch, crouch, and deep crouch) seen during first encounters are associated with *dominance.* Others (tail low and sex crouch) are associated with *defeat.* These postural signals significantly reinforce an established peck order and the learned social rank.

The peck order in domestic fowl is maintained by four major processes: individual recognition, communication (i.e., posture, but probably also vocalization), learning, and the available innate releasing mechanisms for the species. All four must interact if a stable hierarchy is to exist.

Pigs

Relationships are often *bidirectional* rather than absolute, and groups of as many as 18 pigs frequently show linear orders, triangular, and even equal status relationships. In pigs, the three major components of the development of dominance are intraspecific aggression, submission signals, and acceptance of submission.

As in other species, unfamiliar animals first meet and then fight to provide a winner and a loser. The subordinate pig moves away with its mouth open, head held high, and squealing loudly. After repeated interactions, the loser habituates or learns the outcome of aggressive encounters with more dominant pigs. From this experience, the loser retreats at the threat of a dominant animal (in pigs, threats consist of a brief glance and grunt by the dominant animal).

Subordinate pigs are less active, to avoid attracting attention and attack by a dominant pig. Social rank appears to have a measurable effect on general activity and feeding behavior: in an 8-week-old pig, 17 percent of the body weight is attributable to social dominance.

Cattle

As with domestic fowl, the established dominance-submission relationship in cattle seems to persist for some time. In a herd varying from 26 to 44 animals, yearly comparisons of all possible pair combinations over 8 years indicated that the relationships were stable, with a maximum reversal of ranking of about 15 percent.

Seniority is a pertinent concept insofar as it relates to social rank. High-ranking older cows gain "seniority" over other animals solely because of time spent in the herd. The threat-submission encounter ends when the loser lowers its head and turns away. Fighting may occur if threat does not produce a submissive response (Fig. 32–21).

Gonadal secretions are important in the control of agonistic behavior. The expression of agonistic behavior is sexually dimorphic, with males being generally more aggressive than females, presumably because of the testicular an-

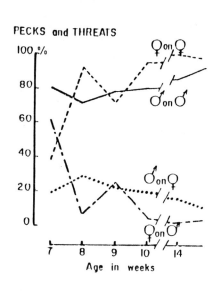

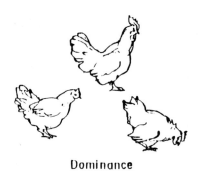

Dominance

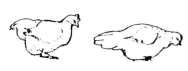

Subordinance

Submissiveness

A   B

Figure 32–20 A, The gradual development of unisexual pecking is shown by the percentage of unisexual and heterosexual pecking that occurs during the establishment and the maturation of peck orders. **B,** The postures associated with dominance, subordinance, and submissiveness.

drogens. However, the effects of castration and of androgen therapy may differ according to time of treatment and sex.

Comparisons of social behavior of bulls and of steers castrated at either 3 or 12 months of age indicate that bulls are not more aggressive than these steers, either to other bulls or toward steers. The steers castrated at 3 months behave as females do, establish dominance relationships quickly, tend to be more aggressive than bulls or steers castrated at 12 months, and show the highest frequency of spontaneous withdrawals. Steers castrated at 12 months show behaviors intermediate between that of bulls and that of steers castrated at 3 months and tend to behave more like bulls than like females.

Sheep and Goat

Sexual priority is important in dominant rams, as pregnancies in a flock of 100 ewes decrease by 26 percent when the dominant ram in a team of three is rendered infertile without affecting its libido (vasectomy). Vasectomy in subordinate rams does not affect the rate of pregnancies. Some females mate exclusively with dominant rams during the period of estrus, which is the optimal time for conception.

During grazing, both sheep and goats show limited territorial and aggressive responses. In goats, unlike in sheep, social dominance seems to affect weight gain and mohair production.

Horses

Dominance in domestic horses is marked by two interesting observations. In contrast with several other animal species (e.g., cattle), seniority in the herd has little effect on social rank. Within dominance hierarchy, well-defined attachments exist and may be related to mutual grooming, which is often initiated by subordinate horses.

CHRONOBIOLOGY

Chronobiology refers to the cyclical view of time held by the ancient Greeks. In its modern acceptation, chronobiology is a science, still in its infancy, that looks for biological patterns or rhythms that repeat themselves cyclically. In other words, it is the study of oscillations in physiological phenomena as a function of time. It has a language of its own to describe the characteristics of a rhythmical function (Fig. 32–22).

In ancient times, observed movements of parts of plants during the day were attributed to movement of the sun, the moon, and the earth. In a similar way, animal behaviors, such as daily activity patterns and migrations, have been tied to astronomic events. Scientists have slowly and gradually accepted that the environment impinges on the functions of organisms, and that biological rhythms represent adapta-

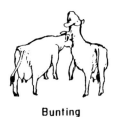

Bunting

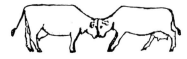

Contact

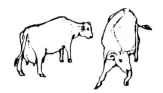

Forceful

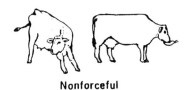

Nonforceful

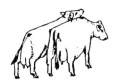

Pushing

Figure 32–21 Postures of cows during encounters. *Bunting,* when a cow uses her head to attack or to displace physically another cow. *Contact,* head-to-head combat with no clear-cut loser or winner. *Forceful,* with a threatening swing of the head in the direction of the subordinate animal, which responds with a submission or avoidance behavior. *Nonforceful,* when a cow purposefully avoids another cow. *Pushing,* A dominant cow physically displacing another cow with some part of the body other than the head.

tions to cyclical events in the physical environment. Findings have supported the conclusion that some biological rhythms are endogenously generated and are not linked to external stimuli.

> Although Greek philosophers of the classical era proposed a central role for the sun, this view was displaced by geocentric speculations. Even Copernicus's "proof" of a heliocentric universe was rejected by many scholars of his day.

The 20th century scholar TCHIJEVSKY emphasized the importance of cosmobiology and of the sensitivity of the biosphere to solar activity.

In the 17th century, the Italian SANCTORIUS weighed himself at every meal for 30 years and established that his weight followed a monthly cycle. A French astronomer observed that leaf movements of plants persisted in complete darkness and occurred at intervals of less than 24 hours. In a cave entirely free of solar and other radiations, humans also continue to exhibit rhythms, which tend to be longer than 24 hours.

The introduction of the clinical thermometer in the 18th century has allowed the repeated measurements needed to establish that the rhythm of the core temperature in humans and other animal species is about 24 hours. Body temperature and sleep-wakefulness rhythms of mammals are examples of conditioned reflexes impressed from without and persisting from within.

Continuous measurement with data recording and computer-assisted processing is necessary today so that statistical evaluation of differences can be made efficiently. Variations can be standardized to define normal basal rhythms and to allow detection of abnormal patterns.

Types of Rhythms

Rhythmical patterns are frequently observed with periods ranging from fractions of a second to very long intervals extending to years. Depending on their periods (i.e., the duration of one complete rhythmical cycle), three classes of domains or types of rhythms have been defined (Table 32–3). These rhythms all continue even when the organism is isolated from normal cyclical environmental cues.

Ultradian Rhythms. With these rhythms, the period (i.e., duration of one complete cycle) is less than 20 hours, ranging from fractions of a second through several hours. The classic example is the heartbeat. Another example is the migrating myoelectrical complexes that recur at regular intervals in the intestinal wall of ruminant animals (90 minutes in sheep). A *circhoral rhythm* recurs at about hourly intervals.

Circadian Rhythms. A biorhythm is considered circadian when it occurs over an arbitrary range from one cycle per 20 hours to one per 28 hours (i.e., about a day in length). An example in chickens is the dramatic fall in basal metabolic rate that occurs during the hours of darkness (Fig. 32–23). The vertebral canal and body temperatures of pigeons also show fluctuations of the circadian type. A mix of sleep mechanisms and circadian rhythm control systems is responsible for these fluctuations, with heat production being lowest when birds are asleep in the dark. In mice, the number of leukocytes rises and falls with the circadian rhythm, which is abolished by adrenalectomy.

Infradian Rhythms. These are longer (28 hours) than the circadian. They may range from one cycle per week

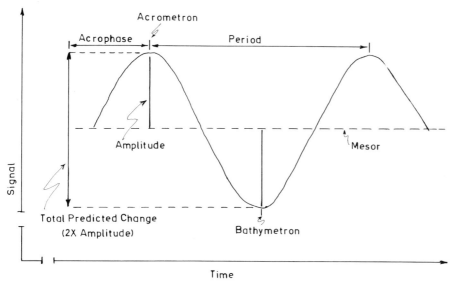

Figure 32–22 In chronobiology, the characteristics of rhythms observed in chemical reactions, cells, organs, organisms, groups, or herds. Terms such as mesor, period, amplitude, acrophase, acrometron, and bathymetron are used to describe the parameters of a rhythmic function. The diagram of an oscillation, which is like a snapshot of a roller coaster, illustrates these basic chronobiological terms. *Mesor* denotes the midline that estimates the statistic of rhythm (i.e., the average value), which is not necessarily the arithmetical mean. *Period* means the duration of one complete rhythmical cycle, measured from peak to peak. *Amplitude* signifies half the total predictable change in a rhythm. *Acrophase* is the lag between the reference time (e.g., 0000 hours or midnight in a 24-hour day) and the time of the rhythm's crest. *Acrometron* denotes the measure of the highest predicted value of a rhythm. *Bathymetron* refers to the lowest measure.

to one cycle per year or season. An example of an infradian rhythm is the estrous cycle, which recurs every 20.5 days in nonpregnant dairy cows, with a range from 18 to 24 days.

A *circaseptan rhythm* occurs once per week. In humans, a cycle of about 7 days (circaseptan rhythm) governs the endocrine metabolites. Rhythms that approximate a month in duration (i.e., that recur monthly) are referred to as *circatrigintan, circamensan,* or *circalunar* rhythms. Yearly or seasonal rhythms are termed *circannual rhythms.*

Circannual (about yearly) rhythms have been shown also to have an endogenous component. In catfish, a rhythm of about a year occurs in the ovarian weight. The Jamuna catfish of India exhibits massive ovarian enlargement (16-fold) during the monsoon season even when it is kept in complete darkness.

TABLE 32–3 Types and Periods of Rhythms

Types of Rhythms	Periods*
ULTRADIAN	Less than 20 hr
Circhoral	About 1 hr
CIRCADIAN	More than 20 hr, but less than 28 hr
INFRADIAN	More than 28 hr
Circaseptan	About 7 days
Circasemilunar	About 15 days
Circalunar	About 30 days
Circasemiannual	About 6 months
Circannual	About 12 months

*Duration of one complete cycle.

Two rhythms can interact to either form a third, when their peaks coincide, or to cancel each other, when their peaks are out of phase. A model is seen in marine animals, which gear their activity, feeding, and reproduction to two different environmental rhythms: the rise and fall of the tides, and the rising and setting of the sun. Both rhythms are related to the earth's turning on its axis, exposing its face to the sun and to the moon during each daily rotation. Twice each lunar month (i.e., every 15 days) at the full moon and the new moon, the sun's gravitational pull is added to the moon's to cause larger tides; this creates a third rhythm.

An example of two rhythms interacting to produce a third one is seen in the New England fiddler crab, which shows rhythmic darkening as protection against sunlight and predators. It darkens during the day and turns lighter at night (i.e., shows a *circadian rhythm*). Also, it turns darker during the day at low tide, which lags by 50 minutes each day, that is, shows a *ultradian rhythm* coincident with the tidal cycle recurring at intervals of 12.4 hours, or twice a day. Together, the two rhythms interact to form a third, 15-day cycle (*infradian rhythm,* or *circasemilunar rhythm*), in which the crab assumes its darkest color at the same hour as it did 15 days earlier.

The Master Timekeeper: The Suprachiasmatic Nucleus

The circadian rhythms are dictated by a master timekeeper. In studies to locate the site of this master pace-

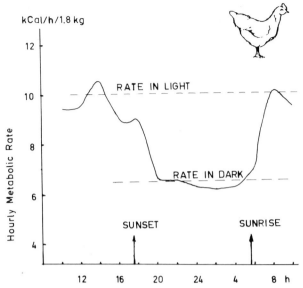

Figure 32–23 Effect of light-dark cycle on metabolic rate in chickens. The hourly metabolic rate decreases by about 35 percent during the period of darkness.

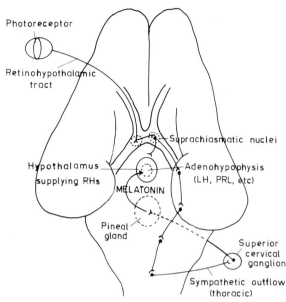

Figure 32–24 Photoneuroendocrine pathway governing biorhythms sensitive to day length in mammals. From the retina, optic impulses transit to the suprachiasmatic nucleus, then to the hypothalamic hormone–releasing neurons and the adenohypophysis. From the suprachiasmatic nucleus, nerve impulses pass to the brain stem and spinal cord to reach the sympathetic nervous system and return to the pineal gland. (LH, Luteinizing hormone, PRL, prolactin.)

maker, rats kept in a treadmill showed a typical running pattern of 12 hours on and 12 hours off. These experiments first indicated that the timekeeper for this marathon behavior resides in the anterior hypothalamus, above the optic chiasma. More than a decade later, the site of the timekeeper has been pinpointed to the tiny bilateral *suprachiasmatic nucleus* (SCN) of the anterior hypothalamus.

The SCN rhythmically produces vasopressin (also known as antidiuretic hormone [ADH]) and vasoactive intestinal peptide (VIP). In the retina, via the optic nerves, specialized cells feed information about day-length cycles to the SCN. Outflow from the SCN descends via the brain stem and spinal cord to the thoracolumbar sympathetic nerves. Preganglionic fibers then run to the superior cervical ganglion (SSG) neurons, which emit postganglionic fibers that reenter the brain and supply the pineal gland (Fig. 32–24). Humoral products of the pineal produced during darkness (e.g., melatonin) then pass to that part of the hypothalamus producing the various releasing hormones (RHs), which drive the adenohypophysis. The effect of RHs is to modulate the production of hormones (e.g., corticotropin, gonadotropins, growth hormone, prolactin, and thyrotropin) that govern breeding cycles and seasonal behaviors. Melatonin also produces drowsiness, and its use has been suggested to reset the "body clocks" after crossing several time zones to offset the jet-lag associated with long distance air travel.

Lighting Cycles

The intensity of solar radiation and the angle at which it reaches different regions of the earth's surface vary with the earth's elliptical orbit around the sun and with the rotation of the earth on its tilted axis. The results are day-night cycles of light and temperature, and seasonal cycles of day-length and temperature. In addition, socioecological external cycles exist in addition to these astronomic phenomena. By changing the pattern of the daily alternation of light and dark periods, a number of physiological rhythms can be modified. These can range from the circadian rhythm of DNA and RNA formation, with the resulting mitosis at the cellular level, through a number of endocrine rhythms, to rhythms in overall behavior such as activity and sleep.

The lighting cycle seems to be linked to the synchronizing of many physiological rhythms, which are then called *"entrained"* rhythms. The german term *Zeitgeber* is often used for this phenomenon, but *synchronizer* is preferable. If the rhythms persist in the absence of the synchronizer, they are called *free-running*, implying that they have an endogenous pacemaker component that assumes its own rhythm.

When circadian coupling to synchronizers is reduced experimentally, ultradian oscillations become more discernable. Examples include

1. destroying the SCN, so that this putative pacemaker no longer emits rhythmic stimuli;
2. eliminating circadian rhythmicity in plasma levels of hormones, which mediate facets of circadian systems;
3. isolating tissues in vitro, in media depriving them of the normal circadian influences to which they are subjected; and
4. placing animals in a constant environment, without circadian synchronizers.

Although circadian rhythms are a ubiquitous feature of biology, they are but one class within an intermodulating spectral distribution of multifrequency rhythms. On several ranges of intermodulating biological frequencies, different levels of rhythmic organization (cellular, endocrine, neural) have been recognized and quantified as "feed sidewards" to distinguish them from classic feedback along axes. The spectrum of biorhythms is considered to be integrative, with each component playing an important part as they interact and affect physiological responses in feed sidewards networks.

A great scope for studies of these processes exists in animals, with the potential for manipulation of the animal's regulatory systems for improved performance, health, and response to treatment. Fundamental molecular genetic studies with type species of *Drosophila* (fruit fly) and *Neurospora* (a mold) are leading to identification of the genes associated with some circadian and other biorhythms. Circaseptan (about 7 days) rhythms are observed in transplant rejection studies. Regardless of the date of the surgery, episodes of threatening rejection recur every 7 days postoperatively (about 7, 14, 21, 28 days and so on).

It is interesting that keeping animals under highly standardized environmental conditions does not completely remove the variations seen in nature. Even specific pathogen-free (SPF) rats that are kept continuously under a rigorously controlled physical environment in climate chambers (constant temperature, humidity, and duration of light period, with external sound-proofing in a Faraday cage to screen out electromagnetic phenomena) manifest significant variations in mean values of many circadian physiological variables. Circadian patterns of enzyme activities are modified in both phase and amplitude during the seasons. These changes override sex and strain differences. Marked differences in environmental light-dark cycles are stressful, and the longevity of mice subjected to 180-degree weekly inversion of this cycle is reduced by 6 percent.

Basic Rest-Activity Cycle

Dreaming is associated with the REM stages of sleep. REM sleep is correlated with cyclical physiological changes, such as loss of muscle tone, rapid eye movement, and characteristic changes in electroencephalographical (EEG) wave amplitude and frequency.

The concept of basic rest-activity cycle (BRAC) initially presupposed a basic cycle length of about 90 minutes. By correlating BRAC to the cyclical gastric contractions in human neonates, the basal BRAC is only of 50 to 60 minutes. However, the actual periodicity of infant feedings is some integer multiplier of the basal value, usually 3 to 4 hours, that is linked to a sleep-wakefulness cycle.

The antral contractions of the stomach of adults occur regularly between feedings in monogastric species (90 to 120 minutes in humans). Known as the interdigestive housekeeper of the gut, they are related to the frequency of the migrating myoelectrical complexes of the intestine but are independent of the REM−non-REM sleep cycles. Several other recognized cyclical processes, such as episodic cortisol secretion pulses, do not appear to be related to the REM stage of sleep. Consequently, the idea of a widespread role for BRAC in physiology is challenged.

REFERENCES

Berman A, Meltzer A. Metabolic rate: its circadian rhythmicity in the female domestic fowl. J Physiol 1978;282:419.

Bouissou MF, Demurger C, Lavenet C. Social behavior of bulls and steers: effect of age at castration. In: Nichelmann M, ed. Ethology of domestic animals. Toulouse: Privat IEC, 1986.

De Lahunta A. Veterinary neuroanatomy and clinical neurology. 2nd ed. Philadelphia: WB Saunders Co, 1983.

Dement WC, Kleitman N. Cyclic variations in EEG during sleep and their relation to eye movements, body motility, and dreaming. Clin Neurophysiol 1957;2:673.

Follet BK. The environment and reproduction. In: Austin CR, Short RV, eds. Reproduction in mammals. 2nd ed. Book 4. Reproductive fitness. Cambridge: Cambridge University Press, 1985.

Halberg F. Circadian (about 24-hour) rhythms in experimental medicine. Proc Soc Med 1963;56:253.

Halberg F. Chronobiology. Annu Rev Physiol 1969;31:675.

Heller HC, Graf R, Rautenberg W. Circadian and arousal state influences on thermoregulation in pigeons. Am J Physiol 1983;245:R321.

Horlein BV. Canine neurology. Philadelphia: WB Saunders Co, 1971.

Jakinovich W, Sugarman D. Sugar taste reception in mammals. Chem Sci 1988;13:13.

Kleitman N. Sleep and wakefulness. Chigago: University of Chicago Press, 1963.

Kleitman N. Basic rest-activity cycle 22 years later. Sleep 1982;5:311.

Kripke DF. Ultradian rhythms in behavior and physiology. In: Brown FM, Graeber RC, eds. Rhythmic aspects of behavior. Hillsdale, NJ: Erlbaum Assoc., 1982.

Lincoln GA. The pineal gland. In: Austin CR, Short RV, eds. Reproduction in mammals. 2nd ed. Book 3. Reproduction. Cambridge: Cambridge University Press, 1984.

Meyers LJ, Redding RW, Wilson S. Abnormalities of the brain stem auditory response of the dog associated with equilibrium deficit and seizure. Vet Res Comm 1986;10:73.

Moore RY. The suprachiasmatic nucleus and mammalian circadian system. In: Hekkens WTJM, Kerkhof GA, Rietveld WJ. Trends in chronobiology. Adv Biosci 1988;73:97.

Moore-Ede M, Czeisler CA, Richardson GS. Circadian timekeeping in health and disease. I. Basic properties of circadian pacemakers. N Engl J Med 1983;309:469.

Richter CP. Biological clocks in medicine and psychiatry. Springfield: Charles C Thomas, 1965.

Sollberger A. Biological rhythm research. Amsterdam: Elsevier, 1965.

Syme GJ. Competitive orders as measures of social dominance. Anim Behav 1974;22:931.

CHAPTER 33

AUTONOMIC NERVOUS SYSTEM

All the efferent axons leaving the central nervous system (CNS) except those innervating skeletal muscles (motor neurons) belong to the autonomic nervous system (ANS). The axons of motorneurons run *without interruption* to the neuromuscular junctions in skeletal muscles, whereas the autonomic axons leaving the CNS make *synaptic connections* with peripheral neurons, which in turn innervate the effector cells of muscles or glands. The cells or soma of these peripheral autonomic neurons occur in clusters, form swellings (or ganglia) on nerve trunks, and are referred to as ganglion cells. The axons that form synapses with the ganglion cells are called *preganglionic* autonomic fibers, and the innervating effector cells are called *postganglionic* autonomic fibers.

The division of the autonomic nervous system into the *sympathetic* (or orthosympathetic) system and the *parasympathetic* system is based on the anatomical location of the neurons that give rise to the preganglionic autonomic axons. The cell bodies giving off the preganglionic axons of the sympathetic division of the ANS are found in the lateral horns of the *thoracic* and of the upper two or three *lumbar* segments of the spinal cord. The sympathetic ganglion cells are 12 to 60 μm in diameter, and their number is estimated at 150,000 to 200,000. The preganglionic axons of the parasympathetic division originate in cell bodies distributed in the brain stem (*cranial* outflow) and in the terminal segment (*sacral* outflow) of the spinal cord. The global distribution of the sympathetic and of the parasympathetic divisions in the horse is impressive (Fig. 33–1).

The phenomenon of chemical transmission at synapses of the nervous system was discovered in 1921 by LOEWI (Germany) who gave the name *Vagusstoff* (later found to be acetylcholine) to a substance released into the perfusion fluid upon vagal stimulation (electrical) of the isolated frog heart.

In 1905, ELLIOTT (USA) observed that injection of epinephrine produced effects similar to stimulation of the sympathetic nerves. CANNON and URIDIL (USA) described the release of *sympathin* by the spleen following stimulation of the sympathetic nerves.

In 1933, DALE and FELDBERG (England) categorized as cholinergic and adrenergic the synapses that released acetylcholine or epinephrine (adrenaline), respectively, as chemical mediators. In 1936, VON EULER (Germany) defined the adrenergic neurotransmitter as norepinephrine (noradrenaline). In 1948, AHLQUIST (USA) identified the receptor sites in adrenergically innervated tissue as predominantly excitatory (α) or inhibitory (β).

THE SYMPATHETIC SYSTEM

In the sympathetic system, the preganglionic axons usually contact a large number of ganglionic neurons located not too far from the preganglionic cells of origin (Fig. 33–2).

The chain arrangement of ganglia permits an entering preganglionic axon to contact a large number of neurons in a given ganglion and a large number of neurons in other ganglia through its ascending or descending paths in the chain. The result is marked divergence of sympathetic motor impulses, with a possibility of generalized effects.

General stimulation of the sympathetic division of the ANS produces responses that prepare the body for emergency while suppressing irrelevant activities. This is described as a *fear-fright-flight syndrome*. Typically, the pupils are dilated, hair is erected, blood sugar level is raised, heart rate is accelerated, and blood flow through muscle is increased, whereas blood is diverted from the gastrointestinal tract and the kidneys.

The same syndrome can be produced by electrical stimulation of the posterior regions of the *hypothalamus*. Removal of the forebrain from animals produces bouts of aggressive behavior known as *sham rage* together with the signs of generalized sympathetic discharge. The appearance of these signs in decorticate animals suggests that higher centers have an *inhibitory influence* over the hypothalamic sympathetic centers.

Sympathetic stimulation produces the following effects on the skin: constriction of cutaneous vessels, dilation of skeletal muscle vessels, contraction of pilomotor muscles and elevation of hair, and secretion of sweat glands. In cattle, alpha receptors are involved, with epinephrine as the principal mediator, to produce inhibition of smooth muscle of the stomach, of the pyloric sphincter, of the small intestine, and of the bladder wall.

THE PARASYMPATHETIC SYSTEM

The efferents of the parasympathetic system are long preganglionic fibers that serve a few ganglionic neurons in the walls of specific organs (Fig. 33–3). The degree of divergence in the parasympathetic system is limited by the diffuse arrangement of the postganglionic neurons and the degree to which a given postganglionic axon can arborize at its effector terminal. Such limited distribution is compatible with the discrete action attributed to the parasympathetic system; however, the parasympathetic system plays an important role in coordinating the specific functional activities of the digestive tract.

Parasympathetic stimulation produces contraction of the smooth muscle of the walls of the gastrointestinal tract, including the rumen and gallbladder. In carnivores (cats, dogs), the parasympathetic activity causes stimulation of the smooth muscle of the sphincters of the gastrointestinal tract (e.g., the pylorus). In contrast, in ruminants both the py-

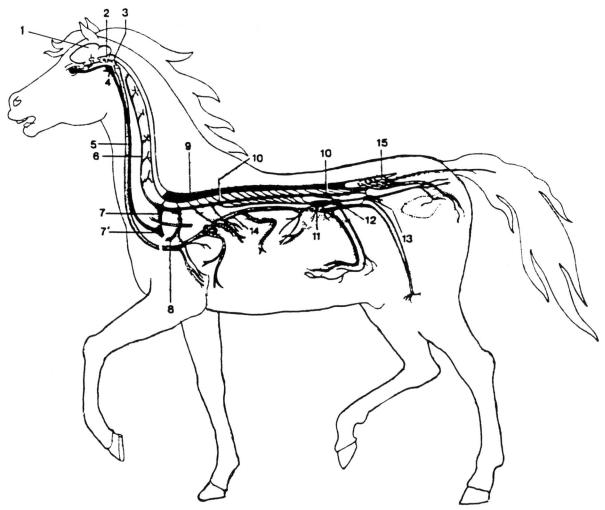

Figure 33–1   General distribution of the sympathetic (——) and parasympathetic (- - -) nervous systems: *1*, parasympathetic oculomotor nucleus; *2*, salivatory nuclei; *3*, dorsal vagal nucleus; *4*, cranial cervical ganglion; *5*, vagosympathetic trunk; *6*, vertebral nerve; *7*, cervicothoracic ganglion; *7'*, middle cervical ganglion; *8*, ansa subclavia; *9*, sacral outflow from spinal cord; *10*, sacral trunk with paravertebral ganglia; *11*, celiac ganglion; *12*, cranial mesenteric ganglion; *13*, caudal mesenteric ganglion; *14*, vagus nerve with distribution to thoracic and abdominal organs; *15*, sacral outflow of parasympathetic nervous system.

loric and the reticuloomasal sphincters are inhibited by parasympathetic activation.

AUTONOMIC REFLEXES

The autonomic reflex arc consists, likes its somatic counterpart, of an afferent (sensory) part and an efferent (motor) part. Visceral sensory fibers entering the dorsal horn send branches rostrad in the spinal sensory columns and make synaptic connections to nearby interneurons. The interneurons transmit impulses to the preganglionic neurons in the cord or the brain stem. Preganglionic axons make up the efferent part and carry the visceral motor stimuli to ganglion cells, from which postganglionic axons innervate visceral effectors.

Some important autonomic reflexes are the peristaltic reflex, the micturition reflex, and the reflexes involving interoceptive receptors.

Peristaltic Reflex

The peristaltic reflex is unusual in that it may be observed in segments of intestine that are completely isolated from the body and so are not under the control of the extrinsic nervous system. In the peristaltic reflex, stretching the walls of the gut stimulates intramural sensory neurons. The axons of these neurons form synapses either directly or through a local interneuron, with postganglionic parasympathetic neurons. In the intact animal, this extraspinal reflex arc is influenced by centers in the brain stem. They exert control through preganglionic vagal, pelvic, and post-

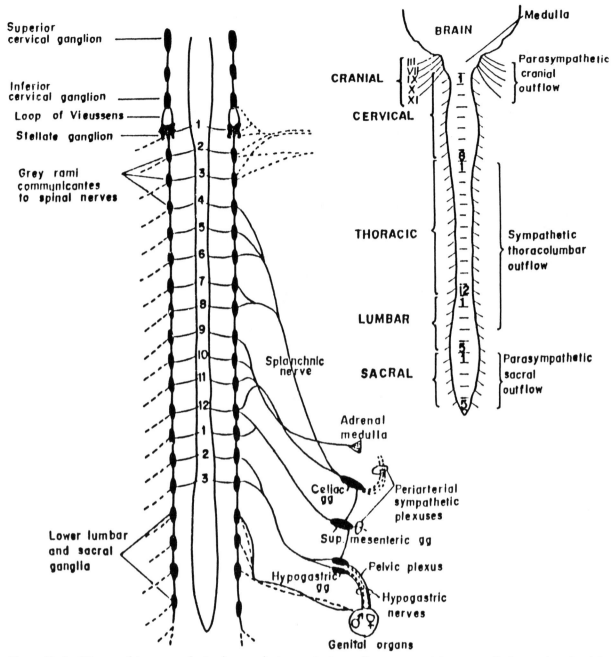

Figure 33-2 Diagram of the paravertebral and prevertebral sympathetic ganglia; nerves containing preganglionic axons (——) and those with postganglionic axons (- - -). The postganglionic outflow from the sympathetic chains in the gray rami communicantes is shown on the left side only. The outflow of other postganglionic axons and of the preganglionic axons traveling to the prevertebral ganglia is shown on the right side only. The insert shows the sympathetic (thoracolumbar) and the parasympathetic (cranial and sacral) divisions.

ganglionic sympathetic axons that terminate also on the peripheral parasympathetic ganglion cells.

Reflex of Micturition

The reflex of micturition, and those of defecation and ejaculation, are under the control of higher centers, but these reflexes persist after transection of the spinal cord. The denervated bladder and spinal cord reflex of the bladder have sensory or motor differences (Fig. 33-4).

Micturition is a complex reflex involving stretch receptors in the bladder wall, primary axons of cell bodies located in the sacral spinal ganglia (general visceral afferent, general proprioception), and the dorsal gray column of the sacral segments of the spinal cord. The afferent axons, carrying the

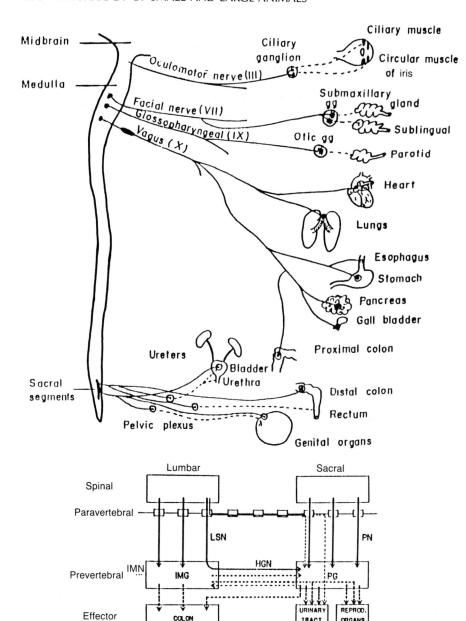

Figure 33–3 Parasympathetic outflow in *cranial* nerves and in the *sacral segments* of the spinal cord shows the pathways of postganglionic neurons to the main effector tissues. Preganglionic axons (———), postganglionic axons (- - -). The diagram indicates only the nerves emerging from the right side of the CNS. **Below,** Arrangement of efferent extrinsic innervation of distal part of the bowel. *LSN,* Lumbar splanchnic nerve; *HGN,* hypogastric nerve; *PN,* pelvic nerve; *IMN,* intermesenteric nerve; *IMG,* inferior mesenteric ganglion; *PG,* pelvic ganglion.

impulses generated by stretching of the bladder, travel to the spinal cord in the pelvic nerves and may either terminate on different types of sacral interneurons or continue rostrad toward the higher centers.

Some sacral interneurons complete the reflex arc by synapsing with preganglionic parasympathetic neurons, which causes the smooth muscle of the bladder to contract. Other interneurons course craniad to the L4 to L1 spinal cord segments to synapse on other interneurons that activate the beta-adrenergic preganglionic sympathetic neurons. In turn, through their postganglionic axons, these sympathetic neurons inhibit the smooth muscle, allowing the bladder to stretch and to contain more urine. Still other sacral interneurons course rostrad in the spinal cord, primarily within

the spinothalamic system. Some of the primary afferent neurons are carried also into the fasciculus gracilis to the medulla, where they synapse in the nucleus gracilis. Both of these pathways (spinothalamic, fasciculus gracilis) relay through the thalamus to reach the somesthetic cortex and give conscious perception of bladder sensation.

Cell bodies of postganglionic parasympathetic axons are located in the pelvic plexus, or more commonly in the bladder wall. Stimulation of these neurons results in contraction of the detrusor muscle, relaxation of the striated sphincter of the bladder, and evacuation of urine via the urethra.

In the bladder neck and in the proximal urethra, sympathetic postganglionic axons terminate on alpha receptors, which facilitate contraction and increase the tone of smooth

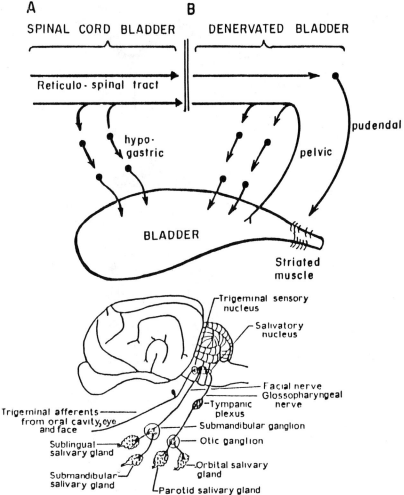

Figure 33–4 Examples of autonomic reflexes. **Top,** The *micturition* reflex requires facilitation of the sacral parasympathetic neurons and inhibition of the sacral somatic neurons to the striated urethral muscle and of the lumbar sympathetic neurons to the urethral musculature. A thoracic lesion results in *spinal cord bladder,* with loss of bladder sensation, distention, and need for frequent voiding anywhere. A lumbosacral lesion causes a *denervated bladder,* with loss of bladder sensation, distention, and incontinence. Small and brief contractions of the bladder muscle occur via intramural reflex activity, but bladder emptying is incomplete. **Bottom,** Salivary reflexes are due to stimulation of the oral or lingual mucosa by foreign substances or by drying. The afferent limb is the trigeminal, facial, glossopharyngeal, or vagal nerve. The internuncial neurons of the reflex arc are located within the reticular formation of the brain stem, and the efferent limb involves neurons of the rostral and caudal salivatory nuclei, which project fibers into the facial nerve (to the lingual and mandibular glands) and the glossopharyngeal nerve (to the parotid gland). The type of saliva produced is related to the type of stimulus applied.

muscle. On the body of the bladder, some sympathetic postganglionic axons end on smooth muscle with beta receptors, which inhibit the motor response of smooth muscle. Their activity permits the bladder wall to expand further to accommodate a greater volume of urine.

Voluntary micturition is mediated from the caudal brain stem by tectospinal and reticulospinal components. These are facilitatory to sacral parasympathetic preganglionic neurons and inhibitory to sacral somatic efferent neurons to the urethral muscle and to the lumbar sympathetic preganglionic neurons.

Interoceptive Receptors

Receptors sensitive to *changes in pressure* (or tension in the walls) occur in specialized regions of the vascular system and cause cardiovascular reflexes. Other receptors respond to internal pressure or wall tension. Normally, they are linked to reflexes concerned with local autonomic control. Unusually high tensions or pressures give rise to pain, often described as "colic" (e.g., biliary colic). The cause may be a

mechanical obstruction opposing the work of the smooth muscle, or it may be a powerful contraction (*spasm*) of the smooth muscle. Contractions of uterine smooth muscle elicit labor pain. Local spasms of smooth muscles are sometimes relieved by sectioning their autonomic and sensory supply or by destroying the nerve with an injection of alcohol or phenol. Such treatment is used particularly for chronic spasms of blood vessels, which result in an insufficient blood flow to the extremities.

Certain *interoceptive chemoreceptors* respond selectively to specific stimuli and ensure specific regulatory function (e.g., oxygen receptors linked to respiratory control). In addition, some diffusely distributed chemoreceptors respond to a wide range of stimuli (e.g., metabolic products such as carbon dioxide), and excessive stimulation of them produces pain (e.g., angina).

Light reflexes and trigeminofacial reflexes are important in the organism's relation with the environment (Fig. 33–5). When a light shines on the retina of either eye, both pupils constrict to reduce the amount of light passing through the pupil. This is known as the *pupillary light reflex.* The afferent limb of the pupillary light reflex is the retina (receptor organ)

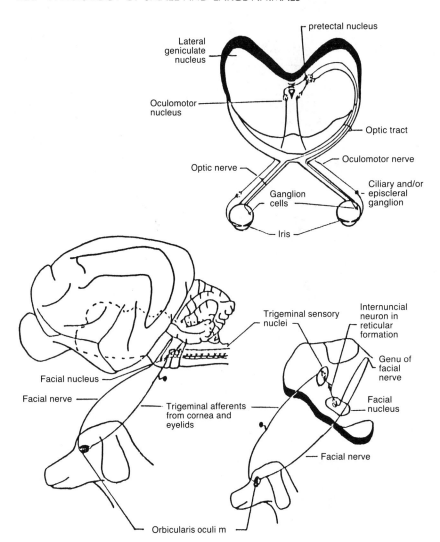

Figure 33-5 Central nervous system pathways involved in light reflexes (**top**) and trigeminofacial reflexes (**bottom**).

with the optic nerves and tracts. The nerve fibers of the optic tracts terminate within the pretectal nucleus. The internuncial neurons of the pretectal nucleus project to the rostral portion of the oculomotor nuclei and initiate excitatory synaptic activity on the neurons of these nuclei. This, in turn, initiates action potentials within the circular smooth muscles of the iris, causing them to contract, and the pupils to constrict. The constriction of the pupil of the eye receiving the stimulus is referred to as the pupillary light reflex, whereas the constriction of the pupil of the opposite eye is referred to as a *consensual light reflex*. The reflex arc does not depend on the integrity of other nuclear structures of the visual pathway, such as the lateral geniculate bodies and the cerebral cortex. The response of the pupil to light is not influenced by control from higher centers.

If the cornea receives a tactile stimulus, a blink is elicited (*corneal blink reflex*), and lacrimation is increased (*lacrimation reflex*). These reflexes protect the cornea from injury by foreign material. The afferent limb of both the blink and the lacrimation reflexes is the ophthalmic division of the trigeminal nerve. Internuncial neurons are involved in both reflex arcs. The cell bodies of these neurons are located within the reticular formation of the brain stem. The efferent neurons for the blink reflex are the alpha motor neurons of the facial nucleus.

AUTONOMIC CENTERS

The gray matter of the brain stem (medulla, pons, midbrain, thalamus, and hypothalamus) is distributed into groups of nuclei separated by fiber systems and by the brain stem reticular formation (BSRF). Extending rostrad from the upper end of the spinal cord into the thalamus and the hypothalamus, the BSRF is made up of a network of nerve fibers projecting in all directions and of neurons scattered throughout this network.

The visceral motor column contains neurons analogous to those of the intermediolateral cell column of the spinal cord and of the parasympathetic nucleus of the sacral spinal cord. The nuclei involved in this visceromotor column are distinct from the rostral and caudal *salivary nuclei,* which are parts of the reticular formation. Other distinctive nuclei of the column are the Edinger-Westphal nucleus (in the third ventricle, near the origin of the aqueduct of Sylvius), which supplies fibers to the intrinsic muscles of the eye, and the *dorsal motor nucleus of the vagus,* which innervates the cervical, the thoracic, and the abdominal regions.

A single structure within the medulla oblongata, the *nucleus of the fasciculus solitarius,* forms the visceral sensory column. This nucleus receives afferent fibers from the oral cavity (pharynx and larynx) and from the thoracic and abdominal viscera. The nerves are the vagus and visceral afferents, which relay information up the spinal cord. In contrast, the somatic sensory column of neurons corresponds to afferents from the trigeminal nerve, supplying the head and face with sensory innervation.

The ANS is sometimes referred to as the "vegetative," the "involuntary," or the "visceral" (as opposed to somatic) nervous system. These terms may be taken to be synonymous, at least as far as the peripheral parts are concerned; however, the word "autonomic" suggests a much greater degree of independence from the rest of the nervous system than in fact exists. Acceleration of heart rate and respiration slightly *precedes and accompanies* increased activity of the skeletal muscles (and thoughts or memories may be accompanied by autonomic responses such as flushing, pallor, and sweating). Functional links between the autonomic and somatic nervous systems have been demonstrated by experiments involving pavlovian conditioning and by the somatic projection of visceral points (e.g., acupuncture). The responses mediated by somatic motor neurons may be conditioned to appear after excitation of sensory receptors that are normally concerned with unconditioned autonomic reflexes. As the frontal areas of the cerebral cortex contain centers that control autonomic activity, it is probable that coordination of autonomic and voluntary activity is brought about by association fibers at the cortical level.

In addition, all the spinal and lower brain stem autonomic centers are controlled and coordinated by nuclei in the hypothalamus, which is the most important subcortical autonomic center. Stimulation of the *posterior* parts of the hypothalamus causes *sympathetic activity,* whereas stimulation of the *rostral or anterior* hypothalamus produces *parasympathetic activity.* This arrangement is found also at the spinal cord level, for erection and ejaculation, which are, respectively, parasympathetic and sympathetic activities. The hypothalamus also has connections with higher centers, especially the limbic system, and with the hypophysis. Through these connections, autonomic activity is coordinated with somatic and endocrine activity to maintain homeostasis.

NEUROCHEMICAL TRANSMISSION

The development of the concept that the nerve impulse is transmitted across synapses and neuroeffector junctions by a chemical mediator arises largely from a study of autonomic nervous functions. The recognition and classification of a neurotransmitter are based on four criteria. First, a neurotransmitter must be synthesized within the neuron from which it is released. Second, a storage mechanism must be present within the neuron from which the neurotransmitter is released. The third criterion appears to be that release of the neurotransmitter is calcium dependent. Fourth, there should be a mechanism for rapid termination of the action of the released neurotransmitters.

Neurotransmission can be interrupted at several sites (Fig. 33–6). The more common mechanisms include the following:

1. Interference of axoplasmic flow of genetic information and substrates (peptide precursor substances).
2. Interference with ionic concentration gradients so that normal depolarization does not occur.
3. Interference with the availability of precursor substances and with their transport to or uptake into a nerve terminal.
4. Interference with the availability of necessary enzymes, cofactors, and ions or alterations in necessary feedback loops for synthesis control.
5. Alteration of storage structures or complexes that protect the neurotransmitter from enzymatic destruction or other forms of inactivation.
6. Other impairments may come from organelles and enzymes, which maintain the processes necessary for metabolic and neurotransmitter activity of the cell. This may be caused by the lack of energy substrates to fuel biochemical reactions, the inhibition or destruction of enzymes necessary for transmitter synthesis, and the inactivation of an excess of neurotransmitter.
7. Interference with calcium-dependent neurotransmitter release or alteration of the presynaptic membrane.
8. At the receptor level, neurotransmission may be modified by either competitive blockade of the receptor site, to prevent access of the neurotransmitter to the receptor (R), or physiological blockade, when the action of substances at other receptors causes an opposing action in the same neuroeffector tissue. Altered receptor sensitivity to the neurotransmitter occurs because of changes in affinity or in receptor numbers.
9. At the postreceptor site, changes in normal ionic responses of target tissue to neurotransmitter receptor may be due to interruption of the systems of enzyme inactivation or of neuronal reuptake by active transport.

Cholinergic Synapses

The rate of spontaneous release of quanta of acetylcholine (ACh) is partly dependent on the calcium ion (Ca^{++}) concentration, but a fraction of the spontaneous release continues even in the absence of this ion. Transmission failure due to nonrelease of acetylcholine is produced by a *lack of calcium or* an *excess of magnesium ions.* Some drugs may

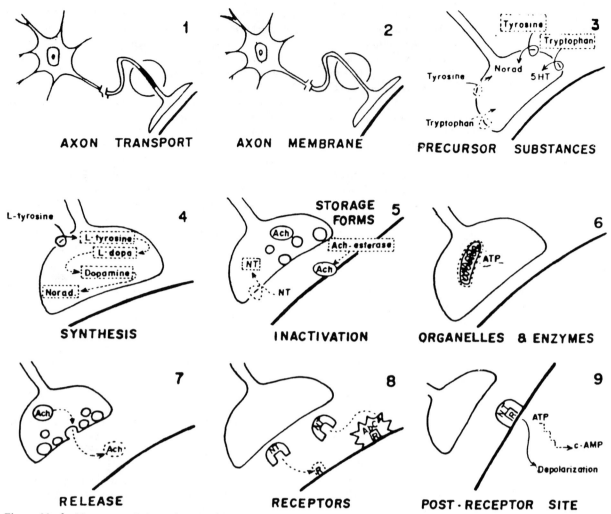

Figure 33–6 Neurotransmission and origin of defective neurotransmission. 1, Interference with axonal transport system, causing failure of transport of vital substrates, enzymes, and organelles from the nucleus to nerve terminals. 2, Interference with axonal membrane permeability to ions, causing inappropriate hyperpolarization or depolarization of plasma membrane. 3, Interference with precursor substances' (e.g., tyrosine, tryptophan) transport to or uptake into the nerve terminal. 4, Interference with availability of necessary enzymes, cofactors, and ions for synthesis of neurotransmitters or alteration of necessary feedback loops for synthesis control. 5, Alteration of storage structure of complexes that protect the neurotransmitter (NT) from enzymatic destruction and other forms of inactivation including reuptake of transmitter. 6, Interference with functions of organelle and enzyme energy system necesary for neurotransmitter synthesis and inactivation. 7, Interference with release of neurotransmitter from nerve terminal. 8, Competitive or physiological blockade of receptor site, preventing neurotransmitter-receptor binding or changes in receptor sensitivity to neurotransmitter, which results in failure of proper response. 9, Interference with normal response in the target tissue to receptor activation.

act at this level (e.g., by complexing with free Ca^{++} or Mg^{++}, by interfering with their binding or their role in the release mechanism of ACh.

In isolated preparations, ethanol and certain drugs such as chloral hydrate, pentobarbital, and paraldehyde increase the release of ACh from cholinergic nerves. This effect at nerve terminals may alter the distribution of charges on the inside of the axonal membrane, with the result that vesicles are no longer repelled from the sites of release.

A component from the venom of a snake and of the black widow spider, *beta-bungarotoxin*, has marked action on synaptic vesicles. When they are applied to a cholinergically innervated tissue, these venoms at first produce an avalanche of miniature *postjunctional potentials*. Subsequently, the miniature postjunctional potentials disappear. At this stage, neuroeffector transmission is blocked, and electron micrographs indicate that the terminals are then devoid of vesicles. At the same time, the terminal axonal membrane is expanded and convoluted, because the empty vesicles have fused with the membrane. These venoms appear to oppose whatever mechanism is normally responsible for separating the vesicular and axonal membranes (Fig. 33–7).

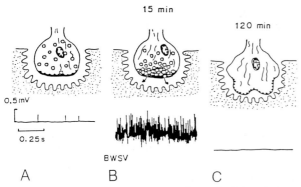

Figure 33–7 Cholinergic junction and record of the miniature junctional potentials (**A**) before hyperactivity (15 minutes after treatment with black widow spider venom (BWSV), (**B**) 2 hours later, and (**C**) when the acetylcholine reserve is exhausted.

The microorganism *Clostridium botulinum* produces one of the most toxic substances known, the *botulinum toxin,* which unlike most bacterial toxins is active by mouth. Six antigenically different types of toxins (A, B, C, D, E, and F) have been identified from strains of the organism, and type C has two subtypes. The basic toxic mechanisms of each of the types are identical. Each toxin possesses two distinct actions: it prevents neurotransmission at all peripheral cholinergic junctions, and it agglutinates erythrocytes by a hemagglutinin. Poisoning by the botulinum toxin is called botulism, and the lethal effect is the result of paralysis of the respiratory muscles. At cholinergic junctions, the toxin prevents the release of ACh. The toxin has no direct effect on the conduction of nerve impulses, on the synthesis of ACh, on cholinesterase, or on the effector cells; however, its effect is very prolonged, and other changes that are secondary to the blockade of transmission may develop in an animal that survives botulism.

Disorders of the ACh system can occur at *muscarinic receptors* (postganglionic parasympathetic, postganglionic sympathetic at sweat glands) and at *nicotinic receptors* (preganglionic sympathetic and parasympathetic or neuromuscular junctions). ACh disorders are the result of inhibition of acetylcholinesterase by organophosphate, of administration of cholinomimetics that are muscarinic receptor blockers, of deficit of choline acetyltransferase in parts of the hippocampus, which is believed to interfere with short-term memory (senile dementia), and of decreased ACh synthesis, especially in the hippocampus (Alzheimer's disease).

For the striated muscle, myasthenia gravis is a major disturbance at the level of the motor end-plate. *Acquired myasthenia gravis* may be due to production of a receptor antibody that blocks receptors by steric hindrance of ACh, reduces synthesis of ACh receptors, or increases the width of the synaptic cleft. *Congenital myasthenia gravis* is an inherited deficiency of ACh receptors in postsynaptic membranes because of possible mechanisms such as failure of synthesis, accelerated degradation, faulty membrane insertion, and low

binding affinity for ACh. The blockade of the junction is also due to plant toxicities (mushrooms: muscarine: deadly nightshade, or *Atropa belladonna:* atropine; henbane, or *Hyoscyamus niger:* hyoscine, or scopolamine), and iatrogenic drug toxicities (inappropriate use of antagonists such as atropine).

Adrenergic Synapses

The precursor of norepinephrine (noradrenaline) is L-tyrosine, obtained from the diet or synthesized from dietary phenylalanine in the liver. In norepinephrine synthesis, *tyrosine hydroxylase* is inhibited by its end-product (norepinephrine) and also by L-dopa, an intermediary product in the synthesis of norepinephrine via L-dopa and dopamine. Increased sympathetic activity accelerates the synthesis of norepinephrine by stimulating tyrosine hydroxylase. Enzymatic *breakdown by monoamine oxidase* (MAO) on mitochondria and by catechol-O-methyltransferase (COMT), a soluble enzyme in the cytoplasm, yields norepinephrine, 3,4-dihydroxymandelic acid, and 4-methoxy-4-hydroxymandelic acid. Disorders of the norepinephrine system include tremor due to beta-adrenergic receptors in the CNS and skeletal muscle. The tremor in Parkinson's disease is reduced by beta-adrenergic receptor blockers, which also correct the phenylpyruvic oligophrenia (congenital lack of enzymes). The enzymes are necessary to convert phenylalanine to tyrosine, and in their absence leads to an accumulation of phenyl derivatives, which are associated with mental retardation.

In the adrenal medulla, by activating the nicotinic receptors of chromaffin cells, ACh causes the opening of the receptor's ion channels, allowing the entry of large numbers of sodium ions (Na^+) and smaller numbers of calcium ions (Ca^{++}). It causes sufficient depolarization of the chromaffin cell membrane to activate the two main voltage-sensitive ion channels (i.e., tetrodotoxin-sensitive fast sodium cation channels and dihydropyridine-sensitive slow calcium (Ca^{++}) channels. The opening of both types of channels results in the firing of action potentials (Fig. 33–8).

Catecholamine secretion may also be elicited by passive depolarization with high extracellular potassium cation concentrations. Such depolarization bypasses the nicotinic receptor. It activates the voltage-sensitive channels directly and produces sodium cation–dependent action potentials. Potassium cation–induced catecholamine secretion needs extracellular calcium (Ca^{++}) and is blocked by calcium-channel antagonists.

The opening of the receptor ionophore is not the only consequence of the interaction of acetylcholine with its receptor. Adenylate cyclase is activated by nicotinic stimulation of chromaffin cells. ACh acts also on chromaffin cell muscarinic receptors, which causes an efflux of cytosolic calcium ions, an increase in cyclic guanosine monophosphate (cGMP), and activation of phosphoinositide breakdown. The influences of these second messengers on exocytosis are largely unknown.

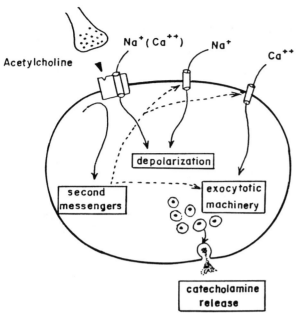

Figure 33–8 Stimulus-secretion coupling in adrenal medullary chromaffin cells.

NONADRENERGIC NONCHOLINERGIC TRANSMITTERS

Powerful nonadrenergic and noncholinergic (NANC) *inhibitory* nerves reach the smooth muscles of the gastrointestinal tract. In addition to contributing to *propulsion* of material through the alimentary canal, these nerves are involved in reflex *opening* of sphincters, in *receptive* relaxation of the stomach, and in descending *inhibition* during peristalsis. The main role of adrenergic nerves is modulation of these activities, mostly at the ganglion level. A purine nucleotide, adenosine triphosphate (ATP), emerges as the most probable contender of neurotransmission.

Autonomic nerves containing enkephalin, substance P, vasoactive intestinal polypeptide (VIP), neurotensin, somatostatin, bombesin, and gastrin/cholecystokinin (CCK) have also been described. On the basis of autoradiographical and electrophysiological studies, evidence indicates that serotonin (or 5-hydroxytryptamine [5-HT]) and gamma-aminobutyric acid (GABA) may be transmitters in some autonomic nerves in the gastrointestinal tract. Some results also suggest the possibility that dopamine (DA) and bradykinin (BK) are autonomic transmitters. In addition, amino acids such as glycine and glutamate may act as transmitters in the enteric nervous system as well as in the CNS. Because of intrinsic neurons in its wall, the gut exhibits behavior patterns independent of the rest of the nervous system, which are modulated by extrinsic parasympathetic and sympathetic nerves.

LANGLEY (England) considered the enteric nervous system, intrinsic to the gut wall, to be a separate division of the ANS.

Regulation of digestive functions is now thought to be operated through neural systems involving not only the classic transmitters norepinephrine and ACh but also the NANC neurotransmitters and the gut hormones. The NANC neurotransmitters are currently the subject of intensive studies to define their roles. It has become apparent that more than one transmitter substance or modulator may be found in the terminal of a single neuron. Since the same peptides occur in gut neurons, gut endocrine cells, paracrine cells, and brain cells, their roles in the body are very complex.

It is becoming clear that neuropeptides commonly extend the actions of the usually short-lived neurotransmitters over a longer time frame. This may be particularly appropriate in more slowly reacting organs with smooth muscle or exocrine gland cells. More specific and precise analytical techniques are necessary to characterize the functions of peptides. One attempt to simplify the peptide story uses a classification based on chemical families such as bombesin–gastrin-releasing peptide, CCK-gastrin, opioid-dynorphin-enkephalin, neuropeptide Y and pancreatic peptide, substance P–tachykinins, somatostatin-neurotensin, VIP-PHI-secretin. Several substances are believed to be transmitters in NANC nerves (Table 33–1).

Serotonin

Serotonin (5-HT) is important in the control of mood and behavior; motor activity; hunger; sleep; thermoregulation; certain hallucinatory states; and possibly some neuroendocrine mechanisms. L-Tryptophan, via tryptophan hydroxylase (Try H), yields 5-hydroxytryptophan (5-HTP) and then 5-HT, which is transformed into 5-hydroxyindoleacetic acid (5-HIAA).

Disorders of the serotonin system include depression, myoclonus, and migraine headache. *Depression* is due to a plasma decrease in free L-tryptophan and an increase in the bound form. *Myoclonus,* in which levels of 5-HIAA in cerebrospinal fluid are low (after anoxia or trauma), is improved with 5-HTP therapy. *Migraine headaches* seem to be helped by methysergide, a 5-HT receptor blocker.

Dopamine

Dopamine (DA) is enzymatically destroyed by MAO, yielding 3,4-dihydroxyphenylacetic acid (DOPAC), and by COMT, yielding homovanillic acid (HVA). L-Dopa is taken up actively and rapidly by dopamine neurons to be converted to dopamine, not to norepinephrine. *Parkinson's disease* is a disorder resulting from degeneration of dopamine neurons in the nigrostriatal pathway and from depletion of GABA. It causes rigidity of limbs, trunk, and face; tremor; abnormal body posture; and inability to initiate voluntary motor activ-

TABLE 33–1 Proposed Nonadrenergic Noncholinergic Transmitters in the Autonomic Nervous System

Nonpeptides
  Adenosine triphosphate (ATP)
  Gamma-aminobutyric acid (GABA)
  5-hydroxytryptamine (5-HT)
  Dopamine (DA)

Neuropeptides
  Adrenocorticotropic hormone (ACTH)
  Angiotensin II (ANG II)
  Bombesin/gastrin-releasing peptide (GRP)
  Bradykinin (BK)
  Calcitonin gene-related peptide (CGRP)
  Cholecystokinin/gastrin (CCK)
  Dynorphin (DYN)
  Endothelin
  Enkephalin (ENK) and beta-endorphin
  Enteroglucagon
  Epidermal growth factor (EGF)
  Gastrin-inhibitory peptide (GIP)
  Luteinizing hormone–releasing hormone (LHRH)
  Motilin
  Neural growth factor (NGF)
  Neurokinins A and B
  Neuropeptide Y and galanin (NPY)
  Neurotensin (NT)
  Pancreatic peptide (PP)
  Peptide with histidine at N terminal and isoleucine amide at C terminal (PHI)
  Secretin
  Somatostatin (SS)
  Substance P (SP)
  Tachykinins (TK)
  Vasoactive intestinal polypeptide (VIP)
  Vasopressin and oxytocin

glion, enkephalin-like immunoreactivity exists in ganglion cells containing norepinephrine. The ACh–rich nerves in cat exocrine glands contain a VIP-like peptide. In some enteric neurons, substance P may be present, together with 5-HT. The list of possibilities is growing rapidly and is becoming almost unmanageable.

Other Peptides

There is some speculation that peptides act as neurotransmitters, as neuromodulators, or as a novel class of neuroactive controllers. The gastrointestinal system contains neuroactive peptides, possibly because peptide-secreting cells arise embryonically from the neuroectoderm. These neuroactive peptides act presynaptically to lower ACh release and thus decrease intestinal motility.

Amino Acids

Among the amino acids, *glycine* and *taurine* are inhibitory, whereas L-*glutamic acid* and L-*aspartic acid* are excitatory. Disorders of the glycine system are tetanus and strychnine toxicity. The tetanus toxin decreases the release of glycine and GABA and lowers the inhibition of spinal alpha motor neurons, with resultant spasticity. In the spinal cord, strychnine toxicity is caused by competitive blocking of sites of inhibitory glycinergic function on alpha motor neurons.

ity. The therapy is L-dopa combined with drugs that inhibit L-dopa decarboxylation. In *Huntington's chorea,* there is a relative overactivity of the dopamine system in the striatum, because of lack of negative feedback by GABA, and increased receptor site response to normal levels of dopamine. *Acute hemiballismus* is due to an increased presynaptic synthesis and release of dopamine, hence an increase in CSF HVA. *Schizophrenia* may be associated with excessive function of dopaminergic pathways in the CNS.

Coexistence of Transmitters

Together with norepinephrine and ACh, ATP is stored in autonomic nerve terminals and is co-released either as a postsynaptic cotransmitter or as a presynaptic modulator of the release of the principal neurotransmitter. Various polypeptides also coexist with traditional neurotransmitters; for example, somatostatin-like immunoreactivity has been observed in about 60 to 70 percent of adrenergic ganglion cells of the inferior mesenteric ganglion and of the celiac superior mesenteric ganglion complex. In the superior cervical gan-

SUMMARY

Taking into account the NANC neurotransmission in the gastrointestinal smooth muscle (including the enteric nervous system), eight roles are possible for neurotransmitters:

1. Intramural inhibitory neurons supplying nonsphincteric circular muscle (ATP)
2. Interneurons, excitatory (5-HT, substance P) or inhibitory (enkephalin)
3. Sensory nerves (substance P)
4. Perivascular inhibitory nerves (VIP)
5. Inhibitory nerves to sphincteric smooth muscle (VIP)
6. Excitatory nerves supplying longitudinal smooth muscle (substance P)
7. Nerves regulating gastrointestinal secretion (somatostatin, VIP)
8. Nerves that modulate the release of transmitter from cholinergic and adrenergic nerve terminals, which can produce presynaptic inhibition of ACh release (enkephalin, 5-HT, ATP, somatostatin) or presynaptic inhibition of norepinephrine (ATP, dopamine).

REFERENCES

Burnsock F, Costa M. Adrenergic neurons, their organization, function and development in the peripheral nervous system. London: Chapman & Hall, 1975.

Callahan SM, Creed KE. Non-cholinergic neurotransmission and the effects of peptides on the urinary bladder of guinea pigs and rabbits. J Physiol (Lond) 1986;374:103.

Cannon WB. Bodily changes in pain, hunger, fear, and rage. New York: Appleton Century Crofts, 1929.

Dyce KM, Sack WO, Wensing CJGI. Textbook of veterinary anatomy. 3rd vol. Philadelphia: WB Saunders Co, 1987.

Janig W. Spinal cord integration of visceral sensory systems and sympathetic nervous system reflexes. In: Cervero F, Morrisson JBF, eds. Progress in brain research. Visceral sensation. Amsterdam: Elsevier, 1986.

Langley JN, Andersson HK. On the innervation of the pelvic and adjoining viscera. Part I. The lower portion of the intestine. J Physiol (Lond) 1895;18:67; 1896; 19:85.

CHAPTER 34

BEHAVIOR, EMOTIONALITY, AND CONDITIONING

Behavior is the result of interactions with the environment by which an animal learns to cope with many kinds of signals or stimuli that indicate success or failure in attaining goals such as food intake and reproduction. This field of study is difficult, since inferences from *subjective experiments* must be used in an attempt to augment limited *objective observations*. Behavior is classified as conditioned behavior or emotional behavior.

CONDITIONED BEHAVIOR

In classical conditioning, innate responses, including changes in salivation, blood pressure, heart rate, and pain withdrawal reflex, are conditioned to be elicited by neutral stimuli that have been associated with the natural stimulus, such as taste of food and sight of food (social or environmental). The concept of *operant conditioning,* or operant learning, is different, as a reward (reinforcer) follows the response and increases the probability of its occurrence.

Learning by observation does not necessarily involve rewards: people and animals can learn by watching others and imitating them. Typical of the evidence of such learning is an experiment in which naive rats are placed in a test chamber adjacent to an identical chamber containing thirsty rats that have already been trained to press a lever for a water reward. The naive rats, able to watch through a Plexiglas partition the trained rats working for their water rewards, also have a lever in their chamber that they are free to press for a water reward. Most naive rats soon start pressing their own lever and obtain water rewards. Naive rats that can see only an empty adjacent chamber learn lever pressing by trial and error, at a much slower rate (Fig. 34–1).

EMOTIONAL BEHAVIOR

The degree of emotionality of an animal can be judged by subjecting it to stress, such as separating the young from the mother, combining strange animals in one group, isolating or overcrowding them, or exposing them to artificial sounds. The frequency and type of vocalization made by the animals, or the heart rate under social stress is used to provide an objective measure of the emotional state. The reaction of an animal to alarm situations is affected by temperament, the presence or absence of young, and experience during early life.

A state of extremely angry behavior known as *sham rage*

is produced in animals by amputating the brain rostrad to the hypothalamus. Nuclear regions and their interconnections around the brain stem and on the medial and the ventral aspects of the brain, which are known as the *limbic system,* are involved in sham rage. An animal with limbic lesions shows periodic displays of rage, with extended claws, opened jaws, and tensed muscles. Upon provocation, or simply gentle restraint, the animal growls, thrashes about, lunges, and snaps. The rage display is not directed specifically to the source of provocation, because the higher centers are lost. An augmented sympathetic discharge shown by the increased heart rate, higher blood pressure, pupillary dilation, and thick hypersalivation is seen if the hypothalamus is intact and has not been destroyed. Limbic brain structures are related to emotions as afferent activity passes from the thalamus to the hypothalamus, then via the mammillary bodies to the anterior thalamic nucleus, and from there to the cingulate cortex.

The *cingulate cortex* is the site of the subjective appreciation of the emotional states not only of rage, but of feeding and of sexual behaviors. These behaviors have been referred to as preservation of the self, and preservation of the species. These two biological goals are necessary for carrying on animal life. Aggressive or placid emotive states connected with hunger and satiety have biological significance in the drive toward these goals or in indifference toward them. The altered behavior produced by a defect in this system, as after bilateral temporal lobectomy, leaves the organism at a disadvantage with regard to its environment.

In the monkey, ablation of the *temporal lobes* brings out the relation of limbic brain structures to behavior. Such monkeys show bizarre behavior patterns, such as loss of normal fear of snakes, and loss of genetically determined "fear" objects. They seem to "explore" their environment orally, by putting edible and inedible objects alike into their mouths. Finally, the animals take as sex partners members of other species, or even inanimate objects.

Domestication causes a marked decline in the degree of emotionality, as measured by changes in heart rate. In rats that are physically restrained, electrocardiographical records show an increase in the heart rate in wild rats but little or no change in domestic rats. The reaction of wild animals to stress may vary from that of their domestic counterparts (e.g., hares versus rabbits).

Animals exposed to artificial *sounds* or *unusual objects* show an alarm reaction upon initial exposure, but auditory or visual memory quickly operates to establish conditioning, or habit formation (Fig. 34–2). Upon first exposure to alternating relative quietness and noises of 115 to 120 decibels (dB) suckling sows rise to their feet and search for the source of the

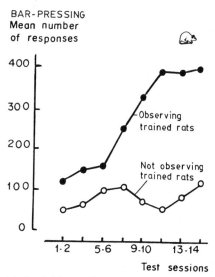

Figure 34–1 Evidence of learning by observation. Rats are allowed to observe other rats in adjacent chambers performing bar-pressing responses for water rewards. The rats (●) that see trained rats operate the bar-press learn more rapidly than those (○) that can see only other naive rats in the adjacent chamber.

sound. This is followed by resumption of suckling, and then apparent indifference to the sounds. In the absence of the dam, piglets exposed to these sounds are alarmed and crowd together. Habituation occurs rapidly in the presence of the dam. At 6 to 7 weeks of age, at the end of the critical period for primary socialization young puppies show more severe emotional reactions when they are exposed to the sounds after a brief separation and in a strange place.

In monkeys, the extent of experimental damage to the *hippocampus* is correlated with the degree of impairment in remembering the external stimuli. On the evolutionary scale, the *striatum* is a more ancient part of the brain than the cortex and the limbic system. Habit formation is mediated by this primitive structure, so even unevolved animals can learn automatic responses to stimuli. Development of habits also seems to be primitive and unrelated to age, since infant monkeys do almost as well as adults in tests of habit formation but do poorly on memory tests.

This chapter presents aspects of conditioning and of memory. It also discusses ingestive and reproductive behaviors.

CLASSICAL CONDITIONING

The fundamental achievement of Pavlov (Russia) was to demonstrate that temporary connections are established in the cortex by the repetition of external stimuli that are linked only by a constant time interval. In his classic experiment with dogs, the repeated sound of a metronome, presented at a fixed interval before food was given, caused salivation to occur at shorter and shorter latency intervals and at an increased rate of secretion. He identified the instability and

temporary character of the conditioned reflex, in contrast with that of the inborn unconditioned reflexes serving instinctual movements. He saw the difference between natural conditioned reflexes, learned in early life, and the artificially conditioned reflexes of the laboratory, both of which are classic examples of conditioning.

The process of classical conditioning involves presenting a *neutral stimulus* immediately prior to the *unconditioned stimulus*. After a number of pairings—perhaps as few as one, depending on the response being conditioned—the neutral stimulus eventually evokes the visceral response alone. Conditioning is most efficient if the neutral stimulus precedes the unconditioned stimulus by an interval of a few seconds or less. Some types of conditioning still occur, however, with a much longer time lag. Several visceral responses can be conditioned (Table 34–1). If the conditioned stimulus (CS) is presented repeatedly to the animal and the response is provoked without giving the unconditioned stimulus (US), the CS loses its strength and its ability to elicit the response (extinction).

Blood glucose level is regulated by an interplay of feedback controls. After a meal, when blood glucose concentration tends to rise, the pancreas secretes *insulin*. In the absence of sufficient insulin, blood glucose levels remain high (diabetes mellitus). When the blood glucose level falls, other hormones, glucagon and corticosteroids, are secreted that cause the liver to convert protein into glucose or to release glucose from stored glycogen. The secretion of these hormones is regulated directly or indirectly via the central nervous system (CNS). These responses are subject to classical conditioning, first the secretion of insulin to lower the blood glucose level and then the secretion of glucagon and corticosteroids to raise it. Repeatedly pairing an *olfactory stimulus* with an injection of *insulin* causes a moderate lowering of the glucose level (which is followed in turn by secretion of glucagon and corticosteroids). Eventually, the olfactory stimulus alone can evoke the secretion of glucagon and corticosteroids.

Localization in the Central Nervous System

In pavlovian studies, an animal is conditioned by first receiving a sensory stimulus—the unconditioned stimulus

TABLE 34–1 Some Visceral Responses That Are Subject to Classical Conditioning

Natural Response	Natural or Unconditioned Stimulus (US)	Conditioned Stimulus (CS)
Asthmatic reaction	Foreign protein	Environment with the protein
Emotional activation	Painful stimulation	Sight of the person
Milk ejection	Massage of the udder by the calf	Banging of milk cans
Nausea	Food poisoning	Taste of food
Salivation	Taste of food	Sight of food
Secretion of insulin	Ingestion of sugar	Smell of food

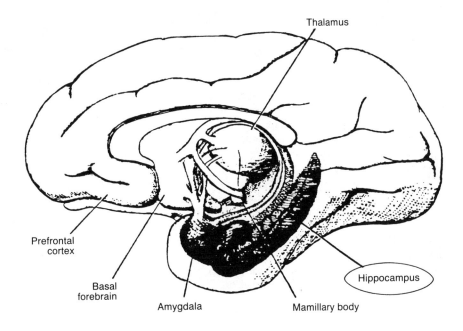

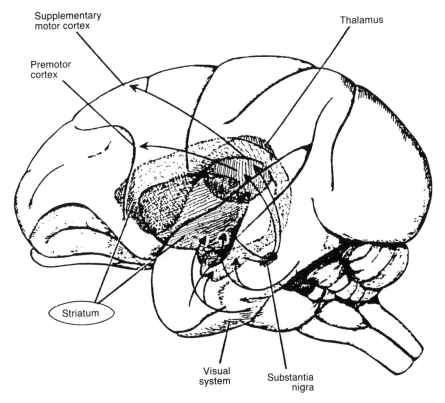

Figure 34–2 Visual recognition memory in monkeys requires two parallel circuits encompassing parts of the diencephalon and of the prefrontal cortex. One circuit is rooted in the amygdala, and the other in the hippocampus. Each structure, in turn, sends signals to the basal forebrain. Through its many connections to the cortex, the basal forebrain can close the loop and cause the perception to be stored there as memory. The development of automatic connections between a stimulus and a response—habit formation—may depend on the striatum. This stucture receives extensive connections from sensory systems in the cortex (here typified by the visual system) and in turn sends fibers to communicate with the premotor cortex and the supplementary motor cortex. Damage to the striatum hampers the performance of the monkey on a visual test that measures habit formation.

(US)—to which it later responds in an unlearned manner. Food juices or vinegar placed in the mouth of a hungry dog are examples of such an unconditioned stimulus. An unconditioned food stimulus causes an *unconditioned response* (UR) (e.g., salivation), and the measure of the response is the amount of saliva produced. If presentation of the US coincides with or immediately precedes the ringing of a bell, after a number of such pairings the animal salivates in response to the ringing of the bell alone. The sound of the bell is termed the *conditioned stimulus* (CS), and salivation in response to it is a *conditioned response* (CR).

After conditioning is established, some neural connections are made in the cerebral cortex and in subcortical structures, so that the CS can take the place of the US with which it has been paired. The original theory held that decorticate dogs could not be conditioned; however, as simple types of classical conditioning are now known to occur in decorticate animals, it seems that subcortical regions may be involved in learning. Since stimulation of *nonspecific thalamic nuclei* causes synchronized widespread discharge in both hemispheres, in addition to loss of consciousness, subcortical structures (thalamus, limbic system) may be at the origin of some CR.

The cortex is critically involved in complex learning tasks, because animals with ablated frontal lobes show a defect in their *delayed response performance*. In a delayed response, an animal is allowed to see a food bait placed under one of two specially marked covers. Then, after a delay, the animal is permitted to select one cover or the other to obtain the bait. A successful performance is the proper choice of the cover over the food bait. Animals with ablated frontal lobes are still able to discriminate one object from another if both objects are presented simultaneously, because the frontal cortex is involved in recent memory. Animals with ablated frontal lobes are more distractable while they wait to choose and may not have a sufficiently prolonged interest in the test object during the time it is out of sight. A fundamental difference in the mechanisms responsible for the acquisition of learned behaviors and for their retention is that once learning has been achieved, disruption of the activity of the frontal lobes does not interrupt delayed responses.

Electrical Correlates of Behavior

Changes in the electroencephalogram (EEG) have been correlated with a classical conditioning procedure that uses the alerting reaction. Shining a light in the eye produces the usual period of low-amplitude fast waves. Also required to show EEG conditioning is a tone signal, which does not by itself produce alerting (Fig. 34–3). This is arranged by *habituation* of the alerting response to the sound signal. A first sound stimulus produces alerting, and with repeated presentations the alerting response diminishes. When the stimulus no longer produces alerting, the animal is habituated to that specific stimulus. Alerting is also caused by the light signal early in the course of conditioning. After a number of such pairings of light and sound as the CS, conditioning to the sound stimulus also occurs.

A type of EEG conditioning is shown when a light (the US) is flashed at a rate of 7.5 Hz to produce a series of evoked cortical potentials. A tone signal to which the animal is habituated is the CS presented in association with the light stimulus. After a number of pairings, the tone signal elicits a CR at the same frequency as that of the light flashes used as the US. This conditioned response is seen in a number of cortical regions, and in a later stage of conditioning the CR becomes localized to the visual cortex (i.e., the unconditioned primary receptor areas).

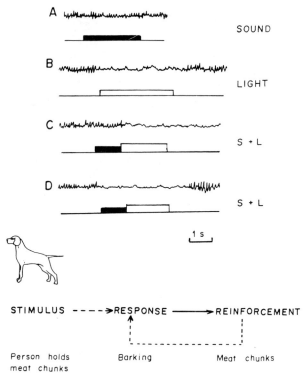

Figure 34–3 Top, EEG desynchronization during conditioning to sound, with light as the unconditioned stimulus. **A,** The record of a resting EEG without an alerting response to a tone signal; **B,** alerting response to a light stimulus; **C,** the tone signal preceding the light signal is not yet conditioned; **D,** After a number of pairings, conditioning is evidenced by the alerting response, which occurs at the onset of the tone signal. **Bottom,** Operant learning for barking. The dog learns to respond (barking) mostly when the stimulus (meat) is present, but the response is not forced (i.e., is voluntary). A response that is followed by a reward, or "reinforcement," tends to be repeated.

OPERANT CONDITIONING

In contrast with classical conditioning, a greater involvement of the cortex in learning is shown by use of *instrumental, or operant,* conditioning. Animals make responses, which at first may be part of their normal repertoire of activity. When the desired response is made, the animal is immediately rewarded (see Fig. 34–3). It soon learns to discriminate between rewarded responses and, if motivated, consistently performs those responses that have been so reinforced.

Food is the *reward* for several experimental protocols of operant conditioning. A common procedure is to place an animal in a box with a small bar that, when it is pressed, activates a food release system. As the naive animal moves about inside the box, it occasionally strikes the bar, and a food pellet is delivered into a food hopper in the box. The animal soon learns to repetitively strike the bar for food. If the reward or reinforcement is removed, the animal gradually decreases its rate of bar pressing and eventually ceases this activity (*extinction*).

In dogs, when barking is followed by a reinforcement, such as a chunk of meat, it tends to be repeated. However, barking is reinforced only when a person is present to deliver meat chunks, and the stimulus, a person holding meat chunks, evokes the barking response. Since the dog may bark as frequently as it pleases, or not at all, it is said that the response is *emitted* rather than *elicited*.

Operant Level

The operant level is the frequency of a behavior that exists before the task is learned. For example, *barking* is natural for dogs and occurs spontaneously at a certain rate. To teach barking requires simply waiting for a dog to bark and then presenting it with meat each time it does. Special procedures can be used to increase the operant level of barking; for example, the researcher may make barking sounds.

Another example is *begging* behavior. A dog lying under the table at dinner smells meat, is aroused, gets up, and begins to walk around. As the dog paces around the table, it may eventually rest its head on the leg of a person, a behavior that was previously a way of soliciting petting. If some meat is given to the dog, it will not require many meat reinforcers before the head resting behavior is firmly established and the dog has learned a type of begging behavior.

In an operant conditioning apparatus, *hens* can be trained to increase the *size of their cage* by means of key pecking (Fig. 34–4). The total number of key pecks delivered to increase the size of the cage is the same whether the cage floor is wood shavings or wire mesh. The operant level of key pecking for access to shavings is greater than that of key pecking for access to wire. Thus, it is inferred that available space is more important to hens than access to litter. Operant conditioning is a valuable method of determining the prefer-

ences of domestic hens for various aspects of the environment considered to be relevant to their welfare.

Comparative Studies

Birds, especially chickens, have been erroneously considered to be inferior to cats in the acquisition of a two-way conditioned avoidance response. In fact, chickens apparently acquire the CR as quickly as cats. The hypothesis was wrongly based on a deficiency in neural structures, the interruption of which by mammillothalamic tractotomy in the cat produces a profound deficit in retention of conditioned avoidance responses.

In dogs, cats, and rabbits, the acquisition of conditioned avoidance responses is very similar. A difference in speed of acquisition in favor of cats and rabbits over dogs could be hypothesized on the basis of the *conditioned response* (a flexion response for dogs, and movement of a rotating wheel for cats and rabbits). On the basis of *neural structure,* it might be hypothesized that the smooth-brained rabbit would condition at a slower rate than either the cat or the dog, each of which has a more convoluted cortex. Nevertheless, the most prominent characteristic of the data obtained is not differences but *similarity* for the three species.

MEMORY, OR ENGRAM, MECHANISMS

Two types of memory are usually distinguished: neuronal activity responsible for *recent memory* and molecular changes in neurons responsible for *long-term memory*. Long-term memories may be stored in the *cortex:* the effects of various cortical lesions on the retention of a learned response indicate a relationship between the amount of cortex damaged and the degree of memory loss. Electrical stimulation of

Figure 34–4 Operant conditioning apparatus used to define floor preference (wire mesh or a solid surface covered with wood shavings) in hens. A movable divider permits four hens to have access to a larger cage (6,100 cm² instead of 1,800 cm²). Food and water dispensers are located on the walls of the minimum-sized cage. The floor is a 10 mm² wire-mesh grid, and either wire or litter is on the floor of the variable sector of the cage.

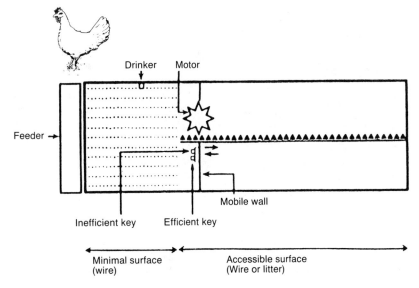

the temporal cortex of conscious patients under local anesthesia elicits vivid memories, but stimulation of cortical areas outside the temporal lobes does not. For this reason, the temporal lobe may be the support for the interpretive function required in remembering external stimuli at the hippocampus level and habituation at the striated level (see Fig. 34–2).

The Split Brain

The use of the split brain preparation is promoting progress in understanding the processes of short-term memory (Fig. 34–5). To produce a split-brain monkey, the optic chiasm–corpus callosum tract connecting the two hemispheres as well as the crossing fibers of the anterior commissure are cut in the anteroposterior plane. The visual information input from each eye can pass only to the ipsilateral hemisphere. With one eye covered, the animal is taught a visual discrimination in the hemisphere on the side of the open eye. After training is completed on that side, the opposite eye is uncovered, and the eye on the trained side is covered. The animal is then unable to perform the visual discrimination that it had learned previously. The habit remains localized to the brain ipsilateral to the eye that was open during training.

The use of this technique makes it possible for two habits to be laid down, one on each side of the brain. On one side, the animal may learn to respond to a square and not to a circle and, on the other side, only to a circle and not to a square. With both eyes open, the animal responds positively to one or the other symbol. At times, one habit dominates, at times the other; the animal does not respond partially to the habits laid down on each side. If the optic chiasm is cut in the midline as usual but the corpus callosum is left intact, sensory information is channeled to the other side. We know this because after such animals are trained with one eye open and the other covered, and then later the previously open eye is closed and the other is opened, the animal readily recognizes the visual stimulus and responds to it.

The Spreading Depression

By the use of spreading depression, one or both cerebral cortices may be functionally incapacitated for several hours. During such functional and *temporary decortication* with potassium chloride, animals may learn a simple type of classical conditioned response. With spreading depression present in one hemisphere, an animal learns an instrumental (operant) response on the side not involved with spreading depression. Localization of the learned response to the cortex that is not depressed during the training sessions is demonstrated by depressing the trained cortex. Such lateralization of the learned response to one hemisphere may remain for a long time, even though the interhemispheric connections present in the corpus callosum may be expected to transfer the habit from the trained side to the other side.

Role of Vasopressin

All memories are present subcortically, but the cortex plays a role in retrieving them. The molecular basis suggested for long-term memories involves changes in the ribonucleic acid (RNA) composition of neuron cell bodies and, in turn, their synthesis of specific proteins. How neuronal activity is transformed into RNA changes remains unknown.

Evidence for a physiological role of vasopressin in learning and memory processes comes from rats (Brattleboro strain) that have hereditary hypothalamic *diabetes insipidus*. Rats that are homozygous for this disease lack the ability to synthesize vasopressin. Avoidance learning is impaired in diabetic rats, compared with their heterozygous littermates. Avoidance acquisition in diabetic rats is retarded, and they show serious learning deficits. Memory functions are more at fault in diabetic rats, as indicated by an impaired retention of one-trial learning of passive avoidance responses.

This behavioral deficit can be normalized by administration or arginine-vasopressin (AVP) or fragments of this peptide, either immediately after the learning or before the retention test. This finding suggests that retrieval of information is impaired because of impaired storage in the absence of vasopressin. In normal Wistar rats, intracerebroventricular administration of AVP antiserum decreases the availability of endogenous vasopressin in the brain and re-

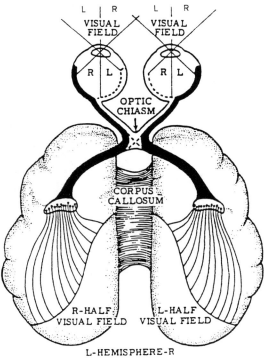

Figure 34–5 A split-brain animal is produced by sectioning the corpus callosum. By analogy, the visual input from one eye can be restricted to one hemisphere by section of the optic chiasm in the midline.

sults in behavioral deficits similar to those observed in the rats with diabetes insipidus. Therefore, lowering of the level of endogenous vasopressin in the brain results in a behavioral deficit similar to that observed in diabetic rats, and endogenous vasopressin may be involved in the formation and expression of memory.

The behavioral deficits of Brattleboro rats with diabetes insipidus and of Wistar rats with decreased availability of central vasopressin may be due to an oxytocin-induced amnesia, which is manifested when little or no vasopressin is available. That centrally available oxytocin is involved in the modulation of memory processes is suggested by the use of antiserum given intracerebroventricularly. The avoidance behavior is improved in Wistar rats by lowering the level of centrally available oxytocin with such antiserum.

INGESTIVE BEHAVIOR

Voluntary intake of food constitutes a discontinuous process in which periods of eating alternate with periods of not eating. Animals eat discrete meals, and within meals some short bouts of eating are separated by short episodes of other activities.

Measurement of food intake include various parameters of meal patterns, such as the number of meals taken over a given period, meal size, meal duration, intermeal intervals, and the ratio of meal size to pre- and postmeal intervals. In addition, certain intrameal characteristics may be assessed, such as the number, size, and duration of eating bouts. These techniques draw attention to the distinction between *food intake* (usually assessed by measuring the weight of food consumed) and *ingestive behavior,* which can be understood only through a close analysis of the details of the eating response (Fig. 34–6). Although measurement of sheer bulk of food consumed may throw light on certain features of energy balance, a more detailed behavioral analysis is required to determine how brain processes exert moment-to-moment control over feeding activities. For a behavioral analysis, it is necessary to provide the animal with the opportunity to display the full range of behaviors in the ingestive repertoire.

Ingestion is not simply the manifestation of an organ-

Figure 34–6 Top, Structure of ingestive behavior showing the relationship between the expression of particular activities and states used to describe changes in voluntary feed intake. **Bottom,** Food intake viewed as an interaction between the *milieu intérieur* and the external environment.

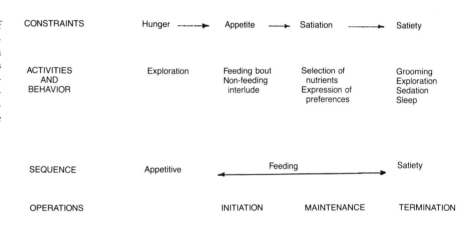

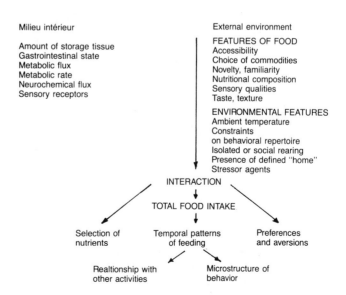

ism's need but is also indicative of the relationship between the animal's *milieu intérieur* and its social environment (i.e., an intimate bond between the organism and the world in which it lives). The puzzle is that feeding appears to be an automatic extension of a bodily need into the external world and occurs with a diverse set of actions that fluctuate from moment to moment and from place to place (see Fig. 34–6, bottom).

The spontaneous *feeding and drinking patterns* of a large omnivorous species like the pig, when an operant conditioning setup for feed and water is in place, seem to be a useful model for studying the factors involved in control of food and water intake. As pigs grow from 10 to 130 kg, daily intake increases nearly threefold, while the number of eating bouts is halved (from 14 to 7). In addition, both the amount of food consumed during an eating bout and the interbout interval increase. However, the amount of food eaten during a bout increases primarily because of an *increased rate of eating,* without any increase in bout duration. Neither premeal nor postmeal intervals correlate with meal size. Of the pig's daily *water intake,* 75 percent is closely associated with eating bouts, and 25 percent is preprandial. About 65 percent of the daily food and water intake occurs during the 12-hour light period.

In pigs fed ad libitum, meal timing and size are not correlated and are random, whereas pigs moderately deprived of food eat large meals related to the duration of deprivation (i.e., via a nutrient deficiency threshold). The puzzle of what determines meal size and meal occurrence may be resolved by considering the disturbances in *hyperphagia* and those in *anorexia nervosa*. In the CNS, the ventromedial and lateral areas of the hypothalamus appear to be involved in satiety and hunger, respectively. Another important hypothalamic area is the paraventricular nucleus, as the intracerebroventricular injections of the neurotransmitters alpha- and beta-adrenergic agonists, serotonin (5-hydroxytryptamine, 5-HT), and gamma-aminobutyric acid (GABA) agonists stimulate feed intake in ruminants. Intravenous administration of benzodiazepines stimulates feed intake in sheep and cattle, possibly by increasing GABA levels in the brain. Neuropeptides of the opioid and cholecystokinin (CCK) families have reciprocal hunger-stimulating and satiety-eliciting effects when they are administered centrally. Furthermore, concentrations of these neuropeptides in specific areas of the hypothalamus change with the state of hunger or satiety. None of the hormones associated with the hypophysis, adrenal glands, pancreas, or gastrointestinal tract is sufficiently effective to control food intake.

Hyperphagia

Genetically obese (ob/ob) rats or mice are hyperphagic, possibly because satiety does not occur. In fact, neural satiety mechanisms triggered via serotoninergic pathways (fenfluramine), vagal afferents (CCK), and the hypothalamic paraventricular nucleus (neurotensin) function in these genetically obese animals. The satiety defect of ob/ob mice resides outside the nervous system. In addition, ob/ob mice have other disturbances (e.g., impaired thermogenesis and increased adipose deposition) before the onset of hyperphagia at weaning. The early manifestations of the *ob/ob syndrome* cannot be attributed to increased food consumption. However, the metabolic hyperglycemia and hyperinsulinemia of hyperphagia are greatly reduced by fasting or prolonged dietary restriction. Hyperphagia is thus a crucial determinant of the full expression of the ob/ob syndrome. Hyperphagic mice are deficient in an axon-nervous satiety factor from a source other than the pancreatic islets, and sufficient putative gastrointestinal satiety signals (hormones) are not generated by feeding.

Anorexia Nervosa

Aphagia in animals is correlated with anorexia nervosa. In fact, the term "anorexia" is a misnomer, because appetite is not impaired, and hunger continues to be perceived. In monkeys, the results of *destruction of the locus caeruleus,* a noradrenergic nucleus, are marked hyperphagia and hyperdipsia. The resultant weight gain is proportional to the reduction in the concentrations of the noradrenergic metabolite 3-methoxy-4-hydroxyphenylethyleneglycol (MHPG) in the nucleus's projection areas in the brain. Anorexia nervosa may be due to overactivity of a norepinephrine-mediated satiety center. The precursor of norepinephrine is dopamine (DA), and anorexia nervosa can be associated also with dopaminergic hyperactivity. Accordingly, reduction of food intake in animals following DA stimulation (e.g., by amphetamine or apomorphine) can be blocked by DA receptor antagonists (e.g., pimozide). Prolonged DA receptor stimulation (e.g., with L-dopa) may cause anorexia and weight loss, whereas chlorpromazine (as a DA antagonist) produces weight gain.

Selection of Nutrients

The composition of the diet may affect the concentration of important neurochemicals. For example, the 5-HT level in the brain of rats is raised after a carbohydrate-rich meal. The process is probably mediated by effects on blood levels of tryptophan and its availability for CNS uptake.

Disturbances

In horses, some behavior disorders such as biting, wind sucking, and crib biting have long been perceived to be genuine impairments that reduce the animal's effectiveness. Biting and kicking can be considered as exaggerated self-protective behaviors. Crib biting and wind sucking can be considered as fragments of innate feeding activity that have become established as habits. These *displacement activities* are adapted from instinctive movements and are substitutes for the appropriate actions when the latter cannot be executed properly at the time.

The pig provides one example of abnormal behavior in the puerperium. When a sow savages its newborn piglets, the behavior is antagonistic to the preservation of the species. This behavioral abnormality responds to treatment with tranquilizers.

In sheep, stereotyped compulsive behavior is induced by CNS excitation by morphine or morphine-like substances.

The CNS structures involved in the regulation of food intake are probably informed continuously about the nutritional state of the body by many positive and negative feedback loops. Hormones such as insulin, glucagon, CCK, glucocorticoids, and many others play a role in these feedback loops to achieve long- and short-term regulation of food intake. Besides these humoral factors, mechanical factors (e.g., information from stretch receptors and chemoreceptors in the digestive tract) contribute to the action of these feedback loops. In addition, learning processes and habits are involved.

REPRODUCTIVE BEHAVIOR

The concept that most sex-related behaviors, including aggression, are influenced by gonadal androgens acting on the CNS is inferred from the effects of *castration*. Research on hormones and reproductive behavior has advanced to a complex level of analysis to explain the role of the brain in puberty, in initiation of the breeding season, and in precoital behavior.

Erection and ejaculation are mediated at the *spinal level*, as such reflexes are elicited in rodents and small ruminants by transrectal electrical stimulation for the collection of semen. The discovery of *neurosecretion* is related to facts about the *hypothalamus* and to the neural (and vascular) connections in the *hypophysial stalk*. The hypothalamus serves as a target organ for the gonadal and hypophysial hormones; it is an integrator of exteroceptive stimuli; and it is part of a feedback loop that controls the release of gonadotropins.

In 1910, RAMON Y CAJAL (Spain) noted an abundance of fine nerve fibers in the posterior pituitary (neurohypophysis), which originated in a group of cells situated behind the optic chiasm (decussation).

The reasonable interpretation of the function of the neurohypophysis came in 1940 from E. and B. SCHARRER (USA), who showed that the peptides (vasopressin, oxytocin) of the neurohypophysis are of hypothalamic origin (supraoptic and paraventricular nuclei). At about the same time (1942), from destruction of extrahypothalamic areas such as the amygdala, BEACH and others suggested a role for limbic structures in the onset of puberty and in hypersexuality in males.

Finally, the group of LERNER (1958 to 1960) discovered melatonin (*N*-acetyl-5-methoxytryptamine) in the bovine pineal gland (epiphysis), which is innervated by two large sympathetic nerve tracts derived from the superior cervical ganglia. The secretion of melatonin increases during the night and influences the onset of reproductive activities, especially in short-day breeders such as sheep.

Sexual Behavior

Libido (a psychic drive or energy particularly associated with the sexual instinct) and general sexual responsiveness are of considerable importance in practical breeding and farming. Communication between the male and the female can take the form of a behavior change such as unwillingness to escape or move away, adoption of a particular stance, or the female seeking out and investigating the male. Bulls and rams spend an increasing amount of time in close proximity to females during proestrus. Field evidence indicates that bulls systematically survey cows several times each day and may be able to identify impending estrus up to 4 days before the cow reaches the receptive state. The obvious interpretation is that the male is initially attracted to the female by the changes he perceives, and shortly afterward the female reaches a *sexually receptive state*. The observed behavior of the male may be used to infer the stage of the female's estrous cycle (Fig. 34–7).

Female Sexual Behavior

Attractivity, proreceptivity, and receptivity are the three distinct features of the female that, respectively, arouse the male, reflect a state of positive sexual motivation, and indicate readiness to participate in the consummatory phase of copulation.

Behavioral estrus occurs, even in seasonal breeders such as ewes and mares, as part of a cycle of events under the influence of sensory stimulation, hormone secretion, and central neural organization. If a young female is spayed, normal sexual behavior does not appear; in a mature female, spaying is followed by permanent anestrus and invariable rejection of males.

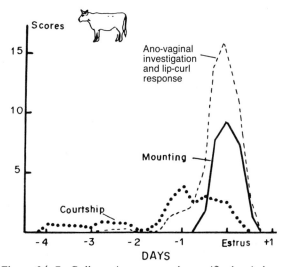

Figure 34–7 Bull reaction scores to the specific chemicals contained in vaginal secretions of a cow near estrus. The result of their action on the vomeronasal, or Jacobson's, organ in the male is the lip-curl, or flehmen response, that terminates an olfactory investigation.

The *hormonal factors* essential for restoring sexual behavior in ovariectomized females vary among species. In sheep, the action of either endogenous or exogenous *estrogens* is greatly facilitated by previous treatment with *progesterone*. A reverse relationship occurs in rodents in which an initial dose of estrogens should be followed by a small amount of progesterone. In dogs and cats, estrogens alone are sufficient to induce sexual receptivity.

Evidence for a *hypothalamic sexual facilitation* mechanism exists in a variety of mammalian species. Lesions in the anterior hypothalamus abolish estrus in the estrous ewe, without producing major changes in the cyclical endocrine relationship between the hypophysis and the ovary. Destruction of an area just dorsal to the anterior median eminence, but not of the *massa intermedia* or optic chiasm, abolishes estrus (Fig. 34–8).

During copulation, to accommodate intromission by the male, the female displays special postural adjustments commonly known as *lordosis* (Fig. 34–9). This pattern is quite marked in female rats. After copulation, mares and cows may exhibit an "orgasm-like" reaction characterized by posture of copulation during which the "galvanic skin response," or electrical resistance of the skin, suddenly drops. Visual, auditory, and olfactory cues play a role in the expression of estrus. The sow shows a characteristic *"mating stance"* (rigidity in the hind legs) when pressure is applied to her back. The rhythm of the boar's courting sound, or song (*chant de cour*), is an important cue to elicit this mating stance. Gilts in estrus that do not respond to hand pressure alone become responsive when a recorded courting sound is broadcast during the test. Both neural and hormonal factors are involved in lordosis behavior, or mating stance.

Male Sexual Behavior

The effects of castration on sexual behavior depend in part on the animal's previous experience. A male cat that has not copulated before is likely to be sexually unresponsive after castration, whereas in experienced males, the mating pattern persists for 6 to 8 weeks after castration. Once the sexual pattern has been organized through experience, it becomes partly independent of hormones (Fig. 34–10).

Central influences on sexual behavior in male mammals are more involved than those in females. Mating performance of the male depends on the neocortex. Copulatory patterns are controlled by complex pathways from the autonomic nervous system. Erection and ejaculation involve cortical coordination, primarily triggered through the sacral autonomic (parasympathetic) nerves for erection, and through the sympathetic system for ejaculation and secretions of accessory glands. Ejaculation is elicited also by stimuli acting on the receptors in the penis (temperature for the bull and the ram, pressure for the stallion). Vasoactive intestinal peptide (VIP) participates in the parasympathetic induction of vasodilation that is the basis of vascular erection. During erection in large animals (bull, stallion), coordinated contractions of the striated muscles increase the intravascular pressure at the penis to very high levels (more than 1,000 mm Hg).

Positive Effects of Behavior at the Time of Mating

A female mouse that is successfully mated with a male, and is then exposed to and mates with another male within 24 hours of the first copulation, tends not to become pregnant from the first male. A pheromone released by the new male seems to cause this effect, the *Bruce effect*. Other similar examples of effects of stimulation of females by males are *induced ovulation* (in which intromission is required for ovulation to occur in some species such as the cat, ferret, rabbit) and the *progestational state* required for pregnancy in rats that is induced by intromission.

In *mice,* the phenomenon of synchronization, or the bringing on of the appropriate state for mating to occur, is known as the *Whitten effect.* As a result of the introduction of a male into a group of mice, the production of young per litter increases (e.g., the number of live young born 23 days after introduction of a male may be about 11 per litter instead of 9 per litter in individually bred mice).

In *sheep* the introduction of rams into the flock induces estrus, and the ovulation rate at this initial estrus is higher than at subsequent estrous cycles. In *pigs,* a component of the boar's courting behavior, the vigorous nosing of the flanks of the sows during courting, increases the farrowing rate (ratio of farrowing to sows mated). The use of this stimulus (i.e., 2 minutes of courting by a boar) is successful in pair-housed sows submitted to artificial insemination but not in single-penned sows. In pair-housed sows, the farrowing rate increases by almost 25 percent, and the number of piglets born alive increases from 8 to 10. In single-penned sows, the negative effect on reproductive success is associated with an initial response of aggression or of fear.

The restriction of male courtship activities to the proestrus and estrus stages of the estrous cycle presents some advantages: (1) a male's energies are not wasted in attempts to copulate with unreceptive females; (2) females in estrus are less likely to be missed; (3) females' activities are not dis-

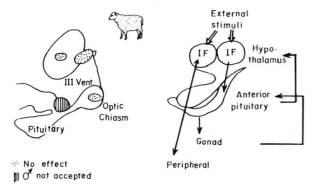

Figure 34–8 In the ewe, hypothalamic lesions in hatched area inhibit estrous behavior, and lesions in dotted areas have no influence. Diagram of both facilitatory (F) and inhibitory (I) hypothalamic mechanisms that influence adenohypophyseal function and sexual behavior in response to external stimuli.

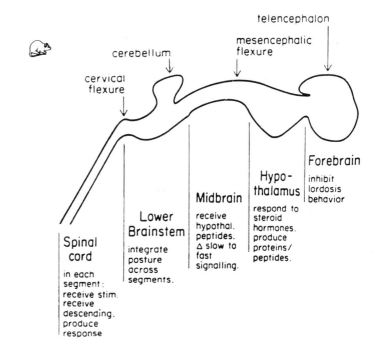

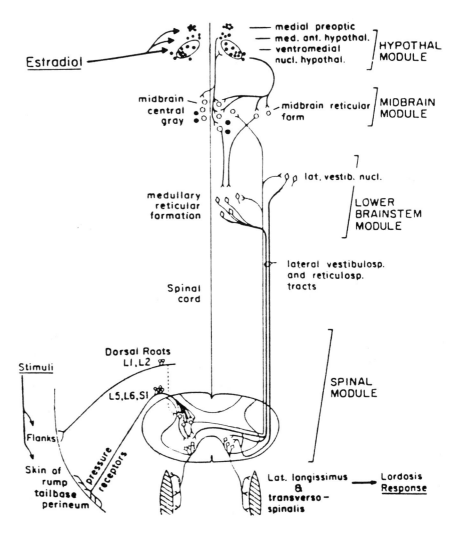

Figure 34–9 Top, Structures involved in neural and hormonal control of lordosis behavior in the rat. **Bottom,** Diagram of neural circuit for the lordosis behavior, including the somatosensory activating stimuli and the sensory and ascending pathways to the ventromedial hypothalamus, where estradiol and progesterone act to facilitate the behavior. Descending pathways from hypothalamus to midbrain, to medullary reticular formation, and to lumbar spinal cord are also shown. The contraction of the deep back muscles (lateral longissimus and transversospinalis) then elicits the behavior.

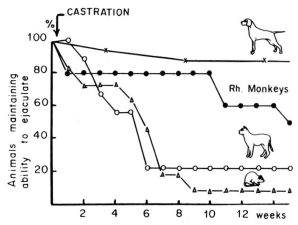

Figure 34–10 Percentage of animals maintaining the ability to ejaculate after castration: data drom rhesus monkeys and dogs are different from those of cats and rats, which lose their ejaculatory ability 6 to 8 weeks after castration.

rupted by the attentions of a persistent male; and (4) one male can mate with more females.

Abnormal Sexual Behavior

Several subnormal patterns of male sexual behavior have been observed: expression of only part of the chain of events of copulation, courtship and mounting without erection or protrusion, licking of a female in estrus without mounting her, lack of interest other than standing near or following a female in estrus, and failure of males reared in isolation from females to detect estrus in a female.

Hypersexuality is seen after the destruction of limbic structures (Fig. 34–11).

Pineal tumors have been associated with precocious sexual development and macrogenitosomia because the pineal gland (epiphysis) has some endocrine functions. The syndrome is the result of failure of inhibition of sexual development. In long-day breeders, the pineal gland is activated by longer periods of darkness to secrete substances that *inhibit gonadotropins* and, in turn, gonadal functions. This prevents these animals from successfully breeding and delivering young during the winter months. After a period of reproductive quiescence, the gonads begin to regenerate and reach full maturity in the spring.

> The golden, or Syrian, hamster (*Mesocricatus auratus*) is a hibernating species. During the long photoperiods of a laboratory (more than 12½ hours of light per day), the golden hamster is a continuous breeder, whereas in its natural habitat it is a seasonal breeder, being reproductively incompetent during the winter hibernating period. Increased activity of the pineal gland accounts for this period of reproductive dormancy.

Maternal Behavior

Reproductive behavior also involves *parental behavior.* Maternal behavior occupies a central position in the social

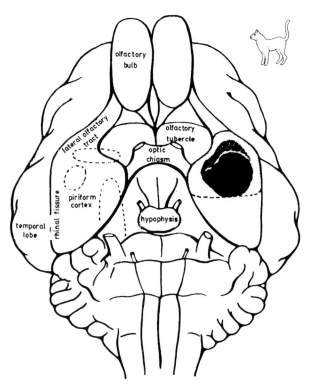

Figure 34–11 Ablation of the pyriform area at the base of the brain produces hypersexuality in male cats.

organization of the species. For the offspring, the behavior of the mother (nest building, care at parturition, nursing, nurturing) is critical for its adjustment to the environment. The preparturient female, which normally lives gregariously in a closely integrated herd, leaves the herd and seeks isolation and shelter. Postures taken by animals during parturition are related to the manner in which they establish care of the young. Rodents, for instance, give birth sitting on the hind legs, with the back arched and the head bent down between the front legs. During birth, the offspring is propelled forward between the hind limbs of the doe, close to her mouth.

Maternal Care

Ewes, cows, and mares stand up very shortly after delivery and start licking the newborn, usually at the head. The birth membranes may be eaten during the cleaning process (a third of the ewes and nearly all cows do so). The dam is initially attracted to her young by the smell and taste of the birth fluids, and it is possible to attract a ewe for short distances with a rag that has been rubbed in the fluids. However, washing the birth fluids off with detergent does not prevent the ewe from accepting her lamb. The birth membranes facilitate but are not essential to the initiation of maternal care. Nevertheless, it is common folklore among shepherds that it is necessary to cover an orphan lamb with the skin of the foster mother's dead lamb to get her to accept the stranger.

Bond Formation

The critical period after parturition during which a mother will form a bond with her offspring is short. For a few hours during this period, maternal behavior is under hormonal control, but after that, the newborn has to provide cues that stimulate the mother to behave in a maternal way. In sheep, the odor of the lamb is crucial but so is active perception of the parturition. For example, lambs born when ewes have spinal anesthesia are not adopted. Only a short period of contact (less than 30 minutes) is needed to establish a bond that enables the mother to discriminate her own offspring from others. It appears also that during this initial period, a ewe, doe, cow, or mare that has given birth approaches any young animal and can become attached to it. This explains lamb swapping between two ewes that lamb close together at the same time. The attachment is learned, not imprinted, as was once thought.

Nursing

During early lactation in the sow, the massage of the udder ends when the piglets fall asleep. In later stages of lactation, the sow brings it to an end by turning over onto her udder or by walking away (Fig. 34–12). Piglets have a fairly fixed "teat order," which is established extremely rapidly, often within an hour of birth, even before the last piglet is born, and some piglets continually receive less milk if a sow has a particular nursing position. The more frequently a sow changes nursing position on the first day after parturition, the longer it takes to establish the teat order. Sight, smell, and recognition of neighbors are involved in the identification of teats and teat order. Rubbing their noses around the teat is suggested to be a marking behavior by piglets for teat recognition. When a sow turns over, it is common to see, for example, a piglet from a front upper teat, confused between this teat (now the lower) and the rear upper teat.

The mechanisms governing nursing behavior are unknown. The decline of lactation is associated with that in nursing behavior, but the hormonal mechanisms involved in the two processes are independent, except for an effect of mammary engorgement. The mother dog or cat spends most of the day with the young during the first week after delivery. One month after whelping, some bitches begin regurgitating their food, which is quickly consumed by the puppies. The response is stimulated if the mother is separated from her litter for several hours and then returned soon after eating (*epimeletic behavior*). Rabbits seem to visit their young only once a day and allow suckling for only a few minutes.

Species differences in duration of the nursing period are correlated with the gregariousness of the species in adulthood. Female rats normally nurse for 25 to 30 days, but nursing behavior can be maintained for a year by providing a succession of foster litters.

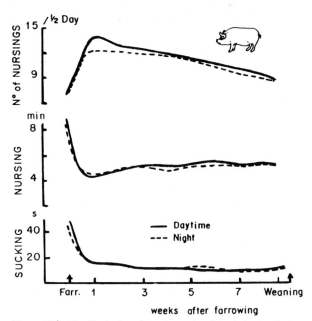

Figure 34–12 Evolution of nursing and sucking behavior during lactation, until weaning. Physical separation of dam and offspring at the 8th week after farrowing not only deprives the young of the mother's milk but also breaks the social attachment between mother and offspring.

REFERENCES

Baile CA, McLaughlin CL. Mechanisms controlling feed intake in ruminants: a review. J Anim Sci 1987;64:915.

Bailey CJ, Flatt PR. Anorectic effect of fenfluramine, cholecystokinin, and neurotensin in genetically obese (ob/ob) mice. Comp Biochem Physiol 1986;84A:451.

Bigelow JA, Houpt TR. Feeding and drinking patterns in young pigs. Physiol Behav 1988;43:99.

Fox MW. Abnormal behavior in animals. Philadelphia: WB Saunders Co, 1968.

Fraser AF. Ethology of farm animals. A comprehensive study of the behavioral features of the common farm animals. Amsterdam: Elsevier, 1985.

Garattini S, Mennini T, Bendotti C, Invernizzi R, Samanin R. Neurochemical mechanism of action of drugs which modify feeding via the serotoninergic system. In: Nicolaidis S, ed. Serotoninergic system, feeding and body weight regulation. London: Academic Press Inc, 1986.

Hart BJ. The behavior of domestic animals. NY: WH Freeman Co, 1985.

Hinde RA. Animal behavior. A synthesis of ethology and comparative psychology. New York: McGraw-Hill Book Co, 1970.

Lagadic H, Faure JM. Preferences of domestic hens for cage size and floor types as measured by operant conditioning. Appl Anim Behav Sci 1987;19:147.

Nichelmann M. Ethology of domestic animals. Toulouse: Privat IEC/Univ Paul Sabatier, 1987.

Steffens AB, Strubbe JH. Regulation of body weight and food intake. Sci Prog Oxf 1987;71:545.

Syme GJ, Syme LA. Social structure in farm animals. Developments in animal and veterinary sciences. Amsterdam: Elsevier, 1979.

CHAPTER 35

THE ENDOCRINE BRAIN

The degree of complexity of functions observed in vertebrates is the result of evolution of the two primary integrating systems, the *nervous* system and the *endocrine* system. Each system participates in the regulation and coordination of the activities of the organism.

The nervous system acts in an immediate, short-term fashion, and the endocrine system provides longer-term regulation. The endocrine system operates to maintain the internal environment (the body fluids) at a relatively constant level of volume and concentration. It also transmits information by means of chemical messengers, the *hormones.* The hormone-secreting elements of the brain are the secretory cells of the hypothalamus, of the pineal gland (epiphysis), and of the hypophysis. Other endocrine organs include the pancreas, the parathyroid glands and derivatives of the ultimobranchial body, the thyroid gland, the adrenal gland (medulla and cortex), the gonads, and the placenta.

In 1849, BERTHOLD (France) probably made the first experimental demonstration of an internal secretion by grafting testicular tissue to prevent atrophy of the comb of a capon. Endocrinology remained almost dormant for the next 50 years. In 1902, BAYLISS and STARLING (England) demonstrated the physiological role of secretin. The term "hormone" was first used by Starling in 1905, and the possibility that constancy of the internal environment might be maintained in part through hormonal mechanisms was suggested.

Modern endocrinology has advanced with chemistry and was stimulated by clinical studies of the endocrine system. The amino acid sequence and chemical structure of insulin were established by SANGER. The active principles of the neurohypophysis (vasopressin, oxytocin) were determined and synthesized (DU VIGNEAUD). Techniques of electrode implantation (HESS) were modified and utilized to gain knowledge of the relationship between the central nervous system (CNS) and the adenohypophysis (SAWYER). HARRIS pioneered the study of the relation between the hypothalamus and the neurohypophysis. NALBANDOV made major contributions to the conception of hypothalamic-releasing hormones, and GUILLEMIN characterized some of them. The radioimmunological techniques introduced by BERSON and YALOW for the assay of polypeptides and protein hormones in the plasma and tissues have contributed much to the understanding of endocrine functions.

Histological and biochemical studies have demonstrated the presence of the various releasing hormones, not only in the hypothalamus but in other areas of the CNS, in peripheral neurons, in the gut, and in the pancreas. In addition, chemical transmitter substances released from hypothalamic neurons influence physiological neural functions as diverse as sexual behavior (luteotrophic hormone–releasing hormone, or LHRH), memory (vasopressin, or antidiuretic hormone [ADH]), and neuronal transmission (thyrotropin-releasing hormone, or TRH). The true significance of these observations is that in the brain, as in the dorsal horn neurons of the spinal cord (Fig. 35–1), the information is not only transmitted but is modulated by several chemical substances. The *final common pathway* for a neuron is then the result of spatial and temporal summation of several excitatory and inhibitory factors.

THE NEUROHYPOPHYSIS

Strictly speaking, the neurohypophysis serves as a storage place for certain hormones secreted by the hypothalamus. Microscopically, the neurohypophysis contains four basic structures: unmyelinated nerve fibers, glial cells, and capillaries surrounded by argyrophilic connective tissue. Cells of the supraoptic and paraventricular nuclei are at the origin of nerve fibers, which give secretomotor innervation to cells called pituicytes. The cells of the *supraoptic* and *paraventricular* nuclei possess stainable cytoplasmic granules, which are regarded as neurosecretory products. These neurosecretory granules, found throughout the extent of the supraopticohypophysial tract, appear as swellings in the fibers and in the interstitial spaces of the infundibular process (Fig. 35–2).

The neurosecretory materials of the neurohypophysis, oxytocin and vasopressin (ADH), are peptides. *Ejaculation* (but not erection) in the male (and genital manipulation of the female) causes release of oxytocin. A sustained (about 30 minutes) increase in the effective osmotic pressure of only 2 percent causes an increase in ADH release and a decrease in free water clearance. Similarly, the ingestion of a large volume of water lowers the global osmotic concentration, and the secretion of ADH is depressed, resulting in diuresis. The injection of hypertonic solutions (sodium chloride, glucose, sucrose) into the carotid artery decreases water *diuresis,* whereas injection of urea, which is ineffective osmotically at the cellular level, does not effectively lower water diuresis.

Hypothalamic receptors near or within the *supraoptic nuclei* are sensitive to differences between the osmotic concentrations of the extracellular and the intracellular fluids. Stimulation of the area around the supraoptic nucleus causes inhibition of water diuresis and increases chloride excretion. The electrical activity of single neurons in or adjacent to the supraoptic nuclei is increased also by the injection of hypertonic saline solution.

Superimposed on this basic mechanism are alterations induced by nervous reflexes. Distention of the *left atrium,* of the pulmonary vein, and of the pericardium is invariably followed by diuresis associated with lowered ADH secretion. The secretion of oxytocin is increased by tactile stimuli from the teat and from the genital canal.

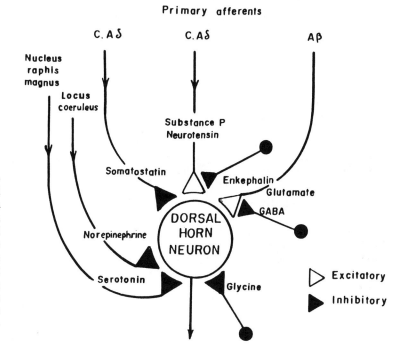

Figure 35–1 Schematic illustration of some presynaptic mechanisms and of known or postulated transmitters, which can modify the activity of a *multireceptive dorsal horn neuron.* The sensitivity of an animal to noxious stimuli can be entirely reduced by electrical stimulation of discrete regions of the brain stem. In addition to the endogenous opioids implicated at brain stem and at spinal levels, caudal inhibition can be mediated via axons containing *serotonin* that have cell bodies in the nucleus raphis magnus of the brain stem, and via *norepinephrine* (noradrenaline) from cells in the nucleus locus caeruleus. (CAδ, Aβ, types of nerve fibers.)

Figure 35–2 Midsagittal section through the hypophysis. Parts of the arterial hypothalamic primary capillary plexus, and the long and short portal vessels of the adenohypophysis are secondary capillary plexuses that drain into the venous outflow. The blood flow of the neurohypophysis is countercurrent to the blood supply to the adenohypophysis. Hypothalamohypophyseal fibers from peptidergic and dopaminergic neurons reach the primary and secondary plexuses. (M, mamillary body; ME, median eminence; OC, optic chiasm; PT, pituitary [hypophysis].)

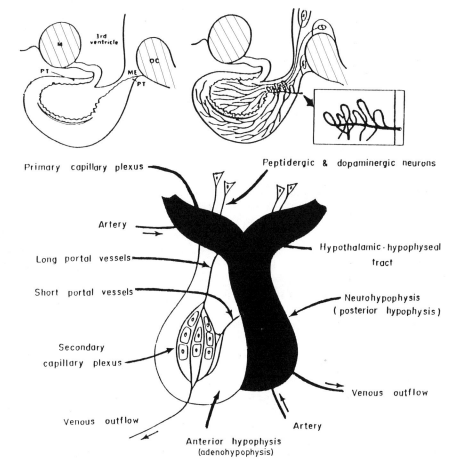

THE HYPOTHALAMOHYPOPHYSIAL SYSTEM

Several functional alterations result from adenohypophysectomy in young animals: (1) *failure of the gonads to mature,* with resultant infantile sexual development and sterility; (2) *atrophy of the thyroid gland* and the characteristics of thyroid insufficiency; (3) *atrophy of the adrenal cortex,* and signs of hypoadrenalism without salt loss; (4) *cessation of growth* and failure to attain adult stature; and (5) a decided *tendency toward hypoglycemia,* hypersensitivity to insulin, and loss of body nitrogen accompanied by diminished catabolism.

The adenohypophysis is under hypothalamic control, as is the neurohypophysis; however, the regulation of the control of the adenohypophysial secretions is not mediated via direct neural connections as are those of the neurohypophysis. The control of adenohypophysial secretion is exerted through hypothalamic neurons, which release specific mediators into the capillary plexus of the portal vessels in the median eminence (see Fig. 35–2).

In 1950, HARRIS reported that the secretion of the hormones of the adenohypophysis is controlled by chemical transmitter substances released from the hypothalamus and conveyed to the hypophysis via the *hypophysial portal* vessels. His experiments are regarded as landmarks in endocrinology.

In conscious rabbits, he showed that electrical stimulation of discrete areas of the hypothalamus causes the release of adenohypophysial hormones, whereas the placement of lesions in the same areas effectively suppressed adenohypophysial function. Destruction of the vascular links between the hypothalamus and the adenohypophysis resulted also in gross hypophysial dysfunction.

Hypothalamic-Releasing Hormones

The first hypophysiotropic hormone characterized, TRH, a *tripeptide* isolated in 1969, stimulates the release of thyroid-stimulating hormone (TSH). LHRH, a decapeptide found 2 years later, is now called *gonadotropin-releasing* hormone (GnRH), since it stimulates release from the adenohypophysis of LH but also of follicle-stimulating hormone (FSH). Another hypothalamic hormone isolated is growth hormone release–*inhibiting* hormone (GHRIH), or somatostatin, a tetradecapeptide. This discovery was surprising, since the hypothalamus exerts mostly a *positive influence* over growth hormone secretion through growth hormone–*releasing* hormone (GHRH), or somatocrinin.

In contrast with the other adenohypophysial hormones, prolactin is secreted under the tonic control of inhibitory hypothalamic hormones (prolactin-inhibiting factors [PIFs]). The major PIF is probably dopamine, since dopaminergic nerve terminals (seen with immunofluorescence techniques) impinge on the portal vessels, and levels of catecholamine are much higher in the blood of the hypophysial stalk than in the peripheral veins.

The first postulated hypophysiotropic hormone, *corticotropin-releasing factor* (CRF), a 41–amino acid polypep-

tide, stimulates the release of equimolar amounts of adrenocorticotropin (ACTH) and of beta-lipotropin (β-LPH), which are adenohypophysial hormones formed from a large precursor molecule (proopiomelanocortin). The action of CRF on the control of ACTH is potentiated by vasopressin (ADH). Like morphine, opioid peptides act on specific hypothalamic opioid receptors, which stimulate the secretion of CRF.

In addition to the neurotransmitter substances of the CNS (i.e., norepinephrine, dopamine, and serotonin), neuronal peptides (mostly from the hypothalamus) are produced with releasing hormones. The endogenous opioid peptides (enkephalins and endorphins) participate in the control of brain endocrine activity in a manner similar to that in which morphine influences hypothalamohypophysial function.

Feedback Regulation

An increase in the rate of secretion of a trophic hormone stimulates a greater rate of secretion from the respective target gland. The secretions of the target gland, in turn, tend to produce countereffects to oppose the secretion of its particular trophic hormone by the hypophysis and to inhibit the source of the initial stimulus. For example, when a lower rate of secretion of TSH by the adenohypophysis is needed, it is because the rate of secretion of thyroxine from the target gland (thyroid) is increased. With secretion of more thyroxine, the output of TSH is inhibited. The end result is first a balance of the forces involved and of the thyroid function, and then a second level of interaction between thyroxine and TRH. A similar example could be illustrated with ACTH, corticosteroids, and CRF.

The secretion of ADH is subject to the integrative effects of the neuroendocrine system, and the hypothalamus correlates neural and humoral signals from the whole organism (Fig. 35–3).

SEX HORMONES AND THE BRAIN

The period early in life when exposure to sex hormones irreversibly alters an animal's brain—and its subsequent sexual behavior—is termed the *critical period.* For example, a *female* rat that is administered *male sex hormones* in the *first few days of life* develops into an adult that fails to ovulate and does not assume the female mating stance (lordosis) when approached by a male rat. A *male rat* that is castrated early in life (deprived of male sex hormones) develops into an adult that assumes the female mating posture when it is given estrogens but does not mount females when it is given testosterone.

Visible synaptic differences between males and females exist in the preoptic area, adjacent to the hypothalamus. The *sexually dimorphic nucleus* is five times larger in males than in females but is much smaller in males castrated during the critical period. Conversely, newborn females that are given testosterone have larger nuclei. Thus, newborn male rats that

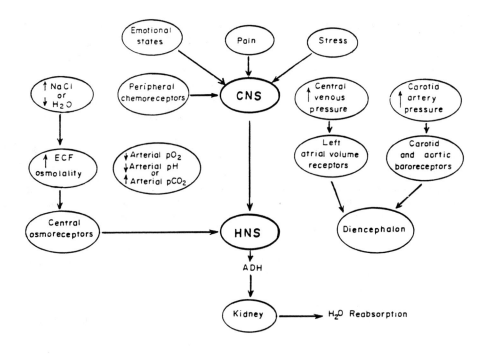

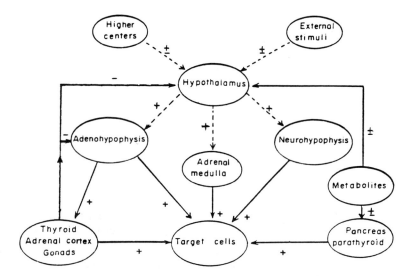

Figure 35–3   Regulation of ADH secretion by the hypothalamoneuro-hypophysial system (HNS), and illustration of the relationship between the endocrine glands and the CNS. Stimulation, +; inhibition, −; neural pathway, - - -; humoral pathway, _____.

are castrated during the critical period develop a female pattern of synaptic connections, whereas females that are given testosterone during the critical period develop a male pattern of synaptic connections.

Injection of radiolabeled estrogen indicates that estrogen binds mainly in the preoptic area, which is rich in estrogen receptors. *Estrogens are the key hormones for male* (not female) *brain development.* Newborn female rats are protected from the effects of estrogen in their blood by alpha-fetoprotein, a protein made by the fetal liver and found in diminishing quantities during the first 3 weeks of life. The newborn male rats synthesize testosterone, but alpha-fetoprotein does not bind testosterone. Thus, testosterone reaches the brain cells of newborn males, where it is converted to estrogen (and

dihydrotestosterone). This estrogen is sufficient to alter the animal's brain and to permit development of normal male sexual behavior. High doses of estrogen, given to females during the critical period, overwhelm the alpha-fetoprotein protection and have a masculinizing effect.

NEUROMODULATION OF PAIN

Three levels of the neuraxis are involved in the perception of pain: the *periaqueductal,* or central, gray (*PAG*) matter of the midbrain, the medullary reticular formation, and the dorsal horn of the spinal cord. Surrounding the cerebral aqueduct of Sylvius, the PAG is a critical locus for the generation of endogenous opiates and the analgesia they produce. The PAG receives an extensive afferent input and contains a variety of opioid peptides (endogenous opiate receptor ligands, such as beta-endorphins and enkephalin) as well as nonopioid peptides (VIP, bombesin, neurotensin, and substance P), several of which generate an analgesia-like state at the dorsal horn.

Descending control of spinal nociceptors is conveyed through axons with relays in *brain stem nuclei*. Several bulbospinal monoaminergic cell groups are important, for example, serotonin-containing nucleus raphe magnus (NRM) in the ventral medulla and the catecholamine-rich nucleus reticularis paragigantocellularis (NRPG) lateral to the NRM. The descending input to spinal nociceptors is not exclusively monoaminergic: an additional population of NRM neurons contain both serotonin and substance P (Fig. 35-4).

In several animal species, a brief period of restraint is accompanied by analgesia and is followed by reflex immobility, which outlasts the original stimulus. In rats intensely restrained for 30 minutes in an acrylic plastic cage, a significant analgesia can be demonstrated with the hot plate test. Immediately following the end of the restraint and 90 minutes after, this analgesia is manifested by an increase in the escape reaction time without any change in the paw lick latency. Repeated daily restraint causes a gradual decrease in the magnitude of the analgesia, which is still present on day

4. The effect is abolished by pretreatment with naloxone (an antagonist) and with hypophysectomy.

The most common immobility response observed in experimental settings is the so-called *animal hypnosis*, or tonic immobility, which may be induced by a few seconds of restraint in the *sitting* (sheep) or in the *inverted* or supine position (rabbit). In rabbits, the tonic immobility is sharply reduced following *denervation of the carotid sinus*. In addition, its duration is increased after ablation of the dorsal *hippocampus* and is decreased by lesions of the dorsal column.

Analgesia is observed during both restraint and tonic immobility, but the mechanisms underlying this analgesic effect are probably different. In the rabbit, the physiological modifications that occur during the restraining period of induction do not necessarily continue once the immobility response is elicited. Restraint stress and tonic immobility are apparently different adaptation responses to potentially threatening situations.

PEPTIDES AS NEUROTRANSMITTERS

Extracts of lungs cause vasodilation that is not due to histamine (Said, 1960). The vasodilator component, named vasoactive intestinal peptide (VIP) by SAID and MUTT, has been found in brain and nerves.

A population of noradrenergic ganglion cells of guinea pig was found to be immunoreactive to somatostatin (HOK-FELT, 1977). Just like monoamines, somatostatin decreased gastric acid secretion.

The coexistence of classic neurotransmitters and peptides is common, the action of the former is to *prolong the effect* of the latter (Table 35-1).

Another challenging aspect of the peptides is the pervasiveness of the opioid peptides in the body. Functional data indicate that opioid peptides have many functions other than modulation of pain perception (Table 35-2).

The current concept is that *sleep* is promoted by peptides instead of by humoral factors. The direct transfer into rats of cerebrospinal fluid (CSF), collected from sleep-de-

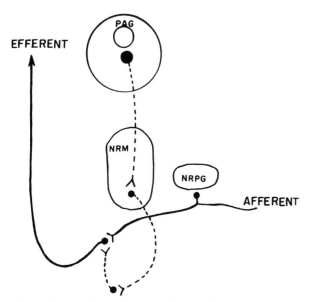

Figure 35-4 Modulation at an afferent-efferent synapse. Antinociceptive projection originating from the periaqueductal gray (PAG) matter on several nuclei located in the rostral medulla (- - -), including the *nucleus raphis magnus* (NRM), and the nucleus reticularis paragigantocellularis (NRPG). Axons from NRM (and NRPG) convey analgesia through the dorsolateral funiculus to inhibit dorsal horn nociceptors. While analgesia generated from NRM involves serotonin-containing axons, analgesia elicited from NRPG is mediated by norepinephrine.

TABLE 35-1 Coexistence of Classic Transmitter with Neuropeptides

Classic Transmitter	Neuropeptides	Tissue
ACh	Enkephalin	Preganglionic nerves
	Neurotensin	Preganglionic nerves
	Somatostatin	Heart
	VIP	Autonomic ganglia
Dopamine	CCK	Brain
	Enkephalin	Carotid body
Epinephrine	BPP	Medulla oblongata
	Enkephalin	Adrenal medulla
GABA	Motilin	Cerebellum
	Somatostatin	Thalamus
Serotonin (SHT)	Substance P	Medulla oblongata
	TRH	Medulla oblongata
Norepinephrine	Enkephalin	Sympathetic ganglia
	Neurotensin	Adrenal medulla
	Somatostatin	Sympathetic ganglia

TABLE 35–2 Evidence for Physiological Functions
of Endogenous Opioid Peptides

Physiological Role	Representative Evidence
Cardiovascular regulation	Beta-endorphin: systemic administration produces hypotension in rats. Naloxone protects rats from hypovolemic shock.
Digestive tract	Naloxone reverses diarrhea in mice induced by prostaglandin $F_{2\alpha}$, bethanechol, or serotonin.
Feeding behavior	Naloxone abolishes overeating in genetically obese (ob/ob) rats.
Glucose metabolism	Enkephalin analog produces hypoglycemia in man.
Mental processes	Naloxone abolishes schizophrenic hallucinations.
Neuroendocrine functions	Beta-endorphin secreted concomitantly with ACTH by the adenohypophysis stimulates secretion of prolactin (PRL) and growth hormone (GH) in vivo.
Renal function	Beta-endorphin stimulates renal ornithine decarboxylase in rats.
Respiratory response	Metenkephalin applied to ventral brain stem of cats depresses respiration. Naloxone increases carbon dioxide–stimulated respiration in rabbits.
Sexual behavior	Naloxone induces copulatory behavior in sexually inactive rats.

prived goats, induces an excess of slow-wave sleep (SWS). In sleep-deprived animals, the amino acid analyses of the sleep-promoting substance "substance S," isolated from CSF or urine, reveal a muramyl peptide comprised of muramic acid, alanine, glutamine, Glu, and diaminopimelic acid in molar ratios of 1 : 2 : 1 : 1 : 1. Other substances also affect sleep or drowsiness following eating, or postcoital nervous exhaustion in males: delta sleep–inducing peptide (DSIP), arginine-vasotocin, (4-10) ACTH, arginine-vasotocin, and VIP.

DSIP is a nonapeptide isolated from the dialysate of cerebral venous blood of rabbits during "hypnogenic" stimulation of the hypothalamus. Systemic administration (30 nmol per kg) or intracerebroventricular administration (7 nmol per kg) is active but not dose dependent in rabbits or cats. *Arginine-vasotocin* (nonapeptide) is synthesized in the pineal gland (epiphysis) and in the subcommissural organ. Its level increases in the CSF after phases of paradoxical sleep (humans), but in the cat it induces only SWS. Both *(4-10) ACTH* and *arginine-vasotocin* alter the frequency of hippocampal (theta) rhythm during paradoxical sleep. Depending on the time of injection, the VIP also has hypnogenic effects. When VIP (100 ng) is administered in the cat during the light period (at 10:00 a.m.), the total duration of paradoxical sleep is increased by 15 hours. When VIP is injected during the dark period (at 6:00 p.m.), it significantly prolongs the duration of SWS by 18 percent and that of paradoxical sleep by 65 percent.

REFERENCES

Amit Z, Galina SH. Stress-induced analgesia. Adaptive pain suppression. Physiol Rev 1986;66:1091.

Bonsfield D. Neurotransmitters in actions. Amsterdam: Elsevier Biomedical Press, 1985.

Porro CA, Carli C. Immobilization and restraint effects on pain reactions in animals. Pain 1988;32:289.

Willer JC, Roby A, Lebars D. Human nociceptive reactions. Brain 1984;107:1095.

THERMOREGULATION AND METABOLISM

CHAPTER 36

BODY TEMPERATURE AND ENERGY EXCHANGE

Under the usual circumstances, the animal body is continually losing or gaining heat by evaporation, radiation, convection, and conduction. To maintain a constant temperature, the homeothermic animal establishes an equilibrium between heat loss and heat production. A slight increase in body temperature causes great changes in chemical reaction rates. For example, a rise of 10°C in body temperature doubles or triples the rate of many physiological metabolic processes. If body temperature is not held nearly constant but varies with that of the environment, as in cold-blooded (*poikilothermic*) animals (e.g., lizards), the subtle neuroendocrine regulatory mechanisms are either not operative or are inadequate.

Homeotherms are animals whose metabolic activities are appropriate to maintaining a nearly constant internal body temperature (Fig. 36–1). As a result, the chemical reactions of the physiological processes occur at constant rates, whatever the environmental temperature. The *hibernators* are exceptions among the homeotherms. During hibernation, to save energy, these animals adjust by lowering their body temperature to just a few degrees above the ambient temperature.

CORE TEMPERATURE

The body of an animal may be considered as having an inner core held at a constant temperature (near 39°C in many mammals) and an outer shell capable of changing its temperature. The body strives to keep a definite core temperature, which is achieved at the expense of the shell (skin) temperature.

About 66 percent, or two thirds, of the body mass is at the core temperature, which is represented by the rectal temperature (T_{re}) or some other measure of internal temperature (e.g., oral). The remaining third of the body mass is composed of the shell or skin and is at skin temperature (T_s). The mean body temperature (T_b) may be expressed by the equation: $T_b = 0.33\,T_s + 0.67\,T_{re}$.

HEAT LOSS

Heat loss occurs by *evaporative*, or *insensible*, heat loss and by *nonevaporative*, or *sensible*, heat loss. Heat is lost by evaporation of the water molecules, which continuously diffuse through the permeable skin. Insensible perspiration represents about 20 to 25 percent of the basal heat produc-

tion lost by evaporation. Evaporative heat loss is increased greatly by sweating, panting, and profuse salivation during heat stress. Convection, radiation, and conduction are the processes of nonevaporative, or sensible, heat loss, which decrease during hot temperatures. Convection is increased by wind or water immersion; radiation heat is lost as a form of electromagnetic waves; and conduction heat loss occurs by direct exchange between the skin and the environment.

METABOLIC HEAT PRODUCTION

The metabolic activities of the entire organism constantly supply heat and may be regarded as the metabolic heat source. Metabolism, or heat production, ranges from a basal level (when the body is resting) to a level that may be 20 times higher (during heavy muscular activity). During exposure to cold temperatures, shivering (which increases skeletal muscle activity) may increase metabolic heat production approximately fivefold. During exposure to heat, the basal metabolic rate cannot be lowered by the temperature-regulating processes.

Cells use carbohydrates, fats, and proteins to synthesize large quantities of adenosine triphosphate (ATP). Since ATP is used as an energy source for many cellular functions, it is a sort of energy "currency." Indeed, cells transfer energy from the different foodstuffs to functional systems mostly through ATP or the very similar nucleotide, guanosine triphosphate (GTP).

Each gram of carbohydrate, since it is oxidized to carbon dioxide (CO_2) and water, yields about 4.1 kilocalories (kcal), which is equivalent to 17.2 kilojoules (kJ), as 1 kcal = 4.185 kJ. The metabolism of 1 g of the average dietary protein liberates about 4.35 kcal (18.2 kJ), as it is oxidized to carbon dioxide, water, and urea. The calorigenic value of 1 g of lipid is about 9.3 kcal (38.9 kJ), about twice that of glucose or amino acids. The metabolism of 1 g of the usual volatile fatty acids generates an energy of 3.5 kcal (14.6 kJ) with acetic acid, 5.0 kcal (20.8 kJ) with propionic acid, and 6.0 kcal (24.9 kJ) with butyric acid.

ATP is highly valuable as an energy currency because of the large quantity of *free energy* (7,300 kcal, or 30,550 kJ, per mole, under physiological conditions) vested in each of its two high-energy phosphate bonds. During muscle contraction, an enzyme, myosin, causes breakdown of ATP into adenosine diphosphate (ADP). During active transport across membranes, ATP provides the energy necessary to oppose the electrochemical gradient. About 70 kcal per $kg^{0.75}$ is required for the chemical processes that make it

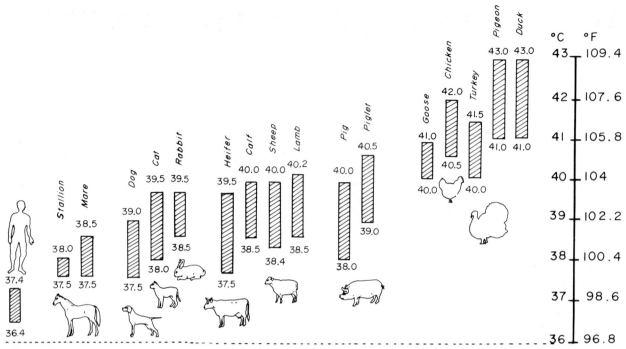

Figure 36–1 Range (Celsius and Fahrenheit) of normal rectal tempertures in domestic animals; man is included for comparison. Temperatures are higher in animals than in man, and the highest are in birds.

possible for the cells of an animal to continue living or to function physiologically.

Fasting Metabolism

The fasting metabolism of homeotherms (from mice to cattle), expressed in kilocalories or kilojoules per day, is about 70 kcal per $kg^{0.75}$, or 293 kJ per $kg^{0.75}$. Slight differences occur among animal species (Table 36–1). The relationship $kg^{0.75}$ is termed the *metabolic weight,* a concept that is used to compute the energy expenditure and requirements, the work of various organs (heart, kidneys, lungs), and various parameters of drug metabolism.

TABLE 36–1   Fasting Metabolism in Animal Species of Various Sizes

Species	Mass (kg)	kcal/day*	kcal/kg	kcal/m²†
Cat	4	285	71	1140
Chicken	2	120	60	750
Cow	600	8500	14	1250
Dog	15	535	36	1160
Horse	500	7400	15	1225
Man	65	1600	25	1020
Mouse	0.02	3.7	185	465
Pig	100	2200	22	1055
Rabbit	2	120	60	750
Rat	0.25	25	100	625
Sheep	50	1300	26	985

*kcal/day = 70 × $kg^{0.75}$
†S (m²) = 0.1 × $kg^{0.66}$

Heat Increment of Food

The factors that increase the heat production of foods are the energy cost of eating, the work of digestion, and the work of nutrient metabolism. The energy value of eating is about 8 kcal per kg per minute in cattle (Table 36–2). The extra energy linked to eating may be only 53 kcal when a sheep is fed concentrates, but it may be as much as 129 kcal when a sheep is eating fresh grass (Table 36–3).

Ruminant animals can be supported entirely by intraruminal infusion of volatile fatty acids, casein, and other essential nutrients (i.e., without any oral feed intake, rumination, and rumen fermentation). In these energy-sparing animals, there is *no energy cost for eating, for rumination, and for fermentation.* In normal animals, the energy costs for these activities amount to about 25 percent of the daily heat expenditure associated with food.

TABLE 36–2   Energy Loss in Cattle at Pasture and in Confined Cattle

	Energy Loss (kcal/day)	
Activity	Confined	At Pasture
Eating	880	1,880
Standing	0	380
Changing position	0	70
Walking	240	1,500

Extra energy cost at pasture 2.5 Mcal/d
Confinement maintenance heat 11.9 Mcal/d
Pasture heat loss 14.3 Mcal/d
Extra heat loss due to activity 9–32%

TABLE 36–3 Heat Increment of Food in a 50-kg Sheep Fed 4,000 kcal (Twice the Maintenance Requirement)

	Chopped Hay (kcal)	Fresh Grass (kcal)
Total heat increment of food	1,800	1,875
Ingestion and digestion heat loss		
Eating	55	110
Fermentation	320	320
Rumination	30	30
Digestion	85	85
Percentage of Total heat increment of food	(27.2)	(29.1)
Heat of nutrient metabolism	1,310	1,330

The *work of digestion*—the mechanical and secretory processes associated with the presence of food in the gastrointestinal tract—accounts for 10 percent of the daily energy requirements. The *work of nutrient metabolism* accounts for about 65 to 70 percent of total heat generated by food. In adult ruminants, the work of nutrient metabolism refers to nutrients used for maintenance requirements and for energy retention (almost entirely as stored fat).

Maintenance Requirement

Maintenance requirement is that amount of food energy that is needed to balance exactly heat production. In adult cattle, the maintenance requirement is about 112 kcal per $kg^{0.75}$ per day, or about 1.4 times fasting metabolism. Animals expend that amount of energy whether they are confined in a calorimeter or sheltered on the farm. The energy cost of activity depends on the energy cost of each activity per unit of time and on the additional time spent in each activity. The extra energy costs of major activities occurring while the animal is in the pasture are about 10 percent more than the cost in confinement (see Table 36–2).

THERMONEUTRAL ENVIRONMENT AND HOMEOTHERMY

An environment that is neither too cold nor too hot is thermoneutral. Metabolic heat production in such conditions is minimal and is not affected by air temperature. At negligible energy cost, the animal regulates its body temperature only by adjusting its heat loss.

Sensible (perceptible) heat loss is determined mostly by climatic factors—air temperature and wind speed (convection), rain or snow (conduction), and radiation exchanges. Protection against sensible heat loss is provided by two layers of thermal insulation: tissue insulation of the body shell, and external insulation by hair coat or wool and the air trapped in and on them. *Tissue insulation* is fixed partly by physical factors (thickness of the skin and subcutaneous fat) but more by the rate of blood flow through the body shell. Tissue insulation is maximal when vasoconstriction is maximal. *External insulation,* related to coat thickness, protects against climatic factors such as wind and precipitation. Food intake, a major determinant of heat production related to metabolic mass ($kg^{0.75}$), is also an important determinant of tolerance to cold. Among animals with similar thermal insulation, the more cold-tolerant and the more productive ones are those with the greatest food intake.

Thermal Neutrality Zone

The thermal neutrality zone (TNZ), or the comfort zone, is the preferred environment for optimal production (i.e., the animal derives maximal benefit from food intake). Metabolic energy cost is minimal in this interval, which is bounded by calorigenic zones on each side (Fig. 36–2).

Homeothermy refers to the maintenance of the core

Figure 36–2 Diagram of heat production (HP) at low and high ambient temperatures. The thermoneutral zone (TNZ) is bounded on each side by the lower and upper critical temperatures (LCT and UCT) at points A and D. The TNZ, in terms of ambient temperature, is between 13 and 25°C for calves, 0 and 15°C for cows, −2 and 20°C for ewes, and 0 and 15°C for pigs.

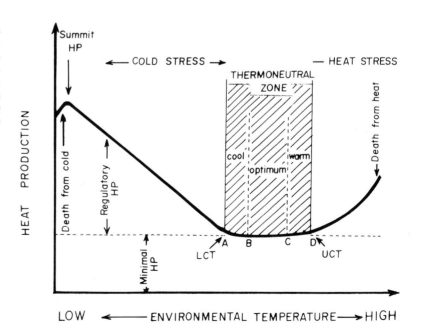

temperature by an increase in *heat production* (HP) corresponding to the *heat loss* (HL) exaggerated by a low ambient temperature (cold stress at the lower critical temperature [LCT]). Above the upper critical temperature (UCT), HP and core temperature are increased because the greater insensible heat loss is still insufficient to compensate adequately (Fig. 36–3). *Direct calorimetry* is the measurement of HL from an animal confined in a respiration calorimeter. *Indirect calorimetry* is the measurement of HP from an animal's respiratory gas exchange.

Direct Calorimetry for Measurement of Heat Loss

Direct calorimetry is used to measure HL by the body and to convert it in terms of heat production or energy production. Energy loss is measured as the sum of sensible and insensible (evaporative) heat loss in the respiration calorimeter.

The *respiration calorimeter* consists of a chamber with insulated walls supporting cold water pipes for cooling, electrical elements for heating, thermocouples for measuring temperature, and meters of air ventilation flow rate and water vapor. Heat flow through the chamber wall is prevented, and the heat generated is absorbed by the circulating water pipes inside the chamber. Nonevaporative heat loss is calculated from the heat removed into the circulating water. This requires finding temperature differences across the water inlet and outlet and measuring flow rate or volume of water. The evaporative water loss is calculated from the ventilation air flow rate and the water vapor content of the ingoing and outgoing air. At an environmental temperature of 25°C, every gram of evaporated water represents a heat loss of 0.6 kcal.

The respiration calorimeter is now replaced by the *thermoelectrical*, or *gradient*, *calorimeter*. The newer gradient calorimeter requires measurement only of the nonevaporative heat loss. This apparatus permits simple, rapid, and reliable measurement of sensible (convection, conduction, and radiation) heat loss. The response time of the gradient calorimeter is less than 1 minute.

Metabolism is expressed in terms of the metabolic size (i.e., kcal per $kg^{0.75}$). As heat loss is related to body surface, metabolism can be expressed in terms of body surface area (kcal per hr per m^2) instead of the more acceptable metabolic size. Meeh's formula for evaluating the surface of animals is

$$S \ m^2 = k \times kg^{0.66}$$

with 0.1 representing the average value of k, which varies slightly between animals (e.g., pig, 0.087; sheep, 0.121).

Indirect Calorimetry for Measurement of Heat Production

Also known as respiratory calorimetry, indirect calorimetry involves estimation of metabolic heat production of an animal from its respiratory gas exchange.

Types of Respiratory Calorimetry

Indirect calorimetry can be an open-circuit or a closed-circuit method.

LAVOISIER (1790) first recognized that animal heat is derived from oxidation of substances in the body and from absorbed oxygen (i.e., indirect calorimetry). Closed-circuit apparatuses to measure oxygen consumption were built for

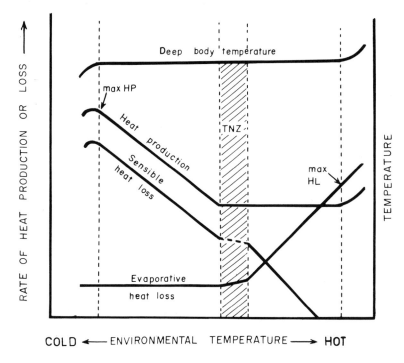

Figure 36–3 The core temperature is stable until the animal reaches its maximum ability to generate heat (summit rate, or max HP) or until the maximum rate of evaporative heat loss (max HL) is attained. The LCT may be −40°C in small arctic mammals with fur thickness of 50 to 70 mm.

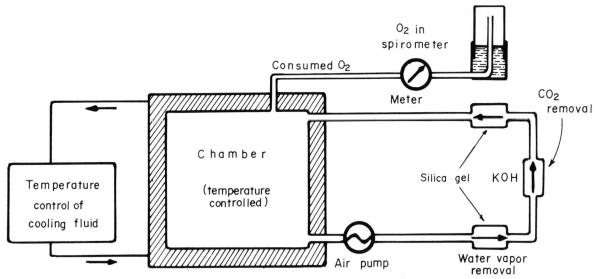

Figure 36–4 Principle of closed-circuit indirect calorimetry for measurement of respiratory exchange. Chamber air is forced through silica gel to remove exhaled water vapor and then through potassium hydroxide and silica gel in tandem to remove carbon dioxide and the reaction water. The quantity of pure oxygen admitted to replace the amount consumed is measured from a spirometer. A temperature control unit pipes cooling fluid in the walls of the chamber to keep the inside temperature constant.

dogs by REGNAULT and REISET in 1849 (Fig. 36–4), for horses by ZUNTZ in 1885, and for cattle by ARMSBY in 1887. In 1886, open-circuit apparatuses (PETTEN-KOFFER and VOIT, and KELLNER) were designed to measure carbon dioxide production. Starch equivalent values were calculated from the results of indirect calorimetry and became the basis of early feeding standards in cattle (1886). A starch unit (also known as a Kellner unit) represents 2,360 kcal.

In the *open-circuit* method, the animal breathes air from the outside, while its exhaled air volume is measured. The volume of oxygen consumed per minute ($\dot{V}O_2$) is calculated by measuring the oxygen in the expired air. Open-circuit calorimetry requires three major steps: (1) collection of the exhaled air, (2) measurement of its volume, and (3) analysis of its O_2, CH_4, and CO_2 content (Fig. 36–5).

In *closed-circuit* calorimetry, the animal is completely cut off from the outside air and breathes from and into a spirometer (a reservoir containing a known volume of O_2). The expired air is circulated over silica gel to remove the water vapor and over a carbon dioxide absorber (silica gel and potassium hydroxide) to remove the carbon dioxide. The volume of pure O_2 lost in this closed system represents the oxygen consumption (VO_2) over a given period of time (Fig. 36–5).

Thermal Equivalents of Oxygen

The utilization of oxygen produces quantities of energy, which vary with the substrate oxidized. The energy produced by 1 L of oxygen when glucose ($C_6H_{12}O_6$) is oxidized is 5.007 kcal; that is, 673 kcal $\div$ (6×22.4) = 5.007 kcal of heat. This is in accordance with the equation in which the oxidation of 1 mole of glucose requires 6 moles of oxygen

(i.e., $C_6H_{12}O_6 + 6 O_2 = 6 H_2O + 6 CO_2 + 673$ kcal). Thus, 134.4 L, or 6×22.4 L, of O_2 yields 673 kcal, and 1 L of O_2 = 5.007 kcal. When a mixture of carbohydrates is oxidized, the thermal equivalent of 1 L of oxygen is 5.047 kcal.

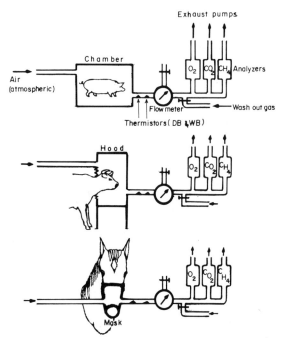

Figure 36–5 Principles of open-circuit indirect calorimetry for measurement of respiratory exchange. Air expired (into a chamber, hood, or mask) by an animal is measured and is forced over thermistors that record dry bulb (DB) and wet bulb (WB) temperatures. Gas analyzers measure the concentrations of oxygen, carbon dioxide, and methane in the expired air.

Whereas oxidation of a mixture of fats generates 4.686 kcal per liter of O_2, the oxidation of tripalmitin (C_3H_5 $(OOC.C_{15}H_{31})_3$) produces 7,657 kcal per 1,624 L or 4.71 kcal per liter of O_2. Tripalmitin requires 72.5 moles of oxygen (1,624 L) to be converted into 51 CO_2 and 49 H_2O and yields 7,657 kcal.

Animals do not obtain energy exclusively from either carbohydrates or fats but from carbohydrates, fats, and proteins in various mixtures. The proportion of each type of compound is globally reflected in the value of the *respiratory quotient* (RQ), the ratio of the volume of CO_2 produced by the animal and the volume of O_2 it uses to oxidize the nutrients. From standard tables, a thermal equivalent value (for 1 L of O_2) can be determined for each value of the RQ; values vary from 0.7 kcal per L for lipids (e.g., tripalmitin, 51 $CO_2/72.5$ O_2) to 1.0 for carbohydrates (e.g., glucose, 6 $CO_2/6$ O_2). The proportions of fat and carbohydrate can also be determined from standard tables. For example, 0.9, which is the RQ for oxidation of a mixture of 32.5 percent fat and 67.5 percent carbohydrate, indicates that the thermal equivalent of oxygen for this mixture is 4.924 kcal per L.

Food mixtures also include protein, which is incompletely oxidized in animals because the body cannot oxidize nitrogen. The average amount of heat produced by the catabolism of 1 g of protein is 4.3 kcal, and 0.77 L of CO_2 is produced as 0.96 L of oxygen is used (Table 36–4). The average RQ associated with utilization of protein is 0.8 kcal per L (i.e., $0.77/0.96 = 0.8$). An estimate of the quantity of protein catabolized is obtained from the nitrogen excreted in the urine (1 g of protein = 0.16 g of urinary N).

Respiratory Calorimetry in Ruminants

In ruminants, anaerobic ruminoreticulum fermentation of carbohydrates yields combustible gases, principally methane (CH_4). A correction for this effect is necessary to calculate heat production with indirect calorimetry methods (i.e., from analyses of respiratory CO_2 production and O_2 consumption). The simplest correction is to deduct 0.5 kcal for each liter of CH_4. An alternative method of overcoming this problem is to calculate heat production by using only oxygen consumption. Using an RQ of 0.82 and a thermal equivalent value of 4.8 kcal per L, which assumes oxidation solely of fat and carbohydrate, introduces an error of less than 3.5 percent.

Another simplification is possible concerning protein metabolism in ruminants. The assumed thermal equivalent of oxygen when protein is catabolized is 4.5 kcal. Because only a small portion of the heat production is from protein oxidation, it is unnecessary to assess it separately, and urinary nitrogen excretion need not be considered.

Body Mechanisms of Heat Loss

Dissipation of heat from the body and maintenance of body temperature within a range that is normal for an animal species involve the skin and the respiratory system. Heat loss occurs through the channels of evaporation (insensible perspiration, sweating, respiratory evaporation, and panting), or radiation (vasomotion), of conduction, and of convection (vasomotion) (Fig. 36–6). Evaporative heat loss operates even when the external temperature is above body temperature, but then nonevaporative heat loss is not possible and the body tends to be warmed instead of cooled.

Evaporative Heat Loss

Evaporation of water is accompanied by loss of heat from the body or a cooling effect in bare-skinned (pig or man) and in short-haired animals (horse). At 25°C, the evaporation of 1 g of water dissipates 0.6 kcal of energy. Loss of energy per unit of time by animals is sometimes expressed in watts: 1 kcal per hr = 1.16 W = 4.185 kJ. In fur-coated animals, evaporation takes heat largely from the surrounding air and does not cool the body efficiently.

TABLE 36–4 Heat Production from Respiratory Gases and Urinary Nitrogen Excretion in a Calf

Experimental results (24 hr)	
Oxygen used (L)	390
Carbon dioxide produced (L)	311
Urine nitrogen (g)	15
Energy from protein catabolism	
Protein metabolized (g) (6.25 × 15)	93.8
Heat production (kcal) (4.3 × 93.8)	403
Oxygen used (L) (0.96 × 93.8)	90
Carbon dioxide produced (L) (0.77 × 93.8)	72
Energy from carbohydrate and fat metabolism	
Oxygen used (L) (390—90)	300
Carbon dioxide produced (L) (311—72)	239
Nonprotein RQ (243.5/306)	0.80
Thermal equivalent at RQ 0.80	4.8
Heat Production (kcal) (4.8 × 300)	1,440
Total energy produced (kcal) (403 + 1,440)	1,843

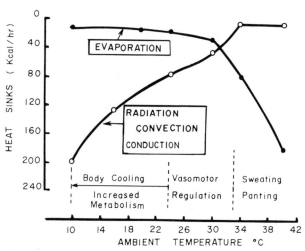

Figure 36–6 Nonevaporative (radiation, convection, and conduction) and evaporative (sweating, panting) partition of heat losses by animals at different ambient temperatures.

Insensible Perspiration

Water diffuses continuously through the skin, which is not waterproof. Sanctorius (1616) observed this *insensible perspiration,* which differs from sweat, during careful body weight studies. Evaporation of this water on the body surface is considered to be a heat sink. An animal can maintain its thermal equilibrium by dissipating all of its heat production by evaporating water from the body surface. For example, a 100-kg animal must produce 240 g of water per hour for cutaneous evaporation to balance its hourly metabolic heat production (i.e., $0.6 \times 240 = 144$ kcal per hr, or 167 W, or 603 kJ). At thermal neutrality, the amounts of energy lost by cutaneous and respiratory routes are about equal. At higher environmental temperatures, the respiratory contribution is usually higher (sheep, pig), except in cattle, in which skin heat losses are twice those of the upper respiratory tract (nasal, tracheal).

Sweating

The evaporation of the watery secretion (apocrine in cattle, eccrine in man) sweat is important for heat loss under hot conditions. Some animals (cattle, horses, camels) can sweat very profusely, whereas others (pig, dog, cat, wildebeest, Grant's gazelle) cannot. Zebu cattle (*Bos indicus*) are more heat tolerant than European cattle (*Bos taurus*). This greater resistance to heat stress, or prostration, is due mostly to more heat loss from their body by evaporation, primarily because of more numerous and larger cutaneous sweat glands. This also helps reflect solar radiation by giving a sheen to the hair coat under hot conditions.

Some animals (mice, kangaroos) wet their hair coat by licking when conditions are very hot. Animals with relatively poor sweating response compensate by panting, which is a type of respiratory evaporative cooling. Animals with wool coats that get wet in rainy or snowy weather benefit from an exothermic reaction between wool fibers and water.

Respiratory Evaporative Loss

Movements of air over the upper respiratory surfaces produce evaporation in a manner similar to the effect of wind on a moist body surface. The mucosa lining the respiratory tract gives up water to saturate the inspired air. When air is expired, some water condenses on the mucosa, and some nonevaporative heat is returned to the mucosa. Because of these savings in heat and water, the temperature of expired air is lower than the core temperature of the body and carries less water vapor. In some desert animals (camel, donkey, kangaroo rat), this respiratory water conservation is considerable.

Panting, or *thermal polypnea,* effects evaporative cooling of the nasal mucosa blood by the rapid movements of air over the wet mucosa of the vasodilated turbinate region of the nasopharynx. Most domestic animals pant when they are overheated to a point where the rectal temperature is elevated above 39 to 41°C (102 to 106°F), depending on the species. The horse is an exception, as it cannot pant. It adapts to heat by increasing the frequency of respiration while reducing the tidal volume.

Availability of water is critical to thermal adaptation because most heat loss mechanisms involve evaporation of body water to enhance cooling. In cattle, the water required to moisten the mucosa of the turbinate is provided by small mucosal glands and a diffuse lateral nasal gland. Dogs have a lateral nasal gland with a duct that opens near the external nares, and its secretion is increased during panting. Dogs, cats, and sheep use panting as their main mode of evaporative heat loss. Sheep can tolerate high environmental temperatures (43.4°C, or 110°F, and above), provided that relative humidity stays below 65 percent. In cattle, which pant with the mouth closed, this thermal hyperpnea is not as efficient as evaporative heat loss by sweating, which is well developed in Zebu cattle.

Pigs are very sensitive to heat and cannot tolerate high temperatures unless the environmental air is very dry. For pigs, neither panting nor evaporative heat loss by sweating is effective in hot conditions. Shade seeking (by most species) and wallowing in water (buffalo) or mud (pigs) are important behavioral adaptations to excessive heat.

In thermal polypnea, panting, or the first phase of rapid shallow breathing, the tidal air volume is small. Air moves from the dead space, increasing the minute volume by 10-fold in cattle, 12-fold in sheep, 15-fold in rabbits, and 23-fold in dogs. The carbon dioxide loss is not excessive and does not disturb the acid-base equilibrium (i.e., no respiratory alkalosis). In cattle under severe heat stress, *thermal hyperpnea,* or second-phase breathing, increases the alveolar ventilation up to five-fold and causes greater losses of carbon dioxide and respiratory alkalosis, with a blood pH of 7.7.

Blood cooled by panting drains into the venous sinuses at the base of the skull, where it joins with blood draining the ears (and horns). From there, this pooled-blood circulates in the *rete mirabile,* a network of small arteries that supply blood to the base of the brain. The *rete mirabile* may function in countercurrent heat exchanges, the blood supplying the brain being cooled by blood draining the nasal mucosa, the ears, and the horns (Fig. 36-7).

Signs of distress from overheating tend to develop suddenly and can be life threatening when rectal temperature exceeds 41.7°C (107°F) in cattle and 40.6°C (105°F) in pigs. Loss of water and of electrolytes leads to hemoconcentration and neurological disorders, with panting and frothy oronasal discharges.

Nonevaporative Heat Loss

Radiant Heat Loss

Some body heat is lost by radiant heat transfer. Radiant heat (long and short waves) emitted by the skin is transmitted easily through polyethylene (used to reduce the convective heat loss due to wind). In contrast, long-wave radiant energy is absorbed by, or does not pass through, opaque cloth and materials such as glass and most plastics.

When the environmental temperature is cold, the radiating surface of the body is reduced to lower the net radiant heat exchange. Also the cutaneous blood flow may be reduced to minimal values, because of *vasoconstriction.* The

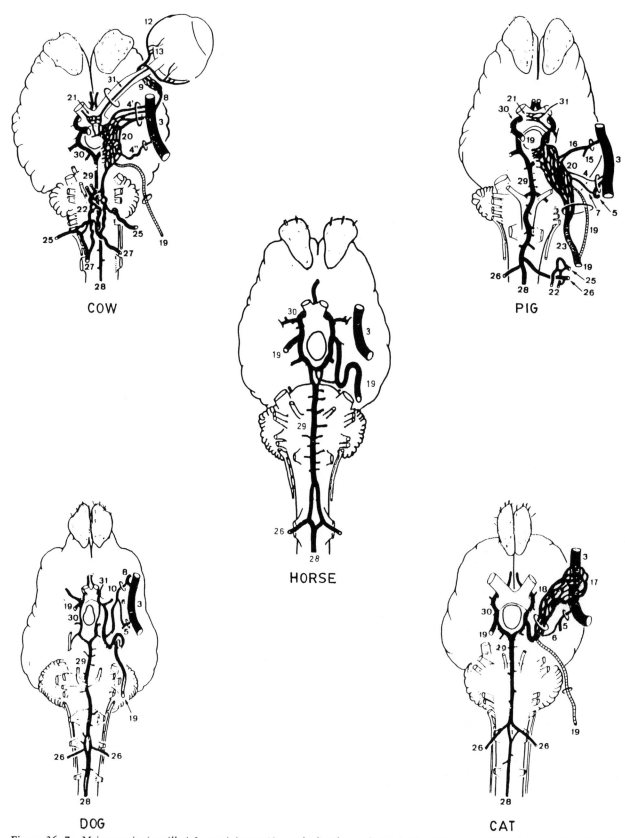

Figure 36–7 Major arteries (*maxillaris* 3, *carotis interna* 19, *vertebralis* 26, *spinalis* 28, *basilaris* 29, and *circulus arteriosus cerebri* 30) to the brain of domestic animals. In horses, the *maxillaris* (3) supplies very little blood (if any) to the cerebral arterial circle (30), in contrast with the other species. Extensive development of the *rami retis* (18) occurs in cats, and the *rete mirabile* (20) is prominent in oxen and pigs.

difference between outgoing and incoming radiant energy becomes minimal and favors absorbing heat.

Cold-induced opening of arteriovenous shunts in some extremities (ear, limbs) of the body results in *vasodilation* that may increase peripheral blood flow by 100-fold to raise skin temperature. This response, which prevents frostbite damage to the tissues, causes increased heat loss by radiation and by convection. It tends to be cyclical in some species, the so-called "hunting reaction." In conditions of heat stress, the overall skin blood flow may increase by 10-fold.

Thermography provides an image of the surface temperatures over the body of an animal. A picture, comparable to one on black-and-white or color television, represents the precise instantaneous flux of thermal radiation energy within the field of view of the thermography camera. For fur-coated animals, the surface imaged by the camera is some layer within the coat. Equilibrium temperature in this layer represents heat lost by radiation and convection, conduction of heat through the coat, and exchange of thermal (long-wave) and short-wave radiation. A thermogram of the surface of a black-and-white cow in the shade shows an almost uniform distribution of heat. Within a few minutes after exposure to weak thermal radiation, the same cow's coat shows a visible difference in radiant heat loss between the white and the black areas: the *black spots are hotter* than the white ones by about 8 to 10°C, because the black coat absorbs heat and the white coat reflects it.

Convection

Convection heat loss, the transfer of heat by redistribution of molecules within a fluid (air or water), is related to properties of the surface of the animal body and of the environmental air. Temperature, shape, hair coat, and body surface area, together with temperature and displacement rate of air, affect the amount of convective heat exchange.

Forced and Natural Convection. The convection movement of molecules in air or water may result from an external force or from a buoyancy force due to temperature differences in the fluid. An example of forced convection is the propulsion of air by a fan, and a special form of forced convective heat loss occurs when cold inspired air passes over structures of the upper respiratory tract. Natural or free convection occurs when air rises from a warmed or heated surface.

Convection is mostly forced when wind impinges on an animal's body, and mostly natural or free at low wind speeds and in still air. In pigs, forced convection dominates when wind velocity is above 0.2 m per second, and natural convection occurs below 0.1 m per second. The convective heat flow around the body may be turbulent with forced convection, or laminar (streamlined) with natural convection. In still air (up to 8 cm per second), the natural convection boundary layer of air around the body is the zone through which convective heat exchange takes place. The movement of air by natural convection over the surface of animals, and the associated boundary layer, can be made visible by Schlieren photography. When air is still, pigs (with sparse hair, fewer than 1000 hairs per cm^2) lose heat by both radiation and convection, in contrast with rabbits and horses (with dense fur), which lose heat mostly by convection.

Conduction

Conductance is the reciprocal of insulation. Heat dissipation by conduction does not involve actual translocation of molecules but contact with a cold substance (solid or liquid). Conduction heat loss may be considerable for animals that lie on the ground or on the floor of enclosures. The rate of heat transfer from an animal body to the floor is determined by thermal diffusibility (i.e., the ratio of thermal conductance to thermal capacity) of the solid surface. Heat is lost until the floor temperature is raised to the body temperature, the lower the diffusibility the more heat is required until thermoequilibrium is attained. A posture that reduces the area of the body in contact with the cold floor and reduced blood flow in the skin area in contact with the cold floor are means used by animals to decrease the conductive heat loss. In this situation, some heat is also lost by convection from the parts of the body facing the floor. Pigs may lose as much heat by conductivity as by radiation and convection combined. In the neonate pig, conduction heat loss is about 15 percent on a concrete floor, 6 percent on a wooden floor, and only 2 percent on expanded polystyrene. Actions to decrease the conductive heat loss on a concrete floor include covering it with wood planking or with a bedding (about 2.5 cm or 1 inch). The thermal quality of such a bedding decreases from woodwool, to straw, to wood shaving. Conduction heat loss by a sheep resting on cold ground may represent 30 percent of its total metabolic energy production. When fur is compressed, wetted, or soiled by urine, it loses the high insulating capacity provided by air trapped between hairs. Consequently, larger conductive transfer of heat occurs from the warm body to the cold solid surface or to water.

In sheep and pigs, small amounts of conductive heat, about 3 percent of the total heat loss, are used to warm ingested food and fluid.

Heat Loss Mechanisms in Different Domestic Animals

The operative mechanisms for heat loss in animals differ according to species.

Cat

Cats and dogs rely mostly on heat loss by panting, since sweat glands distributed over their furred skin do not help with thermoregulation. Cats' sweat glands on the feet and toe pads respond to both thermal and psychogenic activation.

Stimulation of the peripheral end of the medial plantar nerve leads to greater hydration of the stratum corneum of the foot pads and is followed by increased evaporative water loss. Visible sweating does not represent the start of the sudomotor response but indicates the phase in which secretion is more active than its reabsorption into the stratum corneum.

The activity of the sweat glands on the foot pads is estimated by observing the appearance of droplets at the skin surface. In anesthetized cats in air-circulation capsules, objective measurements of skin evaporative loss (water vapor) are used to evaluate the secretion of foot pad sweat glands (Fig. 36–8). In addition, changes in the hydration of the stratum corneum (temperature and composition of perfusion fluid, electrical stimulation) can be studied with electrodes. Besides measuring water vapor, skin electrical potential (SP), and skin electrical conductance (SC) can then be recorded. The appearance of sweat droplets at the skin surface is preceded by a reduction in skin potential, which is then followed by a higher skin electrical conductance (see Fig. 36–8). These electrical changes correspond to the secretion of sweat and to the filling of the ducts. A delayed and slightly positive part of the SP recording is associated with passive reabsorption of sweat into the stratum corneum.

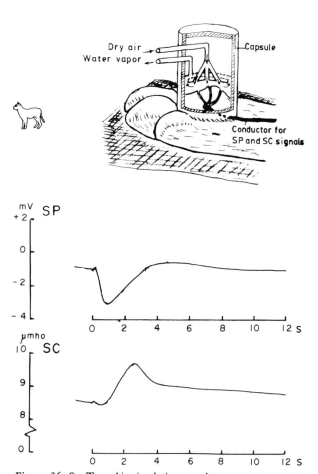

Figure 36–8 **Top,** Air circulation capsule removes water vapor from the foot pad, and electrodes detect and record skin electrical potentials (SP) and skin electrical conductance (SC) from the foot pad. **Bottom,** Foot pad responses to peripheral (medial plantar) nerve stimulation show temporal and functional relationships of SP (millivolts) and SC (micromho). SP precedes SC. SP is lowered, whereas SC is raised.

Cattle

On the body surface of cattle numerous apocrine sweat glands (about 500 per cm^2) are associated with each hair follicle and secrete a fluid with low concentrations of electrolytes. In cattle, evaporation of sweat from the skin provides more heat loss (70 percent) than respiratory evaporation. Eccrine glands, analogous to the thermoregulatory structures of man and to those on foot pads of cats and dogs, are not found on the body surface of cattle.

The apocrine sweat glands of cattle are controlled via an alpha-adrenergic transmitter system, in contrast with the eccrine glands of humans, cats, and dogs, which are regulated by cholinergic nerves. Circulating catecholamines released from the adrenal medulla do not stimulate sweating in heat-exposed cattle.

Evaporative skin heat loss mechanisms are as well developed in newborn calves as at 18 months of age, and sweating is complemented by panting (Fig. 36–9). Results with newborn and with 12-month-old calves exposed to a hot environment (40°C, with 30 percent relative humidity) indicate greater total moisture loss from the skin per metabolic body size ($W^{0.75}$) in the newborns. Young animals can produce more sweat per unit of heat-producing body mass and have a thermoregulatory advantage over older calves. The high rate of evaporation from the skin of these young animals reduces the demand for evaporative cooling from the respiratory tract. Even in an environment with a temperature of 50°C, most young calves do not breathe at the maximal rate and still have a functional reserve.

Horse

In horses exposed to high environmental temperatures, sweating is the principal means of maintaining thermal balance. Profuse sweating results from exercise, excitement, pain, and drug administration. Endurance-trained horses exercising in high environmental temperatures may lose as much as 10 to 15 kg per hr, and develop clinically significant dehydration (i.e., a 7 to 10 percent loss of body weight). For a 450-kg horse, this represents a water loss of about 30 to 45 L. Such a water loss amounts to 30 to 40 percent of the extracellular fluid volume, which is estimated to be about 100 L, or 22 percent of body weight. Water is undoubtedly drawn from the intracellular fluid as well. In such horses, the packed cell volume and plasma protein level increase, whereas serum sodium concentration remains relatively unchanged. However, hypochloremia is manifested.

The concentration of electrolytes in sweat differs according to the cause of sweating. Sweat from exercise is twice as rich in potassium and calcium as sweat resulting from beta₂-adrenergic stimulation, for example, intravenous administration of epinephrine (Table 36–5). The concentrations of other electrolytes of sweat (sodium, magnesium) are relatively increased because of the water loss, and some loss of chloride is reflected in a lower blood level of that salt.

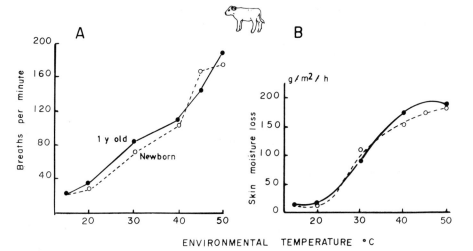

Figure 36–9 **A,** Identical mean respiratory frequencies (20 to 200 breaths per minute) of young calves (○, newborn; ●, 12-months old) exposed to increasing environmental temperatures (10 to 50°C). **B,** Water loss from the skin follows a sigmoid pattern, increasing rapidly (from about 10 to 125 g/m²/hr) in the 20 to 40°C temperature interval. The rise is slightly more sustained in the neonate than in older calves.

Pig

Porcine skin contains sweat glands that respond to alpha-adrenergic agents but not to heat stress (environmental temperature of 34°C). Water vapor diffuses passively through the skin of the pig. The direction of the diffusion across the epidermis is directed by the vapor pressure of the air. Water vapor moves from skin to the environment only at an ambient vapor pressure of less than 25 mbar. Since the maximal rate is only about 30 g per m² per hour, evaporative heat loss from the respiratory passages is required.

The respiratory response to heat stress begins when the pig's skin temperature rises above 35°C. Breathing frequency (f) and the rate of respiratory evaporative heat loss increase, whereas tidal volume, alveolar ventilation (tidal volume minus dead volume), and minute respiratory volume (tidal volume × f) drop. This thermal polypnea augments the quantity of air passing through the upper respiratory passages but not the alveolar ventilation rate. In contrast with cattle, swine are less prone to developing respiratory alkalosis because they do not readily shift from thermal polypnea to thermal hyperpnea (slower, deeper breathing) as heat stress intensifies. Indeed, pigs can raise minute respiratory volume only three-fold, as compared with the five-fold increase of which sheep are capable.

The rationale of the sweat-box, or Turkish bath, piggery system for housing pigs is questionable on physiological grounds. Proponents of this high-humidity, high-temperature, and high–stocking density environment claim that in tropical climates pigs live in high temperatures and humidity without ill effect. They also infer that sweat boxes reduce pneumonia, because disease-carrying microorganisms are adsorbed onto water droplets. Opponents of sweat boxes argue that overheating predisposes pigs to fatal cold draughts, as cold shock induces malignant hyperthermia. In cold shock, pigs overheat because they are unable to stop shivering, even when they have warmed up. Shivering and malignant hyperthermia prevent escape of heat at the surface of the body by high muscle activity and constriction of subcutaneous blood vessels. The rapid muscle activity also leads to a rapid buildup of lactic acid, raising acidity in the bloodstream, which is made worse by the high level of carbon dioxide (1 percent) in the air of sweat boxes. The rapid rise in temperature and in acidity of blood may finally cause heart collapse and dissolution of muscle proteins, producing a typical pale, soft exudative pork meat.

Adaptation to Hot Dry Environment

The kangaroo rats of the Arizona deserts have a remarkable capacity to survive long periods without water. They achieve this goal by several strategies that minimize water loss:

1. They produce very dry fecal pellets in small amounts, which they recycle via coprophagy to recapture nutrients and water.

2. They produce a minimal volume of urine that has a very high osmotic concentration of waste products.

3. They lose little water to respiratory evaporation via a heat exchanger air flow mechanism in the nasal passages that lowers the temperature of exhaled air below body temperature. In this way, about 75 percent of the water vapor in pulmonary gases is recondensed before the expired gas passes out at the nares.

4. Burrowing behavior and nocturnal habit keep them

TABLE 36–5 Concentrations of Electrolytes in Equine Sweat

	Na^+	K^+	Cl^-	Ca^{++}	Mg^{++}
Exercise-induced mEq/L (SD)	132	53	174	6	5
	(43)	(21)	(66)	(3)	(4)
Epinephrine-induced mEq/L (SD)	130	25	149	3	4
	(11)	(5)	(11)	(2)	(2)

out of the solar radiation and excessive heat of the day.

5. They produce sufficient metabolic water to sustain the water content of the body.

The camel cannot enjoy the privilege of daylight escape into burrows or of nocturnal feeding and activity, but it exploits the day-night thermal differentials by allowing its body temperature to rise during the day. The stored heat is dissipated back to the environment by radiation and conduction at night, with its body temperature often falling below normal by daybreak. In hot weather, the body temperature of the camel may fluctuate within a wide range, from 34 to 41°C.

The high daytime temperature of its body reduces the thermal gradient of heat stress. This benefit is supplemented by the insulating effect of the hair coat, which reduces water loss by up to 50 percent. If its body temperature rises above 41°C, the camel must drink, or dehydration will develop.

A remarkable feature of the camel's adaptation to desert living is its ability to tolerate severe dehydration. Unlike the dog, whose lethal limit of dehydration occurs at about 12 percent, the camel's lethal limit is about twice as much.

Finally, camels can literally extract water from pulmonary gases prior to its exhaling, particularly when they are dehydrated. In that state, the membranes of the nasal passages become dried out and coated with hygroscopic mucoid material that takes up much of the moisture in the air to be expired, releasing it again to the next wave of inspired air. When drinking water becomes available, the camel takes on a large volume of water in a short time.

REFERENCES

Adams T. Characteristics of eccrine sweat gland activity in the footpad of the cat. J Appl Physiol 1966;21:1004.

Bianca W, Hales JRS. Sweating, panting and body temperatures of newborn and one-year-old calves at high environmental temperatures. Br Vet J 1970;126:45.

Carlson GP, Ogen PO. Composition of equine sweat following exercise in high environmental temperatures and in response to intravenous epinephrine administration. J Equine Med Surg 1979;3:27.

Dawson WR. Evaporative losses of water by birds. Comp Biochem Physiol 1982;A71:495.

Hensel H. Thermoreception and temperature regulation. Monographs of the Physiological Society No. 38. London: Academic Press, 1981.

Ingram DL, Mount LE. Animals and man in hot environment. New York: Springer-Verlag, 1975.

McLean JA. The significance of carbon dioxide and methane measurements in the estimation of heat production in cattle. Br J Nutr 1986; 55:631.

Owens FN. New techniques for studying digestion and absorption of nutrients by ruminants. Fed Proc 1987;46:283.

Webb NG. Sudden deaths in sweat-box piggeries. Farm Build Prog 1980;51:13.

Yousef MK. Stress physiology in livestock. Boca Raton: CRC Press Inc, 1985.

CHAPTER 37

BODY TEMPERATURE REGULATION

Body temperature is regulated by the thermostatic centers of the hypothalamus. When the temperature of the blood rises, a rostral hypothalamic center is stimulated and reacts by increasing heat loss through evaporation (from panting or sweating) and through vasodilation of cutaneous vessels. In contrast, when the temperature of the tissues in the caudal hypothalamus falls below normal, heat losses are reduced by vasoconstriction and hemoconcentration, both of which lower tissue conductance.

Heat production is increased by thyroxin, sympathetic stimulation (which can almost double basal metabolic rate), and contraction of skeletal muscles. In a resting animal, skeletal muscles contribute about 25 percent of total heat production. Muscle activity can raise heat production as much as 60-fold.

This chapter deals with regulation of the balance between heat loss and heat gain (Fig. 37–1), an integrative function that can be considered in terms of (1) central controls at the hypothalamic level; (2) sensors for detecting hypothermia and adapting or acclimating; (3) effectors for heat loss and heat production, which include both autonomic and behavioral thermoregulatory components; and (4) situations of hyperthermia.

HYPOTHALAMIC THERMOREGULATORY CENTERS

The hypothalamus contains thermoregulatory centers for conservation of heat in its caudal part and for dissipation of heat in its rostral part.

Caudal Hypothalamic Heat Conservation Center

A "warming" center is situated in the caudal hypothalamus, just rostrad to the brain stem. After transection of the diencephalon, an animal is no longer homeothermic and does not respond to an environmental cold temperature or to central or blood thermoreceptors.

When the spinal cord of a dog is transected at the level of the upper thoracic segments, the caudad part of the body is completely isolated from the higher nerve centers. By immersing the hind paws of this animal in cold water, the forelegs and the head are made to shiver. This response cannot be a reflex, as all afferent routes from the hind legs are transected. Its cause is the cooling of the blood flowing through the hind legs. When the cooled blood passes through the hypothalamus, it stimulates a center for heat production, inhibits heat loss, and causes a compensatory rise in body temperature. Similarly, cooling of the blood in

the carotid artery of a normal dog results in a higher body temperature, and conversely, warming of the carotid blood lowers body temperature.

Electrical stimulation of the lateral and caudal parts of the hypothalamus increases the activity of the heat production mechanisms (i.e., piloerection and release of epinephrine); the latter induces glycogenolysis (hyperglycemia). The caudal hypothalamus (Fig. 37–2) contains a warming center that stimulates heat production and raises body temperature. This center is activated directly by a drop in blood temperature and indirectly by cold receptors in the skin.

Extensive destruction of the caudal part of the lateral hypothalamus lowers the body temperature. The animal remains inactive and no longer shivers or reacts to cold by piloerection, even when it is hypothermic (rectal temperature less than 30°C). It behaves as a poikilothermic animal.

Rostral Hypothalamic Heat Dissipation Center

The so-called cooling center situated in the rostromedial hypothalamus (Fig. 37–3) responds to thermal stimulation by causing substantial loss of heat (vasodilation of skin vessels, sweating, panting). Since it also inhibits heat production by shivering, rectal temperature then falls markedly.

The central coordination of heat dissipation mechanisms by the rostral hypothalamic heat loss center is based on the effects of electrical stimulation and of local warming. In conscious goats with implanted brain electrodes, electrical stimulation of the rostral hypothalamus, between the rostral (anterior) commissure and the optic chiasm, evokes polypnea, vasodilation of the skin, and inhibition of shivering. The rectal temperature may even fall by as much as 10°C. In cats, dogs, and monkeys, local warming of the rostral hypothalamic area (preoptic area) also leads to heat loss reactions such as cutaneous vasodilation of the toes, sweating, and polypnea (panting) (Fig. 37–4). In dogs, local heating of the rostral hypothalamus also depresses the somatomotor activity and induces sleep.

HYPOTHERMIA

An animal's tolerance to cold is determined by several metabolic, dietary, and physical factors. The major factors are metabolic heat production (Table 37–1), which varies with the degree of acclimatization, the heat increment of foods, the amount of fat in milk for species in cold countries

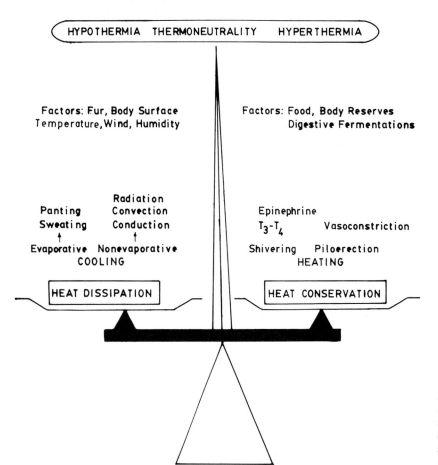

Figure 37-1 Factors that affect the balance between the heat dissipation (loss) and heat conservation (gain) systems. Excessive activity in one of the systems results in either hypothermia or hyperthermia.

(Table 37–2), and the thermal insulation (fur) against the outdoor environment (Table 37–3).

Hypothermia may result from failure of the temperature-regulating mechanisms during exposure of the animal to adverse environmental conditions (cold, humidity, wind), or during anesthesia. Nonacclimatized mammals exposed to extreme cold, such as ice water immersion, are rapidly depleted of readily available body energy stores. Body cooling leads to a reduced rate of metabolic heat production, suppression of central nervous activity, and a reduction in thermoregulatory control (a positive-feedback effect). When metabolic activity is reduced, muscles are weakened, with ensuing respiratory failure and cardiac arrest. At temperatures near 0°C, tissue metabolism is so low that circulation may not be necessary for survival.

Hypothermia is used as a routine technique in *surgical procedures* requiring relatively prolonged arrest of circulation, such as during heart or brain surgery. Through extracorporeal heat exchangers, blood is cooled to decrease metabolism and tissue oxygen demand and to minimize the risk of tissue damage by anoxia.

With anesthesia and external cooling, various degrees of hypothermia are obtained: mild (30 to 32°C), moderate (22 to 25°C), and profound (0 to 8°C). The animal organism is able to return body temperature to normal from above 28°C. Below 28°, this ability is lost, and external heat is necessary to rewarm the animal to normal temperature.

Controlled hypothermia is obtained by inhibition of the hypothalamus-hypophysial system and of the brain stem reticular formation with phenothiazine derivatives, such as chlorpromazine. When these phenothiazine derivatives are given in a therapeutic dose to reduce oxygen consumption and to abolish acidosis, they cause minimal disturbance of

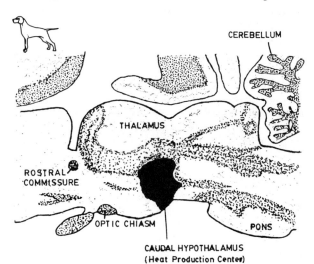

Figure 37-2 The heat gain or heat conservation center of the dog is situated in the caudal hypothalamus. Destruction of this area leads to hypothermia from lack of shivering and piloerection.

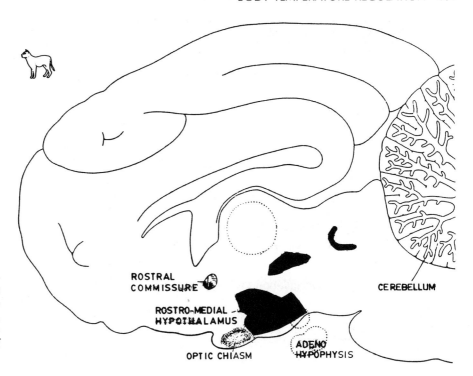

Figure 37–3 In the cat, the rostromedial hypothalamic area for heat dissipation, or heat loss, is associated also with hypersalivation, cutaneous vasodilation, and panting. Destruction or dysfunction of this area leads to hyperthermia.

oxidative processes in the organism. Achievement of hypothermia by neuroplegic agents leads to a new physiological balance resembling that found under normal conditions. With ganglionic blocking agents (e.g., hexamethonium), it is possible to suppress the sympathetic-adrenergic reaction. An efficient functional arrest may be performed (without disturbing the metabolism to any great extent) by blockade at different levels: blockade of the hypothalamus–brain stem by neuroplegics and sympathetic-adrenergic blockade by ganglioplegics. The blocking of visceral reactions by cold allows cooling to 20°C only, as the normal function of isolated tissues (e.g., auricles of the heart) ceases at this temperature.

In *hibernating animals,* cold probably does not uncouple phosphorylations and oxidations. A special metabolism, which affects ion balance, is assumed to operate in hibernators. Thermoregulation in hibernating animals is a very active programmed function that involves reduction of the whole metabolism and of the heart rate. This hibernation mechanism becomes inoperative when the body temperature falls to − 1°C. In hibernating animals, hypothermia increases the activity of brown adipose tissues.

Brown adipose tissue, referred to as the "hibernating gland," exists in all true hibernators. It is an essential source of body heat during the rapid rewarming phase of emergence from hibernation. Brown adipose tissue occurs also in some newborn mammals, serving as a primary defense against body cooling immediately after birth.

Figure 37–4 Rostromedial hypothalamic sites of thermal stimulation in a cat with chronically implanted thermodes. Stimulation at level *C* causes more intense panting than at level *B*.

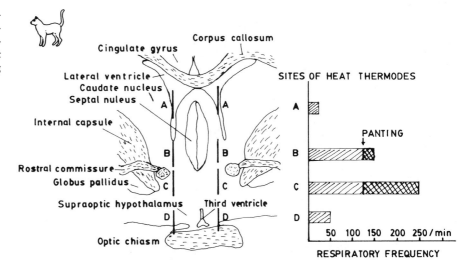

TABLE 37–1 Metabolic Intensity in Cattle in a Thermoneutral Environment

	$Cal/24\ hr/kg^{0.75}$
Beef cows (425 kg), pregnant, maintenance feeding	
Outdoors, midwinter (−26 to 14°C)	103
Calves (150–350 kg), fed ad lib	
Outdoors, winter ($\bar{x}$: −5°C)	119
Steers, growing, 50% grain-fed	
Outdoors, early winter ($\bar{x}$: −6°C)	106
Outdoors, midwinter ($\bar{x}$: −22°C)	119

$\bar{x}$, Average temperature.

AUTONOMIC, BEHAVIORAL, AND ENDOCRINE THERMOGENESIS PROCESSES

Autonomic Thermoregulation Processes

The autonomic processes of heat production include shivering and nonshivering thermogenesis. Shivering thermogenesis, from asynchronous and concurrent contractions of both extensor and flexor muscle fibers, causes a rise in heat production without producing movements of the body relative to its environment. Nonshivering thermogenesis is a rise in the rate of heat production in response to cold stress without any evidence of muscle tremors.

Three types of physiological adaptation are usually considered: habituation, acclimation, and acclimatization. *Habituation* involves a gradual reduction in the elicited response as a result of repeated stimulation. *Acclimation* is an adaptation to a single environmental factor, cold exposure. *Acclimatization* is an adaptation to a complex of natural phenomena such as day length, nutritional changes, and temperature. Adaptation to cold is a change in the normal physiological responses resulting from an experience of cold exposure. It has the effect of improving an animal's ability to thermoregulate, to tolerate hypothermia, and to improve its viability during cold stress (Table 37–4).

Acclimation

Acclimation to a *cold* climate or to an immediate temperature drop in the environment is the process of physiological adaptation of an individual animal as it becomes tougher, or hardened to cold.

Acclimatation, or *acclimatization,* is the result of an es-

TABLE 37–3 Some Factors Affecting Tolerance to Cold of Cattle, Sheep, and Red Deer in a Thermoneutral Outdoor Environment*

	Cattle (500 kg)	Sheep (50 kg)	Red Deer Hind (70 kg)
Heat production	129	97	129†
kcal/kg$^{0.75}$/day			
Mcal/m²‡/day	2.35	1.47	2.01
Thermal insulation (°C/m²/day/ Mcal)	16	30	16
External			
(Wind 0.4 m/sec)			
(Wind 4.5 m/sec§)	8	15	8
Lower critical temperature (°C)	−16	−7	+1
(Wind 0.4 m/sec)			
(Wind 4.5 m/sec)	0	+11	+14

*Maintenance feeding, 15 percent activity increment.
†In winter.
‡Body surface (m²) = 0.1 × kg body weight$^{0.66}$.
§4.5 m/sec = 10 msec/hr.

tablished state of adaptation or higher tolerance of a species *to several factors* in a new environment.

Warm-blooded animals use thermal acclimation to optimize the efficiency of thermoregulation. *Morphological acclimation* consists of seasonal changes in the thickness of fat or fur insulation. *Physiological acclimation* adjusts metabolism, vascular perfusion, and respiratory patterns to approximately current ambient conditions, using thermal environments experienced in the recent past. Behavioral mechanisms finetune the adaptation, as physiological mechanisms cannot anticipate random (stochastic, or aleatory) day-to-day variations in ambient conditions.

In domestic cattle, effective acclimation time is about 9 to 14 days. In elk and male deer, the effective acclimation period is less than 6 days.

Cold resistance (water bath–tested) in lambs is highly heritable and is a selection criterion in the Scottish blackface breed. Genetic selection for cold resistance favors production of more viable lambs in cold environments. In addition, since survival of newborn lambs depends on effective thermoregulation, selection for resistance to hypothermia reduces early mortality in cold environments (see Table 37–4).

TABLE 37–2 Composition of Milk in Cattle, Sheep, Yak, and Red Deer

Substances	Holstein Cattle (%)	Sheep (%)	Yak (%)	Red Deer (%)
Ash	0.7	0.9	0.9	1.2–1.5
Carbohydrates	4.7	4.2–5.4	4.6	2.1–2.7
Fat	3.5	2.6–7.1	6.5	17.1–18.7
Protein	3.1	5.0–6.5	5.4	2.7–5.2
Water	88.0	80.1–83.9	82.6	62.0–68.2

TABLE 37–4 Resistance to Acute Body Cooling* in Different Breeds of Sheep (Waterbath Test)

Subjects	Scottish Blackface (min)	Southdown (min)	Tasmanian Merino (min)	Welsh Mountain (min)
"Naive" (without previous cold experience)	449	294	125	230
Cold-acclimatized	557	374	208	303

*Minutes required for body temperature to fall to 36°C.

Behavioral Thermogeneration Processes

Chilling is directly or indirectly linked to huge wastage of live-born piglets during the initial few days and weeks after farrowing. Piglets born toward the end of parturition tend to be disadvantaged because their liver glycogen is depleted before they are born. In neonate piglets, the rapid first-day increase in cold resistance results more from changes in the metabolic response to cold than from improvement in their thermal insulation.

At birth, thermal insulation is meager in piglets, because even if their bodies are small, their surface:mass ratio is large. They also possess little subcutaneous fat and hair. However, the newborn piglet can respond to cold stress by both peripheral vasoconstriction and piloerection, which reduce heat dissipation to the cold environment. The piglet also reduces the area of its body surface in contact with a cold floor or a cool radiant environment by individual postural adjustments and by huddling with littermates. These behavioral adaptations can lower the environmental heat demand by as much as 40 percent. Despite gains in hair density and subcutaneous fat deposits, the overall insulative response to cold does not improve during the piglet's first postnatal week.

Endocrine Processes of Thermogenesis

After acclimatization to cold, heat production is more the result of metabolic activity than of muscle contractions. In dogs, cooling of the body raises the metabolic rate by 7 percent before there is any manifestation of reflex muscle activity. This neurohumoral activation of heat production involves the liver, the adrenals (medulla and cortex), the thyroid, and the adenohypophysis (thyrotropic hormone [TSH] and adrenocorticotropic hormone [ACTH]).

When the adrenal medulla is stimulated reflexly by cold stimuli acting on the rostral hypothalamus, it secretes *epinephrine.* This hormone minimizes heat loss by causing vasoconstriction on the surface of the skin. The major metabolic functions of epinephrine are activation of cellular metabolism, mobilization of liver glycogen, and enhancement of heat production. The epinephrine thermogenesis is small compared with the massive increase in metabolism (about 60 to 80 percent) obtained with reflex shivering.

Catecholamines (i.e., epinephrine, norepinephrine, dopamine, and serotonin) are important in mammalian thermoregulation. During exposure to heat or to cold, sympathoadrenal activity increases the plasma and urine levels of epinephrine and norepinephrine in different breeds of cattle, sheep, goats, and pigs.

Short-term exposure to cold or heat raises the plasma levels of norepinephrine in all ungulates, but the epinephrine titer increases only in some species and remains unchanged in others. *Long-term* (3 days) *exposure to cold* (16.5°C) has no significant effect on blood levels of norepinephrine and epinephrine in pigs. During cold exposure, Longhorn cattle (a cold-intolerant breed) show a significant rise in norepinephrine and dopamine, but Hereford cattle (a cold-tolerant breed) do not.

Long-term (24 days) *exposure to heat* (35°C) induces high and sustained plasma levels of norepinephrine and epinephrine in *cattle.* Exposure to heat significantly increases norepinephrine and epinephrine in Herefords (heat-intolerant breed) but not in Longhorns (heat-tolerant breed). However, the latter have higher plasma levels of serotonin. In cattle, the plasma levels of biogenic amines can be used as reliable indicators of thermal stress.

The *thyroid* gland of cattle responds slowly (60 hours) to heat exposure, so it plays a minor part in the early period of adaptation. However, the thyroid plays a major role in the later "compensation" stages. After cattle are removed from the heat to a thermoneutral environment, 108 hours must pass before blood thyroxin returns to the control level.

HYPERTHERMIA

Small diurnal variations in temperature (<0.5°C) occur normally in large animals (cows, elephants, horses). The temperature of female primates increases by about 1°C at ovulation. The camel, adapted to large variations in environmental temperature and to restriction of water, easily tolerates diurnal fluctuations in body temperature of as much as 5°C. For most other animals, temperature variations of such magnitude are not compatible with life.

A state of hyperthermia, which may lead to heat stroke, results from reduced heat loss when animals are subjected to an environment of high humidity with intense solar radiation or with high temperature. Such hyperthermia is usually associated with dehydration (loss of water) and thus is corrected by administration of water.

During heat stress or during exercise, when body core temperature rises, it is imperative that the temperature of the brain remain at a lower level. Brain temperature regulation, a process somewhat independent of the rest of the body, is provided by countercurrent heat exchanges at the extremities and in the brain. By means of evaporative panting, returning venous blood is cooled and exchanges heat with neighboring incoming cooler arterial blood.

Heat exchange between venous and arterial blood is probably improved when a species possesses a brain with a *rete mirabile,* a fine capillary network meeting the internal carotid artery as it crosses the *sinus cavernosus.* The roles of both *rete mirabile* and *sinus cavernosus* (Fig. 37–5) had been a mystery until it was realized that they function as heat exchangers.

Humans do not pant, but the intense sweating on the skin of the forehead probably cools the venous blood from the intracranial sinuses. Heat exchanges, as well as modification of tissue conductance in the arms (see Fig. 37–5), also help cool the venous blood in primates.

Animals smaller than the rabbit cannot use evaporative sweating or panting for thermoregulation over long periods. The amount of vaporized water would be too great a percentage of their body weight. Under very severe heat conditions, the rat salivates and licks its fur to induce evaporative cooling. This behavior enables the rat to survive in otherwise

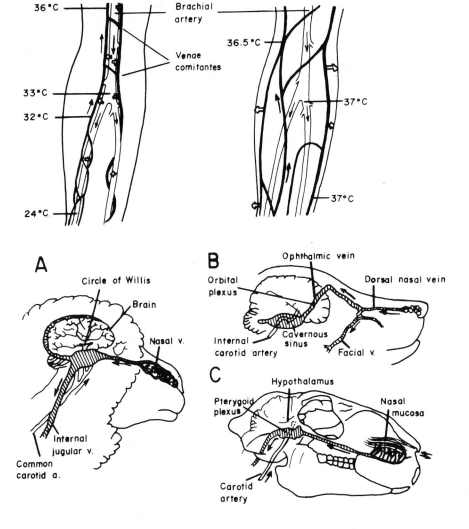

Figure 37–5 Top, Countercurrent heat exchange in the human forearm: arteries (brachial and radial) lose heat to the surrounding veins and peripheral veins conduct heat outside of the body. **Bottom,** In some animals, a vascular countercurrent system helps cool the brain. Venous blood, first cooled at the nasal mucosa, proceeds to exchange heat in sinuses or rete mirabile in the brain (A, Sheep; B, dog; C, rabbit.)

lethal conditions, provided that the high temperatures are of short duration and do not recur too soon.

Cardiac Adjustments in Heat Stress

During heat stress, cardiac output is redistributed in favor of tissues essential for heat dissipation.

When buffaloes experience acute heat stress during which rectal temperature rises from 38.5 to 39.7°C, the frequency of cardiac and respiratory events increases. Heart rate goes from 40 to 50 beats per minute, and breathing rate increases from 25 to 85 breaths per minute. In cattle, short-term thermal stress, caused by discrepancies between actual and acclimated temperatures, results in dwindling feeding activity and reduced feed intake.

The responses of sheep to heat stress, which have been studied in detail, differ from those of dogs. In mildly heat-stressed sheep (<0.5°C rise in deep body temperature), the flow of blood is higher to the skin, the nasal region, and respiratory muscles, whereas the flow of blood is lower in nonrespiratory muscles and in most abdominal organs (Fig.

37–6). The cardiac output of sheep remains unchanged during fever. Redistribution of cardiac output follows a pattern similar to that of *cold-stressed* animals during the phase of *rising* temperature and one similar to that of *heat-stressed* animals during the phase of *disappearance* of fever (defervescence).

In dogs heat stress progressively decreases blood flow to nonrespiratory skeletal muscles, whereas blood flow to these muscles is increased in severely hyperthermic sheep. Blood flow to the internal organs is better in dogs than in sheep, although, in contrast with sheep, dogs must increase cardiac output during heat stress.

Turnover of Body Water during Heat Stress

Body water plays a central role in evaporative cooling. In heat-stressed large ruminants (buffaloes), the flow rate of liquid from the rumen and body water turnover are accelerated. The larger blood volume accompanies greater plasma and erythrocyte volumes. Paradoxically, the elevation of water in plasma coincides with a rise in plasma proteins and

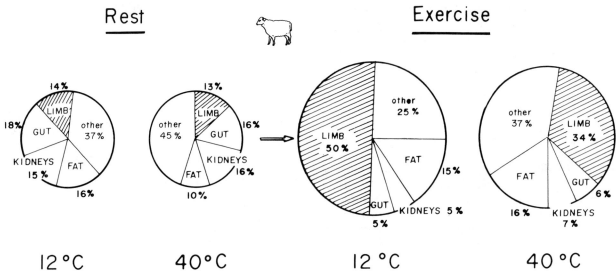

Figure 37–6   Distribution of the cardiac output in various organs, at rest and during exercise, in sheep exposed to a thermoneutral environment (12°C) or to mild heat stress (40°C).

glucose. The water dilution of plasma is due to transfer of water from the extracellular space, especially from the rumen and the lower digestive tract.

The process of evaporative heat loss by panting or by sweating is facilitated in some small mammals such as rats by their spreading saliva on their fur. Pigs achieve similar results by wallowing in mud.

For large animals kept under hot-weather husbandry conditions, a shelter with a roof inclined at an angle is preferable to one with a flat roof. Shelters made with sheets of iron provide shade, but iron exposed to sunlight becomes very hot. Thus, this type of shelter imposes radiant loads on the sheltering animals. Insulation of the inner surface reduces the long-wave radiation, and white paint on the outer iron surface causes reflection of a large part of the short-wave solar radiation (Fig. 37–7).

Malignant Hyperthermia

In cats, cattle, chickens, deer, dogs, horses, humans, rabbits, and mostly in pigs, an increase in body temperature is associated with a hereditary dysfunction in the handling of intracellular Ca^{++}. This syndrome, called *malignant hyperthermia* or *porcine stress syndrome,* is initiated in awake animals by stress (trauma, handling, exercise, mating, transportation). Administration of inhalation anesthesia (e.g., halothane, methoxyflurane, enflurane [Ethrane], fluroxene, chloroform), depolarizing muscle relaxants (e.g., succinylcholine), and amide local anesthesia (e.g., lidocaine) also trigger malignant hyperthermia. The myofibrils (mostly Type II, i.e., myosin ATPase-rich, light, or white, fibers) of affected animals possess an excess of Ca^{++}, which activates myofibrillar ATPase, intracellular glycogenolysis, and hypercontraction with a consequent rapid (1°C every 6 minutes) increase in body heat. The hyperthermia denatures

the proteins (myoglobin) of the myofibers, and the fluid of the metabolically dead cell escapes into the intermyofiber space to cause edema. A characteristic myoglobinuria (rhabdomyolysis) accompanies malignant hyperthermia in horses.

At necropsy of pigs, the aspect of these hyperactivated muscles (pale, swollen, and moist) is described as pale, soft, and exudative (PSE) lesions of pork.

Dantrolene sodium, an intracellular muscle relaxant, interferes with the availability of Ca^{++} in fast contracting (type II) myofibers and prevents malignant hyperthermia.

Fever

The normal body temperature of each animal species is maintained at a set point by thermosensitive neurons in the

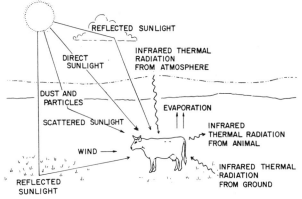

Figure 37–7   Interaction of various factors of the outside environment and their effect on evaporative cooling in cattle. Sunlight (direct, reflected, or scattered), infrared radiation (atmospheric, animal, ground), humidity, and wind act as vectors that enhance or reduce cutaneous evaporative cooling.

preoptic area (rostral, or anterior) of the hypothalamus. During *fever,* or *pyrexia,* this hypothalamic temperature set point is raised abnormally, with subsequent reduction in heat loss (cutaneous vasoconstriction) and additional heat production (shivering).

The preoptic area of the hypothalamus, primed by prostaglandins E synthesized in the central nervous system, reacts to *endogenous heat-labile pyrogen* (a peptide lymphokine from polymorphonuclear leukocytes, monocytes, macrophages, and Kupffer's cells). The endogenous pyrogen interleukin-1 (IL-1) is released after activation of its sources by *exogenous heat-stable pyrogens* such as steroids (metabolites of progesterone) and lipopolysaccharides of infectious agents (gram-negative bacteria, parasites, and viruses). The process of pyrexia is blocked or reversed by substances that inhibit the liberation of prostaglandins (e.g., acetylsalicylate) or the leukocytic release of IL-1 (e.g., cortisol, which inhibits protein synthesis).

REFERENCES

Baker MA. Brain cooling in endotherms in heat and exercise. Annu Rev Physiol 1982;44:85.

Bell AW, Hales JRS. Cardiovascular, respiratory and thermoregulatory function during exercise. Armidale (Australia): University of New England Press, 1982.

Chaiyabutr N, Buranakarl C, Muangcharoen V, Loypetjra P, Pichaicharnarong A. Effects of acute heat stress on changes in the rate of liquid flow from the rumen and turnover of body water of swamp buffalo. J Agr Sci Camb 1987;108:549.

Mount LE. Adaptation to thermal environment. London: Edward Arnold, 1979.

Owens FN. New techniques for studying digestion and absorption of nutrients by ruminants. Fed Proc 1987;46:283.

Simoens P, Lauwerss H, de Geest JP, de Schaepdrijver L. Functional morphology of the cranial *Rete mirabile* in the domestic mammals. Schweiz Arch Tierheilk 1987;129:285.

Yousef MK. Stress physiology in livestock. Boca Raton: CRC Press Inc, 1985.

CHAPTER 38

INTERMEDIARY METABOLISM AND CARBOHYDRATE METABOLISM

The concept of metabolism encompasses all the various sequences or pathways of chemical reactions and interchanges that occur in a living animal. The animal body is a marvelously intricate physicochemical machine that operates on the chemical fuels that it ingests as food. Chemical reactions digest the feed ingredients via the host's enzymes and secretions and via gut microbial enzymes and activities. The absorbed nutrients form the substrates for the enzymatic pathways of intermediary metabolism that are managed to meet the needs of the animal for materials and energy.

Two aspects of overall metabolism can be identified: catabolism and anabolism. *Catabolism* is the breaking down of complex molecules to simpler ones, with the release of energy. *Anabolism* is the formation of more complex molecules from simpler ones. The energy released in catabolism is used to drive the synthetic pathways of anabolism and to meet the mechanical and secretory needs of the body. Some metabolites that are used by the body are processed by specialized mechanisms and are then excreted.

The three categories of organic macronutrients are carbohydrates, lipids, and proteins. The metabolism of these three will be considered separately. In general terms, the major metabolites absorbed by the body and their fate can be represented in a simplified form (Fig. 38–1).

BASIC METABOLIC DRIVES

The fundamental mechanism of the machinery of the body is to unlock and control the energy in chemical bonds and to use it to drive reactions of synthesis or to generate the energy needed to accomplish physiological goals such as muscle contraction, glandular secretions, and nerve potential initiation, amplification, and conduction.

The major strategies used by the body are the release and capture of energy. Sequences of enzymes are deployed as metabolic pathways that release energy by hydrolysis, often involving oxidation. The capture of energy occurs in the form of high-energy bonds and reducing equivalents, which in turn, operate to drive other chemical reactions. Separation by semipermeable membrane barriers is a feature of these systems.

High-energy phosphate compounds are the dynamic "currency" for processing the energy used in anabolism and other cellular work. The type of compound in this class is *adenosine triphosphate*, or ATP. The complete oxidation of glucose to carbon dioxide liberates 686,000 kcal per mole (180 g). This is called the "free energy," or delta F, of the metabolite. The amount of ATP that can be obtained by

hydrolysis of glucose depends on the pathway of metabolism. The last two of the three phosphate radicals in ATP have high-energy bonds. Hydrolysis of each of these bonds can yield about 12,000 kcal per mole under the conditions prevailing in the body, or only 7,300 kcal under standard conditions (Figs. 38–2 and 38–3).

Phosphorylation, a process used to preserve this energy and to control it in syntheses, is used to direct pathways of metabolism. The high-energy phosphate bonds may also be stored as nitrogen-containing phosphagens, such as creatine phosphate. They are also employed in the activation of molecules, particularly in the creation of thioesters involving coenzyme A (CoA). Hydrolysis of ATP generates the energy needed to form CoA derivatives (e.g., acetate → acetyl CoA), which is then utilized for acylation reactions.

The glycolytic pathway generates only modest amounts of ATP. In the absence of oxygen, when pyruvate is not converted to acetyl CoA it is reduced to lactate, thereby oxidizing the reduced form of nicotinamide-adenine dinucleotide to the oxidized form (NADH→NAD$^+$) to keep some energy available during hypoxia.

Another major system for capturing chemical energy for useful work involves oxidation-reduction reactions. Oxidation of substrates generates energy in the form of hydrogen, which can serve for reductive biosynthesis of more complex chemical compounds needed by the body. Alternatively, the hydrogens can be combined with oxygen, thereby forming water, using the large amount of released energy in a coupled way to form ATP. This process is called *oxidative phosphorylation.* The dehydrogenase enzymes are linked to coenzymes containing nicotinamide (NAD, NADP), which can be reduced by the addition of a hydrogen atom and two electrons to yield NADH or NADPH and a hydrogen ion (a hydrogen atom lacking an electron). Conservation of free energy is achieved by a graded series of steps involving a chain of electron carriers with small reduction potentials (E_o^1) and by apposing the sequence of enzymes in an ordered structure in the mitochondria. They are also oriented with respect to the membrane of these organelles to perform transfers.

CARBOHYDRATE METABOLISM

Carbohydrates contain carbon, hydrogen, and oxygen atoms in a ratio equivalent to one carbon (C) to one water (H_2O), or $C(H_2O)$. This diverse group of substances includes, particularly the sugars and their derivatives. The key substance for intermediary metabolism is glucose. Impor-

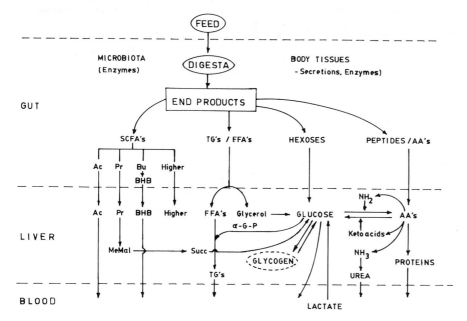

Figure 38–1 General schema of major metabolites entering or mobilized in the body. α-G-P, α-glucose phosphate; AAs, amino acids; Ac, acetate; Bu, butyrate; BHB, β-hydroxybutyrate; BHBA, β-hydroxybutyric acid; FFAs, free fatty acids; MeMal, methylmalonate; Pr, propionic acid; SCFAs, short-chain fatty acids; Succ, succinate; TGs, triglycerides.

tant roles are also played by fructose and galactose (hexoses), by ribose and deoxyribose (pentoses), by glycerol and glyceraldehyde (triose), by sedoheptulose (heptose), and by erythrose (tetrose).

Combined with lipids, carbohydrates from glycolipids, and with proteins they form glycoproteins. Polymerized carbohydrates are also important, including the alpha-1,4–linked glucose storage polymer, glycogen, and heteropolymers such as the glycosaminoglycans that make up the ground substance of connective tissue.

An animal's diet contains a vast range of carbohydrates, including the polymers starch, cellulose, hemicellulose, pectins, and lignin, and the disaccharides maltose, sucrose, and lactose. Ascorbic acid (vitamin C) is an essential nutrient for primates and guinea pigs but not for other species. After digestion and entry into the intestinal mucosal cells, most digestible dietary carbohydrate is absorbed as hexoses. Hexoses must be phosphorylated (Fig. 38–4A) before they can be utilized in metabolism; this requires ATP.

Glucose

After absorption or gluconeogenesis, glucose can undergo catabolism to provide energy or metabolites for synthetic pathways. The first stage of glucose metabolism is *glycolysis*, or *Embden-Meyerhof* fermentation. Under anaerobic conditions, glucose breaks down to lactate, yielding a net 2 mole of ATP per mole of glucose (see Fig. 38–2). Four moles of ATP is generated, but two is used to phosphorylate first glucose and then fructose-6-phosphate.

Under aerobic conditions, the reduced NADPH plus H^+ may be oxidized via oxidative phosphorylation to produce 3 mol of ATP and pyruvate. Pyruvate then enters the tricarboxylic acid (TCA) cycle (*Krebs's cycle*) and becomes

oxidized to carbon dioxide and water while generating 15 mol of ATP (see Fig. 38–3).

During vigorous exercise, muscle cells produce lactate faster than it can be utilized, via pyruvate, by the cells' mitochondria. The excess of lactate diffuses into the capillary blood and is carried to the liver to form the basis for gluconeogenesis. This is called the *Cori cycle* (Fig. 38–4B).

Another route for glucose metabolism is the *pentose phosphate* pathway, which is important in generating the NADPH used in synthesis of fatty acids in adipose tissue, mammary gland, and liver in response to demand. Nutrients or metabolites differ greatly in their relative efficiency as sources of ATP energy (Table 38–1).

Digestion and Absorption of Carbohydrates

In monogastric species, dietary carbohydrates are digested by host enzymes. The alpha-1,4 bonded glucose polymers, starch and glycogen, are hydrolyzed by amylase via dextrins to maltose; the maltose is transformed to glucose with the help of maltase. Sucrase converts sucrose to glucose and fructose. Lactase breaks lactose into glucose and galactose. When these enzymes of the intestinal mucosa are present, these monosaccharide end-products are absorbed (Table 38–2). Some species and strains of animals that are deficient in lactase suffer digestive disturbances if they ingest milk, which contains lactose.

Absorption of glucose can be measured with a *glucose tolerance test*. The test dose of glucose is given orally, then the blood glucose concentration curve is measured over a 3- to 4-hour period. In canine malabsorption syndrome, the characteristic rise in glucose is reduced; dogs with pancreatic exocrine deficiency may show a diabetes-type tolerance curve. The test has been used to a limited extent in horses.

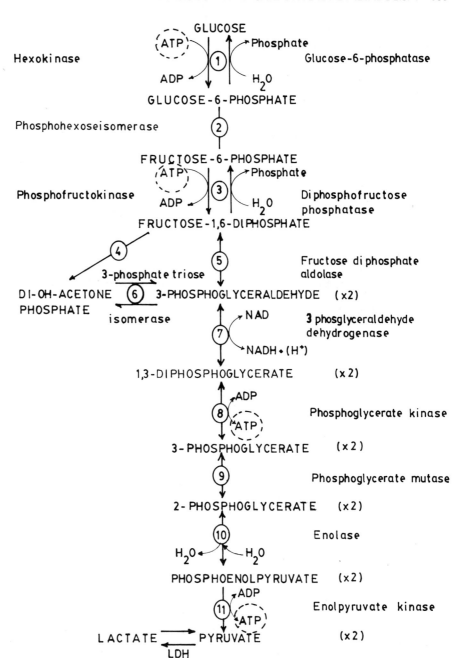

Figure 38–2 The glycolytic (Embden-Meyerhof) pathway is a two-stage process. Two moles of ATP (1 and 3) are used in the initial phosphorylation, and two others are later (8 and 11) produced for each 3-carbon subunit proceeding to pyruvate, which can be anaerobically transformed into lactate.

An alternative test, the D-*xylose absorption test,* uses D-xylose, which is not metabolized. Therefore, the problem of interpreting the variable utilization of glucose by tissues is avoided. Also, the rate of absorption of xylose is proportional to the luminal concentration of this sugar in the intestine, because the dose used is large enough to exceed any active transport effects. A 25-g dose of D-xylose is given via a stomach tube to a dog, then blood is sampled over a 5-hour period. The peak blood level of about 50 mg/dL is reached in 60 to 90 minutes in normal dogs, but a level of about 25 mg/dL is attained in ones that have the malabsorption syndrome.

The beta-1,4–bonded glucose polymer, cellulose, in plants requires that organisms have cellulase enzymes to degrade it. Mammals lack this enzyme, and only those that have microflora that do manufacture it can digest cellulose. Ruminants have this capacity well developed in their forestomachs, and cecocolic fermenters such as horses have it in the cecum and colon. The rumen microflora digest cellulose

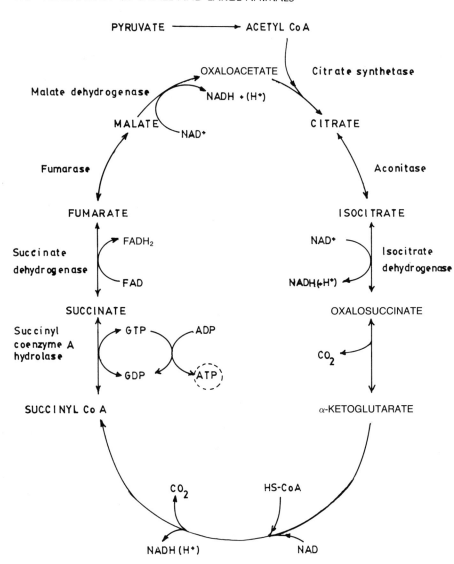

Figure 38–3 In the presence of oxygen, pyruvate is transformed into acetyl CoA, which is metabolized by mitochondrial enzymes through a cyclical system, the *tricarboxylic acid, or citric acid, or Krebs's cycle.* The aerobic tricarboxylic acid cycle produces most of the energy used by cells. An acetyl CoA can generate 12 molecules of ATP from NADH + H$^+$ (3 ATP × 3), FADH$_2$ (2 ATP × 1), and GTP (1 ATP × 1).

and starch to short-chain fatty acids, leaving the host dependent on gluconeogenesis for its glucose needs in intermediary metabolism.

Transport and Storage of Carbohydrates

Blood glucose levels are lower in ruminant species than in monogastric ones; chickens have very high levels. The blood levels of the keto acids, pyruvic acid and alpha-ketoglutaric acid, are higher in most animals than in man (Table 38–3). Glucose is the repeating unit for synthesis of animal starch or glycogen, which is the chief storage form for carbohydrates in the body. Together with galactose, glucose forms the disaccharide lactose, or milk sugar, in the lactating mammary gland.

Glycogen polymers can expand with the addition of more glucose residues or can contract when glycogenolysis is initiated. The starting compound for glycogen formation is uridine diphosphate glucose (UDPG), which in turn forms from glucose-1-phosphate (see Fig. 38–4A). The UDPG reacts with primer molecules, the most effective being glycogen itself. It can react with the simple disaccharide maltose, but the process is slow. The UDPG reacts with the fourth hydroxyl group of the nonreducing end of the primer chain, aided by glycogen synthetase. Glycogen also contains some 1,6 bonds that allow the molecule to branch. This is accomplished by amylo-(1.4→1,6)-transglucosylase.

Gluconeogenesis

Because of the central role of glucose in energy metabolism, the body has mechanisms to keep glucose concentrations in extracellular fluids in an appropriate range. Excess blood glucose leads to glycosuria and the syndrome of dia-

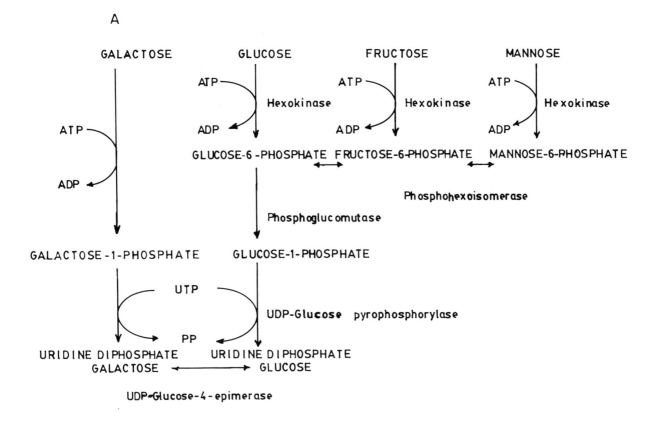

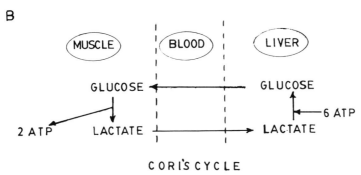

CORI'S CYCLE

Figure 38–4 **A,** Interchanges among monosaccharides, showing the sites of enzyme action and ATP involvement. **B,** Formation of glucose from skeletal muscle–derived lactate (Cori's cycle).

TABLE 38–1 **Relative Efficiency of Some Metabolites as Sources of ATP**

Metabolites	Mol of ATP per Mol	Mol of ATP per 100 g	kJ of Heat per Mol of ATP
Acetate	10	16.7	87.5
Butyrate	25	28.4	87.5
Glucose	38	21.2	74.1
Glutamate	23	15.6	98.8
Palmitate	408	50.6	77.9
Propionate	17	22.9	90.4

TABLE 38–2 **Enzymes Hydrolyzing Glycoside Bonds**

Enzymes	Source	Substrate
alpha-Amylase	Pancreas, saliva (some species)	Glycogen, starch, dextrin
Lactase	Small intestine	Lactose
Maltase	Small intestine	Maltose
Oligo-1,6-glucosidase	Small intestine	Dextrins
Sucrase	Small intestine	Sucrose

TABLE 38–3 Levels of Glucose, Pyruvate, and Alpha-Ketoglutarate in Blood of Domestic Animals and Chickens

Animals	N	Glucose (mmol/dL) Mean (SD)	Pyruvate (mmol/dL) Mean (SD)	Alpha-Ketoglutarate (mmol/dL) Mean (SD)
Cat (Felis catus)	5	75 (9)	0.70 (0.2)	0.22 (0.1)
Bull (Bos taurus)	10	53 (8)	0.92 (0.3)	0.27 (0.1)
Cow	15	54 (8)	0.96 (0.2)	0.28 (0.1)
Dog (Canis familiaris)	7	63 (11)	0.72 (0.2)	0.21 (0.1)
Heifer	11	51 (8)	0.78 (0.2)	0.24 (0.1)
Hog (Sus domesticus)	15	65 (10)	0.76 (0.2)	0.22 (0.1)
Horse (Equus caballus)	15	79 (10)	0.86 (0.2)	0.25 (0.1)
Piglet	11	87 (14)	1.05 (0.3)	0.23 (0.1)
Rabbit (Oryctolagus cuniculus domesticus)	11	152 (26)	1.42 (0.4)	0.29 (0.1)
Sheep (Ovis aries)	15	47 (7)	0.94 (0.3)	0.27 (0.1)
Chicken (Gallus domesticus)	14	173 (31)	1.15 (0.3)	0.35 (0.1)

N, Number of observations; SD, standard deviation.

betes mellitus. This disorder occurs in pet animals and horses but rarely in other species. A greater problem for many animal species, particularly ruminants, is avoiding the other swing of the pendulum to hypoglycemia. All species have metabolic enzyme pathways to synthesize glucose from other substances, but the need of ruminants is much more chronic and continuous because of their general lack of absorbable glucose from the intestine.

Three groups of starting substances are available for gluconeogenesis: carbohydrates, glucogenic amino acids via deamination, and odd-numbered fatty acids. All species have access to the *carbohydrates* (lactate, pyruvate, and oxaloacetate). *Glucogenic amino acids* (especially alanine and glutamate) can be oxidatively deaminated and transferred to the carbohydrate pathways via alpha-keto acids with reduced nicotinamide coenzymes. The reactions are reversible; the hydrogenases are located inside the mitochondria. They are subject to allosteric inhibition by ATP and guanine triphosphate (GTP) but also to activation by ADP and GDP. These reactions exert an autoregulatory role (i.e., they promote oxidative deamination of amino acids in the liver) when energy reserves are low and triphosphate levels are dropping.

The third class of gluconeogenic substrates comprises *odd-numbered fatty acids* (odd numbers of carbon atoms), which yield odd-numbered acyl CoA derivatives, particularly propionate. This is a major and essential contributor to gluconeogenesis in ruminants. The utilization of propionate involves its activation to propionyl-CoA and addition of a carboxyl group to form D-methylmalonyl-CoA (using propionyl-CoA carboxylase, which contains biotin). D-Methylmalonyl CoA is then racemized to the L form, which, in turn, is converted to succinyl-CoA by methylmalonyl-CoA mutase, an enzyme that contains a derivative of cobalamin (vitamin B_{12}). The cobalamin serves as a source of free radicals that allow the removal of hydrogen atoms and subsequent intramolecular rearrangement to succinate.

The glucose formed can itself serve as the source material for the synthesis of other important carbohydrates: glycogen and lactose. Glycogen is the chief storage carbohydrate. Lactose (milk sugar) is specifically synthesized in the mammary glands of lactating animals.

Blood Glucose Concentration and Its Regulation

Insulin: Glucagon Ratio. *Insulin*, secreted by the beta cells of the islets of Langerhans in the pancreas, is the key regulating agent in energy metabolism. It promotes the uptake and utilization of glucose by many peripheral tissues, the uptake and incorporation of amino acids into protein, and lipogenesis. On the other hand, it inhibits gluconeogenesis and glucose release by the liver, proteolysis, and lipolysis. Thus, it governs the overall dynamics of energy metabolism and tissue synthesis.

Glucagon, secreted by the alpha cells of the islets, works primarily in the liver. It stimulates liver glucose output by accelerating hepatic glycogenolysis and gluconeogenesis. The physical proximity of alpha and beta cells suggests that functional interactions probably occur between the two hormones in the push-pull changes that maintain blood glucose levels.

The ratio of insulin to glucagon (I:G) in dogs is an indicator of physiological status (Fig. 38–5). A *low I:G ratio* because of a relatively high rate of glucagon secretion indicates dominance of hepatic glycogenolysis and gluconeogenesis. This is a feature of starvation, diabetes mellitus, and catabolic states seen in certain diseases. A *high I:G ratio* occurs after ingestion of large quantities of readily digestible carbohydrates, which increases insulin secretion, and indicates decreased hepatic gluconeogenesis and increased peripheral uptake of glucose, amino acids, and fatty acids. A high I:G ratio is rare in ruminants, but such a ratio may indicate the degree of gluconeogenesis from propionate and amino acids.

Diabetes has been recognized as a syndrome since time immemorial. The Ebers papyrus of about 2,500 years ago describes it. The most noticeable sign, the passing of large volumes of urine ("the pissing evil" of WILLIS, who also noticed the urine was "wonderfully sweet" in 1684), was accompanied by "unquenchable thirst" and "melting down of flesh and limbs into urine."

In 1788, CAWLEY identified the pancreas as the site of the disorder, but it was 1869 before LANGERHANS described the islets that make up about 2 percent of the pancreatic tissue. It was 1889 before MERING and MINKOWSKI performed pancreatectomy on dogs to produce an experimental model of diabetes. Then, in 1921, BANTING and BEST extracted insulin from the islet tissue that survived after they had destroyed the exocrine pancreas by duct ligation.

Role of the Hypothalamus–Sympathetic–Adrenal System. In 1849, Claude Bernard made the interesting discovery that puncture of the floor of the fourth ventricle of the medulla oblongata (*piqûre*) leads to hyperglycemia and glycosuria. The interpretation is that the action stimulates the efferent pathways from the hypothalamus that pass caudally via the cord, the preganglionic sympathetic nerves, and the splanchnic nerves to the adrenal glands. The resulting

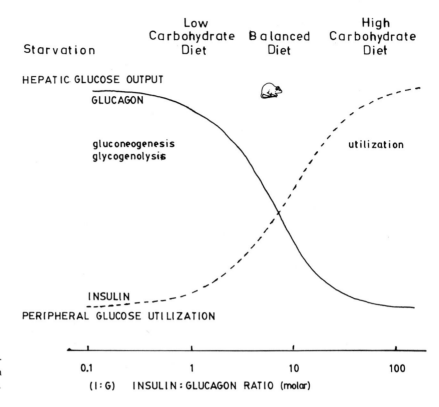

Figure 38–5 The molar I:G ratio is peripheral plasma and glucose metabolism in rats. The principle also applies in dogs.

secretion of epinephrine raises the blood glucose level by activating glycogenolysis in liver and muscle (Fig. 38–6).

Epinephrine secretion by the adrenal medulla is lowest during deep sleep and increases upon awakening. It increases further after emotional upsets, pain, and cold. Extreme exercise and emotional stress, such as from anger or fear, can lead to maximal stimulation of the hypothalamus–sympathetic nerves–adrenal medulla system, raising the blood glucose level. A 10-fold increase in epinephrine secretion can be evoked by electrical stimulation of the caudal paraventricular region of the hypothalamus. Stimulation of different sites in the caudal hypothalamus can lead to selective increases in the secretion of epinephrine or norepinephrine. Similar differentials are seen after physiological stimuli such as hypoglycemia or stimulation of pain afferents leading to epinephrine secretion, while fear or carotid occlusion results in higher norepinephrine output.

Antiinsulin Factors of the Adenohypophysis

From 1925 to 1930, Houssay's group in Buenos Aires showed that, in the dog, diabetes induced by pancreatectomy was improved by hypophysectomy and that extracts of the adenohypophysis had an antiinsulin effect. Prolonged administration of such extracts damaged the islets of Langerhans, inducing hypophysial diabetes. Later, it was found that both adenohypophysial *adrenocorticotropin* (ACTH) and *growth hormone* (GH) can contribute to this effect. Long-term administration of GH damages the islets, but it also inhibits the effects of insulin, causing insulin-resistant diabetes. A

rise in blood glucose level results because of glycogenolysis and of inhibition of glucose phosphorylation. GH and ACTH also stimulate gluconeogenesis. Eosinophilic adenoma of the adenohypophysis leads to hypophysial diabetes. The pancreas also produces *somatostatin* in the delta cells of the islets and *pancreatic polypeptide*. Arterioles enter the islets and perfuse the core containing the beta cells before the cortical areas, which enclose the alpha and delta-cells and supply the venules. Sympathetic fibers reach the islets.

The pancreas has endocrine roles implemented by its islets of Langerhans, which produce insulin in the beta cells. Destruction of the beta cells by alloxan or by pathologic changes causes failure of insulin secretion and diabetes mellitus of pancreatic origin. The islets also contain alpha cells that secrete another hormone, glucagon, which promotes glycogenolysis and gluconeogenesis with resultant hyperglycemia. The secretion of glucagon is increased by GH.

The delta cells of the pancreatic islets produce somatostatin, which inhibits the release of both insulin and glucagon. Hypothalamic production of somatostatin inhibits the release of somatotropic hormone (STH) or GH from the adenohypophysis. Somatostatin also inhibits gastrointestinal functions, including selective reduction in the secretion of the duodenal glands (Brunner's glands). Its general inhibitory action in the gut has been interpreted as a safety mechanism that prevents excessive secretory and motor responses after eating. A synthetic analogue with longer action, minisomatostatin, has shown promise in the treatment of intractable diarrhea caused by tumors of the gastro-

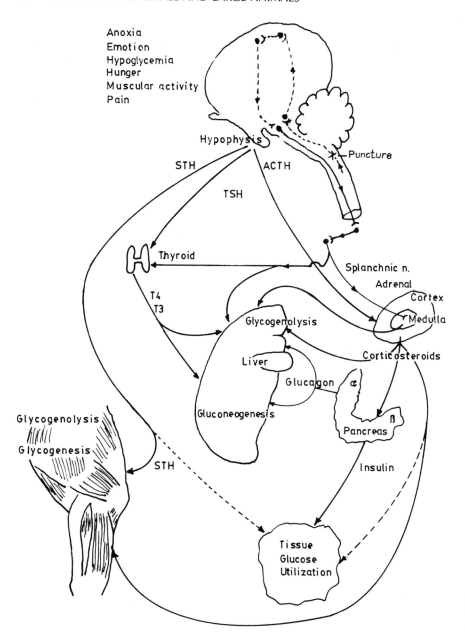

Anoxia
Emotion
Hypoglycemia
Hunger
Muscular activity
Pain

Figure 38–6 Diagram of neuro-humoral control of carbohydrate metabolism.

intestinal tract. The delta cells also contribute pancreatic polypeptide, which inhibits the secretion of enzymes by the pancreas and the contraction of the gall bladder.

Glucose Metabolism in Ruminants

In the diets of ruminants, the carbohydrate precursors of glucose are utilized by ruminoreticular microorganisms in pathways that extend beyond glucose to the short-chain fatty acids (SCFAs), formerly called volatile fatty acids (VFAs). Some dietary ingredients that resist rumen digestion, such as maize (corn), can yield some glucose. The ruminant must supply most of its needed glucose via gluconeogenesis. It does this by using the absorbed nutrient propionate and the

glucogenic metabolic products that can be recycled into glucose. These metabolites come from glycogenolysis (e.g., lactate), from amino acid deamination (e.g., alanine, glutamate), and from triglyceride hydrolysis (glycerol).

Because so much of their dietary energy is derived from SCFAs rather than carbohydrates, ruminants have well-developed pathways for utilizing acetate and beta-hydroxybutyrate for energy oxidation, synthesis, and storage, as well as for gluconeogenesis from propionate and amino acids. The rate of such glucose formation rises as these end-products of digestion are absorbed after feeding. Plasma insulin concentration also increases after feeding, peaking about 4 hours after each feeding is commenced (Fig. 38–7). Preruminant calves and lambs show a more cyclical monogastric-type response.

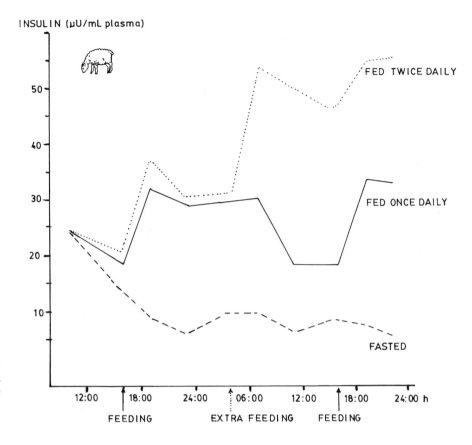

Figure 38–7 Insulin concentrations in plasma of sheep fasted (-- -- --) or fed 800 g (50 percent alfalfa chaff and 50 percent oat grain) once (———) or twice (· · · ·) a day. (N = 6, $\bar{x}$).

Dietary Effects on Somatotropin

Sucking in lambs results in a rapid decline in plasma GH concentration, followed by an increase to high levels by 30 to 90 minutes after ingestion. Speculations are that the following sequence may occur: (1) the anabolic effects of insulin occur alone, without GH involvement; (2) insulin and GH function together to increase protein synthesis; (3) GH acts alone, thereby enhancing lipolysis. Adult sheep show a decrease in plasma GH after feeding, which is followed by a return to oscillating prefeeding values.

Hypoglycemic Ketosis

The adult ruminant's dependence on gluconeogenesis is accommodated mainly by the liver, with some help from the kidneys. Ketone bodies (acetoacetate, beta-hydroxybutyrate, and acetone) arise (1) during absorption of SCFAs via the rumen epithelium mainly as beta-hydroxybutyric acid (BHBA) formed during butyrate absorption in fed animals, and (2) by hepatic cell mitochondrial metabolism.

The liver cannot further oxidize and metabolize ketone bodies once the coenzyme A is removed; however, other tissues (notably brain, skeletal and cardiac muscles) can reconvert acetoacetate to acetyl CoA and thereby use ketones for chemical energy generation. The liver is dependent on the ratio between the acetyl CoA production rate from beta oxidation of fatty acids and oxaloacetate production from the

carboxylation of pyruvate. The oxaloacetate utilizes the acetyl CoA residues in the citric acid cycle.

Diminished carbohydrate availability or utilization results in the accumulation of ketone bodies beyond the capacity of extrahepatic tissues to utilize them. The resulting condition is called *ketosis,* or *acetonemia.* Acetone can be detected by the characteristic odor of this ketone on the breath. Accumulation of acetoacetic acid and beta-hydroxybutyric acid brings metabolic acidosis and ketonuria.

Starvation or diabetes leads to ketosis because of lack of available glucose and because of mobilization of triglycerides. Ruminants are uniquely susceptible, sheep during pregnancy, and cattle during heavy lactation. Ewes in late pregnancy with two or more fetuses have a high requirement for glucose and may develop severe hypoglycemia ("twin lamb disease," or ovine pregnancy toxemia), high plasma free fatty acids (FFAs), and ketosis. A period of starvation increases the risk of occurrence of this disease, because it may trigger a decrease in hepatic gluconeogenesis and a hypoglycemic crisis.

Lactation ketosis in dairy cows that produce large quantities of milk is accompanied by hypoglycemia and increased levels of FFAs, acetate, and ketone bodies. Primary ketosis of metabolic origin usually occurs during the period of heaviest lactation, the first 6 weeks after calving, when the metabolic demand of milk production is greatest (the lactose in 40 kg of milk requires over 2 kg of glucose as a precursor). Secondary ketosis can occur in any disease or condition that causes a

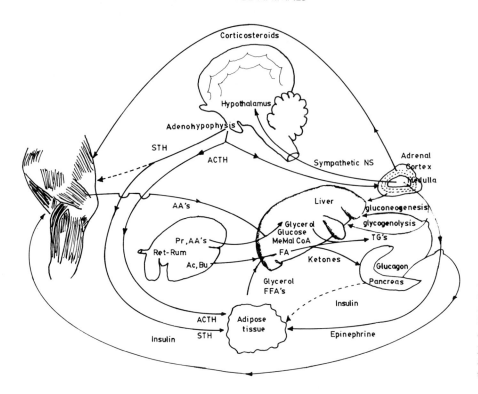

Figure 38–8 Hormonal control of intermediary metabolism in ruminants. Hypoglycemia induces hormonal adjustments in the pancreas, hypothalamus, adenohypophysis, and adrenal cortex and medulla directed at muscle proteins and lipid reserves.

reduction in food intake or depresses gastrointestinal function.

A feature of clinical ketosis is fatty liver, with accumulation of triglycerides. An extreme example of that is seen in the "fat cow syndrome," which differs from classic ketosis in that hypoglycemia does not occur. It seems to be related to obesity in late pregnancy and to postparturient metritis or mastitis.

Portal venous blood flow increases greatly after feeding, in parallel with the higher hepatic glucose production, then it declines again. The blood flow to the rumen epithelium increases as the concentration of SCFAs in the digesta rises after feeding.

The sequence of metabolic and endocrine changes that regulate metabolism in ruminants can be outlined (Fig. 38–8). If hypoglycemia occurs, insulin secretion is reduced and glucagon increases, while the hypothalamus is called upon to increase the secretion of epinephrine. The result is increased hepatic glycogenolysis and mobilization of FFAs and glycerol from adipose tissues. The FFAs serve as an alternative fuel for oxidation, and glycerol is used in gluconeogenesis. The skeletal muscles respond by releasing more amino acids, generating additional precursors (notably alanine and glu-

tamine) for gluconeogenesis. These are the initial short-term responses.

If hypoglycemia persists, longer-range actions take place—increased production of ACTH and GH by the adenohypophysis. The increased ACTH secretion stimulates more glucocorticoid hormones to be secreted by the adrenal cortex. The latter promote protein catabolism in the tissues, yielding more amino acids for gluconeogenesis. Glucocorticoids also reduce milk secretion and inhibit glucose utilization. The increased secretion of GH augments lipolysis, making more glycerol and fatty acids available.

REFERENCES

Edwards AV. The hyperglycaemic response to stimulation of the hepatic sympathetic innervation in adrenalectomized cats and dogs. J Physiol 1972;220:697.

Katz ML, Bergman EN. Hepatic and portal metabolism of glucose, free fatty acids and ketone bodies in sheep. Am J Physiol 1969;216:953.

Kleiber M. The fire of life. NY: John Wiley, 1961.

Van Soest PJ. Nutritional ecology of the ruminant. Corvallis, OR: O and B Books Inc, 1982.

CHAPTER 39

LIPID METABOLISM

Lipid is a term used for organic chemical substances that have low solubility or are insoluble in water but dissolve in nonpolar organic solvents. The latter are used to extract them from plant or animal tissues, which contain a variety of these substances. Lipids carry out a multitude of important functions in the animal body (Table 39–1). These roles and the regulation of lipid metabolism are of considerable interest for animal production, veterinary medicine, and basic biomedical research.

The majority of biological lipids are esters of fatty acids (FAs). FAs are covalently bonded chains of carbon atoms with (unsaturated) or without (saturated) double bonds, the remaining valences being occupied by hydrogen atoms except for a terminal carboxyl group. Most FAs have zero to four double bonds. Palmitic acid (16:0) is the most common fully saturated FA in adipose tissue, while oleic acid (18:1), the most prevalent of the FAs, has one double bond. Animals can form double bonds from the omega-9 position to the end of the chain.

The so-called *essential fatty acids* include the polyunsaturated fatty acids (PUFAs), linoleic acid (18:2, omega-6), linolenic acid (18:3, omega-3), and arachidonic acid (20:4, omega-6). Their essentialness as nutrients stems from the fact that animals cannot synthesize double bonds in the omega-3 or omega-6 position. The PUFAs are vital components of cell membranes throughout the body, and one of their major roles is to generate a group of highly active local hormones (autocrine and paracrine actions), the *eicosanoids*. The synthesis of these 20-carbon compounds (prostaglandins, leukotrienes, and lipoxins) originates from PUFAs, mostly arachidonic acid.

Nonesterified or free fatty acids (FFAs) are not common except as steps in the digestion and metabolism of lipids. Most of the FAs occur as esters, in which the terminal carboxylic group is esterified with the hydroxyl group of an alcohol.

The triglycerides (TGs), the typical fats and oils, are esters between glycerol (which has three alcoholic hydroxyl groups) and FAs (1, 2, or 3, forming mono-, di-, and triglycerides, respectively). When two of the hydroxyl groups are bonded to FAs and the third to a phosphate, which may be also attached to another organic radical (e.g., choline, ethanolamine, serine, or inositol), the resulting compound is a phospholipid (PL).

Cholesterol is another important lipid that is the starting point for steroid hormone synthesis.

DIETARY LIPIDS

Plant and animal products that are used for animal feed contain some lipid components. The largest category of lipids in feeds is the glycerides of fats and oils, which are usually compounds of a sugar or glycerol residue with fatty acids.

The plants ingested by herbivorous animals contain galactoglycerides, triglycerides, and phospholipids. In the fermenters (ruminoreticulum, cecum, colon), the microbes hydrolyze these compounds. Polyunsaturated long-chain fatty acids (e.g., linoleic and linolenic) are major intermediary products; however, polyunsaturated fatty acids are almost completely hydrogenated, and monounsaturated FAs are converted from *cis-* to *trans-* isomer forms. In the ruminoreticulum, the microorganisms also synthesize lipids for their cell walls, and these become another nutrient source when they pass to the intestine. Some of the lipids synthesized de novo have branched-chain forms that are found in the lipids of tissues and milk. It should be noted that bovine milk has a relatively low content of linoleic acid (18:2, omega-6).

QUANTITATIVE ASPECTS OF LIPID ABSORPTION

Several functional tests are available for the clinical evaluation of intestinal absorptive capacity for lipids. Oleic acid and triolein, labeled with iodine-131, have been used in dogs. On the day prior to the test, a small dose of Lugol's iodine is given orally to saturate the thyroid and to protect it against thyroidal uptake of isotope. Trace amounts of the isotope-containing substance are mixed with unlabeled carrier, the mixture is then given orally to provide a known dose of isotope. Subsequent measurement of plasma radioactivity, at intervals, allows estimation of the percentage of the dose that has been absorbed, based on assumptions about plasma volume.

Normal dogs excrete as much as 5 g of fat in the feces daily, a fairly constant amount over a range of fat intake from 15 to 48 g per day. *Intestinal malabsorption syndromes* are characterized by decreased ability to absorb fat, and fecal fat increases and becomes proportional to dietary intake. Excess fecal fat is called *steatorrhea*. It is characterized by bulky gray or tan stools that may have an oily appearance. It is usually accompanied by diarrhea, with loss of water, electrolytes, and fat-soluble vitamins. Four processes are involved in successful fat absorption: (1) hydrolysis by pancreatic lipases; (2) emulsification by bile salts, forming micelles; (3) entry of fatty acids and monoglycerides into epithelial cells of the villi; and (4) reesterification of fatty acids in the intestinal cells, with formation and secretion of chylomicrons.

In swine, absorption of ^{14}C-oleic acid has been studied with a dilution- and leakage-free perfusion of an isolated jejunal loop, with two reentrant fistulas (Fig. 39–1). Absorption of micellar lipid is about 40 percent compared with

TABLE 39–1 Functions of Lipids in the Animal Body

1. To store energy in a mobilizable form
2. To serve as important structural components of cell membranes
3. To serve as insulating material for conducting tissues such as myelin
4. To interact with micronutrients or vitamins that are lipid-soluble and hormones or other regulatory substances that are lipid derivatives
5. To serve as solubilizing agents for other lipids such as bile acids
6. To generate steroid hormones or their precursors and other regulatory substances such as prostaglandins and other eicosanoids
7. To serve as structural units for further synthesis

10 percent for particulate lipid. Absorptive efficiency is about 30 percent higher at low (2 to 4 mL per minute) than at high flow rates (10 mL per minute).

In ruminants, intestinal lipid absorption differs from that of monogastric species in that mostly very low density lipoproteins (VLDL) are absorbed into the intestinal lymph and are transported to the body tissue. Most of the absorption occurs after interaction with bile and pancreatic lipase, so the jejunum is the main site of absorption for long-chain fatty acids (LCFAs). Of course, large amounts of short-chain fatty acids (SCFAs) are produced in the ruminoreticulum as a result of microbial digestion of carbohydrates. These are absorbed mainly from the forestomachs, which can absorb fatty acids of chain length up to 12.

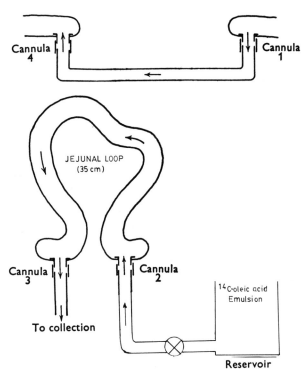

Figure 39–1 In acute studies of lipid absorption in pigs, a 35-cm loop of jejunum is isolated (cannulae 2 and 3), while progress of chyme is established between cannulae 1 and 4. The isolated segment is quantitatively perfused with a radioactive ^{14}C-oleic acid emulsion. The absorption of perfused lipids (at 40°C) is maximal at low flow rates (2 to 4 mL per minute) and is reduced at higher flow rates (10 mL per minute).

Lipids encapsulated with proteins, that have been denatured with formaldehyde, and made resistant to ruminoreticulum microbial digestion pass to the intestine, where they can be digested and absorbed as in monogastric animals. It is a way of protecting lipids from hydrogenation, so host tissue and milk fats can contain more polyunsaturated FAs. In the jejunal mucosa, the resulting triglyceride synthesis proceeds via the monoglyceride pathway rather than via 3-glycerol phosphate. Overall absorption of up to 1,400 g of FAs has been observed in lactating cows fed such protected lipids. The cow can utilize these substantial amounts of absorbed lipids effectively. It is surprising that levels of plasma ketone bodies are consistently lower, whereas concentrations of very low and high density lipoproteins (VLDL, LDL, and LDL$_2$, and HDL) and FFAs are increased in plasma and serum.

TRANSPORT OF LIPIDS VIA THE CIRCULATORY SYSTEM

Most triglycerides in the digestive tract are hydrolyzed to monoglycerides and fatty acids. On passing into the epithelial cells of the intestine they are re-formed into new molecules of TGs, which then coalesce to form minute (<0.5 μm) droplets called *chylomicrons*. These pass into the lymphatic capillaries and are carried with the lymph to enter the vascular system via the thoracic duct. Animals that consume large amounts of fat attain peak values (>1 percent) for chylomicrons in plasma about 1 to 2 hours after a fatty meal. The plasma may become turbid as a result. Since the chylomicrons have a short half-life in plasma (<1 hour), as the fat is removed by hydrolysis, the plasma soon becomes clear again. The removal of chylomicrons occurs mainly in the liver and adipose tissues. Both of these sites are well endowed with lipoprotein lipase. The enzyme is present in the capillary endothelium, where it attacks TGs, forming FFAs and glycerol.

FAT SYNTHESIS IN THE ANIMAL BODY AND LIPOGENESIS

Synthesis of fatty acids occurs in two general systems: cytoplasmic and mitochondrial. The *cytoplasmic system* builds palmitic acid, starting from acetyl CoA. This pathway, which requires NADP$^+$, ATP, carbon dioxide, and Mn^{++}, first transforms acetyl CoA to malonyl CoA. It is a route active in the liver, kidneys, adipose tissue, mammary glands, lungs, and brain. The other pathway, a *mitochondrial* system, elongates existing FAs by adding 2-carbon units via acetyl CoA. It requires ATP and yields saturated FAs with 18, 20, 22, or 24 carbon atoms, usually starting with the 16-carbon palmitic acid synthesized by the cytoplasmic system. Unsaturated FAs with one double bond may be formed in the liver from saturated FAs of the same chain length. Esterification of FFAs requires adequate amounts of

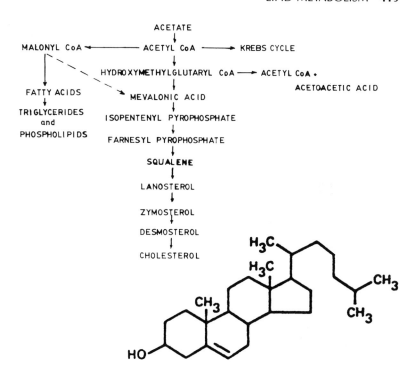

Figure 39-2 Top, Steps in the metabolic transformation of acetate into cholesterol. **Bottom,** Molecular structure of cholesterol.

glycerol in the form of alpha-glycerophosphate, a reduction product of dihydroxyacetone produced in glycolysis. As fat cells have low glycerokinase activity, they are dependent on the glycolytic pathway. Adipose tissue can use circulating FAs from chylomicrons and lipoproteins. Thus, the absorbed FAs and hepatic fats can influence the FA composition of depot fats. Extracellular lipoprotein lipase, formed by fat cells, induces the release of FFAs from lipoproteins. However, adipose tissue cannot effectively utilize the free glycerol released, and it must be returned to the liver for gluconeogenesis or must be metabolized in other tissues. Therefore, adipose cells require a concomitant supply of glucose to generate the alpha-glycerophosphate needed for esterification and for fat synthesis. Fat cells also lack the ability to form lipoproteins, hence their TGs must be stored via the droplets at their interior surfaces. They cannot be exported as TGs. The pentose phosphate cycle generates the necessary $NADP^+$ for cytoplasmic fat synthesis.

An important subgroup of lipids is derived from the condensed complex ring structure of phenanthrene. These substances, called *steroids,* are derived from the parent sterol compound cholesterol (Fig. 39-2). Several important hormones are based on the steroid nucleus. Human health is much concerned with the relationship between dietary lipids and cholesterol or TG concentrations in the blood. Because much cardiovascular disease is attributed to atherosclerosis, cholesterol metabolism has been a focal point for the study of lipid regulation.

Cholesterol has been a source of curiosity and fascination since it was first isolated from gallstones in 1784. In 1964, the Nobel Prize was awarded to K.E. Bloch and F. Lynen for defining the biosynthetic pathway for cholesterol.

Then, in 1985, the Nobel prize went to M.S. Brown and J.L. Golstein for identifying the LDL receptor pathway governing how cells obtain cholesterol. They also showed how an inherited defect in the pathway, seen in familial hypercholesterolemia, can lead to atherosclerosis (i.e., clogging of the arteries with plaques [atheromas] composed mainly of cholesterol).

Efforts continue in the search for safe and effective ways of confining blood cholesterol levels to a range that may prevent the formation of the lesions.

Cholesterol is synthesized de novo in the liver and other tissues, and it is also absorbed from the digesta. In the plasma, it is esterified with an LCFA (long-chain fatty acid [>16 C]) by lecithin-cholesterol acyl transferase. This cholesterol ester is transported to the peripheral tissues via LDL. There, the cholesterol can enter the plasma membranes of cells. The HDL fraction transports cholesterol from the tissues to the liver for excretion in the bile (Fig. 39-3).

The surface of the LDL is made up of the hydrophilic groups of the phospholipids that form the interface between the interior lipids and the aqueous plasma. Each LDL contains about 1,500 molecules of cholesterol esters and a protein molecule called apoprotein β-100. With specific tissue cell receptors, the LDLs form a complex that enters the cell, and lysosomal enzymes release the cholesterol in the cytoplasm. Accumulation of cholesterol in the cell suppresses 3-hydroxy-3-methylglutaryl CoA reductase (HMG CoA reductase), the rate-setting enzyme of cholesterol biosynthesis. A negative-feedback mechanism also results in suppression of LDL-receptor synthesis. Hypercholesterolemic patients cannot bind, internalize, and degrade the LDLs efficiently. The increased level of cholesterol in the blood can lead to its

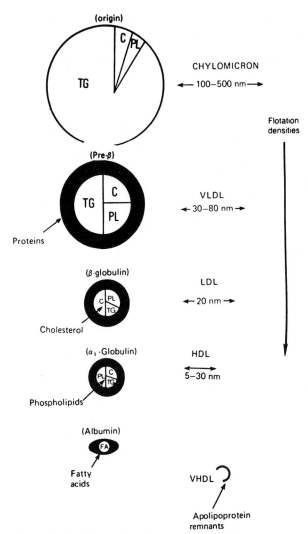

Figure 39–3 Types of blood lipoproteins according to their relative sizes, content of protein (outer layer), and lipid constituents (C, cholesterol; FA, fatty acids; PL, phospholipids; TG, triglycerides) in the central zone. Serum proteins are in parentheses. (HDL, High-density lipoproteins; LDL, low-density lipoproteins; VHDL, very-high-density lipoproteins; VLDL, very-low-density lipoproteins.)

deposition on the vascular endothelium of arterial walls, increasing the risk of heart attacks when the plaques form in branches of the coronary arteries.

MOBILIZATION OF FREE FATTY ACIDS

Mobilization of lipids from the TG stores of adipose tissues occurs when the supply of carbohydrates is inadequate to meet the body's basal energy needs or its increasing demands. Emergency situations that activate the sympathoadrenal system also lead to lipolysis. The key to the switch to lipolysis, or the release of FFAs from adipose tissue,

is hormone-sensitive lipase. The adipose cells contain an internal lipase system that has two components. The first, the rate-limiting step, is the lipase that hydrolyzes TGs, or triacylglycerols, to diacylglycerols (DAGs) upon activation by cyclic AMP (cAMP) produced in response to certain hormones. The second enzyme completes the hydrolysis of DAGs to glycerol and FFAs. The FFAs form a complex with plasma albumin and are carried via the blood to the liver and other organs.

The catecholamines (epinephrine and norepinephrine) increase the formation of cAMP and activate lipolysis. Glucagon, adrenocorticotropin (ACTH), somatotropin, and somatotropic hormone (STH) (also known as growth hormone [GH]) have similar effects. In contrast, insulin counteracts cAMP formation and inhibits lipolysis. In the absence of insulin, marked mobilization of FFAs occurs.

Two general types of adipose tissue are distinguishable visually by color. The cells of *white adipose tissue* have little cytoplasm and few mitochondria. *Brown adipose cells* have many mitochondria, which accounts for their brown color, since these organelles are rich in cytochromes. The brown adipose cells play a vital role in newborn and hibernating animals. The brown fat functions as a protecting thermogenic system surrounding the vital organs of neonates and as a heat-generating system to arouse the hibernators. Cold stress leads to sympathoadrenal stimulation and enhanced lipolysis. The specialized mitochondria of brown adipose tissue contain thermogenin, an unusual protein that responds to increases in FFAs by equilibrating H^+ across the mitochondrial membrane. This prevents the establishment of the proton gradient that couples the oxidation of FAs to ATP formation. The resulting uncoupling of oxidative phosphorylation leads to the energy of oxidative metabolism (cellular respiration) being released as heat. This process is called *nonshivering thermogenesis* and is a truly remarkable example of physiological adaptation.

Compared with control piglets housed at a temperature of 23°C, cold-adapted piglets (kept at 12°C) can attain comparable growth rates and carcass composition but consume 20 percent more feed. Lipoprotein lipase activity is higher in white adipose tissue and the heart. Lipogenesis is greater in white adipose tissue than in the liver. Cytochrome oxidase activity increases in interscapular muscle (75 percent), perirenal adipose tissue (40 percent), and liver (30 percent). Plasma levels of thyroid hormones are also raised.

Other events, such as those leading to anxiety or discomfort, can result in release of epinephrine and norepinephrine, each promoting the release of FFAs into the bloodstream. Rapid mobilization of FFAs, like glucose, might be a part of the overall physiological response to situations that threaten homeostasis. Centrally acting changes, such as respiratory acidosis, induced by breathing a gas mixture high in carbon dioxide, trigger a discharge of the sympathoadrenal system. Asphyxia or anoxia causes stimulation of the hepatic-sympathetic system, leading to a release of K^+ by hepatic cells and increased blood glucose in dogs. In adrenalectomized cats and dogs, stimulation of the peripheral ends of the splanchnic nerves produces a hyperglycemic response that is directly dependent on activation of sympathetic afferent fibers to the liver. Low oxygen tensions also increase sympathetic activity, resulting in tachycardia, hyperglycemia, hypertension, increased FFAs in plasma, and higher hematocrit (packed cell volume). Adrenalectomy or sympathectomy greatly reduces most of these responses (Fig. 39–4). The activity of the sympathetic system, triggered by sudden changes in plasma pH or carbon dioxide, causes a release of FFAs.

When supplies of carbohydrates are adequate to meet the needs of the body, utilization of TGs for energy is depressed. The carbohydrates are used in preference to fats, the so-called *"fat-sparing" effect* of carbohydrates. In adipose tissues, TGs and FFAs are in equilibrium. When a surplus of alpha-glycerophosphate is present, the equilibrium shifts in favor of TG synthesis, leaving very little FFA available for energy. At the same time, FFAs are synthesized more rapidly

than they are degraded, because carbohydrates form large amounts of acetyl CoA, which can be converted into FAs.

The first stage in the synthesis of fatty acids involves the carboxylation of acetyl CoA to form malonyl CoA, a rate-limiting step, via the biotin-containing enzyme acetyl CoA carboxylase, which requires ATP. The added —COOH residue is stripped off as CO_2 later during condensation reactions. This carboxylase reaction is accelerated by the intermediates of the carboxylic acid cycle that increase when carbohydrates are available in excess. The stimulation of fat synthesis can lead to obesity, or "fattening," or to fat sparing.

A lack or undersupply of carbohydrates shifts the TG-FFA equilibrium in favor of FFA formation. This leads to mobilization of TGs from adipose cells and increased use of FFAs for energy in place of the missing carbohydrates.

Figure 39–4 In dogs, changes in blood (femoral artery) free fatty acids during respiratory anoxia, adrenal hypoxia, and anoxia after sympathectomy (section of both splanchnic nerves).

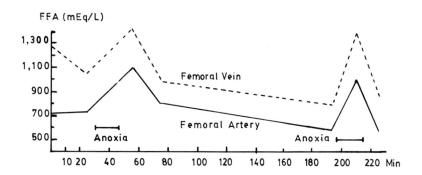

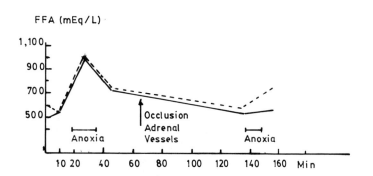

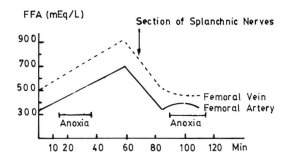

HORMONAL REGULATION OF LIPID METABOLISM

Insulin is the most important hormonal modulator of substrate flows in fat metabolism. It stimulates glucose uptake and utilization by fat cells and accelerates lipogenesis by leading to an increased rate of production of acetyl CoA in their cytoplasm. The formation of acetyl CoA in mitochondria is increased also by triggering dephosphorylation of pyruvate dehydrogenase, converting this enzyme to its active form, and stimulating oxidative decarboxylation. The absence of insulin in diabetes mellitus leads to unrestrained stimulation of intracellular lipase and marked mobilization of FFAs. A similar sequence occurs in starvation, since the lowered blood glucose suppresses the production and release of insulin.

Increased oxidation of FFAs occurs during strenuous exercise and other types of stress. This is attributable mainly to the effects of *epinephrine and norepinephrine* from the adrenal medulla and sympathetic nerves. These mediators activate TG-lipase in fat cells. The concentration of FFAs in the blood can increase up to eight-fold as a result, with a corresponding rise in the use of FFAs for energy.

The adenohypophysis–adrenal cortex system also uses the mechanism of TG-lipase activation. It involves release of *ACTH* that causes the adrenal cortex to secrete glucocorticoid (mainly *cortisol*). Mobilization of FFAs similarly occurs. If these hormones are secreted in excess over a long period, as in Cushing's disease, the chronic fat mobilization may lead to ketosis. This is called the *ketogenic effect*, of interest in veterinary medicine because glucocorticoid hormones and their analogues are used pharmacologically to treat bovine ketosis. *Cortisol* prevents the cytosolic formation of eicosanoids (prostaglandins and leukotrienes) by inhibiting the liberation of arachidonic acid from phospholipids of the plasma membranes.

Growth hormone (or somatotropic hormone) has an action similar to those of corticotropin and glucocorticoids on the hormone-sensitive lipase. It too can have a modest ketogenic effect.

Thyroid hormones triiodothyronine (T_3) and thyroxine (T_4) cause rapid fat mobilization, apparently via an indirect action as part of its overall effect of increasing the rate of energy metabolism. This leads to reduced levels of acetyl CoA and of other intermediates of fat and of carbohydrate metabolism. Equilibria shift in favor of increased mobilization of fats.

FATTY LIVER OR HEPATIC LIPIDOSIS

Abnormal accumulation of fat in the parenchymal cells is a common response of the liver to injury or to metabolic stress. It occurs when the rate of triglyceride accumulation within the hepatic cells exceeds their rate of metabolic degradation and their release as lipoproteins. Despite a multiplicity of etiological factors that can contribute to the patho-

genesis of fatty liver, the lipids that accumulate in the hepatocytes are predominantly triglycerides. Fatty liver is seen in animals with high energy demands (e.g., peak lactation or late gestation), when more fat is mobilized from adipose tissue to the hepatocytes. Obese animals subjected to dietary restriction (anorexia in cats, postparturient stresses in cows) also develop hepatic lipidosis.

In rats, fatty liver can be induced experimentally by administration of toxic substances or by dietary excess. Carbon tetrachloride, phosphorus, ethionine, and puromycin are given to create experimental hepatic lipidosis. Diets deficient in choline or containing added orotic acid also cause hepatic lipidosis. It should be noted that choline is involved in methyl transfer reactions and phospholipid synthesis and also serves as a precursor for acetylcholine synthesis. Adrenalectomy prevents or delays many types of fatty liver.

The basic pathogenetic mechanism of all these appears to be a block in the secretion of hepatic TGs into the plasma. A characteristic feature is that the deposition of TGs is both preceded and accompanied by decreasing concentrations of plasma TGs and lipoproteins. In the hour following intoxication, the level of hepatic TGs rises rapidly, whereas the level of plasma TGs decreases very rapidly at first and then declines more slowly (Fig. 39–5). It appears that the level of TGs in the plasma falls prior to an increase in the level of TGs in the liver. It is presumed that this is because only a fraction of the TGs in the liver are immediate precursors of plasma TGs, the pool of liver TGs is much greater than that of the plasma TGs, and the turnover of plasma TGs is faster than that of liver TGs.

Identification of the primary defect remains elusive. It may be at the level either of conjugation of the various components or of the secretion of preformed lipoproteins. In ethionine-induced hepatic lipidosis, a profound drop in hepatic adenosine triphosphate (ATP) is one of the earliest changes. In orotic acid–fed animals, the synthesis of plasma proteins is not impaired. In the early stages of fatty liver development, the fine lipid droplets often appear surrounded by a membrane that is continuous with that of the endoplasmic reticulum. As the condition progresses, the droplets grow in size and coalesce. The small 'liposomes' mature into giant liposomes composed largely of TGs, and the formation of endoplasmic reticulum is reduced. Defective synthesis or secretion of lipoproteins causes the TGs to build up in the cisternae of the endoplasmic reticulum (Fig. 39–6). Administration of adenine to ethionine-treated rats with hepatic lipidosis leads to rapid disappearance of the liposomes from the endoplasmic reticulum and of the fat agglomerations from the liver cells.

Another nonmetabolic form of hepatic lipidosis follows injury to hepatocytes, and the accumulation of fat within the hepatic cells is then termed *fatty degeneration*.

PHOSPHOLIPID METABOLISM

Phospholipids (PLs) contain phosphorus, glycerol, and FAs. They have the unique property of having a lipid-soluble

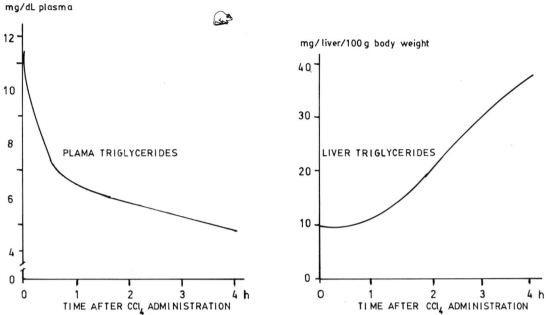

Figure 39–5 Chronology of changes in the triglycerides of hepatic cells and in the plasma of fasting rats after oral administration of carbon tetrachloride.

hydrophobic part (the FAs), and a water-soluble hydrophilic part (the phosphoglycerol moiety). Phospholipids tend to form thin sheets that pair up to create a bilayer with the hydrophobic alkyl FA chains sandwiched between the hydrophilic phosphoglycerol facing the aqueous medium on each side. This is the basic structure of most biological membranes, which also contain protein molecules that provide for the specialized functions of the cell membranes.

Plasma membrane phospholipids are the source of 20-carbon polyunsaturated acids (4 C=C: arachidonic or eicosatetraenoic acid, which can also arise from 3 C=C eicosatrienoic acid; and 5 C=C: eicosapentaenoic acid) for the cytoplasmic enzymes synthesizing the eicosanoids. Phospholipases activated by mechanical, chemical, or radiation insult or by other autacoids released by inflammatory cells liberate 20-carbon acids from the plasma membrane into the cytoplasm. *Autacoids* (e.g., histamine, 5-hydroxytryptamine, bradykinin) are natural agents employed by the animal organism to perform various functions in health and disease. The antiinflammatory effect of cortisol is explained

Figure 39–6 Role of liposomes in hepatocytes during the metabolism of blood lipids (plasma FFAs, chylomicrons) during normal formation of lipoproteins, and dysfunctions associated with excess (ethionine, puromycin, phosphorus, carbon tetrachloride, orotic acid) or deficiency (choline) of substances leading to development of hepatic lipidosis (fatty liver).

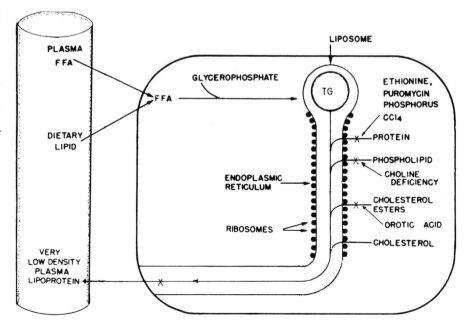

by its inhibition of these phospholipases and of the subsequent synthesis of all eicosanoids. Specific microsomal or cytosolic enzymes use these 20-carbon acids to synthesize the various eicosanoids. The cytosolic lipoxygenase pathways lead to the formation of lipoxins and mostly leukotrienes (LTs or LT_4s), both powerful bronchoconstrictors. The LTs were formerly known as the slow-reacting substances of anaphylaxis (SRS-A, or SRS). The microsomal cyclooxygenase pathway, activated by oxygen free radicals and lipid peroxides, creates first a prostaglandin endoperoxide (PGG_2) and then the endoperoxide PGH_2, which is the common precursor of all biologically active prostaglandins. Some nonsteroidal antiinflammatory agents (NSAIAs) such as acetylsalicylic acid (aspirin) and indomethacin specifically block cyclooxygenase activity and the synthesis of prostaglandins but do not affect the lipoxygenase pathways for synthesis of LTs and lipoxins. By acting on PGH_2, separate synthetases form prostacyclin (PGI_2) and thromboxane (TXA_2), and specific isomerases synthesize prostaglandins E_2 and D_2, whereas a reductase produces $PGF_{2\alpha}$.

The phospholipids also are part of the complex structure of lipoproteins that transport lipids in the blood. In the liver, the phospholipids are metabolized by dephosphorylation to yield diacylglycerols for fat synthesis (TGs). The hepatocytes can also use phospholipids as starting points for synthesis of other more complex phospholipids such as phosphatidyl derivatives with choline, serine, glycerol, inositol, and ethanolamine.

Myelin, the insulating sheath around large nerves, contains cholesterol, sphingolipids (sphingomyelin and cerebroside), and phospholipids (ethanolamine, plasmalogens).

OTHER LIPID COMPOUNDS

A variety of other lipid substances in the animal body do not fit in these general classes. These include the fat-soluble vitamins A, D, E, and K.

REFERENCES

Bergman EM. Energy contribution of volatile fatty acids from the gastrointestinal tract in various species. Physiol Rev 1990;70:567.

Brown MS, Golstein JL. Lipoprotein metabolism in the macrophage: Implications for cholesterol deposition in atherosclerosis. Annu Rev Biochem 1983;52:223.

Durchschlag RP, Robinson JL. Species specificity in the metabolic consequences of orotic acid consumption. J Nutr 1980;110:822.

Freeman CP, Noakes DE, Annison EF, Hill KJ. Quantitative aspects of intestinal fat absorption in young pigs. Br J Nutr 1968;22:739.

Herpin P, Bertin R, Dividich JLE, Portet R. Some regulatory aspects of thermogenesis in cold-exposed piglets. Comp Biochem Physiol A 1987;87:1073.

Lombard B. Considerations on the pathogenesis of fatty liver. Clin Invest 1966;15:1.

McElroy WT, Jr, Spitzer JJ. Mobilization of FFA in dogs during respiratory acidosis. J Appl Physiol 1961;16:339.

Mersmann HJ. Lipid metabolism in swine. In: Swine in cardiovascular research. Boca Raton: CRC Press, 1986.

CHAPTER 40

PROTEIN METABOLISM

Proteins make up the largest percentage (about 75 percent) of the body solids. Structural proteins, contractile proteins, heme and myoglobin, nucleoproteins, enzymes, and regulatory peptides and proteins are a few among the great variety of proteins in the animal body. Specific aspects of protein metabolism in veterinary physiology that require special attention include the unique features of nitrogen metabolism in ruminants. Special considerations relate to protein deposition for growth in meat production and for solids rather than fat in milk production.

Many young animals grow two to three times faster than human babies because they have much higher rates of protein accretion. Ruminants have rather variable conversion rates from forage protein to milk protein, about 23 percent for dairy cows but only about 3 percent for lactating ewes.

Depending on the nature of the dietary proteins in the rumen, a large proportion is degraded to ammonia and organic acids and to nonprotein nitrogen (NPN) compounds such as urea. The rumen microbiota can incorporate nitrogen from urea and ammonia into microbial protein. The biological value of bacterial proteins tends to be lower than that of many feed proteins. Because much of the feed protein is digested by the microbes, the ruminant host has no choice and must accept the resulting "diet" composed of microbial carcasses.

Neonatal animals absorb colostrum proteins intact from the small intestine to provide passive immune protection via gamma-globulin. Plasma gamma-globulin levels rise from very low levels within a few hours after the first ingestion of colostrum. This is the principal mechanism by which the newborn of the major domesticated mammals acquire maternal passive immunity. In the absence of the absorption of colostrum antibody proteins, the risk of infection and serious disease is greatly increased. The intestine of the young of most species can absorb these proteins only during the first day or two after birth.

BASIC PROPERTIES OF PROTEINS

A protein is a string of amino acids (AAs) linked together by the peptide bond between the carboxyl group of one AA and the amino group of another, leaving one of each of the groups free at each end to establish another such bond. The resultant chain can be a small peptide, made up of two or more AA residues, or huge proteins comprising as many as several thousand AAs with molecular weights ranging from 18,000 to 10 million. Special groups on some AAs allow for cross-bridging, as when two sulfhydryl (SH) groups are present and can join as —S—S—. It is very important to recognize that secondary and tertiary arrays of the molecule

occur because these give the structure three-dimensional arrangements in space, which permit the creation of active sites for particular functions. Since 20 or more different AAs are used as building blocks, there is an almost infinite variety of possible combinations to create different polypeptides and proteins. The sequence of AAs is identical in each molecule of a given protein in a particular species or strain. This sequence is determined by the succession of nucleotides in the nucleic acid or the chromosome responsible for its synthesis. Three nucleotides code for each amino acid.

The AAs are the basic currency of protein metabolism. From the dietary viewpoint, an amino acid that cannot be synthesized de novo in the animal body is called essential, whereas one that can is termed nonessential (Fig. 40–1). About 10 different AAs in the body are essential nutrients in the young of most animal species. Thus, these animals are dependent on autotropic plants and certain bacteria that can synthesize the necessary AAs, or they must obtain them by eating the tissues of other animals. The range of concentration of total AAs in the plasma is about 35 to 65 mg per deciliter, an average of about 2 mg per deciliter per AA, but some are present in much higher concentrations than others. Having ionizable weak acidic and basic groups, the AAs are ionized at the pH of the extracellular fluid and account for 2 to 3 mEq of each of the anions and cations in the plasma. Proteins usually form colloidal solutions except for the fibrous ones, which are insoluble. Many proteins exist in conjugated form with nucleic acids, carbohydrates, or lipids.

The plasma protein profile reflects dietary intake of protein and energy-producing substances. For example, when dairy cows are fed 5 to 8 kg of hay and 4 to 6 kg of beet pulp, wheat bran, and concentrate, the ratio of essential (E) to nonessential (N) free AAs in plasma is about 1.08. When the level of feed is reduced by 30 percent, the ratio increases to 1.29, indicating an increase in gluconeogenesis from AAs and a loss of body weight. If digestible protein in the diet is selectively reduced by 30 percent, the E : N ratio is lowered to 0.86 despite high levels of glycine and alanine (Table 40–1).

The plasma levels of glycine and serine are higher, and those of valine, leucine, isoleucine, and phenylalanine are lower in cattle fed purified diets containing urea as the sole source of dietary nitrogen, than for cattle fed soybean protein. Apparently insufficient amounts of branched-chain fatty acids in the rumen lead to lower levels of valine, leucine, and isoleucine. Plasma concentrations of most of the AAs, especially the essential ones, are lower when urea is the only source of nitrogen. Nevertheless, it is remarkable that so much of the protein requirements of ruminants can be met with no proteins or AAs in the diet.

Ammonia is used for microbial protein synthesis in the rumen, but some is absorbed from the forestomachs and

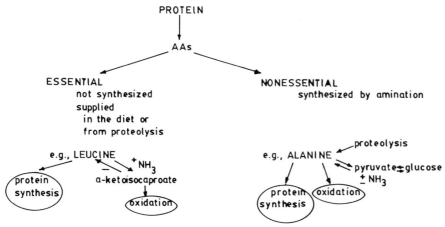

Figure 40–1 Not synthesized in the body of monogastric animals, *essential AAs* are produced by microorganisms in the ruminoreticulum of ruminant animals. Essential AAs are supplied as nutrients in food or from protein degradation. *Leucine,* an essential AA, is metabolized by reincorporation into protein synthesis (75 percent) and deaminated into aketoisocaproate, which may be reaminated into leucine or may be oxidized (25 percent). *Nonessential AAs* are synthesized mostly de novo by amination of a carbon skeleton or are produced from protein degradation. A nonessential AA such as *alanine* can be reincorporated into protein, oxidized, or deaminated into pyruvate, which can be reaminated into alanine.

intestine. Ammonia then passes to the liver, where it is synthesized into urea for recycling to the gastrointestinal tract in saliva or for excretion via the kidneys. The enzymes for the cycle are present in the ruminant liver but do not appear to increase adaptively when high levels of urea are fed. Ammonia is toxic if it accumulates in the body, leading to neurological disorders and acid-base imbalance.

TRANSPORT AND STORAGE OF AMINO ACIDS

Absorption of intact proteins occurs in the first few days or weeks of life, especially of colostrum proteins and antibodies. They can be detected in vacuoles in the cytoplasm and in tubular spaces within the cells. They appear to enter via invagination of the apical plasma membrane, an example of pinocytosis. This process is self-limiting and disappears within a few days or weeks, depending on the species. Administration of cortisone accelerates cell maturation and the "closure" effect; the epithelial cells lose the capacity to absorb intact proteins.

Peptides are absorbed by enterocytes more readily than free AAs. It is uncertain whether they are hydrolyzed to AAs before entering the circulatory system or whether they can pass intact in the peptide form. Conflicting experimental evidence suggests that both routes are used, with peptides constituting very little to as much as 70 percent of the total AAs (free and combined) in the portal plasma.

Individual AAs have different transport systems into the intestinal cells, depending on their chemical structure:

1. Neutral (monoamino-monocarboxylic) AAs show mutual competition for transport and have the greatest requirement for Na^+. This group includes histidine.
2. Acidic (monoamino-dicarboxylic) AAs are not transported actively (i.e., against concentration gradients). After uptake, aspartic and glutamic acids are transaminated. Under physiological conditions, when they are absorbed, nearly all these AAs enter the portal blood as alanine.
3. Basic (diamino-monocarboxylic) AAs and the neutral AA cystine all appear to be absorbed via the same transport system. This group includes lysine, arginine, and ornithine.
4. A miscellaneous group, composed of proline, hydroxyproline, N-methylglycine, N-dimethylglycine, and betaine, has low affinity for the Na^+-dependent pathway of absorption.
5. A gamma-glutamyl cycle, not requiring Na^+ for absorption, has been proposed as a transport system for AAs. The membrane-bound enzyme gamma-glutamyl transferase (GGT) catabolyzes the initial step in glutathione degradation, transferring the gamma-glutamyl moiety to AA receptors forming cysteinylglycine.

Malabsorption of tryptophan, the first clear demonstration of a defect in AA transport, shared by intestine and kidney cells, is responsible for the clinical signs (cerebellar ataxia) and functional disturbances of Hartnup's disease. The blue diaper syndrome is a familial form of hypercalcemia linked to defective intestinal absorption of tryptophan. This defective absorption is identified by techniques used to study Hartnup's disease. The blue color is attributable to oxidative conjugation of two molecules of indican to indigotin, or indigo blue. Administration of neomycin prevents formation of the indigotin.

TABLE 40–1 Levels of Free Essential and Nonessential Amino Acids in Plasma of Dairy Cows, After 6 Months of Experimental Feeding with Diets Adequate in Protein, Reduced in Protein Quantity, and Reduced in Protein Quality

Free Amino Acids in Plasma	Protein Feeding		
	Adequate (mg/dL)	Inadequate Quantity (mg/dL)	Inadequate Quality (mg/dL)
Essential (E)			
Arginine	1.53	1.56	0.97
Histidine	1.30	0.92	1.12
Isoleucine	1.40	1.27	1.17
Leucine	1.49	1.54	1.11
Lysine + ornithine	2.81	2.51	2.41
Methionine	0.39	0.22	0.21
Phenylalanine	1.10	0.66	0.80
Threonine	1.25	1.06	0.83
Valine	2.51	2.50	2.06
TOTAL	13.79	12.24	10.70
Nonessential (N)			
Alanine	2.54	1.53	2.05
Aspartic acid	0.57	0.49	0.17
Citrulline	1.86	1.56	0.38
Glutamic acid	1.16	0.87	1.61
Glycine	2.74	1.60	3.63
Proline	0.69	1.21	1.41
Serine	1.16	0.97	1.71
Taurine	0.64	0.50	0.56
Tyrosine	1.13	0.73	0.90
TOTAL	12.49	9.46	12.42
E : N ratio	1.08	1.29	0.86

Methionine malabsorption results in the appearance of hydroxybutyric acid in the feces. Cystinuria is a defect in intestinal transport of dibasic amino acids (e.g., lysine, arginine).

Most absorbed AAs are removed by the liver, with the exception of some of those that have branched chains. Particularly large hepatic uptake occurs with alanine, glycine, and glutamine, and uptake of arginine, tyrosine, phenylalanine, and serine is substantial. Both free AAs and plasma proteins pass into the circulation from the liver for subsequent uptake, synthesis, or catabolism in the tissues, particularly skeletal muscle and mammary gland (during lactation).

Nucleic acids are required for cell multiplication, but their precursors are usually well represented in the diet. Purines and pyrimidines are degraded, and allantoin is the principal excretory end-product of purine metabolism in ruminants. Urinary purines can account for 14 to 47 percent of purines absorbed from the small intestine. Sheep, for example, show a linear relationship between nucleic acid digestion and allantoin appearance in the urine. The rumen, blood, and urine concentrations of purines decrease rapidly when cattle are fasted. Again, rumen concentrations of nucleic acids are correlated with the levels of allantoin and uric acid in the urine and plasma. The pyrimidines, cytosine and uracil, appear to be degraded with the production of beta-alanine. Similarly, catabolism of thymine involves the production of beta-aminoisobutyric acid.

The nutritive value of various feed sources of nitrogen is

TABLE 40–2 Biological Parameters with Various Sources of Dietary Nitrogen in Sheep

Parameters	Soybean Meal	Milk Casein	Corn Zein	Urea
Biological value (BV)	84.8	78.3	84.3	76.4
Digestibility (True)	88.9	79.8	68.1	88.7
Net protein value	75.4	62.5	57.4	67.8
Nitrogen balance (g/day)				
Calculated*	0.04	−0.68	−1.23	−0.85
Experimental	0.04	−0.53	−1.00	−0.68

*From true digestibility of nitrogen requirement = (endogenous urinary N + 1 + metabolic fecal N) × 6.25 × 100/BV, where 1 is the daily N deposition in wool); or N balance = digestible N intake − (endogenous urinary N + 1 + metabolic fecal N) × 100/BV.

not uniform in animals. In sheep, the biological value (BV) (i.e., the percentage of digested nitrogen retained by the body) ranges from 76.4 for urea to 84.8 for soybean meal (Table 40–2).

PROTEIN REQUIREMENTS AND REGULATION

Sheep nourished only by intraabdominal infusion of enriched casein (BV, 1.0), casein (BV, 0.8), or gelatin (BV, 0.07) are used to estimate endogenous losses of nitrogen. These are about 245 mg nitrogen per kilogram$^{0.75}$ body weight. Urinary nitrogen levels do not change in response to enriched casein (casein plus added methionine, lysine, phenylalanine, and arginine) infusions, but major changes are seen when gelatin is infused (Figs. 40–2 and 40–3).

The maintenance requirement for nitrogen is the amount that needs to be retained to offset the endogenous loss, using the mean value of 245 mg per unit of metabolic

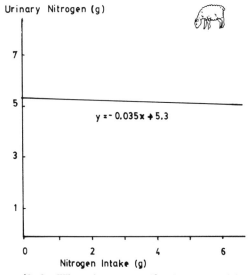

Figure 40–2 When sheep are artificially nourished by intra-abomasal infusion of enriched casein, urinary nitrogen excretion is almost constant regardless of the quantity of protein administered.

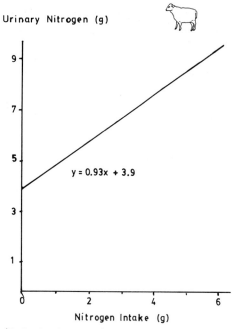

Figure 40–3 In sheep artificially nourished by intraabomasal infusion of gelatin, urinary nitrogen excretion increases with the quantity of protein administered.

body weight (MBW) per day. Matching this level with absorbed nutrients requires 282 mg per MBW per day of casein or 3,500 mg per MBW per day of gelatin. It is virtually impossible to meet the nitrogen needs on a pure gelatin diet.

HORMONAL REGULATION OF PROTEIN METABOLISM

The hormones involved in protein metabolism are growth hormone, insulin, glucocorticoids, anabolic hormones, and thyroid hormones.

Growth hormone (GH) affects a variety of tissues, promoting the growth of bone, muscle, and viscera in young, rapidly growing animals. It can modulate DNA transcription and RNA translation in cells, favoring protein synthesis. It may also increase the uptake of amino acids by muscle cells, by stimulating membrane transport of AAs. Since it promotes lipolysis of depot fats, the increased availability of FFAs for energy reduces the rate of oxidation of AAs, sparing more of them for protein synthesis. GH also promotes sulfate and AA incorporation into collagen, cartilage, and fibroblasts via the polypeptides called *somatomedins* that are produced in the liver.

Insulin stimulates AA uptake into cells, may also regulate translation, and may increase phosphorylation of ribosomal protein. In addition, it increases polyamine formation, which is involved in synthesis of ribosomal RNA. The absence of insulin reduces protein synthesis almost to zero because of the lack of the above effects and because the decreased availability of glucose leads to a greater use of AAs for energy, leaving less for protein synthesis.

Glucocorticoids decrease the quantity of protein in most tissues, raising the levels of AAs in the plasma. An exception is that both liver protein content and plasma protein levels are increased. The general effect is to increase the mobilization of protein from extrahepatic tissues, allowing the liver to step up the synthesis of hepatic cell proteins and plasma proteins. Lack of glucocorticoids leads to inadequate availability of AAs for either significant gluconeogenesis or ketogenesis from proteins.

Anabolic hormones, notably *testosterone and the synthetic steroid stanozolol,* lead to increased protein deposition throughout the body but particularly in contractile proteins of skeletal muscle. Unlike GH, which causes tissues to grow continuously, anabolic hormones cause muscle to enlarge only during several months, then a plateau is reached despite their continued administration. Their action appears to occur via acceleration of RNA and protein anabolism.

Thyroid hormones such as thyroxine (T_4) accelerate cell metabolism generally. If adequate supplies of carbohydrates and lipids are available, along with an excess of AAs, thyroid hormones can increase the rate of protein synthesis. When sufficient carbohydrates and lipids are unavailable, T_4 leads to rapid degradation of proteins and to the use of the liberated AAs for energy.

PYRIMIDINE AND PURINE METABOLISM

Complex nitrogen-containing rings are essential components of the polynucleotides of DNA and RNA and of nucleotide coenzymes. Synthesis of the purine and pyrimidine rings is complex and occurs from AAs, mainly in the liver.

The pyrimidine ring is formed by condensation of aspartic acid and carbamyl phosphate. This complex is oxidized to orotic acid, then converted to a nucleotide by adding phosphoribosyl pyrophosphate (PRPP) and decarboxylated to uridylic acid (uridine monophosphate, or UMP). Addition of an amino group (NH_2) leads to cytidylic nucleotide (cytidine triphosphate, or CTP), whereas adding a methyl group (CH_3) yields the thymidilic series (thymidine monophosphate, or TMP). The latter requires 1-carbon units bound to folic acid and vitamin B_{12}. The TMP series is essential for DNA synthesis in rapidly differentiating blood cells; otherwise, anemia results. The formation of pyrimidines of the thymidylate series may require a coenzyme derived from vitamin B_{12} to reduce and transfer the 1-carbon fragment that is needed. Large doses of folic acid may alleviate the anemia associated with the pernicious anemia syndrome, but they cannot reverse the devastating effect of vitamin B_{12} deficiency on the nervous system.

Purine synthesis starts with PRPP, to which the first nitrogen atom is added and built up in a series of steps to form the purine ring. Two of the steps require a hydroxymethyl transferase tetrahydrofolate and serine to generate and transfer the 1-carbon groups that are needed. The resulting inosinic acid (inosine monophosphate, or IMP) can be converted to either adenylic acid (adenosine monophosphate, or AMP) or guanylic acid (guanosine monophosphate, or GMP) by adding nitrogen at the appropriate site.

Pyrimidine ring structures can be completely catabolized to carbon dioxide and ammonia. Purine bases, which cannot be catabolized to carbon dioxide and ammonia, are either recycled as the free bases or deaminated to xanthine (e.g., guanine) or hypoxanthine (adenosine and inosine). Xanthine oxidase catalyzes their conversion to the end-product uric acid, which is filtered and excreted via the urine. Precipitation of crystals of monosodium urate, which has low solubility, leads to mechanical inflammation of the joints, often accompanied by renal damage with renal calculi. Unsightly swellings, called *tophi,* contain sodium urate deposits. In humans, this painful condition is called gout.

REFERENCES

Aldrete JS, McIlrath DC, Hallenbeck GA. Effect of portal ligation and of Eck's fistula on hepatic blood flow and concentration of blood ammonia. J Surg Res 1967;7:504.

Asplund JM. Amino acid requirements and biological value of protein for sheep. J Nutr 1987;117:1207.

National Research Council. Ruminant nitrogen usage. Washington, DC: National Academy Press, 1985.

Ørskov ER. Possible nutritional constraints in meeting energy and amino acid requirements of the highly productive ruminant. In: Ruckebusch Y, Thivend P, eds. Digestive physiology and metabolism in ruminants. Westport, CT: AVI Publishing, 1980.

Owens FN, Goetsch AL. Digesta passage rates and microbial protein synthesis. In: Milligan LP, Grovum WL, Dobson A, eds. Control of digestion and metabolism in ruminants. Englewood Cliffs, NJ: Prentice-Hall, 1986.

Owens FN, Zinn R. Protein metabolism of ruminant animals. In: Church DC, ed. The ruminant animal. Englewood Cliffs, NJ: Prentice-Hall, 1988.

Wallace RJ. Ecology of rumen microorganisms: Protein use. In: Dobson A, Dobson MJ, eds. Aspects of digestive physiology in ruminants. Ithaca, NY: Cornell University Press, 1988.

Webb KE, Jr. Amino acid and peptide absorption from the gastrointestinal tract. Fed Proc 1986;45:2268.

CHAPTER 41

METABOLISM OF SKELETAL MUSCLE

A metabolically complex tissue, skeletal muscle serves several roles in the animal organism. The primary function of muscle tissue, which comprises about 50 percent of the body mass, is to produce movement and posture. It also provides amino acids to the liver for gluconeogenesis (production of glucose for general body requirements). The working activity of skeletal muscles (W = force × distance) dictates a parallel increase in the work of the striated cardiac muscle and changes in the activities of smooth muscle. Striated cardiac muscle decreases the volume of the chambers of the heart in a coordinated rhythm to propel blood through the vascular system. Smooth muscle in the wall of hollow organs may cause viscera to contract, as in the digestive tract and in the vessels of the circulatory system, and to maintain organ dimensions against applied loads. These changes occur, in association with harder work by the respiratory muscles, to pump and to bring more metabolites and oxygen to the working skeletal muscle fibers.

INTRODUCTION TO MUSCLE FUNCTION

A remarkable feature of skeletal muscle is its ability to change rapidly from a relaxed state to an active state. The chronological processes that occur during skeletal muscle activity include cholinergic transmission of a depolarization signal coming from a spinal motor neuron, propagation of this action potential over the plasma membrane surface and into the muscle cell, release of Ca^{++} from intracellular reserve, and intervention of ATPase for the contraction of the protein myofilaments (actin, myosin). A knowledge of the intimate structure of the skeletal muscle is essential for a clear understanding of the contraction mechanism.

Exercise (i.e., the activity of skeletal muscles associated with locomotion) causes an enormous increase in energy expenditure, which can quickly attain a maximum that may be 100 times that of the resting state. Skeletal, or voluntary, muscles are attached to the bones and the joints of the skeleton in such ways that their contraction leads to movement, mainly locomotion. The *growth* of the locomotor skeleton is programmed genetically to proceed in harmony with the growth of the locomotor muscles.

Classification of Skeletal Muscle

Striated muscles are composed of muscle fibers (myofibers) with different contractile properties. All myofibers innervated by a single motor neuron (a motor unit) in the ventral horn of the gray matter of the spinal cord are of the same fiber type. The classification of these myofibers is based on major physiological features: rates of contraction (fast, slow), rates of fatigue (nonfatiguing, fast fatiguing, fatigue resistant), histochemical staining (oxidative with low myosin ATPase activity, glycolytic with high myosin ATPase activity), biochemical activity of myosin, and color (light, dark).

Three major types of skeletal muscle fibers are recognized: Type I, Type IIA, and Type IIB. A Type-I fiber is characterized as dark (red), slow-contracting (S), low in myosin ATPase, rich in mitochondria, nonfatiguing, and having a slow twitch with a high oxidative capacity (SO). Type-IIA fibers are light (white) and fast contracting and have a fast twitch with both oxidative and glycolytic activities (FOG), intermediate myosin ATPase activity and mitochondrion number, and fatigue resistance. Type-IIB fibers are light (white), fast contracting, fast fatiguing, and have a fast twitch pattern and mainly a glycolytic metabolism (FG), high myosin ATPase activity, and few mitochondria. The metabolic patterns of each of the three main types of mammalian skeletal muscle differ (Table 41–1).

Most muscles contain Type-I (dark) and Type-II (light) fibers in percentages that vary from muscle to muscle and within muscles. The variation in the percentages of Type-I and Type-II fibers affects the color of muscles. Type-I fibers (slow-contracting, slow-fatiguing, oxidative) predominate in muscles that function to maintain posture and slow locomotion (e.g., vastus intermedius) and muscles that contract slowly or continuously (e.g., diaphragm, masticatory muscles). Muscles that contract quickly for sprinting (semimembranosus, semitendinosus) contain more Type-II fibers and are naturally pale.

The proportions and distributions of the three types of muscle fibers vary among animal species and between breeds. The mean proportion of Type-I fibers is only 3 percent in greyhound dogs, 31 percent in mongrel dogs, 7 percent in quarter horses, 12 percent in thoroughbreds, and 31 percent in hunters. In horses, muscle fiber types also vary with breed or genetic background. The mean percentage of Type-II fibers is 93 percent in racing quarter horses, 84 percent in thoroughbreds, and 64 percent in other breeds. Dogs have no Type-IIB fibers, but chiefly Type-I and Type-IIC (moderate ATPase reactivity). Atypical Type-IIB fibers, which have both oxidative and glycolytic capacities and are more fatigue resistant, have been reported in greyhounds. Type-II fibers predominate in the propulsive muscles of greyhounds (97 percent, versus 69 percent for mongrels). A variant of Type-IIC, now designated Type-IIM, is found in canine masticatory muscles (temporalis, masseter, and pterygoideus).

Within one animal species, some muscles may contain different proportions of the various types of fibers. The gastrocnemius muscle of newborn kittens has muscle fibers that are all slow. Later, these fibers differentiate to serve

TABLE 41–1 Differences among the Three Types of Skeletal Muscle Fibers

Characteristics	Type I (Slow, Oxidative)	Type IIA (Fast, Oxidative-Glycolytic)	Type IIB (Fast, Glycolytic)
ATPase pH 4.7	High	None	Low
ATPase pH 10.3	None	High	High
Fatigue resistance	High	Intermediate	Low
Glycogen stores	Intermediate	Intermediate-high	Intermediate-high
Glycolytic capacity	Low	Intermediate	High
Location of nuclei	Peripheral	Peripheral	Central
Oxidative capacity	High	Intermediate	Low
Speed of contraction	Slow	Fast	Fast
Triglyceride stores	High	Intermediate	Low
Vascularity (redness)	High	Intermediate	Low

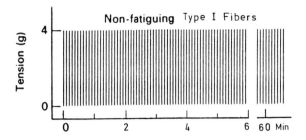

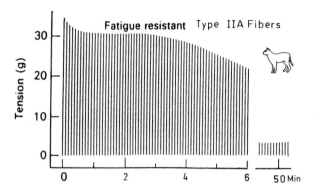

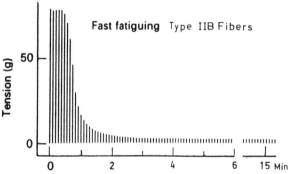

Figure 41–1 Electrical stimulation of the feline gastrocnemius muscle (effective voltage, 40 Hz, every 5 seconds) produces a contraction of greater strength in type IIB fibers than in type IIA or type I. Fatigue appears in less than a minute in type IIB fibers and less rapidly in type IIA. Fatigue does not occur in type I fibers.

various roles according to the neuronal influences and to the uses to which the muscle is put. Some fibers mature into fast fibers that develop a strong force of contraction and fatigue rapidly. Others evolve into fast fibers that are relatively resistant to fatigue. A third group is made up of slow-contracting fibers that do not manifest fatigue at all (Fig. 41–1). Congenital hypertrophy of some Type-I fibers occurs in daft lambs of the border Leicester breed; congenital hypertrophy of some Type-IIB fibers (so-called muscle doubling) is seen in cattle and, occasionally, in sheep. Birds have skeletal fibers of Type IIIA and Type IIIB, which are slow-contracting and have a tonic function.

The vascularity of muscles is increased by athletic training. The proportions of the types of myofibers may even change with intense motor activity; for instance, athletic training causes some Type-IIB fibers to be converted to Type-IIA. Muscles with Type-I fibers, which depend on aerobic metabolism, are more vascular than those with Type-II fibers that are either mixed oxidative-glycolytic or glycolytic. Type-I and Type-IIA fibers are dependent primarily on aerobic oxidative metabolism, whereas Type-IIB fibers are mostly anaerobic. The Type-I fibers are slower to contract, having lower myosin ATPase activity, but they are also slower to fatigue. They are able to meet their energy demand by aerobic metabolism of both glycogen and fatty acids. Also, they have a denser capillary network. Type-II fibers have more myosin ATPase and contract more quickly, but they also fatigue more rapidly because of fewer mitochondria and lower oxidative capacity. Type-II (A and B) fibers differ in their myosin myofilaments. Type-II fibers are forced to be more dependent on glycolysis, and they generate more lactate.

A skeletal muscle is a voluntary muscle because it can be activated by the conscious will of its host; however, some muscles, such as those of respiration, are programmed to cycle rhythmically in contracting and relaxing without conscious intervention. Similarly, the body makes many reflex movements that are not initiated by volition.

Architecture of the Muscle Cell

Each muscle has a distinct architecture designed to accomplish its range of assigned movements. A skeletal muscle is composed of bundles of enormous elongated *cells* (80 μm in diameter; may extend to 30 cm). These cells are referred to as *muscle fibers* or *myofibers*.

When viewed under the photonic (light) microscope, these cells show cross-striations of alternating dark (anisotropic to polarized light) and light (isotropic to polarized light) bands, or disks, along with peripherally located nuclei. With the electron microscope and with x-ray diffraction, the higher magnification reveals a highly organized arrangement of structures inside each muscle cell, or myofiber. These subcellular *membranes, myofibrils,* and *tubules* form the basic contractile unit, the *sarcomere*.

The *sarcolemma,* or outer membrane surrounding each muscle cell, is made up of two components, the plasma membrane proper and a basement membrane rich in glycoproteins and collagen. When the plasma membrane is stimulated to become permeable to sodium and potassium ions, it spreads a wave of depolarization over the entire cell (myofiber) surface. This depolarization arrives at the motor end-plate (i.e., the neuromuscular junction, or synapse, of the myofiber with the axon of a motor neuron from the ventral horn of the spinal cord). Tubular extensions (300 μm in diameter) of the sarcolemma, the so-called *T tubules,* penetrate the myofiber at the level of the Z line to allow rapid penetration of the wave of depolarization into the muscle cell. Mitochondria, sarcoplasmic reticulum, Golgi apparatus, and liposomes are organelles also found in the myofiber. The multiple nuclei of the myofiber are located at the periphery in the differentiated muscle but are situated in the center of the fiber in the embryonic muscle tissue and in Type-IIB fibers.

Myofibrils and Myofilaments

Below the sarcolemma, only cytoplasm separates each myofiber, which contains smaller fibrous structures of a diameter of about 1 μm, the *myofibrils.* These myofibrils, arranged in parallel fashion along the long axis of the muscle cell, are further subdivided into *thick* and *thin myofilaments* (about 1,000/mm^2 in diameter). The thick myofilaments are about 10 to 14 nm wide, and 1.6 μm long, whereas the thin myofilaments are only about 7 nm wide and 1 μm long.

The arrangement of the longitudinal thick and thin myofilaments accounts for the cross-striations, which result from the regular succession of dense anisotropic disks, or bands (A bands) and lighter isotropic disks, or bands (I bands). The A bands contain thick myofilaments, whereas the I bands contain light myofilaments attached on both sides of a denser cross-bar called the Z line.

A *sarcomere,* the fundamental contractile unit of muscle, consists of the region between two consecutive Z lines. It is a region of about 2.6 μm that includes one A band, and one half of an I band at each of the A band (Fig. 41–2). The sarcomere shortens during the muscular contraction and is extended to more than 2.6 μm when the muscle is stretched.

Electron microscopic examination of a cross-section of the myofilaments shows the myofilaments to be arranged like a packet of rods in a cylinder, or arrows in a quiver. The dark myofilaments are anchored in their center (M line) by connections with other dark myofilaments. The extremities of each dark myofilament are surrounded by six equidistant light myofilaments, and each light myofilament is surrounded by three thick myofilaments. The directionally polarized light myofilaments terminate in a free end and are mobile to interdigitate with the directionally polarized stationary thick myofilament, thus reducing the length of the sarcomere to less than 2.6 μm during muscle contraction, and that of the H zone in the center of the A band (Fig. 41–3).

Molecular Basis of Muscle Contraction

At the level of the sarcomere, the process of contraction, or shortening of a myofibril, involves the forced sliding of several myofilaments of actin over a stationary myofilament of myosin. These two motor proteins, myosin and actin, have been known for a long time. The sarcomere is surely one of life's most remarkable and effective mechanisms. It is still premature to present a definitive description of the molecular changes that make contraction possible, but enough progress has been made to suggest some tentative models that have been tested, at least in part. First the molecular components must be described.

The myofibers, or muscle cells, consist mostly (about 75 percent) of *motor proteins* (myosin in the dark filaments; actin in the light filaments) and of about 25 percent *regulatory proteins* (tropomyosin, troponin, enzymes). The term "motor proteins" is preferred over "contractile proteins," because during muscle contraction these proteins do not contract but merely slide past each other to interdigitate.

Motor Proteins of Muscle Contraction

The motor proteins and polypeptides of the myofilaments are complex. Myosin represents a group of proteins found in the thick myofilament of the A band, and actin is another complex protein system present in the I band of each sarcomere.

Myosin occurs in a number of isoforms that are specific for the types (I, IIA, IIB) of fibers. It is one of the heaviest proteins (MW, about 450,000 daltons) with either four polypeptide units (slow muscles) or six polypeptide units (fast muscles) not covalently bonded. Each molecule of myosin has two heavy chains that each have a long hydrophobic *fibrous tail* component and a hydrophilic *globular head* (MW >20,000 daltons). The fibrous tails wind around each other in an alpha helix arrangement. In its general form, a single myosin molecule is reminiscent of a two-headed golf club, with a shaft (tail) that is 2 nm in mean diameter and about 150 nm long and with two contiguous 10-nm heads at one extremity (Fig. 41–4A).

The tails of the neighboring helical pairs cluster in a parallel structure of about 400 molecules of myosin per thick myofilament. In close proximity, the globular structures (heads) of each subunit project at an angle at different points and angles along the thick myofilament (Fig. 41–4B). The tails are fused on the M line, and the heads are oriented away from it.

Actin, a *monomer globular protein (G-actin)* that is about 6 nm in diameter (MW, about 42,000 daltons), is the most abundant protein of the light myofilaments (Fig. 41–5). One molecule of G-actin can bind a Ca^{++} and a molecule of adenosine triphosphate (ATP) or adenosine diphosphate (ADP). In the presence of neutral salts (potassium chloride) and energy from ATP, it binds end to end into a long, fibrous, ellipsoid polymer. An ellipsoid chain binds with another similar one to form a *fibrous polymer (F-actin).* One F-actin fibrous helix chain requires about 350 molecules of G-actin, arranged in an alpha helix with a spiral repeated every 37 nm along the axis. Other proteins in the actin complex are tropomyosin and troponin, which are also considered regulatory proteins of muscle contraction. Actin, in association with other proteins (desmin, vimentin), is also

≂30cm   SKELETAL MUSCLE CELL (Muscle fiber, Myofiber)

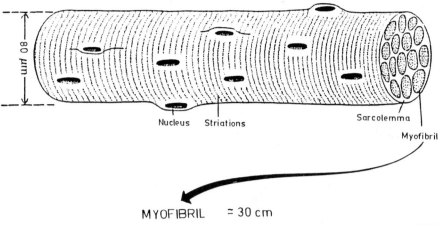

Figure 41–2 The surface of a muscle fiber presents multiple peripheral nuclei and cross-striations. A cross-section of a myofiber reveals bundles of myofibrils encased in sarcolemma, which covers a network of sarcoplasmic reticula and of transverse tubules (T tubules). Each myofibril is composed of a multitude of thick and thin myofilaments, which give rise to functional units (sarcomeres) and various disks or bands (isotropic [I] and anisotropic [A] to polarized light). Within a sarcomere, delimited by two Z lines, are found a wide A band, a narrower H band, or zone, and a central line, or midline (M line). An I band on both sides of an M line is made up by parts of two sarcomeres—each extremity of a sarcomere contains half an I band, and two adjoining halves constitute the I band.

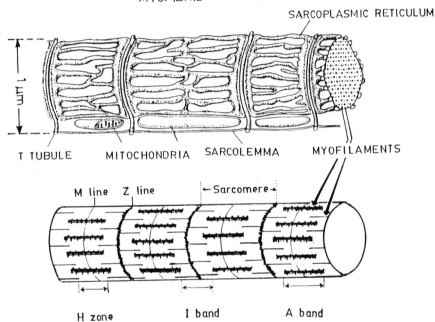

present in the Z lines, which serve as supports for the light myofilaments and as limits of the sarcomeres.

Regulatory Proteins of Muscle Contraction

The motor proteins (actin and myosin) interact only during muscle contractions. In the resting state, when the supply of ATP and Mg^{++} is adequate, a natural inhibition is provided by the so-called regulating proteins of muscle contraction, troponin and tropomyosin, which are both interrelated, present in the thin myofilament, and linked to actin. ATP depletion, an abnormal situation in muscle cells, leads to the formation of permanent actomyosin complexes, producing rigidity. *Rigor mortis* (muscle rigidity after death) occurs because of a lack of ATP.

Troponin, the most important regulatory protein in striated muscles, is a globular protein (MW, 70,000 daltons) made up of three subunits (C, binding Ca ions; I, inhibitory; and T, binding to tropomyosin). It binds to the extremity of a rod-shaped tropomyosin molecule in a 1:1 ratio and to one of the two helical chains forming F-actin. Since troponin occurs about every 40 nm along the F-actin axis, each troponin-tropomyosin complex establishes close contact with up to seven monomers of G-actin (Fig. 41–6).

Tropomyosin is a rod-shaped molecule composed of two separate helical polypeptide chains, each with a molecular weight of about 35,000 daltons, wound around each other in a 40 nm by 2 nm rigid supercoil. On each thin myofilament, about 50 molecules of tropomyosin are attached to the F-actin polymer.

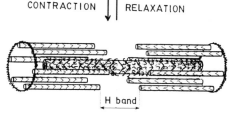

Figure 41–3 The thick and thin myofilaments interdigitate, except in the H-band, where only the thick (myosin) myofilaments are present. The Z lines anchor the thin (actin) myofilaments of adjoining sarcomeres. The myofilaments on either side of the Z lines and M lines are of opposite polarities. The thin myofilaments outnumber the thick ones by 2 to 1. Cross-sections in the I band (a) show that the thin myofilaments are organized in groups of six, in the A band (b) indicate that each thick myofilament is surrounded by these six thin myofilaments, on the M line (c) demonstrate that the thick filaments are self-attached, and in the H band (d) reveal that each thick myofilament is further surrounded by six thick ones and is equidistant from three myofilaments. (Small circles, thin myofilaments; large circles, thick myofilaments; open circles, myofilaments visible only on cross-sections; solid circles, cross-section of myofilaments [thin or thick] also visible longitudinally.) The width of the H band decreases during contraction as the thin myofilaments slide over each of the thick ones, whereas it increases during relaxation.

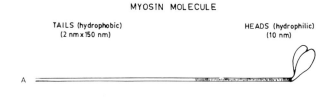

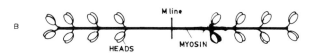

Figure 41–4 **A,** The general form of the myosin molecule is reminiscent of a twin-headed golf club. **B,** The backbone of a thick myofilament is the end-to-end joining of LMM chains, with their heads projecting on either side, away from the central M line. The central portion of the thick myofilament is devoid of projecting heads and contains only fibrous rods.

Conceptual Model of the Motor Process in Striated Muscles

Conceptualizing the contractile, or motor, process in striated muscles may be enhanced by dividing it into four phases: activation, regulation, contraction, and relaxation.

Activation

Stimulation of a motor neuron leads to an axon-conducted nerve impulse, or *action potential*. This impulse arrives at the specialized invaginating end-plate of the neuromuscular junction, where the action potential causes release of acetylcholine into the synaptic cleft. The activation of the *sarcolemma* travels into the myofiber along the *T tubules* (infoldings of the sarcolemma) to the *sarcoplasmic reticulum* (SR) to the terminal lacunae or cisterns, which release *calcium ions*. These cisterns lie adjacent to the Z lines, and the Ca^{++} ions enter the fluid around the myofibrils, where they activate the motor process, excitation-contraction coupling of actomyosin.

One spinal motor neuron may activate only a few myofibers (e.g., ocular muscles) or several thousand (e.g., limb muscles). Whatever the number, the combination of a neuron and myofibers is called a *motor unit,* because all these myofibers, which are of one type, are activated simultaneously by a single nerve impulse.

Regulation

The regulatory proteins, *troponin* and *tropomyosin,* play a crucial role in starting and stopping the motor process in myofilaments. In an animal at rest, the level of Ca^{++} ions in the sarcoplasm is very low and binding does not occur to troponin-C. Troponin-T is united with tropomyosin, and

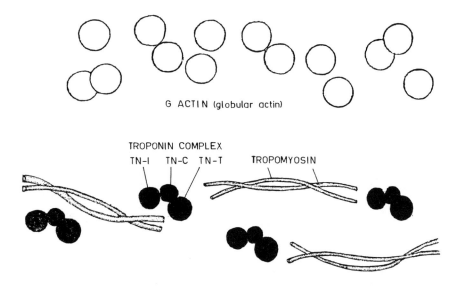

G ACTIN (globular actin)

TROPONIN COMPLEX
TN-I TN-C TN-T   TROPOMYOSIN

Figure 41–5 Arrangement of the molecules of G actin, tropomyosin, and troponins (I, T, and C) resulting in the formation of the helical chains of F actin, which form the myofilaments of the myofibril components of the myofibers.

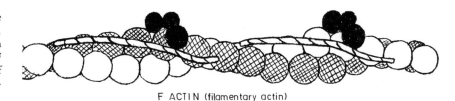

F ACTIN (filamentary actin)

the troponin-I (inhibitory) part of the complex prevents the active engagement of the myosin with the actin complex by inhibiting ATPase in the presence of tropomyosin. It appears that both regulatory proteins are a specialized piece of the mechanism that responds to the incoming surge of Ca^{++} ions.

The Ca^{++} ions entering the myofibrils saturate the binding sites of troponin-C, a specific calcium-binding protein with properties similar to those of calmodulin. This 100-fold surge of Ca^{++} ions triggers a series of rapid changes that are poorly understood. When troponin-C binds Ca^{++}, the inhibition by troponin-I is lifted, allowing the activation of myosin ATPase. The troponin-C–Ca^{++} complexes also

modify the union of troponin-T–tropomyosin complex to the actin myofilaments and unmask the active sites on F-actin. The troponin-tropomyosin mechanism appears to act as an allosteric regulatory unit. Each tropomyosin strand is made to alter its contacts with its six or seven G-actin monomers, so the active sites on the light myofilaments can react with the light (short) polypeptide chains in the heads of the myosin molecule. Each head, or expanded carboxyl terminal, of the myosin molecule has two active sites: an actin-binding site and an ATPase site. These two light polypeptide chains (MW, about 15,000 to 25,000 daltons) are called the alkali (ALC) and phosphate (PLC) chains (Fig. 41–7). Their roles are poorly understood. When the active sites of the

Figure 41–6 Parameters of the components of F actin: each G actin is about 6 nm in diameter, tropomyosin is in contact with seven molecules of G-actin and with troponin T, and the troponin groups recur at about 40-nm intervals along the helical chain.

HELICAL F ACTIN CHAIN

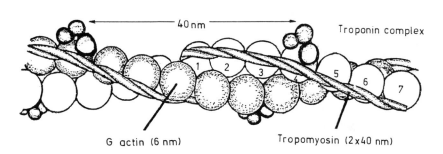

Troponin complex

G actin (6 nm)   Tropomyosin (2 x 40 nm)

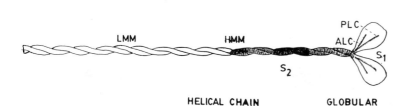

LMM   HMM   PLC

ALC

S_1

S_2

HELICAL CHAIN   GLOBULAR

Figure 41–7 The myosin molecule consists of two fibrous (hydrophobic) chains wrapped around each other (alpha-helix) to form a rodlike portion, which originates at the M line. Each long chain ends as a globular (hydrophilic) structure called a head. Myosin contains six polypeptide chains: two polypeptides of about 200,000 daltons (one in each helical chain), and four shorter polypeptides (two in each globular structure), the so-called alkali (ALC, MW 15,000 daltons) and phosphate (PLC, MW 25,000 daltons) light chains. By trypsin, each helical chain can be divided into two parts, a light meromyosin (LMM) chain and a heavy meromyosin (HMM) chain. In turn, papain separates HMM into an ATPase-containing segment (S_1) and a tight-coiled segment (S_2).

actin are unmasked and the ATPase on the myosin heads is activated, immediate binding occurs between the myosin heads and the actin. Cross-bridges are then formed between the thick (myosin) and the thin (actin) myofilaments.

Contraction

The mechanism of chemomechanical transduction of energy that causes contraction to occur is the most elusive part of the series of molecular events that shorten the sarcomere. One part of the mystery derives from the difficulty of visualizing the extremely quick changes: in the molecular structure of the myosin heads after they bind to actin and in the conformation of the actin-myosin cross-bridges that cause movement. Another part of the problem relates to the peculiar tendency of light myosin subunits to be activated by ATPase and to be inhibited by its products ADP and inorganic phosphate (P_i). This allows the energy of hydrolysis of one of the high-energy bonds to be rapidly deployed on contraction and restored by the oxidative processes of metabolism, supplemented when needed by anaerobic glycolysis. In addition, if mechanical work is not performed, the energy of the high-energy bond is not used.

The crucial ingredient is a molecular device that can be triggered to transfer chemical bond energy into the effective physical movement of folding. The site of this device must involve the myosin heads that move to form cross-bridges to the actin then stretch and swivel to pull the thin myofilament over the thick myofilament. The myosin molecules can be broken at two articulation sites by the proteolytic enzymes trypsin and papain. One of these articulation sites, which is trypsin sensitive, is where each helicoidal strand of the long chains (light meromyosin [LMM]) attaches to a corresponding short chain (heavy meromyosin [HMM]). At the other site, which is papain sensitive, the HMM is separated into HMM S_1 and HMM S_2 segments (Fig. 41–8). The most important HMM S_1 part, which carries ATPase and can bind to both actin and myosin, corresponds to the head. The tight helicoidal HMM S_2 part is the hinge between LMM and HMM S_1.

When the stimulus arrives, some stretching of the LMM chain must occur before the HMM S_1 parts form the cross-bridges between actin and myosin. The heads attach to actin sites then swivel to draw the thin actin myofilaments over the thick myosin ones. However, it has been estimated that the maximum movement of one myosin head would be only about 10 nm. Since the actual shortening of the sarcomere is about 0.75 μm, or 750 nm, a repetitive make-and-break process must occur, with the various cross-bridges sequentially continuing the shortening effect.

Some type of association-dissociation cycle must occur asynchronously to avoid relaxation slippage. It is presumed that the amount of shortening and the tension developed are proportional in some way to the number of bridges that are formed. The explanation may involve the pitch of the helix and the subunit repeat distance, which are different for actin and for myosin. Two analogies are proposed: (1) the pedaling cyclist who imparts repeated bursts of energy, through the moving sprockets, to the links of the drive chain, and (2) the rower who energizes oars that dip rhythmically into the water to propel the boat as force is applied. The latter resembles the myosin head model in which a molecular arm swings out, allowing contact to be made with the fixed medium (myosin bonds on the thin myofilament, which is anchored to the Z line), then the head bends and imparts the propulsive force (Fig. 41–9).

After death, no more ATP is generated, yet a larger proportion of cross-bridges are established and persist. This suggests that bonding generates the tension and that ATPase is needed for the dissociation that allows the cycle to be repeated.

Each thick myofilament is equidistant from six thin myofilaments; each thin myofilament is equidistant from three thick ones. Therefore, there are twice as many thin as thick myofilaments, even though the total mass of the thick ones is considerably greater than that of the thin ones. Every myofilament exhibits polarity, that is, the groups of the thin myofilaments on each side of the Z line point in opposite directions. The same holds for the parts of the thick myofilaments on each side of the M line (Figs. 41–3 and 41–10): the heads of the myosin molecules are always directed away from the midpoint of the thick myofilaments. The three-dimensional arrangement of the myofilaments is such that successive pairs of cross-bridges on the thick myofilament are

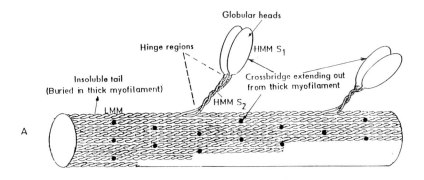

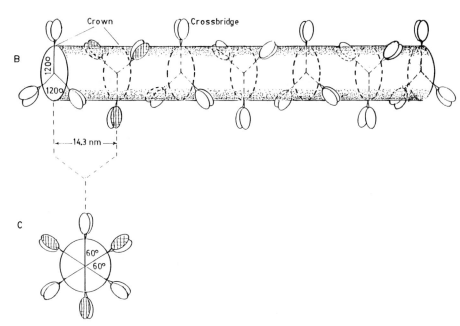

Figure 41–8 A, The hinge between the LMM-HMM S$_2$ chain permits bending of the HMM S$_2$ out of the thick myofilament, whereas the hinge between the HMM segments provides some mobility to the head, or globular part, of each myosin molecule. **B,** Every 14.3 nm, the heads around the thick myofilament form paired three-head units, or crowns. Each crown is rotated by 60 degrees, so that an end view of a cross-section of the thick myofilament shows about 400 rodlike portions and a radial arrangement of the six heads. **C,** Serial cross-sections, at 14.3-nm intervals, demonstrate three groups of radially opposed globular heads, which are separated by a 120-degree angle.

rotated 120 degrees, producing a staggered arrangement with the cross-bridges projecting toward each of the six surrounding thin myofilaments in a geometric lattice. A thick myofilament is of fixed length (about 1.6 μm), carries 300 to 400 cross-bridges, and is made up of many myosin chains that start and stop in a regular pattern at different points along the myofilament.

Myosin reacts with Mg-ATP to form a reactive complex of myosin with ADP and P$_i$. This is the resting form, when the actin sites are blocked. Upon activation by Ca^{++}, the myosin heads (HMM S$_1$ segments) move slightly toward the unblocked sites of the F-actin chains and then bind. Simultaneous activation of ATPase releases bond energy, which causes the cross-bridges to change their conformational angle and forces the myofilaments to slide past each other (see Figs. 41–3 and 41–10).

Resynthesis of the ATP occurs very quickly, and this binds to the actomyosin complex, causing the cross-bridges to break and yield free actin and unreactive myosin-ATP. This scheme is confusing, as under the influence of ATP and

ATPase, it calls for a cycle of metabolic changes in actomyosin bridges at different stages of the cycle. In the presence of ATP, a high-energy reactive intermediate of actin-myosin-ATP is temporarily formed from actomyosin; contraction follows when the bound ATP is hydrolyzed by ATPase. Then, myosin dissociates from actin to bind to ADP and P$_i$, and the cycle is ready to be repeated.

Relaxation

The regulatory effect of the calcium-sensitive proteins (troponin-C, which affects troponin-I, troponin-T, and tropomyosin) is reversed when the levels of myofibril Ca^{++} ions decline. This occurs after the stimulus has passed and as the ATPase-dependent calcium pumps return Ca^{++} ions to the lacunae or cisterns of the sarcoplasmic reticulum. One ATP is hydrolyzed for each pair of Ca^{++} ions pumped back across the membrane of the sarcoplasmic reticulum.

As the concentration of Ca^{++} ions falls past a certain threshold, the troponin-C releases its Ca^{++} ions. This causes

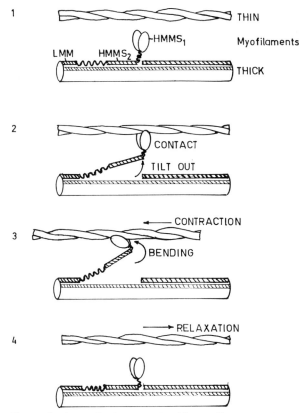

Figure 41–9 *1, Resting state,* the thin myofilament (actin-tropomyosin-troponins complex) is separated from the thick myofilament (myosin). *2, Association* of the thin and thick myofilaments, by projection of the HMM S_2 segment out of the myosin bundle, followed by binding of the HMM S_1 (globular heads) to actin. *3, Contraction,* with pulling of the thin myofilament over the thick myofilament (shortening of the sarcomere) when the globular heads rotate. *4, Dissociation* of the actin and myosin myofilaments and return of the thin myofilament to its original resting position.

the troponin-I to reattach to the actin, pulling the tropomyosin back over the active sites on the G-actin monomers. As further cross-bridge attachment is prevented, the sarcomere relaxes and returns to its resting length. The overall features of the cycle of contraction and relaxation are summarized in Figure 41–11.

Energy for Contraction

Muscle contains only small amounts of ATP, although the high-energy compound is the primary source of energy for muscle contraction. Therefore, muscle tissue has a special system for rapid regeneration of ATP after it is hydrolyzed to release its energy. One source of high-energy bonds to replace ATP in vertebrates is *creatine phosphate,* which serves as a short-term reservoir because there is more of it than ATP. The next high-energy level reservoir compound is *glycogen,* which makes up about 0.5 to 2.0 percent of the weight of resting muscle. This energy store must undergo metabolism

to yield the high-energy bonds, but the muscle stores are equivalent to about 100 times that of creatine phosphate. Even in the absence of oxygen, glycogen can be metabolized to lactic acid, but the energy yield is less than 10 percent of that produced in the presence of oxygen. Finally, there is the oxidation of *fatty acids,* the largest reservoir, as a further source of energy.

Isometric and Isotonic Contractions

When muscle fibers are stimulated to contract, they normally shorten. However, if shortening is prevented by fixation of both ends, force is then applied to both points of attachment. This is termed an *isometric contraction.* If the muscle can shorten while it is working under a constant load, that is an *isotonic contraction.* In practice, neither of these ideal situations usually exists because length and load change continuously. Nevertheless, these terms are useful in arranging laboratory quantitative studies of force and work.

After a stimulus is applied, there is a short lag, or latent period, of a few milliseconds before the force of contraction develops. Then the force rises rapidly, peaks, and declines a little more slowly. This cycle is called a twitch. The time elapsed until peak contraction varies with the muscle.

Force of Muscle Contraction

The *force* of contraction can be increased by applying a second stimulus before the first contraction has completely declined. The refractory period of skeletal muscle is extremely short. If electrical stimuli are applied repeatedly, close together, the twitches become fused into a continuous contraction, or *tetanus.* Overstretching a muscle prior to stimulation prevents it from contracting. Maximum force is developed at a length where all cross-bridges on the thick myofilaments of myosin establish contact with the reactive actin sites on the thin myofilaments.

Work done by muscles isotonically is maximal at an optimal degree of shortening. Further shortening leads to a decline in work, which is the product of the load moved and the distance it is moved. *Power* (i.e., work per unit of time) differs from *work* because there are fast- and slow-contracting muscles. Muscle fibers may be classified as *twitch* (fast) or *tonic* (slow), depending on the speed of their contractile response. Twitch fibers have an all-or-none response and a threshold stimulus level for activation. Tonic fibers exhibit slower, graded contractions and are present in postural muscles.

Heat is produced during muscle contraction. This helps maintain body temperature in cool environments. Over 20 percent of basic metabolic heat production is muscle derived, increasing with exercise. An activation component occurs during excitation of the membrane by the action potential and release of Ca^{++} ions. *Initial heat* is another component that relates to the contractile process and the hydrolysis of ATP. Then *recovery heat* derives from the pumping of Ca^{++} ions back into the sarcoplasmic reticulum and the restoration

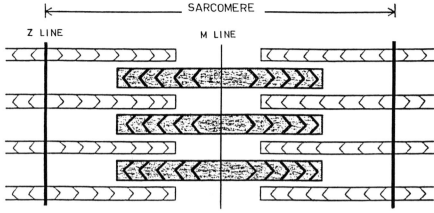

Figure 41–10 Diagrammatic representation of the interdigitation of thick and thin myofilaments with the same polarity on each side of their respective midline (i.e., M line for the thick myofilaments, and Z line for the thin myofilaments).

of the high-energy compounds needed for the next cycle. The overall efficiency of muscle work is about 40 to 45 percent.

Electromyography

The bioelectrical potentials associated with muscle activity can be recorded by surface or needle electrodes conveying the signals via wires (or radio transmitter) to an amplifier-recorder system. The information that can be gained can be very useful clinically and in basic research. Electromyography has been particularly useful in studying the time programs of muscle action and how they correlate with each other and with other activities. An example involves a study of the timing of contraction of each of the muscles involved in swallowing (Fig. 41–12) in the dog.

A constant pattern is observed involving a coordinated pattern of excitation and inhibition among the participating muscles.

After pharyngeal stimulation, the act of deglutition is found to be initiated by nearly simultaneous excitation of a "leading group" of muscles. This group includes the mylohyoideus, geniohyoideus, posterior intrinsic muscles of the tongue, palatopharyngeus, and superior constrictor.

A second group of muscles is inhibited at first and then is excited in a sequential fashion. That sequence is the thyrohyoideus, thyroarytenoideus, middle constrictor, cricothyroideus, and inferior constrictor.

The electromyogram (EMG) can yield clues to defective muscle function. It can be used also to study temporal coordination between muscle activity and other activities that can be recorded, such as stages of sleep, gastrointestinal

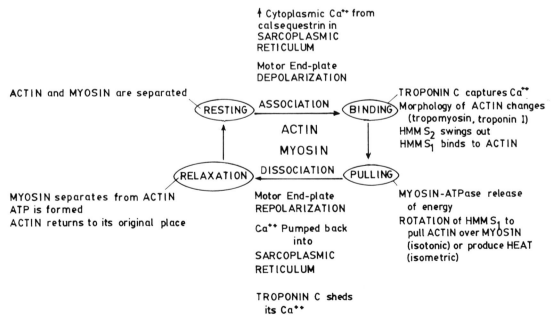

Figure 41–11   Summary of the overall features during a cycle of contraction and relaxation in the skeletal muscle.

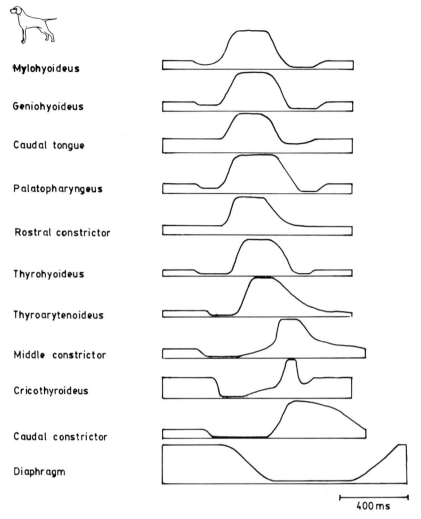

Mylohyoideus

Geniohyoideus

Caudal tongue

Palatopharyngeus

Rostral constrictor

Thyrohyoideus

Thyroarytenoideus

Middle constrictor

Cricothyroideus

Caudal constrictor

Diaphragm

400 ms

Figure 41–12 In the dog, electromyography of the muscles involved in the process of swallowing (deglutition). Analyses of the extremely rapid events indicate the duration of the almost simultaneous contraction of rostral esophageal muscles, the relaxation and delay in the activation of the caudal esophageal muscles, and the relaxation of the diaphragm.

and other visceral activity, neural activity, respiration, and circulation.

EXERCISE IN ANIMALS

Exercise is a term for muscle activity at the level of the whole animal. Movements involve the coordinated activity of the nervous system and of several muscles, require energy derived from chemical sources, and generate heat. Heavy exercise makes enormous metabolic demands on the body, which makes adaptive changes in the functions of many of its systems in an attempt to maintain homeostasis.

In wild animals, movement is necessary in the daily effort of finding food (or suckling) and water, for hunting or for escaping, and for periodic activity such as grooming, playing, fighting for dominance, and mating. Grazing domesticated stock may still have to traverse long distances in search of food or water. Most domesticated animals may be spared some of the dangers and the effort of finding food, but

some may be subjected to greater demands for work. Examples of these work requests are the physical work of traction in draft animals or burden in pack animals, the work of carrying a rider, and the work of competitive racing. The use of three categories of energy is related to movement: energy of the work itself, energy of moving the animal, and energy of heat loss during the work.

In domesticated animals, the most intense demands are made during racing. While draft animals may be expected to pull implements or wagons for 8 to 10 hours per day, the rate at which they can work decreases during the day.

Races tend to be either short and very fast or very long and medium-paced. The former type of race became possible after the domestication of the dog and the development of selected types, or breeds, for helping with the hunt. Coursing wild game became a popular activity: initially to improve the chances of success and later practiced purely for sport. Use of the horse in hunting followed when ways of catching, taming, and mastering it developed. Ultimately, both the dog and the horse were trained for the sport of racing.

Endurance Exercise

One of the avenues of domestication was the development of animals for endurance work, be it for traction (draft horses, oxen, water buffalo), riding, or war. Remarkable endurance feats are regularly accomplished by sled dogs (e.g., Siberian husky, Samoyed, Alaskan malamute, Eskimo dog) in exploration, in Eskimo life, and in sled dog marathon races, usually as a team, or pack.

> John BEARGREASE was a Chippewa Indian who delivered the mail along the north shore of Lake Superior by dog sled from 1887 to 1900. The John Beargrease Sled Dog Race is held every year in his memory from Duluth to Grand Portage on a round trip of 500 miles (800 km). The Iditarod Sled Dog Race, held in Alaska, covers 1,049 miles (1,680 km) over very rugged terrain, often in extremely low temperatures. Human marathon running, an olympic sport, covers 26 miles 385 yards (42.2 km) in a little more than 2 hours. The average energy used is 84 kJ per minute.

The muscles of a long-distance runner such as a husky dog have a predominance of fatigue-resistant Type-I muscle fibers that have a high oxidative capacity and large myoglobin reserves. The energy for this kind of exercise is drawn from stores in the muscles themselves (glycogen and triglycerides) and from stores in other tissues (glucose and free fatty acids [FFAs]). The glucose comes from glycogenolysis and gluconeogenesis in the liver. Hepatic glycogen stores probably provide only as much as about 15 percent of the energy needs of a marathon runner. The biggest single source of energy must be the fatty acids. Horses and dogs show large progressive increases (up to three to five times) in plasma FFA concentrations during prolonged moderate exercise. During very long distance running, there is a drop in the respiratory quotient (RQ, the ratio of the volume of carbon dioxide produced to the volume of oxygen consumed), which may reach 0.7, indicating a nearly complete dependence on fats for energy.

Glycogen phosphorylase "a" activity in the liver is stimulated by mechanisms involving hormones (epinephrine, norepinephrine, glucagon), titers of which rise several fold as glucose uptake by muscle action increases, causing a drop in plasma glucose concentration. The activity of the "b" form of the enzyme also increases, as its substrate levels change. Of course, pancreatic insulin secretion declines.

In adipose tissue, triacylglycerol lipase activity increases greatly under the influence of the varying concentrations of endocrine factors and the changing use of substrates. Maximal performance requires synchronized use of the limited carbohydrate reserves with the more plentiful stores of triglycerides. The carbohydrates are necessary for the most efficient use of the lipid stores and must be deployed at a controlled rate; otherwise, the power output soon drops and fatigue sets in. Muscle glycogen stores are usually the last resort prior to exhaustion. If the oxidative capacity is exceeded, anaerobic metabolism accelerates and acids (especially L-lactic acid) accumulate as pH falls, ATP levels decline, glycogen is depleted, and weakness and incoordination develop.

In racing, the paws and hooves are the parts most stressed, along with the joints of the extremities of the limbs. Variable friction or unevenness of the surface abrades and may twist the feet. The temperature of the ground or snow cover can freeze or scorch the feet. The weight of the animal and the dynamics of the gaits put enormous pressures and strains on the architecture of the distal joints and supporting structures of the limbs. This is particularly evident in horses during the impact of the hoof with the ground and in draft animals pulling heavy loads.

Many adjustments are made to systems other than the locomotor system during exercise. The heart and vascular system must make major adjustments in both the minute volume of the heart (cardiac output) and the proportionate distribution of blood to the different tissues. Increased blood flow is needed not only by the working muscles but also by the supporting systems for increased circulation, respiration, heat loss, and fuel supply.

Supramaximal Exercise

The most remarkable terrestrial spurting machines among the mammals are probably the cheetah, the hot-blooded horse breeds (those breeds produced by interbreeding with the Arabian horse), and racing greyhounds. Cheetahs have been clocked at 70 miles per hour (112 km per hour) during short sprints. Their unusually long legs for their size, combined with the design of the limb muscles for high stride frequency, afford the cheetah this unique capacity for acceleration. The American quarter horse, selected for sprint racing, often exceeds 45 miles per hour (72 km per hour) over short distances, carrying a rider. In greyhound breeding, priority in selection has been given to muscles used in sprinting and their coordination. About 57 percent of a greyhound's body weight is muscle, compared with an average of 43.5 percent for mongrel dogs. Racing greyhounds attain speeds of over 40 miles per hour (more than 64 km per hour) and can maintain this pace over 400 m.

The physiology of exercise in the *greyhound* has been studied at high speed, on a special *treadmill*, for different durations. A very short sprint (of no more than 15 seconds) generates an *oxygen debt* and depletes high-energy phosphates. It appears to create a significant "alactic acid" debt, which oxidative metabolism repays in just 1 or 2 minutes of very heavy breathing. A peak of alactic acid debt capacity of about 42 mL of O_2 per kilogram is reached in about 15 seconds. The *heart rate* of sleeping greyhounds is usually about 42 beats per minute, but it may be as low as 29. In awake greyhounds, the resting heart rate, which is very variable, averages about 100 beats per minute. During a run, the heart rate increases very quickly to reach a peak of about 318 beats per minute. In the 2 minutes following a race, there is an initial rapid decline in heart rate followed (at 9 to 12 minutes) by an increase to a secondary peak of 180 to 200 beats per minute, varying with the length of the race. Then, the slow decline of the heart rate continues for about an hour, when resting values return.

The resting *heart rate* of the *standardbred horse* is about 52 beats per minute in 3-year-olds and 42 beats per minute in 7- to 14-year-olds. With *telemetry monitoring* during *jogging* or light exercise on a racetrack, the heart rate is found to increase rapidly by about three-fold, to 125 to 138 beats per minute. During a *supramaximal exercise* over the distance of a mile (1.6 km) at top speed, the equine heart rate is maximal, about 215 beats per minute. In horses, cardiac recuperation occurs rather rapidly after either type of exercise (Fig. 41–13).

During high-speed runs by greyhounds, the *cardiac output* attains a peak of 914 ± 209 mL per kilogram per minute, from an average of 214 mL per kilogram per minute at rest. *Stroke volume* increases 32 percent, from 2.2 mL per kilogram at rest to 2.9 mL per kilogram during the run. The greyhound's heart weight as a fraction of body weight is 50 percent greater than that of mongrels. At rest, the *packed cell volume* (PCV), or hematocrit, is between 0.42 and 0.48 L per liter, but a supramaximal run increases it to 0.62 to 0.66 L per liter (spleen blood PCV is about 0.80 L per liter). These data indicate the enormity of the circulatory adjustments that the greyhound can and does make when sprinting.

The magnitude of the demands of maximal exercise on body function is illustrated by the fact that, despite these great adjustments in circulatory physiology, marked *acidosis* develops. During the first minute of recovery after running, the jugular venous *pH* falls from 7.4 to approximately 7.1. About 20 to 30 minutes is required for the pH to return to normal or slightly above 7.4. *Base excess* reaches a low point of about 23 mEq per liter by 5 minutes after the end of a 30- to 45-second race then recovers slowly over the first hour following the race. Venous *L-lactic acid* concentration increases greatly during and after a run, reaching a peak 5 to 7 minutes after the race then declining to a normal level within an hour.

From a resting level of less than 1 mM per liter, the L-lactic acid concentration reaches 13 mM per liter in a 15-second race, and 20 mM per liter in a 45-second race. The venous PCO_2 is raised shortly after runs of 15 or 30 seconds (but not after one of 45 seconds); it drops well below normal during recovery, reaching a low point 10 to 15 minutes after the end of the race, then returns to normal by 1 hour. Venous PO_2, which arrives at a peak 5 to 10 minutes after stopping, is back to normal within an hour after exercise.

Adaptation of the greyhound's respiratory function to the demands of sprint racing is one of the most remarkable findings. The average resting *respiratory rate* of 16.5 breaths per minute rises to an average of 188 breaths per minute in a run of 30 seconds and drops back to about 70 breaths per minute when the dog stops. Then, during the first 5 to 10 minutes into the recovery or postexercise period, the respiratory rate steadily increases again, to a peak of about 100 to 130 breaths per minute. From a resting value of about 15 mL per kilogram, the *tidal volume* changes first during the run to 23 to 43 mL per kilogram (with much variation, or high standard deviation) and then during the first minute into recovery (peaking at about 50 mL per kilogram), before it slowly returns to normal. With maximal exertion, the most impressive change is in the *expired volume per unit of time*. From the mean resting expiratory volume of 0.2 L per kilogram per minute, a mean of 6.0 L per kilogram per minute is reached midway through a 45-second race—an incredible 30-fold increase. Individual values over 200 L per minute have been recorded. This expiratory volume declines after the race but remains higher by more than 10-fold for about 10 minutes. Other large changes occur—in oxygen uptake (over 20-fold during the run, from 5.4 mL per kilogram per minute, up to

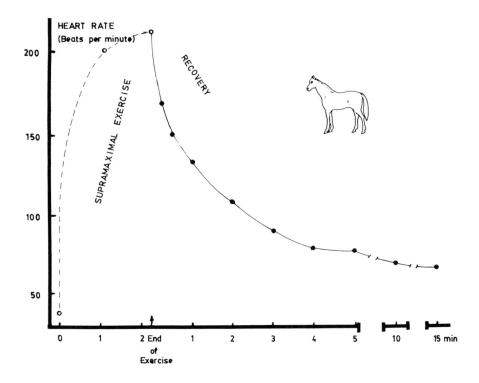

Figure 41–13 Heart rate, as determined by telemetry electrocardiography, in trained standardbred horses during and immediately following supramaximal exercise (workouts) on a 1-mile (1.6-km) racetrack.

143) and in carbon dioxide output (up to 30-fold increase during the run, from 5.2 to 162 mL per kilogram per minute). The respiratory exchange ratio or quotient (RQ) increases from the resting value of 0.95 to levels as high as 2.3 during the first 2 minutes of recovery. This is due in part to the titration by lactic acid, which contributes to hyperventilation, thereby lowering the blood P_{CO_2}.

When greyhounds run, acceleration is very costly in energy. The first segment of the run (the first 7.5 seconds) is three times as demanding in terms of energy and oxygen per meter as the remainder. For each meter of acceleration, about 3.7 kcal per kilogram and 0.7 mL of O_2 per kilogram is required during the first 7.5 seconds, compared with 1.2 kcal per kilogram and 0.2 mL of O_2 per kilogram for each meter of acceleration during the next 7.5-second segment of the run. The first 7.5-second component is also the period during which anaerobic glycolysis (as indicated by lactic acid accumulation) is the predominant source of power (about 59 percent of this segment).

Because horses are compulsory nose breathers, their adaptation to exercise differs from that of other species. Their long soft palate prevents them from panting to lose heat. The countercurrent heat exchanger action of the nasal passages is less effective than the rapid oral breathing and evaporation of panting for promoting heat loss in hot environments. Consequently, horses are much more dependent on sweating for cooling in hot climates and during strenuous exercise. Exercise-induced sweating is evoked by increases in both epinephrine and norepinephrine, which stimulate the beta-adrenoreceptors. The early sweat secretion is rich in glycoproteins, which may have a surfactant effect to disperse the droplets for faster evaporation and give a sheen to the hair coat for solar reflection. Failure to sweat normally in hot climates, a condition called anhydrosis, renders horses unable to race effectively.

When horses are exercised to exhaustion on an inclined treadmill, the $\dot{V}O_2$ values are 131 to 153 mL per kilogram per minute, the mean oxygen debt is 3.24 mL per kilogram, the peak blood lactate is 34.5 mM per liter, and the muscle pH falls from 7.05 to 6.75.

Work Exercise

Other species of domestic animals that are raised mainly for meat production are used for traction in some parts of the world. It is surprising that in spite of scientific genetic improvement and advances in nutritional science to ameliorate the efficiency of meat production, the muscle of meat animal species is a relatively low percentage of their live weight. The explanation probably lies in the fact that they are, in many cases, herbivorous and are often ruminants fed on bulky fibrous fodder or pasture. So they must carry a voluminous load of abdominal viscera and digesta. Cattle, sheep, and pigs have 30 to 40 percent of their body weight as muscle. The muscle-to-bone ratio of cattle and sheep is 4.6 to 4.8, very close to that of greyhounds, 4.7; for mongrel dogs it is only 3.6, and for pigs, 3.5. Greyhounds have very small stores, averaging less than 0.3 percent live weight,

compared with an average of 0.9 percent for other types of dogs.

High respiratory rates, sometimes with panting, are seen in ruminants housed indoors or kept in hot environments. Although draft animals contribute about 85 percent of the power used on farms in developing countries, they have received little attention from scientists, so their power output and work are not yet adequately characterized. Very few scientific metabolic studies of exercise for traction have been carried out. During work, the force exerted by draft animals has been measured with a dynamometer and averaged over short periods of time. Such data are considered inadequate owing to the unevenness of the tractive effort. It is more accurate to integrate the force with respect to distance (distanced-based average draft force [DADF]) than to time, but measurements are usually made over intervals that are too short. In addition, oxen are usually used in a paired yoke harness. One device developed for measurement of draft force includes an odometer and a load cell (capacity 0 to 2,500 Newtons; $1 N = 1 kg \cdot m/s^2$) coupled to an integrate-divide-and-display data processor. Tested on a treadmill, the device shows that oscillating irregular variations (with a frequency of 2 to 4 Hz) occur owing to the alternate forward thrust of the animal's legs (Fig. 41–14). A team of oxen doing heavy work such as plowing in the field exerts an average DADF of 1,210 to 1,740 N, depending on the task performed and the conditions and slope of the soil as well as on the oxen pairs. When using Brahma and criollo oxen, the average speed is almost 1 m per second, and the average power is 1,250 W; $1 W = 1 N \cdot m/s$.

GROWTH OF CELLS, TISSUES, AND ORGANS

Growth, the progressive increase in body size, begins with conception. It first involves the stem cells, before they differentiate to more specialized roles. Then, the different types of cells in the various tissues and organs must proliferate in a balanced way, along with any extracellular materials and water that may be required.

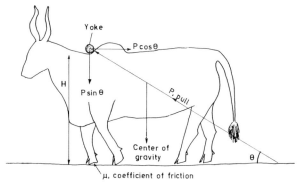

Figure 41–14 Direction of the forces involved in animal traction. Consideration must also be given to inertial forces and to irregularity of forces resulting from the alternating forward thrust of the legs. A majority of the tractive effort, but not all, is developed at the rear hooves.

Cellular kinetics measures the duration of a cell cycle and of its phases (Fig. 41–15) and parameters such as birth rate of cells (BRC) and growth fraction. The cycle time (T_c) is the interval between successive episodes of mitosis. The obligatory and successive components of a cell cycle are the duration of mitosis (M), the phase of growth or gap (G_1), any side extension (G_o) of the gap phase during which cells may be specifically responsive only to stimulation by growth factors, the phase of DNA synthesis (S), and the preparation of mitosis (DNA replication) without any morphological changes (G_2). Interphase comprises the G_1, S, and G_2 phases. Some cells do not reproduce, and they die after the long interphase following the mitosis that caused their occurrence, for example, erythrocytes (T_c, 100 + days) and myofibers (T_c, life of the animal).

The BRC refers to the proportion of cells in mitosis (alpha) divided by the duration of mitosis (delta). The *growth fraction* is the ratio of total number of cells to the number of those proliferating. Proliferating cells that subsequently divide are of two types: clonogenic and nonclonogenic. Clonogenic cells have a potential for differentiation, and some, such as embryonic and epithelial cells, reproduce rapidly. In embryos, the first generations of cells have life cycles almost limited to successive M and S phases only, as the G_1 and G_2 phases are ultrashort because growth does not occur. In these cells, T_c is about 30 minutes in frogs and about 12 hours in mice (G_1, 1 hour; S, 6 hours; and G_2 + M, 5 hours). In epithelial cells (skin, lungs, and gut), the T_c may be as short as 8 hours. Nonclonogenic cells undergo mitosis five or six times before dying.

Tissue growth begins with the ova and spermatozoa and continues to encompass the cell multiplication, differentiation, and organ development stages of embryonic, fetal, and neonatal growth, juvenile growth, puberty, and growth to maturity. The relative growth of tissues varies with species and tissue functions. In addition to growth of tissue, there is production of eggs and milk. Each species has a pattern for its rate of growth and a characteristic typical range of sizes at maturity. Errors can occur, leading to disturbances in the pattern of growth or its end-point or in the distribution of sizes among the various body constituents such as bone, muscle, viscera, and fat.

Growth, which requires energy, involves the increased net production and storage of materials and is the basic goal of animal production and animal science. The rate of growth and efficiency of food conversion to body tissues, particularly muscle, are of great importance in meat production.

The body systems vary within the stages of overall growth in the timing of their peak growth rate. Initially, the nervous system usually grows fastest, followed by the locomotive system, muscle, and viscera, whereas adipose tissue may continue to expand rapidly after the bony framework of the body has attained close to its mature size and protein accretion has reached a plateau. Deposition of adipose tissue requires twice as much metabolizable energy per gram as protein. The number of muscle fibers does not increase significantly after birth in the domestic animals that have been studied, but adipose tissue is different. It exhibits three growth phases: prenatal hyperplasia, postnatal hyperplasia and hypertrophy, and later, hypertrophy alone. In animal species, the tendency is for neural and musculoskeletal systems to be favored in the beginning, but in species in which the young exhibit extremely rapid growth (e.g., goslings), the digestive tract has priority.

Control of Growth

The genotype of an organism contains provision for built-in controls that define the size to which it will grow and its maximal rate of growth. Attainment of "maturity" implies reaching a stable body weight by an animal that has a mature skeletal structure, in a range of values representative of the species, the breed, and the gender. This normal pattern of growth requires balanced development of all the tissues and organs. It also needs specific growth factors, including growth hormone, somatomedins, and a variety of other factors that have permissive, inhibitory, or promotional effects on the growth process. If an individual's normal growth curve is interrupted by disease or food deprivation, a catch-up phenomenon occurs later, involving processes that are not understood yet. This can lead to a several-fold increase in growth rate until the normal curve is reattained. Animals grow most rapidly immediately after birth, after which there is a progressive decline, except for an acceleration during puberty. The pubertal growth spurt begins later and persists longer in males. It targets the musculoskeletal system and the visceral and reproductive organs and is responsible for the development of secondary sexual characteristics.

Selection for large body size in pigs has resulted in animals whose muscles have more myofibril bundles containing more, thinner myofilaments per unit weight. More re-

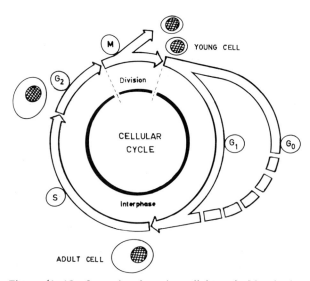

Figure 41–15 Successive phases in a cellular cycle: M, mitosis; G_1, beginning of interphase, with rapid growth; G_0, side extension of interphase, with possible intervention of specific growth factors; S, synthesis of DNA; G_2, end of interphase of endocellular beginning of a mitosis.

cent selection to obtain strains of miniature pigs for research has required reversal of this process, in part by reintroduction of genomes from wild stock. The postural muscles of miniature pigs have a greatly reduced content of Type-I myofibers. Double muscling in some breeds of cattle involves shifting muscle weight distribution away from deep and distal muscles in favor of superficial, fleshy, multidimensional ones, especially those that pass over more than one joint. These include those that have a high proportion of white myofibers.

Differentiating between cell proliferation and hypertrophy in muscles is difficult. Proliferation of the muscle precursor cells (myogenic cells) occurs during embryonic development and continues after birth. This phase of cell multiplication and protein synthesis ends with the maturation of myoblasts that can no longer divide but tend to fuse with one another to form multinucleated myotubes that are transformed into mature skeletal muscle cells. From that point on, any further growth is restricted to hypertrophy of these cells with deposition of myofibrillar proteins.

The body contains a great variety of specialized cells, tissues, and organs. During growth and repair, there must be balance and coordination of multiplication and of maturation among all the different building blocks, the cells. Each individual has a built-in embryonic program for normal growth from fertilization to maturity that is genetically controlled. An adequate, balanced supply of nutrients and freedom from severe disease are prerequisites for animals to attain their full growth potential. Fetuses and young animals reduce growth rate to compensate for deprivation and disease. Complete arrest of growth can occur under extreme conditions. If excess nutrients are available, growth may be distorted, resulting in unbalanced tissue development and obesity.

The study of control systems for the initiation, rate, and termination of growth has required the development of suitable tissue culture techniques in which nutrient supply and composition can be controlled. Then manipulation of the supply can be used to determine which nutrients are necessary for the growth process and the amount required for normal development. The nutrients that cannot be synthesized by the body are the essential amino acids and vitamins, and at least one polyunsaturated fatty acid (linolenic acid). A number of minerals must also be provided for skeletal development, electrolyte composition of body fluids, respiratory pigments, and certain metal-containing enzymes.

Growth-Promoting Substances

Endocrine messengers, including the peptide and steroid hormones and a few other specialized molecules, communicate between organs. Under the overall direction of the nervous system, these signals bring about the sequential changes needed for metabolic development, growth, and sexual maturation.

Growth occurs when the rate of tissue anabolism exceeds that of its catabolism. Stimulation of anabolism in skeletal muscle is mediated by *somatomedins* (a group of compounds released by the liver, acting as "agents" of *growth*

hormone), and by *insulin*. *Thyroid hormones,* as well as *ACTH* and *glucocorticoids* (cortisol), also have roles in normal growth. The *androgenic hormones* cause increased protein synthesis in muscle via their stimulation of a cytoplasmic receptor, with subsequent activation of nuclear ribonucleic acid (RNA) synthesis.

Several *other humoral factors* have been shown to promote protein anabolism. An exciting development in physiological research has been the discovery of a range of polypeptide growth factors that stimulate cells to grow and divide (Fig. 41–16). The first of these, **epidermal growth factor** (EGF), promotes eye opening in newborn mice. It is also produced in digestive glands and inhibits gastric secretion. It is identical to the urogastrone molecule, a substance discovered long ago to be a potent inhibitor of gastric secretion. It has a general effect of causing proliferation of many kinds of cells, especially in epithelial and connective tissues. EGF acts as a cell receptor that causes phosphorylation of proteins at their tyrosine moieties. Some endogenous oncogenes cause excessive cell growth, which surmounts normal constraints such as contact inhibition.

Fibroblast growth factors (FGFs) have been isolated from the brain and the hypophysis. They are heparin-binding mitogens that cause cell migration and growth in mesoderm- and neuroectoderm-derived cells. FGFs promote repair of vascular endothelium, skin, muscle, cartilage, and bone. When FGFs are applied topically with heparin, they accelerate wound closure in mice and also show potential for repair of neural tissue.

Platelet-derived growth factor (PDGF) is an active mitogenic agent. As the name implies, it is stored in platelets and is released when they are activated by contact with damaged endothelium or releasing agents. By a mechanism similar to that of EGF, PDGF evokes proliferation of glial, smooth muscle, fibroblast, and other cells.

Another type of compound that has a similar effect is the **transforming growth factor** (TGF), which is produced by certain kinds of tumor cells and causes them to proliferate and escape normal regulation of cell multiplication. The TGF can also activate untransformed fibroblasts and some other cells to proliferate. Its action appears to be comparable to that of EGF and PDGF. TGF-B was initially called NRK (normal rat kidney) factor because it allows reversible transformation of such cells to anchorage-dependent growth.

Expansion of the vascular tree is a necessary accompaniment to tissue growth. Stimulation of the formation of new capillary beds to serve the growing tissues is accomplished by **tumor angiogenesis factors** (TAFs), so named because they were demonstrated initially in tumor cell extracts. Later, they were shown to occur where needed for normal growth, wound repair or inflammation, and corpus luteum formation.

Nerve growth factor (NGF) stimulates hypertrophy and axon growth in sympathetic ganglion cells and peripheral adrenergic neurons. Some neurons in the central nervous system are stimulated transiently to replicate during a stage of their embryonic development.

Insulin-like growth factors (IGFs), or somatomedins, depend on growth hormone. IGF acts through autocrine and

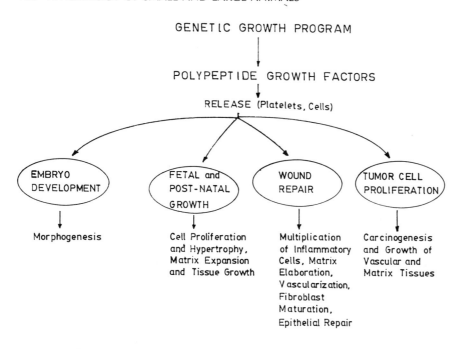

Figure 41–16 Some probable roles of polypeptide growth factors. Some of these regulatory proteins induce cells to grow in tissue culture preparations. They stimulate the synthesis of receptors for matrix proteins (collagen, fibronectin). They may inhibit the secretion of proteases while increasing the production of protease inhibitors.

paracrine mechanisms to stimulate desoxyribonucleic acid (DNA) synthesis in astroglial cells during normal brain development. It is released after ischemic injury in skeletal muscle, possibly inducing proliferation of satellite cells in regenerating muscle tissue.

Interactions between growth-promoting hormones (ACTH, androgens, glucocorticoids, GH by somatomedins, insulin, and thyroxin) and growth factors are being studied. Production of erythrocytes is stimulated by erythropoietin. *T and B lymphocytes' growth factors* participate in immune responses.

All the aforementioned factors are stimulants of either cell replication or growth. Other substances, the chalones or antigrowth factors, are inhibitory to tissue growth. Cell hypertrophy is reversible in some cases (e.g., when a stimulating factor that initiated it in the first place is later withdrawn).

It is recognized that the investigation of the functions of specific growth stimulators and inhibitors is currently in a very dynamic and turbulent stage and is clearly a very active cutting edge of basic and applied biological research. Their discovery has opened the door to investigations of fundamental changes in the development of the ovarian follicle and every stage that follows therefrom. Future developments should be monitored closely, as they will surely lead to important developments in animal science and veterinary physiology.

However, mitogenic agents are two-edged swords. Their necessary and desirable roles in embryonic development, growth, wound repair, and healing depend on coordination so that a balanced anatomical architecture results. In the case of repair, the initial tissue growth spurt must be followed by a remodeling phase. The other side of the coin is that uncontrolled or excessive mitogenesis can lead to unbalanced growth or tumor formation (see Fig. 41–16).

Tumors

The smallest detectable tumor mass (about 1 g) contains some 10^9 cells, but the usual detected mass (about 10 g) holds 10^{10} cells. A mass of 1 cm in diameter has undergone about 30 doublings. The ratio of proliferative tumor cells to resting cells is mostly between 3 : 10 and 6 : 10 but may be only 1 : 10 in a slow-growing mass. Treatment arrests growth at the G_2 phase.

Undifferentiated cancer cells have biochemical profiles resembling fetal immature cells. They reproduce at lower concentrations of growth factors (i.e., "hormonal" factors such as nerve growth factor, angiogenesis factor, epidermal growth factor, somatomedins). These cells exhibit higher rates of anaerobic glycolysis (i.e., they are less dependent on oxygen) as well as less cohesiveness, adhesiveness, and density-dependent growth. On the surface of an undifferentiated cancer cell, the reduction of complex glycolipids improves cell-cell and cell-substrate communications. The power of these tumor cells for invasion and metastasis increases as they gain cell-surface enzymes, and they lose fibronectin (an adhesive) to increase their mobility. The loss of cAMP, a glycoprotein that controls intracellular reaction rates, makes them produce more self-stimulating (autogenic) growth factors (e.g., TAF, sarcoma growth factor, and PDGF). They also synthesize more prostaglandins (local hormones), which help tumor cells escape immune surveillance and allow metastases to become established. Prostaglandin E suppresses T-cell proliferation and killer cell immunity. Prostaglandin

E_2 synergizes with carcinogens to inhibit killer cells. Prostaglandin D stimulates TAF.

REFERENCES

Art T, Lekeux P. Effect of environmental temperature and relative humidity on breathing pattern and heart rate in ponies during and after standardized exercise. Vet Rec 1988;123:295.

Astrand PO, Rodale K. Textbook of work physiology. 3rd ed. New York: McGraw-Hill, 1988.

Beitz DC. Physiological and metabolic systems important to animal growth: An overview. J Anim Sci 1985;61(Suppl 2):1.

Engelhart Wv. Cardiovascular effects of exercise and training in horses. Adv Vet Sci 1977;21:173.

Evans CL, Smith DEG, Ross KA, Weil-Malherbe H. Physiological factors in the condition of "dry coat" in horses. Vet Rec 1957;69:1.

Gill GM. Hormonal regulation of growth and development. In: West JB, ed. Best and Taylor's physiological basis of medical practice. 11th ed. Baltimore: Williams & Wilkins, 1985.

Gillespie JR. Respiratory system: Functions and functional limits of the equine athlete. Proc AAEP 1987;33:251.

Gunn HM. The proportions of muscle, bone and fat in two different types of dog. Res Vet Sci 1978;24:277.

Hammond JM, Hsu CJ, Mandschein JS, Canning SF. Paracrine and autocrine growth factors in the ovarian follicle. J Anim Sci 1988;66(Suppl 2):21.

Jennisch E, Hansson HA. Regenerating skeletal muscle cells express insulin-like growth factor I. Acta Physiol Scand 1987;130:327.

Jones WE. Equine sports medicine. Philadelphia: Lea & Febiger, 1989.

Kerr MG, Snow DH. Composition of sweat of the horse during prolonged epinephrine infusion, heat exposure and exercise. Am J Vet Res 1983;44:1571.

Lawrence PR, Pearson RA. Factors affecting the measurements of draught force, work output and power of oxen. J Agric Sci Camb 1985;105:703.

Parks JR. A theory of feeding and growth in animals. New York: Springer-Verlag, 1982.

Pathak BS. Engineering and draught animal power. In: Copland JW, ed. Draught animal power for production. ACIAR Proceedings Series No. 10. Canberra: Australian Centre for International Agricultural Research, 1985.

Persson SGB. On blood volume and working capacity in horses. 1967; Acta Vet Scand(Suppl):19:1.

Roberts AB, Flanders KC, Kandaiah P, Thompson NL, Van Obberghen-Schilling E, Wakefield L, Rossi P, De Crambrugghe B, Heine U, Sporm MB. Transforming growth factor B: Biochemistry and roles in embryogenesis, tissue repair and remodelling, and carcinogenesis. Recent Prog Hormone Res 1988;44:157.

Robertshaw D, Taylor CR. Sweat gland function in the donkey. J Physiol 1969;205:78.

Rose RJ. Endurance exercise in the horse. A review. Br Vet J 1986;142:532.

Rose RJ, Hodgson DR, Kelso TB, McCutcheon LJ, Reid TA, Bayly WM, Gollnick PD. Maximum O_2 uptake, O_2 debt and deficit, and muscle metabolites in thoroughbred horses. J Appl Physiol 1988;64:781.

Schlessinger J. Allosteric regulation of the epidermal growth factor kinase. J Cell Biol 1986;103:2067.

Shakin KA, Berg RT. Growth and distribution of individual muscles in double-muscled and normal cattle. J Agric Sci Camb 1985;105:479.

Snow DH. Identification of the receptor involved in adrenaline-mediated sweating in the horse. Res Vet Sci 1977;23:246.

Snow DH. The horse and dog, elite athletes—why and how. Proc Nutr Soc 1985;44:267.

Snow DH, Persson SGB, Rose RJ. Equine exercise physiology. Cambridge: Granta Editions, 1983.

Staaden R. The exercise physiology of the racing greyhound. PhD Thesis. Perth, Australia: Murdoch University, 1984.

Stickland NC, Handel SE. The numbers and types of muscle fibers in large and small breeds of pigs. J Anat 1986;147:181.

Thomas KA. Fibroblast growth factors. FASEB J 1987;1:434.

CHAPTER 42

VITAMINS AND MINERALS IN METABOLISM

Food is the total alimentary intake of an organism used for energy, growth, repair, and vital processes. Today this can be extended to encompass parenteral nutrition in the event that sufficient food cannot be taken or tolerated orally. *Nutritional and metabolic physiology* is the branch of physiology and biochemistry that deals with the fate of the energetic, structural, and catalytic (micronutrients) ingredients absorbed from the digestive tract. A relatively new field within physiology, it has grown rapidly, particularly the science of animal nutrition and, more recently, its human counterpart. The link between nutrition and health is an extremely important one that provides a sound basis for preventive medicine. The diet of animals usually contains some indigestible ingredients that pass through the tract, serving only as filler. Otherwise, the bulk of the food can be classified into macronutrients and micronutrients.

Macronutrients are substances that yield *energy* for use or for storage in the form of carbohydrates or fats, of proteins for movement or support, and of materials that can contribute to structural and productive demands (e.g., fetal development, lactation, reproduction). Some *minerals* fit into the category of macronutrients because they are required in substantial amounts for growth or milk secretion (e.g., *calcium, phosphate, magnesium, sodium, potassium, and chloride*). The physiological roles of these substances have been studied since the middle of the 19th century.

The *micronutrients,* the *vitamins and trace minerals,* play important but less obvious parts in the tapestry of body function. Their identification and role definition took much longer to determine and are still not completed. Tracking some of their functions required prior establishment of the effects of their lack, their presence in specific pathways of intermediary metabolism, and their molecular mechanisms.

Ancient history had identified two diseases of mysterious causation that we now know to be caused by vitamin deficiency: *beriberi,* observed in the Orient (circa 2,000 B.C.), and *night blindness,* described by Hippocrates around 500 B.C. The empirical approach to problem solving had some success in controlling *scurvy,* which plagued the crews of the oceanic explorers of the 15th and 16th centuries at a cost of tens of thousands of lives.

In 1747 James LIND, a British Naval surgeon, showed that scurvy could be reversed rapidly by daily consumption of citrus fruits (oranges and lemons). The Navy then prescribed the juice of limes and lemons for its British sailors (hence the nickname limeys).

The syndrome known as *beriberi* was identified in the rice-growing regions of the Orient. The disease is characterized by polyneuropathy (widespread peripheral nerve dysfunctions), muscle weakness, and sometimes cardiac failure with edema.

This neurological and cardiac disorder has been recognized as a disease for 4,000 years. Its name is derived from a Sinhalese word meaning inability or great weakness. It results from a preference for eating polished rice, which has the germ and coats removed by milling, leaving almost pure starch.

The Dutch physician Christiaan EIJKMAN investigated the cause of beriberi in the Dutch East Indies (part of Indonesia today), where it was then widespread and believed to be an infectious disease. He observed (1888) a similar condition in chickens fed on polished rice that was cured if their diet was switched to unpolished rice or if the millings were added to the feed. He showed that some factor in the unpolished rice also prevented human beriberi. This discovery was of enormous importance for human health in those areas of the world where rice is a staple food.

It is interesting to note that a surgeon in the Japanese Navy, Admiral TAKAKI, who trained at Guy's Hospital in London, noted that British sailors did not suffer from beriberi, while its incidence then in the Japanese fleet was a shocking 60 percent. He made the empirical observation that the British received a high-protein diet, whereas his countrymen were fed mainly rice. He wrongly attributed the disease to protein deficiency, but by adding meat and fish to the Japanese navy kitchens, he eliminated the problem.

In 1929, Eijkman shared the Nobel Prize with Frederick Gowland HOPKINS. A professor in chemical physiology at Cambridge University, Hopkins made enormous contributions to nutritional and metabolic chemistry, including the general concept of accessory food factors that must be added to synthetic diets in small amounts if normal growth is to be achieved (Fig. 42–1).

The name vitamines was coined by the Polish nutritional scientist Casimir Funk (it was then erroneously believed they were all amines). As awareness of Hopkins' accessory food factors grew and research expanded in the early decades of the 20th century, McCollum and Davis (USA) in 1915 proposed a classification of these substances. They noted that there were at least two vitamins, one fat-soluble and necessary for growth in rats, which they called A, and the other water-soluble, which they christened B, the antiberiberi factor. However, it was not long before B had to be subdivided to provide for C, the antiscurvy factor. Then A had to make room for fat-soluble D, the antirickets substance. Later, the original B was found to include several factors. One, the anti-beriberi agent, was shown to be heat labile and became B_1. The others were heat stable and were grouped as vitamin B_2, the antipellagra factor. When corn (maize) became a dietary staple, pellagra created havoc in

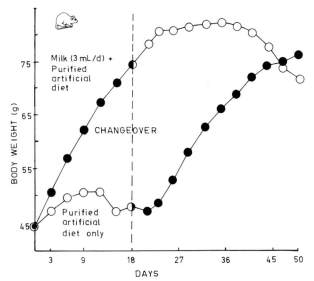

Figure 42–1 Hopkins's experiment on accessory food factors (1912) showed that then-undiscovered dietary factors, different from the basic nutrients (carbohydrates, fats, and proteins), are necessary for growth. The protocol follows the growth of rats on a purified diet (blank dots), on a purified diet supplemented with 3 mL of milk per day (black dots), and during the cross-over treatment. The content of milk in macronutrients is too small to affect the outcome, and the micronutrients postulated to be contained in the milk are essential for growth.

Europe and in the southern United States among poor people. Later the spectrum of water-soluble B vitamins had to be expanded again to include riboflavin, niacin, pyridoxine, pantothenic acid, and biotin. The antipellagra activity was found to reside in niacin. Some proposed B vitamins were considered and counted for a while but were later discarded, hence there are gaps in the B-vitamin numbering system. So far, the last of the series is vitamin B_{12} (cyanocobalamin, or cobalamin). However, there is also folic acid, which has not been accorded a number within the B complex. Nutritionists have also discovered two other categories of fat-soluble vitamins, E and K, and some different forms of A (beta-carotene, vitamins A_1 and A_2) and of D (D_2 and D_3).

To complete the saga, several of the established vitamins have been found to be toxic when they are consumed in large amounts. Cats fed high doses of A are susceptible to tooth loss. Vitamin D is also toxic in high doses because of its effect on calcium metabolism. Its use as an agent to manipulate mineral metabolism, with a view to preventing milk fever by administering high doses prior to parturition, has revealed its potential for toxicity. Similarly, errors in feed formulation have led to overdosage toxicity.

The classic example of vitamin toxicity is the case of the arctic explorers who became very ill after dining on the unusual gourmet dish of polar bear's liver. Vitamin A is stored in the liver, and the level is unusually high in these bears because of the cumulative food chain effect of their diet of seals, which eat large marine fish whose livers are very high in vitamin A.

The status of an animal with respect to a given micronutrient (vitamin or trace element) at a point in time may lie within a normal range compatible with function. Alternatively, it may be in a state of undersupply or oversupply. Excess leads to accumulation and eventual toxicity. Undersupply starts with a negative balance that leads to depletion of the tissues. At some critical point, dysfunction occurs and a deficiency status is revealed; if it continues disease results. For each nutrient, there are circumstances that can predispose to vulnerability, such as the stage of development or growth, the season, the cycles of reproduction and production or effort, environmental stress, and the presence of other diseases. Information is accumulating on the dietary and tissue levels of micronutrients and on the range of factors that affect the latter. This information will help improve the accuracy of interpretations of nutritional status and their consequences, and the prescribing of corrective or preventive actions.

FAT-SOLUBLE VITAMINS

Vitamin A

Although the syndrome of night blindness and the value of liver in its reversal was known to the ancients, the first "vitamin A" was not isolated and characterized until 1913. Vitamin A does not occur in plant tissues, so herbivorous animals must depend on carotenoids, especially the *provitamin* beta-carotene, in plants as their source.

Beta-carotene is cleaved by a mucosal dioxygenase in the gut, forming two molecules of *retinaldehyde*. The enzyme activity requires bile salts and lecithin as well as oxygen. Cattle and chicken (strains having yellow fat) may absorb the beta-carotene and cleave it in the liver. Unlike cats, dogs can utilize beta-carotene. Cats lack the mucosal cleavage enzyme, and it is essential that they ingest their vitamin A, which they obtain from the animal tissues in their diet.

The *retinal* entering from the gut is esterified, usually with palmitate, and travels via lymph chylomicrons to the liver. There, the ester bond is hydrolyzed and the aldehyde is reduced to *all-trans-retinol*. This complexes with *retinol-binding protein* (RBP) for transport to the tissues. There are two forms of dietary vitamin A (as well as beta-carotene). These are *vitamin A_1*, the form in mammalian and avian tissues, and *vitamin A_2*, with two double bonds in the ring instead of one, found in fish liver oils. The vitamin A_2 form is active in fish but not in mammals or birds. It is interesting to note that chickens tend to be night blind.

Even after more than 75 years, all the metabolic roles of vitamin A are not well understood. The most refined knowledge of its function is in the area of *vision*. The photoreceptor cells of the retina are activated by light. Vitamin A aldehyde, retinal, is involved in the transduction of the incoming light energy to chemical energy that can be conveyed by the fibers of the optic nerves to the cerebral cortex for integration and image assembly. The *rod* and *cone* cells of the retina with their layers of disks must surely rank among the most sophisticated of all physiological mechanisms and are the basis of the photographic sensory organ of vision.

The metabolic aspect of rod vision requires that vitamin A, or all-*trans*-retinol, be oxidized from the alcohol form to 11-*cis*-retinal, the aldehyde form, and be changed from a *trans* to a *cis* isomer. In the rods, 11-*cis*-retinal complexes with the protein opsin to form the photosensitive molecule, *rhodopsin* (visual purple); in the *cones* a different protein, *iodopsin*, is involved. In a deficiency of vitamin A, insufficient 11-*cis*-retinal is formed, and night blindness results.

An incoming photon of light causes remarkable changes to occur, switching the 11-*cis*-retinal group back to the all-*trans*-retinal form. The molecular changes, through some fleeting intermediary steps, lead to dissociation of rhodopsin into *trans*-retinal and opsin, to reconversion from the *trans* to the *cis* form of retinal, and recombination of *cis*-retinal with opsin. During the conformational change of retinal and opsin, the plasma membrane becomes hyperpolarized. With the cumulative stimulation of sufficient photons, it appears that the graded response reaches a threshold for activation of the synapse. The latter process may involve a light-sensitive protein named transducin, which binds guanosine diphosphate (GDP) and, when it is exposed to light, triggers conversion of the bound GDP to guanosine triphosphate (GTP), and subsequent activation of cyclic guanosine monophosphate (cGMP) phosphodiesterase. The resulting reduction of cGMP and concurrent increase in calcium ions may have the combined effect of closing sodium channels in the plasma membrane, leading to postsynaptic activation.

It should be noted that the aminosulfonic acid taurine is an essential amino acid for photoreceptor and cardiac cell functions in cats. Cats deficient in taurine are susceptible to cardiomyopathy.

Although extraordinary progress has been made in gaining an understanding of the molecular mechanisms of vision, the other roles of vitamin A have not yet been explained to a satisfactory degree. Its participation in growth, epithelial integrity, bone strength, reproduction, and disease resistance is not well understood, but these aspects of vitamin A functions are extremely important in animals.

Slow adaptation to night vision and the eventual loss of it are the earliest signs of vitamin A deficiency. Xerophthalmia, which involves drying, thickening, and clouding of the cornea and conjunctiva, associated with a loss of the protective film over the eyeball, is a widespread problem among malnourished young children with vitamin A deficiency. It also occurs in young animals, notably puppies and calves. Daytime blindness with dilated pupils occurs in cattle lacking vitamin A. The eye lesions may progress to keratinization and corneal ulceration, especially in horses.

The secretory mucosal surfaces are susceptible to vitamin A deficiency. In cattle lacking vitamin A, the parotid duct shows marked squamous metaplasia. Epithelial atrophy followed by stratification and keratinization occur, accompanied by reduced resistance to infection and decreased growth rate. (Already in 1928, vitamin A had been christened the antiinfective vitamin.)

Vitamin A deficiency impairs the development of undifferentiated epithelial and mesenchymal cells. These cells have two characteristics in common: (1) they undergo continuous replacement and progressive differentiation, and (2) they produce mucopolysaccharides (MPS). Dysfunction of such cells explains many of the features of vitamin A deficiency:

1. Failure of differentiation and reduced secretions of the conjunctiva and periorbital glands coupled with keratinizing changes of the cornea lead to xerosis.
2. Failure of goblet cell differentiation leads to suppression of secretion of protective mucus in airway and intestine, increasing susceptibility to pneumonia and enteritis.
3. Impairment of bone resorption and remodeling results from decreased differentiation of osteoclasts, resulting in deposition rather than resorption. Bones are thicker but less dense.
4. Arrest of fibroblast differentiation leads to continuation of secretion of MPS ground substance rather than the normal maturation to less active forms (fibrocytes). In the central nervous system, the arachnoid epithelium secretes abnormal amounts of MPS and the dura mater becomes thickened, resulting in compression of the arachnoid villi and impaired reabsorption of cerebrospinal fluid (CSF).
5. Differentiation of mesenchyme-derived cells of the adrenal cortex may be inhibited (i.e., zona glomerulosa cells fail to transform to zona fasciculata cells, which secrete steroids). Estrogens have effects antagonistic to vitamin A and the drop in progesterone levels in late pregnancy increases requirements for the vitamin. A combination of vitamin A deficiency with increased estrogen and decreased progesterone leads to regressive changes in the placenta and fetal death and resorption. Retinol alone does not prevent these changes, nor does it sustain the differentiation of spermatogonia into spermatozoa. It disappears rapidly in the testis. In addition, the Sertoli cells secrete estrogen, disturbing the hormonal balance. Vitamin A is not stored in, and disappears rapidly from, chicken eggs and embryos.

Vascular development requires mesenchymal proliferation and differentiation, so it fails in vitamin A deficiency. Degenerative lesions of the placenta may lead to abortion or delivery of nonviable young, often with retained placenta. Defective organogenesis may produce congenital defects.

Defective bone structure leads to thickened, porous, and weakened bones. The incoordinated growth of the bones of the skull distorts the development of the central nervous system. Failure of the skull to meet the space demands of the developing brain leads to elevated CSF pressure and encephalopathy with papilledema in cattle. Decreased reabsorption of CSF, which accompanies the thickening of the meninges, is followed by bouts of syncope and convulsions. In cattle, convulsions and optic nerve constriction occur with serum vitamin A levels below 5 μg per deciliter, whereas ataxia and blindness are associated with levels between 5 and 9 μg per deciliter. Pigs also show signs of neurological dysfunction and myelin degeneration that may be accompanied by osteodystrophy, elevated CSF pressure, and paralysis. Puppies born to vitamin A–deficient dams may have degeneration of the middle ear resulting from stenosis of the foramina.

Underlying the pathological and clinical manifestations of vitamin A deficiency may be a specific function of the vitamin in membrane glycoprotein synthesis. Vitamin A is phosphorylated then acts as a carrier for carbohydrates that are incorporated into the oligosaccharide structure of plasma membrane glycoproteins. Because these compounds play a major role in surface recognition and differentiation of cells, the impact of a deficiency of vitamin A could be profound.

Other pathways involving vitamin A include cholesterol synthesis. Deficient cholesterol synthesis leads to diversion of mevalonate to ubiquinone (coenzyme Q), which acts as a carrier to shuttle electrons from flavoproteins to the cytochromes. The effect of the deficiency is to reduce overall steroid synthesis, and it may also impair the formation of progesterone from pregnenolone. There are flow-on effects to the steroid endocrine system, including suppression of cortisol-dependent gluconeogenesis.

After beta-carotene is absorbed, it is an efficient quencher of oxygen-free radicals and appears to have significant antioxidant effects. This is not the case with vitamin A. Since it is lipid soluble and enters cell membranes, including lysosomes, beta-carotene may act synergistically with vitamin E in protecting against peroxidation and in reducing the incidence of cancer.

Vitamin D and Calcium Metabolism

Although a treatise on rickets had been written as early as 1650 (Glisson), it was a long time before scientific understanding of the nutritional physiology of the disease started to develop. In the 20th century, the idea of accessory food factors (Hopkins), including vitamins, emerged. The awareness that something in fats was important for body formation led to the discovery of vitamin A. Dietary fats were also found to contain a protective factor against rickets in dogs. After vitamin A was shown to be inactivated by aeration and heat, which did not affect the antirachitic factor, it was possible to establish a clear distinction between vitamin A and the antirickets factor (vitamin D). Besides rickets, two other dysfunctions are attributable to vitamin D deficiency, osteomalacia and tetany (or paresis).

Vitamin D is unique among the vitamins in that it is only a true dietary vitamin for animals that do not receive adequate exposure to sunlight (ultraviolet radiation of 290 to 310 nm wavelength) to allow them to form it from its precursor 7-*dehydrotachysterol* in the *skin* (Fig. 42–2). If this photoproduction of the vitamin in vivo is inadequate and if dietary supplementation with vitamin D is inadequate also, rickets may occur in young animals and osteomalacia in mature ones. People living at high latitudes (toward the polar regions) are more susceptible during the solarless winter months.

In *plants,* the "provitamin" *ergosterol* is converted to

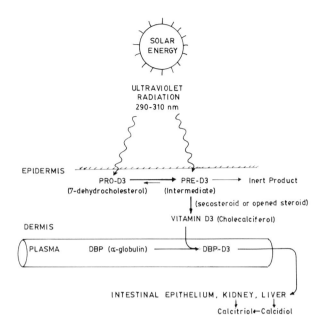

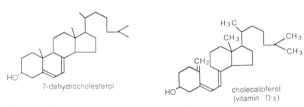

Figure 42–2   Synthesis of vitamin D_3 in skin by photochemical conversion of epidermal stores of 7-dehydrocholesterol. This D_3 precursor is picked up by the plasma D-binding protein and directed first to the liver cells, which convert it to *calcidiol,* and then to the kidney for formation of the active *calcitriol* (vitamin D hormone, vitamin D_3, or $1\alpha,25$-dihydroxy-D_3).

vitamin D_2 by ultraviolet radiation (this occurs in sun-dried hay). By convention, the two terms vitamin D and calciferol today encompass both D_2, which is *ergocalciferol*, and D_3, which is *cholecalciferol*. Other forms, D_4 and D_5, occur in some fish oils. In birds, the naturally occurring form in animals, D_3, is much more potent than D_2, although in mammals the two forms are about equipotent. It is very important to note that D_3 is more than ten times as *toxic* as D_2.

The three main metabolic functions of vitamin D are to control calcium homeostasis, to participate in the regulation of bone growth and metabolism, and to help coordinate phosphate metabolism. Ingested vitamin D is absorbed into the lymph via chylomicrons in mammals, but it is absorbed directly into the portal circulation in birds and fish. The liver enzyme alpha-25-hydroxylase converts vitamin D_2 to 25-hydroxy-D_3, *calcidiol,* which passes via the circulation to the kidney, where a 1-alpha-hydroxylase converts it to 1,25-dihydroxy vitamin D_3 (Fig. 42–3). The 1-hydroxylase is a regulatory enzyme that must be activated to cause this conversion. If it is not activated, the calcidiol is metabolized

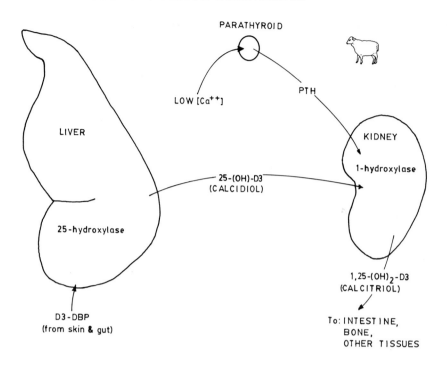

Figure 42–3 Through the stimulus of parathyroid hormone (PTH) and hypocalcemia, the body adapts to higher demands for calcium ions by increasing the production of calcitriol (vitamin D hormone). (DBP, D-binding protein.)

to 24,25-dihydroxy-D₃ instead. Control of the 1-alpha-hydroxylase activation involves calcium and phosphate concentrations and may require parathormone (PTH). There is also feedback inhibition of the enzyme by its product, 1,25-dihydroxy-D₃ or *calcitriol*, which is the metabolically active form of the vitamin for promotion of calcium absorption, the vitamin D hormone.

Calcitriol is carried to the intestine, where it is transferred to a receptor attached to the nucleus of the epithelial cells. There, it stimulates the synthesis of an mRNA that codes for a special protein with a very high affinity for calcium ions, the *calcium-binding protein* (CBP) (Fig. 42–4). Renal tubular cells produce a very similar CBP, perhaps to avoid excretory loss of the increased calcium ions absorbed from the gut or to protect the cells from undesirable effects of high calcium concentration. One unexplained piece of the mechanism is that the increase in calcium absorption slightly precedes the burst of CBP formation. This implies that there

may be an additional calcitriol-sensitive process that triggers the accelerated pumping of calcium. This may involve increased activity of a calcium-stimulated ATPase. Separate enhancement of phosphate absorption also occurs, perhaps via a Ca, Mg-ATPase sensitive to calcitriol.

The activated vitamin D₃ also acts in conjunction with PTH and other factors to induce some resorption of bone, after a lag period, with solubilization of the calcium and phosphate from bone mineral. The roles of calcitriol and 24,25-dihydroxy-D₃ in bone deposition and resorption have not yet been clarified sufficiently.

Deficiencies of vitamin D₃ are more common in intensively housed animals than in animals kept outdoors. The decreased rate of mineral deposition in young animals that are growing rapidly with vitamin D₃ deficiency or phosphorus deficiency in the diet leads to bent and deformed limb bones with enlarged ends and increased susceptibility to fractures. In young chickens, even the beak softens. In ma-

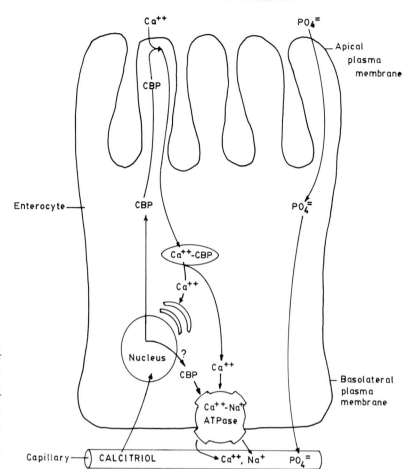

LUMEN   VILLUS EPITHELIUM

Figure 42–4 Diagram of possible mechanisms for enhancement of intestinal absorption of calcium, under the stimulating influence of calcium-binding protein (CBP). The formation of CBP in enterocytes is increased by circulating calcitriol. CBP facilitates the apical entry of calcium cations (Ca^{++}) into the cytosol and the organelles of enterocytes. It also may promote the access of more calcium ions into blood by reacting with a calcium-ATPase located at the basolateral portion of the plasma membrane.

ture animals, when bone is already shaped and cartilage is mature, D_3 deficiency is manifested by demineralization of the bone, leading to osteomalacia or osteoporosis. Vitamin D–deficient hens lay fragile eggs that have thinner shells than normal.

The third type of syndrome involving vitamin D_3 is the hypocalcemic crisis that may result from the sudden onset of—or rapid increase in—milk production around the time of parturition or early in lactation. Three hormones participate in the *regulation* of the level of *calcemia: PTH, calcitriol, and calcitonin*. Their actions must be integrated and must also allow for changes in the function of other organs. The manifestation of this situation may take the form of *parturient paresis,* or milk fever, in dairy cows, or *puerperal tetany* with convulsions in bitches (rarely in queens), especially those of small excitable breeds and poodles. These breeds also have the highest incidence of spontaneous hypoparathyroidism. There is a spectrum of responses ranging from paresis to tetany that varies with species and strains and among individuals. Milk fever is a very important disease of high-yielding dairy cows: the overall incidence exceeds 5 percent.

All mammals must struggle to adapt to the mineral and energy drain when they start a new *lactation,* but for *dairy cows*

the drain is far greater than for most other animals because of their selection for high yields (equivalent to the *needs of ten or more calves*). The colostrum flow may involve a loss of about 3 g of calcium per hour, more than all the calcium normally present in the entire blood volume!

It is apparent that enormous metabolic adaptations must take place in the phase immediately prior to, during, and after parturition to increase the supply of calcium and nutrients, or a crisis is inevitable (Fig. 42–5). Accelerated absorption of calcium from the intestine under the influence of vitamin D_3 hormone is an essential part of this. In mineral metabolism, phosphorus is linked to calcium. It is absorbed from the intestine and is returned to the rumen via the copious salivary flow in cattle and sheep. Any surplus is excreted via the urine and is regulated by PTH and calcitriol. The content of phosphorus in milk is close to that of calcium. The readily exchangeable pools of calcium and phosphorus have been estimated to be 35 and 100 times larger, respectively, than the plasma pool. Dairy cows are very dependent on increased absorption of calcium from the intestine under the influence of calcitriol to help them through the early stages of the onset of lactation around the time of parturition. Bone calcium resorption usually plays a lesser role until the

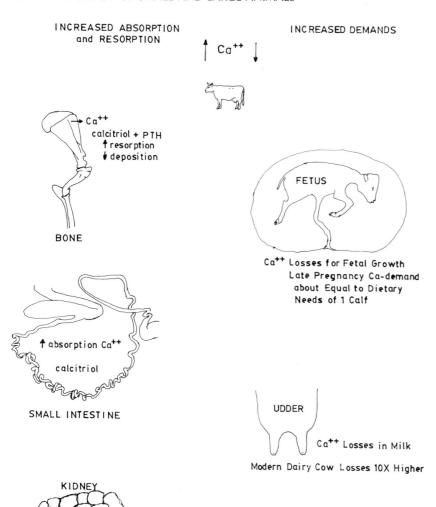

INCREASED ABSORPTION
and RESORPTION

INCREASED DEMANDS

↑ Ca⁺⁺ ↓

Ca⁺⁺
calcitriol + PTH
↑ resorption
↓ deposition

BONE

FETUS

Ca⁺⁺ Losses for Fetal Growth
Late Pregnancy Ca-demand
about Equal to Dietary
Needs of 1 Calf

↑ absorption Ca⁺⁺

calcitriol

SMALL INTESTINE

UDDER

Ca⁺⁺ Losses in Milk
Modern Dairy Cow Losses 10X Higher

KIDNEY

↑ retention of Ca⁺⁺
But ↑ excretion if
[Ca⁺⁺] >10 mg/dL

Figure 42–5 The end result of increased production of calcitriol is hypercalcemia associated with improvement in intestinal absorption, in bone resorption, and in plasma retention (by the kidney) of calcium ions.

second week postpartum, unless the cows have been fed low-calcium diets prepartum, a technique that activates the mobilization process. If a hypocalcemic crisis with parturient paresis occurs, calcium administered as the borogluconate salt intravenously is often an effective treatment to get the animal through the crisis and give the mechanisms of calcium homeostasis more time to adapt.

There is a long-term problem of providing enough calcium for the entire lactation period. A modern cow yielding about 9,000 kg (20,000 pounds) per year over a 300-day lactation period must secrete about 11 kg of calcium and 8.6 kg of phosphorus into milk. Since the calcium availability from the diet is estimated to be only 38 percent, the cow must ingest about 100 g of calcium per day to replace the 37 g per day secreted in the milk plus another 30 g for nonlactational maintenance, for a total intake of 130 g per day. Attainment of this level usually requires supplementation of

the diet with calcium and phosphorus, particularly during the early months of lactation. Estimated needs vary but are in the range of 3 to 5 g per kilogram of milk for calcium and about half that amount of phosphorus to achieve the desired balance. Currently available data suggest that the dietary calcium level of high-yielding cows should be 0.75 percent for the first 4 months at least.

The ultimate goal of health management of dairy cows must be the prevention of periparturient paresis and of postpartum negative balance of calcium and phosphorus. Not only is milk fever a major health setback for a cow facing the long lactation ahead, but also it tends to be followed by a high incidence of other problems of disease. Genetic selection against milk fever susceptibility should be practiced. The use of calcitriol or its precursors as a preventive has not been very effectively deployed yet, because these vitamin D_3 metabolites cause feedback suppression of hormonal response to low plasma calcium. It does raise plasma calcium levels in lactating cows, and further study is indicated. It is essential to avoid high dietary calcium prepartum. A low-calcium diet can be beneficial by activating bone calcium resorption. At the time that lactation is initiated, anorexia often occurs, with a fall in plasma calcium, which increases PTH and calcitriol formation, leading to increased intestinal absorption of calcium and the start of bone resorption. A major difference between normal and milk fever–prone cows may be an impairment of osteoclast function in the latter group. This may be the result of a failure to activate their precursor cells monocytes and macrophages. High cortisol levels at parturition may suppress monocyte numbers and their differentiation.

It is interesting that both the tetanic spasms and convulsions seen in lactating bitches or queens and the paresis of milk fever cases in cows respond to parenteral calcium therapy. In the bitch, the biggest challenge to homeostatic calcium controls occurs when multiple puppies are developing large appetites, usually from the second to the fourth weeks of lactation. The onset is more gradual than in cows and appears to be associated with a lower threshold for activation of nerve connections and neuromuscular junctions leading to tetanic contractions and convulsions (eclampsia). The cow's syndrome results from the sudden onset of very high levels of colostrum and milk secretion at parturition. This can lead to such a dramatic fall in plasma calcium concentration that smooth muscle function is compromised. Loss of gastrointestinal motility at this critical stage may prevent the increased calcitriol secretion from becoming fully effective in increasing calcium absorption from the intestine. If, at the same time, there is defective osteoclast formation with failure to promote bone calcium resorption, the homeostatic response fails. Intravenous calcium restores intestinal function and gives homeostatic controls another chance. The kidneys provide protection against hypercalcemia by excreting calcium if plasma calcium levels exceed 10 mg per deciliter (5 mEq per liter, or 5 mmol per liter).

Bone Resorption and Osteomalacia

Osteoporosis is a condition in which bone mass and density are reduced, while bone architecture is preserved. *Osteomalacia,* deficient mineralization of the osteoid tissue with softening of the bone, may be the result of phosphorus deficiency in herbivores. *Rickets* is a form of osteomalacia with defective mineralization of growth plate cartilage in young animals.

The development of osteomalacia involves a complex chain of reactions at the cellular and molecular levels that govern the activities of the bone cells. Calcitriol (1,25-dihydroxy-D_3) and PTH cause monocytic cells to differentiate into osteoclasts aided by T cells that release lymphokines. PTH and calcitriol suppress the activity of osteoblasts in collagen formation while enhancing their release of paracrine resorption factors such as osteoblast-derived resorptive factors (OBDRF). These two effects accelerate bone remodeling. Coupled release of a skeletal growth factor helps maintain the bone structure. Glucocorticoids also suppress

collagen formation, an effect that progesterone opposes. Estrogens and androgens have an important protective effect on bone, increasing collagen matrix production by osteoblasts and suppressing the cell differentiation in osteoclasts. Transforming growth factor beta released by osteoblasts has a similar effect on osteoclasts. Calcitonin also suppresses osteoblast activation. Thus, there seems to be a system of checks and balances between the forces that cause bone resorption and those that promote bone deposition. This system is governed by endocrine systems that respond to the demands of the body (Fig. 42–6).

When bone deposition exceeds the rate of resorption, osteopetrosis may result. This is a condition occasionally seen in male animals, particularly bulls, which may develop it if they are fed high-calcium diets. Sustained excessive intake of calcium leads to hypercalcitoninism, which arrests bone resorption, with hypophosphatemia and osteopetrosis. The resulting hypocalcemia, hyperparathyroidism, and hypophosphatemia are analogous to parturient paresis.

Vitamin E and Selenium in Metabolism

Vitamin E is the generic name for the biologically active compounds among the tocopherols and tocotrienols. Vitamin E was originally designated as the antisterility factor, because rats fed diets lacking in plant oils failed to reproduce. Its name, *tocopherol,* was chosen because it means "to bear offspring." Several naturally occurring substances have vitamin E activity. Among these related compounds, *alpha-tocopherol* (5,6,7-trimethyltocol) is most potent. When animal feeds are supplemented with the vitamin, the racemic form is used as the acetate salt, which resists oxidation.

A compound with multiple roles in body function, tocopherol may be most important for its chain-breaking *antioxidant* effect. This protects molecules that are vulnerable to oxidation, such as the polyunsaturated fatty acids (PUFAs) of cell membranes (Fig. 42–7). In the presence of oxygen, such components undergo progressive peroxidation, which may cause hepatic necrosis as one outcome. Free radicals and metallic ions expedite these reactions. Tocopherol donates the hydrogen of its 6-OH group to *reduce free radicals* ($OH^\bullet$). (Chemical nomenclature uses a dot superscript to show the presence of the single unpaired electron that is a feature of these reactive molecules or molecular fragments.) The tocopherols provide a shield for the PUFAs in the membranes, such as arachidonic acid. They prevent the abstraction of a hydrogen atom from a PUFA molecule by a free radical that initiates peroxidation and may start an autocatalytic chain reaction called lipid peroxidation.

Formation of free radicals may be stimulated by salts of transition metals, by redox reactions that involve transfer of an electron, or by certain types of radiation or photosensitization:

$$H_2O_2 + Fe^{++} \rightarrow Fe^{+++} + OH^- + OH^\bullet$$

Iron dextrose, once commonly injected into piglets to prevent iron-deficiency anemia, may cause hindlimb paral-

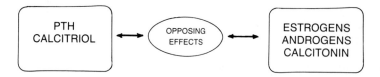

1. Promote multiplication and maturation of osteoblasts but suppress their formation of collagen (i.e., decrease the matrix for bone deposition)

2. Promote differentiation of monocytic cells into osteoblasts, while inducing release of paracrine resorption factors from osteoblasts (i.e., activate the machinery for bone mineral resorption)

NET EFFECT:
    Acceleration of bone remodeling, with increased resorption of bone minerals

1. Promote increased production of collagen matrix by osteoclasts (i.e., increase the matrix for bone deposition)

2. Suppress differentiation of monocytic cells into osteoclasts and decrease release of resorption factors from osteoblasts (i.e., deactivate the mechanisms for bone resorption)

NET EFFECT:
    Deceleration of bone remodeling, with decreased resorption of bone minerals

Figure 42–6 Opposing effect of the PTH-calcitriol and the sex calcitonin-steroids systems on bone mineral resorption and deposition.

ysis in a vitamin E–deficient animal. It can produce a syndrome involving hypercalcemia with massive mobilization of calcium ions, hyperphosphatemia, diarrhea and vomiting, hyperkalemia and hyperglycemia, increased transaminases, and peroxidation of muscle lipids with high malonyldialdehyde.

Cell membranes contain PUFAs. The enzymes cyclooxygenases and lipoxygenase act on PUFAs to produce a series of compounds called eicosanoids, tissue hormones that have profound effects on local tissue function. However, these enzymes also give rise to detrimental peroxides and free radicals that must be neutralized. In cattle, a combination of deficiencies of vitamin E and *selenium* (Se) and an excess of PUFAs appears to be responsible for the pathogenesis of nutritional degenerative myopathy (NDM), or white muscle disease. This disease affects many species, causing myopathy of skeletal and cardiac muscle. In some species, there are degenerative changes in other organs such as hepatic necrosis (swine), mulberry heart disease (swine), encephalomalacia (chick), and steatitis (most species). In cats, high fatty acid intake (from diets excessive in tuna, in canned cat foods, and in cod liver oil) may cause steatitis (yellow to orange sub-

cutaneous masses) similar to vitamin E deficiency. In dogs, excess fatty acids or a deficiency of vitamin E is associated with a cutaneous syndrome resembling demodicosis (*Demodex* mite infestation of the skin). It appears that linolenic acid (18:3, i.e., 18 carbon atoms and 3 double bonds) and PUFAs with 3 double bonds are responsible for initiation of NDM, and the lesions it causes can be prevented by pretreatment with vitamin E or selenium.

The enzyme *glutathione peroxidase* (GSH-Px) contains *selenium* and destroys peroxides as they are formed in the body, oxidizing glutathione in the process. Therefore, the presence of an adequate supply of selenium to keep this enzyme fully operational is an important complementary mechanism to that of vitamin E, which helps prevent lipid peroxide formation (Fig. 42–8). However, it must be kept in mind that selenium has a rather narrow safety margin, so there is a risk of intoxication (e.g., blind staggers), especially in areas where high-selenium forages grow. As the GSH-Px does not occur in the cell membranes, but only in the cytosol and mitochondria, this may limit its protective action to the interior of cells, unlike that of vitamin E.

The body's defense mechanisms use free radicals to

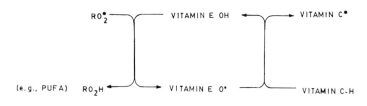

Figure 42–7 Some examples of antioxidant effects that protect the body's cells from damage by free radicals (`•`). **A,** The water-soluble vitamin C can continuously regenerate the reduced (antioxidant) form of the lipid-soluble vitamin, which acts in the cell membranes. **B,** Vitamin C can also regenerate glutathione.

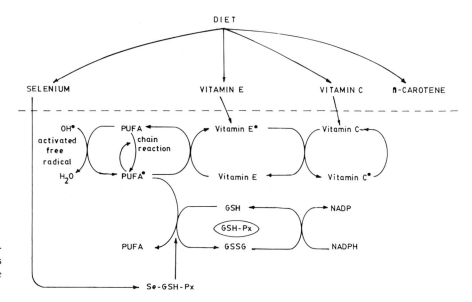

Figure 42–8 Examples of antioxidant defense mechanisms against free radical and progressive lipid peroxidation.

destroy invading microorganisms. For example, the polymorphonuclear leukocytes (PMNs) use little oxygen in the resting state. When they are stimulated by phagocytes that have encountered foreign antigens, the PMNs can show a 100-fold increase in oxygen consumption, the so-called respiratory burst. This process is catalyzed by NADPH (nicotinamide-adenine dinucleotide phosphate) oxidase, a flavoprotein enzyme that leads to a one-electron reduction of oxygen to superoxide in the cell membrane, releasing the radical outside the cell:

$$NADPH + 2O_2 \rightarrow NADP + H^+ + 2O^{\bullet -}$$

The oxygen radical is only weakly bactericidal until it is changed into a peroxide, H_2O_2. The NADPH is regenerated via two hexose monophosphate (HMP) shunt enzyme steps:

1. Glucose-6-phosphate dehydrogenase
2. 6-Phosphogluconate dehydrogenase

The HMP shunt shows a 20-fold increase in PMNs after phagocytic stimulation. The cytoplasm of leukocytes contains superoxide dismutase that destroys this free radical to protect the host cells:

$$O_2^{\bullet -} + O_2^{\bullet -} + 2H^+ \rightarrow H_2O_2 + O_2^{\bullet -}$$

The H_2O_2 is then detoxified by the GSH-Px (glutathione peroxidase) cycle.

Alternatively, catalase can protect the cells:

$$2H_2O_2 \rightarrow 2H_2O + O_2$$

The iron-containing hemeprotein catalase occurs only in peroxisomes and is thought to be less important than superoxide dismutase under most conditions. Other vitamins, notably vitamin A, beta-carotene, and vitamin C, make important peroxy radical–scavenging protective contribu-

tions, as do the metalloenzymes containing manganese, zinc, or copper.

Muscular dystrophy is seen in rapidly growing young animals that are deficient in vitamin E. It involves degeneration of skeletal and cardiac muscle, with replacement by whitish-colored connective tissue (white muscle disease of calves, stiff-lamb disease of sheep). Sudden death occurs occasionally in acute cases, in foals, turkeys, and ducks. Deficient feeder pigs may develop a syndrome with mulberry heart disease or hepatic necrosis accompanying the muscular dystrophy. Deficient chicks exhibit a specific form of encephalomalacia, as well as exudative diathesis. They develop ataxia, tremors, retraction or twisting of the head, clonic spasms of the legs, and stupor. The lesions include edema and hemorrhage, massive necrosis, and a very large and distinct area of encephalomalacia in the cerebellum. Dogs may show seborrhea and cats steatitis. Reproductive disorders include degeneration of the testicular germinal epithelium and damage to placental attachments. Toxic contaminants in food, such as fungal toxins that cause liver injury, can lead to accumulation in the skin of porphyrin photosensitizers, which normally would be excreted in the bile. This can lead to photosensitization damage to the skin, particularly in light-colored areas.

Some of the subtleties of species differences in the manifestations of pathologic conditions from vitamin E and from selenium deficiencies can be explained by differences in the selenium requirement of enzymes, particularly GSH-peroxidase (GSH-Px). This enzyme occurs in both selenium and nonselenium forms. Deficiency is more likely to cause liver necrosis in animals that have mainly the Se-GSH-Px (e.g., cats) than in those that depend on the nonselenium enzyme (e.g., sheep). This is not a complete explanation of the situation, however. It is of great current interest that antioxidant molecules have shown protective effects against some cancers.

Vitamin K and Blood Coagulation

A hemorrhagic syndrome was observed in chicks fed diets extracted with fat solvents, and later a protective fat-soluble factor was isolated from alfalfa and characterized to be 2-methyl-3-phytyl-1,4-naphthoquinone. This was christened vitamin K_1 (for *koagulation,* in Danish) or phylloquinone. Another agent, isolated from fish meal in the first instance, was labeled K_2. Synthesized by bacteria, it has an unsaturated polyisoprenoid side chain at the three position of the naphthoquinone ring. This is one of several menaquinones (MKs) that have been isolated (MK_6 to MK_{13}, depending on the length of the side chain).

Menadione (2-methyl-1,4-naphthoquinone), a synthetic substance without a side chain, can be converted to a biologically active form of vitamin K in mammalian tissues, mainly as MK_4. Menadione is widely used in animal feeds, especially for poultry, which are susceptible to a hemorrhagic syndrome. The preferred form is a complex with sodium bisulfite, which is both stable and water soluble.

The bleeding disorders of vitamin K deficiency are attributable to reduced production of prothrombin and other clotting factors in the hemostasis cascade. Vitamin K acts as a coenzyme for a carboxylase, a hepatic cell microsomal enzyme, that forms gamma-carboxylglutamyl residues from their plasma protein precursors (glutamyl proteins). These carboxy derivatives or activated proteins (prothrombin, factor VII, factor IX, and factor X), in the presence of calcium ions, are necessary for hemostasis. As clotting factors, the latter interact with phospholipid surfaces for clot formation and adhesion.

Deficiency or defective absorption of vitamin K or its precursors leads to a hemorrhagic syndrome. Since the vitamin is synthesized microbially in the gastrointestinal tract, it is not required normally in the ruminant diet. Other species vary in their requirements, depending on whether, like rabbits, they practice coprophagy (cecotrophy) or to what degree absorption occurs from the gut. Pigs may show a vitamin K–responsive bleeding disorder.

Moldy sweet clover hay causes a severe acute hemorrhagic syndrome if ingested by calves. This finding has led to the isolation of the toxin (competitive inhibitor) dicoumarol, which is formed from coumarin (a structural analogue of vitamin K) by microorganisms. Also a group of anticoagulants with antivitamin K activity was developed. Warfarin, the first one in a series of antagonists, is used in medicine and for rodent control. The major function of dicoumarol anticoagulants is to prevent the formation of the normal active prothrombin.

WATER-SOLUBLE VITAMINS

Thiamine (Vitamin B₁)

As for scurvy, which was prevented by citrus (vitamin C), the discovery of vitamin B_1, or thiamine, is associated with the disease beriberi, which responded to dietary ther-apy. A protective agent was first isolated and characterized in 1926 from rice polishings and rice bran. Later, other dietary sources of the vitamin, wheat germ and yeast, were identified, and a decade after its initial discovery, thiamine was synthesized in the laboratory.

It is surprising that the animal kingdom has not acquired a way of synthesizing thiamine de novo, given the importance of this substance to intermediary metabolism. Animals are dependent on plant and microbial synthesis for vitamin B_1. They ingest it in the diet, which may be supplemented by microbial synthesis in the forestomachs in ruminants. Carnivores obtain most of it from animal tissues, and pig tissues contain higher levels of thiamine than those of the other domestic species.

Dietary thiamine is the essential precursor of the active *coenzyme* known as *thiamine diphosphate* (TDP) or thiamine *pyrophosphate* (TPP). Although the metabolically active form of thiamine is TPP, at least four forms are present in the animal body. These are free thiamine (T), thiamine monophosphate (TMP), TDP, and *thiamine triphosphate* (TTP). TDP plays a crucial catalytic assistant role in oxidative decarboxylation reactions that set the stage for ATP production, in the tricarboxylic cycle, and for synthetic activities, in the pentose phosphate pathway.

Role of Thiamine in ATP Production

A critical switching point in metabolism is the *pyruvate decarboxylase complex* comprising three interacting enzymes and their cofactors. The first stage involves pyruvate dehydrogenase, with TPP as a cofactor, to expedite the conversion of pyruvate to hydroxyethyl TPP and carbon dioxide. The second enzyme in the complex is dihydrolipoyltransacetylase, for which lipoamide is the coenzyme. The reactive disulfide group of lipoamide oxidizes the hydroxyethyl group attached to the TPP, producing an acetyl group that bonds to lipoamide to form acetyl lipoamide and releasing the TPP as a carbanion. The acetyl group is then transferred from acetyl lipoamide to form acetyl coenzyme A (AcCoA), which has a high-energy thioester bond. Finally, the third enzyme, dihydrolipoyldehydrogenase (with its FAD prosthetic group) regenerates oxidized lipoamide, the reduced FADH being reoxidized by NAD^+. The three enzymes and their prosthetic groups are closely associated structurally, thereby facilitating this amazingly complex mechanism for generating acetyl CoA to fuel the tricarboxylic acid cycle (Krebs's cycle) and many synthetic pathways.

A similar TPP-requiring complex and mechanism provide for the oxidative decarboxylation of alpha-ketoglutarate within the Krebs's cycle.

Role of Thiamine in Synthetic Activities

Thiamine diphosphate is a coenzyme in another major metabolic pathway called the *pentose phosphate pathway.* A primary role of this metabolic chain is the generation of reducing power for *synthetic activities* rather than oxidation for ATP production. The biochemical vehicle for this is NADPH (TPNH), which serves as a hydrogen and electron donor for the enzyme pathways leading to reductive biosynthesis. The activity of this pathway is low in skeletal muscle and very high in the adipose tissue cells, which form fatty acids from acetyl CoA. It is also important in brain metabolism.

One of the enzymes in the pathway is transketolase, which has TPP as its prosthetic group. In a fashion resembling that of the pyruvate dehydrogenase complex, the active carbanion form of TPP bonds to the carbonyl group of a ketose substrate, such as xylose-5-phosphate, retaining the activated 2-carbon glycoaldehyde part while shedding the rest. The activated unit condenses with an aldehyde acceptor such as ribose-5-phosphate, then dissociates from the TPP. Regulation of flow of substrate through the pentose phosphate pathway is largely a function of the availability of $NADP^+$, which accepts the electrons in the initial step, the oxidation of glucose-6-phosphate. There is a reversible linkage between the pentose pathway and glycolysis involving the transketolase and transaldolase enzymes, since ribose-5-phosphate can be converted to glycolytic intermediates. This allows for adaptation to changing demands between fat synthesis and energy release. The activity of transketolase in erythrocytes and the effect of adding TPP can be measured as a diagnostic test for thiamine deficiency or inadequacy. In thiamine deficiency, erythrocyte precursors disappear from the bone marrow.

Types of Thiamine Deficiencies

An equilibrium exists between free thiamine and TDP. TTP occurs in the membranes of nerves cells in a tightly bound form that appears not to exchange rapidly with the other forms. Normal blood thiamine levels in sheep and cattle are in the range of 75 to 185 nmol per liter, and levels below 50 nmol per liter are indicative of vitamin B_1 inadequacy. A *deficiency* leads to a slow decline in thiamine and TDP. It appears that a critical stage is reached if TDP in brain tissue falls to about 20 percent of normal.

Thiamine Deficiencies in Ruminants. A deficiency of thiamine may be the result of its lack in the food; this usually requires 4 to 7 weeks of a deficient diet. *Polioencephalomalacia* (PEM) can be induced in very young lambs by depriving them of dietary thiamine. In this experimental model, after 4 to 7 weeks the characteristic clinical signs are accompanied by an extreme depletion (to less than 20 percent) of free thiamine and TDP in affected parts of the cerebral cortex. The severe brain damage leads to dysfunction of the ocular muscles, blindness, head pressing, anorexia, tremor, often opisthotonus, weakness, and collapse with clonic convulsions. It is reversible if large parenteral doses of thiamine are given at an early stage of the signs, but there is irreversible brain damage if treatment is delayed. Oral B_1 or thiamine propyl disulfide may be effective as a preventive in young lambs.

High intake of sulfates in feed or water is implicated in a neurological disorder of ruminants resembling PEM. It is intriguing that the thiamine levels in tissues are then normal or elevated, and it may be that this is another route of pathogenesis to a common neurological lesion.

Substances that *inhibit thiamine,* present in the *food* or in the *gastrointestinal tract,* can induce a lowered blood level of thiamine. The process may be accelerated when ruminants are fed certain diets, usually ones that are *high in readily fermentable carbohydrates,* where the extracellular enzyme *thiaminase I* may be formed in the ruminoreticulum. Since this enzyme is a transferase, its action is accelerated in the presence of substrates that can participate in the exchange reaction (e.g., nicotinic acid) with the thiazole moiety. It is possible, but has not been proved, that a toxic antithiamine agent could be formed in the process.

A neurological disorder that occurs in feedlot cattle fed very high levels of molasses in Cuba, called locally *barrachio* (drunkenness) resembles PEM, but it does not respond to thiamine therapy. It may be due to deranged metabolism of fatty acids in the rumen with increased levels of VFAs (SCFAs) having chain lengths C4 or higher, which are the usual sequel to a bout of lactic acid fermentation lasting 2 days.

In parts of eastern Australia, a monocrop of a plant rich in thiaminase occurs following flooding in some seasons. This plant, called nardoo (*Marsilea drummondii*) may cause a thiamine-related disease in sheep, similar to the PEM described in North America. The result of the disease in ruminants is dramatic deterioration of parts of the cerebral cortex, cerebral cortex necrosis (CCN), and degeneration of some lower nuclei in the brain.

The enzyme thiaminase I is frequently present in the gastrointestinal tract of animals that do not manifest signs of disease (PEM). This is not surprising, as it takes several weeks of total deprivation of vitamin B_1 to induce the disease. The origin of the enzyme may be a bacterium, *Bacillus thiaminolyticus,* found in the rumen and gastrointestinal tract. As mentioned previously, fern-like plants such as *Marsilea drummondii* in Australia, and bracken fern (*Pteridium aquilinum*) also contain thiaminase. Other microbes may produce the enzyme in the rumen.

Thiaminase I is a transferase, and when thiamine is broken down, new compounds are formed, depending on which cosubstrates are present to participate in the exchange reaction in the rumen. One hypothesis is that toxic antimetabolites of thiamine might be formed in this exchange reaction. One of these substances, delta-pyrrolinium, has been detected in cases of CCN. This attractive idea would help explain the unpredictable nature of the disease, but it has not yet been possible to confirm it. Thiaminase activity reaches a peak in the gut of young lambs during the first few weeks of life and then declines rapidly. The enzyme may build up within a functioning rumen if there is a dietary change that increases the readily fermentable carbohydrates. This occurs in feedlot diets or grazing stubbles where a considerable amount of grain has been spilled on the ground or when supplementary grain is fed.

The antibiotic feed additive *monensin* suppresses the rumen synthesis of vitamin B_1, which is correlated with microbial protein synthesis (microbial growth and multiplication).

Thiamine deficiency can also be induced by chronic oral dosing with the thiamine antimetabolite *amprolium* (commonly used as a coccidiostat). The signs of this thiamine dysfunction are anorexia, gastrointestinal dysfunction, and neurological disorders. The electroencephalogram shows unusual bursts of long-lasting (up to 90 seconds) high-amplitude spindle activity, which appear several hours before signs of disease become detectable. Depression, loss of visual reflexes, involuntary eye movements, decreased rates of rumen and intestinal contraction during slow-wave sleep, passage of loose feces rather than formed pellets, knuckling of the fetlocks of the front legs, and sleep disturbances are also noted. The manifestations of thiamine deficiency and amprolium toxicity are quite different.

Thiamine Deficiencies in Carnivores. Fur-bearing animals raised commercially are affected by *Chastek's paralysis* if their diet is deficient in thiamine. Domestic carnivores are susceptible to a syndrome similar to PEM, resulting from thiamine-destroying compounds and enzymes in fish-based diets. *Cats* are particularly vulnerable. The signs include neurological disorders, but the neck musculature responds in a manner different from that of ruminants (torticollis instead of opisthotonus).

In *young dogs,* thiamine deficiency leads to slower growth rates, then progressive inappetance with weight loss; some exhibit coprophagy during this asymptomatic phase. Eventually, there is abrupt onset of clinical signs of a neurological disorder. Concentrations of L-lactate and pyruvate in the blood are high during the presymptomatic stages and decline in the terminal phase with low blood glucose levels in some cases. An unusually wide stance of the rear limbs, with rigid tail flexion between the legs, may be seen. Along with emesis, defective limb reflexes, sensory ataxia with knuckling, kyphosis, nystagmus, and trismus may be observed. Torticollis may be present. These signs are followed by recumbency, tonic-clonic convulsions, and death. Occasionally an affected dog develops tachycardia and cardiac failure with sudden death. Low levels of erythrocyte transketolase with a high TPP effect are found. Severely affected animals show marked pathological changes in part of the gray matter. Spongiosis with vacuolation of the neuropil and myelin sheaths is followed by demyelination, neuronal cell body necrosis, endothelial cell proliferation, and neutrophil infiltration. Phagocytes containing lipids are observed in the late stages. Of the two patterns of distribution of lesions seen, one is limited only to the caudal colliculi, whereas in the other, damage is widespread. The latter type involves the suprasplenial gyri, and frequently the caudal colliculi, the claustra, nodulus of the cerebellum, and medial vestibular nuclei.

Riboflavin (Vitamin B₂)

Vitamin B_2 (riboflavin) is a heat-stable, light-sensitive, yellow pigment that was discovered during studies of enzyme reactions involved in the oxidation-reduction pathways of intermediary metabolism. It is an organic compound formed by bonding D-ribitol to isoalloxazine. Both riboflavin and its 5′-phosphate are selectively absorbed from the small intes-

tine. B_2 is an essential nutrient for all animal species except those that can obtain it from microbial synthesis in the gut (e.g., mature ruminants, and coprophagic rabbits, which eat their morning soft feces).

Riboflavin is the starting point for two of the crucial coenzymes in animal tissues, *flavin mononucleotide* (FMN), and *flavin adenine dinucleotide* (FAD). These serve as prosthetic groups in flavoprotein enzymes, which include several oxidases and dehydrogenases. The flavin coenzymes are the intermediaries for electron transfer to the pyridine nucleotides in the chain that releases chemical bond energy in tissue respiration. Unlike the pyridine nucleotides, FAD accepts both of the hydrogen atoms given up by the substrate.

Deficiency of riboflavin causes a specific curled-toe paralysis in *chickens* that is accompanied by dermatitis, retarded growth, and reduced embryo survival. *Pigs* show a peculiar muscle stiffness and twisting of the limbs, ocular lesions, and dermatitis with a sebaceous exudate; they may have cardiovascular and kidney lesions. *Dogs* manifest dermatitis, anemia, weakness, and cardiovascular problems. Preruminant *calves* may exhibit salivation and lacrimation accompanied by anorexia, slow growth, scours (diarrhea and dysentery), and alopecia and dermatitis at stress points.

Niacin

Originally isolated in the quest for the anti-beriberi factor and then discarded, niacin was rediscovered as the coenzyme diphosphopyridine nucleotide. This set the stage for characterization of the pyridine nucleotide coenzymes that contain nicotinamide and form part of the catalytic electron and hydrogen transfer chain that facilitates many oxidation-reduction reactions in the tissues of the animal body.

Nicotinic acid and nicotinamide are two dietary forms of niacin. They are converted to the two active forms of coenzyme, *nicotine adenine dinucleotide* (NAD), and *nicotine dinucleotide phosphate* (NADP). Synthesis of the coenzymes from nicotinic acid involves adding ribose phosphate to form nicotinate ribonucleotide, which is converted to desamido-NAD^+ by addition of AMP. The completion of NAD^+ synthesis requires transfer of an amide group to the niacin carboxyl group. $NADP^+$ is formed from NAD^+ by phosphorylation of the 2′-hydroxyl of the adenine ribose.

A major acceptor of electrons and hydrogen ions in the oxidation pathways that yield free energy, each NAD^+ molecule accepts one hydrogen ion and two electrons, forming $NADH + H^+$. $NADP^+$ acts mainly in the reduced form, NADPH, because it participates mainly in reductive biosyntheses.

The human disease called pellagra ("rough skin") was known long before the role of niacin had been clarified. It swept through the poor people of southern Europe like an epidemic after corn (maize), introduced by Columbus from the New World, became a staple food in the 18th and 19th centuries. Early in the 20th century, countless cases developed in the American corn belt and southern United States.

The symptoms included dermatitis of the exposed skin, diarrhea, and dementia. Again it occurred primarily in poor people.

Niacin deficiency proved to be one of the most complex of the vitamin-related problems to unravel. Joseph Golberger, of the Public Health Service, had established that the disease was of nutritional origin.

> An anomaly revealed early was that the people of Central America did not seem to be affected like those of Europe and North America. It emerged that the different systems of corn preparation and cooking offered one explanation. It was the custom throughout most of that region to treat the corn with lime (alkali), which has the effect of making more of the niacin available.
>
> A veterinarian first proposed (in 1916) that canine black tongue disease was analogous to human pellagra. This triggered research into the nutritional cause of the disease, using dogs as the experimental model. The animal model of black tongue in dogs was used to investigate the protective and curative effect of various foods.

A wave of nutritional experimentation was conducted in dogs but was frustrated in the early days by the dogs' indulging in coprophagy, which protected them by supplying some microbially formed niacin.

A third complicating factor was the later (1945) discovery that niacin is synthesized in mammalian tissues from the amino acid tryptophan. It takes about 50 times as much tryptophan as dietary niacin to achieve the same effect in meeting the animal's needs. It should be noted that cats lack this pathway.

> As corn contains the low-quality protein zein, which is deficient in lysine and tryptophan, it fails to provide enough tryptophan to compensate for a niacin deficiency. To furnish enough niacin, the tryptophan level in the diet must be about 150 mg per gram of diet. Though they may contain less niacin than corn, other grains, except rice, supply this amount.

The role of niacin is still not fully understood. There are still unanswered questions, because much of the earlier research was done prior to a thorough understanding of the vitamin B complex. The implications of amino acid imbalances or deficiencies were unknown, and the roles of trace elements such as zinc had not been discovered. Other discoveries are likely to be made concerning the interactions of these various classes of nutrients and metabolites with receptors on cells and in enzyme reactions.

In animals, niacin deficiency features epithelial lesions affecting the skin, oral cavity, and digestive tract. Anorexia and retarded growth are observed, accompanied by diarrhea and dermatitis. Affected chicks have a malformation of the legs called *perosis*. Pigs are particularly susceptible; they show severe gastroenteritis, scaly dermatitis with alopecia, microcytic anemia, and a neurological disorder with posterior paralysis and lesions of malacia. Ruminants are resistant because they obtain niacin from their commensal rumen microflora. In dogs, the characteristic stomatitis is known as *black tongue*.

Black tongue in dogs was a very unpleasant disease. Affected dogs manifested anorexia, vomiting, apathy, and prostration. Some convulsed and died.

The inner surface of the cheeks and lips and the edges of the tongue were so covered with pustules as to resemble rotten flesh. There was a foul odor to these lesions, and fusospirochetal organisms were isolated from them. Gentle swabbing caused the friable mucosa to come off in shreds. There was intense salivation and bloody fluid diarrhea of low volume accompanied by straining and discomfort.

At postmortem, large ulcers were common in the colon and rectum, and sometimes were present in the duodenal mucosa. Occasionally, large pustules were observed on the skin of the thorax and anterior abdominal wall.

The effect of niacin in reducing lipolysis while increasing glucose and insulin has been advocated for treatment and prevention of primary ketosis in lactating cows.

Pyridoxine (Vitamin B₆)

Three forms of vitamin B_6 have been identified—*pyridoxine, pyridoxal, and pyridoxamine*. All can be converted to the active coenzyme pyridoxal phosphate (PLP). It is a cofactor in a wide range of reactions involving amino acids, including transamination decarboxylation, nonoxidative deamination, desulfhydration, and other reactions that bring about molecular rearrangements such as those induced by racemases.

Additionally, B_6 participates in the synthesis of catecholamines and the metabolism of gamma-aminobutyric acid (GABA). As coenzyme for delta-aminolevulinic acid synthetase, it contributes to porphyrin synthesis. It also interacts with glycogen phosphorylase, which is responsible for glycogen catabolism. A reactive chemical, PLP attracts electrons from amino acid substrates, thereby serving as an electrophilic facilitator of various reactions involving amine groups.

In dogs and the pigs, a deficiency of PLP precursor vitamins leads to retarded growth, weakness, dermatitis, and anemia. More specific changes occur as a result of CNS dysfunction. These include hyperirritability and epileptiform convulsions. Strains of Fayoumi fowl have been identified as being genetically susceptible to these neurological disorders.

Pantothenic Acid

Pantothenic acid is one of several vitamins in the B-complex group that has not been assigned a number, but its status as an essential dietary nutrient is securely established. Its name was selected because it means "everywhere."

Pantothenic acid is known best as a key constituent of coenzyme A (CoA). Synthesis of CoA involves phosphorylation of the pantothenic acid. The 4'-phosphopantothenate then forms a peptide bond with cysteine, which loses a carboxyl group to yield 4'-phosphopantetheine. AMP is added, then another phosphate group, resulting in CoA. This remarkable substance plays a pivotal role in fatty acid metabolism through its capacity to transfer acyl (acetyl or other) groups after combining with them (e.g., acetyl CoA). It is also the avenue for oxidative decarboxylation of pyruvate.

As a constituent of acyl carrier protein (ACP), which is a peptide chain of 77 amino acid residues, a form of pantothenic acid is also involved in intermediary metabolism. The phosphopantetheine acts as a prosthetic group attached to the protein via a serine residue. This is the form of pantothenic acid that participates in the synthesis of fatty acids; CoA is the form of panthothenic acid used for their degradation.

Deficiency of pantothenic acid leads to retarded growth as well as pathological changes in many organs. *Chicks* show impaired feather development; ocular and oral dermatitis; degeneration of lymphoid cells in the crypts of Lieberkühn, the bursa of Fabricius, the spleen, and the thymus; vacuolation with hyaline deposits in the acinar cells of the pancreas; myelin degeneration in the nervous system; and degeneration in the adrenal cortex.

Deficient weanling *pigs* exhibit decreased growth rate, diarrhea, a characteristic goose-stepping gait, and pathological changes in afferent neurons. The crypts of Lieberkühn show cystic mucoid dilatation, hyperplasia of the lymph nodules, and a lymphocytic cell reaction. The large intestine harbors some degenerative changes, colitis, and ulceration. Reproductive performance is impaired. Deficiency can be induced in young *calves,* but mature ruminants can meet their requirements from bacterial synthesis in the rumen.

Biotin

D-Biotin occurs as biocytin, a form that is covalently bonded to lysine, and serves as a prosthetic group for carboxylases. The reactions it expedites involve the use of ATP's bond energy to activate carboxyl groups. Ruminants and rabbits obtain sufficient amounts from microbial synthesis in the gut unless this is suppressed by chronic oral chemotherapy. *Avidin,* a heat-labile protein constituent of raw egg whites, complexes with biotin to render it unabsorbable. Dietary requirements for chickens are known.

Deficiency of biotin leads to skin and oral mucosal lesions. There is growing evidence that it may lead to specific lesions of the hoof in swine. Lameness is a major cause of culling and economic loss in hoofed animals, particularly swine. Biotin, which has a direct effect on the epidermis responsible for horn formation and its quality, improves the mechanical properties of the hooves. By increasing the number of tubules in the horn by up to 50 percent, oral biotin supplementation also reduces the incidence of claw lesions.

Dietary biotin helps sows attain their full reproductive potential. More sows return to estrus and conceive within 10 days of weaning. Also the total weight of weaners per sow per year is increased. It is estimated that breeding sows need 175 μg of available biotin per kilogram of diet for optimum performance. The feeding of biotin supplements is reported to increase litter size.

Vitamin B$_{12}$ and Folic Acid

The syndrome of pernicious anemia (PA) was described first around 1834 and in greater detail in 1849. As the adjective "pernicious" implied, it was incurable and almost invariably fatal until the life-saving discovery was made of the value of feeding liver (1926). This finding triggered a search for a vitamin. It proved to be more complicated than expected, for in 1929 it was found that the body produced an *intrinsic factor* (IF), which was shown to be a protein essential for absorption of the *extrinsic factor* (EF) in liver.

PA patients had achlorhydria, and their gastric juice was deficient in IF. Their anemia was megaloblastic and progressive, often being accompanied by neuropathy.

Folic acid, or folacin, a substance named after foliage from which it was first isolated in 1941, was another complicating factor. It was shown to be a growth factor for some bacteria and was characterized in 1943. Malabsorption or deficiency of folacin leads to defective erythrocyte development and macrocytic anemia in man.

The search for the extrinsic factor was completed in 1948 with the isolation of crystalline vitamin B$_{12}$, or cyanocobalamin. This was shown to be the animal growth factor (AGF), and its chemical structure was defined in the next few years.

Since the molecule contained the trace element *cobalt,* another twist of the tale was able to be unraveled. The fascinating history of the development of human research in this field has been thoroughly recorded.

In 1936, trail blazing research on trace minerals showed that important wasting diseases of sheep (bush sickness) and cattle in some parts of Australian range lands, featuring normocytic normochromic anemia, were attributable to cobalt deficiency. The advances in the physiology and biochemistry of intermediary metabolism then allowed the assembly of a clearer picture of the roles of the dietary factors, *B$_{12}$, folic acid, and cobalt.* This knowledge could be integrated with that of microbial synthesis in the rumen and the intestine, the presence of B$_{12}$-binding substances and intrinsic factor in gut secretions, and the storage mechanisms in the liver (Fig. 42–9). The pathways of intermediary metabolism and the sites where the coenzymes acted were determined.

Using germ-free animals, it was found that feces could be one source of methyl groups, which otherwise must be synthesized in the tissues from methionine or homocystine plus choline and vitamin B$_{12}$.

Vitamin B$_{12}$ and Cobalt

The extrinsic factor, or *cobalamin,* contains the metallic element cobalt, bonded in a porphyrin-type tetrapyrrole ring with a hydroxyl or water group attached to the cobalt atom. The resulting cobalt-containing nucleus is called a *corrin.* There are a number of side chains, one of which is linked to a nucleotide via its phosphate group.

Though vitamin B$_{12}$ was initially obtained by extraction from liver and subsequent purification, it soon became possible to prepare it via microbial fermentation, then from

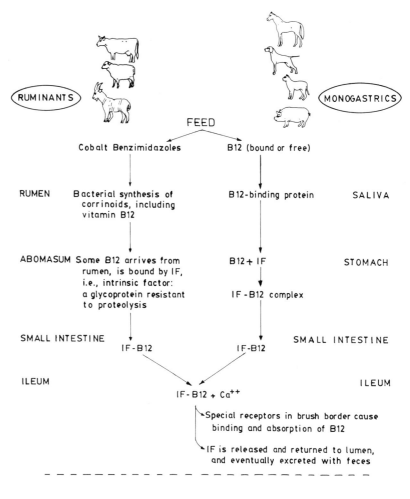

Figure 42–9 Illustration of the different types of synthesis and intermediary substances in ruminant and monogastric species meeting their requirement for vitamin B_{12}.

B12 enters plasma, binds to transcobalamin-2 (TC-2), also to TC-1 and TC-3, and is transferred to LIVER and other tissues, for conversion to coenzymes and storage

---

cultures of *Propionibacterium shermanii*. The coenzyme that is formed from B_{12} in vivo and its molecular functions at specific steps have been characterized.

Vitamin B_{12} is synthesized in the rumen contents by bacteria, provided that there is sufficient cobalt in the diet or in forage plants. A variety of corrinoids are formed that vary in their metabolic value to their animal host. The chemistry of the corrinoids is extremely complex because of their intricate structure and of the large numbers of natural and synthetic compounds now known. *Cobamides and cobiamides* occur in ruminant blood and liver, but the cobiamides, which lack a nucleotide moiety, are inactive in man and animals.

Among the cobamides, cyanocobalamin (CN^+Cbl) is the artificial cyanide derivative of aquacobalamin ($AqCbl$) or hydroxycobalamin ($OHCbl$), the two naturally occurring forms produced by bacteria, which are the true anti–pernicious anemia factor (APAF) or extrinsic factor, or animal protein factor (APF), or *Lactobacillus lactis Dorner factor*

(LLDF). The KCN-derivative is preferred because of its stability. All three cobamides are absorbed from the intestine, and are active in mammalian metabolism, and the term vitamin B_{12} encompasses all three. The mammalian form of B_{12} or cobalamin (Cbl) contains 5,6-dimethyl-benzimidazole.

Several species of rumen bacteria synthesize B_{12} and related analogues, particularly *Selemonas, Peptostreptococcus,* and *Butyrivibrio* species. The corrinoids are growth factors for some rumen bacteria and are coenzymes for their metabolism. Only a small fraction (3 to 15 percent) of the total production is in the form of the active B_{12}, cobalamin. The animal daily requirement of sheep for B_{12} is about 11 pg; this can be supplied by supplementing a cobalt-poor diet with cobalt salts at a cobalt dose equivalent to 1 mg per day. Forage levels below 0.07 ppm (70 μg/kg) cobalt, which are considered deficient in this trace element for ruminants, occur in regions where the soil is cobalt deficient (e.g., parts of Australasia, southern Africa, and large areas of central and western North America). High levels of cobalamin are found in the rumen epithelium and other parts of the gastrointestinal tract, but these are thought to be absorbed from the intestine and returned to the epithelium via the blood in the case of the forestomachs. The highest levels among tissues are found in the liver and kidneys. Levels of B_{12} in healthy ruminants' livers substantially exceed those of other species. The milk of cows and ewes is relatively high in vitamin B_{12} (3 to 12 and 1 to 6 μg per liter, respectively).

The vitamin itself is not valuable as a dietary additive for ruminants. Supplementation with cobalt or use of trace-mineralized salt or a slow-release cobalt oxide bolus in the rumen is effective. Also, more effective utilization of cobalt can be obtained by adding benzimidazole to feed.

Vitamin B_{12} is singularly important for animals that derive much of their nutritional energy from fermentation end-products of gut bacteria, short-chain fatty acids (SCFAs or VFAs). Ruminants are particularly dependent on propionate (3-carbon SCFA) for gluconeogenesis. Metabolism of propionyl-CoA via methylmalonyl-CoA mutase to succinyl-CoA requires mitochondrial adenosylcobalamin as a coenzyme. This pathway is compromised in B_{12} deficiency, with serious consequences.

The more general requirement of B_{12} in all animal species is for the pathways that require generation of methyl groups to allow synthesis of methionine, choline, and thymine. The methyltransferase system requires methylcobalamin as a coenzyme. The absorbed vitamin becomes methylcobalamin and is bound to a special protein in plasma, transcobalamin II (TC2), which transports it to the liver and other tissues (other binding proteins, TC1 and TC3 occur, the latter being formed by granulocytes). In the liver, coenzyme B_{12} may be stored by attachment to a storage protein. It must be modified into an active coenzyme form. This conversion requires formation of the 5′-deoxyadenosyl derivative of B_{12} or 5′-deoxyadenosylcobalamin, a process using ATP, FAD, and NADH that replaces the methyl group with a deoxyribose-adenine group. This is the form that is active for conversion of methylmalonyl-SCoA to succinyl-SCoA via a mutase enzyme. In vitamin B_{12} deficiency, MeMalCoA builds up and is excreted in the urine. In monogastric animals, it comes from valine or (via propionylCoA) from leucine.

Another function of B_{12} does not require prior conversion to the coenzyme form. This involves the affinity of cobalamin for methyl groups. A cyclic reaction is primed by B_{12}, forming methylcobalamin, which transfers the methyl group from methyltetrahydrofolate (MeTHF) to homocysteine, forming methionine, with the B_{12} being restored to its original state, able to repeat the cycle having returned a methyl group to THF. This is an important link between the roles of B_{12} and folic acid. In B_{12} deficiency, the MeTHF cannot be restored to THF and builds up in the plasma (Fig. 42–10).

The critical consequence of deficiency of B_{12} or folic acid appears to be impairment of DNA synthesis and elongation of bone marrow cells. Neurological sequelae may be attribu-

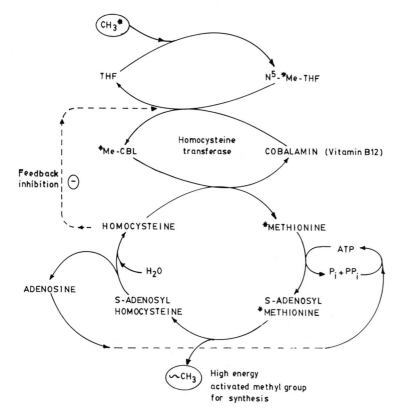

Figure 42–10 Activation of methyl groups for syntheses (e.g., purines, pyrimidines). Illustration of the flow of one-carbon units (asterisk) and their activation via ATP and of the interaction between folic acid and vitamin B_{12}.

table to disturbances in lipid metabolism, with decreased capacity to elongate and further desaturate PUFAs. The lack of sufficient long-chain PUFAs with four or more double bonds could lead to impaired nerve function.

Folic Acid

Folic acid consists of a pteridine moiety linked through para-aminobenzoic acid to one or more glutamic acid residues.

Folic acid functions as a coenzyme in the form of tetrahydrofolic acid in reactions involving one-carbon atom transfers for the formation of specific amino acids and purines. In addition, it is involved in hydroxylation of other amino acids, leading to the formation of catecholamines and serotonin. For monogastric species and poultry, it is a growth factor, and it is required also for optimum reproductive performance.

Inadequate diet, impaired absorption, increased demands for folic acid, or defective hepatic storage can lead to deficiency. The end result of folic acid deficiency is impaired DNA synthesis and depleted formation of blood cells. A form of macrocytic anemia that occurred in India was associated with malabsorption resulting from flattened and shortened intestinal villi (tropical sprue). This disease could be cured by administration of folic acid.

If the dietary form contains more than one glutamate residue, the other residues must be deconjugated by special folate conjugase enzymes that can break the gamma-glutamyl linkages in the membranes of the intestinal epithelium. The folate is absorbed and may be methylated for transfer to the liver for use or storage. Folate is reduced by folate reductase enzymes to tetrahydrofolate (THF), the active coenzyme. The THF can bind on the N-5 and N-10 positions of the pteridine moiety various one-carbon units, such as formyl (—CHO), methyl (—CH$_3$), and form-imino (—CH=NH). Alternatively, it can carry a one-carbon unit bridging these two nitrogen atoms (e.g., methylene [>CH$_2$] or methenyl [>CH]). Thus, the special role of THF is to give and receive methyl or formyl groups, which are necessary for synthesis of purines, thymidine, and some amino acids.

Microbial synthesis in the intestine is the primary source of folate for monogastric nonherbivorous species. Poultry not allowed access to their droppings need dietary supplementation or may show defects in feather development.

From measurement of folate and B$_{12}$ blood levels in horses, it seems desirable to feed supplementary folic acid, but B$_{12}$ is not necessary.

Choline

Choline (trimethylethanolamine) was first identified as a constituent of the bile of pigs. It is a component of lecithin, or phosphatidyl choline, a building block for cell membranes that participates in lipid metabolism. Choline undergoes oxidation, forming betaine, which yields methyl groups for

synthesis of methionine and creatine from their precursors. It is also a precursor of the important and ubiquitous neurotransmitter acetylcholine. Although choline is not classed as a vitamin, it is an essential nutrient for young, growing mammals and birds. All mammalian species develop the capacity to meet their choline needs by synthesis from ethanolamine, but young swine, carnivores, lagomorphs, and rodents have a dietary requirement. Dogs are susceptible to overdose, showing hyperchromic anemia at quite low oral doses of choline.

Absence of choline in the diet of *chicks and poults* leads to perosis or chondrodystrophy and reduced growth rate. Progressive damage to the tibiometatarsal joint leads to rotation of the metatarsus and displacement of the Achilles tendon from the supporting condyles. Experimentally, deficient neonatal *calves* show anorexia, extreme weakness, and hyperpnea. *Pigs* appear to be particularly susceptible, developing fatty liver and ataxia, which are frequently fatal.

Vitamin C (L-Ascorbic Acid)

Historically, the oldest known confirmed vitamin therapy was that of an unidentified factor in fresh fruits and vegetables that prevented the early oceanic explorers' and mariners' disease known as scurvy. The recognition of the protective role of citrus fruits dates to James Lind in 1732. It was almost 200 years later that the chemical factor responsible was identified, as L-ascorbic acid.

The human race and some primates are almost uniquely susceptible to a deficiency of this vitamin, as they lack the terminal enzymes needed for its synthesis. Exceptions include guinea pigs (the only laboratory animal able to show signs of vitamin C deficiency) and some bats and fish. All other mammals need L-ascorbic acid, but most can synthesize it.

Ascorbic acid has a special place in metabolic pathways as a very powerful redox compound, participating in hydroxylation reactions and collagen synthesis. Vitamin C acts as a strong reducing agent, supplying electrons to activate oxygen so that it will form a transient peroxide on the proline ring. Rapid oxidation by alpha-ketoglutarate then leaves a hydroxyproline residue and succinate. Ascorbic acid also expedites bonding of one-carbon groups to the N-5 or N-10 position of tetrahydrofolates. In vivo, it antagonizes the anticoagulant effect of dicoumarol.

Susceptible animals that are fed a vitamin C–deficient diet are unable to synthesize stable collagen effectively. The basic defect of ascorbic acid deficiency appears to be inability to synthesize hydroxyproline. Without it, the collagen that forms lacks the ability to form a triple helix. This leads to the signs characteristic of the syndrome of scurvy: defective blood vessels, bleeding, skin ulcers, swollen gums, weak bones, loose teeth, and anemia.

Navel bleeding in newborn piglets is prevented by giving ascorbic acid to pregnant sows (1 g per day) for 1 week prior to parturition (vitamin K is ineffective).

Other functions of vitamin C include its role as a reducing agent, aiding iron absorption (while decreasing copper absorption), and its transfer to the ferritin molecule from transferrin. Ascorbic acid is readily oxidized to dehydroascorbic acid, during this absorption process protecting other molecules from oxidation. It also expedites the formation of the neurotransmitters norepinephrine and 5-hydroxytryptamine. In high doses, it influences tyrosine metabolism, preventing the accumulation and favoring the excretion of intermediary compounds.

High levels of vitamin C are found in the adrenal cortex, but this level falls if adrenocorticotropic hormone (ACTH) is administered.

INORGANIC ELEMENTS IN METABOLISM

A very large number of elements are found in the animal body, including several that participate mainly in the organic chemical structures and processes of the body. A few examples of organometallic complexes are important, such as hemoglobin, myoglobin, cyanocobalamin, and metal-containing enzymes. Sulfur, phosphorus, and iodine are nonmetallic elements that are often tied up in organic structures.

Many inorganic elements take part in metabolism, usually in ionized form as metallic cations, anions, or more complex ionized minerals. All these body constituents interact in the body, and it is desirable to highlight some of the important physiological roles of minerals that may easily be overlooked.

Cations in the Body

The metals can be classified into those that are present in large amounts ("major" metals) and those that are there in lesser amounts ("minor" metals). Because some elements are found in the body in very small amounts, they are often referred to as trace elements. These adjectives apply only to the relative *amounts* of the substances, not the level of importance for body function, which often depends on their availability. Dysfunctions result when the amounts of trace elements in the diet are too low; in some cases, toxicity results if too much of a trace element is provided.

The four *major* metals of the animal body, in rank order of amount per unit of body weight, are calcium, potassium, sodium, and magnesium. Calcium is by far the most prevalent metal in the body, but most of it is in the skeletal tissues and teeth. Nevertheless, it has very important functions in the soft tissues as well. Bone tissue, comprised of the salt of calcium and phosphate known as hydroxyapatite, contains other minerals such as magnesium and must receive special consideration. The aspects of skeletal metabolism that are different from calcium metabolism presented with vitamin D are considered in this section. Magnesium is very important in herbivorous animals, particularly ruminants, and this aspect merits some special attention. The interactive effects of sodium and potassium, not previously considered with the body fluids (as electrolytes), are looked at in this section.

The *trace* metals that have established functional roles in the animal body include iron, copper, cobalt, zinc, and manganese. Some elements are more important in ruminant animals (e.g., cobalt and selenium). Many others are present but do not appear to have important physiological functions, and some are even toxic in excess.

Anions in the Body

Among the anions, chloride has been considered previously with sodium and potassium in the body fluids and in digestive physiology (gastric secretion). Phosphate surfaces in several sections, including body fluids, digestion, vitamin D and calcium, skeletal metabolism, and endocrinology. Discussion of the important and essential iodide is reported with the thyroid gland. Fluoride, not considered essential, plays an important protective role in preserving and protecting tooth and bone structures. An excess of fluoride anions is toxic. Sulfate is a special case; the anion does not appear to have a function and is excreted; however, sulfur is necessary to provide sulfhydryl groups in some amino acids and specific molecules and is important for wool and tissue growth. Carbonate is an important buffer and is also a metabolic end-product.

Skeletal Metabolism

The skeleton comprises bone and cartilage arranged in architectural units connected by joints to permit the appropriate movements of animals to occur. Thus, the skeleton is the supporting structure of the animal body that provides its framework and a system of levers for posture and movement as well as the armor for protection of delicate organs. The locomotor system is designed so that the skeletal muscles can apply their forces in effective and coordinated ways for movement.

During embryonic development, cartilage and bone start to appear. Migratory cells, called *osteoblasts,* synthesize and array collagen fibers and proteoglycans into a matrix of osteoid tissue. These cells tend to form a single-cell layer over the surface of sites for new bone formation. The resulting fibrous matrix subsequently calcifies. Other cells derived from osteoblasts, called *osteocytes,* infiltrate the forming bone and become entrapped in it in islands called lacunae. These cells have filamentous projections and seem to keep open channels of communication within the bone, perhaps allowing for mineral exchanges. *Osteoclasts,* a third type of cell, are large multinucleated cells that can cause bone resorption to occur, with mobilization of the calcium and phosphate for return to the plasma.

The bone minerals exist in the form of crystallites that resemble those of the mineral substance fluoroapatite, the bone form being hydroxyapatite. Bone is not a pure substance but contains small amounts of other minerals such as carbonate, sulfate, silicates, and magnesium. Over two thirds of the body's magnesium occurs in the bones, and some other metals accumulate in bone. Large crystals of calcium phosphate also occur on surfaces such as those of dentine in the teeth. The calcium cations in bone tissue are at equilibrium with phosphate and hydrogen phosphate anions. The product of the concentration of calcium multiplied by that of the phosphate gives a value that determines the tendency for mineral precipitation to occur or for solubilization to begin. This outcome is subject to modification by proteins, by other minerals, and also by specific effects of some hormones.

As the anion fluoride, fluorine can become part of the apatite crystalline structure in the place of hydroxyl anion in teeth and bones. In susceptible species, fluoride protects teeth to a certain extent against dental caries. In mature animals, it may protect the bones against osteoporosis and osteomalacia. Excessive intake of fluoride-containing minerals can cause fluorosis, with tooth discoloration and tooth and bone deformities, resulting in anorexia and lameness. Manganese deficiency also can lead to skeletal deformities.

Collagen

It is surprising to learn that the most prevalent protein in the animal body is collagen. This fibrous protein is the structural material for the extracellular framework of the body—in bone, cartilage, fascia, skin, and specialized tissues such as the glomerular filters. The alpha-chains are combined into a triple helix rod-like structure having high proportions of glycine, proline, and hydroxyproline. In addition to the calcified bone minerals and the collagen, bone contains ground substance and water. The ground substance consists of mucopolysaccharides, low-molecular-weight molecules, and ions.

Nutritional secondary hyperparathyroidism is a syndrome that affects animals fed a diet low in calcium but high in phosphate or in calcium-binding agents such as oxalate. Horses are particularly susceptible because of some dietary practices. The resulting syndrome was called "miller's or bran disease," or big head, because wheat bran has an unfavorable ratio of calcium to potassium (about 1:11). Affected animals exhibit maxillary and mandibular swelling accompanied by loosening of the teeth and dysphagia.

The imbalanced or deficient diet, often grain and bran with no legumes or legume hay (which have high Ca:P ratios), leads to serum calcium levels in the lower end of the normal range. The parathyroid glands hypertrophy and secrete excess parathormone (PTH). This causes increased reabsorption of calcium ions in the renal tubules, greater phosphate excretion, and activation of calcitriol formation in the kidneys. The 1,25-dihydroxy-D$_3$ favors increased intestinal absorption of calcium and calcium reabsorption from bone, the latter aided by PTH and other factors. The end result is weak bones, and a tendency to fractures, torn ligaments, and swollen joints.

Magnesium Depletion

Hypomagnesemic tetany of calves in the first months of life, and lactation tetany of cows are important clinical syndromes. The former is attributable to low efficiency of absorption of magnesium ions, which leads to a progressive decline in levels of magnesium ions in bone, plasma, and cerebrospinal fluid (CSF). Tetany may occur if the magnesium titer drops below 0.33 mmol per liter; a drop in magnesium is often accompanied by hypocalcemia. Affected calves exhibit neurological disorders progressing from hyperesthesia, with an apprehensive manner accompanied by repetitive ear movements, to exaggerated reflex responses, ataxia, abnormal head movements, and muscle tremors. Clenching of the teeth, with foaming at the mouth, and spasticity may follow. Ultimately, an epileptic fit–like crisis may feature head retraction, jaw champing, falling with respiratory arrest, and convulsions.

Lactation tetany occurs in milking cows and ewes, particularly those grazing on lush spring pastures. Magnesium intake is then low, and very little magnesium is absorbed owing to the laxative effect of the grass. Increased rumen ammonia levels and the high potassium levels may contribute to the syndrome by their negative impact on magnesium absorption.

A syndrome similar to lactation tetany has been observed in cattle and sheep that are underfed when on poor winter pastures in harsh, cold environments. So-called wheat pasture poisoning occurs when cattle are grazed on young cereal crops. This may involve the consequences of fertilizer use and the composition of the green plant material. High levels of potassium and nitrogenous salts may be present in these herbages, and very little sodium.

During prolonged droving or shipment, transit tetany, a tetanic syndrome, is seen in late pregnant ruminants and in lactating mares. The syndrome is accompanied by hypomagnesemia and hypocalcemia. Affected late pregnant ewes may have hypoglycemia.

The signs of hypomagnesemic disease are related to increased sensitivity of excitable tissues, nerves, and neuromuscular junctions associated with low magnesium concentrations in the extracellular fluid (ECF). The level of magnesium ions in the CSF is reduced, which may reflect changes in the composition of brain ECF underlying the signs of CNS disturbance. Low magnesium inhibits the process of collagen resorption, making bone resorption less responsive to mineral depletion. Cold exposure and undernutrition activate adrenergic responses, increasing lipolysis and reducing magnesium ion concentrations in extracellular fluids. Marked hyperglycemia, not accompanied by a rise in insulin, is observed in hypomagnesemic cows. Clearly, hypomagnesemic tetany is a complex metabolic disturbance that is susceptible to environmental and nutritional decisions.

Iron and Copper in Metabolism

Iron is an essential element that makes possible many of the functions of the animal organism by its roles in oxygen-transport and oxidation-reduction reactions. Over two thirds of the iron in the body is in the form of hemoglobin in erythrocytes that ferry oxygen from the pulmonary capillaries to tissues throughout the body. Muscle also contains additional iron in the oxygen-storage compound myoglobin. Iron is also bound to its storage protein apoferritin, to form ferritin.

Absorbed iron enters from the intestinal lumen as ionic ferrous iron (Fe^{++}) or in a heme or porphyrin complex. Ascorbic acid promotes iron absorption within the mucosal cells. After transient binding to a small carrier protein, iron crosses the serosal surface and enters the plasma, where it binds to the transport protein transferrin as ferric iron (Fe^{+++}). Transferrin is a glycoprotein that migrates in the beta-globulin fraction. Changes in the percentage saturation of transferrin with ferric iron affect the rate of absorption of iron from the intestine. Normally, about one third of the iron-binding sites are occupied, but many fewer may be occupied in iron-deficiency anemia, or many more with excessive intake with hemochromatosis. Surplus iron may bind to apoferritin and remain in the intestinal mucosa, to be sloughed off later when the cells age in a few days.

Via two types of complex iron-storage proteins called apoferritins, the main storage sites for iron in the body are the liver and spleen. Apoferritins exist as complexes of 24 subunits, one (H) being specific for heart and the other (L) for liver and spleen. One of these complexes binds about 20 percent of its weight as iron in the form of a ferric hydroxide–ferric phosphate complex surrounded by protein subunits. Part of the *ferritin* store is more labile than the rest and can be mobilized more readily. Another storage form of iron in cells is in agglomerated iron oxide particles called *hemosiderin* that appear after iron overload.

Body iron exists in a dynamic equilibrium. The macrophage (reticuloendothelial) system scavenges aging erythrocytes, releasing their iron so it can be recaptured by transferrin for transfer to the bone marrow. In the marrow, this iron is taken up in the reticulocytes for erythropoiesis. The ferritin stores act as a buffer to protect the body from surplus iron or to release it in times of need. Only relatively small amounts enter the system daily from the gut. Copper-containing proteins, called ferroxidases, are involved in the redox reactions that oxidize ferrous iron to ferric iron for incorporation into transferrin and ferritin. Reduction of ferric iron to ferrous iron for hemoglobin production requires a flavoprotein and NADH. Ceruloplasmin is a plasma protein that deposits copper in the liver; if it is deficient owing to a low level of dietary copper, transferrin cannot take up absorbed iron, and anemia may result.

Iron-deficiency anemia is an important syndrome in many animal species. It can result from dietary deficiency of absorbable iron or from chronic blood loss through parasitism or hemorrhage. Young, fast-growing animals are particularly vulnerable, as they have a high demand for iron-containing compounds and lack reserves. A major contributing factor is the low level of iron in milk. Piglets housed in buildings that allow no access to earth require supplemental iron if anemia is to be avoided, but iron toxicity can result, especially if vitamin E deficiency is present. The common denominator of iron deficiency leads to inadequate heme production for hemoglobin formation in erythrocytes. Iron-deficient piglets show impairment of gastric acid secretion with atrophic gastritis, accompanied by villous atrophy in the mucosa of the small intestine, together with changes in gut pH and microflora. There is an increased incidence of diarrhea and malabsorption. Safer formulations (than iron-dextran) for iron administration have been developed.

Other iron-containing proteins and enzymes play essential roles in metabolism, such as the iron-sulfur proteins, the cytochromes, and catalase. Although their iron content is only a very small fraction of body iron, their significance to the body's function is enormous. Cytochrome oxidase and several other metallooxidases are copper-containing enzymes.

Copper deficiency in young ruminants leads to poor growth, diarrhea, lameness, and anemia. Ewes grazing copper-deficient pastures may deliver lambs that become afflicted with swayback or neonatal ataxia. This disease, resembling multiple sclerosis in humans, is characterized by cerebral demyelinization, degeneration of motor nerves in the cord, and necrosis of large neurons in brain stem and spinal cord. Ruminants grazing copper-deficient pastures occasionally have spontaneous fractures of long bones. Excess copper becomes very toxic after a certain threshold level is exceeded.

Molybdenum occurs in some metalloenzyme systems involving redox reactions; however, its functional significance is best known in its interaction with sulfur to influence copper retention. Unusually low levels of molybdenum ions and sulfur in the diet render animals much more susceptible to copper toxicity. High levels of molybdenum and sulfur may provoke signs of copper deficiency at dietary copper ion levels that would otherwise be considered adequate. Thiomolybdates may be mediators of the induced deficiency by sequestering copper in a copper-thiomolybdate complex.

Zinc ions have some energy roles in brain transmitter function, endocrine activity, energy metabolism, respiration, gastric secretion, and RNA function. Zinc deficiency or unavailability contributes to parakeratosis, alopecia, hoof deformities, and lameness. The basic signs are failure of keratinization, arrest of wool and hair growth, coronary band dysfunction, and skeletal abnormalities.

The fetus obtains all its copper, manganese, and sulfur from the dam. Acute maternal hypocuprosis leads to brain lesions in developing lambs. Similarly, manganese deficiency results in abnormal fetal epiphyseal cartilage and deformed lambs. Both organic and inorganic sulfur pass to the fetus, where it is incorporated into chondroitin sulfate of cartilage.

REFERENCES

Austad R, Bjerkas E. Eclampsia in the dog. J Small Anim Pract 1976;17:795.

Baird GD. Primary kesosis in the high producing dairy cow: Clinical and subclinical disorders, treatment, prevention, and outlook. J Dairy Sci 1982;65:1.

Booth A, Reid M, Clark T. Hypovitaminosis A in feedlot cattle. J Am Vet Assoc 1987;190:1305.

Boxer LA. Regulation of phagocyte function by alpha-tocopherol. Proc Nutr Soc 1986;45:333.

Braham JE, Villareal A, Bressani R. Effect of lime treatment of corn on the availability of niacin for cats. J Nutr 1962;76:183.

Brewer NR. Comparative metabolism of copper. J Am Vet Med Assoc 1987;190:654.

Carpenter KJ. Effects of different methods of processing maize on its pellagragenic activity. Fed Proc 1981;40:1531.

Carrigan MJ, Glastonbury JRW, Evers JV. Hypovitaminosis A in pigs. Aust Vet J 1988;65:158.

Chittenden RH, Underhill FP. The production in dogs of a pathological condition which closely resembles human pellagra. Am J Physiol 1917;44:13.

Dunlop RH, Bueno L. Molasses neurotoxicity and higher volatile fatty acids in sheep. Ann Rech Vét 1979;10:462.

Edwin EE, Jackman R. Ruminant thiamin requirement in perspective. Vet Res Comm 1982;5:237.

Edwin EE, Jackman R. Thiaminase I in the development of cerebrocortical necrosis in sheep and cattle. Nature 1970;228:772.

Evans HM, Emerson OH, Emerson GA. The isolation from wheat germ oil of an alcohol, alpha-tocopherol, having the properties of vitamin E. J Biol Chem 1936;113:319.

Gooneratne SR, Olkowski AA, Klemmer RG, Kessler GA, Christensen DA. High sulfur—related thiamin deficiency in cattle: A field study. Can Vet J 1989;30:139.

Halliwell B. Free radicals and metal ions in health and disease. Proc Nutr Soc 1987;46:13.

Haussler MR, Mangelsdorf DJ, Komm BS, Terpening CM, Yamaoka K, Allegretto EA, Baker AR, Shine J, O'Malley BW, Pike JW. Molecular biology of the vitamin D hormone. Recent Progr Hormone Res 1988;44:263.

Herbert V. Nutrition science as a continually unfolding story: The folate and vitamin B-12 paradigm. Am J Clin Nutr 1987;46:387.

Hidiroglou M, Knipfel JE. Maternal-fetal relationships of copper, manganese and sulfur in ruminants. J Dairy Sci 1981;64:1637.

Holler H, Breves G, Lebzien P, Rohr K. Effect of monensin on net synthesis of thiamin and microbial protein in the rumen of cows. Proc Nutr Soc 1985;44:146A.

Hopkins FG. Feeding experiments illustrating the importance of accessory factors in the normal dietaries. J Physiol (Lond) 1912;44:425.

Horst RL. Regulation of calcium and phosphorus homeostasis in the dairy cow. J Dairy Sci 1986;69:604.

Kempson SA, Currie RJW, Johnston AM. Influence of biotin supplementation on pig claw horn: A scanning electron microscopic study. Vet Rec 1989;124:37.

Krehl WA. Discovery of the effect of tryptophan on niacin deficiency. Fed Proc 1981;40:1527.

Larkin HA, Hannan J. Gastrointestinal flora of iron-deficient piglets. Res Vet Sci 1985;39:5.

Lean IJ, Troutt HF, Boermans H, Moller G, Webster G, Tracy M. An investigation of bulk tank milk selenium levels in the San Joaquin Valley of California. Cornell Vet 1990;80:41.

Levine M, Morita K. Ascorbic acid in endocrine systems. Vitamins Hormones 1985;42:1.

Loew FM, Martin CL, Dunlop RH, Mapletoft RJ, Smith SI. Naturally occurring and experimental thiamin deficiency in cats receiving commercial cat food. Can Vet J 1970;11:106.

Luecke RW. Domestic animals in the elucidation of zinc's role in nutrition. Fed Proc 1984;43:2823.

Machlin LJ, Bendich A. Free radical tissue damage: Protective role of antioxidant nutrients. FASEB J 1987;1:441.

Mason J. Thiomolybdates: Mediators of molybdenum toxicity and enzyme inhibitors. Toxicology 1986;42:99.

Moate PJ, Schneider KM, Leaver DD, Morris DC. Effect of 1,25-dihydroxyvitamin-D_3 on the calcium and magnesium metabolism of lactating cows. Austral Vet J 1987;64:73.

Peters JP, Bergman EN, Elliot JM. Influence of vitamin B_{12} status on hepatic propionic acid uptake in sheep. J Nutr 1983;113:1221.

Ramberg CF, Johnson EK, Fargo RD, Kronfeld DS. Calcium homeostasis in cows with special reference to parturient hypocalcemia. Am J Physiol 1984;246:R698.

Rammell CG, Hill JH, Forbes S. Blood thiamin levels in normal cattle and sheep at pasture. NZ Vet J 1988;36:49.

Read DH, Harrington DD. Experimentally induced thiamin deficiency in beagle dogs: Pathologic changes of the central nervous system. Am J Vet Res 1986;47:2281.

Rice DA, Kennedy S. Assessment of vitamin E, selenium and polyunsaturated fatty acid interactions in the etiology of disease in the bovine. Proc Nutr Soc 1988;47:177.

Roberts MC. Serum and red cell folate and serum vitamin B_{12} levels in horses. Aust Vet J 1983;60:106.

Seawright AA, Hrdlicka J. Pathogenetic factors in tooth loss in young cats on a high daily oral intake of vitamin A. Aust Vet J 1974;50:133.

Sharma GL, Johnston RL, Luecke RW, Hoeffer JA, Gray ML, Thorp F. A study of the pathology of the intestine and other organs of weanling pigs when fed a ration of natural feedstuffs low in pantothenic acid. Am J Vet Res 1952;13:298.

Simming PH, Brooks PH: Supplementary biotin for sows: Effect on reproductive characteristics. Vet Rec 1983;112:425.

Slater TF, Cheeseman KH, Davies MJ, Proudfoot K, Xin W. Free radical mechanisms in relation to tissue injury. Proc Nutr Soc 1987;46:1.

Spencer TN. Is black tongue in dogs pellagra? Am J Vet Med 1916;11:325.

Suttie JW. The metabolic role of vitamin K. Fed Proc 1980;39:2730.

Suttle NF. Copper deficiency in ruminants, recent developments. Vet Rec 1986;119:519.

Thomas KW. Oral treatment of polioencephalomalacia and subclinical thiamin deficiency with thiamin propyldisulfide and thiamin hydrochloride. J Vet Pharmacol Ther 1986;9:402.

Thomas KW, Griffiths FR. Natural establishment of thiaminase activity in the alimentary tract of newborn lambs and effects on thiamin status and growth rates. Aust Vet J 1987;64:207.

Thornber EJ, Dunlop RH, Gawthorne JM, Huxtable CR. Induced thiamin deficiency in lambs. Aust Vet J 1981;57:21.

Willson RL. Vitamin E, selenium, zinc and copper interactions in free radical protection against ill-placed iron. Proc Nutr Soc 1987;46:27.

CHAPTER 43

THE LIVER AS A METABOLIC ORGAN

The liver, the hub of the body's metabolic activities, is an indispensable component of the body's homeostatic system. In the embryo, the liver plays an important role in the synthesis of blood cells. After birth, its primary role as the body's central metabolic unit develops along with its specialized functions of bile acid formation and excretion of the by-products of metabolism. Because it produces somatomedins or insulin-like growth factors associated with the hypothalamus-hypophysis axis, the liver is also an endocrine organ involved in regulating growth.

The core of liver activity is metabolic processing of the incoming nutrients and compensating for the impacts of the competing demands by the various tissues of the body for maintenance, growth, milk production, and reproduction. The liver acts as an emunctory or excretory organ, like the kidneys, for xenobiotics (dyes, drugs, and toxins), for the by-products of heme metabolism, and for certain other metabolites via the bile. This concurrent excretion includes the formation of important components for protecting the body (by oxidation and conjugation) from hazardous substances that may have been absorbed; however, a few agents may be made more toxic.

Several of its numerous metabolic functions have already been referred to, but some deserve special focus. They include (1) the formation of bile salts and their enterohepatic recycling, both necessary for digestion of lipids; (2) the excretion of pigments (biliverdin and bilirubin) issued from the hemoglobin of erythrocytes that have lived out their life span; (3) the filtration and limited storage of blood draining the intestine through a venous portal system before it flows from the liver into the systemic circulation (Fig. 43–1); (4) some metabolic transformations of nutrients (e.g., vitamin D_3, carbohydrate, lipid, protein) induced by resident enzymes; and (5) synthesis of plasma proteins to help repair wear and tear in tissues, and of clotting factors to correct any effraction or breakage in the wall of blood vessels.

Selective storage functions, which can be drawn from an examination of the hepatocyte structure (Fig. 43–2), are that of iron as ferritin, especially at the level of the macrophages (Kupffer's cells) and that of vitamins (liposoluble A and D; water-soluble B_{12}).

BLOOD IRRIGATION AND ARCHITECTURE OF THE LIVER

Most of the blood irrigating the liver is under low pressure (<10 mm Hg) because it has already passed through one set of capillaries in the other abdominal organs. The venous portal blood flow, which varies among species but represents about 15 percent of the cardiac output, is increased after ingestion of food. The portal blood travels in a vessel with capillaries at both ends and serves as the main supply for incoming nutrients from the digestive tract. The remaining blood comes from the hepatic artery, which supplies oxygenated blood under high (arterial) pressure. The higher pressure arterial supply serves to filter large molecules from blood into the hepatic lymphatic fluid. The vascular outflow from the liver is the hepatic vein, which has very low hydrostatic pressure (about 0 mm Hg), close to that of the central venous pressure in the vena cava.

The architecture of the liver is in the form of a very large number of microscopic lobules, tiny cylinders of tissue up to a few millimeters long and about 2 mm in diameter. The features include a central vein that drains each lobule emptying into the outgoing venous system that supplies the hepatic vein. Around the periphery of the lobule are "triads" of the three tubular systems, that is, incoming vascular branches from the portal vein and the hepatic artery, and outgoing branches or canaliculi that convey bile to the terminal duct that ends in the wall of the duodenum. Blood and bile travel in opposite directions. In addition, a less readily visible network of outgoing lymphatic vessels carries lymph from the lobule, where it is formed, into the central lymphatic return channels.

Adjacent liver lobules are separated by septa containing small *portal venules* that receive their blood from the portal veins draining the intestine. Upon leaving these portal venules, blood flows, as a flat film, between the hepatic plates into branching *hepatic sinusoids* and from these into the *central vein*. *Hepatic arterioles* also present in the septa supply arterial blood to the septal tissues and may empty directly into the hepatic sinusoids mixing arterial with venous blood to raise the hydrostatic pressure within the sinusoids.

Between these clusters of vessels and the central vein lie hepatic plates made up of sheets of hepatic cells and sinusoids that receive both portal venous and hepatic arterial blood. A sheet of endothelium-like cells composed of protective tissue macrophage cells (Kupffer cells [reticuloendothelial cells]) separates the blood in the sinusoids from the lymph bathing the hepatic cells. These endothelial formations of littoral macrophage cells line a microscopic extracellular space (space of Disse) between them and the sheet of hepatic cells, where lymph collects and passes to the peripheral lymphatics via fine terminal lymphatics. Within the sheets of hepatic cells are other tiny spaces, bile canaliculi, where the bile forms and passes back to the periphery of the lobule via small vessels that merge to form the bile duct system.

The lining of the venous sinusoids shows wide pores (1 μm) between and within the walls of the endothelial cells. Because of these large pores in the walls of the sinusoids and of the higher intrasinusoid pressure due to the arterial blood supply, the large molecules in the plasma can easily filter

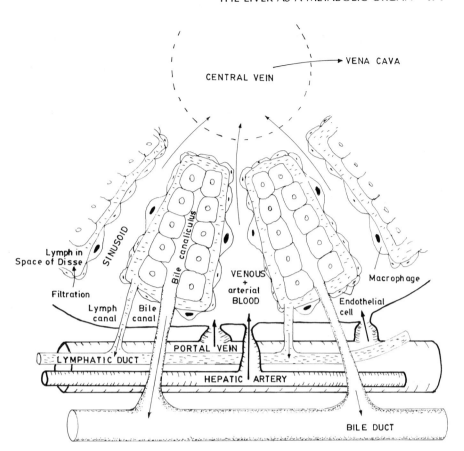

Figure 43–1 Basic structure of a liver lobule showing two hepatic cellular plates, each bathed by lymph in the space of Disse, which drains into lymphatic vessels. A bile canaliculus between the hepatocytes of each plate transports bile in the same direction as lymph, but in the direction opposite to blood (in the hepatic artery and the portal vein), which is directed into the sinusoids. Pores between the endothelial cells and macrophages facilitate the formation of lymph in the space of Disse.

into the space of Disse and move in close proximity to the plasma membrane of the hepatocytes. It is very important to note that the very porous lining of the sinusoids even allows plasma proteins to pass into the lymph in the space of Disse and to join the proteins newly formed by the hepatic cells. Thus, the lymph leaving the liver tends to have an unusually high protein content.

EXCRETION OF SUBSTANCES IN BILE

Bile Pigments, Biliverdin and Bilirubin

An understanding of the formation and excretion of bilirubin is useful for the diagnosis of blood and liver diseases. When erythrocytes become old (3 to 4 months), they break up and are phagocytosed by macrophages throughout the body. The hemoglobin is split into heme and globin, then the heme structure is opened to release iron that is picked up by transferrin for transport in the blood. The residue, a straight chain comprising four pyrrole nuclei, is the substrate for bile pigment formation.

The initially formed biliverdin is soon reduced to bilirubin, which is slowly released to the plasma to be conveyed in the blood by plasma albumin. Normal plasma bilirubin levels are below 0.5 mg/dL, except in horses (1 to 2 mg per deciliter) and pigs (1 mg/dL). The plasma membrane of the hepatocyte takes up the bilirubin by trapping it onto two proteins that have high affinity for it. Most is conjugated with glucuronic acid to form bilirubin glucuronides (80% of conjugates); 10% of conjugates are with sulfate, and the remaining 10% combines with other substances such as glucose and xylose. These conjugated forms pass to the bile canaliculi and to the biliary tree for excretion into the duodenum. Owing to reduced hepatic uptake of the pigment, horses show little conjugation and manifest hyperbilirubinemia after anorexia. In other species, most of the bilirubin is conjugated (e.g., about 75% in dogs).

The greenish-yellow pigment *bilirubin*, an end-product of hemoglobin catabolism, gives bile its characteristic color in most animal species. The pigment initially produced after the breakdown of hemoglobin, *biliverdin*, is an almost pure green substance coloring the bile of most birds, and bilirubin is the reduced form of biliverdin. Since bilirubin is highly soluble in all cell membranes and is also quite toxic, its excretion is one of the important blood detoxification functions of the liver. Accumulation of bilirubin in the body leads to the yellowish discoloration of the tissues known as jaundice or icterus. This can occur as a result of an increased rate of hemolysis or by reduced hepatic uptake and conjugation.

Bacteria in the intestine convert a large part (50%) of the bilirubin to soluble urobilinogen, some of which is

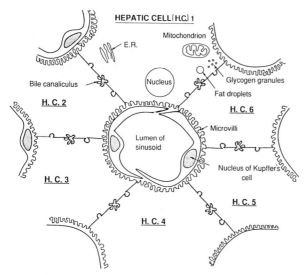

Figure 43–2 Cross-section of a single layer of a liver lobule showing the arrangement of hepatic cells around sinusoids whose walls are made up of littoral Kupffer's cells and contain pores but no collagen. Bile canaliculi are shown. The sinusoids receive blood from both the portal venous system and the hepatic artery, discharging into the hepatic vein. The three-dimensional architecture requires envisioning the system of tubes and layers of cells that extend above and below the plane of the page. (E.R., Endoplasmic reticulum.)

absorbed and mostly reexcreted by the liver, except for a small percentage (about 5%) that is excreted in the urine.

Hormones and Xenobiotic Substances

Several of the hormones secreted by the endocrine glands are either chemically altered or excreted by the liver. Thyroxine and essentially all the steroid hormones (e.g., estradiol, cortisol, and aldosterone) are processed mostly in the liver. In the cat, the excretion of steroid is exclusively biliary, and none of the metabolites of adrenal and sex steroids appear in the urine.

Many drugs are excreted into the bile, including antibiotics (ampicillin, chloramphenicol, erythromycin, penicillin, tetracyclines and sulfonamides). An index of the total hepatic blood flow and of the ability of hepatocytes to remove xenobiotic substances from blood is provided by the administration of a known quantity of a dye, bromsulfonphthalein (BSP), which is selectively excreted in bile. The concentration of the dye is plotted against time to give its rate of disappearance from plasma. Indocyanine green, a dye not conjugated in the liver, may be used as an alternative to BSP.

BSP binds to plasma albumin, and the complex is taken up by hepatic cells, which release the dye and conjugate it with glutathione for passage into the bile canaliculi. In cats, which excrete BSP very rapidly, a prolonged BSP half-life indicates some dysfunction of the hepatic cell mass that may be reversible.

A substance excreted in bile reaches the small intestine and may be reabsorbed, usually in the ileum, and returned to the portal circulation. A fraction of the reabsorbed substance presented to the liver cells is reexcreted in the bile, and the remains reappear in the systemic circulation. Such a cycle, known as the enterohepatic circulation of a substance, occurs with bile salts, endogenous steroids, and several drugs. The enterohepatic circulation of an endogenous substance (e.g., bile salts) or of a drug (e.g., tetracyclines) may delay its elimination and may extend the duration of its effective blood level. During the digestive process of a meal, through successive enterohepatic cycles, the bile salts of an animal are recirculated several times. The absorbed bile salts are conjugated with taurine or glycine prior to reexcretion. New methods for determination of bile salts in plasma have made their assay a useful indicator of hepatic dysfunction.

Many foreign chemicals and drugs (*xenobiotics*) are transported bound to plasma proteins, some in lipoprotein complexes. Such protein-bound compounds, also insoluble in water, escape filtration by the renal glomeruli. The hepatocytes contain a microsomal enzyme system that utilizes cytochrome P450 to introduce oxygen (*hydroxylation*) into xenobiotics. A wide range of reactions can then occur involving *reduction, oxidation, hydrolysis,* and *removal* or *addition (conjugation)* of chemical groups. A common hepatic detoxification mechanism is hydroxylation followed by conjugation with groups (e.g., glucuronide, sulfate, glycine or benzoate), which render the xenobiotics water soluble.

It is likely that this hepatic system evolved as an adaptation to detoxify plant alkaloids and other toxic natural substances. Today it serves to cope with a wide variety of man-made chemicals, which have also an inducing effect on these mixed function oxidases, that typically increase the rate of detoxification metabolism of some classes of foreign chemicals. Occasionally, instead of accomplishing its usual role of detoxification, the system transforms a foreign substance into a more toxic agent.

METABOLIC FUNCTIONS OF THE LIVER

The liver is involved in the metabolism of the primary nutrients: carbohydrates (glycogen), lipids (triglycerides), and proteins (amino acids). Transamination between amino acids and keto acids (carbon radicals) of various origins (carbohydrate or lipid), saturation and desaturation of fatty acids, as well as synthesis of proteins (albumins, alpha-globulins) and of urea are some of the major metabolic processes taking place in the liver. As a target organ stimulated by growth hormone from the hypophysis, the liver responds by secreting somatomedins, peptidic hormones necessary for growth.

Metabolism of Carbohydrate

In carbohydrate metabolism, the primary goal of the liver appears to be to serve as a *glucostat* system, ensuring adequate availability of glucose for the tissues. The liver has the necessary enzymes to contribute to the supply of glucose by (1) converting into glucose any hexose such as fructose and galactose (*glucogenesis*) absorbed from the small intestine, (2) transforming into glucose (*gluconeogenesis*) several metabolites (e.g., propionate, lactate, glucogenic amino acids), (3) producing glucose from its substantial store of glycogen (*glycogenolysis*) to provide a short-term supply of glucose, and (4) storing any surplus of glucose as glycogen (*glycogenesis*), a readily available source of glucose.

> The Cori cycle involves breakdown of muscle glycogen to L-lactic acid, which is conveyed to the liver to be reconstituted into glucose and then glycogen.

In ruminants, special metabolic pathways are required, because dietary hexoses are utilized by the flora and fauna in the ruminoreticulum and fewer hexoses are available and absorbed from the intestine. In adult ruminants, where hypoglycemia (relative to monogastric species, and to preruminant lambs and calves) is a normal state, considerable liver gluconeogenesis occurs from a three-carbon short-chain fatty acid (SCFA), propionate. A great quantity of glucose is made from propionate via the methylmalonyl coenzyme A pathway. Also, many glucose-sparing strategies have evolved in the tissues of ruminants where lipogenesis develops from acetate, beta-hydroxybutyrate, and lactate instead of from glucose. The bridging of energy metabolism between carbohydrate and lipid sources is a critical component of ruminant metabolism. Ensuring an adequate supply of glucose for the ruminant brain is a high priority, and a constant challenge, but the relatively small size of the brain (only 110 g in a sheep, versus 1,400 g in humans) simplifies the task. Whether gluconeogenesis from propionate is normal or depressed can be detected by measuring blood glucose levels after intravenous propionate loading (2.5 mmol/kg).

Metabolism of Lipids

> The role of the liver secretion (bile) in the digestive and absorptive processes of lipids in the intestinal tract was shown by Claude Bernard (1859), who gave oil to rabbits.
>
> The lymphatics, outlined by their milkiness or lactescence, are apparent beyond the entrance of the pancreatic duct, caudad to the duct (20 cm from the pylorus). The lymphatics in the proximal duodenum, before the point where bile is delivered, are not visible and show no signs of lipid digestion and absorption.
>
> When the bile duct is transposed surgically 40 cm beyond the pylorus, the lymphatics become milky (a sign of lipid absorption) only beyond this level.

The liver is a primary site of lipid metabolism. Excessive accumulation of triglycerides in hepatocytes (lipidosis, fatty liver) is a well-known nonspecific change. Hepatic lipidosis is even induced by forced feeding in birds such as geese, to produce the gourmet's pâté de foie gras.

Very large amounts of lipid substances can be metabolized by the healthy liver. Some lipids specialized for the functions of individual tissues are synthesized in those body systems or organs. Thus, long-chain fatty acids are formed in adipose tissue cells, whereas SCFAs are made in the cells of the mammary gland. The liver is a major site of fatty acid synthesis in nonruminants, but this function is less significant in ruminant species. This is because there is less glucose available to spare for formation of the glycerophosphate and acetyl-CoA precursors in ruminants, and they must depend on lactate and absorbed acetate and butyrate.

The liver splits triglycerides into their components, fatty acids and glycerol. Then, by beta-oxidation, the fatty acid molecules are subdivided into two-carbon acetyl radicals to form the acetyl-CoAs, which combine as water-soluble acetoacetic acid, a distribution form to deliver substrate to the tissues.

An important bridge between lipid and protein metabolism is the liver's role in forming lipoproteins, which attach to and transport lipid substances around the body. In addition, amino acids can be deaminated to provide carbon skeletons for fatty acid synthesis, and glucogenic amino acids can provide the glycerol components for triglyceride synthesis.

Circulating nonesterified fatty acids (NEFAs) and glycerol are used by the ruminant liver to make very low density lipoproteins (VLDLs). This is very important in early lactation and late pregnancy to meet the higher needs of mammary gland or fetus for VLDLs. If the cow or ewe is deficient in glucose and other glycerol precursors, the ruminant liver esterifies circulating NEFAs and oxidizes them to form ketones. These processes contribute to the development of ketosis, an important disease of early lactation in high-producing cows and of late pregnancy in ewes carrying twin lambs.

The liver must also synthesize the polyunsaturated fatty acids (PUFAs) to meet the body's needs. Calves and lambs have low reserves of these at birth, yet PUFAs are required for adaptation to the environment. For instance, the lower melting points of these PUFAs help provide the antifreeze effect for extremities exposed continuously to cold winds and snow and for maintaining circulation in hibernating animals. The PUFAs are also important for further synthesis of essential compounds; for example, arachidonic acid is the starting point for synthesis of eicosanoid hormones (prostaglandins and leukotrienes).

Cholesterol is absorbed from the intestine and is also synthesized in the liver. Much of the cholesterol is used to make bile salts, which are conjugated with some amino acids (taurine, glycine). The remainder is transported on lipoproteins to tissues, where it serves as a substrate for steroid hormone synthesis and for structural applications.

Essential for production of cell membranes and some organelles, phospholipids are processed and synthesized in the liver. From there, they are transported on the lipoproteins to meet the body's needs.

The liver is also associated with another important group of lipid substances, the fat-soluble vitamins (A, D, E, and K). Large amounts of vitamin A are stored in the liver; in some species (e.g., polar bear) so much that the liver is rendered toxic to humans. The liver transforms the inactive vitamin D_3 into a more active substance, calcidiol, which reaches its full activity after modification to calcitriol in the kidney.

The liver facilitates the absorption of dietary vitamin E, which has an important antioxidant role in the body, and interacts with selenium to prevent muscular dystrophy in animals (white muscle disease). The common form of vitamin E, alpha-tocopherol, also protects against free radicals, which convert lipids to peroxides and to reactive intermediates that harm enzymes and receptor sites on the extracellular surface of the plasma membrane.

The liver plays an essential role in maintaining the coagulability of the blood. Provided by dietary or bacterial synthesis sources, absorbed vitamin K is required for the hepatic synthesis of prothrombin and other factors that participate in the cascade of blood coagulation. In several liver diseases, laboratory tests for coagulability show a reduction in clotting factors in plasma and impaired clotting.

Metabolism of Nitrogenous Compounds

A vital function of the liver is to control the anabolism and catabolism of the proteins. Synthesis of proteins, especially the plasma proteins, is a major hepatic function. Most of the plasma proteins, except the gamma-globulins (formed by cells of the lymphocyte series), are made in the liver.

The liver also balances the proportions of the various amino acids needed to meet the needs of the body. It uses transamination to synthesize all the so-called nonessential amino acids. A keto acid with the same chemical composition as that of the desired amino acid is first formed. Then, by transamination, an amino radical from an available amino acid is transferred to the keto acid to take the place of the keto oxygen. The necessary "mix" of essential and nonessential amino acids can then be made available for protein synthesis and for meeting specific amino acid requirements in the tissues. If liver function is impaired, the levels of branched amino acids (leucine, isoleucine, valine) decrease, whereas those of aromatic amino acids (phenylalanine, tyrosine) increase. Thus, the ratio of branched to aromatic amino acids is low in hepatic insufficiency and toxic hepatopathy.

Catabolism of nitrogenous compounds occurs in the gut and the tissues, with production of ammonia, which is toxic for nerve cells. In the tissues, glutamine synthetase catalyzes the fixation of ammonia on glutamic acid for the formation of glutamine, which is carried in blood to the kidney and the liver. In encephalopathy problems, blood ammonia concentration is helpful in detecting clinical portosystemic shunts.

In dogs, experimental surgery has been used to demonstrate the role of the liver in the metabolism of ammonia (Fig. 43–3). Eck's fistula, or end-to-side portacaval shunt, which allows portal blood to bypass the liver and drain directly into the vena cava, produces signs of portal systemic encephalopathy, because of an increase in peripheral blood ammonia. The ligation of the portal veins, which excludes the flow of venous blood into the liver and leaves only the flow of hepatic arterial blood, also raises peripheral blood ammonia to almost the same level. In both experimental situations, the increase in peripheral blood ammonia results in signs of portal encephalopathy (hepatic coma, hepatic encephalopathy).

> The characteristic signs of "portal systemic encephalopathy" include weakness, ataxia, weight loss, convulsions, and coma. Most animals succumb within a few months.

Mostly in the liver, but also in the kidney, enzymes add two ammonia molecules to amino acids (ornithine, then citrulline) to form arginine, which is eventually hydrolyzed into ornithine and urea (Fig. 43–4). This is Krebs's urea cycle. It protects the body from accumulation of toxic end-products of nitrogen metabolism. In the kidney, glutaminase separates ammonia from glutamine for its excretion as ammonium ions in the urine.

In most animals, urea is excreted in the urine. In ruminants, some urea is recirculated into the ruminoreticulum via saliva and the ruminoreticulum wall, where it serves, with other nonprotein nitrogen compounds (e.g., amino acids, ammonium salts, and nitrates), for bacterial protein synthesis; the remainder is excreted via the kidney.

In cattle, an inborn error of amino acid metabolism affecting the urea cycle, citrullinemia, is attributed to a lack of argininosuccinate synthetase. Acute neonatal citrullinemia, which appears 1 to 5 days after birth and is followed by death within 12 hours, is accompanied by signs of cerebral edema and hepatic lipidosis.

> Plasma levels of the amino acid citrulline may reach 2,200 to 13,000 $\mu M/L$ (i.e., 40 to 200 times normal levels, respectively). Signs include depression, blindness, aimless walking, head pressing, opisthotonus, hyperthermia, hyperpnea, tremors, convulsions, recumbency, and coma. This finding may serve as an awakening or an early warning to the risks of inbreeding for high milk production, using semen from a few high-performance bulls.

In animals, the end-products of purine metabolism include uric acid, which is converted to allantoin by uricase. Lacking uricase in their kidneys, Dalmatian dogs eliminate high concentrations of uric acid as the end-product of purines and are prone to urate calculus formation. Chickens also excrete uric acid.

PLASMA ENZYMES AS INDICATORS OF HEPATOCELLULAR DAMAGE

In diseases that cause damage to organs containing cytosolic enzymes, the levels of these enzymes increase in the plasma. Tests for these plasma enzymes are less rewarding as diagnostic tools than was first hoped; nevertheless, some valuable knowledge can be obtained using assays of plasma enzymes. Organ specificity and species differences are very important aspects, and the findings in human dysfunctions cannot be transferred to domestic animals without testing in the species being studied.

In ruminants and horses, though its instability in samples causes variations in assays, plasma *sorbitol dehydrogenase*

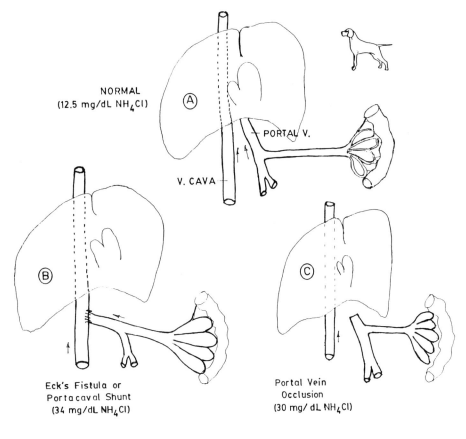

Figure 43–3 To study the effects of experimental surgical modifications of the liver blood supply on the hepatic removal of ammonium from the blood, ammonium chloride (0.25 mEq per kg hour) is infused into the femoral vein. After the infusion (40 minutes), the blood levels of ammonium (μ per dL) are higher (and almost similar) in the animals with Eck's fistula (**B**), and with portal occlusion (**C**), than in the normal animals (**A**). Both surgical animal preparations interfere with the elimination of ammonium by preventing portal blood from reaching the hepatocytes. The portal blood is transferred directly into the vena cava in the portacaval shunt preparation, whereas it remains in the portal veins and dilates these vessels in the portal obstruction preparation.

The histogram demonstrates that, during continuous infusion of BSP (0.05 mg per kg per minute) in the same experimental groups, the blood flow (mL per kg per minute) into the vena cava and the theoretical outflow from the liver (total hepatic blood flow) are similar in the normal dogs (**A**) and in those with end-to-side portacaval shunts (Eck's fistula) (**B**). However, both these parameters are markedly reduced in the dogs with occluded portal circulation (**C**). The portacaval shunt returns portal blood to the systemic circulation, but the portal occlusion prevents the access of portal blood to the general circulation.

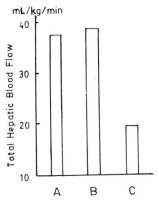

(SDH) is considered to be a relatively specific indicator of hepatic cell damage. In small animals (carnivores, primates, rodents), measurement of plasma *alanine aminotransferase* (ALT) is a valuable test of hepatocellular dysfunction. ALT was formerly known as glutamic-pyruvic transaminase (GPT). In dogs, horses, ruminants, and rats, plasma *glutamate dehydrogenase* (GDLDH, or GD) titer, a mitochondrial enzyme, is a successful indicator of hepatic necrosis.

Many other plasma enzymes have been considered for diagnostic value but were rejected because of a lack in specificity or of difficulty in assay. In the liver, *alkaline phosphatase* (ALP) occurs mainly in cells lining the bile ducts and duct-

ules, but it is also present in other organs. Damage to these structures by obstructive or proliferative biliary disease results in a higher level of plasma ALP. In dogs, abnormally high levels of circulating corticosteroids are associated with marked elevations in plasma ALP. In horses and ruminants, plasma *gamma-glutamyl transpeptidase* (GGT) is used to detect chronic liver diseases and toxicities. GGT indicates hepatobiliary disease, even if it is more widely distributed within the liver than ALP.

With advances in physical imaging techniques, such as ultrasound, magnetic resonance imaging, and scintigraphy of isotope-labeled cholephilic agents, noninvasive assessment

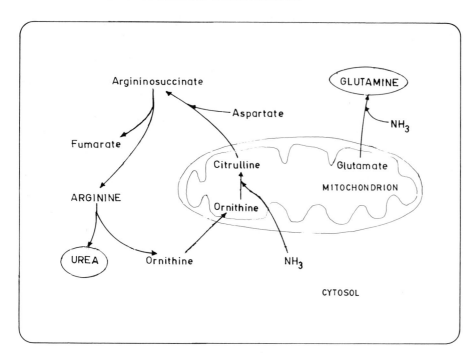

Figure 43–4 The so-called urea cycle in the hepatic cell. From the cytoplasm, ammonia crosses the mitochondrial membrane and unites with ornithine, then with citrulline. After migration into the cytosol of the hepatocyte, citrulline undergoes changes leading to formation of arginine. By hydrolysis, arginine is divided into urea and ornithine. Urea leaves the hepatocyte to be excreted from the renal blood into the urine, whereas ornithine reenters the mitochondrion for another urea cycle.

of hepatobiliary function is becoming a reality. The bottom-line, or ultimate test for determining the presence of liver pathologic conditions, still requires biopsy and histologic examination.

THE LIVER AS AN ENDOCRINE ORGAN

As the main relay for growth hormone activity, the liver of the adult animal produces polypeptides called somatomedins (SMs), or insulin-like growth factors (IGFs). Almost solely of liver origin, somatomedin C (SM-C; also called IGF-I) and IGF-II (also called MSA [multiplication-stimulating activity]) are single chains of 70 and 67 amino acids, respectively. They have some structural similarities with the A and B chains of proinsulin. Each is transported bound to plasma proteins, which considerably decrease their insulin effect to 1 to 2 percent, even if their plasma concentration is 1000 times higher than that of insulin. The hepatic production of IGF is stimulated by growth hormone (GH) and during pregnancy by prolactin. Somatomedins exert a negative feedback on the synthesis of adenohypophysial GH.

In vitro, IGFs stimulate the proliferation of chondrocytes and fibroblasts and exhibit only a mitogenic effect in the presence of other growth factors (e.g., platelet-derived growth factor [PDGF]). In vivo, IGFs can mimic the effects of insulin: they stimulate the entrance of glucose into the cytoplasm of cells and the synthesis of glycogen or lipid. IGFs increase the growth of tissues, the transport of amino acids, and the synthesis of proteins (collagen) in smooth, skeletal, and cardiac muscle cells and in chondrocytes and bone tissue. Steroidogenesis (of progesterone) by granulosa or luteal cells is also stimulated by the IGFs of the liver.

REFERENCES

Abdekkader SV, Hauge JG. Serum enzyme determinations in the study of liver disease in dogs. Acta Vet Scand 1986;27:59.

Abe H, Molitch ME, van Wyk JJ, Underwood LE. Human growth hormone and somatomedin C suppress the spontaneous release of GH in unanesthetized rats. Endocrinology 1983;113:1319.

Aldrete JG, McIlrath DC, Hallenbeck GA. Effects of portal ligation and of Eck's fistula on hepatic blood flow and concentration of blood ammonia. J Surg Res 1967;7:504.

Allison AC. Turnovers of erythrocytes and plasma proteins in mammals. Nature 1960;188:37.

Badylak SF, Dodds WJ, van Fleet JF. Plasma coagulation factor abnormalities in dogs with naturally occurring hepatic disease. Am J Vet Res 1983;44:2336.

Berelowitz M, Szabo M, Frohman LA, Firestone S, Chu L, Hintz RL. Somatomedin C mediates GH negative feedback by effects on both the hypothalamus and the pituitary. Science 1981;212:1279.

Billing B. Twenty-five years of progress in bilirubin metabolism (1952–1977). Gut 1978;19:481.

Boyer JL. New concepts of mechanisms of hepatocyte bile formation. Physiol Rev 1980;60:303.

Center SA, Baldwin EH, Dillingham S, Erb HN, Tennant BC. Diagnostic value of serum gamma-glutamyl transferase and alkaline phosphatase in hepatobiliary disease in the cat. J Am Vet Med Assoc 1986;188:507.

Center SA, Baldwin EH, Erb HN, Tennant BC. Bile acid concentrations in the diagnosis of hepatobiliary disease in the dog. J Am Vet Med Assoc 1985;187:935.

Clampitt RB, Hart RJ. The tissue activities of some diagnostic enzymes in ten mammalian species. J Comp Pathol 1978;88:687.

Engelking LR, Anwer MS, Lowstedt J. Hepatobiliary transport of indocyanine green and bromsulfophthalein in fed and fasted horses. Am J Vet Res 1985;46:2278.

Ford EJH. The activity of sorbitol dehydrogenase in the serum of sheep and cattle after liver damage. J Comp Pathol 1967;77:405.

Ford EJH. Activity of gamma-glutamyl transpeptidase and other enzymes in the serum of sheep with liver or kidney damage. J Comp Pathol 1974;84:231.

Grohn Y. Propionate loading test for liver function in spontaneously ketotic dairy cows. Res Vet Sci 1985;39:24.

Harper PAW, Healy PJ, Dennis JA, O'Brien JJ, Rayward DH. Citrullinaemia as a cause of neurological disease in neonatal Friesian calves. Aust Vet J 1986;63:378.

Jungermann K, Katz N. Functional specialization of different hepatocyte populations. Physiol Rev 1989;69:708.

Kaneko JJ. Clinical biochemistry of domestic animals. 4th ed. New York: Academic Press, 1989.

Keller P. Enzyme activities in the dog: Tissue analyses, plasma values and intracellular distribution. Am J Vet Res 1981;42:575.

Kraus-Friedmann N. Hormonal regulation of hepatic gluconeogenesis. Physiol Rev 1984;64:170.

Mullen PA. The diagnosis of liver dysfunction in farm animals and horses. Vet Rec 1976;99:330.

Richardson PDI, Withrington PG. Physiological regulation of the hepatic circulation. Annu Rev Physiol 1982;44:57.

Rothuizen J, van den Ingh TSGAM, Voorhout G, van der Luer RJT, Wouda W. Congenital porto-systemic shunts in sixteen dogs and three cats. J Small Anim Pract 1982;23:67.

Schaeffer MC, Rogers QR, Buffington CA, Wolfe BM, Strombeck DR. Long-term biochemical and physiologic effects of surgically placed portacaval shunts in dogs. Am J Vet Res 1986;47:346.

Strange RC. Hepatic bile flow. Physiol Rev 1984;64:184.

Strombeck DR, Weiser MG, Kaneko JJ. Hyperammonemia and hepatic encephalopathy in the dog. J Am Vet Med Assoc 1975;166:1105.

van den Ingh TSGAM, Rothuizen J, van den Brom WE. Extrahepatic cholestasis in the dog and the differentiation of extrahepatic and intrahepatic cholestasis. Vet Quart 1986;8:150.

van Wyk JJ, Underwood LE, Lintz RL, Clemmons DR, Voina SJ, Weaver RP. The somatomedins: A family of insulinlike hormones under growth hormone control. Rec Prog Horm Res 1974;30:259.

Washizu T, Koizumu I, Kaneko JJ. Postprandial changes in serum bile acids concentration and fractionation of individual bile acids by high-performance liquid chromatography in normal dogs. Jpn J Vet Sci 1987;49:593.

Weibel ER, Staubli W, Gnagi HR, Hess FA. Correlated morphometric and biochemical studies on the liver cell. I. Morphometric model, stereologic methods and normal morphometric data for rat liver. J Cell Biol 1969;42:68.

ENDOCRINE AND REPRODUCTIVE FUNCTIONS

Metabolic activity, or homeostasis, is coordinated by communications through the nervous system and the endocrine system. These systems allow normal growth and development to proceed and provide effective adaptations to stress. The nervous system generally operates swiftly by transmitting information or commands through chemically interconnected nerve fibers originating in neurons. At intercellular junctions (synapses), various chemical *neurotransmitters* are liberated to link the nerve fibers. The endocrine system functions with some delay through *hormones,* another type of chemical messenger. Specialized cells secrete and excrete hormones, which may act on some target receptors of the secreting cells (*autocrine action*), on neighboring target cells (*paracrine action*), or on distant target cells (*endocrine action*) after traveling in extracellular fluids (blood, interstitial fluid).

The two systems are partly or entirely regulated by the central nervous system, particularly by a neuroendocrine organ, the hypothalamus. The nervous system and the endocrine system actually form the *neuroendocrine system,* which integrates the metabolic activities of the living organism. Contrary to the nervous system, the endocrine system cannot store information.

CHAPTER 44

FUNDAMENTAL PRINCIPLES OF ENDOCRINOLOGY

This chapter presents the general organization and functions of the endocrine system. Some concepts of hormonal types, blood levels, secretory and synthesis mechanisms, metabolism, and target cells are also discussed.

ORGANIZATION AND FUNCTIONS OF THE ENDOCRINE SYSTEM

The endocrine system of higher vertebrates comprises the following anatomical structures (Fig. 44–1): (1) the endocrine glands (internal secretions), including the adenohypophysis, thyroid, parathyroids, adrenals, and gonads; (2) the parts of the nervous system, including nuclei in the hypothalamus, neurohypophysis, and other components of the central nervous system; (3) temporary tissues—corpus luteum, ovarian follicles, and placenta; (4) disseminated cellular masses—islets of Langerhans, peptidogenic duodenal and jejunal cells, and some hepatic and endothelial cells; and (5) other organs, including the thymus and leukocytes, epiphysis (pineal gland), heart, brain, kidneys, and skin.

The cells of all these endocrine structures synthesize *hormones,* that is, *chemical messengers* that transport and provide information between different cellular populations in the animal organism. The cells upon which these hormones exert their single or multiple actions are called *target cells,* which contain a *secondary messenger* reaching the nuclear protein synthesis mechanisms. The endocrine system is essentially composed of *emitters* and *receptors,* with feedback communications through specialized messengers, hormones. These messengers transmit information only to *complementary receptors.*

The proper functioning of the endocrine system is dependent on (1) the quantity of circulating hormones, which may be either too high or too low; (2) the number of receptors; (3) the quantity of secondary messenger produced within the target cell; (4) the quantity of metabolites or of hormones synthesized by the target cells; and (5) the proper operation of the feedback mechanisms.

Principal Functions

The main functions of the endocrine system are centered on four domains: (1) homeostasis of interstitial fluid; (2) response to urgent situations; (3) integration of the mechanisms of growth; and regulation of metabolism; and (4) regulation of sexual reproduction and lactation.

For each function under hormonal control, several hormones may be needed to regulate this function, and a single hormone may be needed for several functions. Endocrine physiology is concerned with the interactions between the hormones, between some metabolic regulators, and between some neuroendocrine regulators such as: the hypothalamus, acting on the adenohypophysis; the autonomic nervous system, controlling vascularization; and the central nervous system, providing perception.

Classification of Hormones

The classifications of hormones may refer to the organ of origin or to the chemical composition of the endocrine secretions. On the basis of the *tissues of origin,* hormones may be termed hypothalamic, adenohypophysial, thyroid, parathyroid, pancreatic, adrenocortical, adrenomedullary, gastrointestinal, gonadal, and placental.

On the basis of their *chemical composition,* hormones belong either to lipid-related groups (steroids, eicosanoids) or to nitrogen-related groups (amines or amino acid derivatives, peptides or polypeptides, proteins) (Table 44–1). *Steroid* hormones are lipid-soluble substances synthesized from the cholesterol nucleus in the gonads and adrenal cortex. In blood, their half-life is about 1 hour, and they circulate bound to carriers. *Eicosanoids,* which include prostaglandins and leukotrienes, are unsaturated fatty acids (20-carbon) derived from arachidonic acid (eicosatetraenoic acid). They have hormone-like properties and influence the actions of other hormones.

Peptide hormones, made up of 3 to 200 amino acids, are water soluble and true regulators of organic activities. In blood, their half-life is from 5 to 60 minutes, and they circulate freely without the need of carriers. *Amine* hormones, all derivatives of tyrosine, have characteristics of both steroids and peptides, their half-life is from a few seconds to 7 days, and they are either free or bound to a carrier in blood plasma.

The adrenal hormones may also be classified according to their actions on specific receptors. Adrenocortical hormones then have predominantly glucocorticoid (e.g., gluconeogenesis) or mineralocorticoid (Na^+ retention and K^+ loss) actions. The adrenergic actions of adrenomedullary catecholamines then reflect their binding to $alpha_1$, $alpha_2$, $beta_1$, and $beta_2$ receptors.

Blood Concentrations of Hormones

The blood hormone levels that produce physiological effects are usually expressed in nanograms (10^{-9} g, or ng), but the possible range goes from the microgram (10^{-6} g, or

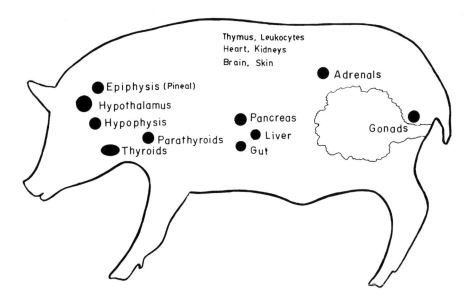

Figure 44–1 Diagrammatic representation of the hormone-secreting tissues in animals.

μg) to the picogram (10^{-12} g, or pg) of hormones per mL of plasma or blood. As an illustration, the blood glucose in monogastric animals represents one million ng, whereas the level of growth hormone is only about 2 ng/mL.

Hormone levels are measured by radioimmunoassay (RIA), nonradioactive immunoassay (enzyme-linked immunosorbent assay [ELISA]), competitive protein-binding and radioreceptor assays, and high-performance liquid chromatography (HPLC).

> RIA is based on the specificity of an antibody and its affinity for binding the free and radiolabeled forms of a hormone. It usually yields accurate information, but false high values may result from cross-reactions with related hormones or with precursors and metabolites of the hormone.
>
> In ELISA, hormone-antibody complexes are made to react with antiantibody antibodies to which enzymes are linked. The enzyme activity following the reaction provides an estimate of the hormone concentration.
>
> The competitive protein-binding and radioreceptive assays depend on the availability of a protein (mostly a carrier or, less often, a receptor) that binds the hormone with high affinity and specificity.

Transport of Hormones

Peptidic hormones, catecholamines, and prostaglandins are free in blood and circulate without carriers. In contrast, for their transport, steroid and some amine hormones bind with proteins, called carriers. A balance exists between bound and free hormones, but *only free hormones are physiologically active.* The regulatory mechanisms for hormone production and release are more sensitive to the free than to the total hormone blood level.

Steroids, not very soluble in water and able to filter at the renal glomeruli, must bind to a carrier to stay in the circulating blood. Two steroid carriers are recognized: *transcortin,* or *cortisol-binding globulin (CBG),* which specifically binds corticosteroids and progesterone, and *sex hormone–binding globulin (SHBG),* the carrier for estradiol and for testosterone.

The iodinated thyroid hormones (amines) in blood are also associated with plasma proteins: mostly with *TBG (thyroxine binding inter-alpha-globulin (TBG),* less so with thyroxine-binding prealbumin (*TBPA*), and to a lesser extent with albumin. Melatonin binds to plasma albumin.

Drugs can change the blood levels and the binding affinity of carriers. Estrogens increase the plasma levels of SHBG and TBG, whereas synthesis of these binding proteins tends to diminish with androgens. Acetylsalicylic acid (aspirin) decreases the affinity of TBG for thyroxine and lowers the synthesis of prostaglandins.

MECHANISMS FOR HORMONE PRODUCTION AND RELEASE

Endocrine glands synthesize and, to some extent, store their hormones for subsequent release into the circulation. This occurs in anatomically separate glands (adenohypophysis, thyroid, adrenal, parathyroid) or in specialized cells or cell clusters within host tissues (testis, ovary, small intestine, kidney, islets of Langerhans, liver).

Cells that are said to contain *a regulated secretory pathway* release some polypeptide hormones (insulin, glucagon, growth hormone) by active exocytosis of granules. Other proteins, mostly insensitive to regulatory stimuli, are released by *a constitutive secretory pathway* shortly after their synthesis (e.g., somatomedins). Steroid hormones diffuse down concentration gradients, whereas thyroid hormones are released by proteolysis of thyroglobulin.

The pattern of release of hormones shows much variation. Adrenocorticotropic hormone (ACTH) and cortisol as well as gonadotropin-releasing (GnRH), luteinizing (LH), and follicle-stimulating (FSH) hormones appear in pulses. These irregular bursts of hormones reflect changes in either synthesis or release.

TABLE 44–1 Classification of Hormones According to Source Organ and Chemistry

Organ	Hormones	Chemical Group		
		Amine	Peptide	Lipid*
Adenohypophysis	Corticotropin (adrenocorticotropic hormone [ACTH])		X	
	Follicle-stimulating hormone (FSH)		X	
	Growth hormone (GH)		X	
	Luteinizing hormone (LH)		X	
	Prolactin (PRL)		X	
	Thyrotropin (thyroid-stimulating hormone [TSH])		X	
Adrenal cortex	Aldosterone			S
	Androgens			S
	Cortisol			S
Adrenal medulla	Dopamine	X		
	Epinephrine	X		
	Norepinephrine	X		
Gastrointestinal tract	Cholecystokinin (CCK, or pancreozymin)		X	
	Gastric inhibitory peptide (GIP)		X	
	Gastrin		X	
	Vasoactive intestinal peptide (VIP)		X	
Gonads	Estrogens (E)			S
	Inhibin		X	
	Progesterone (P4)			S
	Relaxin		X	
	Testosterone			S
Heart	Atrial natriuretic factor (ANF)		X	
Hypothalamus	Antidiuretic hormone (ADH)		X	
	Corticotropin-releasing hormone (CRH)		X	
	Gonadotropin-releasing hormone (GnRH)		X	
	Growth hormone inhibitory hormone (GHIH), or somatostatin (SS, or SRIF)†		X	
	Growth hormone–releasing hormone (GHRH)		X	
	Oxytocin		X	
	Prolactin-inhibitory hormone (PIH), or dopamine	X		
	Thyrotropin-releasing hormone (TRH)		X	
Kidney	Erythropoietin		X	
	Vitamin D_3			S
Liver	Angiotensinogen		X	
	Somatomedins		X	
Pancreatic islets	Glucagon		X	
	Insulin		X	
	Pancreatic peptide (PP)		X	
Parathyroids	Parathyroid hormone, or parathormone (PTH)		X	
Pineal	Melatonin	X		
Placenta	Gonadotropin		X	
	Somatomammotropin		X	
Thymus and leukocytes	Cytokines		X	
	Lymphokines		X	
	Thymic hormones		X	
Thyroids	Calcitonin		X	
	Tetraiodothyronine (T_4, or thyroxine)	X		
	Triiodothyronine (T_3)	X		
Tissues	Leukotrienes			E
	Lipotoxins			E
	Prostaglandins			E

*S, Steroid; E, eicosanoid.
†Also in the stomach, pancreas, small intestine, and central nervous system.

Basal Secretion

The precise evaluation of the basal secretion rate of a hormone is difficult because of its extremely low concentration. Nervous stimuli probably influence the basal secretion rate of some hormones. For these hormones, a nycthemeral (day-night) rhythm limits their production to a moment during the day or during the night. For other hormones, the basal secretion is restricted to or varies during a period of the estrous cycle, or periods of growth. Through hypothalamic nuclei, the central nervous system controls all these rhythms and cycles, which are modulated by feedback effects of products secreted down the line.

Stimulation of Hormonal Secretion

When a hormone maintains the concentration of a metabolite within physiological limits, excessive changes (deficit or excess) in the blood level of this *metabolite* modify its secretion rate. Usually, a deficit of the metabolite triggers the hormonal secretion, and conversely, an excess of metabolite decreases or inhibits the production of hormone. The opposite rule may apply, when the function of the hormone is to lower the level of the metabolite; for example, an excess of metabolite (glucose, Ca^{++}) stimulates the output of the hormone (e.g., insulin, calcitonin), whereas a deficit of the metabolite (glucose, Ca^{++}) inhibits the production of that hormone and induces the output of another one, such as glucagon or parathormone (PTH).

A hormone or several hormones may be involved in the control of the production of another hormone; this is the situation with tropic hormones (e.g., thyrotropic hormone). The simplest relation implicates a tropic hormone dedicated to stimulating or inhibiting the processes of synthesis in an endocrine structure secreting another hormone. A more complex interrelation requires that a tropic hormone produces two effects on target cells, or that two tropic hormones are needed to trigger the production of the desired hormone.

> The names of adenohypophysial hormones are composed by adding the suffix "tropic" or "tropin" (tropea in Greek: toward or in the direction of) to the root designating the target tissue (e.g., thyrotropin). The suffix "trophic" or "trophin" (trophikos in Greek: to nourish), once prominently used, is now less favored.

The central nervous system regulates hormone release in several ways. Through the hypothalamus, changes occur in the delivery of releasing hormones to the adenohypophysis. The sympathetic nervous system also influences the hormonal part of the "fight or flight" response (e.g., insulin, renin, and epinephrine release).

Negative or Positive Feedback

Inhibition of hormonal secretion, a critical aspect of endocrine functions, is provided by humoral negative feedback. This major mechanism may be either a *direct negative feedback* following a change in the level of a metabolite or a more complex *indirect negative feedback,* through a tropin.

A typical example of a simple direct negative feedback involves the parathyroids, the source of the hypercalcemic hormone (PTH). An elevated blood calcium level exerts a direct inhibitory action on the production of PTH by the parathyroids.

A simple indirect negative feedback is represented by the adenohypophysis, producing thyrotropic hormone (thyroid-stimulating hormone [TSH]), which is itself controlled by a hypothalamic peptide, thyrotropin-releasing hormone (TRH). TSH induces a negative feedback on the hypothalamus (short-loop negative feedback) and stimulates the thyroid to secrete thyroxine (tetraiodothyronine, or T_4). The T_4 output from the thyroid is regulated by two long-loop negative feedbacks (i.e., a major one for TSH production by the adenohypophysis, and a secondary one for the production of TRH by the hypothalamus) (Fig. 44-2).

A more complex humoral negative feedback is exemplified by the regulation of the estrous cycle. The level of a hypothalamic peptide (gonadotropin-releasing hormone [GnRH]) influences the rate of its output from the hypothalamus (ultrashort negative feedback). Also, GnRH regulates the pulsatile liberation of two hormones from the adenohypophysis: follicle-stimulating hormone (FSH) or luteinizing hormone (LH) according to the long-loop negative feedback provided by the plasma levels of two steroid ovarian hormones estradiol (E_2) and progesterone (P_4).

During the estrous cycle of most adult females a *positive feedback* occurs to *change* the normal *pulses* of some hypothalamic and adenohypophysial hormones into a tremendous preovulatory *surge.* Instead of the usual braking action, higher estrogen blood levels then exert a facilitatory effect on the release of hypothalamic GnRH, which brings a sudden rise in plasma adenohypophysial LH that is about 100-fold.

METABOLISM OF HORMONES

Chemical modifications or degradations of circulating hormones are means of regulating the turnover of active hormones and their supply to target cells. In blood, steroid and thyroid hormones are bound to plasma proteins. These carriers protect the hormones from catabolic enzymes or postpone their interaction with these plasma enzymes. The carriers, by delaying or making difficult the meeting of hormones and target cells, are also involved in regulating hormonal maturation.

Biliary or renal excretion is the usual avenue for removal of free hormones. A reduction in the loss of the thyroid hormones (T_3 and T_4) via biliary excretion is caused by their ileal reabsorption for an enterohepatic circulation. Similarly, the urinary excretion of the hydrophobic steroids is slowed by tubular reabsorption in the kidney.

Thyroid and steroid hormones, mostly active in long-term metabolic regulation, are eliminated slowly (more than a week for thyroxine). In contrast, peptidic hormones, which produce almost immediate responses, are eliminated rapidly from plasma (a few minutes). The plasma level of prostaglandins is very low, as the action of these eicosanoids is limited to sites within or adjacent to their production cells.

Amine and steroid hormones are generally inactivated

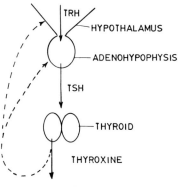

TARGET CELLS

Figure 44–2 Examples of stimulatory and inhibitory actions of the endocrine secretions of several organs. A stimulating action occurs successively along the hypothalamic-adenohypophysis-thyroid axis (TRH, TSH). Then the secretory response of the last organ of the series (e.g., thyroid) stimulates some effect on specific target cells and exerts an inhibitory feedback on the output of hormones from the adenohypophysis and from the hypothalamus.

or altered in the liver. Some eicosanoids (prostaglandins) are extracted from blood in one passage through the lungs. The metabolism of peptidic hormones is more intricate, many of them undergo proteolysis in blood plasma in the process of being changed into a range of active, partially active, and inactive fragments (e.g., PTH).

BIOSYNTHESIS OF HORMONES

Peptidic Hormones

The complex endocellular process of peptidic hormone synthesis involves four phases: transcription and post-transcription, which occur within the nucleus, and the cytoplasmic phases of translation followed by posttranslation processing and modification (Fig. 44–3).

Transcription of DNA leads to the formation of complementary RNA or pre-mRNA. Genes contain more genetic information than is classically recognized by the genetic dogma: the formation of each amino acid requires three bases. According to this dogma, a peptide of 39 amino acids (e.g., ACTH) should be coded on the DNA by 117 bases. However, recent findings indicate that the ACTH molecule comes out of a sequence of 7,300 bases. Transcription of DNA thus yields a molecule of complementary RNA (pre-mRNA) that has to be matured.

Posttranscription marks a series of events causing specific modifications of the complementary RNA (pre-mRNA) to form messenger RNA. It is done by cleavages of pre-mRNA, excisions and rejoining of RNA segments (introns and exons). The RNA segments (introns) that will not be in the mRNA are excised (eliminated), and only the RNA segments (exons) carrying the essential genetic information are joined into mRNA, which passes into the cytoplasm. Two important biochemical modifications at the ends of the mRNA molecule are (1) polyadenylation at the 3' end and (2) addition of a 7-methylguanine "cap" to the 5' end.

During *translation,* the nucleotide triplets (anticodons) and amino acids carried by transfer RNAs (tRNA) find corresponding codons on the mRNA-ribosome complex. The result is the sequential assembly of amino acids, and their polymerization into polypeptide chains.

Posttranslation processing and modification appears when the preprohormone polypeptide enters within the endoplasmic reticulum and is cleaved to become a prohormone. In addition, the prohormone is glycosylated, phosphorylated, acetylated, and cross-linked with disulfur bonds. The modified molecule is then directed to the Golgi apparatus, where additional cleavages mature the prohormone into the active peptidic hormone, which is then packaged into secretory granules. Through secretion, or exocytosis, these secretory granules are transferred into the extracellular fluid.

Steroid Hormones

Steroid hormones are synthesized in the adrenal cortex (corticosteroids) and in the gonads (sexual steroids). Cholesterol, either intercepted by endocrine cells or synthesized in these cells, is the chemical precursor of all steroids. Its side chain is cleaved to yield the 21-carbon pregnenolone, which then undergoes a series of specific enzymatic hydroxylations, placement of double bond (progesterone, testosterone, cortisol, aldosterone), or aromatization (estrogens) in the A ring.

The adrenal cortex is the main source of glucocorticoids (*zona fasciculata and zona reticularis*) and of mineralocorticoids (*zona glomerulosa*), and to a lesser extent of sexual steroids (*zona reticularis*). ACTH stimulates mitochondria to change cholesterol into pregnenolone. Transformation of pregnenolone into glucocorticoids, mineralocorticoids, or sexual steroids is performed by three different enzymatic pathways localized in microsomes and mitochondria.

Stimulated by a hormone from the hypothalamus and by two trophins from the adenohypophysis, the gonads produce most of the sexual steroids. Estradiol originates in cells of the ovarian follicles, progesterone in the cells of the corpus luteum. In the *testicles,* androgenic steroids (androstenedione, testosterone) are synthesized in Leydig cells. Two female steroid hormones are also produced by these cells: estradiol (physiologically in very limited quantity) and progesterone.

The skin, the liver, and the kidneys contribute to the synthesis and activation of vitamin D, a steroid that helps raise blood calcium levels.

Amine Hormones

This group includes the iodinated thyroid hormones (tetraiodothyronine [T_4] and triiodothyronine [T_3]) and the catecholamine hormones of the adrenal medulla (epinephrine, norepinephrine, and dopamine). The thyroid hormones are formed from tyrosine in the thyroid follicles with the assistance of a macromolecule, thyroglobulin. The major thyroid hormone (T_4) serves largely as a prohormone, since it

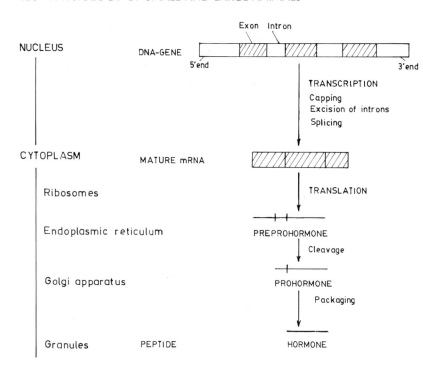

Figure 44–3 The synthesis of a peptide hormone is the result of a specific nuclear stimulation. The changes in the DNA are followed by transcription, capping at the 5' and 3' ends, excision of introns, and splicing of exons, with formation of messenger RNA (mRNA). The mRNA then reaches the ribosomes in the cytoplasm for assembly of amino acids (i.e., translation into prepropeptides). In the endoplasmic reticulum, these prepropeptides, or preprohormones, are then cleaved of the prehormone segment to form prohormones. In the Golgi apparatus, prohormones and hormones are packaged into granules, which are ready for extrusion across the plasma membrane into the extracellular fluid. The hormone can then act on the cell of origin itself (autocrine effect), on neighboring target cells (paracrine effect), or on distant target cells.

is converted to the more active T_3 in the peripheral tissues. Free tyrosine is also at the basis of the enzymatic synthesis of catecholamines.

Eicosanoids

The prostaglandins and leukotrienes are synthesized from polyunsaturated (4 or 5 C=C) long-chain fatty acids that reach the cytoplasm from phospholipids located in the plasma membranes. The immediate precursor for synthesis of the eicosanoids is arachidonic acid (20:4, i.e., 20 carbons, 4 double bonds). The enzymes that convert the precursor to the prostaglandins (cyclooxygenase, synthetases) and the leukotrienes (lipooxygenases) are located in the cytoplasm.

SECRETORY MECHANISMS

Proper functioning of the endocrine system requires a sufficient number of secretory cells able to liberate, on adequate command, a physiological quantity of active hormones. The secretory mechanisms as such are unable to evaluate the proper time for liberating hormones and cannot calculate the quantity of hormones needed. The secretory cells must receive information to evaluate properly the condition of their environment. Because the endocrine cells are subjected to numerous and often contradictory influences, an integration system is needed to regulate the intensity of the signals triggering their secretion. Active stimulation and inhibition of the secretory mechanisms are necessary.

The general secretory mechanisms of polypeptide hormones include (1) their synthesis on the polyribosomes of the endoplasmic reticulum and their transfer inside the membranous saccules; (2) their transport to the Golgi complex; (3) their enclosure in secretory granules; and (4) their liberation outside the plasma membrane by exocytosis. Some secretory granules contain immature or inactive peptides, and several granules are destroyed in the cytoplasm by the lysosomes (crinophagy).

Catecholamines are secreted somewhat like the peptidic hormones. The catecholamines contained in the secretory granules in chromaffin cells of the adrenal medulla enter the bloodstream after crossing the plasma membrane by exocytosis. In sympathetic nerves, the release of catecholamine-containing secretory granules is limited to the interneuronal space.

Steroids are not produced in secretory granules but are concentrated into lipid droplets that are secreted outside the endocrine cells. The lipid-soluble prostaglandins cross cell membranes to act locally, either on the plasma membrane of the cells that have produced them (autocrine) or on that of neighboring cells (paracrine).

RECEPTORS ON OR IN TARGET CELLS

In order to act on a cell, an active molecule of a hormone must be identified from among 10^5 to 10^9 other competing molecules. This very specific recognition mechanism operates through receptors and results in diverse hormonal actions. Generally, receptors are cellular proteins, reversibly saturable, that have great affinity for their substrate. They are responsible for recognition of a specific hormone, and transduction of a message. Receptors hold the entire program for activation of a cell, and it is experimentally possible to activate a cell without using a hormone. Like other cellular proteins, receptors regenerate continually. Under normal physiological conditions, the processes of synthesis and catabolism are in equilibrium, and the number of receptors remains constant. The turnover of receptors is very rapid; for example, most of the insulin receptors are replaced every 24 hours.

The role of hormones is limited to letting the receptor give the information it carries. Hormones do not bring energy or new metabolic orientation to target cells. Some changes in endocrine activity may involve changes in the number of receptors as well as changes in the availability of a hormone. According to the classes of hormones, the specific hormonal receptors are localized either on the plasma membrane (for peptides) or in the cytoplasm (for steroids).

Examples of hormonal effects following stimulation of receptors include the regulation of intermediary as well as mineral and water metabolism, and the coordination of cardiovascular and respiratory systems. Some hormones also control growth as well as development and differentiation of structures and can modify the reproductive functions.

SECOND MESSENGER HYPOTHESIS

Calcium ions and *cyclic AMP* (cAMP) are considered as the second messengers implicated in the hormonal activation of target cells. *Prostaglandins* may also be considered as a type of intracellular second messenger, since they diffuse through cellular membranes. They modify the reactivity of plasma membrane receptors and modulate the effects of peptidic hormones within target cells.

In most endocrine tissues, such as the adenohypophysis, pancreas, and adrenal medulla, Ca^{++} is considered to be the most important *second messenger,* whereas *cAMP* is relegated to a secondary role. In addition to calcium's effects on the contractile elements and the permeability of the plasma membrane, it is an important regulator of enzymatic activity. Adenylate cyclase, cAMP, phosphorylase kinase, and ATPase all are Ca^{++}-dependent enzymes. Calmodulin (calcium-dependent regulatory protein) is a protein with four calcium-binding sites. It functions to provide an adequate supply of Ca^{++} to calcium-dependent enzymatic systems. These enzyme systems are activated only upon binding to calmodulin, already provided for with Ca^{++}.

In tissues under adenohypophysial control (adrenal cortex, gonads, thyroid), the production of cAMP results from the action of *adenylate cyclase.* Present in the internal lipid layer of the plasma membrane, this enzyme transforms cytoplasmic ATP into *cAMP.* The action of peptidic hormones and catecholamines is mediated by cAMP. All the actions of cAMP in cells are expressed by the transformation of inactive phosphokinases into active enzymes. The results are phosphorylations of specific protein substrates to cause responses by the target cells.

Adrenal Cortex. The catecholamine hormones from the adrenal medulla reach the adrenergic receptors on the plasma membrane of adrenocortical cells. The catecholamine-receptor complex activates adenylate cyclase to produce (from ATP) the second messenger (cAMP), which induces nuclear activities for synthesis of proteins (enzymes) needed for adrenocortical hormone production.

Steroids. Lipid-soluble steroids passively cross the plasma membrane of all cells. Target cells have intracellular receptors that can freely traverse the nuclear membrane but show affinity for chromatin only in the presence of a steroid. When this condition is satisfied, the activated receptor attaches on an acceptor site of the chromatin and enhances the expression of a gene to produce mRNA. The potential of steroids to activate genes is limited to 1 percent of the "genetic library."

Thyroid Hormones. In target cells, the cytoplasmic receptors to thyroid hormones are not essential to evoke a response. The functional receptors are on chromatin, as they are for steroid hormones, and a thyroid hormone–receptor complex induces the production of mRNA. A deficiency of thyroid hormones can reduce synthesis of mRNA by 50 percent in target cells.

Regulation of Adenylate Cyclase

This enzyme is made up of a receptor subunit and a catalytic subunit. The enzyme is activated by adding a third component to the system, which then includes (1) the hormone-receptor complex (H-R), (2) the enzyme (adenylate cyclase), and (3) the regulator (nucleotide regulatory protein [NRP]). Activation of adenyl cyclase happens after hormone-receptor coupling, activation of the regulator by the H-R complex, recognition of the regulator by the receptor subunit, and activation of the catalytic subunit of adenylate cyclase.

Mechanism of Action of cAMP

Hormones do not modify any of the intrinsic metabolic pathways in cells. They may alter the speed of the biochemical reactions or may activate dormant metabolic processes that are already present in the cells. Enzymes involved in numerous metabolic pathways are then present in the cellular cytoplasm but are inactive. For these enzymes to be activated, they (proteins) must be phosphorylated by protein-kinases. The mechanism is as follows:

1. The protein-kinases are in two parts: a regulator and a catalyzer.
2. When these parts are together, the enzyme is inactive.

3. cAMP separates the two parts of protein-kinases, letting the catalyzer portion phosphorylate inactive metabolic enzymes.
4. The phosphorylated enzymes participate in biochemical reactions of the metabolic pathways.

The formation of eicosanoids is inhibited by cAMP, which prevents the action of phospholipase-A_2 on the plasma membrane structure and the subsequent release of free arachidonic acid in the cells.

REFERENCES

Felig P, Baxter JD, Broadus AE, Frohman LA. Endocrinology and metabolism. 2nd ed. New York: McGraw-Hill Book Co., 1987.

Norman AW, Litwack G. Hormones. New York: Academic Press, 1987.

Wilson JD, Foster DW. Williams' textbook of endocrinology. 7th ed. Philadelphia: WB Saunders, 1985.

Yalow RS. Radioimmunoassay: a probe for the fine structure of biologic systems. Med Phys 1978;5:247.

CHAPTER 45

THE HYPOTHALAMIC-HYPOPHYSIS COMPLEX

In animal species, the hypothalamus and the hypophysis (pituitary) form a physiological unit that is most important for peptidic hormone syntheses. Some of the major functions of the hypothalamus-hypophysis complex are achieved through control of somatic growth, of gonads for the reproductive cycles, of adrenal cortex for adaptation to the various stresses constantly challenging the organism, of milk secretion, of thyroid hormone output, and of renal water excretion. This system also contributes to blood pressure regulation, control of liquid and food intake, and regulation of energy expenditure by the organism. All these functions involve the use of peptidic biochemical messengers, and an intricate feedback system from peripheral hormones.

Although the hypothalamus and the hypophysis are adjoining organs, it took almost 25 years of research to prove their biochemical relationship. Since 1982, most of the chemical mediators associated with the major functions of the hypothalamus-hypophysis complex have been isolated and chemically characterized. Some of these are even used clinically (e.g., gonadoliberin, or gonadotropin-releasing hormone [GnRH]).

Because of its numerous nervous connections with the higher brain centers and its location in close proximity to the cerebrospinal fluid canals, the hypothalamus is strategically situated. The hypothalamus is specifically responsible for control of body temperature and of food intake. It is probably the major intermediary between the central nervous system and the major hypophysial endocrine controls (Fig. 45–1). As a "neuroendocrine transducer" it translates neural activity into hormonal output.

The endocrine secretions of the adenophypophysis are regulated by the peptidic hormones, produced in the cranial and midportion of the ventral hypothalamus. These regulatory peptidic hypothalamic hormones reach the adenohypophysis via the portal vessels, which convey blood from the hypothalamus to the adenohypophysis. The cranial hypothalamus is also the site of synthesis of the hypophysial neurohormones (antidiuretic hormone [ADH], or vasopressin; and oxytocin [Ot]). These peptidic neurohormones pass via the axons of the hypothalamic neurons to the pituicytes of the neurohypophysis, where they are stored in a form that is releasable into blood.

The hypophysis, because it supervises several of the biological functions of the organism, has been characterized as the master gland or "conductor of the endocrine orchestra." Today, this role might be more appropriately assigned to the hypothalamus.

ARISTOTLE considered the pituitary gland (adenohypophysis) to be the transfer point for one of the four humors, phlegm or pituita, to pass from brain to body.

MORPHOLOGY OF THE HYPOTHALAMIC-HYPOPHYSIS COMPLEX

This section is limited to a description of the neuroendocrine components, the terminology, and the relationships of the hypothalamus-hypophysis complex. To help understand the operation of the hypothalamic-hypophysis complex, the anatomical relationship between the two structures and of circumscribing organs is briefly reviewed. Some highlights are given on the hypothalamus, hypophysis, hypophysial portal system, nervous communications between hypothalamus and hypophysis, and circulation of cerebrospinal fluid.

Hypothalamus

The hypothalamus, a structure situated near the third ventricle, is limited cranially by the *optic chiasma* (crossing of the fibers of the optic nerves), caudally by the *mammillary bodies,* dorsally by the *thalamus,* and ventrally by the the *median eminence.* The median eminence, the result of the medial junction of both hypothalami, is a structure of major importance in the working of the neuroendocrine hypothalamic-hypophysis complex and of the organism. It contains nerve terminals with concentrations of releasing and inhibitory hormones that are about 10 to 100 times higher than elsewhere in the hypothalamus.

Each half of the hypothalamus contains neurons (or transducer cells), with both neuronal and endocrine characteristics, that are grouped into defined masses known as nuclei (Table 45–1). A nucleus is formed of neurons able to synthesize substances, which are candidates for the functions of hormones or chemical mediators. Some nuclei have neurons with over 10,000 connections with other parts of the central nervous system. The hypothalamic nuclei have several functions and contribute to many biological processes.

The nuclei are located in the cranial, lateral, medial, and caudal areas of the hypothalamus. The *cranial* (anterior) area of the hypothalamus is concerned with regulation of body temperature, and synthesis of releasing hormones (liberins) such as GnRH; thyreoliberin, or thyrotropin-releasing hormone (TRH); and somatoliberin, or growth hormone–releasing hormone (GHRH), or somatocrinin. The *lateral* area is a crossroad joining the limbic system, the other hypothalamic regions, and the mesencephalon (midbrain). This lateral hypothalamus and the median eminence contain individual neurons, not organized as separate nuclei, and unmyelinated nervous fibers (i.e., not covered with myelin).

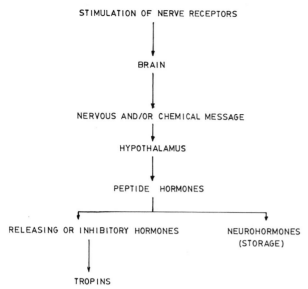

STIMULATION OF NERVE RECEPTORS

↓

BRAIN

↓

NERVOUS AND/OR CHEMICAL MESSAGE

↓

HYPOTHALAMUS

↓

PEPTIDE HORMONES

RELEASING OR INHIBITORY HORMONES   NEUROHORMONES (STORAGE)

↓

TROPINS

Figure 45–1 Synopsis of the neuroendocrine communications between the central nervous system, hypothalamus, adenohypophysis, and neurohypophysis.

The lateral nuclei are separated from the third cerebral ventricle by the *medial* nuclei. The hypothalamus is also a regulator of complex metabolic and behavioral activities, including feeding, drinking, sleep, and sexual activity.

Hypophysis

The former name of the hypophysis was the "pituitary," a medieval term indicating its supposed role in lubricating the nasal mucosa.

RATHKE (1793–1860) first showed that the pituitary consists of two separate parts, anterior and posterior.

In domestic mammals, the hypophysis is formed by three distinct anatomical structures, which are, craniocaudally, the adenohypophysis, the intermediary lobe, and the neurohypophysis. This glandular and secretory complex is at the base of the cranium, in a depression (saddle) of the sphenoid bone, the *sella turcica.*

The hollow space of the *sella turcica* cavity, of varied depth in different species, is covered by a thickened reflection of the dura mater, the *diaphragma sellae.* The external layer of the dura mater lines or faces the inside of the cavity. The diaphragma sellae gives passage to the hypophysial stalk and associated blood vessels.

The size of the hypophysis varies with species, gender, and physiological conditions (e.g., gestation). It is usually between 500 and 2,000 mg in large domestic species. During gestation, the adenohypophysis, which is 75 percent of the glandular mass, may double in size because of larger and more numerous prolactin-secreting cells.

MARIE noted that pituitary tumors were associated with acromegaly, a condition marked by excessive and unbalanced growth of the extremities. CUSHING obtained improvement of the acromegaly symptoms by surgically removing part of the pituitary (1909).

Anatomical Terminology

An international commission on the anatomical nomenclature recommends the following terminology for the parts of the hypophysis:

1. The adenohypophysis should be referred to as *lobus glandularis;* the anterior lobe as *pars distalis* and *pars tuberalis;* and the posterior lobe as *pars intermedia* and *processus infundibuli.*
2. The neurohypophysis should be called the *lobus nervosus;* and the infundibulum, *pediculis infundibularis, bulbus infundibularis,* and *labrum infundibularis* or median eminence of *tuber cinerum.*

The *pars intermedia* is found in all domestic animals, but only during the fetal life in humans.

TABLE 45–1 Major Hypothalamic Nuclei—Their Hormones, Functions, and Pathology

Nuclei	Hormones	Functions	Pathology
Anterior or cranial area	GnRH	Estrous cycle; temperature control	Infertility; fever
	TRH	TSH control	Energy; goiter
	GHRH	GH control	Growth
Arcuate	GHIH	GH inhibition	Growth problem
Lateral area		Appetite center	Aphagia
Median eminence	All	Concentrates all hormones	
Paraventricular	Oxytocin	Uterine contraction; milk secretion	Uterine inertia; agalactia
Supraoptic	ADH	Arterial pressure; water retention	Diabetes insipidus
Ventromedial area		Satiety center	Obesity; hyperphagia

Embryology

The fetal development of the hypophysis can help explain the complexity of this tissue, which originates from two ectoderm structures. The first ectoderm structure starts at the oropharynx and develops as the adenohypophysis (*pars distalis*). The second ectoderm structure is a growth of nervous tissue from the diencephalon (interbrain), at the base of the third ventricle, that develops into the neurohypophysis. When the two structures are in contact, the glandular cells of the oropharyngeal sheath differentiate into the intermediary lobe.

In summary, the *neurohypophysis* is a nervous tissue (not a glandular tissue) and is strictly dependent on the central nervous system. The *hypophysial stalk,* which results from the growth of the diencephalon (midbrain), is also a nervous structure. The *third ventricle* penetrates the hypophysial stalk. The *glandular parts* have a common origin, and the anatomical terminology considers the spatial distribution rather than the biochemical differentiation of the tissues.

Hypophysial Portal System and Vascularization

Arterial supply to the hypophysis is through vessels coming from the internal carotid: the dorsal (superior), middle, and ventral (inferior) hypophysial arteries. Ramifications of the dorsal hypophysial artery subdivide in a complex network of capillaries irrigating the external surface of the infundibulum at the level of the median eminence. This external plexus comes in contact with the internal plexus of the median eminence (primary plexus) and travels in long portal vessels crossing the hypophysial stalk toward a capillary plexus (secondary plexus) in the pars distalis. The middle and ventral (inferior) hypophysial arteries nourish the hypophysial stalk and the processus infundibuli, without irrigating the anterior lobe. All the arterial blood of the anterior lobe must pass through the hypophysial portal vessels after having drained the infundibular region of the median eminence.

It appears that veins do not exist to drain the voluminous anterior lobe; most of the venous blood is directed into the capillary network of the posterior lobe, which is connected to the hypophysial portal system. The main exit for venous blood is through the hypophysial veins, which emerge from the posterior lobe to direct venous blood into a cavernous sinus at the base of the hypophysial complex. The intermediary lobe is apparently avascular. The direction of blood circulating in the hypophysial portal system is still a disputed question. A flow of blood from the primary plexus to the secondary plexus is very probable. A retrograde system should exist to bring adenohypophysial and neurohypophysial chemical messengers to the median eminence and the higher nervous centers.

Innervation of the Hypophysis

The hypophysis is practically without innervation. A few postganglionic sympathetic fibers, which accompany the arterioles, terminate in the walls of blood vessels. Sympathetic influence on the flow of blood in the hypophysis is unknown.

Nervous Communications between the Hypothalamus and the Hypophysis

Nervous signals occur essentially between the hypothalamic supraoptic and paraventricular nuclei and the neurohypophysial processus infundibuli. These neurons are of the "peptidergic" type (i.e., they synthesize and secrete peptides). The cell bodies of these neurons are in the hypothalamus. Their axons end at the processus infundibuli, where secretory granules of peptides are stored. Nervous cell bodies are absent in the neurohypophysis, which is limited to function as a reservoir. Unlike the anterior and intermediary lobes of the hypophysis, the posterior or neural lobe is not an active center for syntheses.

Cell Types in the Adenohypophysis

About 20 percent of the cells of the adenohypophysis cannot be stained by antibodies and can be considered as either resting degranulated cells or undifferentiated primitive secretory cells. However, immunochemical stains have been used to distinguish and to identify six specific cell clusters in the adenohypophysis: corticotrope, gonadotrope, mammotrope or lactotrope, melanotrope, somatotrope, and thyrotrope. The cytoplasmic secretory granules of mammotrope and somatotrope cells are acidophilic, whereas those of the others are basophilic.

The *corticotrope* (15 to 20% of the adenohypophysis) yields a precursor molecule, or prohormone, proopiomelanocortin (POMC), which can be fragmented to produce adrenocorticotropic hormone (ACTH), and endorphins and lipotropin. The pulsatile production of ACTH, which depends on corticotropin-releasing hormone (CRH), is highest in early morning and lowest in the evening (the norm is opposite in rats, nocturnal animals). The *melanotrope* is morphologically similar to the corticotrope, with cytoplasmic granules of 100 to 200 nm. Also, since melanocyte-stimulating hormone (MSH) is a breakdown product of ACTH, it is possible that the corticotrope and melanotrope are the same (i.e., corticomelanotrope).

The *gonadotrope* (about 15% of the adenohypophysis) contains two types of cells with cytoplasmic granules of different size (e.g., 300 to 700 nm in the large rounded type A, or I; and 200 to 250 nm in the ovoid type B, or II). These multihormonal cells, which are more numerous after castration, produce both luteinizing hormone (LH) and follicle-stimulating hormone (FSH) in a pulsatile fashion modulated by GnRH. The *mammotrope, or lactotrope,* carries a substantial number (40 to 50% of the 6×10^6 cells of rat adenohypophysis) of polymorphic cells producing and releasing prolactin (PRL). Type I cells have small spherical granules (130 to 200 nm); type II have medium-sized spherical or polymorphic granules (250 to 300 nm); and type III of the lactotrope cells have large polymorphic granules (400 to 800 nm). The basal synthesis and release of PRL is under the pulsatile inhibitory control of dopamine (prolactin-inhibiting hormone [PIH]).

The *somatotrope* harbors more cells (10 to 25 percent of the adenohypophysis) that produce rather large (300 to 400 nm) secretory granules of growth hormone (GH). Bursts of GH secretion are regulated by a balance between the stimulatory GHRH and the inhibitory somatostatin (SS). The *thyrotrope* is composed of small elongated cells (3 to 6 percent of the adenohypophysis) with few small secretory granules (125 to 200 nm). The output of thyroid-stimulating hormone (TSH) is rapidly enhanced by TRH and then is swiftly inhibited by a rise in thyroid hormones, which have negative feedback on both TRH and TSH.

HYPOTHALAMIC HORMONES THAT ACT ON THE ADENOHYPOPHYSIS

In close communication with the central nervous system, the hypothalamus receives impulses from the limbic system, the cerebral cortex, the thalamus, the spinal cord, and the visual center. Via neurotransmitters (acetylcholine, dopamine, norepinephrine, epinephrine, serotonin, histamine, and gamma-aminobutyric acid), nervous stimuli from these structures influence secretion of hypothalamic hormones. This section presents the hypothalamic peptides that act on the adenohypophysis, the so-called *hypophysiotropic* hormones.

Considerable studies have been done with dopamine, norepinephrine, and serotonin, three major monoamines present in the anterior and ventromedial areas of the hypothalamus. In response to these neurotransmitters, the hypothalamic neurons secrete specific chemical messengers (a single one is a nonpeptide: dopamine) toward definite cells in the adenophypophysis, which in turn produces the tropic hormones that are aimed at specific endocrine target cells (Fig. 45–2).

> Dopamine and norepinephrine, both catecholamine neurotransmitters, are derivatives of tyrosine. Dopamine synthesis requires the hydroxylation of tyrosine to L-dopa, and the decarboxylation of the latter to 5-OH-tryptamine. Besides being a neurotransmitter, dopamine also inhibits the release of prolactin. The formation of norepinephrine is by hydroxylation of dopamine.
> Serotonin, an indolamine neurotransmitter, is a derivative of tryptophan. After its hydroxylation to 5-OH-tryptophan, a subsequent decarboxylation yields serotonin.

The hypothalamus is essential to the hypophysis. The hypothalamic peptidic hormones, secreted in pulses, constantly control the activity of the adenohypophysis by either stimulating or inhibiting the syntheses of adenohypophysical hormones. The hypophysial portal venous blood contains at least ten times more hypothalamic peptides than peripheral blood. These hypophysiotropic regulators are now considered as full-fledged hormones and no longer just as "factors." Of nine identified hypothalamic peptides able to enhance or to inhibit the secretion of hypophysial tropins, the structures of only six hypophysiotropic hormones have been defined.

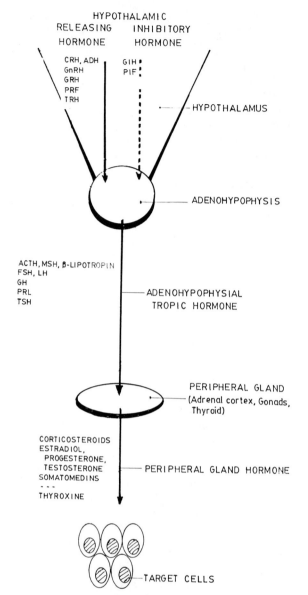

Figure 45–2 Upon nervous or chemical stimulation, the secretory neurons of the hypothalamus synthesize specific adenotropic hormones. Some hypothalamic hormones (e.g., corticoliberin, or corticotropin-releasing hormone [CRH]; vasopressin, or antidiuretic hormone [ADH]; gonadoliberin, or gonadotropin-releasing hormone [GnRH]; growth hormone–releasing hormone [GRH]; prolactin-releasing factor [PRF]; and thyrotropin-releasing hormone [TRH]) induce the release of other peptide hormones from the secretory cells of the adenohypophysis. Other hypothalamic secretions are inhibitory (e.g., growth hormone–inhibiting hormone [GIH]; dopamine, or prolactin-inhibiting factor [PIF]. The response of the adenohypophysis is a selected output of substances related to preproopiomelanocortin (adrenocorticotropic hormone [ACTH], melanocyte-stimulating hormone, and beta-lipotropin), gonadotropins (follicle-stimulating hormone [FSH] and luteinizing hormone [LH]), growth hormone (GH), prolactin (PRL), and thyroid-stimulating hormone (TSH). These chemical messengers act on the target cells of peripheral glands. They stimulate the adrenal cortex to produce corticosteroids; the gonads to synthesize estradiol, progesterone, and testosterone; the liver to supply somatomedins; and the thyroid to yield thyroxine (i.e., tetraiodothyronine).

The terminology of the hypothalamic hormones is based on their major physiological action; for example, corticotropin-releasing hormone (CRH), gonadotropin–releasing hormone (GnRH), growth hormone–releasing hormone (GHRH), growth hormone–inhibiting hormone (GHIH), prolactin-releasing factor (PRF), prolactin-inhibiting factor (PIF), and thyrotropin-releasing hormone (TRH). Melanocyte-stimulating hormone–releasing factor (MSH-RH) and melanocyte-stimulating hormone–inhibiting factor (MSH-IF), which influence melanin coloration of skin, are not considered important in mammals. The suffixes *liberin* (for substances that stimulate the adenohypophysial cells) and *statin* (for those that inhibit adenohypophysial cells) are gaining some acceptance. It was originally presumed that each adenohypophysial hormone had a set of both "liberin" and "statin" substances, but the reality is much more complex. The structures of CRH, TRH, GnRH, GHRH, GHIH (somatostatin), and PIF are known (Table 45–2).

The main steps in the synthesis of the hypothalamic peptides include

1. *transcription* of the hormone's gene into RNA;
2. *processing* of this pre-RNA within the nucleus into mature mRNA;
3. *translocation* of the mRNA to the cytoplasm;
4. *attachment* of the mRNA to ribosomes, and *translation* into the prehormone;
5. *discharge* into the lumen of the rough endoplasmic reticulum during which the leader sequence of the prehormone is removed;
6. *concentration and packaging* of the hormone, within the Golgi apparatus, into secretory granules;
7. *storage* of the hormone in secretory granules; and
8. *transport* of the secretory granules into the terminals of the peripheral cytoplasm by axonal flow, and extracellular release by exocytosis.

The release of hypothalamic hormones is regulated by complex nervous and hormonal feedback mechanisms. For example, hypothermia, detected by hypothalamic thermoreceptors, causes stimulatory signals for release of TRH. In contrast, hyperthermia not only inhibits the release of TRH but also increases the output of GHRH. Humoral negative-feedback mechanisms also modulate the liberation of hypothalamic hormones (Fig. 45–3). These retroactions may be induced by the blood level of the hormones liberated from the action of adenohypophysial tropins on their target cells (*long-loop feedback*), by the hypophysial tropins (*short-loop feedback*), and even by the hypothalamic hormones themselves (*ultra-short-loop feedback*). For instance, a low concentration of thyroid hormones induces an output of TRH, and a high blood content of thyroid hormones inhibits the release of TRH. GH, produced from the action of GHRH on the hypophysial somatotropic cells (somatotropes; formerly called somatotrophs), has an inhibitory feedback effect on the hypothalamic cells that release GHRH.

Hypothalamic peptides bind to plasma membrane receptors on the hypophysial tropic cells (thyrotropic, gonadotropic, somatotropic, corticotropic, mammotropic). They operate through calcium ions and phospholipids (diacylglycerols, inositol phosphates, and arachidonic acid) (Fig. 45–4). Still unknown specific proteins are phosphorylated by activated kinase A or C. With cAMP acting as the second messenger, the synthesis of tropic hormone is stimulated by increasing the levels of mRNA, and exocytosis of the secreted granules occurs from the target adenohypophysial tropic cells.

Corticotropin-Releasing Hormone

Corticotropin-releasing hormone (CRH), or *corticoliberin*, has been characterized as a molecule of 41 amino acids (in sheep) only since 1981. However, the role of this hypothalamic peptide has been studied for over three decades. In fact, CRH was the first hypothalamic hormone discovered, although its structure was not sequenced until 1981.

The physiological function of CRH is to stimulate the release, but not the synthesis, of ACTH from cells in the adenohypophysis. By exocytosis, ACTH is co-released, in equimolar amounts, with beta-lipotropin (β-LPH), another segment of its preproopiomelanocortin precursor. Production of cortisol by the adrenal cortex also results from the increased secretion of ACTH induced by CRH.

Synthesis and liberation of CRH is increased by stress. The output of CRH is also influenced by circadian light-darkness cycles. In diurnal animals (e.g., cattle, dog, horse),

TABLE 45–2 Major Hypothalamic Hormones

Hormones	No. of Amino Acids	Major Action
Corticotropin-releasing (CRH)	41	ACTH
Gonadotropin-releasing hormone (GnRH), or gonadoliberin	10	LH, FSH
Melanotropin-inhibiting factor (MIF), or melanostatin	3	MSH
Melanotropin-releasing factor (MRF), or melanoliberin	5	MSH
Prolactin-inhibiting factor (PIF) (dopamine)	1	PRL?
Prolactin-releasing factor (PRF)	?	PRL?
Somatocrinin (GHRH)	44, 40, 37	GH, TSH
Somatostatin (SRIF, GHIH)	14	GH
Thyrotropin-releasing hormone (TRH)	3	TSH, PRL

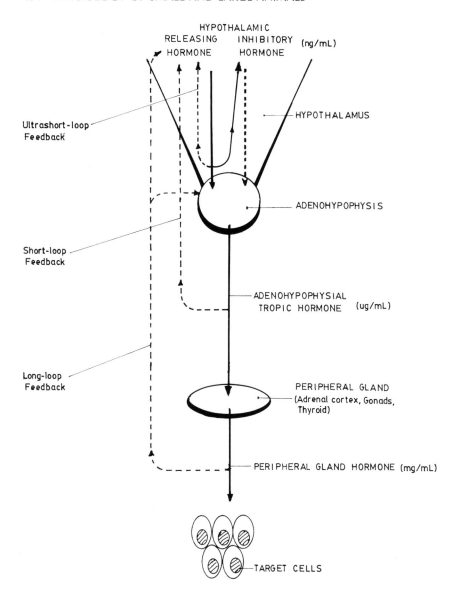

Figure 45–3 Several types of negative-feedback loops act on the releasing hormones of the hypothalamus. In the ultrashort loop, the releasing hormone itself inhibits (dashed line) its liberation. In the short loop, it is the hypophysial proteins (tropins) that exert inhibition on the hypothalamus. Finally, in the long loop, the hormone produced by the target cells depresses the production of hypothalamic peptide.

ACTH levels are highest in the morning and lowest at night, whereas the reverse is true in nocturnal animals (e.g., rat). The genes that direct the synthesis of prepro-CRH are homologous with those for preproneurohormones and for preproopiomelanocortin. It explains the CRH-like action of oxytocin and of vasopressin, which potentiate the effect of CRH during conditions brought on by certain types of stress.

Through a negative short-loop feedback, ACTH inhibits the release of CRH from the median eminence. Glucocorticoids (natural: cortisol; synthetic: dexamethasone, for example) block the hypothalamic release of CRH (not its synthesis). They also prevent the stimulatory effect of CRH on the hypophysis; that is, the liberation of ACTH and other preproopiomelanocortin products (beta- and gamma-lipotropin, and beta-endorphin). A reduced output of CRH leads to secondary adrenocortical failure (Addison's syndrome). In hyperadrenocorticism (Cushing's syndrome, adrenocortical tumor) the synthesis and the release of CRH are inhibited.

Produced in limited amounts for clinical use, ovine CRH has been suggested as a tool to evaluate adrenal cortex function in dogs. CRH increases ACTH and cortisol levels in normal dogs and those with Cushing's syndrome but does not increase levels of these substances in dogs with adrenocortical tumors.

Gonadotropin-Releasing Hormone

In mammals, the hypothalamic decapeptide (10 amino acids) gonadotropin-releasing hormone (GnRH), also known as *gonadoliberin* (formerly known as FSH/LH-RH, LH-RH, or luliberin), is secreted by neuronal perikarya in the rostral

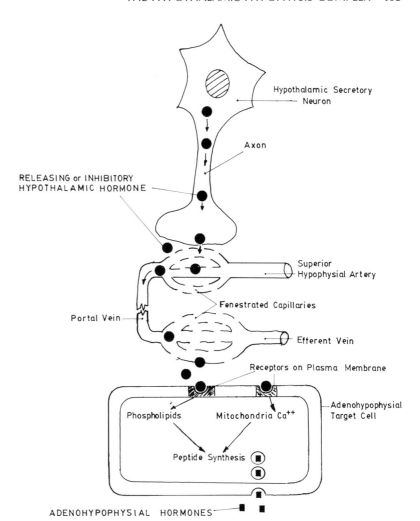

Figure 45–4   Once they are synthesized in the hypothalamic neurons, the granules of releasing or inhibitory peptides progress in the axons to reach the nerve ending terminals for ultimate expulsion into the extracellular space. Fenestrated capillaries permit their passage into the hypothalamic-adenohypophysial portal circulation and their transport to the vicinity of receptors on the adenohypophysial target cells. Their binding to the receptors then induces the liberation of intermediaries, either phospholipids (diacylglycerol, inositol phosphates) with arachidonic acid from the plasma membrane, or calcium ions from the mitochondria. With cyclic adenosine monophosphate (cAMP) as the second messenger, adenohypophysial peptide granules are produced, transported by exocytosis into the extracellular fluid, and brought into the general circulation through penetration of fenestrated capillaries.

hypothalamus, transported by axonal flow, and stored (small granules, about 40 to 130 nm) mostly in terminals in the median eminence. GnRH is released in pulses (about every 2 hours) and causes the liberation of two hormones from the adenohypophysis: LH and FSH. These two gonadotropins participate in the control of reproduction in male and female mammals. As GnRH release cannot be measured in intact animals (a 500-fold dilution occurs from the hypophysial portal to the jugular veins), LH pulse frequency is used as an index of GnRH secretion.

Physiological Actions.   GnRH increases the adenohypophysial secretion of LH and FSH, which influence the production of sexual steroids by the gonads and ultimately affect spermatogenesis, ovogenesis, and ovulation. The production of either LH or FSH is controlled mostly by the nature and the quantity of circulating sexual steroids. When *estradiol* predominates, GnRH favors the liberation of *LH* (e.g., ovulatory peak with twice as many GnRH pulses) from the adenohypophysis, whereas GnRH induces the release of *FSH* when *progesterone* prevails. This mechanism explains in part the rhythm of the estrous cycle, as GnRH can induce ovulation on an ovary prepared by administration of FSH.

Secretion of GnRH is increased during coitus in the cat and is followed by a LH surge after 15 minutes. In small animals, secretion of GnRH is also stimulated by administration of a synthetic, nonsteroidal estrogen analog (clomiphene citrate) or an antiestrogen (tamoxifen). Release of GnRH by the hypothalamus is increased by norepinephrine, estradiol (which inhibits dopamine and facilitates the action of norepinephrine), and opioid antagonists (naloxone).

Examples of neural inputs that influence the hypothalamic output of GnRH are pheromones (airborne or water-borne chemical exciters or inhibitors) that stimulate the olfactory bulb and light-track cycles that act on the retina. Production of GnRH, marked by induction of puberty by overcoming the inhibitory photoperiod effect and decreasing the estradiol negative feedback, is caused by the odor (pheromones) of a ram suddenly introduced among sexually immature ewe-lambs (9-month-old). In sheep and goats, a circadian (about 24 hours) increase in the melatonin (an indolamine), formed during the longer nocturnal periods of the shortening days of autumn, initiates GnRH production. Lambs or kids that have grown sufficiently reach puberty and are then sexually mature, whereas adults begin the annual breeding season when the daylight periods shorten. In wild animals and horses, GnRH release coincident with the breeding season starts during the lengthening days of spring, when circannual melatonin production is minimal.

Dopamine, opioids, and endorphins inhibit the discharge of GnRH from the median eminence into the hypophysial portal blood. Suppression of GnRH by administration of high levels of steroids (testosterone, estrogen, progesterone), the basis of oral contraceptive programs in humans, is probably mediated by endorphin-producing neurons in the hypothalamus. Prolonged treatment with corticosteroids, corticotropin-releasing factor (CRF), and stress have a negative feedback on GnRH output by the hypothalamus. *Inhibin,* a glycoprotein from ovarian follicles and testicular seminiferous tubules, reduces GnRH secretion by hypothalamic cells. Prolactin and LH, via short-loop negative feedback, can also inhibit GnRH. Immunization against GnRH causes disappearance of LH pulses in both female and male adult sheep.

Distribution. As with TRH, the highest GnRH concentration is in the median eminence. Some is also found in the arcuate and the ventromedial nuclei. The half-life of GnRH is 6 to 7 minutes.

Clinical Uses. GnRH and several synthetic analogs are used to trigger the appearance of estrus in domestic animals. GnRH is also useful in assessing the performance of the adenohypophysis by causing the release of its gonadotropin reserve, which can be measured in the peripheral blood.

Prolactin-Inhibiting Hormone

Prolactin-inhibiting factor or hormone (PIF or PIH), which seems identical to *dopamine,* is the only nonpeptide hypophysiotropic hormone. Hypothalamic dopamine (a monoamine, catecholamine neurotransmitter) exerts a pulsatile braking action on the spontaneous or basal (without stimulation by the hypothalamus) secretion of prolactin by the lactotrope cells of the adenohypophysis.

Bromocriptine (a dopamine agonist) and norepinephrine also have a PIF-like effect (i.e., they inhibit output of hypophysial prolactin). The output of dopamine is increased by serotonin. Prolactin inhibits its own secretion by increasing the synthesis and release of dopamine. In contrast, the release of dopamine is decreased by suckling, stress, estrogens, or tranquilizers (chlorpromazine, reserpine).

Growth Hormone–Releasing Hormone

The latest hypothalamic peptide to be recognized, *somatocrinin,* growth hormone–releasing hormone (GHRH or GRH) is a linear peptide that may include 44, 40, or 37 amino acids. The three forms are biologically active, with about similar activity produced by the two larger forms and less activity generated by the smaller form.

Pulsatile (cyclical) secretion of GHRH (formerly somatotropin-releasing factor [SRF]) is linked to the release of growth hormone and some prolactin (PRL) by the adenohypophysis (Fig. 45–5). The response of the hypophysis is increased by glucocorticoids but is reduced with age and by somatostatin, a competitive inhibitor. When GHRH output is continuous (tonic), it inhibits the release of GH.

The pulsatile output of GHRH by the median eminence is increased by estradiol (E_2) and progesterone (P_4), ADH and ACTH, catecholamines (alpha-adrenergic [e.g., clonidine] and dopaminergic agonists), serotonin, stress, and deep sleep. Conversely, melatonin, morphine, antiserotonin and anti–alpha-adrenergic substances, beta-adrenergic agonists, and rapid eye movement (REM) sleep prevent the liberation of GHRH from the hypothalamus. Somatomedin C (mostly from the liver) and GH inhibit,

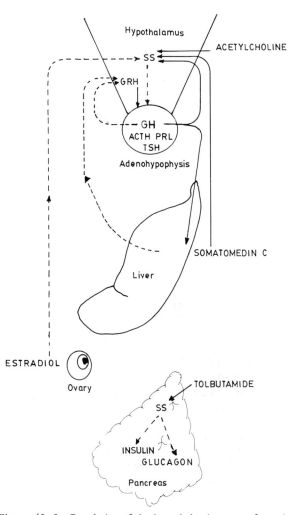

Figure 45–5 Regulation of the hypothalamic output from the median eminence of somatocrinin, or growth hormone–releasing hormone (GRH), and of somatostatin (SS), for the control of adenohypophysial growth hormone (GH). Somatomedin C exerts a double long-loop negative feedback, which simultaneously stimulates the production of SS and inhibits the production of GRH. Through a double short-loop negative feedback, GH accelerates the release of SS and depresses the output of GRH.

respectively, the release of GHRH by a long-loop and a short-loop negative-feedback mechanism.

In lactating cows and ewes, repeated intravenous injections of GHRH cause a galactopoietic response. The milk yield, total milk fat, protein, and lactose increase by about 10 percent in cows and 25 percent in ewes. The milk composition and the feed intake remain normal. The higher milk yield is probably due to GH, which acts on the postabsorptive use of nutrients.

Growth Hormone–Inhibiting Hormone

Growth hormone–inhibiting hormone (GHIH), or *somatostatin* (SS or S) (formerly known as somatotropin-release inhibitory factor [SRIF]), has a tetradecapeptide (14 amino acids) structure and a short half-life. This peptide is produced in the hypothalamic arcuate nuclei and also in the spinal cord and the delta cells of the islets of Langerhans.

Somatostatin inhibits the secretion of several adenohypophysial hormones in a consistent fashion; for example GH and TSH; and in an opportunistic way, PRL and ACTH. It also interferes with the secretion of insulin and of glucagon from the endocrine pancreas and exerts important actions on the gastrointestinal tract.

Hypothalamic release of somatostatin is activated by GH from the adenohypophysis, by somatomedin C produced by the liver, and by acetylcholine (see Fig. 45–5). Estradiol decreases the liberation of SS from the nerve fibers in the anterior hypothalamic periventricular system. Tolbutamide (an oral hypoglycemic drug) favors the release of SS from pancreatic delta cells.

In target cells, somatostatin inhibits the capture of Ca^{++} by reducing the extrusion of potassium (Ca^{++} entry is associated with extracellular movement of K^+), and reduces as well as prevents the stimulatory effect of intracellular cAMP. Somatostatin also decreases the intensity of nerve impulses in the central nervous system.

Thyrotropin-Releasing Hormone

Thyrotropin-releasing hormone (TRH), or *thyreoliberin,* was the first hypothalamic peptide to be completely characterized. A total of 500 tons of sheep brain, providing 50 tons of hypothalamus fragments, was used to get a yield of 1 mg TRH from 300,000 hypothalami.

TRH, a tripeptide, Pyro-Glu-His-Pro-NH$_2$, without structural changes in different mammals, is now commercially synthesized and available (although expensive). It is suggested as a stimulation test to distinguish rare (5%) types of hypothyroidisms (tertiary from secondary) due to hypothalamus-adenohypophysis dysfunction in small animals. Physiological actions are observed with 10 pg/kg, and the in vivo dosage is between 50 and 500 ng/kg.

Tertiary hypothyroidism, a hypothetical condition in animals, is due to inadequate TRH stimulation of the adenohypophysis with consequent lack of thyroid hormones. This hypothalamic dysfunction produces signs of atrophy in the hypophysial thyreotropic cells (thyreotropes) and in the thyroid follicles.

Secondary hypothyroidism is associated with insufficient TSH stimulation of the cells producing the thyroid hormones.

Physiological Actions. The main function of TRH is to stimulate the synthesis and liberation of TSH by the adenohypophysis. It can also influence the liberation of PRL, a mammotropic hormone, from the adenohypophysis. Results indicate that TRH could be one of the oligopeptides used as a neurotransmitter in the higher brain centers. The importance of the contribution of TRH in cellular communications, and its role in carrying and treating information, are still unclear.

Distribution. TRH is found in all vertebrates, in the gastrointestinal system, and in all nervous tissues, but mostly in the median eminence. Notable but decreasing amounts accumulate in the following hypothalamic nuclei: ventromedial, paraventricular, dorsomedial, and arcuate.

Plasma Levels. The level of TRH in circulating plasma is technically difficult to measure. Results from different sources give values between 10 and 20 pg per milliliter. The half-life of the peptide is about 4 to 6 minutes. Chronic exposure to cold is the only situation known to cause a slight increase in the plasma TRH level.

Other Hypothalamic Hormones of Unknown Structure

The as yet uncharacterized hypothalamic prolactin-releasing factor appears to be related to TSH or vasoactive intestinal peptide (VIP), both of which increase the secretion of PRL. The release of prolactin-releasing factor is favored by dopamine antagonists (phenothiazines), opioid peptides (enkephalins, endorphins, dynorphin), serotonin, slow-wave sleep and REM sleep, suckling, and stress of various sorts.

Other substances of unknown structures and of questioned functions are MSH-IF (melanostatin) and melanocyte-stimulating hormone–releasing hormone (MSH-RH or melanoliberin). In animals (frogs) in which mimetism to the environment is important, these substances seem to influence skin coloration by decreasing, or increasing, the melanin contents of certain cells (melanophores).

NEUROHORMONES SYNTHESIZED IN THE HYPOTHALAMUS AND STORED IN THE NEUROHYPOPHYSIS

In addition to the neurons that produce the adenohypophysiotropic peptides, the hypothalamus contains some large (magnocellular) and densely packed neurons that have axons running to the neurohypophysis in a well-defined bundle. These magnocellular neurons synthesize two neuropeptides, antidiuretic hormone (ADH), also known as vasopressin, and oxytocin (Ot). Together with specific neurophysins (I and II), these neurohormones migrate in axonal vesicles, which can be stained and become visible (Herring's bodies, about 20 μm) in the neurohypophysis, where they are stored. The sole role of neurophysins is to reduce the osmolality inside the axonal vesicles. The axonal transport of the neurosecretions from the hypothalamic cell bodies to the neurohypophysis, which is 50 times faster than axonal flow, can be disrupted by colchicine (an alkaloid).

Under specific nervous stimuli from the hypothalamic neurons, each neurohormone and its corresponding sulfur-rich *neurophysin* protein are excreted (secreted) from the neurohypophysis by exocytosis (reverse pinocytosis). Both the neurohormone and the neurophysin enter the very permeable (fenestrated endothelium) neighboring systemic capillaries (Fig. 45–6). The neurophysins serve no further function in the peripheral blood, whereas each neurohormone seeks specific receptors on the plasma membrane of target cells in various organs. ADH combines with V_2 receptors on kidney cells or with V_1 receptors on vascular smooth muscle cells. Oxytocin occupies receptors on smooth muscle cells in the walls of the alveoli of mammary glands or of the uterus.

The large size and the dense grouping of the magnocellular neurons in the supraoptic nuclei (SON) and paraventricular nuclei (PVN) of this hypothalamo-neurohypophysial axis make them suitable for electrophysiological investigation.

In magnocellular hypothalamic neurons of nursing rats, neural activity (e.g., the production of an action potential) is associated with the suckling stimulus. Each action potential generated in these magnoneurosecretory cells in the PVN causes the secretion of a measured quantity of oxytocin, which enhances intramammary pressure and causes maternal milk ejection.

Biosynthesis of ADH and Oxytocin

Both neurohormones are synthesized in bilateral magnocellular (giant neurons) nuclei of the hypothalamus (see Fig. 45–6), ADH in the supraoptic nuclei (SON) and oxytocin in the paraventricular nuclei (PVN). Traveling with neurophysin II in the nonmyelinated supraoptico-hypophysial nerve tract, ADH is directed toward the neurohypophysis and the primary plexus. The paraventriculo-neurohypophysial nerve tract carries oxytocin and neurophysin I into the neurohypophysis and in the proximity of the dorsal motor nucleus of the vagus. The "vasopressinergic" and "oxytocinergic" contents of these pathways show circadian rhythms regarding neurohormone levels independent of those in the peripheral blood. The peripheral concentration of ADH reflects only the secretion of the neurohypophysis in response to stress, blood volume changes, and modification of plasma osmolality, and not the rate of hypothalamic ADH synthesis.

Each neurohormone and its neurophysin are synthesized as prohormones (*pro-pressophysin, pro-oxyphysin*) in the magnocellular bodies. The prohormones, or neurohormone-

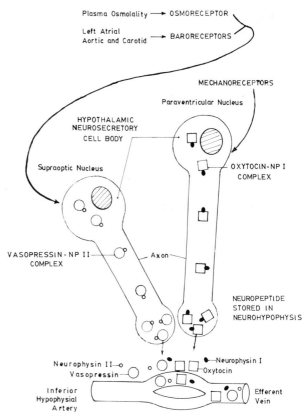

Figure 45–6 Biosyntheses of neurohormones and neurophysins (NP) in magnocellular neurons of the hypothalamus. Syntheses and membrane packaging of neurohormone-neurophysin complexes into granules occur in the body of the neurons. By axonal transport in the nonmyelinated nerve tracts, the granules migrate from the hypothalamic nuclei to the neurohypophysis. The supraopticohypophysial tract carries ADH–neurophysin II, and the paraventriculohypophysial tract oxytocin–neurophysin I. Osmotic, pressure, or mechanic stimuli increase the synthesis of neurohormones. Through depolarization of the neurons in the pars nervosa, the stored granules are released by exocytosis into the peripheral circulation. The capillary plexus contains neurohormones (vasopressin, ○; oxytocin, □) and neurophysins (NP I, ●; NP II, ○).

neurophysin combinations, are transported in membrane-bound vesicles through the axons (less than 1 μm) to the neural lobe of the hypophysis for storage. Processing of the prohormones to the products to be secreted in equimolar amounts (ADH and neurophysin II, oxytocin and neurophysin I) occurs in the vesicles during the course of the axonal migration (see Fig. 45–6).

Cattle, pigs, and mice have a third minor neurophysin (neurophysin C).

Homozygous Brattleboro rats, which are without propressophysin (ADH and its neurophysin), show diabetes insipidus, producing an abundant and dilute (hypoosmotic) urine (i.e., hyposthenuric polyuria (from the Greek, *stenuria*, meaning strength).

Release of ADH or of Oxytocin from the Neurohypophysis

Release by exocytosis of each nonapeptide (octapeptide, if cystine is counted only as one instead of two amino acids) with its neurophysin is calcium dependent and sodium dependent. Influx of extracellular Ca^{++} is necessary for fusion of the neurosecretory vesicle with the plasma membrane at the axon terminals. Calcium channel–blocking agents (e.g., verapamil, nifedipine) inhibit exocytosis of ADH and oxytocin. Depolarization impulses from the hypothalamic magnocellular perikarya require the intracellular influx of Na^+, which is prevented by the sodium channel blocker tetrodotoxin. The neurohypophysial neurons react to cholinergic and to noradrenergic neurotransmitters as well as to several peptides.

Acetylcholine, the synaptic transmitter between the receptors and the magnocellular neurons, stimulates secretion of either ADH or oxytocin. In contrast, alpha-adrenergic agents inhibit the electrical depolarization that triggers the secretion of each hormone, whereas beta-adrenergic agonists (e.g., isoproterenol) cause antidiuresis. Angiotensin II releases ADH (prevented by captopril, a converting enzyme inhibitor) and is dipsogenic. Morphine and some endogenous opioids (beta-endorphins) activate the supraopticoneurohypophysial neurons for exocytosis of ADH. Naloxone, an opiate antagonist, hinders the release of ADH. Endogenous brain prostaglandin E (PGE) favors ADH secretion, whereas indomethacin, by inhibiting the hypothalamic synthesis of PGE, prevents the release of ADH after osmotic stimulation. Halothane anesthesia, and stimulation of arterial chemoreceptors ($PaO_2 < 60$ torr, and higher PCO_2), facilitate ADH release.

Physiological Regulation of ADH Release

ADH maintains a constant blood water concentration by lowering water loss in urine. The neurohypophysial release of ADH is regulated mostly by plasma osmolality and "effective" circulating blood volume. Low blood pressure, hypovolemia, hypoglycemia, angiotensin II, and nausea enhance exocytosis (secretion) of ADH.

Depolarization of osmoreceptors outside of the blood-brain barrier (in the *organum vasculosum* of the *lamina terminalis,* a circumventricular organ), and of the large hypothalamic supraoptic neurons, is caused by an increase in plasma osmolality (less than 2 percent), or by a higher blood sodium or potassium concentration. In contrast, urea or glucose may increase plasma osmolality without stimulating hypothalamic osmoreceptors and increasing the output of ADH. Ingestion of water diminishes the release of ADH.

A 10 percent reduction in the circulating extracellular volume (hemorrhage, shock) causes neurogenic signals, from low-pressure baroreceptors in the atria and high-pressure baroreceptors in the aortic arch, which trigger the neurohypophysial liberation of ADH. Low-pressure receptors are more effective than high-pressure receptors for the release of ADH. Stimulation of low-pressure volume receptors by fluid depletion also lowers the osmotic threshold and augments the osmotic sensitivity for ADH secretion.

Physiological Effects of ADH

In the systemic circulation, the unbound arginine-ADH (lysine-ADH in the pig) has a biological half-life of about 20 minutes. Proteolytic cleavages by peptidases in the liver, brain, and kidneys account for about 75 percent of the metabolic clearance of ADH. The remaining ADH is eliminated in the urine.

Arginine-ADH has comparable vasoconstrictor and antidiuretic activities, which are 100 times that of oxytocin. Generally, addition of 0.1 pg per milliliter of ADH to blood raises urine osmolality by about 30 mOsm per liter, or about $30/300$ (i.e., 10 percent of normal plasma osmolality). In contrast the action of oxytocin on the uterus and on the mammary gland is 20 times greater than that of arginine-ADH. Within the brain, ADH acts as a corticotropin-releasing factor (CRH-like) or enhances the action of CRH, and it functions as a neurotransmitter that facilitates long-term memory.

ADH exerts its effects by binding to V_1 receptors of vascular smooth muscles and to V_2 receptors on renal plasma membranes. By uniting with V_2 receptors, ADH avoids metabolic cleavage, and it stimulates the adenylate cyclase system.

The effects of ADH on medullary renal water and urea as well as on sodium chloride and potassium chloride transport are mediated by intracellular generation of the second messenger cyclic adenine monophosphate (cAMP). ADH binds to specific receptors (V_2) on the basolateral plasma membrane of some medullary renal cells (thick ascending limb of Henle, collecting duct) to activate adenylate cyclase, which then releases cAMP from the cytoplasmic side of the plasma membrane.

> The ADH-V_2-receptor complex activation of adenylate cyclase occurs in two phases: (1) with a guanine nucleotide–binding *regulatory subunit* (N_s) (inhibited by cholera toxin), and (2) with a *catalytic subunit* (C) of adenylate cyclase stimulated by the ADH-V_2-N_s combination.

Through phosphorylation of a cell-specific protein kinase A, cAMP modifies the transport processes at the luminal (apical) plasma membrane of some medullary renal cells. Cytoplasmic vesicles fuse to form microtubule subunits, which are inserted within the apical plasma membrane of those medullary renal cells. Apical membrane transport of *water and urea* in the medullary collecting duct cells, and of *sodium chloride and potassium chloride* in the cells of the medullary thick ascending limb of Henle, can then occur in these additional specialized units of microtubules. The biological action of ADH on kidney cells terminates when it is cleaved by cytosolic phosphodiesterase (PDIE), which is inhibited by theophylline.

The high level of sodium chloride in the medullary interstitium stimulates local interstitial cells to produce PGE_2, which operates two negative-feedback loops against

ADH. PGE$_2$ inhibits sodium chloride absorption in the thick ascending limb of Henle, and it decreases the permeability to free water in the collecting ducts. In contrast, the higher urea level in the interstitium inhibits both PGE$_2$ release, and sodium chloride absorption in the thick ascending limb of Henle (Fig. 45–7).

Diabetes insipidus is a dysfunction of the reabsorption of water (hypoosmotic polyuria) resulting from an insufficient production of ADH (neurohypophysial form) or from an inadequate biochemical response of collecting duct cells to ADH (nephrogenic form). The hypophysial form follows destruction of the supraoptic nucleus in the hypothalamus, of the supraopticoneurohypophysial nerve tract, or of the neurohypophysis.

Physiological Release and Action of Oxytocin

Oxytocin is released from the neurohypophysial vesicles as a result of a *neuroendocrine reflex* that involves a nervous afferent limb and a hormonal efferent limb. Mechanoreceptors in the reproductive tract (vagina, cervix, uterus) and in the teats (nipples) are at the origin of the nervous signals. Distention and touch generate bioelectrical impulses that are relayed in the spinothalamic tract, brain stem, and midbrain before they reach the paraventricular nuclei in the hypothalamus.

Application of a gentle intermittent suction to the nipples of lactating females increases the spontaneous firing rate of almost all the neurons in the PVN. The faster unit firing and concomitant rise in intramammary pressure can serve to demonstrate that the electrical activity of magnocellular hypothalamic neurons correlates with the secretion of a neurohypophysial hormone, oxytocin. An elegant demonstration of the chronological events of this neuroendocrine reflex uses an anesthetized lactating rat during suckling of the pups, since periodic (every 5 to 10 minutes) milk ejection occurs only in somnolent (slow-wave sleep) mothers. The analytical demonstration also requires a recording of the individual evoked depolarization activity at the neurosecretory (magnocellular) hypothalamic cells, a serial measurement of the induced plasma oxytocin levels, the detection of the generated intramammary pressure coinciding with milk-ejection, and observation of the stretching response of the pups at initiation of milk ejection, which usually happens about 15 seconds after the burst of spike potentials (Fig. 45–8).

The magnocellular PVN cells, identified by antidromic stimulation techniques, have a firing rate of about 2 spikes per second (i.e., 2 Hz). In response to sucking by the pups, the neural activity of the maternal PVN cells rises suddenly to about 40 to 50 spikes per second (i.e., 40 to 50 Hz) for about 2 to 4 seconds and then declines exponentially to a period of after-inhibition that is usually less than 1 minute.

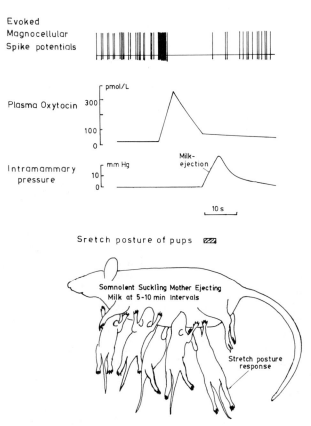

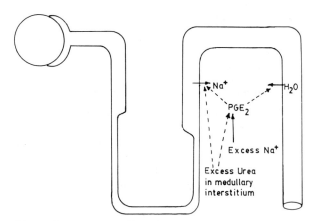

Figure 45–7 The net effect of ADH is antidiuresis (i.e., production of a concentrated urine). The specific action of ADH is to increase the absorption of sodium chloride from the lumen of the ascending loop of Henle into the interstitium, and the permeability of the collecting ducts to water. In the interstitium, the higher sodium chloride concentration has a negative-feedback effect on sodium chloride absorption in the ascending loop of Henle. Components of this negative-feedback loop are urea and PGE$_2$. The latter also makes the collecting ducts less permeable to water.

Figure 45–8 First demonstration of the correlation between electrical activity of hypothalamic magnocellular neurons and the release of oxytocin by the neurohypophysis. Maternal milk ejection, indicated both by a stretch response from the pups and by a rise in intramammary pressure, occurs when the electrical activity of the neurosecretory magnocellular cells is about 40 spikes per second (or 40 Hz), following either suckling or experimental electrical stimulation.

THE HYPOTHALAMIC-HYPOPHYSIS COMPLEX **501**

The sudden burst of neural activity coincides with the secretion of a pulse of oxytocin and precedes by about 15 seconds the simultaneous increase of intramammary pressure and stretch response of the pups.

To release oxytocin, the neurosecretory cells depend on physiologically evoked depolarizations or experimental electrical stimuli occurring at a firing rate exceeding 30 spikes per second (i.e., 30 Hz). The quantity of oxytocin released prior to each milk ejection is about 0.5 mU (i.e., nearly 0.2 percent of the total quantity of oxytocin in the neurohypophysis). Each milk ejection represents the release of about 1 in 1,000 secretory granules. (1 mU oxytocin = 2.2 ng = 2.2 pmol).

The term Ferguson's neurohumoral reflex refers to stimulation of mechanoreceptors in the vagina, cervix, and uterus by mechanical distention. The oxytocic response may be uterotonic (ecbolic, contraction of the uterus) or milk letdown (contraction of myoepithelial cells of the alveoli).

Hypothalamic synthesis of oxytocin is stimulated, and concomitant cholinergic, sodium-dependent, and calcium-dependent processes release oxytocin already stored in vesicles at the extremity of the paraventriculoneurohypophysial nerve tract. Catecholamines prevent the release of oxytocin and inhibit the action of oxytocin that has already been released.

Once oxytocin is in the peripheral blood plasma, it circulates unbound. Its biological half-life is less than 5 minutes, and it is degraded by endopeptidases in liver and kidney cells. In male animals, the blood oxytocin level is comparable with that of females, but its physiological role is not known and may be limited to excitation of hippocampal neurons.

Oxytocin modifies the resting potentials and the excitability threshold of the myometrium of the uterus that has additional oxytocin receptors because of estradiol stimulation. According to its concentration, oxytocin causes the uterus to contract rhythmically (low level) or tonically (high level). With regard to the mammary glands, oxytocin triggers contraction of myoepithelial cells of the alveoli, forcing milk into the lacteal ducts. The action of oxytocin occurs during parturition (expulsion of the fetus and contraction of the umbilical vessels) and during the postparturient period (lactation, and contraction of the uterus for hemostasis).

Pharmacologically, administration of oxytocin is used to induce abortion or parturition in most animals except the sheep. In the mare, foaling occurs within an hour after administration of oxytocin. In the agalactic sow, administration of oxytocin soon establishes lactation.

Production of Luteal Peptides

During the estrous cycle of ruminants, the luteinized granulosa cells produce peptides similar to hypothalamic oxytocin and vasopressin (ADH). Up to the midluteal phase, the active corpus luteum (CL) produces 1,000 times more oxytocin than ADH mRNA and about 250 times more oxytocin mRNA than the hypothalamus. The maximal luteal oxytocin content is about 1 μg per gram of CL in the cow

and 2 μg per gram of CL in the ewe. Thereafter, oxytocin levels decrease and remain low after luteal regression as well as during pregnancy.

Gonadotropins have a stimulating effect on the CL production of oxytocin but do not exert direct control on the output of luteal oxytocin. Insulin-like growth factor (IGF-I) is a potent stimulator of the production of progesterone and of oxytocin by the large luteal cells, which may increase in number by 400 percent during the early luteal phase in the cow. Large luteal cells develop initially from granulosa cells, and later from theca-derived cells. In addition, injection of prostaglandins (cloprostenol, $PGF_{2\alpha}$, PGE_2) causes a significant increase of luteal oxytocin in cows and ewes.

The local effect of oxytocin on the ovary seems to be the delay of synthesis of progesterone during the early luteal phase. Consequently, the life span of the corpus luteum is extended, and the length of the estrous cycle is prolonged. Near the end of the luteal phase, when the effect of progesterone on the uterus is reduced, oxytocin has the opposite effect on the corpus luteum. Oxytocin then induces luteolysis by initiating the release of $PGF_{2\alpha}$ from the uterine endometrium.

MELATONIN, A HORMONE OF THE PINEAL BODY

Situated near the hypothalamus, the pineal body (*epiphysis cerebri*) is a circumventricular organ made up of neuroepithelial (pinealocytes) and glial cells. The usual blood-brain barrier is absent in the pineal and the other periventricular organs (subcommissural organ, subfornical organ, and organum vasculosum of the lamina terminalis). Because of this lack of blood-brain barrier and because of the relatively wide interstitial spaces between their cells, these tissues are easily penetrated by large molecules from blood.

The pineal receives signals from the sympathetic autonomic nervous system, in postganglionic nonmyelinated sympathetic nerve fibers, but is without direct connection with the central nervous system. Capillaries pass in proximity of its true secretory cells, the pinealocytes, which are rich in biogenic amines (norepinephrine, dopamine, serotonin, and histamine). The pineal cells also contain some hypothalamic peptides (e.g., GnRH, TRH, somatostatin, neurophysins with ADH and oxytocin, and an analog of oxytocin called vasotocin). The inhibitory neurotransmitter gamma-aminobutyric acid (GABA) is also found in the pineal, as well as several proteins (e.g., a renin-like enzyme, two proteins that resemble neurophysins, and a protein termed epiphysin). With age, the pineal gland calcifies as deposits of calcium, magnesium, phosphate, and carbonate invest its capsule and septa.

Light impinging upon the retina induces visual and nonvisual responses, the latter affecting the pineal and endocrine regulation. In mammals, the pineal serves as a neuroendocrine transducer, transforming light signals into hormonal signals. The duration of the circadian period of darkness influences the activity of pinealocytes. During the darkness period of a 24-hour interval, pinealocytes are the site of intense metabolic activities involving RNA, enzymes, cAMP, and mostly serotonin.

Through nervous pathways, the lack of photosignals from the retina promotes the release of norepinephrine, which stimulates the uptake of tryptophan, the common precursor of serotonin and melatonin. Norepinephrine also activates the pinealocytes to produce the major indolamine hormone of the pineal *melatonin*. During darkness, this noradrenergic stimulation of postganglionary sympathetic fibers is conducted by the suprachiasmatic nuclei, just above the optic chiasm. The suprachiasmatic nuclei are believed to serve as an internal "clock" (or biological oscillator) that regulates several endogenous endocrine rhythms. A sudden lowering of blood cortisol level (e.g., by administration of metyrapone) also increases the secretion of melatonin.

> The nervous network involves the retina, the optic nerves with the direct retinohypothalamic projection to the suprachiasmatic nuclei, and relays to the adenohypophysiotropic control area of the hypothalamus, to the spinal cord, and to the cranial cervical ganglion.

The decrease in pineal serotonin indicates that it is used for the synthesis of melatonin (Fig. 45–9). Norepinephrine induces the activation of serotonin N-acetyltransferase, with formation of N-acetylserotonin, the first of several enzymatic steps leading to formation of 5-methoxy-N-acetyltryptamine, or melatonin. The pinealocytes probably release melatonin, a very lipid-soluble substance, by diffusion instead of by exocytosis. Nocturnal peak levels of melatonin occur in blood, cerebrospinal fluid, and urine.

The synthesis of melatonin is inhibited by daylight and by beta-adrenergic blocking agents. The release of melatonin is directly inhibited by light. Some of the enzymes involved in the synthesis of melatonin are inactivated by drugs (e.g., actinomycin D, cycloheximide).

The pineal hormone melatonin, transported bound to plasma albumin, is captured by the brain and the gonads. Melatonin operates on the brain to produce drowsiness. In some mammals, melatonin is associated with the inactivity of hibernation. The action of melatonin on the hypothalamus inhibits either or both the secretion and the release of GnRH, with a consequent arrest of LH and FSH secretion by the adenohypophysis. In addition, by stimulating the hypothalamic output of somatostatin, melatonin also inhibits the adenohypophysial release of growth hormone. Melatonin also activates cicatrization of wounds and influences sexual impulses in a complex manner. Administration of melatonin, to mimic the circadian short photoperiods of autumn, advances the onset of the breeding season in sheep.

> In humans, pinealomas, often associated with precocious puberty, occur almost exclusively in males.

It is evident that the daily production of melatonin is higher during the winter than during the summer. This alteration in the output of melatonin, which is associated with changes in the length of daylight and darkness periods during a 24-hour interval, modifies the occurrence of breeding cycles in animals. Melatonin intervenes to restrain or to

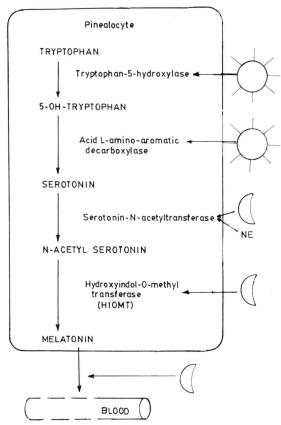

Figure 45–9 In the pinealocyte in diurnal animals, the initial steps in the synthesis of melatonin (N-acetyl-5-methoxytryptamine) are induced by light. The completion of the synthesis, and the transfer of melatonin from the pinealocyte to the peripheral blood, occur in darkness. Norepinephrine is also an activator of serotonin N-acetyltransferase.

stimulate the gonads of different animals under photoperiodic control. It participates in the regulation of sexual development (appearance of puberty) and of sexual function during either spring (long photoperiod: mare) or autumn (short photoperiod: sheep) breeding seasons in animals. In some species (rat, hamster, and mare), melatonin delays puberty, decreases the weight of the ovaries, and reduces the frequency of estrous cycles. In others (sheep and goat), melatonin induces puberty and establishes periodic estrous cycles during autumn (i.e., when periods of daylight become shorter, and those of darkness longer).

> The pineal is involved in the special reproduction of marsupial animals (e.g., wallaby [*Macropus agilis*]), which allow two young at very different stages of maturity to be nursed simultaneously.
> An embryonic diapause, comprising succeeding lactational and seasonal components, suppresses the corpus luteum and maintains the blastocyst in a quiescent state. The lactational diapause is caused by the suckling joey. The seasonal diapause operates through a nervous retinal-cranial cervical ganglion-pineal pathway.

Melatonin is metabolized in the brain, which is permeable to melatonin but not to serotonin, and mostly in the liver, which contains a microsomal enzyme that catalyzes 6-hydroxylation. It is cleared in the urine as an esterified sulfate.

In amphibians, the activity of pineal cells is directly photoreceptive. In batrachians, the action of melatonin is restricted to lightening the color of the skin.

REFERENCES

Antoni F. Hypothalamic control of ACTH secretion: advances since the discovery of 41-residue corticotropin-releasing factor. Endocr Rev 1986;7:351.

Austin CR, Short RV. Reproduction in mammals: 3. Hormonal control of reproduction. 2nd ed. Cambridge: Cambridge University Press, 1984.

Ben-Jonathan N. Dopamine: a prolactin-inhibiting hormone. Endocr Rev 1985;6:654.

Bittman EL, Kaynard AH, Olster DH, Robinson JE, Yellon SM, Karsch FJ. Pineal melatonin mediates photoperiodic control of pulsatile luteinizing hormone secretion in the ewe. Neuroendocrinology 1985;40:409.

Broadwell RD, Oliver C, Brightman MW. Localization of neurophysin within organelles associated with protein synthesis and packaging in the hypothalamoneurohypophysial system: an immunocytochemical study. Proc Natl Acad Sci USA 1979;76:5999.

Brownstein M, Russel JT, Gainer H. Synthesis, transport and release of posterior pituitary hormones. Science 1980;207:373.

Dacheux F. Ultrastructural immunocytochemical localization of prolactin and growth hormone in the porcine pituitary. Cell Tissue Res 1980;207:277.

Dacheux F, Dubois MP. Ultrastructural localization of prolactin, growth hormone, and luteinizing hormone by immunocytochemical techniques in the bovine pituitary. Cell Tissue Res 1976;174:245.

El Etreby MF, Fath El-Bab MR. Localization of gonadotropic hormones in the dog pituitary gland. Cell Tissue Res 1977;183:167.

Enright WJ, Chapin LT, Moseley WM, Zinn SA, Tucker HA. Growth hormone–releasing factor stimulates milk production and sustains growth hormone release in Holstein cows. J Dairy Sci 1986;69:344.

Frohman L. Growth hormone–releasing factor: a neuroendocrine perspective. J Lab Clin Med 1984;103:819.

Gibbs DM, Vale W, Rivier J, Yen SSC. Oxytocin potentiates the ACTH-releasing activity of CRF(41) but not vasopressin. Life Sci 1984;34:2245.

Handler JS, Orloff J. Antidiuretic hormone. Annu Rev Physiol 1981;43:611.

Hart IC, Chadwick PME, James S, Simmonds AD. Effect of intravenous bovine growth hormone or human pancreatic growth hormone–releasing factor on milk production and plasma hormones and metabolites in sheep. J Endocrinol 1985;105:189.

Jackson IMD. Thyrotropin-releasing hormone. N Engl J Med 1982;306:145.

Karsch FJ, Bittman EL, Foster DL, Goodman RL, Legan SJ, Robinson JE. Neuroendocrine basis of seasonal reproduction. Recent Prog Horm Res 1984;40:185.

King JC, Anthony ELP. LHRH neurons and their projections in humans and other mammals: species comparisons. Peptides 1984;5(Suppl 1):115.

Krieger DT. Brain peptides: What, where, and why. Science 1983;222:975.

Lehman MN, Robinson JE, Karsch FJ, Silverman AJ. Immunocytochemical localization of luteinizing hormone–releasing hormone (LHRH) pathways in the sheep brain during anestrus and the midluteal phase of the estrous cycle. J Comp Neurol 1986;244:19.

Li WI, Chen CL, Tiller AA, Kunkle GA. Effects of thyrotropin-releasing hormone on serum concentrations of thyroxine and triiodothyronine in healthy, thyroidectomized, thyroxine-treated, and propylthiouracyl-treated dogs. Am J Vet Res 1986;47:163.

Lincoln DW, Hill A, Wakerley JB. The milk-ejection reflex of the rat: an intermittent function not abolished by surgical levels of anaesthesia. J Endocrinol 1973;57:459.

Lincoln GA, Short RV. Seasonal breeding: nature's contraceptive. Recent Prog Horm Res 1980;36:1.

Nakane PK. Classification of anterior pituitary cell types with immunoenzyme histochemistry. J Histochem Cytochem 1970;18:9.

Page RB. Pituitary blood flow. Am J Physiol 1982;243:E427.

Paull WK, Scholer J, Arimura A, Meyers CA, Chang JK, Chang D, Shimizu M. Immunocytochemical localization of CRF in the ovine hypothalamus. Peptides 1982;1:183.

Reiter RJ. The mammalian pineal gland: structure and function. Am J Anat 1981;62:287.

Renfree MB. Marsupials: alternative mammals. Nature 1981;293:100.

Schams D. Luteal peptides and intercellular communication. J Reprod Fert (Suppl) 1987;34:87.

Smith PF, Luque EH, Neill JD. Detection and movement of secretion from neuroendocrine cells using a reverse hemolytic plaque assay. Methods Enzymol 1986;124:443.

Tamarkin L, Baird CJ, Almeida OFX. Melatonin: a coordinating signal for mammalian reproduction? Science 1985;293:714.

Vale W, Greer M. Corticotrophin-releasing factor. Fed Proc 1985;44:145.

Zimmerman EA, Robinson AG, Husain MK, Acosta MA, Frantz AG, Sawyer WH. Neurohypophysial peptides in the bovine hypothalamus: the relationship of neurophysin I to oxytocin, and neurophysin II to vasopressin, in supraoptic and paraventricular regions. Endocrinology 1974;95:931.

CHAPTER 46

HORMONES OF THE ADENOHYPOPHYSIS

The adenohypophysis (anterior pituitary) secretes six hormones recognized by specific and sensitive radioimmunoassays. They can be grouped into three general categories: corticotropin and related peptides, glycoprotein hormones, and somatomammotropin hormones. Each group has from two to eight individual hormones or products with some hormonal effect (Table 46–1).

This chapter presents the general characteristics of the adenohypophysial hormones secreted by the corticotrope, the gonadotrope, the lactotrope, the thyrotrope, and the somatotrope groups of cells.

CORTICOTROPIN-RELATED, OR ADRENOCORTICOTROPIC, HORMONES

The corticotrope cells of the adenohypophysis synthesize the corticotropin-related peptides as a single precursor molecule, *proopiomelanocortin,* a protein of about 29,000 to 31,000 daltons. This protein gives rise to, or matures into, all the corticotropin-related hormones.

The main steps in the maturation of the 31K precursor molecule, which take place in the adenohypophysis, are

1. Splitting of the 31K precursor into a *high molecular weight form of adrenocorticotropic hormone (ACTH)* (23K) and a molecule of *beta-lipotropic hormone (beta-LPH)* (11.7K), and
2. Cleavage of the 23K molecule into a 16K peptide (*N-terminal*) and the *normal ACTH* (4.5K, 39 amino acids).

Because of this maturation, the peptides of the adrenocorticotropic group originating in the adenohypophysis are ACTH, beta-LPH, and N-terminal.

In the intermediary lobe of the hypophysis, where practically all the neurons are able to synthesize peptides of the adrenocorticotropic group, the maturation process is furthered. ACTH splits into two peptides: *alpha-melanocyte-stimulating hormone (alpha-MSH)* and *corticotropin-like intermediate-peptide* (CLIP). Beta-LPH also divides into two peptides: *gamma-LPH* and *beta-endorphin.* Little is known on the maturation process of N-terminal.

The peptides of the adrenocorticotropic group all are derivatives of the common 31K precursor (Fig. 46–1). The maturation of beta-endorphin into enkephalins (metenkephalin and alpha-endorphin) is still hypothetical.

Since the early 1960s, the existence of different molecular forms of ACTH has inspired studies on the process of ACTH maturation. Immunologic and kinetic tagging techniques have revealed that the product of mRNA translation is a molecule of 31,000 daltons.

The 31K molecule contains a "signal peptide," or "pre-sequence," of 26 amino acids. Once the 31K molecule enters the reticulated endothelium, its "signal peptide" is excised, leaving a molecule termed "pro-sequence" of 250 amino acids, which is later glycosylated in the Golgi complex. During its storage period in the secretory granules, this "pro-sequence," or pro-hormone, matures into all the peptides of the adrenocorticotropic group.

To summarize, the peptides of the ACTH group are
1. *ACTH,* a 39 amino acid molecule found in the center of the 31K precursor. In the adenohypophysis it remains in the 39 amino acid form, but in the intermediate lobe it is transformed into alpha-MSH and CLIP, which are the amino-terminal and the carboxy-terminal parts of ACTH.
2. *Beta-LPH,* which corresponds to the 93 amino acids at the carboxyl-terminal of the 31K precursor. It contains gamma-LPH, beta-MSH, and beta-endorphin. The maturation of beta-LPH into gamma-LPH and into beta-endorphin occurs only in the intermediary lobe. The maturation process of beta-MSH is still unknown.
3. *N-terminal,* or 16K, which represents the amino-terminal part of the 31K. This glycopeptide contains the sequence of gamma-MSH, a peptide of still unproven physiological significance.

Physiological Actions

The corticotropin-related group of hormones includes corticotropic, or adrenocorticotropic, hormone (ACTH); beta-lipotropin (β-LPH); N-terminal; alpha-, beta-, and gamma-melanocortin; and beta-endorphin.

ACTH

The major effects of ACTH are stimulation of steroid (glucocorticoid, mineralocorticoid, and androgenic) secretion from the adrenal cortex. ACTH also stimulates adrenal protein synthesis, which leads to cellular growth and hyperplasia.

ACTH binds to specific receptors on the plasma membrane of adrenocortical cells and activates adenylate cyclase to produce cAMP, which induces the formation of several steroidogenic proteins (enzymes). These enzymes transform cholesterol into pregnenolone, the common precursor of all

TABLE 46–1 Classification of Adenohypophysial Hormones

Groups and Hormones	MW (daltons)	Amino Acids (Number)
CORTICOTROPIN, or ADRENOCORTICOTROPIC, GROUP		
Adrenocorticotropic hormone (ACTH)	4,500	39
alpha-Melanocyte-stimulating hormone (alpha-MSH)	1,800	13
beta-Endorphin	4,000	31
beta-Lipotropic hormone (beta-LPH)	11,200	91–93
beta-MSH	2,000	18
Corticotropin-like intermediate peptide (CLIP)	2,700	21
gamma-MSH	?	
N-Terminal	12,000	80
GLYCOPROTEIN COMPLEX		
Follicle-stimulating hormone (FSH)	29,000	alpha: 92 beta: 118
Luteinizing hormone (LH)	29,000	alpha: 92 beta: 115
Thyroid-stimulating hormone (TSH)	29,000	alpha: 92 beta: 112
SOMATOMAMMOTROPINS		
Growth hormone (GH)	21,800	191
Prolactin (PRL)	22,500	198

corticosteroids. ACTH can thus evoke the production of all types of corticosteroids (i.e., glucocorticoids, mineralocorticoids, and sexual steroids).

Other actions exerted by ACTH are lipolysis in adipose tissue, insulin-releasing effects on the pancreatic B cell, stimulation of growth hormone secretion, acceleration of glucose and amino acid transport into muscles, and prolongation of cortisol half-life in plasma. Its role in the complex dispersion of melanin pigments in melanocytes is less potent than alpha- or beta-MSH. ACTH affects neither behavior nor the central nervous system.

Beta-LPH

In rabbit perirenal adipose tissue, this β-LPH has a weak lipolytic action, which is probably of negligible importance in vertebrates. The importance of beta-LPH seems to lie in its role as a precursor of endorphin. Controversy still persists over whether beta-MSH and gamma-LPH are maturation products of beta-LPH, or simply artifacts.

N-Terminal

A precise role for N-terminal is not definitely recognized, but in humans this peptide seems to increase aldosterone production in adrenal tumors. Physiologically, N-terminal would be a mitotic agent increasing cellular growth in the adrenal cortex.

Alpha-, Beta-, and Gamma-MSH

These three molecules share an almost identical primary chemical nucleus. Their designation is related to their chronological discovery and their homologous structure. Alpha-MSH is a component of ACTH, beta-MSH comes from beta-LPH, and gamma-MSH is a still not isolated segment of N-terminal. All these peptides disperse melanin granules found in the melanophores of amphibians. In mammals, their role is uncertain, and the existence of beta-MSH and gamma-MSH is doubtful.

Beta-Endorphin

In animals, as implied by its name, this peptide acts as an endogenous morphine by binding to the same receptors as morphine. In fact, beta-endorphin has five to ten times more affinity for these receptors than morphine. Interest in this peptide is motivated by its potential to decrease pain and also by the inclusion of a neuropeptide in its structure. This neuropeptide, methionineenkephalin, made up of only five amino acids, is found in various areas of the brain.

Intracerebral (into the cavities or ventricles containing cerebrospinal fluid) injection of beta-endorphin produces a deep general analgesia lasting 3 to 4 hours that is reversible

Figure 46–1 In the corticotropes of the adenohypophysis, prepromelanocortin is at the origin of several peptides. Through successive cleavages, it yields substances that are secreted into plasma: melanocyte-stimulating hormone (gamma-MSH); a joining peptide; ACTH; gamma-lipotropin, or lipotropic hormone (LPH); and beta-endorphins.

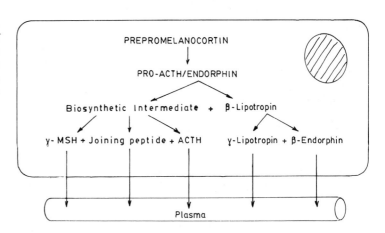

and without any sequelae. The effects of beta-endorphin disappear a few minutes after an intravenous injection of naloxone (narcotic antagonist). Intravenous injection of beta-endorphin (20 mg in a 200-g rat) is without effect, whereas intracerebral injection of 5 to 10 μg in identical subjects induces all the endorphin responses. Clinical use of endorphin has shown the development, as for morphine, of a dependence syndrome. It is recognized that beta-endorphin is not the precursor of enkephalins, contrary to a hypothesis based on studies of the chemical structures of these peptides. Enkephalins are synthesized in the adrenal medulla.

Mechanism of Action of ACTH

ACTH triggers the production of cAMP, through adenylate cyclase, to activate the cellular mechanisms of the adrenal cortex for synthesis of corticosteroids. By binding to the plasma membrane of target cells in the adrenal cortex, ACTH energizes adenylate cyclase in the inner lipid layer to transform ATP into cAMP. As a second messenger, cAMP awakens protein-kinases to cause phosphorylation reactions that activate the enzymes for steroid synthesis.

Blood Level of ACTH

In a healthy animal, the lowest ACTH level is about 10 pg per milliliter of plasma (at night), and the highest is near 50 pg per milliliter (in the morning). Techniques for measurement of ACTH are slow, and expensive to perform and cannot detect levels below 50 pg per milliliter. It is fortunate that the blood level of cortisol (a glucocorticoid), which parallels the ACTH concentration, is ten times higher and much easier to measure. The measurement of ACTH in plasma is difficult. Its assay by a specific antibody represents the sum of the various forms of ACTH circulating in blood, including 31K (precursor) and 23K (high molecular weight) ACTH. The level of cortisol is used as a marker to evaluate ACTH hypophysial secretory activity. However, measurements of both ACTH and cortisol are necessary to determine whether the etiology of a pathologic condition is hypophysial or adrenal.

The appearance of ACTH in blood is not uniform but fluctuates during the day. Its maximum rate of secretion occurs early in the morning, whereas its minimum rate is late in the evening. It is a pulsatile secretion lasting 5 to 10 minutes, occurring every 10 to 25 minutes. The reported half-life of ACTH in plasma varies, with low values of about 3 to 9 minutes and high values between 20 and 25 minutes. Most of it is degraded in the liver and kidneys, a very small amount is utilized by the adrenal cortex. Urine excretion is negligible.

In response to all types of stimulation, beta-LPH, endorphins, and other corticotropin-related peptides are secreted in a ratio equimolar to ACTH. However, the plasma levels of these corticotropin-related peptides are higher than those of ACTH, because of slower metabolic clearance rates.

Control of ACTH Secretion

The regulation of ACTH secretion is related to the activity of the central nervous system (CNS) and of the adrenal cortex.

Influence of the Central Nervous System

The CNS, responsible for the daily metabolic rhythm, influences the production of corticotropin-releasing hormone (CRH) by the hypothalamus. Nonspecific stimuli (stress) and light-darkness cycles modify the activity of the CNS on the hypothalamic neurons that produce the corticotropin-liberating or corticotropin-inhibiting peptides. In animals, a "short-loop" negative feedback causes ACTH to inhibit its own secretion, the retroaction is from the adenohypophysis to the hypothalamus.

The organism is challenged by the nonspecific stimuli of *stress*, which can change circulating ACTH levels. The major ones are physical activity, pain, fever, hypoglycemia, and emotions (depression, anxiety). In these stress situations, the liberation of ACTH is not much influenced by cortisol, except in long-term treatments with glucocorticoids. Prolonged stress greatly disturbs the daily variations in the ACTH secretion rates. A change in the cycle of sleep-activity perturbs the usual daily ACTH secretion rhythm for nearly 7 days.

"Long-loop" Negative Feedback by Cortisol

Cortisol exerts its effects on the CNS and the adenohypophysis. At the hypothalamic level, cortisol inhibits the liberation of CRH. Cortisol also decreases the response of the adenohypophysial target cells to CRH. At this level, cortisol similarly lowers the synthesis of mRNA associated with the assembly of the common precursor (31K molecule) of the adrenocorticotropic group of hormones. Long-term treatments with glucocorticoids may cause involution of the corticotrope cells in the adenohypophysis. In domestic mammals, the intermediary lobe is not influenced by the blood cortisol level.

Evaluation of the Hypophysial-Adrenal Axis

Normally, the adenohypophysis stimulates the adrenal cortex to produce cortisol, which in turn decreases the production of ACTH by a negative feedback. Measurements of cortisol levels should be made on blood samples taken when the ACTH level is high and detectable.

Simultaneous measurements of cortisol and ACTH give a tool for primary evaluation of the workings of the adenohypophysis and of the adrenal cortex. Usually, the results are plotted with the cortisol values on the X-axis, and the ACTH values on the Y-axis. In primary adrenal insufficiency, cortisol values are low and those of ACTH are high (above 300 pg per milliliter.) The high ACTH level is due to the lack of negative feedback by cortisol. In secondary adrenal insufficiency, the levels of both ACTH and cortisol are low (i.e., the adrenal functions normally but is not receiving enough ACTH stimulation). This method cannot differentiate normal animals from animals with adrenal insufficiency. Administration of metyrapone (a drug that inhibits 11-beta-hydroxylase, an enzyme required in cortisol synthesis) elevates the blood levels of 11-deoxycortisol, which does not have a negative-feedback effect on ACTH production, and of ACTH. In animals with deficient adrenals, metyrapone administration only raises ACTH levels in primary adrenal insufficiency, whereas both ACTH and 11-deoxycortisol levels are reduced in secondary adrenal insufficiency.

HYPOPHYSIAL GLYCOPROTEIN HORMONES

Several glycoprotein hormones originate from the adenohypophysis. This group of glycoprotein hypophysial hormones includes TSH and the hypophysial gonadotropins (LH, and follicle-stimulating hormone [FSH]). The structure of this group of hormones is characterized by the presence of two peptidic chains (alpha and beta) or subunits, which are synthesized separately. Each peptidic subunit has branched carbohydrate side chains, which are needed for biological activity and stability in plasma. The biological activity of glycoprotein hormones is linked to the presence of both chains (Fig. 46–2). The isolated subunits are not considered to be biologically active, although the beta-sub-

unit of ovine luteinizing hormone (LH), or lutropin, seems bioactive.

The alpha-chain, nearly identical for all the hormones of the group, is involved in the penetration of the plasma membrane and in the stimulation of adenylate cyclase. The immunologically active beta-chain, which accounts for most of the surface of the hormones, determines the individuality and the specific biological action of each hormone. The presence of cross-species homologies (in the alpha and beta chains) explains the fact that bovine or ovine glycoprotein hormones (e.g., bovine thyroid-stimulating [bTSH] or ovine TSH [oTSH]) are effective in both species.

Thyroid-Stimulating Hormone, or Thyrotropin

Thyroid-stimulating hormone (thyrotropin), synthesized and released from the adenohypophysis after stimulation by thyrotropin-releasing hormone (TRH), binds to plasma membrane receptors (a glycoprotein and a ganglioside) of thyroid cells (Fig. 46–3). TSH then induces production of cAMP, and protein synthesis in the cytoplasm of these cells. It also promotes growth, blood flow, and all the functions of the thyroid gland. E.g., TSH enhances iodine trapping, transport, and binding to protein, and proteolysis of thyroglobulin to release thyroid hormones (thyroxine [T_4] and triiodothyronine [T_3]) in the blood. Fetal TSH production is essential, since maternal TSH cannot cross the fetomaternal border to reach the fetal thyroid cells.

The secretion of TSH is relatively stable (changing in terms of several hours rather than minutes) compared with

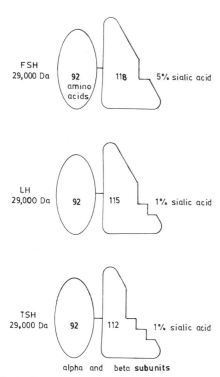

Figure 46–2 Diagrammatic representation of the similarity of the alpha subunits in the three adenohypophysial glycoprotein hormones. The specific biological activity of each hormone is provided by the glycosylated beta subunits. The isolated subunits have no intrinsic biological activity.

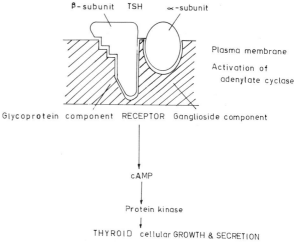

Figure 46–3 The basolateral aspect of the plasma membrane of follicular cells of the thyroid contains specific receptors for TSH (100 receptors per cell). The ganglioside component of the receptor binds with the alpha subunit of the TSH molecule, whereas the glycoprotein component unites with the beta subunit of the hormone. Activation of adenylate cyclase near the cytoplasmic surface of the plasma membrane induces production of cAMP from ATP. The second messenger stimulates protein kinase and results in the production of cellular growth, secretion of iodotyrosines, thyroglobulin, peptidases, and the release of metabolic thyroid hormones into the general circulation.

the fluctuations in output of growth hormone and corticotropin. This stability is the result of a balance of stimulation by TRH and inhibition by thyroid hormones (mostly T_3), which also decrease the hypothalamic production of TRH. In a typical negative-feedback loop, the thyrotrope is very sensitive to minute increases or decreases in plasma thyroid levels, which can suppress or stimulate TRH and, consequently, TSH secretion.

In animals, a decrease in the secretion of TSH occurs during starvation (to lower the metabolic rate) and after an increase in the levels of the adenohypophysial growth hormone, of the hypothalamic peptide somatostatin, of the neurotransmitter dopamine, and of cortisol from the adrenal cortex. The levels of TSH are raised upon exposure to cold (to increase thermogenesis) and at night. The half-life of TSH is about 75 to 80 minutes.

In hypothyroidism, when there is chronic deficiency of thyroid hormones, the plasma concentration of TSH is high and may be 10 to 15 times greater than the normal value, which is about 3 to 6 μU per milliliter. Conversely, in hyperthyroidism, when the thyroid hormones are in excess, the plasma TSH level is lower.

Hypophysial Gonadotropins

In female and male animals, FSH and LH are synthesized and released from the adenohypophysis upon stimulation by hypothalamic gonadotropin-releasing hormone (GnRH). The *basal,* or tonic, output of FSH and LH is *pulsatile* (with modulation of frequency and amplitude of the pulses) during most of the reproductive life of females and males. However, in females, a *massive surge of LH,* which is associated with ovulation, is produced by a precise and intricate positive-feedback cascade.

The basal pulsatile secretion of FSH regulates follicular growth in females and controls spermatogenesis in males. The synthesis and release of FSH is under the negative feedback of *inhibin* (glycosylated A-chain and B-chain polypeptides united by disulfide bonds) and of sustained high plasma levels of estradiol. A rise in progesterone enhances the output of GnRH, stimulating the production of FSH. LH synthesis and release are not influenced by inhibin. The basal pulsatile output of LH functions mainly for maintenance of follicular luteinization in the ovulated female. In the male, tonic LH stimulates the interstitial (Leydig) cells of the testicles to produce testosterone. The basal pulsatile secretion of LH is regulated by GnRH, which is kept in check by the negative feedback of gonadal steroids (mostly estradiol). The GnRH/LH surge near ovulation is associated with the positive feedback of high estradiol levels. Both gonadotropin hormones initiate and maintain the reproductive processes in females and contribute to the periodical event known as the estrous cycle.

The Estrous Cycle

In most animal species, the estrous cycle recurs every 3 weeks throughout the year (e.g., cow and sow) or seasonally (e.g., spring, or long-day, breeders: mare). Shorter estrous cycles occur throughout the year in rodents (5 days in rat and mouse) and seasonally (fall, or short-day, breeders) in small ruminants (17 days).

In primates, the cyclical events in the reproductive organs terminate with menstruation (shedding of the uterine endometrium and accompanying bleeding), which recurs at about 28 days.

> In primates, the functions of the reproductive tract also involve an additional glycoprotein, *chorionic,* or *placental, gonadotropin* (e.g., hCG, which has effects similar to the adenohypophysial LH).

The seasonal appearance of gonadotropins affecting the reproductive cycles is linked with the duration of the daylight and darkness periods, the latter influencing the production of melatonin by the pineal. Besides the length of the daylight and darkness periods, other factors in the external environment influence the secretion of gonadotropins: temperature, odors (pheromones), availability of food, sighting of receptive subjects of the opposite sex, and sounds produced by these receptive subjects. Factors in the "internal" environment (such as body metabolism, weight, and fat) also modify the secretion of gonadotropins.

Phases. The estrous cycle is divided into two phases, with each depending on the growth of tissues and the production of steroids by the ovaries. The follicular phase is marked by follicular growth and an increased secretion of estradiol. The subsequent luteal phase is characterized by the growth of the corpus luteum and the secretion of progesterone (Fig. 46–4).

The *follicular phase* includes the proestrus and the estrus parts of the estrous cycle. During *proestrus,* the corpus luteum degenerates, the circulating progesterone level decreases, and primary follicles gradually develop in the ovary. *Estrus* is a *behavioral* period of female receptivity to the advances of the male, with an increase in physical activity near ovulation time (rupture of the mature follicles). It is not seen in human females but occurs in nonhuman primates.

The *luteal phase* comprises the other two parts of the estrous cycle: metestrus and diestrus. *Metestrus* follows ovula-

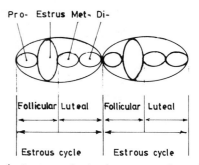

Figure 46–4 In most animals, the estrous cycle can be divided into four periods: proestrus, estrus, metestrus, and diestrus. Proestrus and estrus are parts of the follicular growth phase, or follicular phase, during which LH promotes the production of androgens and their conversion into estrogens. Metestrus and diestrus occupy the luteal phase, during which FSH and progesterone are the predominant hormones.

tion except in the cow, in which ovulation occurs during metestrus and is devoted to the development of the corpus luteum. In *diestrus,* the established and very active corpus luteum secretes progesterone.

Physiological Actions

Interactions between ovaries, adenohypophysis, and hypothalamus are essential for the transformation of each primary ovarian follicle into a mature follicle, which ruptures (ovulates) and eventually yields an ovum. During proestrus and estrus, the basal level of FSH promotes the secretion of estradiol by the granulosa cells as well as growth and maturation of the ovarian follicles. Simultaneously, the basal production of LH activates the internal theca cells to turn out more androgens, which are destined to be transformed into more estradiol by the granulosa cells. The consequent drastic rise in the circulating estradiol level enhances the hypothalamic output of GnRH and results in a higher hypophysial production of both FSH and LH, a rare example of a *positive feedback.* LH is also known as the ovulatory hormone, since a sudden massive surge of LH, very different from the basal or tonic LH production, accompanies ovulation. This surge of LH is associated with ovulation, whether the latter is spontaneous (in most animal species) or is a reflex to mating (e.g., cat, ferret, rabbit, 13-lined ground squirrel, and vole).

After ovulation, during metestrus and diestrus, the basal secretion of FSH and LH causes the granulosa cells to proliferate and to undergo structural and biochemical changes that lead them to produce large amounts of both estradiol and progesterone. However, a sustained elevation of the blood estradiol (E_2) concentration decreases the adenohypophysial basal output of FSH, an usual *negative feedback.*

Doubts still surround the relationship between the release of gonadotropins and the blood levels of ovarian steroids, E_2 and progesterone (P_4). One of the hypotheses used to explain the production of hypophysial gonadotropins by GnRH stimulation is based on the estradiol blood level. When estradiol levels are high, GnRH favors production of LH instead of FSH. During the follicular phase, near the time of ovulation, an elevated estrogen concentration triggers a short burst of GnRH, triggers a sudden surge or maximal output of LH, and progressively decreases the basal production of FSH. Anesthetic agents (e.g., ketamine hydrochloride, pentobarbital sodium, urethane, alpha-chloralose, phencyclidine hydrochloride, alphaxalone) block the hypothalamic neurons that produce this sudden surge of GnRH and of adenohypophysial LH.

In the male, the absence of ovaries rather than the neonatal exposure to androgens, which would anatomically modify the brain and hypothalamus, explains the lack of LH surge and insensitivity to high estradiol levels. This is supported by the appearance of such a LH surge in castrated males after injection of estradiol.

In contrast, high progesterone and low estrogen levels support a hypothalamic output of GnRH, giving a higher priority to FSH production than to LH. Following ovulation,

the quantity of progesterone in blood increases and reflects the progressive transformation of follicular cells into luteal cells. During the luteal phase, the abundance of progesterone induces the hypophysis to produce FSH for the next cycle.

This simple explanation of the complex mechanism that regulates the estrous cycle presumes that each of the two adenohypophysial gonadotropins is influenced by the circulating plasma levels of estrogens and progesterone. A complicating factor is the production of gonadal proteins (activin, inhibin), which exert an influence on the release of hypophysial FSH. *Inhibin,* a protein from the gonads (ovary and testicle), selectively inhibits hypophysial FSH secretion in females and males (Fig. 46–5).

A different mechanism explains the regression of the corpus luteum, and the beginning of another cycle, in the event of lack of pregnancy. An eicosanoid (prostaglandin) synthesized in the uterus is the luteolytic hormone *luteolysin* (Fig. 46–6). This eicosanoid, prostaglandin $F_{2\alpha}$, constricts the uteroovarian vessels and causes corpus luteum ischemia, which interferes with the synthesis of progesterone. The eicosanoid also competes with LH for available receptors on the corpus luteum or destroys the LH receptors.

In humans and some other species of animals, the production of gonadotropins and ovulation are blocked by suckling or high concentrations of prolactin. The probable mechanism is inhibition of the release of GnRH or reduction of the responsiveness of the adenohypophysis to GnRH.

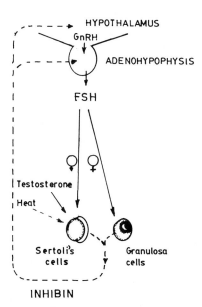

INHIBIN

Glycoprotein (a-ß), 31 amino acids, 32,000 Da, unbound in plasma

Figure 46–5 The output of FSH by the gonadotrope is specifically depressed by inhibin, an unbound glycoprotein hormone originating from the gonads (ovarian follicles, Sertoli's cells of the testes). Testosterone increases the production of inhibin, whereas the application of heat to the testis lessens the output of inhibin by the Sertoli's cells.

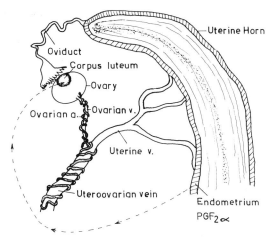

Figure 46–6 In ruminants, near the end of diestrus, the production of prostaglandin F$_{2\alpha}$ by the endometrium of the nonpregnant uterus has a luteolytic effect on the corpus luteum. Luteolysis, brought about by vasoconstriction of the luteal arterioles, terminates the production of progesterone by the corpus luteum during an estrous cycle. To exert this negative-feedback effect, PGF$_{2\alpha}$ is transferred from the utero-ovarian vein to the ovarian artery, a process facilitated by the intimate contact between the two sets of blood vessels.

ADENOHYPOPHYSIAL SOMATOMAMMOTROPIC HORMONES

The somatomammotropic hormones include growth hormone (GH) and prolactin (PRL). Both hormones display intrinsic growth-promoting and lactogenic activities. The globular structure of PRL and of GH is very similar (Fig. 46–7), but their amino acid homology is very limited (about 15 percent).

In most cases, PRL and GH are stored in and released from separate cells: the adenohypophysial somatotrope cells secrete GH and the mammotrope, or lactotrope, cells produce PRL. However, in a minority of cases, both hormones can be secreted by the same cell. Interconversion from one cell type to the other seems possible, as both PRL and GH genes may be derived from a common ancestral gene.

> In a lactating cow, and in a virgin cow, a population of multinucleated cells of the bovine adenohypophysis was found to contain both PRL and GH in separate granules. However, in a few of these multinucleated somatomammotropes, PRL and GH were *colocalized* in the same granules.

Growth Hormone

The growth hormone (GH) protein (191 amino acids, about 21,800 daltons), which shows considerable variation in structure from species to species, is secreted by the adenohypophysial somatotrope cells after stimulation by growth hormone–releasing hormone (GHRH, or GRH). The circa-

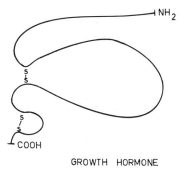

GROWTH HORMONE

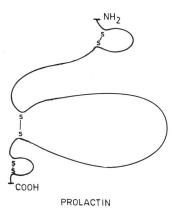

PROLACTIN

Figure 46–7 Diagrammatic illustration of the structural similitude of the two adenohypophysial somatomammotropins GH and PRL. Each polypeptide chain is folded to form a globular shape, and the folds are connected by disulfide bridges.

dian secretion of GH fluctuates according to stimulating and inhibiting influences.

Exercise, fasting (hypoaminoacidemia, hypoglycemia), sleep, and stress are factors that increase GH output. Estradiol, insulin, and some peptidic hormones (ACTH, antidiuretic hormone [ADH], alpha-MSH) enhance the output of GH. Neurotransmitter substances that stimulate production of GH include alpha-adrenergic agonists (clonidine), beta-adrenergic antagonists (propranolol), dopaminergic agonists (apomorphine, bromocriptine, L-dopa), gamma-aminobutyric acid (GABA) agonists (muscimol), and serotonin precursors (5-hydroxytryptamine).

In contrast, GH secretion is inhibited by production of somatostatin (SS, SRIF), which occurs with elevated plasma free fatty acids, glucocorticoids, or postprandial hyperglycemia. Other hormones that also have a suppressive action on GH secretion include progesterone and somatomedin C, or insulin-like growth factor I (IGF-I). Some neurotransmitters also repress the output of GH; for example, alpha-adrenergic antagonists (phentolamine), beta-adrenergic agonists (isoproterenol), cholinergic (muscarinic) antagonists (pirenzepine), dopamine antagonists (phenothiazines), and serotonergic antagonists (methysergide).

GH operates on all cells in the body through a GH-dependent growth factor found in several tissues, but primarily in the liver. The most important of these factors is *IGF-I*, which was formerly called somatomedin C or somatomedin A. Other growth factors are not GH dependent, including epidermal growth factor (EGF) (the former somatomedin B); erythropoietin; estromedins; fibroblast growth factor (FGF), which is also known as insulin-like growth factor II (IGF-II) or platelet-derived growth factor (PDGF); glial growth factor (GGF); mammary growth factor; nerve growth factor (NGF); ovarian growth factor (OGF); thymosin; and transforming growth factor (TGF).

GH binds to specific plasma membrane receptors to stimulate IGF-I production, which is even considered to be a GH second messenger rather than a true hormone. GH and IGF-I are needed for cell differentiation and growth. GH directs the precursor cell to a specific pathway of differentiation, and IGF-I enhances growth and replication by either or both autocrine and paracrine effects. The production of IGF-I is also increased by insulin and hyperproteinemia but is inhibited by estradiol and by glucocorticoids.

IGF-I (somatomedin C or somatomedin A), a peptide of about 7,500 daltons, is reminiscent of insulin by its structural resemblance to proinsulin and by its binding to insulin receptors. On receptors present in many tissues (liver, cartilage), IGF-I seems to have an autocrine action (same cell for synthesis and action) and a paracrine action (cell for synthesis is adjacent to cell for action).

GH regulates linear growth and metabolic processes, stimulates hypertrophy of cardiac and renal cells, induces production of specific hormones (renin, aldosterone), and promotes conversion of thyroxine to T_3. The effects of GH that are mediated by IGF-I or somatomedin include chondrogenesis, cellular differentiation and proliferation, and protein synthesis. In contrast, cellular uptake of amino acids, erythropoiesis, insulinogenesis, and lipolysis are direct actions of GH (i.e., not mediated by IGF-I). Besides contributing much IGF-I, the liver participates in rapid metabolism of GH, which has a half-life of about 25 min.

The effects of GH administration include

1. *Acute effects.* GH increases amino acid uptake and incorporation into protein, stimulates synthesis of new RNA, and enhances glucose utilization. GH antagonizes the lipolytic effects of catecholamines in adipose tissues.
2. *Delayed effects* (after 3 to 4 hours, or diabetogenic effects). GH enhances triglyceride lipolysis and inhibits glucose uptake and utilization secondary to impaired pyruvate decarboxylation.
3. *Multiphasic effect on insulin secretion.* GH produces acute direct stimulation of the pancreatic B-cell, a subsequent inhibitory effect, and a late and persistent stimulation of insulin release that occurs secondary to the impairment of carbohydrate utilization.

Bovine somatotropin (BST), a term for synthetic bovine growth hormone (bGH), has been produced by biotechnology. In ruminants, administration of BST causes a galactopoietic response; that is, it increases milk production or yield (up to 20 percent) without affecting milk composition (milk fat, protein, or lactose) or feed intake. Similarly, repeated daily intravenous administration of GHRH produces a galactopoietic response in cows, goats, and ewes. It is particularly effective in reducing the rate of decline in milk yield after peak production is attained. In cows, BST also prevents a decrease in milk yield due to heat stress. In ewes and cows, since GH has no direct effect on mammary cells, the galactopoietic action of GH is mediated through an extramammary intermediary (IGF-I, also called somatomedin C, and identical to somatomedin A). The situation is different in goats, in which the increased milk yield is a consequence of increased blood flow to the mammary gland. The administration of GH must nevertheless affect the mammary cells, granting them priority in the nutrient-partitioning phenomenon among competing tissues. This is in conformity with homeorhesis or homeorhetic controls (long-term regulation of nutrient-partitioning), which alter and coordinate the responsiveness of growing tissues to homeostatic signals.

Growth hormone enhances the linear growth of bones and anabolism of proteins in young animals. In swine, this positive protein balance effect may lead to the formation of larger-size animals with increased body mass, yielding more meat with a lower fat content.

In cats and dogs, the prepuberal (i.e., before closure of the epiphyses) excess of GH and IGF-I results in *gigantism* of long bones. When chronic excess of GH occurs after closure of the epiphyses (postpuberal), the result is *acromegaly,* a condition consisting of enlarged extremities, enlarged liver (hepatomegaly), and hyperglycemia (diabetes mellitus). In contrast, a deficiency in GH and IGF-I produces *dwarfism,* which is often complicated by metabolic and cutaneous problems arising from an associated lack of ACTH and TSH.

Prolactin

The lactotrope cells in the lateral part of the adenohypophysis secrete prolactin (PRL), a single-chain, folded polypeptide (198 amino acids) that circulates in three major forms: "big-big" (100,000 daltons), "big" (50,000 daltons), and "little" (22,500 daltons). The low molecular weight form accounts for about 80 percent of the total PRL.

The secretion of prolactin is under tonic inhibitory control by dopamine, the prolactin-inhibiting hormone (PIH). Blood prolactin levels fluctuate, with about 6 pulses per day. Exercise, sleep, stress, and hypoglycemia bring about physiological changes in the output of PRL. During the estrous cycle, the high plasma level of estradiol induces the preovulatory surge of gonadotropins (LH and FSH) by the adenohypophysial gonadotropes. A paracrine action of the gonadotropes stimulates the lactotropes to produce also a surge of PRL.

In all animals, lactation and suckling are associated with high plasma levels of prolactin. In ewes, the plasma concentration of PRL is low during the breeding season but high during the period of anestrus in response to daylight. In the cow, the secretion of prolactin increases with day length and temperature.

Dopaminergic antagonists (butyrophenones, phenothiazines, metoclopramide) promote the formation of pro-lactin. A similar stimulative action on PRL secretion is exercised by catecholamine depletors and synthesis inhibitors (alpha-methyldopa, reserpine), GABA agonists (muscimol), histamine H_2 antagonists (cimetidine), opiates (enkephalin analogues, morphine), and serotonin precursors (5-HTP). Estradiol, TRH, TSH, and vasoactive intestinal peptide (VIP) can also pharmacologically contribute to increase the secretion of PRL.

The dopamine agonists (apomorphine, bromocriptine, L-dopa) stimulate dopamine receptors and inhibit the secretion of PRL. Prolactin enhances the hypothalamic secretion of dopamine, which inhibits the adenohypophysial secretion of PRL; that is, PRL produces a negative-feedback loop to inhibit its own secretion. The output of PRL is reduced by serotonin antagonists (methysergide) and by thyroxine. Hyperglycemia and glucocorticoids also suppress the secretion of PRL.

Prolactin receptors are present on the plasma membrane of mammary, liver, kidney, adrenal cortex, heart, brain, and gonad cells. The liver, more than the kidneys, takes care of removing PRL from plasma. The half-life of PRL is about 50 minutes.

In females, the most obvious roles of PRL are to start the differentiation of mammary gland cells into producers of milk proteins and constituents and to initiate and maintain lactation. The function of PRL in male animals is unknown; it may consist of an action on the testis to enhance the activity of LH and to stimulate production of testosterone.

During pregnancy, in conjunction with estradiol, progesterone, and placental lactogen, PRL levels rise constantly, stimulating the growth of the secretory elements of the mammary glands. Following parturition, the abrupt decrease in estradiol and progesterone (derived from the placenta) and the maximal high levels of PRL permit initiation of lactation. Once lactation is initiated, the maximal PRL secretion (about 10 to 15 times the normal level) gradually declines as lactation progresses. Prolactin is required to maintain lactation and to provoke the synthesis of milk constituents, including lactalbumin, casein, lipids, and carbohydrates.

In primates and rodents, hyperprolactinemia of lactation prevents the liberation of GnRH, together with gonadotropins, and the return of the reproductive cycles.

REFERENCES

Clarke IJ, Cummins JT. The temporal relationship between gonadotropin-releasing hormone (GnRH) and luteinizing hormone (LH) secretion in ovariectomized ewes. Endocrinology 1982;111:1737.

Dacheux F. Ultrastructural immunocytochemical localization of prolactin and growth hormone in the porcine pituitary. Cell Tis Res 1980;207:277.

Denef C, Andries M. Evidence for paracrine interaction between gonadotrophs and lactotrophs in pituitary cell aggregates. Endocrinology 1983;112:813.

Dufy-Barbe L, Franchimont P, Faure JMA. Time course of LH and FSH release after mating in the female rabbit. Endocrinology 1973;92:1318.

Eigenmann JE. Acromegaly in the dog. Vet Clin North Am (Small Anim Pract) 1984;14:827.

Eigenmann JE, Patterson DF. Growth hormone deficiency in the mature dog. J Am Anim Hosp Assoc 1984;20:744.

Farnworth ER, Kramer JKG. Fat metabolism in growing swine: a review. Can J Anim Sci 1987;67:301.

Foxcroft GR, Hunter MG. Basic physiology of follicular maturation in the pig. J Reprod Fertil (Suppl) 1985;30:1.

Froesch ER, Schmid C, Schwander J, Zapf J. Action of insulin-like growth factors. Annu Rev Physiol 1985;47:443.

Fumagalli G, Zanini A. In cow anterior pituitary, growth hormone and prolactin can be packed in separate granules of the same cell. J Cell Biol 1985;100:2019.

Gosselin SJ, Capen CC, Martin SL, Targowski SP. Biochemical and immunological investigations on hypothyroidism in dogs. Can J Comp Med 1980;44:158.

Grollman EF, Lee G, Ambesi-Impiombato FS, Meldolisi MF, Aloj SM, Coon HG, Kaback HR, Kohn LD. Effects of thyrotropin on the thyroid cell membrane: hyperpolarization induced by hormone-receptor interaction. Proc Natl Acad Sci 1977;74:2352.

Guillemin R, Vargo T, Rossier J, Minick S, Ling N, Rivier C, Vale W, Bloom F. Beta-endorphin and adrenocorticotropin are secreted concomitantly by the pituitary gland. Science 1977;197:1368.

Isaksson OGP, Eden S, Jansson JO. Mode of action of pituitary growth hormone on target cells. Annu Rev Physiol 1985;47:483.

Kalfelz FA. Observations on thyroid gland function in dogs: response to thyrotropin and thyroidectomy and determination of thyroxine secretion rate. Am J Vet Res 1973;34:535.

Kesner JS, Leung K, Convey EM. Effect of milking and ambient temperature on thyrotropin concentration in serum of cattle. Proc Soc Exp Biol Med 1979;161:38.

Knobil E. On the control of gonadotropin secretion in the rhesus monkey. Recent Prog Horm Res 1974;30:1.

Matsushita N, Kato Y, Shimatsu A, Katakami H, Hanaihara N, Imura H. Effects of VIP, TRH, GABA, and dopamine on prolactin release from superfused rat anterior pituitary cells. Life Sci 1983;32:1263.

Miller WL, Eberhardt NL. Structure and evolution of the growth hormone gene family. Endocr Rev 1983;4:97.

Moudgal NR, Li CH. Beta-subunits of human choriogonadotropin and ovine lutropin are biologically active. Proc Natl Acad Sci 1982;79:2500.

Peel CJ, Bauman DE. Somatotropin and lactation. J Dairy Sci 1987;70:474.

Quinlan WJ, Michaelson S. Homologous radioimmunoassay for canine thyrotropin: response of normal and X-irradiated dogs to propylthiouracil. Endocrinology 1981;108:937.

Reimers TJ, Concannon PW, Cowan RG. Changes in serum thyroxine and cortisol in dogs after simultaneous injection of TSH and ACTH. J Am Anim Hosp Assoc 1982;18:923.

Seidah NG, Rochemont J, Hamelin J, Lis M, Chretien M. Primary structure of the major pituitary pro-opiomelanocortin NH2-terminal glycopeptide. J Biol Chem 1981;256:7977.

Walton JS, McNeilly JR, McNeilly AS, Cunningham FJ. Changes in blood levels of prolactin, LH, FSH, and progesterone during anoestrus in the ewe. J Endocrinol 1977;75:127.

Webb R, Lamming GE. Patterns of plasma prolactin in postpartum suckled cows. J Endocrinol 1981;90:391.

CHAPTER 47

THYROID METABOLIC HORMONES

Found in all vertebrates, the thyroid gland is unique in being entirely endocrine, producing only hormones. These hormones contribute to regulating the metabolic rate of tissues and to the phosphorus-calcium metabolism. The iodinated metabolic thyroid hormones (*thyroxine and tri-iodothyronine*) are produced by the follicular cells bordering each of the millions of follicles. These follicular cells are polarized to secrete toward the lumen of the spherical follicles. In addition to these follicular cells, the thyroid also carries another type of cell, the C-cells, or *parafollicular cells,* which produce *calcitonin,* or thyrocalcitonin, the hypocalcemic hormone. These C-cells, found in the follicular wall or in the interfollicular spaces, are polarized to secrete toward the interfollicular capillaries.

This chapter presents the iodinated hormones that are related to the amino acid tyrosine and synthesized in the thyroid gland: tetraiodothyronine (T_4) and triiodothyronine (T_3). Calcitonin is discussed with the regulation of calcium, which also involves parathormone, secreted by the parathyroid glands.

DEVELOPMENT OF THE THYROID GLAND

The embryonic development of the thyroid gland is similar in all species. Since the thyroid is derived from the gastrointestinal tract, it shares several similarities with salivary glands, especially the ability to concentrate iodine. The *glandular body* of the thyroid develops from an invagination of the pharynx, which also forms a transitory *thyroglossal conduit.* About one of two adult dogs have accessory thyroid tissue located mostly in the fat on the intrapericardiac aorta, but also anywhere in the mediastinum from the larynx to the diaphragm. Some developmental anomalies of the thyroglossal conduit have a clinical importance in dogs, pigs, and occasionally other animals.

From the thyroglossal conduit, functional thyroid tissue may develop in the ventral aspect of the root of the tongue. When such thyroid tissue is present, it is often the *only* tissue able to synthesize thyroid hormones, and its removal results in hypothyroidism because of the prompt increase in hypophysial thyrotropin (TTH) or thyroid-stimulating hormone (TSH). Frequently, remnants of the thyroglossal conduit evolve into functional cysts or into thyroid tissues that migrate into the mediastinum. In such cases, the thyroid gland remains nonetheless functional.

It is essential that fetal thyroid tissue be active because maternal thyroid hormones cannot cross the placental barrier. Fetal thyroid hormones are required for the proper development of the lungs and of the nervous system, as well as for normal growth and bone maturation in young animals.

In humans, the absence of thyroid hormone during this period results in irreversible mental retardation, a syndrome known as *cretinism.* Measurement of plasma thyroxine is used for early detection of neonatal hypothyroidism.

Morphology

In most species, the thyroid gland, which has two lobes connected by an isthmus, is located laterally on the cranial part of the trachea. In the pig, the thyroids are located much lower on the trachea, near its entrance into the thoracic cavity. In neonate dogs and cats, the isthmus disappears before weaning. An abundant conjunctive tissue encases the gland, and in several animal species, it also encloses the parathyroid glands. The recurrent laryngeal nerves are located between the thyroid lobes and the trachea.

The second best nourished gland (after the adrenal glands), the thyroid receives blood at a rate of 5 mL per minute per gram of tissue. The thyroid gland is irrigated by the cranial thyroid arteries, a ramification of the external carotid arteries, and the caudal thyroid arteries, branching from the subclavian arteries (Fig. 47–1). An extensive network of inter- and intrafollicular capillaries provides an abundant blood supply to the *structural and functional units for secretion of the metabolic thyroid hormones*—the follicles (diam.: 20 to 250 μm). A copious supply of lymphatic fluid, rich in iodinated proteins, ensures a large iodine supply. The sympathetic innervation originates from the cervical ganglion and terminates near the basal membrane of the follicles and in the wall of the arterial vessels. The parasympathetic nerves reach the thyroid via the recurrent laryngeal nerve and contribute to regulation of thyroid blood circulation.

The histologic structure of the thyroid is unique for an endocrine gland. Each of the 20 to 30 million spherical *follicles* contains a central lumen filled with a secretion representing a storage form of T_4 and T_3 called *colloid* (consisting mostly of thyroglobulin) produced by the surrounding wall or epithelium of cuboidal (follicular) cells. It must be signaled that the synthesis of the thyroid hormone occurs extracellularly, within the follicular lumen (Fig. 47–2).

> When the follicles are *active,* they have rectangular bordering epithelial cells and a scanty volume of colloid. When the follicles are *inactive,* they have flattened epithelial cells and an abundance of colloid. Evaluation of thyroid activity on the basis of these morphological criteria is risky, since several regions of the gland show simultaneously different degrees of activity.

The cellular epithelium of each follicle rests on a basal membrane that separates follicles from capillaries. A septum may enclose from 20 to 40 follicles to form a *thyroid lobule.* The secretion of the metabolic hormones by the follicular

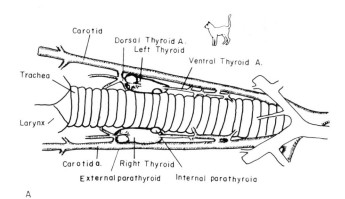

A

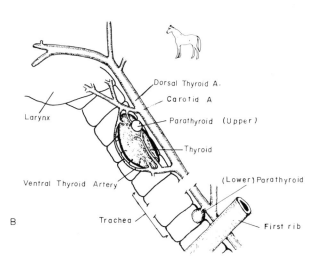

B

Figure 47–1 The oval-shaped thyroid gland is situated on both sides of the first segments of the trachea. **A,** Both the upper and the lower feline parathyroids are on the external and internal aspects of each thyroid gland. **B,** In the horse, only the upper parathyroids are contiguous to the thyroid, since the lower parathyroids are found near the entrance of the trachea into the thorax.

cells of the thyroid gland is controlled by the adenohypophysis in most vertebrates and even by the hypothalamus in higher vertebrates.

The assembly of the thyroid hormones within the follicular lumen is made possible by a special protein, the *prothyroid hormone* called *thyroglobulin*, which is synthesized only by the follicular cells. The raw materials (tyrosine and other amino acids, and carbohydrates such as mannose, fructose, and galactose) for the synthesis of thyroglobulin are derived from plasma. From the plasma, the follicular cells also trap iodide (I^-), concentrate it, then actively and rapidly transport it into the follicular lumen, and oxidize it to iodine (I_2) with a peroxidase found in the extracytoplasmic microvilli of their apical plasma membrane (Fig. 47–3). Thyrotropin, or thyroid-stimulating hormone (TSH), which binds to the basilar aspect of the follicular cell, activates adenylate cyclase and increases the rate of the biochemical reactions for synthesis and for release of the thyroid hormones into the circulation. The thyroid hormones act on many types of tissues (skeletal and cardiac muscles, liver, kidney) by entering into the target cells and binding to a cytosolic receptor protein.

An important action of TSH is to induce the formation of numerous cytoplasmic pseudopodia at the apical membrane. By endocytosis, these pseudopodia engulf some of the follicular colloid and bring it into the cytoplasm of follicular cells, which release the preformed hormones through the plasma membrane at their basal aspect.

In contrast, by repressing the output of thyrotropin-releasing hormone (hypothalamic) and of thyrotropin (adenohypophysis), an excess of thyroid hormones causes an enlargement of the follicles and an involution of the follicular cells.

IODINE METABOLISM IN THE THYROID GLAND

The thyroid gland traps and concentrates iodine, an oligoelement, to synthesize iodinated hormones. Generally, additional iodine is supplied by nutritional additives such as iodinated salt, containing potassium iodide (0.007 percent).

In the animal organism, the reserves of iodine are strictly regulated. Very little of this element is eliminated by

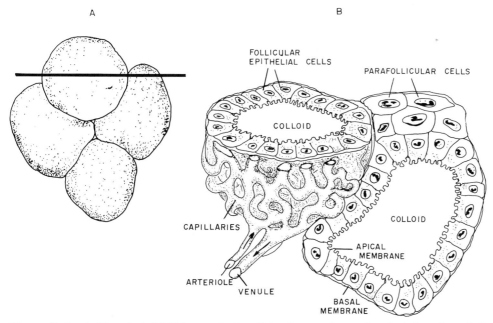

Figure 47–2 **A,** The spherical follicles contain the cellular elements that produce the iodinated metabolic hormones of the thyroid gland. **B,** The follicular cells form a hollow sphere around a central lumen that is covered by their apical plasma membrane and contains colloid. The basal aspect of the follicular cells is surrounded by an extensive network of capillaries that bring raw material for synthesis and receive the thyroid hormones. The enzyme-rich apical membrane of follicular cells, a much folded surface, participates in the transfer of substances from the follicular cytoplasm into the colloid and in the reabsorption of thyroid hormones from the colloid. The parafollicular cells form calcitonin.

the digestive system or the urinary system, and several mechanisms exist for its reabsorption and recycling. In the kidneys, iodine is almost completely reabsorbed by a passive mechanism that is almost completely unaffected by changes in the compositions of plasma and urine. Iodine excretion is higher than absorption in chronic diarrhea, and in renal or lactation problems, which are situations requiring that an additional supply of iodine be given to an animal.

In extracellular fluid, the iodine reserve exists as ions in inorganic compounds (iodide, 1 μg per deciliter). Another important iodine reserve is in the follicles of the thyroid gland, where it is concentrated as molecules in organic compounds (iodine). Besides the kidneys, the thyroid gland plays an important role in the extraction of iodide from plasma. In contrast with that of the kidneys, the extraction mechanism is active and requires energy, since the level of follicular iodine is 20 times higher than that in plasma. Under adenohypophysial activation (TSH), the ratio of iodine levels in the follicles and the plasma may reach 300.

The thyroid adapts to the supply of iodine. In areas with iodine-poor soil, the trapping of iodine is facilitated by a more active transport mechanism in the cellular epithelium of the follicles. Clinically opposite situations create more problems. Animals that have access to plentiful sources of iodine have much less active thyroid glands. If for some reason such animals are suddenly deprived of iodine, the risk of hypothyroidism is greater.

SYNTHESIS OF IODINATED THYROID HORMONES

The synthesis of the iodothyronines and final assembly of the thyroid hormones actually occur extracellularly, within the lumen of the follicle or in the colloid. The transformation of iodide into thyroid hormones may be summarized in these steps (see Fig. 47–3):

1. The active transport (trapping) of iodides (iodine ions) by follicular cells,
2. Iodination of tyrosyl residues of thyroglobulin (in the colloid),
3. Coupling of iodotyrosines (in the colloid),
4. Proteolysis of thyroglobulin (in the follicular cells),
5. Deiodination of iodotyrosines (in the follicular cells), and
6. Recovery of iodine ions (in the follicular cells).

Trapping of Iodine Ions

At the basal membrane of follicular cells, active transport of iodides, catalyzed by a sodium-potassium-ATPase, occurs through a still uncharacterized carrier. The trapped iodine ions, concentrated in the cytoplasm, then oxidized by a peroxidase of the apical plasma membrane, are incorpo-

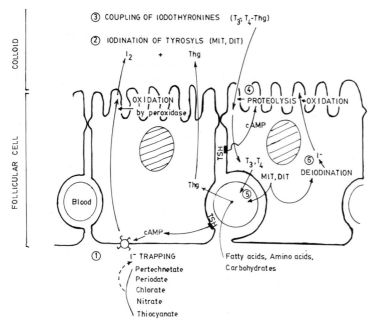

③ COUPLING OF IODOTHYRONINES (T₃, T₄-Thg)

② IODINATION OF TYROSYLS (MIT, DIT)

Figure 47–3 The synthesis of metabolic thyroid hormones takes place in both the cytosol of follicular cells and the colloid of the central lumen. The process is initiated with the (1) absorption of iodide (active) and of raw materials (passive) at the basal aspect of the plasma membrane of follicular cells. The iodide is transferred from the basal to the apical plasma membrane and is oxidized into iodine. In the meantime the fatty acids, amino acids, and carbohydrates in the cytosol are used to form thyroglobulin (Thg). Both iodine and Thg cross the apical cellular border into the colloid, and (2) unite at tyrosyl sites on the Thg to form mono- and diiodotyrosine units (i.e., MIT and DIT). (3) In a subsequent phase, mono- and diiodotyrosines couple and rearrange into tri- and tetraiodothyronines (i.e., T_3 and T_4) still bound to Thg. (4) By pinocytosis, the complex of Thg with MIT, DIT, T_3, and T_4 is reabsorbed from the colloid into the follicular cell and undergoes proteolysis to release MIT, DIT, T_3, and T_4 into the cytoplasm. (5) A small quantity of these substances is admitted into the general circulation by capillaries at the basolateral aspect of the follicular cells. (6) Most of the iodotyrosines and iodothyronines

are deiodinated to recover and recycle the iodide, which is again oxidized and returned into the colloid. TSH binds to specific surface receptors to produce cAMP and to exert a rate-limiting effect on the synthesis of thyroid metabolic hormones. Through cAMP, TSH activates the trapping of iodide at the basal aspect of the plasma membrane, and the reabsorption and proteolysis of the iodine-Thg complex at the apical aspect of the plasma membrane. Some substances impair the trapping of iodide (e.g., pertechnetate, nitrate), whereas others lessen the proteolysis (e.g., thiocarbamides) of the iodinated-Thg complex.

rated into tyrosyl residues of organic molecules (e.g., thyroglobulin) or diffuse at the apical membrane into the follicular lumen fluid.

A number of monovalent anions compete with iodide for active transport into the follicular cells and interfere with iodide trapping. The anions that can be concentrated within the thyroid include biiodate, chlorate, nitrate, perchlorate, periodate, and pertechnetate. Thiocyanate, which is not concentrated in the thyroid, is 10 times less active than perchlorate.

Thiocyanate and naturally occurring goitrogenic (thyroid-enlarging) substances may be eaten with plants of the Brassicaceae family. These vegetables include cabbage, rutabagas, and turnips.

Iodination of Tyrosyl Residues of Thyroglobulin

Thyroglobulin (Thg), the major constituent of colloid, is a glycoprotein (5,800 amino acids, 600,000 to 750,00 daltons) with tyrosyl residues. Thg reacts immediately, through an iodinase, with oxidized iodine to form monoiodotyrosines and diiodotyrosine (i.e., iodotyrosines). Several compounds related to thiourea, the thiocarbamides, inhibit the iodination of monoiodotyrosine (organic binding of iodide), since they compete with the tyrosyl residues for iodine and become iodinated.

Coupling of Iodotyrosines

Within the Thg molecule, the coupling of iodotyrosines (mono and diiodo) forms iodothyronines. The coupling of two diiodotyrosines results in a tetraiodothyronine, or thyroxine (T_4), while the coupling of a monoiodotyrosine (MIT) with a diiodotyrosine (DIT) produces a triiodothyronine (T_3). Structurally, a triiodothyronine may be either T_3 (biologically active) or reverse T_3 (rT_3 or rT'_3) (biologically inactive). The percentages of these intra-Thg molecules are 45 percent, MIT; 35 percent, DIT; 19 percent, T_4; and 1 percent, T_3. The iodinated Thg secreted into the follicular colloid serves as a reserve of thyroid hormones. The thiocarbamides (methimazole, propylthiouracil) that inhibit the iodination of tyrosyl residues also block the coupling of iodotyrosines.

Proteolysis of Thyroglobulin

Before thyroid hormones can be liberated from the Thg, the iodinated protein in the colloid must be reabsorbed by the follicular cells. Apical pinocytosis leads to formation of iodinated Thg–containing endocytotic vesicles, which then fuse into phagolysosomes and migrate near the basal membrane for proteolysis by proteinases. The iodinated Thgs are digested and the T_4, T_3, rT_3, DIT, and MIT molecules are released into the cytoplasm, for either intra-cytoplasmic deiodination or exocytosis from the basal plasma membrane of the cell into the circulation.

Deiodination of Iodotyrosines and Recovery of Iodides

Some of the T_3 and T_4 liberated in the cytoplasm is excreted into the blood by the basal plasma membrane of the follicular cells. However, most of the iodotyrosines of the Thg never become iodothyronines and never exit from the follicular cells. Instead, a deiodinase enzyme within the cells cleaves the iodine and recycles it for synthesis of other molecules of iodotyrosines. This recycling of iodine is two to three times more important than active iodine pumping or trapping by the basal membrane.

Thg, a very important molecule during the synthesis of thyroid hormones, binds T_3 and T_4 by covalent links. A reserve of bound thyroid hormones, which is sufficient to meet euthyroid requirements for the next 50 to 120 days, remains in the colloid of the follicular lumen. In the blood, the thyroid hormones normally attach to protein carriers through noncovalent links. However, during pathological thyroid conditions, Thg is liberated into the blood, and an increased blood level of Thg reflects an inflammation of the thyroid or a form of hyperthyroidism.

SECRETION OF THYROID HORMONES

Besides the secretion of T_4 and of T_3, which is of physiological importance, the thyroid also brings some di-iodotyrosine and some monoiodotyrosine into the blood. A high plasma concentration of MIT and DIT indicates thyroid hyperactivity or a deficiency of iodotyrosine deiodinase, a condition associated with hereditary goiter (abnormal hypertrophy of the thyroid gland).

In all animal species, secretion of T_4 is more important than that of T_3. The secretion of iodothyronines is controlled by the adenohypophysis (TSH, or thyrotropic hormone [TTH]) which acts through cAMP to stimulate cellular apical endocytosis of Thg, and basal plasma membrane exocytosis of iodothyronines. In domesticated animals, sympathetic stimulation increases the secretion of all iodinated hormones.

TRANSPORT OF IODOTHYRONINES

Thyroid hormones circulate in the blood bound to plasma proteins: thyroid-binding globulin (TBG), thyroid-binding prealbumin (TBPA), and albumin. TBG carries 75 percent of the T_3. TBPA transfers 20 percent of the T_4 and none of the T_3. The remaining thyroid hormones are bound to albumin. When the thyroid hormones are attached to

carriers, they are biologically inactive and they can neither influence nor be affected by the hypothalamus-adenohypophysis. The concentration of TBG increases with estrogens, infectious hepatitis, and hypothyroidism. Conversely, the level of TBG decreases with androgens, glucocorticoids, malnutrition, kidney problems, and hyperthyroidism.

Only non–protein-bound or free thyroid hormones can diffuse into tissues, can penetrate cell membranes, can be available to cells, and can have physiological actions by interacting with tissue receptors. Logically, the concentrations of free T_4 and T_3 should be used for evaluation of thyroid gland function. It is unfortunate that procedures for such measurements can be performed only in very specialized laboratories, and current methods measure total concentrations (free and protein-bound) of iodothyronine hormones (T_3 and T_4). Changes in the concentration of plasma protein carriers have only slight repercussions on the levels of free T_4 and T_3. Free iodothyronines exert a negative feedback on the hypothalamus-adenohypophysis, which regulates their blood concentration by producing TSH and thyroid-releasing hormone (TRH).

TRANSFORMATION OF IODOTHYRONINES

All thyroxine in the plasma is secreted by the thyroid. In contrast, the thyroid is at the origin of only a fraction of plasma triiodothyronine, as several extrathyroidal tissues concur to convert T_4 into T_3.

In most domesticated animals, the total concentration of T_4 (3,200 ng per milliliter of plasma) is about 40 times higher than that of T_3 (80 ng per milliliter of plasma). Since the total plasma concentration of T_4 is much lower in the dog and horse (about 1,500 ng per milliliter), the T_4 to T_3 ratio is about 15 and 20, respectively. The free T_4 and free T_3 constitute about 0.2 percent of the total T_4 or T_3; that is, about 640 ng per deciliter for T_4 and 16 ng per deciliter for T_3. At equivalent concentrations, T_3 is five to ten more times more active than T_4, a fact that makes T_3 the primary iodothyronine in replacement of T_4.

Thyroxine is now considered to be a precursor or prohormone without any intrinsic activity, since only T_3 binds to specific intracellular receptors. Formerly, until it was established that enzymatic monodeiodination of T_4 to either rT_3 or T_3 occurs within cells, T_4 was considered as the thyroid hormone.

Active T_3 is 3,5,3'-triiodothyronine, while inactive or reverse rT_3 is 3,3',5'-triiodothyronine (Fig. 47–4). T_3 is produced during normal metabolic states, whereas the biologically inactive and rapidly excreted rT_3 is formed during illness, starvation, or excessive endogenous catabolic states.

The half-life of T_4 is 6 to 7 days, while that of T_3 is less than 1 day. The conversion of T_4 into T_3 or into rT_3 is performed by reactions with either T_4-5'-deiodinase or T_4-5-deiodinase, which occur mostly in the kidneys and the liver.

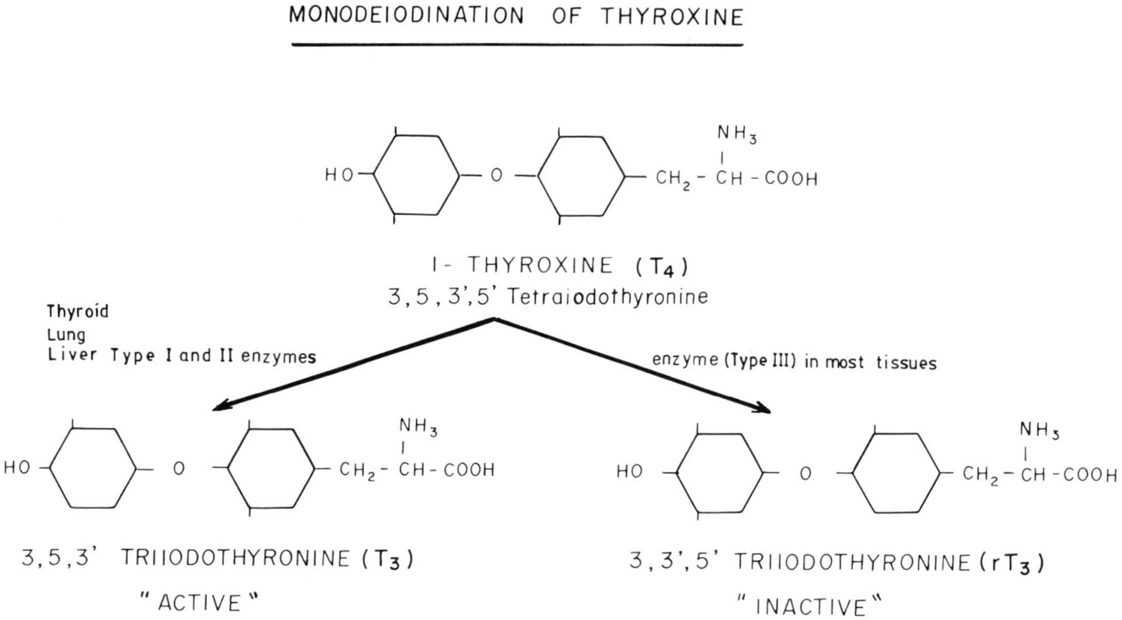

MONODEIODINATION OF THYROXINE

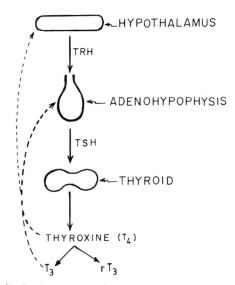

$l-$ THYROXINE (T_4)
3,5,3',5' Tetraiodothyronine

Thyroid
Lung
Liver Type I and II enzymes

enzyme (Type III) in most tissues

3,5,3' TRIIODOTHYRONINE (T_3)
"ACTIVE"

3,3',5' TRIIODOTHYRONINE (rT_3)
"INACTIVE"

Figure 47–4 The thyroid produces all the tetraiodothyronine found in the blood but is not the exclusive source of triiodothyronine. Active triiodothyronine also originates in the lungs and the liver, from deiodination of tetraiodothyronine. Most of the other tissues can perform deiodination of tetraiodothyronine to form reverse triiodothyronine (rT_3), which is biologically inactive.

One of the thiocarbamide compounds, propylthiouracil (but not methimazole), inhibits the conversion of T_4 to T_3 in extrathyroidal tissues. Urine and feces are almost devoid of iodothyronines, since these hormones are deiodinated to recycle the iodine and are transformed into metabolites of tyrosine (glucuronides), which are excreted into bile and urine.

REGULATION OF IODOTHYRONINE SECRETION

The negative-feedback mechanism that regulates the secretion of the iodothyronines operates through the adenohypophysis and the hypothalamus. The hormones TSH (or TTH) and TRH are produced by these tissues.

TRH stimulates the synthesis and the secretion of TSH by thyrotropic cells (thyrotropes) of the adenohypophysis. T_4 inhibits this adenohypophysial function but does not exert a negative feedback on the synthesis of TRH by the hypothalamus. The rapid action of TRH (1 minute after intravenous injection) on thyrotropin is through cAMP and requires an adequate supply of ionized calcium. TRH, which may be mimicked by cAMP, provides a minimal secretion of TSH, but its major control is brought by the levels of T_3 (Fig. 47–5). It is recognized that thyrotropic cells of the hypophysis can transform T_4 into T_3, which is responsible for activation of a gene involved in the synthesis of a protein that inhibits the production of TSH. Triiodothyronine can also decrease the number of TRH receptors found in thyrotropic hypophysial cells.

A thyroid autoregulation mechanism ensures a constant reserve of iodothyronines. Because of this mechanism, the animal organism can adapt to sudden short-term changes in the supply of iodine.

Figure 47–5 An overview of the regulation of the production of the thyroid metabolic hormones. The hypothalamic TRH influences the output of TSH by the thyreotropes of the adenohypophysis. The activating effect of TSH on the follicular cells determines the quantity of iodothyronines released by the thyroid. In turn, the iodothyronines, ultimately mostly triiodothyronine, adjust the hypothalamic and adenohypophysial production of the specific hormones, which have the final objective of stimulating the hormone-producing follicular cells.

Most of the thyroid follicular metabolic processes are regulated by TSH. A long-term stimulation by TSH causes hypertrophy and then hyperplasia of the thyroid gland. TSH binds to receptors on the plasma membrane of follicular cells and activates adenylate cyclase to produce cAMP. Enzymes stirred by cAMP result in

1. enhanced transport of iodine through the basal and apical membranes of the follicular cells,
2. greater iodination of thyroglobulin,
3. higher oxygen consumption and intermediary metabolism in follicular cells, and
4. increased formation of colloidal droplets and a hypertrophy of follicular cells.

MECHANISMS OF ACTION OF IODOTHYRONINES

The numerous physiological actions of iodothyronines occur through activation of intranuclear receptors, which stimulate syntheses of messenger RNAs. Most of these receptors appear specific for T_3. The cytoplasmic receptors for T_3 and T_4 are not essential but are useful as intracytoplasmic reservoirs of these iodothyronines. In contrast with steroids, the cytoplasmic iodothyronine-receptor complex cannot cross the nuclear membrane.

Inside the nucleus of target cells, the T_3-intranuclear complex increases the synthesis of RNA polymerase, which eventually stimulates the synthesis of mRNA, and the transcription of DNAs in target cells. The receptors are localized on chromatin and, in contrast with steroids, are not essential to permit access to the nucleus. The higher production of RNAs accelerates protein syntheses, particularly respiratory enzymes. T_3 stimulates mitochondria to use more oxygen. Administration of T_3 causes an increase in the number of mitochondria and of inner mitochondrial crests. Iodothyronine enhances cellular respiratory events by (1) excitation of mRNAs, causing synthesis of respiratory enzymes, and (2) mitochondrial development.

Mitochondrial membranes have T_3 receptors that cause T_3 to modify the lipid and protein contents of mitochondria and to increase their oxygen consumption.

Plasma membranes have some specific T_3 receptors that favor the trapping of absorption of amino acids by cells.

METABOLIC ACTIONS OF IODOTHYRONINES

Calorigenic Effect. Basal metabolism is increased a few days after administration of T_3 or T_4. T_3 accelerates oxidation reactions (higher consumption of oxygen). The fundamental mechanism probably involves some displacements of Na^+ and K^+ across the plasma membrane and an important contribution of Na^+-K^+ATPase.

Effects on Protein Metabolism. Iodothyronines accelerate protein synthesis and lower the excretion of nitrogenous products. Numerous biochemical reactions occur because of an increase in the synthesis of specific enzymes. Synthesis of proteins is favored only when sufficient quantity of an adequate ration is fed to an animal. When excess feed is given, T_3 induces protein catabolism, particularly that of muscle proteins.

Effects on Carbohydrate Metabolism. T_3 influences all the aspects of carbohydrate metabolism. Intestinal absorption of glucose and galactose, and gluconeogenesis reactions, are stimulated. Many other effects come about by the combined action of triiodothyronine with either insulin or epinephrine. For instance, glycemia remains normal even if insulin is administered, because T_3 increases trapping of glucose by adipocytes and muscular cells.

Effects on Lipid Metabolism. By increasing lipid catabolism, T_3 diminishes the lipid reserves. Lipolysis occurs in adipocytes by making these cells more reactive to catecholamines, glucagon, and glucocorticoids. From these lipolytic reactions, more fatty acids and glycerol become available to hepatic cells for greater synthesis of triglycerides. In hyperthyroidism, the plasma concentrations of cholesterol and triglycercides are reduced.

Effects on Vitamin Metabolism. By accelerating several biochemical processes, iodothyronine forces the animal organism to consume a high proportion of its vitamin reserves. In hyperthyroidism, deficiencies in vitamins D and E should be prevented.

ACTIONS OF IODOTHYRONINES ON SOME SYSTEMS

Iodothyronines stimulate all the systems of the organism and are essential for development and maturation of the central nervous system. Regarding the cardiovascular system, iodothyronines accelerate the rhythm and increase the output and the strength of the heart; they also potentiate the cardiac effects of catecholamines. Peripherally, the iodinated thyroid hormones cause a vasodilation, which permits better dissipation of heat. Concerning the digestive tract, they augment intestinal motility and secretion of digestive enzymes. Physiologically, the iodothyronines facilitate growth of the muscular mass and accelerate the formation of epiphysial conjugation centers in bones.

EVALUATION OF THYROID FUNCTION

Measurements of total, bound, and free iodinated thyroid hormones are often used for clinical evaluation of the thyroid gland. Simple, inexpensive kits are commercially available for measuring levels of T_4 and T_3. Tests that esti-

TABLE 47–1 Approximate Radioimmunoassay Values (Mean and Range) for T_4 and T_3 in the Serum of Domestic Animals

	T_4 (μg/dL)	T_3 (ng/dL)	T_4:T_3 Ratio
Bovine	6.0 (3.6–9)	90 (40–170)	65
Canine	1.5 (0.7–2.2)	95 (60–130)	15
Caprine	3.5 (3.5–4.2)	45 (90–190)	75
Equine	1.5 (1.5–2.4)	75 (30–160)	20
Feline	2.0 (1–3)	65 (40–110)	30
Ovine	4.5 (3–6)	100 (60–150)	45
Porcine	3.5 (1.7–4.7)	90 (40–140)	35
Approx. means in these species	3.2	80	40

mate the metabolic effects of iodothyronines are approximative and complicated.

Methods for Evaluation of Total Concentrations of Iodothyronines

The *concentration of serum iodine* is a measure of the total quantity of iodine (organic and inorganic) in the circulation. Only about 6 percent of the iodine occurs in the form of iodides.

Protein-bound iodine (PBI) is a measure of the iodine bound to precipitable serum proteins. Since T_4 represents about 90 percent of PBI, and the other forms of iodines (T_3, rT_3, MIT, and DIT) account for only 10 percent, the method has been used to estimate the level of T_4. This test has been replaced by more direct methods because of overestimated results due to exogenous sources of iodine (e.g., in food or in iodinated antiseptics), to thyroid iodoproteins produced during chronic thyroiditis, and to some metals reacting with organic solvents.

Radioimmunoassays are based on the principle of the competition between the measured substance (S) and a chemically identical radioactive substance (S') for the sites on an accepting or binding protein (BP) (Table 47–1). The quantity of S' that binds to BP is inversely proportional to the quantity of S, the unknown value. By adding known quantities of S to a standard mixture of BP and S', it is possible to establish a standard curve of the correlation between the quantity of precipitated S' and the quantity of S added.

REFERENCES

Anderson JH, Brown RW. Serum thyroxine (T_4) and triiodothyronine (T_3) uptake values in normal adult cats as determined by radioimmunossay. Am J Vet Res 1979;40:1493.

Blackmore DJ, Greenwood RES, Johnson C. Observations on thyroid hormones in the blood of thoroughbreds. Res Vet Sci 1978;25:294.

Blum JW, Kunz P. Effects of fasting on thyroid hormone levels, and kinetics of reverse triiodothyronine in cattle. Acta Endocrinol 1981;98;234.

Brennan MD. Thyroid hormones. Mayo Clin Proc 1980;55:33.

Cavalieri RR, Pitt-Rivers R. The effects of drugs on the distribution and metabolism of thyroid hormones. Pharmacol Rev 1981;33:55.

Chen CL, Riley AM. Serum thyroxine and triiodothyronine concentrations in neonatal foals and mature horses. Am J Vet Res 1981;42:1415.

Cooper DS. Antithyroid drugs. N Engl J Med 1984;311:1353.

Kaufman J, Olson PN, Reimers TJ, Allen TA, Soderberg SF, Nett TM, Wheeler SL, Wingfield WE. Serum concentrations of thyroxine, 3,5,3'-triiodothyronine, thyrotropin, and prolactin in dogs before and after thyrotropin-releasing hormone administration. Am J Vet Res 1985;46:486.

Larsen PR. Feedback regulation of thyrotropin secretion by hormones. Thyroid-pituitary interaction. N Engl J Med 1982;306:23.

Larsen PR, Silva JE, Kaplan MM. Relationships between circulating and endocellular thyroid hormones. Physiological and clinical implications. Endocr Rev 1981;2:87.

Li WI, Chen CL, Tiller AA, Kunkle GA. Effects of thyrotropin-releasing hormone on serum concentrations of thyroxine and triiodothyronine in healthy, thyroidectomized, thyroxine-treated, and propylthiouracil-treated dogs. Am J Vet Res 1986;47:163.

Oppenheimer JH. Thyroid hormones action at the nuclear level. Ann Intern Med 1985;102:274.

Rosychuk RAW. Thyroid hormones and antithyroid drugs. Vet Clin North Am (Small Anim Pract) 1982;12:111.

Sestoft L. Metabolic aspects of the calorigenic effect of thyroid hormone in mammals. Clin Endocrinol 1980;13:489.

Thoday KL, Seth J, Elton RA. Radioimmunoassay of serum total thyroxine and triiodothyronine in healthy cats: assay methodology and effects of age, sex, breed, heredity and environment. J Small Anim Pract 1984;25:457.

Wilson O, Stone JM, Monty DE. Long-term study of thyroid function in healthy beagle dogs, using [125]I. Am J Vet Res 1983;44:1392.

CHAPTER 48

CALCIUM-REGULATING HORMONES

The metabolism of calcium ions is regulated mainly by three hormones: two hypercalcemic hormones (1,25-dihydroxycholecalciferol, or vitamin D_3, and parathormone [PTH]) and an antihypercalcemic (hypocalcemic?) hormone (calcitonin [CT]). The major target tissues of these hormones are the *intestine* (vitamin D_3, PTH), for the entrance of Ca^{++} into the liquids of the organism; the *bones,* for minute-by-minute regulation of storage (CT, vitamin D_3) or of availability (PTH) of Ca^{++}; and the *kidneys* for reabsorption (PTH) or for excretion (CT) of Ca^{++}.

The three calcium-regulating hormones contribute differently to calcium homeostasis. The development of hypocalcemia is prevented by vitamin D_3 and by PTH. Vitamin D_3 causes sufficient retention of minerals (Ca^{++} and PO_4^{---}) to ensure mineralization of bone matrix, whereas PTH maintains the proper blood calcium for an adequate ratio of calcium to phosphate in extracellular fluids. CT prevents the development of hypercalcemia and functions more as an emergency hormone. Other hormones that also modulate the metabolism of calcium include estrogens, glucagon, glucocorticoids, growth hormone, insulin, prolactin, and thyroxine.

BONE PHYSIOLOGY

Most (95 percent) of the calcium (Ca^{++}) is in the crystalline structure of bones, combined with phosphate. Only a small amount of Ca^{++} is present in *plasma,* about 1 percent, or 10 mg per deciliter (5 mEq per liter, or 2.5 mmol per liter), and in the cytoplasm of cells.

Bones are composed of cells, minerals, and organic matrix. Three types of cells are found in bones: osteoblasts, osteocytes, and osteoclasts. The *osteoblasts* synthesize the collagen and glycoprotein of bone matrix, contain bone alkaline phosphatase, and secrete a noncollagen bone protein that contains glutamic acid (osteocalcin), which may initiate mineralization of the uncalcified organic matrix (osteoid). In bones that are already formed, *osteocytes* within the haversian systems promote local resorption, accretion, and transport of nutrients and waste products. Multinucleated *osteoclasts* contribute to local bone dissolution by elaborating lytic enzymes and organic acids (e.g., citric acid).

In general, bone is of two types: cancellous, or spongiosa, and cortical, or compact. The cancellous bone, found in the metaphyseal (junction of diaphysis and epiphysis) region of long bones, is composed of spicules (pointed bodies) known as trabeculae and is the most metabolically active region. The compact bone, occurring in the cortex and diaphysis, is highly calcified but less metabolically active.

Bone is constantly in a process of "remodeling," as previously calcified bone is absorbed and replaced by new bone deposition or accretion. Physiological factors that influence this remodeling include the following:

1. Changes in blood flow in response to anatomical, biochemical, and nervous influences.
2. Hormones (CT, PTH, vitamin D_3) and growth factors (beta-transforming growth factor).
3. Ion concentrations (e.g., an increase in plasma phosphate promotes the deposition of calcium in bone and inhibits bone resorption. Plasma calcium and phosphate are inversely related. Fluoride affects both the solubility and the size of the crystals of hydroxyapatite.
4. Mechanical stress generates local differences in piezoelectrical fields on bones, at the sites of muscle insertion, and affects the distribution of osteoclasts and osteoblasts in bone.
5. Pyrophosphate inhibits both bone accretion and bone resorption by replacing phosphate in the crystal surface.

CALCIUM METABOLISM

The calcium in the plasma exists in three forms: free (ionized); complexed (chelated, but ultrafiltrable) to bicarbonate, citrate, and phosphate; and bound to plasma proteins (albumin, globulin). The predominant (55 percent of total plasma) free, or diffusible, fraction is in constant exchange with the extracellular fluids. Most of the intracellular calcium is stored in the endoplasmic reticulum or in inositol-responsive organelles (the so-called calciosomes). Stimulation of cell surface receptors results in formation of inositol lipids that become part of a complex inositol phosphate-Ca^{++} intracellular messenger system, which is operative in all mammalian cells.

Calcium ions are involved in blood coagulation (enzyme cofactors), muscle contraction, membrane permeability, nerve conduction, milk secretion, and the structure of the eggshell of birds. In animals, a constant excretion of calcium ions occurs principally in urine, and to a smaller extent in the feces. During growth, pregnancy, and lactation, considerably more calcium ions are drained by tissues, fetus, and milk. The minimal intake requirements for calcium ions must balance this urinary and fecal excretion but must be higher in pregnant and lactating females.

In animals, chronic intake of small quantities of calcium, of high quantities of phosphorus (beef heart or beef liver), or of insufficient amounts of vitamin D can induce compensatory excessive PTH secretion with consequent bone resorption and decalcification (osteoporosis). Chronic high levels of *glucocorticoids* also cause osteoporosis by inhibiting protein synthesis and decreasing the intestinal absorption of bone-forming minerals. Similarly, hyperglycemia (*glucagon*) and excess of *thyroxine* both decrease the normal formation of bone. In contrast, *estrogens* prevent osteoporosis during pregnancy by possibly increasing plasma levels of both CT (for bone mineralization) and vitamin D_3 (for improved intestinal absorption of bone-forming minerals). *Growth hormone* has a net hypercalcemic action, since it enhances intestinal absorption more than it promotes the renal excretion of Ca^{++}.

Lactation hypocalcemia in whelping bitches (termed eclampsia or puerperal tetany) and in postpartum cows (termed milk fever or parturient paresis) is related to calcium nutrition and mobilization. Eclampsia is characterized by excitement and tetanic muscle contractions, whereas parturient paresis is marked by depression and flaccid paralysis.

HYPERCALCEMIC PARATHYROID HORMONES

The two hypercalcemic hormones are quite different. PTH is a polypeptide secreted by the parathyroid glands, whereas vitamin D_3 is a steroid produced from the successive transformation of a metabolite (7-dehydrocholesterol) in the liver and in the kidneys.

Parathormone

In most mammals, parathormone (PTH) is the principal hormone involved in the fine (minute-to-minute) regulation of calcium homeostasis. The hypercalcemic biological action of PTH is by direct influence on target cells in bones (osteoclasts, osteocytes) and kidney (proximal and distal tubules) and by indirect action on the duodenum. In bones, PTH causes bone resorption by mobilizing calcium from the center to the surface of bones and helps solubilize the minerals from the bone by producing an acid environment in the adjacent extracellular fluid. PTH directly and rapidly affects the tubular cells, preventing reabsorption of phosphate by the proximal tubules (causing phosphaturia), while favoring reabsorption of calcium in the distal tubules. It also enhances the renal conversion of 25-hydroxyvitamin D_3 into 1,25-dihydroxyvitamin D_3. By this additional 1,25-dihydroxyvitamin D_3, PTH indirectly increases the absorption of calcium ions in the duodenum and of phosphate ions in the jejunum.

Acting in concert, CT and PTH maintain the blood calcium level within narrow limits and provide a dual negative-feedback mechanism for control of extracellular Ca^{++}. In pregnant cows, the maintenance of calcium homeostasis varies with the calcium composition of the prepartal diet. In cows fed high-calcium prepartal diets, CT becomes the major hormone near parturition and during the early postpartum period. The hypocalcemic effect of CT predominates and causes the blood calcium level to fall to less than 50 percent of the normal concentration (parturient paresis, or

hypocalcemia associated with parturition) in spite of an increase in the release of PTH. In cows fed the high-calcium prepartal diet, the PTH response to hypocalcemia is an unsuccessful increase of intestinal absorption rather than the corrective measure of bone resorption. An increased secretion of CT prepartum, when the cows are fed the high-calcium diet, may be a factor contributing to the postpartum failure of increased PTH to raise the blood calcium level. In contrast, when cows are fed a balanced or relatively low-calcium prepartal diet supplemented with pharmacological doses of vitamin D, the incidence of parturient paresis is reduced, and calcium homeostasis remains under the fine control of PTH.

Development and Morphology of the Parathyroid Glands

All vertebrates with a pulmonary system have parathyroid glands. On the evolutionary scale, parathyroids are seen in developed species that have passed from the aquatic type to the terrestrial type of life. Animals living in the terrestrial environment, which is rich in phosphorus but poor in calcium, require a calcium-conserving mechanism to prevent hypocalcemia and to maintain the integrity of their skeleton.

Parathyroid glands are derived from embryonic pharyngeal pouches III and IV and develop in association with the thymus. Usually, the parathyroids include two pairs of glands located in the cranial cervical region. Internal parathyroid glands (IPTg, parathyroids III, caudal parathyroids) are located near each thyroid and are associated with vestiges of thymus. External parathyroids (EPTg, parathyroids IV, cranial parathyroids) are lateral to the thyroid lobes and smaller than the internal parathyroids. Internal parathyroids receive blood from the cranial thyroid artery, and the external parathyroids are fed by numerous ramifications of the thyroid arteries.

Pigs are without internal parathyroids, and the external parathyroids are embedded either in the thymus in piglets or in adipose tissue in adult animals. In goats, sheep, and cattle, the larger external parathyroids are located a considerable distance cranial to the thyroid, in loose connective tissue, along the carotid artery. In the horse, the larger lower parathyroids are situated caudal to the thyroid, near the bifurcation of the carotid trunk, at the level of the first rib (Fig. 48–1; see also Fig. 47–1).

Microscopic Structure of the Parathyroids

Parathyroid tissue contains chief cells and oxyphilic cells. Actually, only the chief cells are secretory cells, elaborating a single hormone, PTH. Oxyphilic cells would be the final maturation stage of the chief cells of the parathyroids.

Certain fine structural characteristics of chief cells are associated with different stages of protein synthesis and secretion. Inactive or resting chief cells predominate in the parathyroid glands of most animal species. These resting cells are cuboidal, with interdigitations between neighboring cells, and have a cytoplasm with poorly developed organ-

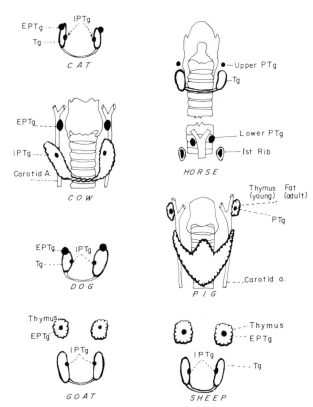

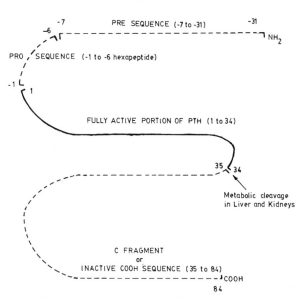

Figure 48–1 Diagrammatic representation of the relationship between the thyroid (Tg) and the parathyroid glands in domestic animals. In small animals (cats, dogs), both internal and external parathyroid glands (IPTg; EPTg) are attached to the thyroid. In ruminants (cows, goats, sheep) only the internal parathyroid glands are united to the thyroid gland. In horses, pigs, and ruminants, the external parathyroids are located cranial to the thyroid. The internal (lower) parathyroids are near the entrance of the trachea in the thorax in horses but are absent in pigs.

Figure 48–2 During the synthesis of parathormone, intracellular cleavages occur at the −7 position, to remove the presequence (−7 to −31), and the prosequence hexapeptide (−1 to −6). The biologically active parathormone (PTH) secretory granules delivered into the circulation are packets of a polypeptide (84 amino acid residues), which is catabolized in the liver and the kidneys. The metabolic cleavage of PTH occurs at the 34 to 35 position, yielding a still fully active portion of PTH (1 to 34), and an inactive COOH sequence (35 to 84). (- - -, Inactive peptide; ——— active peptide.)

elles and few secretory granules. During the active stage of PTH secretion, chief cells have a less dense cytoplasm, which contains fewer organelles, secretion granules, glycogen particles, and lipid bodies. Oxyphilic cells are larger than chief cells, have an abundant cytoplasm with several oddly shaped mitochondria, and increase in number with advancing age.

During thyroid migration, embryonic pharyngeal pouch V contains some cells of neural origin (C cells), which fuse with thyroid parenchyma during the postnatal period. The C cells synthesize CT, a hormone with effects opposite to those of PTH from the parathyroid.

Synthesis of Parathyroid Peptides

The secretion of the chief cells of the bovine parathyroids is a polypeptide chain of 84 amino acid residues. A similar sequence has been found in porcine (p), murine (m), and human (h) *PTH*. A third of the PTH molecule (the amino-terminal residues 10 to 27 and 25 to 35) is essential for its recognition by receptors on target cells, for activation of adenylate cyclase, and for biological activity (Fig. 48–2).

Synthetic PTHs containing the biologically active sequence (1 to 34) produce effects equivalent to those of natural PTH molecules (1 to 84).

The biosynthesis of PTH occurs with the formation of several intermediary molecules, such as pre pro-PTH (115 amino acid residues) and pro-PTH (90 amino acid residues) (see Fig. 48–2). The pre-PTH sequence is enzymatically separated in the rough endoplasmic reticulum. The remaining pro-PTH, which has 0.2 percent of the biological activity of PTH, is transformed in the Golgi apparatus into an 84 amino acid sequence, which is stored in secretion granules. This is the major molecule secreted by the chief cells.

Two other molecules, segment 1 to 34 (biologically active) and segment 35 to 84, are also released into the peripheral circulation. The latter does not exert any significant biological action. Since they are immunoreactive, their presence in blood causes problems with radioimmunological assays for PTH, and clinical interpretations.

The inactive carboxy-terminal peptide (segment 35 to 84) accounts for about 80 percent of the immunoreactive material present in the peripheral circulation. The remaining 20 percent of activity is equally shared by the amino-terminal peptide (1 to 33 segment) and the intact hormone (1 to 84). Because of differences in the ability to distinguish these biologically active peptides from the inactive one, radioimmunoassays for PTH are still too unreliable for practical uses.

PTH has a half-life of about 10 minutes before it is enzymatically fragmented in the kidneys and the liver. The kidneys separate PTH into an N-terminal fragment, which is reabsorbed, and a C-terminal fragment, which is excreted. In Kupffer's cells of the liver, the same fragmentation of PTH occurs, but both residues remain in the circulating blood. The biologically active N-terminal residue has a half-life similar to that of PTH (i.e., about 10 minutes). The circulating C-terminal fragments, accounting for 80 percent of the plasma immunoreactivity, have a half-life of 60 minutes and are excreted by glomerular filtration.

Control of Parathormone Secretion

The plasma concentration of ionized Ca^{++} regulates the secretion of the parathyroids. Calcium ions diminish the capture of amino acids and prevent exocytosis of PTH, that is, stop the fusion of secretion granules with the cytoplasmic aspect of the plasma membrane of chief cells. Parathyroids store relatively small amounts of preformed PTH but respond to minor fluctuations in Ca^{++} (0.1 mg per deciliter in the dog and cat) in either direction from the set normal value. In the cow, the parathyroid reserve is adequate to supply PTH for 7 hours at the normal (physiological) secretion rate or for 1.5 hours at maximal output (i.e., five times normal) (Fig. 48–3). Lactation severely challenges mineral homeostasis, and incomplete compensation of calcium losses may lead to continued hypocalcemia, which ultimately results in parathyroid hyperplasia and PTH output at 10 to 50 times the normal secretory rate.

Glucocorticoids, lithium, magnesium, and vitamin D metabolites modulate the elaboration of PTH. *Glucocorticoids* transiently increase PTH secretion, directly by stimulating the parathyroid glands, and indirectly by lowering the plasma calcium level by inhibiting bone resorption and decreasing duodenal calcium absorption. *Lithium* increases the secretion of PTH by reducing the sensitivity of the parathyroid chief cells to calcium (i.e., hypercalcemia no longer depresses the output of PTH). An excess of *magnesium* ions inhibits the secretion of PTH, but paradoxically, a severe magnesium deficiency results in hypocalcemia, because of impaired secretion of PTH or end-organ response. *Metabolites of vitamin D* have both direct and indirect effects on the secretion of PTH. Vitamin D_3 directly decreases PTH gene transcription, whereas the hypercalcemia of vitamin D_3, due to increased bone resorption and calcium absorption, indirectly inhibits the release of PTH.

HYPERCALCEMIC VITAMIN D_3 (CALCITRIOL OR CHOLECALCIFEROL)

Although cholecalciferol is designated as a vitamin (Latin, *fero,* to carry), it is a secosteroid hormone (Latin, from *secare,* to cut; i.e., open B-ring) synthesized from a precursor (7-dehydrocholesterol) furnished by dietary intake or produced in the epidermis. To achieve biological potency, 7-dehydrocholesterol must undergo further hydroxylation in the liver and in the kidneys. When these active forms of vitamin D are provided as food supplements, their jejunal absorption, by chylomicron formation, is facilitated by bile salts, fatty acids, and monoglycerides.

In the liver, the precursor is activated to 25-hydroxycholecalciferol (also known as calcidiol). In the kidneys, the activation of 1-alpha-hydroxylase for formation of 1,25-dihydroxycholecalciferol (also known as calcitriol) occurs in the proximal tubules. The two major mechanisms of generation of calcitriol are a PTH-mediated one in which cAMP is a

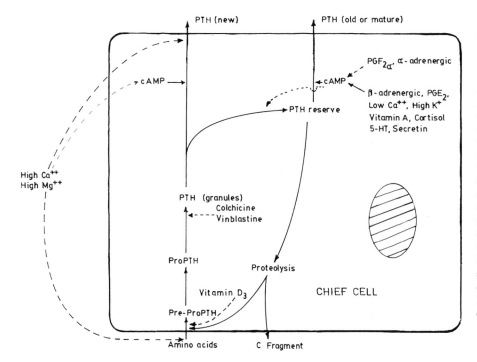

Figure 48–3 Hypercalcemia and hypermagnesemia inhibit the release of newly formed PTH and the trapping of amino acids by the chief cells of the parathyroid. Vitamin D_3 prevents the synthesis of preproparathormone. Factors inducing production of cAMP (e.g., hypocalcemia, beta-adrenergic agonists) cause the release of PTH in reserve in the cytosol and also prevent the formation of such a cytosolic reserve of parathormone. Formation of cAMP can also be depressed by alpha-adrenergic agonists and by $PGF_{2\alpha}$. Proteolytic degradation of cytosolic PTH gives rise to amino acids that are reused in preproPTH synthesis and to inactive C fragments, which enter the circulation. The cleavage of proPTH into PTH is prevented by colchicine and by vinblastine.

second messenger, and a calcitonin-dependent one that uses Ca^{++} as a second messenger. Stimulation of 1-alpha-hydroxylase takes place in mitochondria of cells in the proximal convoluted tubule with PTH and in cells in the proximal straight tubule with CT. The renal output of calcitriol is also enhanced by cortisol, estradiol, growth hormone, and prolactin by still unknown mechanisms. Little if any 1-alpha-hydroxylase is present outside the kidneys, except in the placenta and tumor cells, which can serve as other sources of 1,25-dihydroxyvitamin D_3.

This final step in the formation of vitamin D_3 is complex and is related to the blood levels of calcium, phosphates, and PTH. When the blood calcium level is normal or elevated, the kidneys produce the inactive 24,25-dihydroxycholecalciferol instead of calcitriol. A high level of PO_4^{---} inhibits the renal 1-alpha-hydroxylase, whereas estrogens and prolactin increase the activity of this enzyme during lactation. Metabolic acidosis and insulin deficiency also depress the production of calcitriol.

As vitamin D_3 enters the blood, from the jejunum or from the kidneys, it binds to a protein carrier (vitamin D–binding protein [DBP]) for transport. Protein bound–vitamin D_3 is directed to the primary target cells in bones, intestine, and kidney, where it acts in concert with PTH. Secondary targets for vitamin D_3 are receptors in activated lymphocytes (thymocytes), brain, hypophysis, pancreas, parathyroid, tumors, and skin cells.

DBP blood levels, which usually exceed those of vitamin D_3 and its metabolites, are further increased by pregnancy and estradiol, whereas liver disease and proteinuria decrease them. The affinity of DBP for calcidiol and 24,25-dihydroxy vitamin D_3 is greater than for 1,25-dihydroxyvitamin D_3.

In the cells, vitamin D_3 behaves like a steroid; that is, it penetrates the plasma membrane and combines with a cytosolic receptor to form a complex that reaches the nuclear chromatin to activate the expression of genes. In synergy with PTH, vitamin D_3 influences target cells in the mucosa of the small intestine, where it increases the active absorption of calcium (duodenum) and of phosphorus (jejunum). Vitamin D_3 increases the permeability of the apical brush border membrane to calcium ions, stimulates the subcellular accumulation of these calcium ions into organelles (mitochondria) to avoid toxic cytosolic calcium concentrations, and induces the production of a unique calcium-binding protein (CaBP), which facilitates the active crossing of Ca^{++} at the basolateral border membrane of the enterocyte.

In the bones, with help from PTH, calcitriol seeks osteoclasts to actively move Ca^{++} and phosphate (PO_4^{---}) ions from the cytoplasm into the extracellular fluid. Calcitriol also facilitates Ca^{++} reabsorption in the kidneys. In contrast, glucocorticoids have an anti–vitamin D_3 effect on intestinal absorption and on renal reabsorption of Ca^{++}. Vitamin D_3 inhibits the synthesis and release of PTH, by impairing PTH gene expression in the chief cells of the parathyroids. Strontium, magnesium, and phosphorus inhibit vitamin D_3 metabolism.

Hypovitaminosis D.   In young animals, because of vitamin D_3 deficiency, poor absorption of Ca^{++} causes failure of the mineralization of new bones, a condition known as *rickets*. In adults, an analogous hypovitaminosis D condition of softening (demineralization) of the bones (i.e., *osteomalacia*) occurs mostly without (*isoostosis*) and sometimes with (*hyperostosis*) exaggerated osteoid formation, the latter leading to swelling of bones.

Hypervitaminosis D.   In cows near parturition, the continued feeding of massive doses of vitamin D_3 (e.g., 30 million U for more than 7 days) to prevent parturient paresis may produce toxicity. One of the signs is extensive mineralization of the cardiovascular system.

ANTIHYPERCALCEMIC HORMONE: CALCITONIN

The second population of cells in the thyroid, the parafollicular or clear cells, secrete calcitonin (polypeptide), or thyrocalcitonin, instead of thyroxine and triiodothyronine (tyrosine derivatives). The continuously secreting clear cells (C cells) store calcitonin in secretory granules and release them directly into the circulation upon stimulation (i.e., an elevation of the blood calcium level).

In contrast, the soluble thyroid metabolic hormones are first driven directly from the follicular cells into the follicular lumen for storage. Upon stimulation, the same cells take the metabolic thyroid hormones from storage in the lumen of the follicle and release them into the peripheral circulation at the opposite cellular plasma membrane.

Synthesis

Calcitonin contains 32 amino acid residues, which are of different combinations in the animal species. The cleavage by hydrolysis of *preprocalcitonin* produces calcitonin along with C-terminal and N-terminal peptides. The C-terminal polypeptide made up of 21 amino acid residues, called *katacalcin,* can also lower blood calcium. Calcitonin is degraded in the kidney and has a half-life of about 10 minutes.

The secretion of calcitonin is mainly from the parafollicular cells of the thyroid, but other extrathyroid sources are recognized: adrenal medulla, pancreas, and pars intermedia of the hypophysis. Thyroid C-cell hyperplasia and C-cell tumors occur in aged males (bulls, stallions), but not in aged females. In Guernsey bulls, the occurrence of thyroid C-cell tumors associated with pheochromocytomas seems to be gene-linked.

Release

In addition to calcium (at high blood levels), several other substances increase the output of calcitonin. Beta-adrenergic agonists and dopamine stimulate the release of calcitonin; estradiol, glucagon, and most of the gastrointestinal hormones (e.g., gastrin, cholecystokinin [CCK], and secretin) enhance the production of calcitonin.

Action

The main action of calcitonin is to prevent the occurrence of hypercalcemia, rather than to cause hypocalcemia. Free calcitonin binds to receptors on bone and kidney cells. It decreases the permeability of the plasma membranes of osteoclasts to Ca^{++}, thus inhibiting bone resorption and preventing hypercalcemia. It also increases the urinary excretion of Ca^{++}, Na^+, and PO_4^{---}. These calcium-lowering effects are associated with similar phosphate-lowering actions.

The secretion of calcitonin may protect against postprandial hypercalcemia. Also, in association with higher levels of vitamin D_3, calcitonin may prevent bone resorption in females during gestation and lactation. In these physiological events, the additional maternal Ca^{++} needed for bone formation in the fetus and for milk production is derived from an improved intestinal absorption of Ca^{++}, rather than from an increased demineralization of bones.

REFERENCES

Austin L, Heath H III. Calcitonin: physiology and pathophysiology. N Engl J Med 1981;304:269.

Bell NH. Vitamin D—endocrine system. J Clin Invest 1985;76:1.

Canalis E. The hormonal and local regulation of bone formation. Endocr Rev 1983;4:62.

Capen CC. Functional and fine structural relationships of parathyroid glands. Adv Vet Sci Comp Med 1975;19:249.

Cohn DV, MacGregor RR. The biosynthesis, intracellular processing, and secretion of parathyroid hormone. Endocr Rev 1981;2:1.

DeLuca HF, Schnoes H. Vitamin D: recent advances. Annu Rev Biochem 1983;52:411.

Fraser DR. Regulation of the metabolism of vitamin D. Physiol Rev 1980;60:551.

Habener JF, Rosenblatt M, Potts JT Jr. Parathyroid hormone: biochemical aspects of biosynthesis, secretion, action, and metabolism. Physiol Rev 1984;64:985.

Haussler MR. Vitamin D receptors: nature and function. Annu Rev Nutr 1986;6:527.

Hillyard C, Abeyasekera G, Craig RK, Myers C, Stevenson JC, MacIntyre I. Katacalcin: a new plasma calcium—lowering hormone. Lancet 1983; 1:846.

Kumar R. Metabolism of 1,25-dihydroxyvitamin D_3. Physiol Rev 1984;64:478.

Maloney C, Nissenson R. Canine renal receptors for parathyroid hormone: down-regulation in vivo by exogenous parathyroid hormone. J Clin Invest 1983;72:411.

Meuten DJ. Hypercalcemia. Vet Clin North Am (Small Anim Pract) 1984;14:891.

Norman AW, Roth J, Orci L. The vitamin D endocrine system: steroid metabolism, hormone receptors, and biological response (calcium-binding proteins). Endocr Rev 1982;3:331.

Potts JT, Kronenberg HM, Rosenblatt M. Parathyroid hormone: chemistry, biosynthesis, and mode of action. Adv Prot Chem 1982;35:323.

Putney JW, Takemura H, Hughes AR, Horstman DA, Thastrup O. How do inositol phosphates regulate calcium signaling? FASEB J 1989; 3:1899.

Raisz LG, Kream BE. Regulation of bone formation (parts I and II). N Engl J Med 1983;309:29 and 83.

Reichel H, Koeffler PH, Norman AW. The role of the vitamin D endocrine system in health and disease. New Engl J Med 1989;320:980.

Rosenblatt M. Pre-proparathyroid hormone, proparathyroid hormone, and parathyroid hormone: the biologic role of hormone structure. Clin Orthop 1982;2170:260.

Sherwood LM, Russell J. The role of 1,25-(OH)$_2$D$_3$ in regulating parathyroid gland function. Proc Soc Exp Biol Med 1989;191:233.

Talmage RV, Cooper CW, Toverud SU. The physiological significance of calcitonin. Bone Min Res 1983;1:74.

CHAPTER 49

PANCREATIC HORMONES

The pancreas is both an exocrine and an endocrine gland. The exocrine pancreas synthesizes and secretes major digestive enzymes, for example, proteases (chymotrypsin and trypsin), amylase, and lipase, as well as bicarbonate. The endocrine pancreas produces the peptide hormones glucagon, insulin, gastrin, pancreatic peptide (PP), somatostatin (SS) and vasoactive intestinal peptide (VIP).

The polypeptide hormones secreted by the pancreas originate from roughly a million nests (approximately just less than 0.2 mm in diameter) of endocrine cells, the islets of Langerhans, dispersed in the exocrine pancreatic tissue. The islets, miniature organs themselves, have a distinctive organization of individualized cells, each producing one or several hormones. A cells produce glucagon, B cells form insulin, D cells are the source of SS and of gastrin, and F cells are at the origin of PP. The insulin-containing B cells represent about 60 percent of the islet and form its core, which is surrounded by a rim of A, D, and F cells. Other cells, which are not yet precisely defined, yield VIP.

The secreted insulin has an anabolic action, enhancing the storage of amino acids, fatty acids, and glycogen. In contrast, glucagon has a catabolic action, preventing the storage and promoting the mobilization of these substances. In addition to inhibiting the release of several hypophysial (e.g., growth hormone [GH], thyroid-stimulating hormone [TSH], and prolactin [PRL]) and gastrointestinal (e.g., gastrin, VIP, pancreozymin) hormones, somatostatin decreases the pancreatic output of glucagon, insulin, and somatostatin. Gastrin directly increases gastric acid secretion into the gastrointestinal tract. The precise function of PP is still unknown, although it stimulates gastric secretion, as does gastrin.

PANCREATIC ISLETS, OR ISLETS OF LANGERHANS

The islets, representing about 1 to 2 percent of the mass of the normal pancreas, develop from the endodermal pancreatic ducts. Arranged along fenestrated capillary channels (four to seven times more permeable), the islets receive an abundant blood supply, which drains into the portal venous circulation. The liver, the major target organ of pancreatic hormones, directly receives the full undiluted output of pancreatic islet hormones. The direct sympathetic and parasympathetic innervation, reaching the different types of cells in each islet, is used to modulate the output of specific hormones. Predominance of beta-sympathetic activity increases the output of both the insulinogenic B cells and the glucagonogenic A cells. In contrast, alpha-sympathetic activity is inhibitory to both A and B cells. Parasympathetic

stimulation results in a higher release of glucagon and of insulin (Fig. 49–1).

In close proximity with one another for paracrine effects, the A, B, and D cells seem to function as a tricellular microhormonal secretory unit, regulating the minute-to-minute blood glucose levels and modulating glucose anabolism and catabolism according to physiological needs. The SS from D cells exerts a direct local inhibitory action on the endocrine output of both A and B cells. Similarly, insulin from B cells inhibits the output of the A cells, whereas glucagon from the A cells stimulates the release of insulin from the B cells (Fig. 49–2). The B cells have a basolateral portion that "senses" arteriolar blood and an apical portion that secretes into the venular blood. A similar polarity remains to be demonstrated for A, D, and F cells.

Tight junctions (linear lines of fusion) between plasma membranes of adjacent cells create intercellular lacunae, which are isolated from extracellular fluids and are used to store extracellular insulin.

Gap junctions (bridging channels through adjacent plasma membranes) permit the direct cytosol-to-cytosol passage of small molecules from a B cell to a tightly coupled B or A cell.

In the dog, the cytoplasmic secretory granules of the islet cells show distinctive morphological characteristics. The granules of the more abundant insulinogenic B cells possess a dense internal core surrounded by a wide clear halo, or aura (Fig. 49–3). This zinc-carrying core is pleomorphic (many shapes: circle, bar, Y, or V) and may be central or eccentric. The more abundant bar-shaped internal cores represent mature secretory granules. From studies of islet tumors, it appears that B cells are absent from the pancreatic body or angle joining the two limbs (lobes) of the boomerang-shaped canine pancreas. Each of the granules of A cells has a spherical electron-dense core, with a narrow clear aura. The secretory granules of D cells have a low electron density core, without any clear halo.

Specific types of islet cells are at the origin of different preprohormones, which are enzymatically fragmented first into the various prohormones and then into the pancreatic hormones, which are stored in the diverse secretory granules. Upon adequate stimulation, the pancreatic hormones are released by exocytosis from the islet cells into the extracellular fluid, where they easily diffuse through the walls of the fenestrated capillaries and enter into the plasma of the portal blood.

INSULIN

Insulin is one member of a family of related peptides that also includes the insulin-like growth factors (IGF-1 and IGF-2), formerly known as somatomedins. This hormone

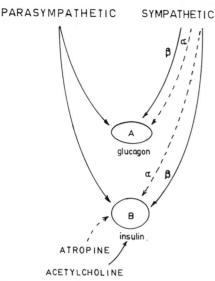

Figure 49–1   General effects of the autonomous nervous system on the release of pancreatic hormones. Parasympathetic stimulation increases the output of glucagon (A cells) and of insulin (B cells). The administration of acetylcholine causes a similar activation of B cells, whereas atropine (muscarinic, sympatholytic) prevents and inhibits this effect. Beta-sympathetic activity, predominant in exercise and conditions of stress, causes a higher output of glucagon and of insulin. In contrast, alpha-sympathetic stimulation has a negative action on the release of both glucagon and insulin.

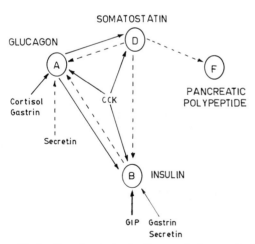

Figure 49–2   Paracrine, or local, effects on the hormonal cells of the pancreatic islets. Somatostatin from D cells inhibits the secretion of the A, B, and F cells. Glucagon stimulates the synthesis of the D and B cells. The insulinogenic B cells depress the output of the glucagonogenic A cells. The gastrointestinal hormones influence the activity of the major endocrine cells of the pancreas. Cholecystokinin (CCK) stimulates the secretion of the A, B, and D cells. Among the gastrointestinal peptides, gastric inhibitory polypeptide (GIP) is the strongest stimulus to B cells, although gastrin and secretin are also insulinogenic. The output of glucagon, which is enhanced by cortisol and by gastrin, declines under the influence of secretin.

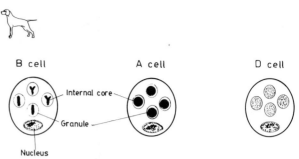

Figure 49–3   The cytoplasmic secretory granules of the different canine pancreatic islet cells differ in their electron density, their shape, and the space between the internal core and the limiting membrane. The internal cores of the granules of A and B cells are electron-dense compared with those of the D cells. The internal core of B cells are bar- or Y-shaped and are surrounded by a wide clear zone inside the limiting membrane. The circular core of an A-cell secretory granule leaves little submembranous space, since it constitutes most of the granule. Each of the granules of D cells has an internal core of low electron density, which adheres to the limiting membrane.

from the B cells directly influences three principal target organs: adipose tissue, liver, and skeletal muscles. It also affects almost every organ of the body (e.g., adenohypophysis, aorta, bone surface, cardiac muscle, cartilages, fibroblasts, leukocytes, mammary glands, and peripheral nerves).

The main function of insulin is to stimulate anabolic reactions involving substances used as biological fuels (i.e., carbohydrates, lipids, and proteins). It regulates many cell functions and catalyzes processes that result in the formation of macromolecules, which are needed to build tissues and to store energy. At the plasma membrane of target cells, it enhances the intracellular entrance of sugars (mostly glucose), amino acids, fatty acids, and potassium and magnesium ions. The overall results are increased glucose oxidation, glycogenesis, lipogenesis, and formation of ATP, DNA, and RNA. In contrast, insulin decreases gluconeogenesis, lipolysis, ketogenesis, and proteolysis.

Synthesis and Release

The synthesis and the release of insulin are responses to an excess of fuel, particularly an increase in the extracellular levels of glucose, which is the major source of calories. The B cells are stimulated to release the insulin stored in secretory granules in a modulated fashion, according to the specific needs. Intake of oral glucose or ingestion of proteins or amino acids (arginine, leucine) evokes a greater response of insulin than when these substances are injected. Anticipatory signals (known as *incretins*) from the gastrointestinal tract to the pancreas, the gastropancreatic axis, induce an increased output of insulin during, rather than after, the intestinal absorption of glucose. Several of the gastrointestinal hormones stimulate insulin release, including gastrin, secretin, cholecystokinin (pancreozymin), intestinal glucagon, vasoactive intestinal polypeptide, and particularly gastric inhibitory peptide (GIP).

The output of insulin by B cells is also increased by beta-adrenergic stimulation, drugs (cAMP, sulfonylurea, theophylline), fatty acids, hormones (adrenocorticotropic hormone [ACTH], cortisol, estradiol, GH, glucagon, progesterone, thyroxine), ketone bodies, and other sugars (fructose, mannose, ribose). In contrast, the release of insulin by the B cells is inhibited by fuel deficiency, somatostatin (during meals), agents that restrict movements of calcium across membranes (phenytoin or dilantin), beta-adrenergic blockers (propranolol), parasympathetic stimulation, and thiazides that are either diuretic (chlorothiazide) or nondiuretic (diazoxide) (Table 49–1).

Glucose stimulation induces the translation of preexisting mRNA for synthesis of insulin in ribosomes that are attached to the surface of the endoplasmic recticulum. The initial synthesis starts with a polypeptide chain of preproinsulin, which is cleaved into a peptide with only 81 to 86 amino acid residues, proinsulin. This prohormone contains the A and B chains of the insulin molecule and the connecting (C) chain.

In the Golgi complex, proinsulin is converted to insulin by enzymatic removal of the C chain, prior to its concentration and its packaging into membrane-limited secretory granules. After budding from the Golgi apparatus into the cytoplasm, the granules await an appropriate stimulus for their release by exocytosis into the extracellular fluid. Lysosomes can also destroy the granules in the cytoplasm of the B cells.

The stimulating substance binds to specific receptors on the plasma membrane of B cells, activates adenylate cyclase, and leads to formation of cAMP from ATP-magnesium. The generated cAMP increases the permeability of the plasma membrane to extracellular calcium ions, and of membranes of organelles to liberate calcium ions from the cytosolic reserves of the B cells. These calcium ions act as second messengers to activate the contractile elements in the microtubule-microfilament system for the equimolar release of the insulin-laden cytosolic granules and of the biologically inactive C chain, or C peptide. The membrane of the granules returns into the cytosol to be either recycled or degraded. Some proinsulin, which has about 5 to 10 percent of the activity of insulin, is also released into the peripheral blood and can add 20 percent to the total insulin immunoreactivity. In cows with parturient paresis (parturient hypocalcemia), insulin release is inhibited by the lack of extracellular calcium, and a hyperglycemia is added to the hypocalcemic dysfunction.

The structure of insulin (about 6,000 daltons), with 51 amino acids distributed in the disulfide-linked A and B chains (Fig. 49–4), is identical in cats, dogs, and pigs. In most other animal species, the differences in the insulin from cattle, horses, humans, rabbits, and sheep are mostly in the amino acids in positions 8, 9, and 10 of chain A (length: 21 amino acids) and in the last position (30) of chain B.

In plasma, insulin circulates unbound to any carrier protein, and its half-life is about 5 to 8 minutes. About half the secreted insulin that reaches the portal blood is immediately degraded by the liver during its first pass. The kidneys are another, but less important, site for the catabolism of insulin (less than 20 percent). A specific glutathione-dependent transhydrogenase separates the disulfide bonds that unite the A and B chains, and a protease fragments the two polypeptide chains. Very little unchanged insulin is excreted in the urine.

The inactive C peptide, which has a longer half-life in blood than that of insulin, can be measured and used to assess blood insulin level in animals receiving insulin therapy, which induces the production of antiinsulin antibodies that hinder the radioimmunoassay measurements.

Porcine insulin can exist as a monomer or as a dimer. The dimers can unite around a single zinc atom to form a tetramer or around two zinc atoms to form a hexamer.

Hypoinsulinemia due to lack of synthesis of insulin causes a metabolic dysfunction known as *diabetus mellitus,* which is characterized mostly by hyperglycemia, glucosuria, polyuria, polydipsia, polyphagia, and emaciation. The hyperglycemia results from a reduced transfer of glucose across the plasma membrane of cells and from increased gluconeogenesis from lipids and proteins of the tissues. In animals (dog), where the hypoinsulinemia is absolute with little functional islet cells, oral hypoglycemic agents are not efficacious. The insulins currently being used therapeutically (100 USP units (U) per milliliter; about 26 to 30 per milligram of insulin) are extracted from the pancreas of cows and pigs obtained at abattoirs. Porcine insulin also serves as the starting point in the synthesis of human insulin, which only requires the replacement of an alanine by a threonine residue at position 30 of the B chain. On a commercial basis, human insulin is produced also by the newer technology of cloning of DNA in *Escherichia coli.*

TABLE 49–1 Substances That Modify Output of Pancreatic Insulin

Enhancers	Inhibitors
Acetylcholine	
Alpha-adrenergic blocker chlorpromazine	Alpha-adrenergic agonist norepinephrine
Beta$_2$-adrenergic agonist epinephrine	Beta-adrenergic blocker propranolol
Amino acids arginine and leucine	Ca^{++} blocker phenytoin
cAMP	Destroyers of beta cells alloxan, streptozocin
Fatty acids acetoacetate	
Hormones ACTH, cortisol, estradiol, progesterone, gastrin, GIP, secretin, glucagon, GH, thyroxine	
Ketone bodies	
Sugars fructose, glucose, mannose, ribose	2-Deoxyglucose Thiazides diuretic (chlorothiazide) nondiuretic (diazoxide)

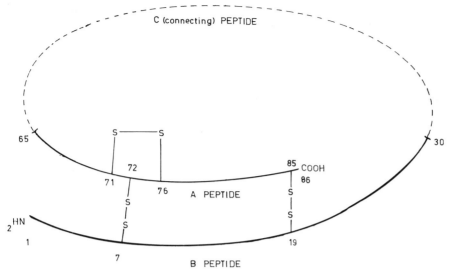

Figure 49–4 The structure of pro insulin is a polypeptide of 86 amino acid residues. After intragranular separation of the connection, or C, peptide from the biologically active insulin, both are extruded in equimolar amounts from the B cells and enter into the portal circulation. In most species, the insulin molecule consists of only 51 amino acid residues, distributed in two peptide chains. The A-peptide chain (21 amino acids, with an intrachain disulfide bridge) is linked with the B-peptide chain (30 amino acids) through two disulfide bonds. Less than 10 percent of the insulin-like activity in plasma is due to the original molecule of pancreatic insulin. A variety of insulin-like growth factors and large molecules (dimers to hexamers of insulin) account for the remaining bioassayable but not immunoassayable material in plasma.

The original insulin, extracted by BANTING and BEST, was of canine origin. The experimental obliteration of the exocrine ducts of the pancreas caused atrophy of the pancreatic secretory units, or pancreatons (acini cells and excretory duct). The remaining endocrine islet tissue was then harvested and was the source of a crude extract that had therapeutic efficacy in hypoinsulinemia dysfunctions, despite the presence of contaminant substances and hormones.

Experimental selective destruction of the B cells of the pancreatic islets is caused by several agents. When the major products for this procedure, alloxan and streptozocin, are injected, they break the DNA strands in B cells. Streptozocin has displaced alloxan as the preferred agent for producing a diabetic state in experimental animals, and it can be useful in treating insulinomas (insulin-secreting tumors). The destruction of B cells by streptozocin is accompanied by hypertrophy of D cells and an increase in the content of somatostatin. Other substances that also induce hypoinsulinemia include dehydroascorbic acid, dehydroisoascorbic acid, dialuric acid, some quinolones, and a rodenticide, pyriminil (Vacor).

In normal animals, more glucose binds to hemoglobin as the erythrocytes become older (average life: 120 days), and about 5 percent of the hemoglobin is glycosylated. With hypoinsulinemia, the resulting hyperglycemia raises the level of glycosylated hemoglobin about five times (i.e., to about 15 percent).

Hyperinsulinemia, causing profound hypoglycemia, occurs with tumors of the islet tissue (insulinoma) that have been reported in dogs and cows.

Intracellular Action

Insulin is effective when specific plasma membrane protein receptors are free and available. The average half-life of a free insulin receptor is about 7 hours. An adipocyte can carry about 10,000 insulin receptors, but the plasma membrane of a hepatocyte can have fives times as many insulin receptors (about 50,000, or 5 receptors per μm^2). The number of insulin receptors on the target cells is increased by a lack of insulin, by starvation, and by oral hypoglycemic agents (sulfonylurea). Conversely, the number of insulin receptors is decreased by large amounts of insulin (downregulation) and by obesity. The affinity of receptors for insulin is inversely related to the plasma levels of adrenal glucocorticoids (i.e., enhanced by their lack and reduced by their excess).

The insulin receptor is a glycoprotein with two symmetrical units connected by a disulfide bond (Fig. 49–5). Each unit is made up of an alpha-subunit (135,000 daltons) and a beta-subunit (90,000 daltons) that are also linked by a disulfide bond. Insulin binds to the alpha-subunits on the extracytoplasmic (glycoprotein) surface.

Other effects of the sulfonylurea are the facilitated release of insulin and glucagon in blood, by increasing the influx of Ca^{++} into the B and A cells, and an increase in the concentration of cAMP in the pancreatic islets. In animals, large doses of these agents have teratogenic effects.

In response to formation of the insulin-receptor complex, the beta-subunits in the plasma membrane induce the multiple effects of insulin. Stimulation of kinases (glu-

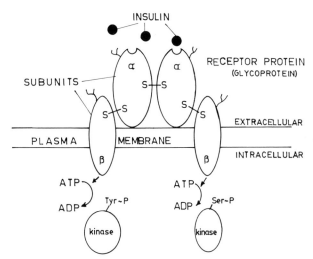

Figure 49–5 The receptor on the plasma membrane of insulin target cells is a complex protein. It is made of two pairs of glycoprotein subunits (alpha and beta), all linked by disulfide bonds. Insulin binds to the extracellular alpha subunits, which are linked to the intracellular beta subunits. The insulin-alpha subunit complex activates the phosphorylation of cytosolic kinases or proteins (at serine or tyrosine sites), which induce the insulin effects on growth and on metabolism of carbohydrate, lipid, and protein.

cokinase, phosphokinase, and pyruvic kinase) may result in phosphorylations of some enzymes, whereas activation of phosphatases may cause dephosphorylations of other enzymes. Transport systems of ions (Mg^{++}, PO_4^{---}, K^+) and of nutrients (glucose, amino acids) are facilitated in most cells except the hepatocytes, and intracellular enzymatic activity is stimulated in nearly all cells. Cytosolic lysosomes destroy the internalized insulin-receptor complex.

The pleiotropic (multiple effects) intracellular aptitude of insulin can be triggered by other mechanisms (e.g., receptor autoproteolysis, phospholipase C activity). Insulin then contributes to the rapid generation of membrane products, which are also able to activate still other intracellular enzymes (e.g., glycogen synthetase). It can also inhibit cAMP-dependent protein kinase A, and it can influence

nuclear mechanisms of cells in the liver and kidneys, suppressing the synthesis of fructose diphosphatase, glucose-6-phosphatase, phosphoenolpyruvate carboxykinase (PEP-CK), and pyruvate carboxylase, all major gluconeogenic enzymes.

Metabolic Actions

Insulin can modify the metabolisms of carbohydrates, lipids, and proteins. It can also affect the functions of major target organs (liver, muscles, and adipose tissue).

The metabolism of carbohydrates is greatly influenced by insulin. The easiest action that can be demonstrated is the decrease in glucose level, which is the culmination of several biochemical reactions. In summary, insulin inhibits the degradation of glycogen and activates its synthesis from glucose in the liver and in the muscles. Glucose storage is stimulated, but the destruction of glucose by glycolysis and its oxidation by the pentose-phosphate pathway is also increased. Likewise, gluconeogenesis is decreased (i.e., less glucose is formed from nonglucidic substances such as amino acids). Finally, insulin inhibits the release of glucose from the liver (and the kidneys), which is the only organ that can practically return glucose into the blood from its reserves, and promotes the entry of glucose into the muscles (Fig. 49–6).

Lipid metabolism also depends on insulin. Insulin enhances the entrance of glucose into cells of the adipose tissue and its transformation to triglycerides. The penetration of fatty acids with lipoproteins into adipocytes, and their incorporation into triglycerides, are also favored by insulin. Lipolysis is inhibited by insulin, and instead, storage of lipids as well as carbohydrates is enhanced. In synergy with glucagon, insulin promotes the delivery of hepatic glucose into the blood and its uptake by muscle cells.

Regarding protein metabolism, insulin increases the entry of plasma amino acids into muscular cells, which hold about 50 percent of the fuel reserve of an animal organism. Insulin activates the posttranslation stage for the synthesis of some tissue proteins (e.g., muscle proteins, collagen by chondrocytes in cartilage). Insulin inhibits the action of intracellular proteolytic enzymes.

Figure 49–6 Insulin promotes the anabolism of fatty acids, glucose, and amino acids. When the supply of insulin is adequate, adipocytes transform fatty acids and glycerol into lipids, preventing the occurrence of gluconeogenesis and of ketogenesis. Glucose then penetrates the plasma membrane to be stored as glycogen (muscles and liver) or to be used as a supply of energy for growth of tissues. In addition, some mechanisms induce the transformation of amino acids into proteins, inhibiting gluconeogenesis and reducing ureagenesis.

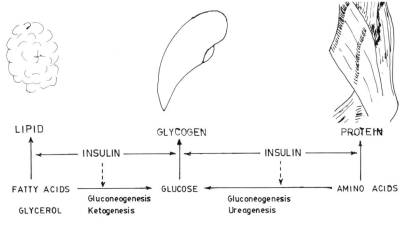

GLUCAGON

Knowledge of the existence of the endocrine secretion of the A cells of the pancreas can be traced back to 1923, which makes it contemporary to insulin. However, since glucagon has little therapeutic importance, its detailed investigation occurred only much later. Structurally related to secretin, the first hormone ever discovered, glucagon is a member of a family of hormones (secretin family) that also includes VIP and gastric inhibitory peptide (GIP).

Glucagon serves as a catabolic hormone used for fuel mobilization during periods of fuel starvation or injury (insult, illness) of the animal organism. It may be considered to function as an antagonist to anabolic insulin, whose primary objective is to store biological fuels during periods of fuel abundance.

Synthesis and Release

Glucagon is synthesized by A cells found in the pancreas, and glucagon-like immunoreactive factors are produced in the walls of the stomach and of the intestine, upon stimulation by low levels of blood glucose. With adequate insulin, the diurnal variations in the plasma glucagon level are small, and the glucagon output as a response to a glucose meal is a relatively small increase. In the absence of insulin, the same stimulus causes a greater release of glucagon. Ingested proteins, and some amino acids (arginine and alanine), are also powerful activators of the output of glucagon. Triglycerides have less stimulatory effect on the genesis of glucagon by A cells. Except for secretin, the gastrointestinal hormones seem to augment glucagon production just as much as they do for insulin. Fasting for a few days, intense exercise, vagal stimulation and acetylcholine, stress (burns, infections, surgery, toxemia), catecholamines, glucocorticoids, GH, and alpha-adrenergic stimulation all increase the synthesis and the release of glucagon. In contrast, hyperglycemia, an increase in the level of free fatty acids or ketones, insulin, and somatostatin suppress the synthesis and the release of glucagon.

Proteolytic enzymes process preproglucagon (18,000 daltons) into a proglucagon (12,000 daltons), which finally occupies the halo, whereas glucagon (29 amino acid residues, 3,500 daltons) is located in the central dense core of the A-cell granules. Upon adequate stimulation, the stored proglucagon is cleaved, and glucagon is released by exocytosis into the portal circulation. Among mammals (bovine, human, porcine), the structure of glucagon is identical.

The ratio of the concentration of glucagon in the portal circulation to that in the peripheral blood (about 1.5:1) is much lower than the 10:1 ratio for insulin. In the blood, glucagon circulates unbound to any protein carrier. The half-life of glucagon, between 5 and 10 minutes, is slightly longer than that of insulin. Its degradation occurs primarily in the liver, in the kidneys, and in the plasma membrane of target cells. Glucagon is inactivated by enzymatic proteolysis (e.g., cathepsin C and muscle proteinase) and removal of its amino-terminal histidine. Urine contains less than 1 percent of the secreted glucagon.

Hyperglucagonemia seems associated only with hypoinsulinemia dysfunction, and a glucagonoma has not been found in animals.

Intracellular and Metabolic Actions

Target cells provided with specific receptors for glucagon include hepatocytes, adipocytes, and islet B cells. The receptor system for glucagon consists of a binding subunit, a modulatory (filtering, intermediary) protein that carries the stimulus only if it is bound to guanosine triphosphate (GTP), and an adenylate cyclase. It is analogous to the beta-adrenergic receptor system but differs by its protein structure.

The intracellular action of glucagon is mediated via stimulation of adenylate cyclase and activation of cAMP-dependent protein kinase. The latter causes hepatic glycogenolysis by simultaneous activation of phosphorylase (via phosphorylase kinase), and inactivation of glycogen synthetase. For gluconeogenesis in the hepatocytes, glucagon deactivates pyruvate kinase, stimulates the conversion of pyruvate to phosphoenolpyruvate, and increases the cellular uptake of amino acids to provide adequate amounts of substrate. In the adipocytes, cAMP stimulates the triglyceride-lipase to fragment triglycerides into glycerol and fatty acids. Glycerol is taken up by hepatocytes for gluconeogenesis. In the islet B cells, glucagon receptors induce the entry of Ca^{++} and exocytosis of insulin-carrying granules.

Contrary to the effects of insulin, glucagon tends to raise plasma glucose levels, mostly by hepatic glycogenolysis and gluconeogenesis. It can also enhance lipolysis in adipose tissue.

SOMATOSTATIN

Somatostatin has a much broader biological significance than its name implies (i.e., inhibition of the output of GH from the adenohypophysis). It also inhibits the release of adenohypophysial thyrotropin, or thyroid-stimulating hormone (TSH), corticotropin, or ACTH, and prolactin (PRL); of the other endocrine peptides (insulin, glucagon, and PP) produced by the pancreatic islets; and of many gastrointestinal hormones (secretin, cholecystokinin-pancreozymin, GIP, and VIP). Somatostatin even depresses intestinal motility and absorption and some of the digestive exocrine secretions (gastric, pancreatic).

Synthesis of Pancreatic Somatostatin

In the D cells (of the islets and of the epithelium of the gut), the synthesis of somatostatin starts with a pre-prosomatostatin (116 amino acid residues). Intracellular proteolyses yield a prosomatostatin (92 amino acid residues) concentrated into secretory granules. Upon adequate stimulation, prosomatostatin and two of its carboxyterminal residues (with 14 and 28 amino acids) enter the portal blood by exocytosis. Quantitatively, the output of the islet D cells is mostly (96 percent) a 14–amino acid somatostatin (tetradecapeptide, S-14 or SS-14). This is accompanied by small equivalent amounts (2 percent) of prosomatostatin and of a 28–amino acid somatostatin (S-28 or SS-28) that is ten times more potent in inhibiting insulin release.

In the islet D cells, the synthesis of somatostatin may be increased by different types of stimuli. A hypersecretion of SS occurs in response to (1) ingestion of all three basic nutrients (fat, carbohydrates, and proteins) in the gut, with an even greater increase after protein or fat-rich meals; (2) a rise in the blood levels of glucose or of amino acids; (3) a higher output of glucagon in the neighboring A cells; and (4) gastrointestinal hormones (gastrin, VIP, secretin, and CCK). In addition, secretion-stimulating nervous signals, mediated by acetylcholine or by beta-adrenergic receptors, may directly reach the D cells.

The secretion of pancreatic somatostatin is inhibited by alpha-adrenergic stimuli, dopamine, and possibly insulin. Cysteamine blocks somatostatin release without affecting the output of insulin and glucagon.

Biological Effects of Pancreatic Somatostatin

The major actions of pancreatic SS are probably mediated through its tonic paracrine inhibition of the release of glucagon and PP from the neighboring A and F cells, with a little local effect on the output of insulin by B cells. In the dog, somatostatin is concerned mainly with inhibition of the intestinal assimilation of triglyceride and xylose. The half-life of somatostatin is very short, about 2 minutes.

PANCREATIC POLYPEPTIDE

Pancreatic polypeptide contains 36 amino acid residues; it has been sequenced in several mammals (cattle, sheep, pigs, humans) and can combine to form dimers, like insulin. The normal plasma level of PP is about equal to that of glucagon but is raised by protein-containing meals. The gastrointestinal hormones are secretagogues to PP, since the output of PP is higher after ingested than after injected glucose or amino acids. Not much is known regarding the role of PP, except that it stimulates gastric secretion of hydrochloride and pepsin and may also act as a satiety factor, like CCK.

REFERENCES

Banting FG, Best CH. The internal secretion of the pancreas. J Lab Clin Med 1922;7:251.

Blundell TL, Humbel RE. Hormone families: pancreatic hormones and homologous growth factors. Nature (Lond) 1980;287:781.

Brockman RP, Laarveld B. Hormonal regulation of metabolism in ruminants: a review. Livest Prod Sci 1986;14:313.

Cheng K, Lerner J. Intracellular mediators of insulin action. Annu Rev Physiol 1985;47:405.

Czech MP. New perspectives on the mechanism of insulin action. Recent Prog Horm Res 1984;40:347.

Czech MP. The nature and regulation of the insulin receptor: structure and function. Annu Rev Physiol 1985;47:357.

Delack JB, Stogdale L. Glycosylated hemoglobin measurement in dogs and cats: implication for its utility in diabetic monitoring. Can Vet J 1983;24:308.

Maruyama H, Hisatomi A, Orci L, Grodsky GM, Unger RH. Insulin within islets is a physiologic glucagon release inhibitor. J Clin Invest 1984;74:2296.

Reichlin S. Somatostatin. N Engl J Med 1983;309:1495 and 1556.

Ribes G, Blayac JP, Loubatieres-Mariani MM. Differences between the effects of adrenaline and noradrenaline on insulin secretion in the dog. Diabetologia 1983;24:107.

Robinson AM, Williamson DH. Physiological roles of ketone bodies as substrate and signals in mammalian tissues. Physiol Rev 1980;60:143.

Sorenson RL, Grouse LH, Elde RP. Cysteamine blocks somatostatin secretion without altering the course of insulin or glucagon release. Diabetes 1983;32:377.

Trent DF, Schwalke MA, Weir GC. Pancreatic and gut hormones during fasting: insulin, glucagon, somatostatin. Hormone Res 1984;19:70.

Unger RH. Glucagon physiology and pathophysiology in the light of new advances. Diabetologia 1985;28:574.

Unger RH, Orci L. Glucagon and the A cell. N Engl J Med 1981;304:1518.

Weigle DS. Pulsatile secretion of fuel regulatory hormones. Diabetes 1987;36:764.

Weir GC, Bonnerweir S. Pancreatic somatostatin. Adv Exp Med Biol 1984;188:403.

CHAPTER 50

HORMONES OF THE ADRENAL CORTEX AND MEDULLA

The paired adrenal glands found on the craniomedial aspects of each kidney contribute to the homeostasis as endocrine and as neurosecretory organs. Their cross-section shows a firm, narrow, golden-yellow, uniform outer rim—the *cortex* (mesodermal origin)—and a soft, reddish-brown to dark-brown core—the *medulla* (neurodermal origin). The ratio of the surface area of the cortex to that of the medulla is about 2:1 in the normal dog, although the mass of the medulla represents only about 15 to 25 percent of each adrenal gland. An unexplained local adrenocortical mineralization, causing no evident adrenal dysfunction, occurs in adult monkeys (50 percent), cats (30 percent), and dogs (6 percent).

Each gland is supplied with a rich arterial plexus that sequentially brings blood into the capsule, the cortex, and the medulla, before converging toward a single vein. This particular arrangement of the adrenal blood circulation creates an intimacy between the cortex and the medulla. Some of the endocrine secretions of the adrenal medulla are stimulated and regulated by the incoming hormones of the cortex.

The adrenal gland is innervated by autonomic fibers. Preganglionic sympathetic fibers run directly to the secreting medullary cells, which are termed chromaffins because they color brown with dichromate stains.

> Accessory adrenocortical tissue is seen frequently near the equine testis and in the reproductive tract of the mare. In dogs, rabbits, rodents, and nonhuman primates, accessory cortical tissue occurs frequently in the adrenal capsule and in the adipose tissue surrounding the kidneys and the adrenal.
>
> The development of the adrenal cortex requires the tropic action of the adenohypophysial corticotropin.

The cortical cells secrete steroid hormones, whereas the medullary chromaffin cells produce tyrosine derivatives, known as catecholamines. The main adrenocortical steroids (corticosteroids) contribute to responses that maintain the balance of electrolytes (mineralocorticoids), of carbohydrates (glucocorticoids), and of sex hormones. The adrenomedullary catecholamines (epinephrine, norepinephrine, and dopamine) act as neurotransmitters between cells, or as chemicals for communications between tissues. The adrenal cortex is essential to maintaining life, unless replacement therapy for glucocorticoids and mineralocorticoids is provided. Ablation of the adrenal medulla does not endanger survival.

HORMONES OF THE ADRENAL CORTEX

The adrenal cortex contains three histological zones that are not always distinct, each producing a definite type of adrenal steroid. The outermost, the *zona glomerulosa* (zona multiformis or zona arcuata), represents about 15 percent of the cortex and secretes *aldosterone,* the principal mineralocorticoid. The middle zone, the *zona fasciculata,* makes up 70 percent of the cortex and produces mainly *cortisol,* the major glucocorticoid. The innermost zone, the *zona reticularis,* accounts for the remaining 15 percent of the cortex and synthesizes adrenal *androgens,* or adrenal sex steroids, which are important in female animals but are trivial in males. In dogs, the ratio of the combined zonae fasciculata and reticularis to zona glomerulosa is about 8:1. Functionally, the zonae fasciculata and reticularis are sometimes considered as a single unit involved in producing glucocorticoids and sex steroids.

The morphology of the adrenal cortex is influenced by corticotropin (ACTH), angiotensin II (Ang II), and potassium. Elevations in ACTH levels increase the blood flow to the adrenal within minutes, and the mass of the zona fasciculata as well as its secretion of cortisol within hours. Prolonged corticotropin stimulation results in hyperplasia and in hypertrophy that can double the mass of the adrenal. Similar increases in Ang II and potassium levels cause hyperplasia and hypertrophy of the zona glomerulosa and raise the output of aldosterone. In contrast, a deficiency in ACTH leads to a reversible atrophy of the zonae fasciculata and reticularis, whereas a lack of Ang II and potassium induces a reversible atrophy of the zona glomerulosa.

Synthesis

The synthesis of adrenal steroids follows a pathway that begins with cholesterol, which contains the *cyclopentenoperhydrophenanthrene* nucleus, like bile acids, vitamin D, as well as ovarian and testicular steroids (Fig. 50–1). Some of the cholesterol is synthesized from acetate, but most of it is taken up from low density lipoproteins (LDL) in the blood.

> Adrenal steroids are either of the C19 or of C21 type, depending on the nature of the side-chain attached at position 17 of the D ring.
>
> The C19 type of steroids has a keto or a hydroxyl group at position 17, and since most have a keto group, they are known as 17-ketosteroids.
>
> The C21 steroids have a 2-carbon side-chain, and those that also have a hydroxyl group at position 17 are termed 17-hydroxycorticoids or 17-hydroxycorticosteroids. The androgen steroids are of the C19 type, and the mineralocorticoids and glucocorticoids are of the C21 type.

Cholesterol is converted to *pregnenolone,* which is then enzymatically transformed into steroids with androgen, glu-

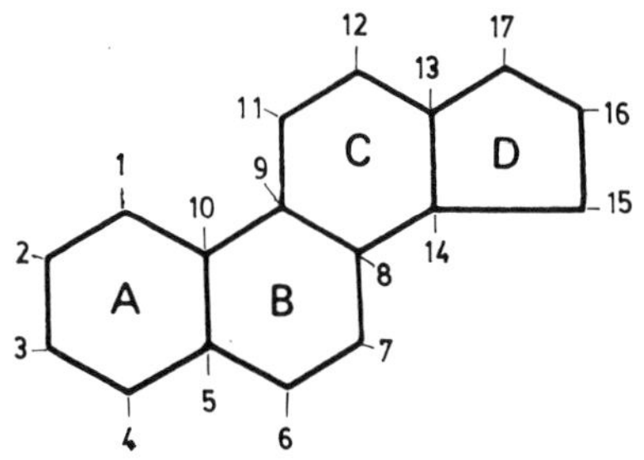

Figure 50–1 The cyclopentanoperhydrophenanthrene nucleus is found in bile acids, cholesterol, steroids (adrenocortical, ovarian, and testicular), and vitamin D. The letters A, B, C, and D identify the rings, while the numbers indicate the positions in the basic steroidal structure.

cocorticoid, and mineralocorticoid activity. Some of the pregnenolone can be converted to *17-alpha-hydroxypregnenolone,* which serves as the major gateway to formation of cortisol, and to a lesser extent for that of adrenal sex hormones (Fig. 50–2). Pregnenolone can also be changed into *progesterone,* which is mostly modified to aldosterone (via corticosterone, only in the zona glomerulosa), and to some cortisol and sex hormones. Adrenocorticosteroids are not stored within the adrenal, and their rate of biosynthesis is equivalent to their rate of release or of secretion.

Animals do not show the congenital enzyme defects of adrenocortical steroidogenesis seen in humans (e.g., 3-hydroxycorticosteroid dehydrogenase or 18-hydroxydehydrogenase).

Drugs can inhibit adrenal steroid biosynthesis at various steps (e.g., metyrapone, aminoglutethimide, mitotane {*o,p′*-DDD}, and spironolactone). Metyrapone depresses mainly 11-beta-hydroxylation and to a lesser extent 21-hydroxylation. Aminoglutethimide blocks the early conversion of cholesterol to pregnenolone. By inhibiting the operation of adrenal mitochondria, mitotane suppresses all adrenal steroidogenesis and causes adrenal atrophy. At high doses

(pharmacological action), spironolactone (an antimineralocorticoid) stops the biosynthesis of aldosterone by inhibiting the 11-beta and 18-hydroxylation steps.

Aldosterone

In most species, aldosterone is the principal and most potent mineralocorticoid regulating sodium and potassium homeostasis. About 60 percent of the total plasma aldosterone is bound to albumin, and only the free plasma aldosterone seems to be physiologically active. *Desoxycorticosterone* (DOC), which also has important mineralocorticoid activity (300 times less than that of aldosterone), has plasma levels similar to those of aldosterone. However, except in the rat, in which it is the only mineralocorticoid, DOC is not physiologically important because 95 percent of it is bound to plasma proteins and its free level is much lower than that of aldosterone.

Normal (nonstressed) aldosterone production is episodic or pulsatile and shows a tendency to circadian rhythm that is less marked than that of cortisol. The sustained period of rest during human monophasic sleep precedes the highest levels of aldosterone (i.e., maximum level around 6:00 AM), whereas the lowest levels are seen after diurnal activity (i.e., minimum at 8:00 PM). Similar circadian variations are recognized in horses, pigs, sheep, and birds (chickens, pigeons), but their existence is still debated in adult dogs. In the cat, as the highest corticosteroid levels occur at night and the lowest in the morning, this reversal of the circadian pattern of secretion supports the notion that the cat is a nocturnal animal.

Aldosterone production is increased predominantly by the renin-angiotensin system (angiotensin II) and by potassium (Fig. 50–3). In the horse, exercise augments plasma renin activity and results in a marked rise in blood aldosterone. Angiotensin II stimulates both the early phase (conversion of cholesterol to pregnenolone) and the late steps (transformation of corticosterone into 18-hydroxycorticoste-

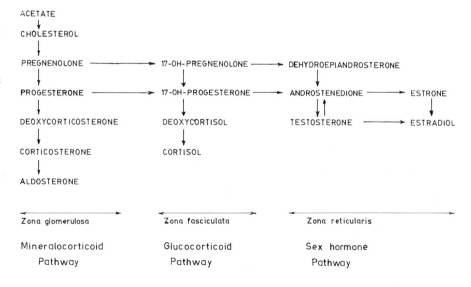

Figure 50–2 Outline of the synthesis of adrenocortical hormones in the zona glomerulosa (mineralocorticoid pathway), the zona fasciculata (glucocorticoid pathway), and the zona reticularis (adrenal sex steroid pathway).

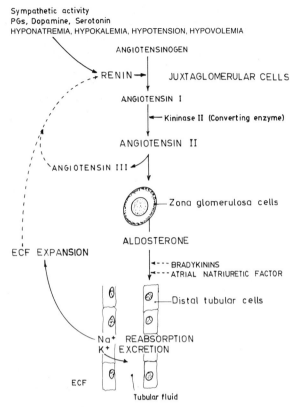

Figure 50–3 Diagrammatic representation of the action of aldosterone and of the factors stimulating (——) or inhibiting (- - - -) the production of renin, which is the principal modulator of aldosterone synthesis by the adrenocortical cells of the zona glomerulosa.

rone) in aldosterone biosynthesis. An increase in the level of plasma potassium (by as little as 0.1 mEq per liter, or 0.1 mmol per liter) enhances aldosterone production independently of sodium or Ang II. Other substances that also promote aldosterone secretion are ACTH, dopamine, serotonin, and sodium.

The *renin-angiotensin system* is composed of renin, angiotensinogen, and converting enzyme. Renin acts on angiotensinogen to yield Ang I, which is transformed into Ang II by the converting enzyme.

Renin, a glycoprotein (274 amino acids), is a proteolytic enzyme produced in the juxtaglomerular cells of the afferent renal arteriole by cleavage from a precursor protein (prorenin). Its release into the circulation is stimulated by lowering the blood pressure (e.g., hemorrhage), salt depletion, beta-adrenergic or central nervous system stimulation, and some prostaglandins. Its output is inhibited by increasing blood pressure, salt loading, Ang II, ADH, K^+, Ca^{++}, beta-adrenergic antagonists, alpha-methyldopa, clonidine, and inhibitors of prostaglandin synthesis (e.g., indomethacin).

Renin release can also be stimulated by other influences: (1) sodium receptors in the *macula densa* of the distal tubule (a specialized segment that is in contact with the juxtaglomerular cells) activated by loss of plasma sodium and chloride (e.g., dehydration, fluid loss); (2) baroreceptors

sensible to changes (decrease) in renal perfusion pressure rather than to the absolute pressure; (3) beta-adrenergic receptors stimulated by norepinephrine from renal sympathetic nerves (ending in the juxtaglomerular cells and smooth muscle cells of the renal afferent arteriole), an action inhibited by propranolol (beta-adrenergic blocker).

Angiotensinogen is a protein (over 400 amino acids) secreted by the liver. Its plasma level is raised by estrogens and glucocorticoids. Angiotensin I only serves as a substrate for production of AgII.

Converting enzyme, present in several tissues but predominantly in the lungs, catalyzes the conversion of Ang I into Ang II. It also catalyzes the inactivation of bradykinin. In humans, inhibitors of the converting enzyme (captopril, enalapril) are widely used as vasodilators and antihypertensive agents.

Angiotensin II acts directly on arterioles as a potent vasoconstrictor hormone, which has a half-life of only 1 or 2 minutes.

The major effects of aldosterone are on renal target cells (distal tubular) and nonrenal target cells (gastric, salivary, and sweat glands; ileal and colonic secretory cells). Aldosterone easily penetrates their plasma membrane and binds to a receptor protein in the cytoplasm. This cytosolic complex then acts on nuclear chromatin to allow expression of the specific genes responsible for production of the enzymes that catalyze the active reabsorption of sodium in exchange for H^+ and K^+. The sodium reabsorption leads to an increase in the acid and potassium content of the secretion of these cells, and to an aldosterone-induced alkalosis. By increasing the extracellular sodium level and causing water retention, aldosterone contributes to an expansion of the extracellular fluid volume and to maintaining the arterial pressure.

Aldosterone has a half-life of between 15 and 30 minutes. Its catabolism is by successive hydrogenation (in the liver and in the kidneys), and the metabolites are conjugated with glucuronic acid. In the liver, this conversion to metabolites is so effective that very little aldosterone survives a single passage through the portal circulation of this organ, which forms tetrahydroaldosterone glucuronide. The urine contains only about 1 percent of free aldosterone, and 99 percent of aldosterone glucuronides (mostly as the tetrahydro derivative).

In young female dogs, a hypoaldosteronemia, associated with chronic immune-mediated adrenocortical insufficiency or with acute hemorrhagic adrenocortical necrosis, may cause a urinary sodium loss (hypernatruria) and a reduced urinary potassium (hypokaluria). The decrease in plasma sodium (hyponatremia) and retention of plasma potassium (hyperkalemia) induce lethal circulatory dysfunctions, which are associated with shock due to the loss of extracellular fluid.

Aldosterone replacement therapy is by intramuscular administration of desoxycorticosterone acetate (DOCA), or by oral fludrocortisone acetate (a synthetic mineralocorticoid, 20 times more active than DOCA). Aldosterone is not effective orally, as it is poorly absorbed by the gut and is immediately destroyed in the liver.

A physiological hyperaldosteronemia occurs during pregnancy, because of an increase in plasma estrogens. Hyperaldosteronemia (Conn's syndrome) with dysfunctions such as hypernatremia, hypokalemia, hypertension, and edema is rarely seen in dogs and cats.

By binding to aldosterone receptors, spironolactone acts as a specific antagonist to the effects of aldosterone.

Cortisol

The cells of the zona fasciculata secrete glucocorticosteroids, *cortisol* and *corticosterone,* that are primarily involved in carbohydrate metabolism. The predominant glucocorticosteroid secreted by most mammals is cortisol, which is considered as one of the few hormones essential for life and is more potent than corticosterone. The cortisol-to-corticosterone ratio is about 5 in dogs, 7 in adult cats, less than 1 in kittens, and 24 in horses. Some cortisol is converted to cortisone, which has a similar metabolic fate. In contrast, corticosterone is the only glucocorticoid secreted by birds and rodents, although some cortisol is produced by chicken embryos.

The activity of the zonae fasciculata and reticularis is controlled mostly by ACTH. The production of ACTH is under neuroendocrine control, that is, cytokines and incoming nervous signals to the hypothalamus (e.g., stress, lactation, anticipation of feeding) induce production and release of corticotropin-releasing hormone (CRF), which is destined to stimulate the adenohypophysial secretion of corticotropin. Within minutes after stimulation by ACTH, the fasciculata cells secrete and release cortisol and corticosterone into the adrenal vein. By a negative-feedback control, the higher levels of cortisol and corticosterone in plasma react on receptors to inhibit the output of CRH by the hypothalamus and of corticotropin by the adenohypophysis. The output of cortisol is pulsatile and follows a circadian pattern, plasma levels decreasing with physical activity (minimum attained in evening) and increasing after a period of continued rest (maximum in morning).

In horses, an antiserotonin drug (cyproheptadine), with antihistamine and anticholinergic effects, blocks the serotonin-mediated release of CRH and ACTH in the hypothalamus-adenohypophysis complex.

In dogs and horses, a dopamine receptor agonist (bromocriptine) suppresses the output of ACTH.

In blood, most (70 percent) of the cortisol binds to an alpha-globulin called transcortin or corticosteroid-binding globulin (CBG), about 20 percent is albumin-bound, and about 10 percent is free. CBG limits the amount of cortisol available for target organs, for inactivation, and for urinary excretion. The binding of cortisol is reversible and produces a reservoir of glucocorticoids that keeps a readily available supply of potential free cortisol in the plasma. Unbound blood cortisol is ultrafiltrable and appears in saliva and milk, after having entered salivary and mammary gland cells. The glucocorticoids also appear in the intestine (via bile) and undergo ileal absorption as part of an efficient enterohepatic circulation, which allows only 15 percent of the secreted cortisol to be lost in the feces. Free cortisol can also find its way into the glomerular filtrate. However, most of this free

cortisol (about 80 percent) is reabsorbed, and only 20 percent is lost in the urine. Cortisol levels in saliva and milk (60 percent of the total ultrafiltrate) are used as an indication of the free cortisol in blood. Total cortisol level is a poor indicator of the true cortisol activity, as some conditions augment the CBG plasma level (e.g., estrogens, postpartum) and bound cortisol without raising the available quantity of active unbound glucocorticoid. In contrast, stress increases the level of free plasma cortisol.

CBG production in the liver is increased by estrogens and pregnancy. It is reduced by cirrhosis and nephrosis.

Although glucocorticoids may act on many cells of the body, their major target cells are in the liver and the thymus. In the liver, the hepatocytes (about 65 percent of total liver cells) are induced to produce gluconeogenic enzymes such as fructose-1-6-diphosphatase, glucose-6-phosphatase, and pyruvate carboxylase. These enzymes enhance the conversion of proteins into glucose, which is utilized during physical and metabolic activity. In addition, an increase in the plasma free fatty acid levels reflects the higher content of lipolytic enzymes in adipocytes of fat deposits (triglycerides). By suppressing thymocytes (similar to lymphocytes in blood of other lymphoid organs), glucocorticoids also impair the production of endocrine-immunological interleukin 2 (lymphokines and monokines) by T lymphocytes. A lack of these hormones reduces the fight against bacteria, viruses, fungi, as well as parasites, and may contribute to their dissemination throughout the body. The number of eosinophils and of basophils in the circulation is depressed by glucocorticoids, which sequester them in the lungs and spleen. However, glucocorticoids cause more erythrocytes (by activation of erythropoietin), neutrophils, and platelets to appear in the circulation. In the fetus, glucocorticoids accelerate the synthesis of lung surfactant by type II granular pneumocytes. This dipalmitoyl lecithin forms a liquid film that lines the interior of the alveolar walls and is critical to maintaining the stability of the alveoli and preventing their collapse.

By causing the synthesis of a protein (named lipocortin, lipomodulin, macrocortin, and remodulin) that blocks the release of phosphatase A_2, which is responsible for the release of arachidonic acid from plasma membrane, glucocorticoids also prevent the formation of eicosanoids (prostaglandins). The glucocorticoids exert an antiinflammatory effect by suppressing the formation of prostaglandin E.

However, in pregnant (near term) ruminants, the formation of prostaglandin $F_{2\alpha}$ (and estradiol) by the endometrium is increased by glucocorticoids. This effect is used to induce parturition a few days (maximum, 14 days) before term, in a functional fetoplacental unit (i.e., living fetus). Massive doses of short-acting (USA) or long-acting (Europe, Australia) forms of synthetic glucocorticoids (e.g., dexamethasone) are administered. The response occurs rapidly (about 48 hours) with the short-acting treatment, and after about a week with the long-acting medication. Placental retention is a frequent sequela.

The half-life of cortisol is longer (60 to 90 minutes) than that of corticosterone (about 50 minutes). The catabolism of cortisol occurs in the liver and to some extent in the kidneys. In dogs, sulfate derivatives are often seen in bile, but most of the urinary metabolites are glucuronides. The urine of the cat contains almost no cortisol or any other steroid metabolite.

Hypocortisolism or lack of glucocorticoid, because of the long-loop negative feedback on the hypothalamus-adenohypophysis complex, causes a higher output of ACTH. Measurement of high concentrations of ACTH is diagnostic of hypofunction of the adrenal cortex (Addison's syndrome). The dog may present a syndrome resembling Addison's syndrome, caused by atrophy of the adrenal cortex, which may be reduced to one tenth its normal thickness.

Among the synthetic steroids, dexamethasone is 25 times more potent as a glucocorticoid and has a lower mineralocorticoid activity than cortisol. Its presence in plasma does not interfere with measurements of cortisol. The metabolism of dexamethasone is enhanced by phenytoin (Dilantin).

Another synthetic glucocorticoid, prednisolone, is four times more potent than cortisol and has about the same mineralocorticoid activity. Like cortisone, a derivative of cortisol formed by oxidation of the 11-beta-hydroxyl group to ketone, prednisolone lacks glucocorticoid activity before its conversion in the liver into biologically active 11-hydroxyl steroids. This conversion may be hindered by hepatic dysfunctions.

For replacement therapy, cortisol or cortisone is short-acting, whereas both prednisolone and dexamethasone are long-acting.

Chronic excess of glucocorticoids (hypercortisolism, or Cushing's syndrome) leads to catabolic effects (skin atrophy, muscle wasting, osteoporosis) and a tendency to hyperglycemia. As a consequence, a higher output of insulin occurs to favor glucose storage, or energy storage, by fat synthesis and fat deposition. In dogs, and rarely in cats and horses, an excess of glucocorticoid consecutive to excessive secretion of ACTH also increases the secretion of PTH and alkaline phosphatase, and androgens, while decreasing the action of growth hormone and calcitriol (or vitamin D_3). Two agents can lower the amount of glucocorticoids in the circulation, metyrapone and aminoglutethimide. Metyrapone inhibits 11-beta-hydroxylation and decreases the adrenocortical production of cortisol. Aminoglutethimide inhibits the desmolases and the aromatases involved in adrenosteroid syntheses and conversions (e.g., androstenedione → estrogens) and creates an accumulation of cholesterol in the gland.

Adrenal Sex Hormones

The zona reticularis produces mostly androgens (e.g., androstenedione) and minor quantities of glucocorticoids and of some other steroid'hormones (e.g., progesterone and estrogens). This production of adrenal androgens is usually initiated at the time of the pubertal period called *adrenarche*. In the plasma, most of the adrenal sex steroids are bound to a sex hormone–binding globulin (SHBG).

Adrenal Androgens.   In healthy animals, the secretion of androstenedione (one fifth the potency of testosterone) is usually trivial in comparison with the production of glu-

cocorticoids and mineralocorticoids. Their action is to promote protein anabolism, growth, and erythropoiesis, without masculinizing effects. It is estimated that the adrenal cortex produces about 10 percent of the circulating androgens in males and about 50 percent of those in the blood of female animals. The catabolism of androgens is not very well understood in domesticated animals. Very little of the secreted adrenal androgens can be measured in urine, and most of them are excreted via bile.

The production of adrenal androgens is controlled by ACTH, not by gonadotropins. An excessive and abnormal output of adrenal androgens (adrenogenital syndrome) is more noticeable in female than in male animals, because of the masculinizing effect (e.g., clitoral enlargement in the mare).

Adrenal Estrogens.   The adrenal-related estrogens come from the zona reticularis and also from the irreversible conversion of circulating androstenedione to estrogens. Their quantity is too small to have any obvious physiological effect.

HORMONES OF THE ADRENAL MEDULLA

The adrenal medulla is composed of modified postganglionic neurons, which are without axons or nerve endings and are essentially neuron cell bodies that have adapted to a secretory function. These cells are called chromaffin cells, because of their affinity for chromium stains and for ferric chloride. They receive stimulation signals through cholinergic synapses with axons from neurons of the sympathetic nervous system (i.e., located in the lateral gray matter of the thoracolumbar cord). For these reasons, it is called the sympathochromaffin system, a component of the autonomic central nervous system. The chromaffin cells function as modified postganglionic sympathetic neurons, somewhat like the second neurons of this system. However, they release catecholamines (hormone and neurotransmitters) into the circulation instead of synapsing with effector organs or tissues (Fig. 50–4).

The chromaffin cells respond by producing *catecholamines*, which are derivatives of tyrosine that is consumed in the diet or converted from phenylalanine (by phenylalanine hydroxylase) in the liver. Synthesized by enzymes of the chromaffin cells, these catecholamines are stored in large cytosolic neurosecretory granules (100 to 300 nm in diameter) and are released by exocytosis directly into the synaptic cleft or into the blood circulation. In the central nervous system, the catecholamines of physiological importance (*dopamine, epinephrine,* and *norepinephrine*) are neurotransmitters, whereas in the periphery, epinephrine serves as a hormone.

Besides the catecholamines (about 20 percent by weight), the neurosecretory granules contain magnesium, adenosine triphosphate (ATP, 15 percent), a specific protein (chromogranin, 35 percent), lipids (20 percent), and peptides (enkephalins, beta-endorphin, proopiomelanocortin). Most (80 percent) of the granules store epinephrine, but some granules contain only norepinephrine (20 percent). In dogs and horses, this ratio of epinephrine secretion to nor-

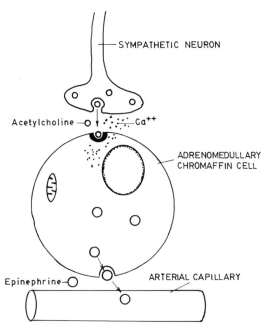

Figure 50–4 The production of epinephrine by the adreno-medullary chromaffin cells is stimulated by the entry of calcium ions, which coincides with the release of acetylcholine at the endings of sympathetic (presynaptic) neurons.

chain. The on-going process of catecholamine synthesis (Fig. 50–5) starts with diffusion of *extracellular tyrosine* (or phenylalanine) into the cytoplasm of chromaffin cells. In the *cytosol*, tyrosine hydroxylase (the rate-limiting enzyme) converts tyrosine to *dopa* (dihydroxyphenylalanine), which is then transformed into *dopamine* by an L-amino acid decarboxylase. Afterwards, dopamine must actively enter within the *neurosecretory granules* to be changed into *norepinephrine*, a reaction catalyzed by the intragranular beta-hydroxylase. To be transformed into *epinephrine*, norepinephrine must move out of the secretory granules into the cytoplasm, as the final enzyme (phenylethanolamine-*N*-methyltransferase [PNMT] is present only in the cytosol. The return of epinephrine from the cytosol into the secretory granules, for storage until release, is an active process that requires ATP and magnesium. In the chromaffin granules, a nondiffusible complex is formed by the catecholamines, ATP, and specific proteins (called chromogranins).

In the chromaffin cells, the production of cytosolic tyrosine hydroxylase and of intragranular dopamine beta-

epinephrine secretion (about 1:1 in the newborn animal) becomes stabilized at about 3:1 to 4:1 within a few weeks after birth. In rabbits, the adrenal production of norepinephrine is minimal, and the epinephrine:norepinephrine ratio is as high as 49:1. In other animals, the adult adrenomedullary output ratio of epinephrine:norepinephrine is also lower (e.g., about 1:1 in pigs, 2:1 in ruminants, and 3:2 in cats).

Nerve growth factor (one of the insulin-like growth factors) stimulates the development of the sympathetic nervous system, which activates the induction of the synthesis of these neural hormones. Catecholamines, also produced by adrenergic neurons, are used as one of the major media—the other is acetylcholine—for rapid chemical neuronal or synaptic communication.

Almost immediately upon entering the circulation, epinephrine functions as a hormone that mediates some of the stress or "fight-or-flight" reactions. The rapidity of its metabolic effects is comparable with that of insulin and glucagon but is quite different from that of the slower-acting adenohypophysial and thyroid hormones. In most animals, the adrenal medullary output of norepinephrine is greater than that of the dog, the horse, and primates. Dopamine and mostly norepinephrine act primarily as local synaptic neurotransmitters released at sympathetic postganglionic neuron-axon terminals.

Synthesis

Epinephrine, norepinephrine, and dopamine are compounds containing a benzene ring with two adjacent OH groups (catechol) attached to an amine-containing side-

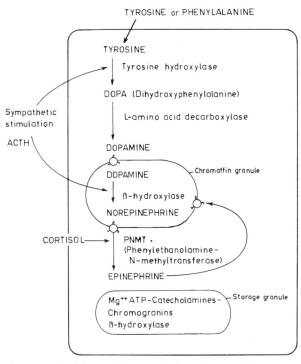

Figure 50–5 The production of the adrenomedullary catecholamines starts with the transfer of tyrosine into the chromaffin cells. Successive cytosolic enzymes transform tyrosine into dopamine, which can actively penetrate into the secretory granules. An intragranular enzyme transforms dopamine into norepinephrine. After actively returning into the cytosol, norepinephrine is modified to epinephrine, which actively returns to the granules for storage, awaiting the releasing stimulus. Sympathetic stimulation and ACTH stimulate tyrosine hydroxylase and dopamine beta-hydroxylase. Cortisol enhances the formation of phenylethanolamine-*N*-methyltransferase (PNMT). Glucagon, histamine, and reserpine stimulate the release of the entire contents of the chromaffin granules. The storage granules contain a nondiffusible complex of Mg^{++}-ATP-catecholamines-chromogranins, lipids, opioid peptides, and dopamine beta-hydroxylase.

hydroxylase is stimulated by sympathetic nerve impulses and by ACTH. Corticotropin augments the intracellular level of cAMP, which activates the protein kinases that in turn accelerate the rate of synthesis of both the hydroxylases. The quantity of PNMT in the cytosol is increased by cortisol, which unites with a cytoplasmic glucocorticoid receptor to form a complex that activates the nuclear transcription for synthesis of this enzyme.

The activity of tyrosine hydroxylase and of dopamine beta-hydroxylase is stimulated by nerve impulses. In contrast, the activity of tyrosine hydroxylase is suppressed by an excess of norepinephrine in the cytosol. Norepinephrine accumulates in the cytoplasm when its transfer for metabolism into the secretory granules is impaired.

Release

The release of the entire contents of the chromaffin granules (catecholamines, ATP, Mg^{++}, chromogranins, dopamine beta-hydroxylase, lipids, and peptides [enkephalins, beta-endorphin, proopiomelanocortin]) is related to the activation of the sympathetic nervous system. The neurosecretion usually coincides with or anticipates the stimulation of the sympathetic nervous system, which comes in direct contact with the adrenal medulla chromaffin cells via splanchnic nerve fibers. Glucagon, histamine, and reserpine (a drug) also induce exocytosis or release of adrenal medullary catecholamines.

Upon stimulation, the acetylcholine released from the sympathetic axon terminals depolarizes the chromaffin cell, increasing the permeability of its plasma membrane to sodium. An influx of Ca^{++} in the cytosol induces the microfilaments to contract and pull the neurosecretory granules close to the cytoplasmic aspect of the plasma membrane. After fusion of the granules with the plasma membrane, their content is discharged by exocytosis. The granular membrane is retained and recycled, whereas the now extracellular compounds enter the local fenestrated arteriolar capillaries and then join the general venous blood circulation.

Actions

In the plasma, most (about 70 to 95 percent) of the catecholamines are inactive sulfate conjugates, and only the free catecholamines are active. In various tissues, dopamine, epinephrine, and norepinephrine exert their effects on target cells through specific plasma membrane receptors. Little is known about dopaminergic receptors, but it should be mentioned that dopamine is the prolactin-inhibiting factor. Several concepts have been established for adrenergic receptors. On the basis of different actions, adrenergic receptors are classified into types alpha and beta, with subtypes (e.g., alpha$_1$, alpha$_2$, beta$_1$, beta$_2$).

Postsynaptic alpha$_1$-receptors mediate vasoconstriction in vascular smooth muscles, whereas the presynaptic alpha$_2$-receptors facilitate reuptake of released norepinephrine and inhibit its further release. Alpha$_2$-receptors are found on nerve endings, platelets, adipose tissue, and smooth muscle.

The postsynaptic beta$_1$-receptors are activated by norepinephrine and mediate positive inotropic (strength) and chronotropic (frequency) effects on cardiac muscle. Beta$_2$-receptors, activated by free epinephrine in the general circulation, mediate smooth-muscle relaxation in the bronchi, blood vessels, and uterus.

> Other hormones, by binding to the receptors, can alter the interaction between catecholamine agonist and adrenergic receptor.
>
> For example, iodinated thyroid hormones increase the quantity of myocardial beta-receptors. Also, the absence of glucocorticoids results in an increase in the number of beta-receptors without any change in the number of alpha-receptors.

The alpha$_2$-, beta$_1$-, and beta$_2$-receptors are structurally similar single-unit glycoproteins (64,000 daltons), whereas alpha$_1$-receptors are glycoproteins of 80,000 daltons. Beta$_1$- and beta$_2$-receptors are coupled to and *activate* adenylate cyclase, and cAMP is the second messenger stimulating protein kinase A and a cascade of changes in enzyme activities. The alpha$_2$-receptor inhibits adenylate cyclase, so cAMP and protein kinase A activity is suppressed. The alpha$_2$-receptors are antagonists to beta$_1$- and beta$_2$ receptors. Alpha$_1$-receptors are coupled to the phosphatidylinositol membrane system, with protein kinase C and Ca^{++} mediating the hormone effects. Propranolol is the traditional antagonist to beta-receptors, and phentolamine to alpha-receptors.

> Selective antagonists exist for alpha$_1$ (prazosin), alpha$_2$ (yohimbine), beta$_1$ (metoprolol), and beta$_2$ (butoxamine) receptors.

Receptors constitute important sites for regulation of adrenergic activity. The quantity of target tissue receptors can be reduced by the binding of an agonist, a process called *down-regulation*. The effect is to reduce the sensitivity of a target cell to high levels of circulating agonist. The reverse occurs with a low level of agonist, in which "*up-regulation*" of receptors occurs, increasing the sensitivity of the target cells. Another aspect of the regulation of both alpha- and beta-adrenergic receptors is *desensitization*, which decreases the response of subsequent doses of an agonist after an acute exposure to a catecholamine hormone (e.g., epinephrine).

The catecholamines, especially epinephrine, stimulate carbohydrate metabolism to cause quick changes and to provide an immediate energy source for "fight-or-flight" responses. The effects of epinephrine on tissues include increases in glycogenolysis and gluconeogenesis in the liver, augmented gluconeogenesis in skeletal muscles, stronger and faster myocardial contractions, relaxation of the uterine musculature, lipolysis or conversion of triglycerides to free fatty acids and glycerol in adipose tissue, elevation of arterial pressure and of cardiac output, and dilation of bronchial musculature.

Metabolism

The degradation of circulating epinephrine and norepinephrine occurs in many tissues, but mostly in the kidney and liver. The metabolic inactivation pathways use two key enzyme systems: catechol-O-methyl transferase (COMT) and a combination of monoamine oxidase (MAO) and aldehyde oxidase (AO). COMT catalyzes the conversion of norepinephrine and epinephrine to normetanephrine and metanephrine, which, under the successive actions of MAO and AO, are in turn transformed into 3-methoxy-4-hydroxymandelic acid. This compound is the major end-product of catecholamine degradation and is usually known as vanillylmandelic acid (VMA). The alternative metabolic route also uses MAO and AO to convert the catecholamine 3,4-dihydroxymandelaldehyde, which is transformed to VMA by COMT.

Epinephrine and norepinephrine have very short life spans in plasma, and their dramatic effects are rapidly turned off because their half-life is only 1 to 3 minutes.

Deficiency of catecholamines is unknown. Synthetic catecholamine agonists (e.g., epinephrine, norepinephrine, dopamine) are used in subcutaneous injections to delay local absorption (by vasoconstriction), to treat shock due to decreased circulating plasma volume, and to increase renal perfusion.

Excess of catecholamines associated with an adrenal medullary tumor (pheochromocytoma) is seen in dogs and, rarely, in cats and horses.

REFERENCES

Anderson MG, Aitken MM. Biochemical and physiological effects of catecholamine administration in the horse. Res Vet Sci 1977;22:357.

Ariens EJ. The classification of beta-adrenoceptors. Trends Pharmacol 1981;2:170.

Critchley JAJH, Ellis P, Ungar A. The reflex release of adrenaline and noradrenaline from the adrenal glands of cats and dogs. J Physiol 1980;298:71.

Feldman EC, Peterson ME. Hypoadrenocorticism. Vet Clin North Am (Small Anim Pract) 1984;14:751.

Goldberg AL, Tishler M, DeMartino G, Griffin G. Hormonal regulation of protein degradation and synthesis in skeletal muscle. Fed Proc 1980;39:31.

Gustafsson JA, Carlstedt-Duke J, Poellinger L, et al. Biochemistry, molecular biology, and physiology of the glucocorticoid receptor. Endocr Rev 1987;8:185.

Guthrie GP, Cecil SG, Kotchen TA. Renin, aldosterone, and cortisol in the thoroughbred horse. J Endocrinol 1980;85:49.

Hardee GE, Lai JW, Semrad S, Trim CM. Catecholamines in equine and bovine plasmas. J Vet Pharmacol Ther 1983;5:279.

Hullinger RL. Adrenal cortex of the dog (*Canis familiaris*). Histomorphological changes during growth, maturity, and aging. Zbl Vet Med C Anat Histol Embryol 1978;7:1.

Insel PA. Indentification and regulation of adrenergic receptors in target cells. Am J Physiol 1984;247:E53.

Kemppainen RJ. Effects of glucocorticoids on endocrine function in the dog. Vet Clin North Am (Small Anim Pract) 1984;14:721.

Kryvi H. Comparison of the ultrastructure of adrenaline and noradrenaline storage granules of bovine adrenal medulla. Eur J Cell Biol 1979;20:76.

Landsberg L, Young JB. The role of the sympathetic nervous system and catecholamines in the regulation of energy metabolism. Am J Clin Nutr 1983;38:1018.

Leftkowitz RJ, Caaron MG. Adrenergic receptors: molecular mechanisms of clinically relevant recognition. Clin Res 1985;33:395.

Lothrop CD, Oliver JW. Diagnosis of canine Cushing's syndrome based on multiple steroid analysis and dexamethasone turnover kinetics. Am J Vet Res 1984;45:2304.

Marver D. Aldosterone action in target epithelia. Vitam Horm 1980;38:57.

Munck A, Guyre PM, Holbrook NJ. Physiological functions of glucocorticoids in stress and their relation to pharmacological actions. Endocr Rev 1984;5:25.

Peterson ME. Hyperadrenocorticism. Vet Clin North Am (Small Anim Pract) 1984;14:731.

Richkind M. Cushing's syndrome in dogs: treatment with bromocriptine and cyproheptadine. Vet Med Small Anim Clin 1981;76:1301.

Rossdale PD, Burguez PN, Cash RSG. Changes in blood neutrophil/lymphocyte ratio related to adrenocortical function in the horse. Equine Vet J 1982;14:293.

Santen RJ. Adrenal of male dog secretes androgens and estrogens. Am J Physiol 1980;239:E109.

Schiebinger RJ, Albertson BD, Barnes KM, Cutler GR, Loriaux DL. Developmental changes in rabbit and dog adrenal function: a possible homologue of adrenarche in the dog. Am J Physiol 1981;240:E694.

Schmidt TJ, Litwack G. Activation of the glucocorticoid receptor complex. Physiol Rev 1982;62:1131.

Toutain PL, Alvinerie M, Ruckebusch Y. Pharmacokinetics of dexamethasone and its effect on adrenal gland function in the dog. Am J Vet Res 1983;44:212.

Toutain PL, Brandon RA, Depomyers H, Alvinerie M, Baggot JD. Dexamethasone and prednisolone in the horse: pharmacokinetics and action on the adrenal gland. Am J Vet Res 1984;45:1750.

Winkler H, Westhead E. The molecular organization of adrenal chromaffin granules. Neuroscience 1980;5:1803.

Yarrington JT, Capen CC. Ultrastructural and biochemical evaluation of adrenal medullary hyperplasia and pheochromocytoma in aged bulls. Vet Pathol 1981;18:316.

Yovich JV, Horney FD, Hardee GE. Pheochromocytoma in the horse and measurement of norepinephrine in horses. Can Vet J 1984;25:21.

CHAPTER 51

EICOSANOIDS AND HORMONES OF THE THYMUS AND LEUKOCYTES, OF THE HEART, AND OF THE KIDNEYS

Several naturally occurring humoral compounds, with various structures and activities, are secreted in small amounts from sources not generally considered as endocrine. Sometimes called *autacoids,* these substances are lipids (eicosanoids) or polypeptides (angiotensin, atrial natriuretic factor, erythropoietin, interleukins, kinins, renin, and thymosin). Their production occurs in cells disseminated in various organs (angiotensin, eicosanoids, interleukins) or in specific cells in organs such as the heart (atrial natriuretic factor) and the kidneys (erythropoietin, renin).

EICOSANOIDS

The eicosanoids represent a heterogenous family of 20-carbon derivatives (eico), such as prostaglandins (PGs), thromboxanes (TXs), leukotrienes (LTs), and lipoxins (LXs). These substances have hormonal or modulating activities on the cells at their origin (autocrine effect), on neighboring cells (paracrine effect), or on distant cells (endocrine effect). A common characteristic is their link to essential fatty acids having three, four, or five double bonds, such as dihomo-gamma-linolenic (eicosatrienoic, or C20:3), arachidonic (eicosatetraenoic, or C20:4), and timnodonic (eicosapentaenoic, or C20:5) acids.

The *prostaglandins,* or prostanoids, are secreted by many cells in most of the tissues of the organism. Their nomenclature takes into account the position of the oxygen radicals on the five-peaked saturated cycle, or cyclopentane nucleus (*classes* A, B, C, D, E, F, G or H, and I), and the number of residual double bonds after the loss of 2 double bonds (C=C) by cyclization of the nucleus (*series* 1, 2, and 3). For PGF, as only the *trans* (alpha) isomer that is physiologically active, this designation is added in subscript after that of the class and of the series. Because of a O—O bond between positions 9 and 11 of the nucleus, PGG and PGH qualify as endoperoxides that have either a perhydroxyl or a hydroxyl group on position 15 (Fig. 51–1). Prostacyclins (PGIs) have a different type of oxygen bridge, between carbon 9 of the nucleus and position 6 of the lateral chain.

Thromboxanes, which carry a six-peak radical instead of the cyclopentane nucleus, are known as epoxides, since an oxygen bridge unites two carbons of this heterocycle. Classes (A and B) and series (1 to 3) are considered for their nomenclature (Fig. 51–2).

Leukotrienes, first discovered in leukocytes, may sequentially be of classes A, B, C, D, and E and are usually of series 4 (i.e., derived from arachidonic acid with 4 C=C) (Fig. 51–3), although some may contain 5 C=C and be derived from timnodonic acid. Except for LTA$_4$ and LTB$_4$, leukotrienes link to a molecule of di- or tripeptide, or to an amino acid, and are called peptidoleukotrienes or sulfidoleukotrienes. LTF$_4$ is an interchangeable derivative of LTE$_4$, formed by addition of gamma-glutamic acid to LTE$_4$.

Lipoxins A and B (LXA, LXB), or lipoxygenase interaction products, are eicosanoids possessing three hydroxyl and four C=C (Fig. 51–4).

Biosynthetic Pathways

The formation of the precursor fatty acids for eicosnaoid synthesis is obtained by chain elongation of the essential fatty acids linoleic and alpha-linolenic acid. Linoleic acid can be transformed into dihomo-gamma-linolenic acid, and the latter into arachidonic acid. Alpha-linolenic acid is at the source of timnodonic acid, which is found mostly in marine animals.

Dihomo-gamma-linolenic acid can give rise to series 1 prostaglandins and arachidonic acid. Arachidonic acid can be the precursor of series 2 prostaglandins, of leukotrienes, and of lipoxins. Timnodonic acid usually leads to the formation of series 3 prostaglandins (Fig. 51–5) but may be at the origin of leukotrienes with 5 C=C.

The intracellular synthesis and the release of eicosanoids from the cytoplasm of their cells of origin are activated by various types of stimulations. These stimuli may be dysfunctional (anaphylaxis, inflammation), hormonal (glucagon), mechanical (distention, parturition), and neurochemical (catecholamines, histamine, tryptamine, serotonin). With calcium ions and calmodulin acting in concert, these stimuli activate enzymatic pathways to liberate the fatty acid precursors and induce the formation of specific eicosanoids.

The biosynthesis of eicosanoids starts with the action (hydrolysis) of phospholipase A$_2$ on plasma membrane phospholipids for liberation of arachidonic acid (Fig. 51–6). The next steps involve the addition of oxygen to arachidonic acid through cytosolic enzymes either of the cyclooxygenase or of the lipoxygenase pathways.

The cyclooxygenase pathway first causes the formation

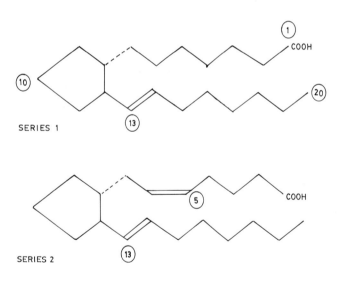

CLASSES OF PROSTAGLANDINS

Figure 51–1   **A,** Classes of prostaglandins according to the position of the oxygen radicals on the cyclopentane nucleus. (---, trans [behind the horizontal plane of the ring].) **B,** The number of double bonds is one in series 1, two in series 2, and three in series 3 of prostaglandins.

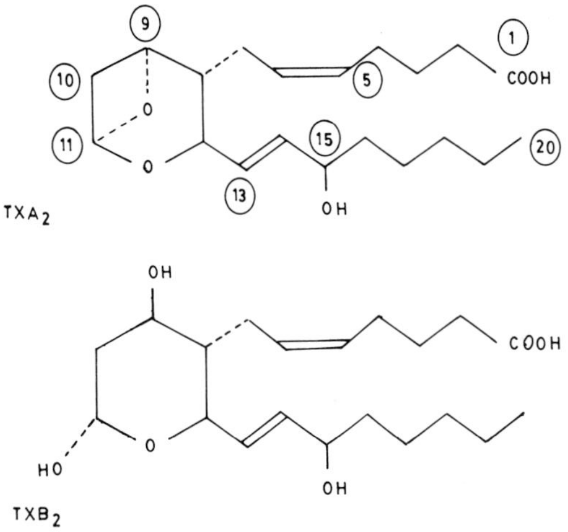

Figure 51–2 Thromboxanes have a six-peaked nucleus instead of the five-peaked nucleus of prostaglandins. The unstable thromboxane A_2 is biologically active, whereas its stable derivative, thromboxane B_2, is inactive.

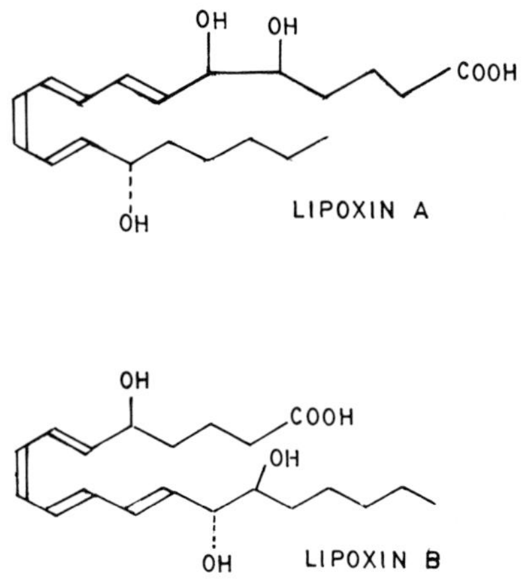

Figure 51–4 Derivatives of arachidonic acid (i.e., 4 C=C), lipoxins A and B carry three OH groups on different positions.

of the unstable endoperoxide PGG_2, which is then transformed into the labile PGH_2 by a peroxidase. Serum albumin or specific prostaglandin-endoperoxide isomerases can then convert PGH_2 to PGD_2, PGE_2, PGI_2, and TXA_2. Chemically unstable, TXA_2 is rapidly converted to the chemically stable and biologically inactive hydration product TXB_2. In contrast, the action of prostaglandin-endoperoxide reductase or of PGF synthase results in the transformation of PGH_2 into $PGF_{2\alpha}$ (Fig. 51–7).

The lipoxygenase pathway catalyzes the transformation of arachidonic acid into a variety of leukotrienes and lipoxins (Fig. 51–7). Leukotrienes result from the enzymatic (arachidonate 5-lipoxygenase) oxygenation of arachidonic acid into an unstable or labile epoxide intermediate, leukotriene A_4 (LTA$_4$). This derivative can be enzymatically hydrated to

leukotriene B_4 (LTB$_4$) or can be conjugated with gluthathione to form the sulfidopeptide leukotriene C_4 (LTC$_4$). Further enzymatic noncatabolic reactions rapidly transform LTC$_4$ into leukotriene D_4 (LTD$_4$), which can in turn be converted to leukotriene E_4 (LTE$_4$) (Fig. 51–8).

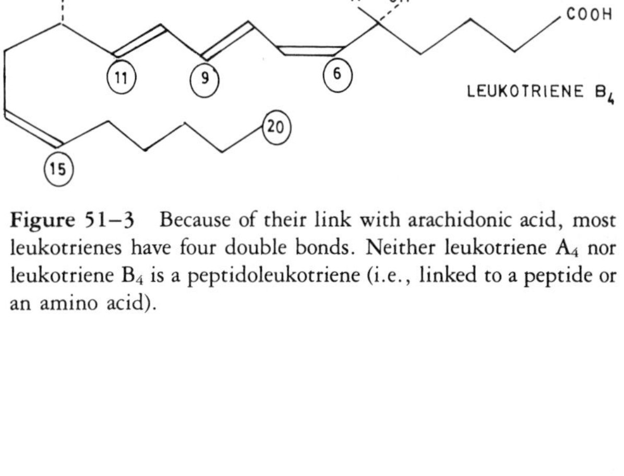

The lipoxins, or *lipox*ygenase *in*teraction products, are the result of lipoxygenations (arachidonate 15- and 5-lipoxygenases) of arachidonic acid at the C-15 position and the C-5 position and of additional reactions (Fig. 51–9). The bioactive compounds are lipoxin A (LXA), or 5,6,15L-trihydroxy-7,9,11,13-eicosatetraenoic acid, and lipoxin B (LXB), or 5D,14,15-trihydroxy-6,8,10,12-eicosatetraenoic acid.

Inhibition of Eicosanoid Synthesis

The initial liberation of fatty acid precursors from the plasma membrane phospholipids is inhibited by cAMP and by cortisol. Elevated levels of cortisol induce the intracellular production of a polypeptide called "lipocortin" or macrocortin, which inhibits phospholipase A_2 and the production of arachidonic acid.

The action of prostaglandin endoperoxide synthase (fatty acid cyclooxygenase) is inhibited by nonsteroidal anti-inflammatory compounds (NSAIs) (e.g., acetylsalicylic acid, or aspirin) and by extracts of onion, garlic, and ginger. Because of their richness in timnodonic acid, which is a poor substrate for cyclooxygenase, fish oils inhibit the synthesis of prostaglandins. Aromatic amides from naturally occurring cinnamic acid, and fatty acids from seed oil, are also strong inhibitors of prostaglandin synthesis. This inhibition of the cyclooxygenase pathway contributes a greater amount of arachidonic acid for formation of leukotrienes and lipoxins by the lipoxygenase pathways. Specific inhibition of thromboxane synthase by analogs of imidazole, such as dazoxiben, reduces the formation of TXA_2. This TX-synthase inhibition increases the amount of cyclic peroxides (PGH_2 and PGH_2) available for formation of PGE, PGF_α, PGD, and PGI (of series 2) by various types of cells.

Inhibitors of arachidonate 5-lipoxygenase, such as di-

Figure 51–3 Because of their link with arachidonic acid, most leukotrienes have four double bonds. Neither leukotriene A_4 nor leukotriene B_4 is a peptidoleukotriene (i.e., linked to a peptide or an amino acid).

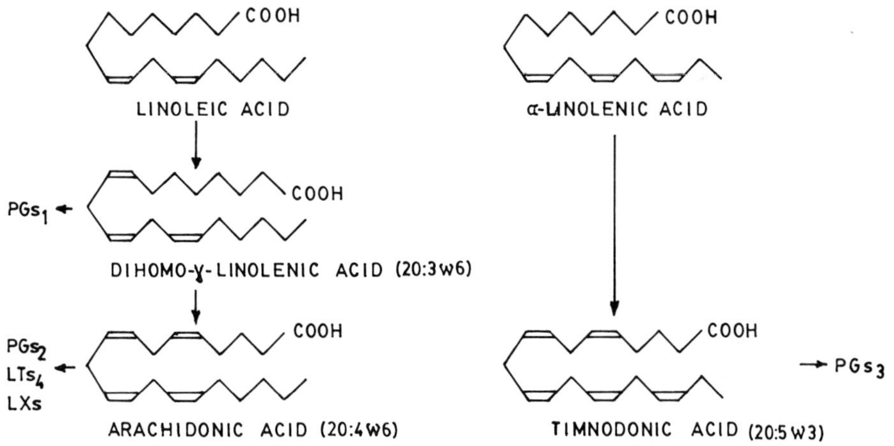

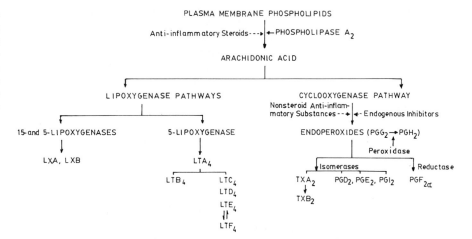

Figure 51–5 The biosynthesis of eicosanoids starts with substances that are formed from the essential fatty acids linoleic acid or alpha-linolenic acid. In marine animals, timnodonic acid (eicosapentaenoic acid), the precursor derived from alpha-linolenic acid, forms prostaglandin compounds of series 3, and leukotrienes with 5 C=C instead of 4 C=C. In mammals, linoleic acid forms dihomo-gamma-linolenic acid and arachidonic acid. Dihomo-gamma-linolenic acid is the precursor of prostaglandins of series 1. Arachidonic acid is the precursor of numerous substances, such as prostaglandins of series 2, leukotrienes of series 4, and lipoxins.

ethylcarbamazine and benoxaprofen, are not very specific but reduce the synthesis of leukotrienes.

Biological Effects

A few PGs (e.g., PGE_1, PGI) can be active within their cells of formation, modulating the effects of hormones or performing as a type of second messenger. As an example, PGI inhibits the cytosolic release of inositol-triphosphate (IP_3) in thrombin-activated platelets.

Most PGs leave the cytoplasm of the cells that produce them and enter the extracellular fluid to act locally, during a short half-life. PGI, synthesized in blood vessels, persists in the blood stream for a longer period of time and can exert its effects on distant targets (e.g., platelets), somewhat like a traditional hormone.

The small amount of PGs in plasma seems to be retained by strong monovalent interactions. The fixation is in

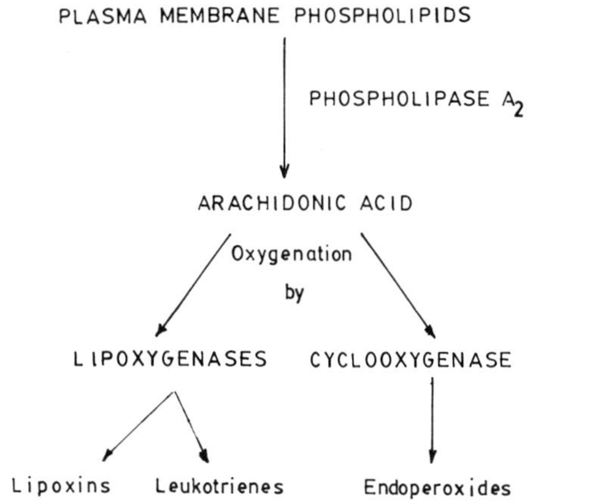

Figure 51–6 The biosynthesis of eicosanoids is initiated by stimuli activating phospholipase A_2 in plasma membranes. The released arachidonic acid is then oxygenated by either the cyclooxygenase or the lipoxygenase pathway.

Figure 51–7 A synopsis of the biosynthesis of eicosanoids, with the major inhibitory processes that can limit either the release of arachidonic acid from the plasma membrane sources or the formation of prostaglandins (PGs) and thromboxanes (TXs) by the cyclooxygenase pathway.

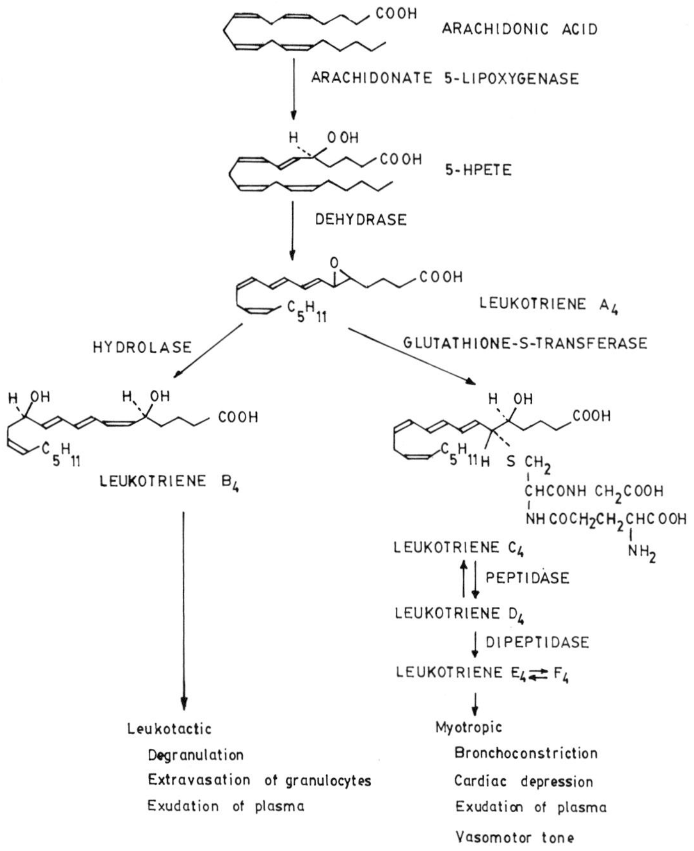

Figure 51–8 A summary of the biosynthesis of the different types of leukotrienes and their biological effects in animals.

inverse relation to the polarity or water solubility of the PGs (i.e., PGA > PGE > PGF_α). Thus, the clearance of PGA is the slowest, that of PGE is more rapid, and that of PGF is the fastest.

Receptors

Binding to receptors specific for the various families of eicosanoids takes place on the plasma membranes of target cells. These receptors are on the plasma membrane of their cells of origin (autocrine effect), on neighboring cells (paracrine effect), or on distant cells (endocrine effect). Two types of receptors for PGs are usually recognized: one for PGEs, with cAMP as the second messenger, and one for $PGF_{2\alpha}$, with cGMP as the second messenger. The PGE receptors, which also bind PGI in platelets and vascular smooth muscles, are present in adipocytes, adrenal medulla, corpus luteum, gastric mucosa, kidney, liver, macrophages, platelets, skin, thymocytes, and uterus. Two different types of PGE and PGI receptors explain the bimodal behavior of these PGs in some tissues and cells. It seems that PGD receptors (different from PGI) would also exist at the level of the central nervous system and the respiratory system. In platelets, vascular and bronchial smooth muscle, and glomerular mesangial cells, membrane proteins (e.g., G protein) interact with TXA and PGH. In the processes activated by the TXA-protein complex, phospholipid metabolites (inositol phosphates, diacyglycerol) initiate signals for subsequent intracellular events (e.g., release of calcium ions from stores).

Even if considerable biological mimicry exists between LTC_4 and LTD_4, different sulfidopeptide leukotriene receptors seem to be present for these LTs in ileal longitudinal muscles. In contrast, the receptors for LTD_4 coincide with those of LTE_4 and involve a greater phosphatidylinositol turnover. By inhibition of calmodulin, calcium-channel blockers (e.g., nifedipine) reduce the release of LTs and PGs.

Prostaglandin D_2

PGD_2 is a pulmonary vasodilator in the fetus and the newborns immediately after birth. Shortly after birth (less than 1 week) its effect on pulmonary circulation changes from dilation to constriction. Regardless of age, PGD_2 is a systemic constrictor.

Prostaglandin E_2

In the adenohypophysis, corpus luteum, and pancreas, micromolar levels of PGE_2 act as a transducer to stimulate the release of hormones. According to this concept, PGE_2 would bring an increased output of adrenocorticotropic hormone (ACTH), growth hormone (GH), gonadotropins, prolactin (PRL), and thyroid-stimulating hormone (TSH) by the adenohypophysis, and glucagon from the pancreas. An effect of PGE_2, similar to that of luteinizing hormone (LH), augments the secretion of progesterone by the corpus luteum. Excessive blood PGE_2 levels are associated with bone resorp-

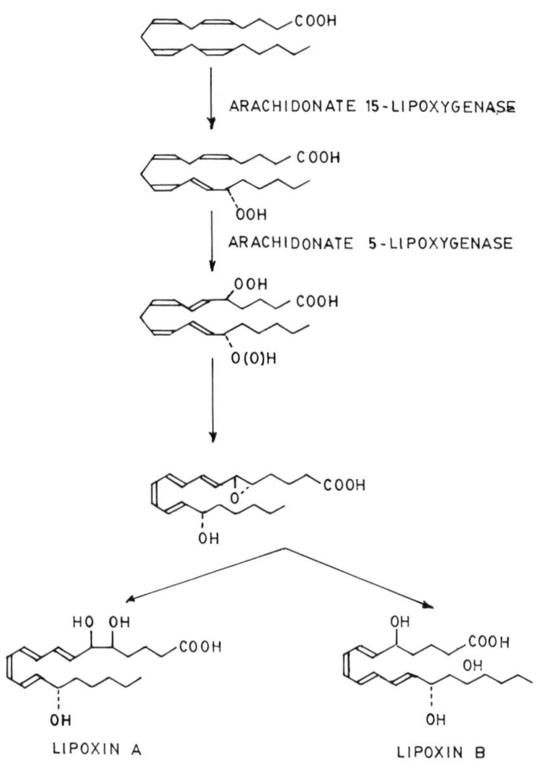

Figure 51–9 An overview of the biosynthesis of lipoxins, through the successive action of arachidonate 15- and 5-lipoxygenases.

tion and hypercalcemia. PGE_2 stimulates the biosynthesis of aldosterone by the adrenal cortex. PGAs and PGEs induce erythropoiesis by releasing erythropoietin from the renal cortex.

In the nervous system, the stimulation of sympathetic nerves increases the output of PGEs, which inhibit adrenergic transmission by depressing the responses at nerve terminals. In contrast, PGFs amplify the responses of effectors to norepinephrine.

Like bradykinin, PGEs are "algesic substances," or pain-producing agents, when they are applied to the skin. PGE_2 can lower the threshold of nociceptors (pain receptors) to other stimuli, such as heat.

By relaxing smooth muscles, PGEs, PGAs, and PGIs are arterial vasodilator and hypotensive substances. By increasing renal perfusion, PGEs, PGAs, PGHs, and PGIs contribute to raise the water, chloride, sodium, and potassium content of urine. PGEs also relax the uterus of nonpregnant animals.

With regard to the digestive system, PGEs and PGFs enhance the contraction of longitudinal muscles of the gut. The sphincters are relaxed by PGEs but are made to contract by PGFs. PGEs, PGAs, and PGIs inhibit gastric secretion, raise the the production of mucus by the stomach and small intestine, and augment intestinal secretions somewhat like the cholera toxin to cause diarrhea. The overall PG effects on the simple or secretory stomach are to thicken the protective mucus layer, to increase HCO_3^- secretion, and to maintain the extensive microcirculation, preventing ischemia.

Prostaglandin F_{2α}

$PGF_{2\alpha}$ facilitates the release of epinephrine from the adrenal medulla. PGFs and TXAs stimulate the replication and growth of hepatocytes.

$PGF_{2\alpha}$ produced by the uterus of animals (cow, ewe, guinea pig, mare, sow) is recognized as "uterine luteolysin," the luteolysis factor that controls the life span of the corpus luteum. In the nonpregnant cow, at about day 14 or 15 of the estrous cycle, a coincident release of $PGF_{2\alpha}$ and oxytocin by the corpus luteum causes the degeneration of the corpus luteum and prepares the ovary for the return of estrus on day 0 (i.e., the twenty-first day of the estrous cycle). The absence of uterine $PGF_{2\alpha}$ permits the persistence of the corpus luteum and the development of the embryo and fetus.

> The luteolytic action of synthetic analogs of $PGF_{2\alpha}$ is used (e.g., cloprostenol) to synchronize estrus in cattle. Two injections are administered at a 10- to 12-day interval (e.g., at days 5 and 18 of the estrous cycle). Estrus appears at about the third day following the second injection.

At the termination of normal pregnancy, determined by a "clock" of still unknown nature, the production of fetal cortisol increases the levels of $PGF_{2\alpha}$, along with those of estradiol and oxytocin. $PGF_{2\alpha}$ binds to receptors on cells of the uterine myometrium, increases the Ca^{++} in their cytoplasm, depresses their contractile mechanism threshold, and contributes to the contractions of the uterus to expel the fetus.

> Administration of analogs of $PGF_{2\alpha}$ to a cow is used to initiate expulsion of a dead or mummified fetus. Glucocorticoid treatment is ineffective in such conditions because it requires a functional fetoplacental unit or viable fetus and placenta.

Prostaglandin I_2

By inhibiting platelet aggregation, by dilating the coronary arteries and pulmonary vessels, by relaxing the muscles of the bronchi, and by lowering blood pressure, PGI_2 produces effects opposite to those of TXA_2.

Thromboxanes

TXAs and all PGs (except PGIs) constrict the pulmonary vessels. TXA and PGH contract the muscles of the bronchi, whereas PGE and PGI dilate the bronchi.

Leukotrienes

LTA_4 is an unstable epoxide intermediate. The other LTs all have proinflammatory effects, participating in host defense reactions and pathophysiological conditions such as immediate hypersensitivity and inflammation.

LTB_4, the dihydroxy derivative of LTA_4, is a calcium, ionophore that causes adhesion and chemotactic movement of polymorphonuclear leukocytes. It stimulates the aggregation of neutrophils, the release of some of their enzymes, and the generation of superoxide in their cytosol. Although it has no direct effects on blood flow, because it stimulates these inflammatory mediators, LTB_4 promotes the local exudation of plasma.

LTC_4, LTD_4, and LTE_4 are considered the most potent bronchoconstrictors, reducing the volume of the lungs and peripheral airways. On a molar basis, their effect is several hundred times more powerful than that of histamine and is comparable with that of the platelet-activating factor (PAF). They increase microvascular permeability in the airways and stimulate mucus secretion in the airways. The peptidoleukotrienes constitute the slow-reacting substance of anaphylaxis (SRS-A). Besides causing constriction of most smooth muscles, and causing exudation of plasma in post-capillary venules, LTC_4 is present in the hypothalamus in the same neurons as luteinizing hormone–releasing hormone (LHRH) or gonadotropin-releasing hormone (GnRH) and contributes to the adenohypophysial release of LH. LTD_4 is involved in smooth muscle contraction, and it is a pulmonary constrictor regardless of age, although its effectiveness increases with age.

Lipoxins

LXA causes arteriolar dilation, which induces glomerular hyperperfusion, hypertension, and hyperfiltration. In the glomerular hemodynamics, LXA produces a selective fall in afferent, but not efferent, arteriolar resistance. LXA activates kinase C more than diacylglyceride. Both LXA and LXB inhibit the cytotoxicity of natural killer cells.

Catabolism of Eicosanoids

PGs and TXs are rapidly inactivated through metabolism either at the site of production, or as they pass through adipose tissue, intestine, kidneys, lungs, liver, and spleen. The half-life of PGG_2, PGH_2, and TXA_2 is about 5 minutes, and that of PGI_2 is about half as long (2 to 3 minutes).

In the plasma, the remnants of PGEs and PGFs are 15-ketodihydro-$PGF_{2\alpha}$ metabolities. The catabolism process occurs in two steps, the first one involving oxidation at C-15, and the second a reduction of a $C=C$ at position 13. Mostly in the liver, but also in the intestine, kidneys, and the lungs, a further degradation by one or two steps of beta- and omega-oxidation of the carbonyl side-chain yields dinor (18C) or tetranor (16C) metabolites. The shorter (16C) metabolites, called "11-ketotetranor PGF metabolites," remain in the plasma for a long time before excretion in the urine.

The catabolism of the unstable PGI_2 and TXA_2 is by conversion to the stable but inactive $PGI_{1\alpha}$ and TXB_2 derivatives. Dinor-TXB_2 is the most abundant urinary metabolite of TXAs.

HORMONES OF THE THYMUS AND OF LEUKOCYTES

A variety of soluble factors (polypeptide molecules known as cytokines, lymphokines, and thymic hormones), considered as putative hormones, are produced by cells in the epitheliolymphoid thymus (a primary lymphoid organ) and in secondary lymphoid organs (spleen, Peyer's patches, lymph glands, as well as the mucosae-associated lymphoid tissues {MALT}). They modulate the induction ($G_0 \rightarrow G_1$), proliferation, differentiation, and maturation of adjacent (autocrine effect) and distant (endocrine effect) hematopoietic and nonhematopoietic cells. These putative hormones thus initiate and control cell-mediated and humoral immunological responses against pathogens and mitogens foreign to the body.

Morphology of the Thymus

In cats, dogs, mice, and rats, the thymus is a paired mediastinal organ (Fig. 51–10). In ruminants (cattle and sheep), horses, pigs, and chickens, an additional cervical extension may reach as far as the thyroid. The thymus is provided with afferent and efferent blood vessels, but it carries only outgoing lymphatics (i.e., it is devoid of incoming lymphatics). During the lifetime of an animal, the thymus undergoes successive major morphological changes, such as rapid growth in the fetus, greater relative size at puberty, and gradual regression during the postpuberal life.

Similar to the other lymphoid organs (spleen, lymph nodes, gut-associated lymphoid tissue {GALT}), the thymus receives noradrenergic postganglionic sympathetic innervation. Norepinephrine is produced in this "hard-wiring" system connecting the central nervous system to the lymphoid organs. Neuropeptides (e.g., vasoactive intestinal polypeptide {VIP}, somatostatin, and substance P) also provide diffuse intercellular signals between the cells of the immune system.

In response to stress, the thymus atrophies rapidly. Nude mice, having a congenital aplasia of the thymus, lack the cellular immunity provided by T lymphopoiesis. A genetic hypoplasia of the thymus, seen in Arabian foals and basset hound puppies, results in failure of T and B lymphopoiesis. This genetic complete immunodeficiency is fatal at an early age in these young animals, which are very susceptible to infections (adenoviral, bacterial, or protozoal). Thymic hypoplasia can result from virus infections, intoxications (lead, mercury, polychlorinated biphenyls), neoplasia and protein malnutrition. The primary and secondary lymphoid tissues are targets of bovine virus diarrhea, canine distemper, equine rhinopneumonia, and feline leukemia and panleukopenia.

Histology of the Thymus

The mammalian thymus originates embryonically from the ventral portions of the third and fourth pharyngeal pouches. The organ is made up of several lobes, which are encapsulated. Each lobe comprises (Fig. 51–11) many lobules that are partially separated by connective tissue septa and are divided into distinctive cortical and medullary parts. The cortex is occupied by dense collections of lymphoid cells, whereas the medulla groups more diffuse lymphoid tissue and also contains Hassall's corpuscles. The latter consist of laminated layers of epithelial cells. The functional roles of the

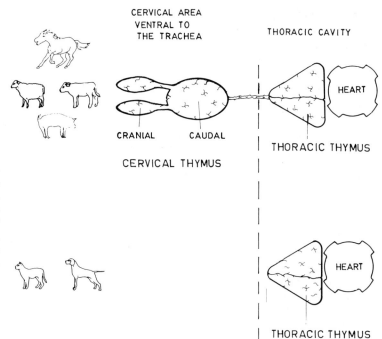

Figure 51–10   In ruminants (calf, lamb, kid), colts, and piglets, the thymus comprises a mediastinal (thoracic) part and a cervical part. The cervical thymus is found along the ventral aspect of the trachea, and its two horns may reach as far as the level of the thyroid. An isthmus (or narrow bridge) between the first ribs connects the thoracic and cervical parts of the thymus. In piglets, the relatively large thymus may be nearly 0.45 percent of the body mass and roughly equals the total lymph node mass. With age, the cervical part and the isthmus regress, leaving only some thoracic thymic tissue. Only the mediastinal thoracic thymus (the right side of which is usually larger than the left) is present in puppies and kittens.

cortex, the medulla, and Hassall's corpuscles are still obscure.

The initial thymus of the fetus is epithelial, but it is soon colonized by lymphoid stem cells (prethymic stem cells) that migrate in blood from extrathymic sites (yolk sac, liver). In the fetus and the developed animal, the lymphoepithelial thymus serves as a primary lymphoid organ for T lymphopoiesis. The primary lymphoid organs for B lymphopoiesis are the Peyer's patches (sheep), bone marrow (mouse, rat), or bursa of Fabricius (chicken).

The maturation of white blood cells is complex and is not identical for polynucleated (neutrophils, eosinophils,

THYMIC LOBULE

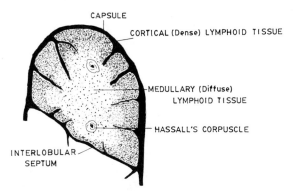

Figure 51–11   Schematic arrangement of the thymic lobules, which are separated by connective tissue septa. Each lobule has a cortical (dense lymphoid) and a medullary (diffuse lymphoid and Hassal's corpuscles) portion. The grouping of several lobules forms a lobe, and the lobes of the thymus are covered by a capsule.

and basophils) and for lymphoid or mononucleated (lymphocytes and monocytes) leukocytes.

After the prethymic cells (stem cell progenitors, prothymocytes) enter into the thymus through afferent blood vessels, they become intrathymic cells (thymocytes), and their surface, or plasma membrane, receptors are rearranged. The immature T cells migrate from the subcapsular, cortical, and medullary zones of the thymus, to differentiate into T lymphocytes.

The cortex contains 85 to 90 percent of the thymocytes, the medulla accounts for the remaining 10 to 15 percent. The thymocytes can be divided into subpopulations on the basis of the reaction of their plasma membrane to some markers (T1, T3, T4, and T8 in humans).

Small cortical $T4^+8^+$ thymocytes (70 percent), dividing typical $T4^+8^+$ cortical blasts (10 percent) and cortical "precursor" $T4^-8^-$ cells (5 percent) populate the cortex, whereas intermediate medullary thymocytes are $T4^+8^-$ (10 percent) and $T4^+8^+$ (5 percent) cells. The small cortical thymocytes are deficient in immune function, while the intermediary-size cells of the medulla are immunocompetent and are very similar to peripheral (in blood, lymph, secondary lymphoid organs) T lymphocytes.

The cortical thymocyte is an inert, unresponsive cell destined for intrathymic death. Intrathymic death seems to be the fate of the majority of cortical thymocytes, which appear to die within the thymus rather than to exit into the peripheral T-cell pool.

The differentiation of leukocytes responsible for immunity in the animal's body, the B lymphocytes or immunoglobulin-positive lymphocytes (Ig^+) and the T lymphocytes or immunoglobulin-negative ones (Ig^-), requires the successive action of several factors (Fig. 51–12). The close contact with cortical epithelial cells, and changes in the

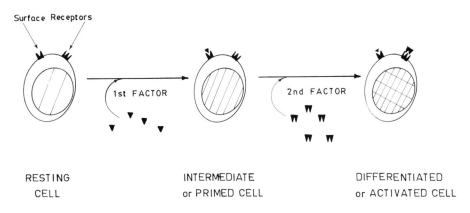

Surface Receptors

1st FACTOR   2nd FACTOR

RESTING   INTERMEDIATE   DIFFERENTIATED
CELL   or PRIMED CELL   or ACTIVATED CELL

Figure 51–12 The differentiation of leukocytes requires at least two factors, which selectively bind with distinct receptors on the surface of the plasma membrane. Through stimulation of the nucleus or derepression of genes, the cytoplasm is made to produce the cytokines or lymphokines required for the proper activity of specific leukocytes (e.g., T cells, including helper, cytotoxic, and suppressor; B cells; macrophages; and granulocytes).

soluble factors in the thymic microenvironment (lymphokines, thymic hormones), influence this induction, development, differentiation, and maturation into the various types of T lymphocytes (T-helper, T-suppressor, and T-cytotoxic). The thymic lymphocytes (thymocytes) are extremely sensitive to stress. Almost any experimental manipulation results in some degree of thymocyte depletion, and major stress (anesthesia, viral infections, surgery) can deplete thymocytes from the cortex and medulla of the thymus.

> Cell depletion of the thymus occurs by *apoptosis* (i.e., without signs of dying cells or of necrosis). It appears to reflect the activation of endogenous endonucleases. Apoptosis is triggered by various soluble mediators and hormones (e.g., lymphotoxin and corticosteroids).

In large animals (pig, sheep), more postthymic cells are released from the thymus in the efferent lymphatics rather than in the efferent veins. These postthymic cells (T lymphocytes) find their way into the peripheral or secondary lymphoid organs (i.e., spleen, lymph nodes, and mucosae-associated lymphoid tissue [MALT]). GALT and bronchus-associated lymphoid tissue (BALT) are parts of the MALT. Established in these secondary lymphoid organs, the critical population of T lymphocytes reproduces and recirculates between these organs and the blood. During the life of the animal, T lymphocytes normally account for about 70 to 80 percent of the peripheral blood lymphocytes.

Hormones of the Thymus

The peptides obtained from the thymus, the "putative thymic hormones," include *thymosin, thymic humoral factor (THF), thymostimulin (TS),* and *facteur thymique sérique (FTS).* They seem to influence the transformation of prethymic stem cells into T lymphocytes. As their precise mechanism of action is still unclear, their involvement in the stepwise process of thymocyte maturation and T-cell differentiation in the primary (thymus) and peripheral (spleen) lymphoid organs is contested. In addition, these thymic hormones seem to stimulate hypothalamic cells to secrete gonadotropic hormones and growth hormone.

These numerous thymic hormones may be related to the diversity of the population of thymocytes and to the complex and multiple interdependent steps conferring immunological maturity on T lymphocytes. They may function as regulators of the differentiation process of the various subsets of T cells. Each hormone may command a specific and defined phase to meet the needs for T-helper, T-cytotoxic, and T-suppressor lymphocytes.

Possibly all or most of the thymic hormones are the cleavage products of a common precursor, still to be discovered. The lack of amino acid homology among the thymic peptides militates against this hypothesis, and supports the more probable existence of a phylogenetically common hormonal control mechanism. This is supported by the isolation of these hormone-like peptides from the thymus of individuals of many animal species (mice, rabbits, sheep, calves, humans).

The adenohypophysial growth hormone (GH) and thyrotropin, or TSH, the latter through the thyroid hormones triiodothyronine (T_3) and thyroxine (T_4), stimulate the growth of the thymus gland. In chickens, T_4 increases the size of the thymus, whereas GH enlarges the size of the bursa of Fabricius.

Steroid hormones tend to cause involution of the gland. Indeed after puberty, the substantial increase in the level of steroid sex hormones contributes to reducing the size of the thymus. Prolonged stress, producing a higher output of ACTH from the adenohypophysis and cortisol from the adrenal cortex, also induces a regression of the thymus. In contrast, a deficiency of adrenal cortical hormones or sex hormones is associated with hypertrophy of the thymus or its failure to involute.

Thymosin

From the calf thymus, a family of polypeptides can be obtained from an extract, the so-called *thymosin fraction 5* (Fr 5). Subsequent purification yields acidic alpha (N = 7) and beta (N = 4) thymosins, and a basic gamma-thymosin. Thymosins alpha$_1$, alpha$_5$, and alpha$_7$ are peptides of about 28 amino acids with molecular mass near 3,000 daltons. A prothymosin alpha may be the true thymic hormone, whereas thymosin alpha$_1$ may be a proteolyzed fragment. Polypeptide beta$_1$, and thymosins beta$_3$ and beta$_4$ (peptides of about 43 amino acids), have also been characterized. Thymosin beta$_4$ appears in many tissues besides the thymus, and thymosin beta₃ is probably a proteolytic fragment of thymosin beta₄.

Thymosins alpha₁ and alpha₇ cause differentiation and maturation of early thymocytes and immature T cells. Thysomin alpha₁ (1.5 to 2 ng per milliliter of plasma) induces differentiation of helper T cells and enhances interferon-gamma (IFN-γ) production by lymphoid cells. Thymosin alpha₇ increases the number of suppressor T cells. With age, a decrease of thymosin alpha₁ in serum would explain the reduction in the T-cell pool and the decline in the cell-mediated immunity. The beta-peptides seem to act selectively upon prethymic stem cells, and thymosin beta₄ induces secretion of LHRH from isolated hypothalamus (rat).

Thymic Humoral Factor

Isolated from calf thymus, this 31–amino acid polypeptide (molecular weight, 3,220 daltons) restores T-cell impairment associated with severe viral infections, and with intensive chemotherapy in malignant diseases. THF enhances T-helper cell activity, promotes interleukin-2 release, and stimulates cytotoxic T-cell activity.

Thymopoietin

Thymopoietin I and II, two closely related polypeptides (49 amino acids) that may be isohormonal variants, have been isolated from bovine thymus. Thymopoietin III, having a largely identical amino acid sequence, has been obtained from bovine spleen. *Ubiquitin,* which is present in all tissues, is a peptide with biological activity similar to that of synthetic thymopoietin II. Similarly, a pentapeptide (TP-5) has only the 32–36 residues of thymopoietin II but retains its biological activity. While increasing the proliferation activity of T lymphocytes already present in lymphoid tissues, thymopoietin inhibits early B-cell differentiation in bone marrow.

Thymostimulin

Prepared from calf thymus, thymostimulin (TS) consists of a group of polypeptides of less than 12,000 daltons. Further purification reveals two fractions: 68 and 78, the latter being similar to ubiquitin. TS increases the survival rate of mice with transplanted tumors and delays the appearance of the latter.

Facteur Thymique Sérique

Absent from the serum of nude mice, the serum thymic factor reappears after thymic grafting. Facteur thymique sérique (FTS) obtained from pig serum is a 9-C or nonapeptide (molecular weight >10,000 daltons), which has been synthesized. The serum levels of FTS are reduced in conditions of immunodeficiency and malnutrition and seem to decrease with age. Similar to the case with THF in humans, natural killer T cells are mobilized by injection of FTS in mice. The active form of FTS, which requires chelated zinc, is called *thymulin.*

Hormones of Helper T Lymphocytes

In the body (blood and lymphoid organs), the total quantity of leukocytes, which equals that of erythrocytes, provides forceful evidence of the importance of lymphoid tissue to the animal organism. In addition to their traditionally recognized functions, leukocytes secrete cellular proteins, or polypeptides, the so-called *cytokines.* These soluble substances bind to specific receptors on other cells or on the secretory cells themselves. These proteins, or polypeptides, stimulate processes such as cellular division, respiration, energy metabolism, and secretion of specific proteins (enzymes). A cytokine produced by a monocyte or from a macrophage used to be known as a *monokine,* and that coming from a lymphocyte as a *lymphokine.* The term lymphokine, now extended to all cytokines produced by leukocytes, includes the interleukins (ILs), lymphotoxin (LT), met-enkephalin, granulocyte-macrophage colony stimulating factor (GM-CSF), neuroleukine (NLK), tumor necrosis factor (TNF), and interferons (IFNs).

Interleukins are lymphokines that facilitate interactions between leukocytes. *Interleukin-1* (IL-1) is synthesized by macrophages and sometimes by B lymphocytes, providing humoral immunity (i.e., antibodies) as well as by epidermal cells, renal mesangial cells, astrocytes, and epithelial cells of the cornea. IL-1 causes many responses: hyperthermia or fever (it is a pyrogen), increased production of interleukin-2, an endocrine effect on activated B lymphocytes (promotes their growth), and enhancement of the action of neutrophils and of their production by the bone marrow.

In mice, helper T lymphocytes (T$_H$) cells produce several lymphokines, which affect the proliferation, differentiation, and maturation of lymphocytes and hematopoietic cells. Two subsets of helper T cells are known, T$_H$1 and T$_H$2. Both subsets produce interleukin-3 (IL-3), GM-CSF, met-enkephalin, and TNF. Subset T$_H$1 cells specifically secrete IL-2, lymphotoxin, and IFN-γ, whereas T$_H$2 cells are unique producers of interleukin-4 (IL-4) and interleukin-5 (IL-5).

The lymphokines from T$_H$1 cells mediate complex cytotoxic responses by macrophages (cell-mediated immunity) against viruses and foreign cells, and optimal production of antibodies by B lymphocytes.

The lymphokines from T$_H$2 cells stimulate key steps in the production of the major cellular and humoral components of allergic and immediate hypersensitivity responses. They enhance interactions among eosinophils, mucosal mast cells of the GALT, and IgE antibodies against pathogens (such as multicellular parasites) and various nonpathogenic allergens.

Interleukin-2 (formerly called TCGF for T-cell growth factor) has an autocrine effect on the growth of T lymphocytes (providing cellular immunity) and stimulates the proliferation of activated B lymphocytes as well as the differentiation and lymphokine secretion of T lymphocytes. *Interleukin-3* (known earlier as multi-colony stimulating factor [MCSF] or as mast cell growth factor-1 [MCGF-1]) is produced only by activated T cells and by tumor or leukemic cells. IL-3 greatly increases the proliferation of bone marrow stem cells, which may differentiate into monocytes, granulocytes, erythrocytes, and megakaryocytes. *Interleukin-4* (once called B-cell growth factor-1 [BCGF-1] and B-cell stimulatory factor-1 [BCSF-1] is a multifunctional lymphokine capable of stimulating T cells, thymocytes, B cells, mast cells, macrophages, and other hematopoietic cells. *Interleukin-5* (formerly known as B-cell growth factor-2 [BCGF-2], T-cell–replacing factor-1 [TCRF-1], killer helper factor [KHF], and eosinophil differentiation factor [KHF]) can also stimulate proliferation and differentiation of B cells and eosinophils. *Interleukin-6* (IL-6), also called B-cell stimulatory factor-2 (BCSF-2), contributes to the production of immunoglobulins.

The *interferons* are a family of cytokines, or soluble glycoproteins (15,000 to 20,000 daltons), secreted by various types of cells upon stimulation by bacterial and viral infections. Considered as lymphokines, interferon-alpha and interferon-gamma regulate interactions between the cells of the immune system. Interferon-alpha is secreted by macrophages and lymphocytes, whereas interferon-gamma is produced by lymphoid cells. Foreign antigens (mitogens, malignant cells) increase the activity of natural killer (NK) cells to secrete interferon-gamma, which has an autocrine stimulatory effect on the NK cells. Interferon-beta, which comes from fibroblasts, binds and destroys free radicals.

ATRIAL NATRIURETIC HORMONES

Several peptides have been isolated from atrial muscles (more were found in the right side than the left side), sequenced, and named according to minor structural variations. In the literature, atrial natriuretic peptides (ANPs), or atrial natriuretic vasorelaxant peptides, are referred to as *atrial natriuretic factors* (ANF 1–33, 2–33, 3–33, and 8–33); *atriopeptin* I, II, and II; *auriculin* A and B; and *cardionatrin* I.

These peptides are found in atrial cardiocytes, but not in the cells of ventricular muscles, in response to stimuli such as expansion of the extracellular fluid volume, sodium loading, and alveolar hypoxia. Through their potent vasorelaxant, diuretic, and natriuretic properties, they participate in the homeostasis of salt, circulatory volume, and arterial blood pressure by the kidneys. ANPs are part of an integrated system involving renin-angiotensin, aldosterone, (antidiuretic hormone [ADH]), vasopressin, and the adrenergic (sympathetic) nervous system.

Derived from a preprohormone of 152 amino acids (preproauriculin), the prohormone of ANPs (126 amino acids) is stored in perinuclear granules in the atrial myocytes. Various types of stimuli activate enzymatic proteolyses to cleave the prohormone into many fragments. Examples of such stimuli are atrial stretch or blood volume expansion, constrictor agents that elevate the arterial blood pressure, high-salt diets, and atrial tachycardia. They all induce the intragranular cleavage of the ANF-prohormone, and the transfer of biologically active ANF into the blood. Several

carboxy terminal fragments, with 23 to 33 amino acids, represent the biologically active forms of ANPs released into the circulation. The half-life of ANPs is less than 1 minute, and they rapidly are excreted in the urine.

Atrial distention also elevates Na^+ excretion by reducing sympathetic neural discharge, which reduces proximal tubular reabsorption of Na^+.

Specific target cells of ANPs are in the kidneys, in arterial smooth muscles, in the adrenal glands, and in some structures of the central nervous system.

Biological Actions

The effects of ANPs can be divided into those dealing with (1) renal hemodynamics and electrolyte excretion, (2) precontracted smooth muscle, (3) arterial pressure and systemic circulation, and (4) the renin-angiotensin-aldosterone axis.

Renal Hemodynamics and Sodium Excretion

ANPs rapidly augment glomerular filtration to improve the extraction of sodium from blood. ANPs selectively constrict the smooth muscles of efferent glomerular arterioles, producing a sustained improvement in glomerular filtration, which is triggered without raising the renal blood flow. The intrarenal blood flow is modified, so more blood is allowed into the usually sluggish circulation in medullary and papillary vessels. This causes a washout of urea and sodium from this medullary zone and decreases the species-characteristic hyperosmolality that drives the ADH-mediated reabsorption of water. In addition, ANPs directly inhibit the proximal and distal tubular reabsorption of sodium. These combined actions lead to natriuresis, to an increased urine volume, and to a reduction in extracellular fluid volume.

Precontracted Smooth Muscles

The second major effect of ANPs is to relax precontracted vascular smooth muscles in the renal vasculature, large arteries (e.g., aorta), and other vascular beds. This is brought about by a direct effect on specific receptors on the plasma membrane of the smooth muscle cells, by activation of guanylate cyclase, which increases the level of cyclic guanosine monophosphate (cGMP) in these cells. The result of this action of ANPs is to counteract the hypertension and to return blood pressure to lower values. ANPs also block the vasoconstrictive action of angiotensin II and the hypertensive action of catecholamines.

Preconstriction of canine renal arterioles occurs after administration of angiotensin II, norepinephrine, vasopressin (ADH), and ouabain.

The vasorelaxant effect of ANPs is more effective on rabbit aorta preconstricted by angiotensin II than by norepinephrine.

Arterial Pressure and Systemic Circulation

In normotensive dogs, ANPs immediately lower the arterial blood pressure. The hypotension is not due to a decrease in peripheral resistance but to a lower cardiac output associated with the less voluminous return of venous blood to the heart. This effect is consequent upon the loss of extracellular fluid caused by diuresis and natriuresis.

The Renin-Angiotensin-Aldosterone Axis

Concerning the renal juxtaglomerular cells (Fig. 51–13), ANPs suppress the renal secretion of renin and the formation of angiotensin II, thereby decreasing the stimulus for aldosterone release from the adrenal cortex. In addition, ANPs directly block the adrenocortical secretion of aldosterone. Because of this lack of aldosterone, renal tubular sodium reabsorption dwindles, reinforcing the concomitant natriuresis process. The ANPs influence the renin-angiotensin-aldosterone axis on four fronts: (1) suppressing renin formation, (2) blocking aldosterone secretion, (3) blocking the vasoconstrictive effects of angiotensin II, and (4) antagonizing the sodium-retaining effect of aldosterone.

HORMONES OF THE KIDNEYS

The kidney is the production site of several hormone-related enzymes (1-alpha-hydroxylase, kallikrein, and renin) and of hormones (prostaglandins and erythropoietin).

Hormone-Related Enzymes

Renal 1-alpha-Hydroxylase

The proximal tubule of the nephron contains the mitochondrial enzyme for the final hydroxylation of 25-hydroxyvitamin D_3 into the biologically active hormone 1,25-dihydroxyvitamin D_3, or calcitriol. The activity of 1-alpha-hydroxylase is increased by dietary and hormonal factors.

Deficiencies of calcium, phosphate, and vitamin D stimulate 1-alpha-hydroxylase, which is also aroused by hormones (e.g., estrogens, placental lactogen, parathormone [PTH], PRL, and somatotropin). In contrast, calcitonin depresses 1-alpha-hydroxylase and reduces the transformation of 25-hydroxycalciferol into calcitriol. Calcitriol exerts a negative feedback on the activity of renal 1-alpha-hydroxylase.

Kallikreins

The kallikreins are a family of kininogenases or serine proteases, which also include various proteolytic enzymes such as trypsin and plasmin. Kallikreins found in plasma and in tissues (mostly in kidney, but also in pancreas and salivary gland) catalyze the transformation of proteins (kininogens) into peptide kinins. Tissue kallikreins are smaller proteins (about 50,000 daltons) than plasma kallikreins (107,000 daltons).

Renal kallikrein, present in the distal tubule, increases renal blood flow, mediates the conversion of prorenin to renin, and causes the release of the decapeptide *kallidin,* or lysyl-bradykinin. Renal kallikrein decreases the production of prostaglandins, whereas renal kallidin (renal kinin) increases the production (and renal excretion) of prostaglandins.

A polyvalent protease inhibitor, aprotinin, inhibits the action of several kininogenases (e.g., kallikrein, trypsin).

Plasma kallikrein exists in an inactive form, as prekallikrein (zymogen), that must be activated. The Hageman's factor (factor XII) changes prekallikrein into its enzymatic form, plasma kallikrein. In turn, plasma kallikrein releases small polypeptide kinins, notably a nonapeptide, bradykinin, from plasma proteins known as kininogens. *Bradykinin,* the most potent vasodilator substance known, increases vascular permeability and induces pain. It brings about the warmth, redness, swelling, and pain of inflammation. It slowly (brady-) contracts some smooth muscles and also stimulates the synthesis of PGA_2, probably by activating phospholipase A_2 and thus increasing the availability of arachidonic acid from plasma membrane phospholipids.

Figure 51–13 Opposite effects of hypertension and hypotension on the release of renin. The angiotensinogen-angiotensin-aldosterone cascade, during which renin and kininase II (converting enzyme) act in concert. The inhibitory effects of atrial natriuretic peptides (ANPs) on Na^+ absorption, secretion of aldosterone, vasoconstrictive action of angiotensin II, and secretion of renin.

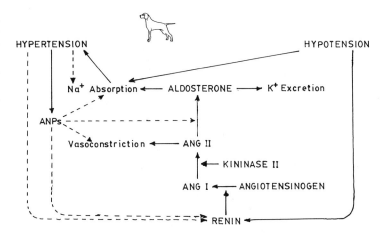

The kinins all have very similar biological actions: they (1) stimulate renal blood flow, (2) reduce blood pressure, (3) depress the reabsorption of sodium by the tubular cells or increase the excretion of sodium (natriuresis), and (4) increase urine flow. Their half-life is very short (15 seconds), as they are catabolized by enzymes (kininase I and kininase II) during a single passage through vascular beds (e.g., lungs). The action of kininase II (also known as angiotensin-converting enzyme and dipeptidyl carboxypeptidase) is rapid, whereas that of kininase I (carboxypeptidase-N) is slower.

Renin-Angiotensin System

The kidneys are the source of renin and the target organ for transformation of the renin substrate angiotensinogen into angiotensin I and into a small amount of angiotensin II. As an excretory organ, the renal tissue also carries the enzymes (angiotensinases) to catabolize any local excess of angiotensin I and angiotensin II.

Renin, a glycoprotein-containing enzyme (about 42,000 daltons), acts on a plasma alpha$_2$-globulin to produce a decapeptide (angiotensin I) that is converted into a octapeptide hormone, angiotensin II, by the ubiquitous converting enzyme. As the tropic stimulatory factor on the zona glomerulosa of the adrenal cortex, angiotensin II induces the biosynthesis and secretion of aldosterone. After systemic transport of the kidneys, aldosterone produces the proteins and enzymes necessary to effect the renal tubular reabsorption of sodium.

A protein (347 amino acids), renin is biosynthesized in the juxtaglomerular cells as a preprorenin (406 amino acids) and as a prorenin (393 amino acids). Its secretion is influenced by several mechanisms related to extracellular volume (Na$^+$) and arterial blood pressure (K$^+$, catecholamines) (Table 51–1). Angiotensin II, the ultimate result of the action of renin, exerts a negative feedback on the renal output of renin.

Renin can be selectively inhibited by some aldehyde peptidic compounds.

Angiotensinogen, the natural substrate of renin, is a plasma glycoprotein (alpha$_2$-globulin, about 57,000 daltons) synthesized in the liver and, to a lesser extent, in the kidneys. Its hepatic biosynthesis is increased by estrogens and by glucocorticoids.

In the renal circulation, renin catalyzes the cleavage of plasma angiotensinogen into a biologically inactive decapeptide, *angiotensin I* (Ang I). In the capillaries of various tissues, another enzyme, appropriately called the converting enzyme, rapidly converts this decapeptide into the biologically active octapeptide angiotensin II (Ang II).

The *converting enzyme,* or dipeptidyl carboxypeptidase, is a zinc-containing protein found mostly in the vascular epithelium of the lungs. Plasma and several other tissues (e.g., adrenal cortex, kidney, liver, neurohypophysis, pancreas, spleen) also carry the converting enzyme. It is also known as kininase II, because it inactivates bradykinin, an autacoid with very potent vasodilator properties.

TABLE 51–1 Factors Influencing the Juxtaglomerular Biosynthesis of Renin

Stimulatory	Inhibitory
Arterial Pressure	
Hypotension	Hypertension
Catecholamines	
Beta-adrenergic agonists	Alpha$_2$-adrenergic agonists
Concentration of Na$^+$ at the Macula Densa	
Decreased	Increased
Extracellular Fluid Volume	
Reduction	Augmentation
Level of Blood Potassium (K$^+$)	
Hypokalemia	Hyperkalemia

Inhibitors of converting enzyme (e.g., captopril, enalapril) suppress the production of angiotensin II and the catabolism of bradykinin.

Angiotensin II binds to specific receptors on plasma cell membranes and acts in concert with cytosolic Ca^{++} to increase the secretion of ADH by supraoptic neurons and the release of ADH from the neurohypophysial stores, to contract smooth muscle, to induce the synthesis and release of aldosterone by the zona glomerulosa of the adrenal cortex, and to increase the output of eicosanoids by some cells. Ang II exerts a dipsogenic (drinking) effect by an action on the preoptic area of the hypothalamus. The adrenomedullary secretion of catecholamines is increased by Ang II, and besides promoting the production of norepinephrine, it amplifies the responses of adrenergic effectors. Ang II is hydrolyzed by angiotensinase (aminopeptidase) and is degraded to Ang III (heptapeptide) and other smaller (hexapeptides) and less active peptides.

A partial agonist of angiotensin II, saralasin, competes for the same receptors and causes an overall depressor effect in sodium-deficient or normal animals (i.e., decreases arterial pressure). In contrast, the Ang II–agonist (hypertension) effect of saralasin predominates in sodium-replete animals.

Angiotensin III retains less than half of the pressor activity of Ang II, and its ability to enhance the secretion of aldosterone is equipotent to that of Ang II.

Renal Prostaglandins

Renal eicosanoids are produced in multiple renal sites (glomeruli, papillae). Their synthesis is increased by Ang II, vasopressin, bradykinin, and catecholamines, which stimulate the phosphatases that liberate arachidonic acid from their plasma membrane stores. The composition of the diet (rich in essential fatty acids, and proteins), tissue ischemia, mechanical trauma, osmotic pressure, and the levels of Na$^+$, urea, and K$^+$ also increase the activity of plasma membrane phosphatases and renal eicosanoid synthesis.

These biologically active autacoids act locally to modulate release of renin, renal blood flow, glomerular filtration, and sodium extraction. They are called into action via the adrenergic autonomic nervous system, once the renin-angiotensin-aldosterone system is in operation (e.g., during fright). An increased blood pressure results from production of more renin by the juxtaglomerular apparatus in response to norepinephrine. A late rise in arterial pressure also follows the reabsorption of sodium and the concomitant increase of fluid in the circulation. The higher renal blood flow, sensed in the medullary zone, causes the interstitial cells to release PGA_2 and PGE_2 into the circulation. Upon reaching the cortical zone, the PGs exert a tonic natriuretic action to prevent sodium-related hypertension. This effect is obtained by inhibition of the peritubular Na-K-ATPase pump and of the reabsorption of Na^+ from the primitive urine into the peritubular vessels.

Erythropoietin

The renal biosynthesis of erythropoietin (EPO) involves a preproerythropoietin and a proerythropoietin, which is cleaved by a proteolytic lysosomal enzyme, erythrogenin. The precise anatomical unit of the kidney responsible for producing EPO is still unknown, but likely candidates are the epithelial cells of the glomerular tufts or of the proximal tubule. The mature erythropoietin present in blood is a glycoprotein produced in mitochondria of cells in the cortical zone of the kidney. It exists as a monomer (e.g., human EPO [hEPO] has 166 amino acid residues; 18,399 daltons) or as a dimer of about 30,000 daltons. The concentration of erythropoietin in blood is increased by hypoxia caused by a decrease in the number of erythrocytes (anemia, hemorrhage), an impaired oxygenation of hemoglobin (pulmonary dysfunction), or a reduction in the quantity of available oxygen (high-altitude habitat).

The targets of erythropoietin are two types of undifferentiated cells in the bone marrow, the pluripotent stem cells and the erythron, or pronormoblast, cells. By binding to specific plasma membrane receptors, erythropoietin induces stem cells to divide and differentiate into erythroid-committed precursor cells and stimulates the replication of pronormoblast cells. Erythropoietin acts as a growth-like factor for these target cells, activating each pronormoblast to undergo four cell divisions and to synthesize the bulk of its hemoglobin in 3 days. Then, at that stage, each cell, now known as a reticulocyte, loses its nucleus and, after 2 days, matures into a young nonnucleated erythrocyte that leaves the bone marrow to enter the blood circulation for a life span that may extend to 120 days. The production of erythropoietin needs to be continuous to support the biosynthesis of about 2 million erythrocytes per second. EPO is excreted in the urine.

Erythropoietin has some properties of the somatomedins, or growth factors. It has analogies with corticotropin-releasing factor (CRF), vasopressin (ADH), and oxytocin (OT). It mediates the inotropic effects of OT on the myometrium, and like CRF, it mediates the action of ADH on the adenohypophysis.

REFERENCES

Andrews P, Shortman K, Scollay R, Potworowski EF, Kruisbeek AM, Goldstein G, Trainin N, Bach JF. Thymus hormones do not induce proliferative ability or cytolytic function in PNA$^+$ cortical thymocytes. Cell Immunol 1985;91:455.

Baertschi AJ, Teague G. Alveolar hypopxia is a powerful stimulus for ANF release in conscious lambs. Am J Physiol 1989;256:H990.

Coe JY, Olley PM, Coceani F. A fetal-instrumented model to study age-specific responses to leukotriene D_4 and prostaglandin D_2 in unsedated newborn lambs. Can J Physiol Pharmacol 1989;67:587.

Degen MA, Breitschwerdt EB. Canine and feline immunodeficiency—Part I. Comp Cont Educ 1986;8:313.

Hawkey CJ, Rampton DS. Prostaglandins and the gastrointestinal mucosa: Are they important in its function, disease, or treatment? Gastroenterology 1985;89:1162.

Inglis JR. T lymphocytes today. New York: Elsevier, 1983.

Laragh JH. Atrial natriuretic hormone, the renin-aldosterone axis, and blood pressure–electrolyte homeostasis. N Engl J Med 1985;313:1330.

Levenson DJ, Simmons CE, Brenner BM. Arachidonic acid metabolism, prostaglandins, and the kidney. Am J Med 1982;72:354.

Lewis RA, Austen KF. The biologically active leukotrienes. J Clin Invest 1984;73:889.

Luckey TD. Thymic hormones. Baltimore: University Park Press, 1973.

Maack T, Marion DN, Camargo MJF, Kleinert HD, Laragh JH, Vaughan ED, Atlas SA. Effects of auriculin (atrial natriuretic factor) on blood pressure, renal function, and the renin-aldosterone system in dogs. Am J Med 1984;77:1069.

Margolius HS. The kallikrein-kinin system and the kidney. Annu Rev Physiol 1984;14:209.

Marsh JA, Gause JA, Sandhu S, Scanes CG. Enhanced growth and immune development in dwarf chickens treated with mammalian growth hormone and thyroxine. Proc Soc Exp Biol Med 1984;175:351.

Miller TA. Protective effects of prostaglandins against gastric mucosal damage: current knowledge and proposed mechanisms. Am J Physiol 1983;245:G601.

Miyasaka M, Trnka Z. Lymphocyte migration and differentiation in a large-animal model: the sheep. Immunol Rev 1986;91:87.

Monroe WE, Roth JA. The thymus as part of the endocrine system. Cont Educ 1986;8:24.

Morris B. The ontogeny and comportment of lymphoid cells in fetal and neonatal sheep. Immunol Rev 1986;91:219.

Needleman P, Greenwald JE. Atriopeptin: a cardiac hormone intimately involved in fluid, electrolyte, and blood pressure homeostasis. New Engl J Med 1986;314:828.

Nicosia S, Patrono C. Eicosanoid biosynthesis and action: novel opportunities for pharmacological intervention. FASEB J 1989;3:1941.

Perryman LE. Comparative pathology of immune deficiency disorders. Comp Pathol Bull 1984;16:1.

Perryman LE, McGuire TC. Evaluation for immune system failure in horses and ponies. J Am Vet Med Assoc 1980;176:1374.

Robertson RP. Characterization and regulation of prostaglandin and leukotriene receptors: an overview. Prostaglandin 1986;31:395.

Roth JA, Kaeberle ML, Grier RL, Hopper JG, Spiegel HE, McAllister HA. Improvement in clinical condition and thymus morphologic features associated with growth hormone treatment of immunodeficient dwarf dogs. Am J Vet Res 1984;45:1151.

Samuelsson B, Dahlen SE, Lindgren JA, Rouzer CA, Serhan CN. Leukotrienes and lipoxins: structures, biosynthesis, and biological effects. Science 1987;237:1171.

Srivastava KC. Isolation and effects of some ginger components on platelet aggregation and eicosanoid biosynthesis. Prost Leuk Med 1986;25:187.

Weigent T, Blalock JE. Interactions between the neuroendocrine and immune systems: common hormones and receptors. Immunol Rev 1987;100:79.

CHAPTER 52

HORMONES OF THE TESTES

The initial role of testicular hormones is to stimulate male development during embryogenesis. This primordial function causes the differentiation and development of target tissues with a specific intranuclear protein receptor for testosterone. The testosterone-receptor complex attached to the nuclear chromatin induces the transcription of specific genes that affect the growth and morphology of male reproductive organs. At puberty, the testicular hormones determine the changes of sexual maturation associated with spermatogenesis. Testicular hormones are important regulators of the reproductive life of mature males.

THE TESTES AND ACCESSORY SEX ORGANS

Development

Determination of sex and sexual differentiation are sequential processes that involve the establishment of the *chromosomal (genetic) sex* (XX or XY) in the zygote at the instant of fertilization. In response to the genetic sex, *the gonadal (primary) sex* (ovaries or testes) is determined. In turn, the gonadal sex regulates the differentiation and development of the genital apparatus and the manifestations of *phenotypic sex.*

Chromosomes control the direction of the development of the indifferent gonad into either a testis or an ovary. In placental mammals, maleness is associated with heterogametic sex (i.e., XY). A gene on the Y chromosome, the *testis-determining factor,* determines that the gonadal anlage (first accumulation of cells destined to develop into a distinct organ) is to differentiate into a testis.

The chromosomal sex determination in birds (ZW/ZZ species) is more complicated, since the cock is homogametic (ZZ), whereas the hen is heterogametic (ZW) and is positive for the Y-chromosome antigen.

> Because of repression of one of the X chromosomes, the somatic cells of genetically male mammals do not have the lump of chromatin, the sex chromatin or Barr body, that characterizes the cell nucleus of genetically female embryos.

The early fetal gonad is indifferent (i.e., bipotential in sexual differentiation), since at that stage of gestation, males and females have the two sets of primitive genital tracts, the wolffian and müllerian ducts. Male sexual development, associated with regression of the müllerian ducts, requires the presence of testes. In contrast, female sexual development (with regression of the wolffian ducts) occurs in the absence of masculinizing factors, since the undifferentiated gonad has an inherent tendency to feminize and form a reproductive tract.

A *müllerian-inhibiting substance* (MIS) produced by fetal Sertoli's cells of the testes has a paracrine effect (local, ipsilateral), causing regression of the adjacent müllerian (paramesonephric) ducts (Fig. 52–1). MIS is a dimeric glycoprotein (about 140,000 daltons) that also has a role in testicular descent, as a lower testicular level of MIS accompanies cryptorchidism (incomplete descent or abnormal retention of one or both of the testes in the abdomen).

Testosterone secreted from the fetal Leydig's cells (interstitial cells) directly promotes the differentiation of the wolffian (longitudinal mesonephric) ducts linking the mesonephric kidney to the urogenital sinus. The portions of the wolffian ducts adjacent to the testes are transformed into the epididymis, the central portions become the muscular vas deferens, and the portions near the urogenital sinus develop into the seminal vesicles (absent in the cat and dog). Later, testosterone intervenes through dihydrotestosterone (DHT), a product that results from the local action of an enzyme (5-alpha-reductase), to transform the early external genitalia, which also have sexual bipotentiality. Under the influence of DHT, the pelvic portion of the urogenital sinus becomes the prostate, the bulbourethral (Cowper's glands), and the membranous portions of the urethra. The genital tubercle elongates to form the glans penis. The genital swellings first move away from the genital tubercle and then fuse to form the scrotum, which is destined to enclose the testes. Finally, the elongated urogenital cleft closes to form the penile urethra.

> Once the placental membranes and fluids have developed, the level of testosterone in allantoic fluid is higher in male embryos.

General Morphology

All species present the basic male reproductive tract (i.e., two testes, two epididymides, two ductus deferens, and a prostate). However, considerable variation exists regarding the other accessory glands: seminal vesicles, ampullary glands, bulbourethral glands, and small mucus-secreting urethral glands (glands of Littré).

Testes

The *testes* are paired encapsulated ovoid organs made up of seminiferous tubules separated by interstitial tissue. In ungulates, the mass of the testes is about 1% that of the body weight, but in the gerbil (*Tatera afra*) the proportion can be as high as 8 percent. The testis is enveloped by a dense connective-tissue capsule, the tunica albuginea, which carries smooth-muscle fibers responsive to adrenergic stimuli.

In most animals, the testes migrate from their origin in the abdomen to a subcutaneous evagination of the perito-

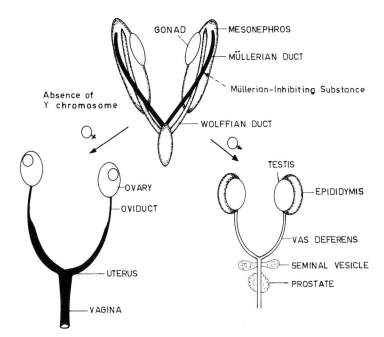

Figure 52–1 Diagram of the undifferentiated ambisexual duct system, with both wolffian and müllerian ducts, in the early embryo. After the onset of the genetic male sex (Y chromosome, and müllerian-inhibiting substance), both the müllerian ducts regress, whereas the wolffian ducts undergo growth and transformation into the accessory structures that link the testes to the urethra.

neum, the scrotum. The final stage of this transabdominal transfer involves the regression of the extraabdominal part of the gubernaculum under the stimulating influence of androgens (masculinizing hormones). Testicular descent occurs during fetal life in large animals (e.g., bull, ram), but only after birth in other animals such as rats and dogs. Cryptorchidism (the incomplete descent of a testis) is seen in horses and dogs.

> Testicond (from the Latin: *testis,* and *condere,* hidden) animals, for example, elephants and armadillos, do not experience migration of the testes, even intraabdominal. Without a scrotum and a spermatic cord, testicond animals have a straight instead of a coiled testicular artery.

Invested by a serosa (*tunica vaginalis*) that is an evagination of the parietal peritoneum, the spermatic cord contains the coiled testicular artery, the tortuous testicular vein plexus (pampiniform), lymphatic vessels, nerves, smooth muscles, and the ductus deferens. The ductus deferens, with the deferential artery and veins, forms a parallel but distinctly separate entity, which can be dissected for vasectomy (i.e., removal of a portion of the ductus deferens).

The testicular artery, issued from the abdominal aorta, is extensively coiled. In bulls and boars, the coiling is so tight that as much as 5 m of artery is crammed into a length of about 10 cm. Gradually decreasing in thickness and carrying fewer layers of smooth muscle cells as it progresses to the periphery, the testicular artery has a flattened profile as it courses on the surface of the testis and ramifies into an arterial rete (network) penetrating the testis. The testicular capillaries are unfenestrated, similar to those found in muscles. The veins from the surface and from within the testis anastomose into a valveless venous plexus, called the *pampiniform plexus,* that surrounds the coiled testicular artery and eventually empties into the central veins (vena cava; hypogastric, common iliac, or renal vein). The coiling of the testicular artery eliminates the arterial pulsations in the spermatic cord without changing the mean arterial pressure. In addition, the incoming arterial blood to the testes is cooled (a loss of about 5° C), whereas the steroid-rich outgoing venous blood is warmed (a similar gain of about 5° C) in the spermatic cord. This is explained by the close proximity of the coiled artery and of the pampiniform plexus, both forming a very efficient countercurrent heat exchanger.

> In bulls, the pampiniform plexus is formed by three networks of veins (200 μm in diameter and covering the artery; 50 μm in diameter and with an unorganized pattern; and smaller periarterial and interarterial veins).
>
> In sheep and pigs, arteriovenous anastomoses in the spermatic cord permit as much as 40 percent of the blood flowing into the testicular artery to bypass the testis and return to the venous system.

Testicular lymph production is highest in the boar (10 μL per gram per hour), intermediate in the ram and ferret (1 μL per gram per hour), and lowest in the rat (0.5 μL per gram per hour), which has the largest lymphatic vessels. In all species, lymph returns a peptide-rich (inhibin) fluid to the circulation. In some species (pigs, horses), the concentration of steroids (testosterone, dehydroepiandrosterone, and total unconjugated estrogens) in testicular lymph is higher than that in testicular venous blood. In the boar, the lymph content of the "*boar-taint*" steroid, 5-alpha-androstenone, is equimolar to that of testosterone. The testicular lymph of vasectomized rams and boars is without erythrocytes but contains spermatozoa, in addition to a normal count of leukocytes (80 percent lymphocytes) of about 250 cells per microliter.

The nervous structures accompanying the testicular artery are distributed to the capsule (very developed in the cat) and the interstitial tissue. Adrenergic fibers exert vasomotor action, stimulate the production of testosterone by

Leydig's cells, and activate cAMP production with aromatization (testosterone → estradiol) in Sertoli's cells. Cholinergic fibers are found in the testicular capsule of rabbits and sheep, whereas peptidergic (vasoactive intestinal peptide, or VIP) ones occur in that of the cat. Sensory receptors (mechano-, chemo-, and thermo-) in the testis and in the scrotum are responsible for pain associated with trauma to the testis.

Beneath its white outer connective-tissue capsule, the testis is separated into lobules separated by interlobular septa containing blood vessels, lymphatics, and nerve fibers. Inside each lobule, the U-shaped seminiferous tubules account for much more of the testicular volume than the interspersed loose connective tissue. The seminiferous tubules have a central lumen, a stratified epithelium composed of spermatogenic and Sertoli's cells, and a thin outer basement membrane. The loose connective tissue stroma between the tubules contains Leydig's (interstitial) cells.

The interlobular septa extend to the mediastinum, an area of connective tissue within which the distal segments of the seminiferous tubules open and drain into the *rete testis* (i.e., an anastomotic network of ducts). The rete testis carries spermatozoa and the fluid in which they are suspended. A system of 12 to 20 *efferent ducts,* or *ductuli efferentes,* links the rete testis to the epididymis. A highly convoluted duct applied to the surface of the testis, the *epididymis,* or *ductus epididymidis,* is held to the tunica albuginea by connective tissue and ends in the ductus deferens. The *ductus deferens* is much more than a simple conduit leading sperm from the epididymis to the urethra, since it possesses a complex epithelium capable of both absorptive and secretory functions.

Accessory Sex Organs

The *ampulla,* which is present in the bull, camel, elephant, jackass, rabbit, ram, red deer, and stallion, is a spindle-shaped thickening of the terminal portion of the ductus deferens. It is a well-developed structure in the stallion (25 × 2 cm), the camel (12 × 0.5 cm), the bull (10 × 1.5 cm), the elephant (8 × 6 cm), and the ram as well as the red deer (7 × 0.5 cm). Ampullary glands exist on the dorsal wall of the urethra in the male hamster, mouse, and rat. In the bull, the secretion from the ampulla is very rich in electrolytes (Na^+, Ca^{++}, and Mg^{++}) and contains much citric acid. The ampulla fluid of jackasses and stallions is characterized by the presence of ergothionine.

The *seminal vesicles,* absent in cats and dogs, are paired, bag-shaped glands in guinea pigs, rats, and stallions. In bulls, boars, and rams, they consist of multiple lobes containing a system of ramified secretory ducts.

The *prostate* is a tubuloalveolar gland that may be diffuse (or disseminate) if it is confined around the urethra, or discrete if it forms a definite body outside the urethral muscle. In rams the prostate is of the diffuse type, whereas both types exist in boars and bulls. The only sexual accessory gland in dogs, the prostate, frequently undergoes an endocrine-related hypertrophy in old animals.

The *bulbourethral glands,* especially large in boars, are absent in bears and dogs. They contain sialomucin, which causes the gelation reaction in boar semen.

The *urethral glands* (glands of Littré), present in boars, do not store their mucous secretion, which is produced during coitus.

HORMONES OF THE TESTES

The major hormones produced by the testes are testosterone (by Leydig's cells) and inhibin (by Sertoli's cells). Their synthesis is regulated by the gonadotropins, luteinizing hormone (LH) and follicle-stimulating hormone (FSH), which are both synthesized and stored in the adenohypophysis. The adenohypophysial release of LH and FSH is regulated by the hypothalamic decapeptide gonadotropin-releasing hormone (GnRH). Neurotransmitters (biogenic amines) in the central nervous system control the output of GnRH, secreted and released in pulses at about 90-minute intervals. GnRH seeks protein receptors on the plasma membrane of gonadotrope cells and causes normal episodic secretion of LH (about 16 pulses per 24 hours) and of FSH. In small ruminants, the period of reproductive rest (long solar days) is marked by less frequent gonadotropin pulses.

LH stimulates Leydig's cells to secrete a steroid, *testosterone.* FSH binds to and activates Sertoli's cells to secrete a polypeptide hormone, *inhibin,* that induces the maturation and growth of the tubule cells, and the aromatization of androgens into estradiol. FSH also causes Sertoli's cells of mice, guinea pigs, pigs, rabbits, rats, and sheep to secrete *androgen-binding protein* (ABP, 90,000 daltons). By binding to the testosterone present in the seminal tubule fluid, ABP inhibits its absorption by cells in the wall of the ductules and ensures the arrival of sufficient testosterone into the epididymis. In addition, FSH supports Sertoli's cells for the morphological maturation of spermatids into spermatozoa.

The hypothalamic-adenohypophysial-testicular axis is a closed-loop system, that is, a system in which the control action depends on (is a function of) the output. It has a negative-feedback system in which testicular hormones (testosterone and inhibin) depress the adenohypophysial secretion of LH and FSH. Castration results in an elevation of both LH and FSH in the circulation, whereas selective germ cell damage produces an elevation in the level of serum FSH alone. The negative feedback of testosterone on the hypothalamic GnRH makes it the primary regulator of gonadotropin secretion (Fig. 52–2), whereas the other testicular hormone, *inhibin,* would suppress mostly FSH release. Testosterone decreases the frequency and the amplitude of the LH pulses. Also, it interacts with endorphin neurons, which depress the GnRH neurons of the median eminence and the discharge of their decapeptide secretion into the hypothalamo-adenohypophysial portal system.

Synthesis and Release of Steroids

Since the mechanism for steroid synthesis in the testes is similar to that occurring in the adrenal cortex, several other testicular steroid metabolites are also produced besides

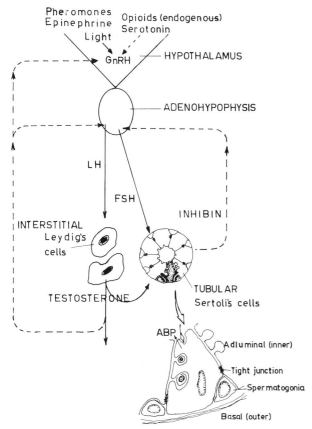

Figure 52-2 In males, the pulsatile hypothalamic secretion of GnRH regulates the release of FSH and LH from the adenohypophysis. LH induces the production of testosterone by Leydig's cells. FSH acts on the Sertoli target cells, stimulating spermatogenesis and the output of inhibin; the testosterone from Leydig's cells stimulates the endoluminal production of androgenbinding protein (ABP). In turn, inhibin suppresses the release of FSH through a direct adenohypophysial negative feedback. In contrast, testosterone has an inhibitory action at the level of both the adenohypophysis (against LH) and the hypothalamus (against GnRH).

testosterone (Fig. 52-3). From cholesterol, with enzymatic reactions giving various intermediary metabolites, Leydig's cells synthesize testosterone from either or both androstenediol and androstenedione.

Some of the *testosterone* released appears in the seminiferous tubule fluid, bound to ABP in order to prevent its absorption by sperm. However, most of the testosterone is released into the lymph and the venous blood draining the testes. About 98 percent of the circulating testosterone is bound to albumin and to testosterone-estradiol-binding globulin (TEBG, 94,000 daltons) produced by hepatic cells. The rate of hepatic secretion of this protein (also called sex steroid–binding globulin {SSBG}) is decreased by androgens, whereas estrogens increase its synthesis. This explains why the plasma concentration of the sex globulin in females is about twice that of males. The SSBG-bound fraction of testosterone serves as a circulating reserve, somewhat like the thyroxine and cortisol bound in plasma. Only unbound testosterone, a small fraction of the total, is available to the androgen target cells.

The concentration of testosterone in the plasma of males is relatively high during three periods of life: the phase of embryonic development in which male phenotypic differentiation takes place, the neonatal period, and adult sexual life. Plasma testosterone levels decline prior to birth and prior to puberty. These levels follow a circadian rhythm, with a trend for higher (by about 25 percent) values in the morning than at night, and circhoral very small pulses.

Males of species that are seasonal breeders (e.g., deer, goat, sheep) lapse into a period of complete sexual quiescence for part of the year. However, sheep can produce sperm all year round in the climate of warm latitudes. The secretion of testicular steroids then declines to a low point, causing a halt in spermatogenesis and libido.

> Seminal vesicle cells synthesize fructose from blood glucose (not in stallions and jackasses). This synthesis of fructose is strictly regulated by androgenic hormones, and the concentration of seminal fructose gives an indication of the androgenic status of an animal.

A pathway that accounts for estrogen synthesis in males is the aromatization of the A-ring of testosterone (but not dihydrotestosterone). This conversion of testosterone to estradiol can occur in Sertoli's cells (about 15 percent, which accounts for more than 95 percent of gonadal estradiol) but occurs mostly (85 percent) in a variety of extraglandular tissues (adipose tissue, brain, and liver).

Synthesis and Release of Polypeptides

Sertoli's cells may secrete several other proteins and peptides that have autocrine and paracrine effects on the testis. Gonadocrinins, a family of peptides structurally similar to GnRH that inhibit the function of Leydig's cells, and both alpha-melanocyte-stimulating hormone (MSH) and beta-endorphin, all secreted by Sertoli's cells, probably have paracrine and autocrine functions. Transferrin (an iron-binding protein), ceruloplasmin (a copper-transport protein), testicular plasminogen activators (important in fibrinolysis), and growth factors (somatomedin C, fibroblast growth factor, epidermal growth factor) are some of the other proteins extracted from cultures of Sertoli's cells.

A few testicular nonsteroidal substances also enter the general circulation to act as endocrine mediators on extragonadal tissues. Under the stimulation of FSH and testosterone, Sertoli's cells of the seminiferous tubules secrete the glycoprotein inhibin, also called Sertoli's cell factor (SCF). The chemistry of male-derived inhibin is not as well known as that of female-derived inhibin, which is produced by the granulosa cells of the ovarian follicles. A precursor of inhibin in the ovarian follicle is a high molecular weight protein (56,000 daltons) that is cleaved to a smaller-size protein before exocytosis. A highly purified inhibin, believed to be the circulating inhibin, has a molecular weight of about 32,000 daltons and is a dimer, that is, contains two polypeptide chains (alpha, or A, and beta, or B) united by disulfide bonds. The alpha-inhibin, or A subunit, is glycosy-

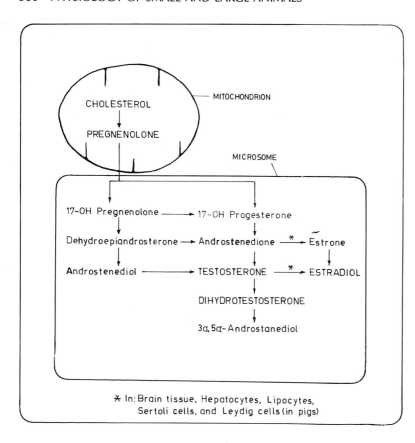

Figure 52–3 Synthesis pathways of the major testicular steroids; testosterone, dihydrotestosterone, and estradiol. The synthesis starts from cholesterol esters in lipid droplets within the cytoplasm. Under LH stimulation, the cholesterol is taken to the inner mitochondrial membrane and converted to pregnenolone, which then moves to the microsomal compartment. The microsomal enzymes operate rapidly and complete the synthesis of testicular steroids.

lated (18,000 daltons) and the beta-inhibin, or B subunit (14,000 daltons), has two forms: B_a and B_b. Consequently, the configuration of inhibin can be A,B_a (inhibin A) or A,B_b (inhibin B). The B_aB_b combination is called *activin*.

Hypophysectomy reduces the production of inhibin in seminiferous fluid (after 7 days), and in cultures of Sertoli's cells (after 3 weeks) as well as that of ABP. In cryptorchids, the elevated temperature causes a reduction in the secretion of inhibin and of ABP besides reducing the number of germ cells.

Actions

Active *androgens* diffuse freely into target cells and bind to a single cytoplasmic receptor. The androgen-receptor complex moves into the nucleus to interact with chromosomal DNA and nuclear protein, with the resultant synthesis of proteins (enzymes).

Testosterone activates target cells devoid of 5-alpha-reductase to induce androgenic (male characteristics) and anabolic (growth-promoting) effects. Besides stimulating the differentiation of the wolffian ducts during embryogenesis, testosterone is directly responsible for growth of the penis and of accessory glands and for initiation as well as maintenance of spermatogenesis. Other androgenic actions ascribed to testosterone include aggressiveness, sexual drive (libido, erection), appearance of spicules on the feline penis or of bones in the canine penis, growth of a mane (in bison, horse,

lion), and growth and shedding (calcification) of antlers in male deer. The anabolic actions of testosterone include greater proliferation of the larynx and of the kidney as well as of muscle mass.

Testosterone accounts for biochemical effects such as nitrogen retention and protein anabolism, antinatriuresis, hematopoiesis, and suppression of hepatic synthesis of carrier-plasma proteins (e.g., cortisol-binding protein, sex steroid–binding globulin, thyroxin-binding globulin). Testosterone also has a negative-feedback effect on the hypothalamus and on the adenohypophysis to regulate the output of LH.

The production of male pheromones (i.e., substances that modify the reproductive behavior of female congeners) is stimulated by testosterone. In sows in estrus, the smell of boars' urine or saliva containing delta-16-steroid pheromones (androstenone and androstenol) produces a typical immobility. The odor of caproic or capric acid in the secretion of the sebaceous scent glands of goats (mediocaudal aspects of the horns), the musk odor of the glands on the abdomen of male musk deer, and the pungent odor of the urine (lipids of renal origin) of male cats and sheep all are androgen related. Likewise, the production of musth, a dark-brown ichor or sanies (i.e., watery fluid) from tiny holes above the eyes of the male elephant is androgen-dependent.

With regard to some target cells, testosterone is not the active form of the hormone but a prohormone. In these target tissues, testosterone must be converted, by a 5-alpha-reductase, to the more active *dihydrotestosterone,* or aromatized to *estradiol* (Fig. 52–4). This is reminiscent of thyroxine serving as a prohormone for triiodothyronine. Dihydrotestosterone serves as the intracellular mediator of most actions of the hormone. The greater androgenic potency of dihydrotestosterone is explained by its binding more tightly (about ten times) to the cytoplasmic androgen-receptor protein than testosterone. In addition, this dihydrotestosterone-receptor complex changes more readily to the activated, or DNA-binding, state than the testosterone-receptor complex. The estrogens enhance some androgenic effects and block others.

Dihydroxytestosterone intervenes during fetal life for the differentiation of the genital tubercle, genital swellings, genital folds, and urogenital sinus into the penis, scrotum, penile urethra, and prostate. At puberty, it induces the growth of the scrotum and prostate, whereas it stimulates secretion by the prostate in adult male animals.

The polypeptide testicular hormone *inhibin* is believed to attach to specific protein receptors on the plasma membrane of the gonadotropes, decreases the level of cyclic adenosine monophosphate (cAMP) and selectively reduces the adenohypophysial output of FSH. Inhibin possibly also acts on the hypothalamus, on the pineal gland, and locally (paracrine effect) on the testis. Also, it may inhibit the development of a female-type reproductive tract in male animals.

Metabolism

After a half-life of about 10 to 20 minutes, free or unbound testosterone is inactivated primarily in the liver. The hepatic catabolism of testosterone first involves oxidation of the 17-OH group, then reduction of the A ring of androstenedione leading to formation of a product with markedly reduced androgenic activity, androst*a*nedione, which has a 3-keto group that is later reduced to form androsterone. Alternatively, androstenedione can be reduced in the 5-beta position and can undergo 3-keto reduction to form etiocholanolone. In the liver, free dihydrotestosterone is also converted to androsterone, androstanedione, and androstanediol.

After oral administration, testosterone or dihydrotestosterone is absorbed into the portal blood. These free androgens are promptly degraded by the liver, so only an insignificant amount of androgen reaches the systemic circulation. Likewise, after parenteral administration as free androgens, they are also rapidly metabolized, unless their molecules are modified to retard the rate of hepatic catabolism or to enhance the androgenic potency of these testicular steroids. One such modification is alkylation at the 17 position, which markedly retards their hepatic metabolism and permits such analogs to be effective orally. Such alkylated androgens have the inconvenience of causing hepatotoxicity.

With radioactive testosterone, about 90 percent of the radioactivity appears in the urine, and about 6 percent in the feces, after it has passed through the enterohepatic circulation. The major metabolites of androgens in urine are physiologically inactive (either as free steroids or water-soluble conjugates). They are predominantly etiocholanolone and androsterone. Etiocholanolone is a 5-beta-reduced metabolite of testosterone and of other 3-keto androgens, and androsterone is a metabolite of dihydrotestosterone. Small amounts of androstanediol and estrogens are also excreted, largely as glucuronide and sulfate conjugates.

The metabolism of inhibin is still unknown.

Figure 52–4 A synopsis of the different transformations of testosterone, which can be considered as a prohormone for active metabolites (dihydrotestosterone and estradiol). The catabolism of testosterone yields inactive metabolites (androsterone and etiocholanolone).

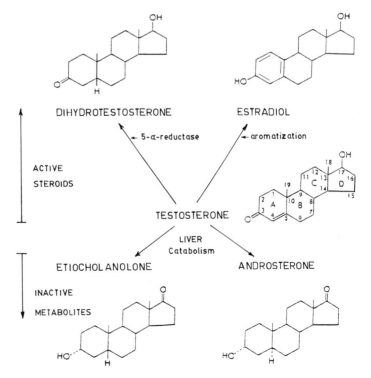

REFERENCES

Depalitis L, Moore J, Falvo RE. Plasma concentrations of testosterone and LH in the male dog. J Reprod Fertil 1978;52:201.

Frey HL, Raijfer J. Role of the gubernaculum and intraabdominal pressure in the process of testicular descent. J Urol 1984;131:574.

Ganjam VK, Kenney RM. Androgens and oestrogens in normal and cryptorchid stallions. J Reprod Fertil 1975;23:67.

Hall PF. Cellular organization for steroidogenesis. Int Rev Cytol 1984;86:53.

Hees H, Leiser R, Kohler T, Wrobel KH. Vascular morphology of the bovine spermatic cord and testis. I. Light and scanning electron-microscopic studies on the testicular artery and pampiniform plexus. Cell Tiss Res 1984;237:31.

Johnson CA. The role of the fetal testicle in sexual differentiation. Compendium Contin Educ Pract Vet 1983;5:129.

Johnstone IP, Bancroft BJ, McFarlane JR. Testosterone and androstenedione profiles in the blood of domestic tom-cats. Ann Reprod Sci 1984;7:363.

Kenagy GJ, Trombulak SC. Size and function of mammalian testes in relation to body size. Mammalogy 1986;67:1.

Miyamoto A, Ishii S, Furusawa T, et al. Serum inhibin, FSH, LH and testosterone levels, and testicular inhibin content in beef bulls from birth to puberty. Anim Reprod Sci 1989;20:165.

Moger WH. Stimulation and inhibition of Leydig cell steroidogenesis by the phorbol ester 12-0-tetradecanoylphorbol-13-acetate. Life Sci 1985;37:869.

Nyman MA, Geiger J, Goldzieber. Biosynthesis of estrogens by the perfused stallion testis. J Biol Chem 1959;234:16.

Saez JM, Sanchez P, Berthelon MC, Avallet O. Regulation of pig Leydig cell aromatase activity by gonadotropins and Sertoli cells. Biol Reprod 1989;41:813.

Setchell BP, Laurie MS, Flint APF, Heap RB. Transport of free steroids from the boar testis in lymph, venous blood and rete testis fluid. J Endocrinol 1983;96:127.

Sharpe RM. Intratesticular factors controlling testicular function. Biol Reprod 1984;30:29.

Wichmann U, Wichmann G, Krause W. Serum levels of testosterone precursors, testosterone and estradiol in 10 animal species. Exp Clin Endocrinol 1984;83:283.

Wilson JD, Griffin JE, George FW, Leshim M. The endocrine control of male phenotype development. Aust J Biol Sci 1983;36:101.

Wright WW, Musto NA, Mather JP, Bardin CW. Sertoli cells secrete both testis-specific and serum proteins. Proc Natl Acad Sci USA 1981;78:7565.

CHAPTER 53

OVARIAN HORMONES

During the reproductive cycles of animals, the female gonads (ovaries) simultaneously provide for the maturation of female gametes (oocytes), for the growth of female reproductive follicular cells (follicles), and for the orderly secretion of several hormones. The ovary secretes two major steroid hormones, estradiol and progesterone, and also produces lesser amounts of other steroids (androstenedione, testosterone) and of nonsteroidal hormones (eicosanoids, inhibin, oxytocin, relaxin).

The adenohypophysial gonadotropins, luteinizing hormone (LH) and follicle-stimulating hormone (FSH), regulate the sequence and the quantity of these ovarian hormones. In turn, the production of these gonadotropins occurs in response to signals from the nervous system and from the ovarian hormones. It is unfortunate that the reproductive cycles of adult females of different species are very different and cannot be described for a standard or typical female. However, known correlations between the nervous system, the adenohypophysis, and the ovaries make it logical to consider the ovary as part of a hypothalamo-adenohypophysio-ovarian system.

GENERAL MORPHOLOGY OF THE OVARY

In contrast with the development of the male organs, which differentiate from the sexually indifferent embryo after steroid (testosterone) stimulation, the development of the ovaries does not require any hormonal stimulus. The ovary is seeded with thousands of primary oocytes, a minority of which will ultimately reach maturity after puberty. The müllerian (paramesonephric) ducts develop, whereas the wolffian (mesonephric) ducts become vestigial. According to the species, the müllerian ducts change to become the oviducts of a duplex uterus (rodents), of a bicornuate uterus (pig), of a bipartite uterus (ruminants), or of a simplex uterus (mare, primates) (Fig. 53–1). The genital tubercle develops into the clitoris, the genital fold into the urethral orifice, and the genital swelling into the borders of the vulva.

In general terms, each of the paired ovaries is an intra-abdominal ovoid organ encased in a *serous basement membrane* (formerly termed the germinal epithelium) that is continuous with the peritoneum. The presence and the size of the ovarian structures found near and under the serous epithelium are not identical in prepuberal and in postpuberal females. The arterial supply to each ovary is provided by an anastomotic group of vessels coming from the ovarian artery (a branch of the aorta) and from the uterine artery. Near the ovary, the arterial vessels are spiraled and imprinted over the converging ovarian and uterine veins. These arterial spirals accommodate cyclical changes in ovarian size and contribute

to maintain a constant ovarian arterial pressure. The close contact of veins with the artery provides an efficient system for exchange of substances between the two countercurrent circuits. Each ovary carries extensive networks of lymphatics, and of sympathetic and parasympathetic nerves, but their importance in controlling ovarian functions remains to be established.

In prepuberal female animals, the ovary is relatively static, apart from undergoing growth, compared with the postpuberal animal. The serous epithelium covers a thin layer of dense connective tissue (*tunica albuginea*), a peripheral zone (*cortex*) interspersed with thousands of *follicles* that each contain a female gamete or *primary oocyte,* and a central zone (*medulla*). Each oocyte that is enveloped by a single layer of cells is termed a *primordial follicle.* The female puppy, unlike the young of other species, does not have primordial follicles at birth, but only after about 3 weeks. Because of a meiotic division that occurs only during fetal life, an oocyte contains only half the number (haploid) of chromosomes that is characteristic of the animal species (Table 53–1). In contrast, this meiotic halving of the chromosome number in the male gametes (spermatozoa) is performed during the entire postpuberal or adult life of the animal.

In adult females, the ovary is in a dynamic state that begins during puberty and continues thereafter during the reproductive cycles that are characteristic for the animal species. The ovarian arteries become more developed and coiled. The serous epithelium covering the ovary is periodically broken at ovulation to permit extrusion of one (monotocous) or several (polytocous) mature eggs, or oocytes, into the reproductive organs linked with the ovaries (oviducts, uterus). During the maturation process of each oocyte, the cells of the single layer surrounding the female gamete divide to form several layers. These granulosa cells secrete an estrogen-rich fluid that fills a cavity or antrum and bathes the egg–cumulus oophorus promontory. The adjacent interstitial cells (theca interna and theca externa) also proliferate, and the vascularization of the theca interna is particularly improved.

The morphology of the primary follicle progressively changes into that of a graafian (mature) follicle. Ovulation is marked by the physical rupture of a mature follicle and the release of the egg–cumulus oophorus complex into the female genital tract.

After ovulation, the cells remaining in the follicle (mostly granulosa) increase in size (hypertrophy) to form the corpus luteum (CL). The CL acquires one of the richest blood flows per gram of any tissue in the body, the renal cortex included. This temporary ovarian endocrine organ is responsible for the secretion of progesterone, a major female steroid hormone, and of oxytocin. If fertilization and implantation do not occur, the corpus luteum undergoes degeneration or

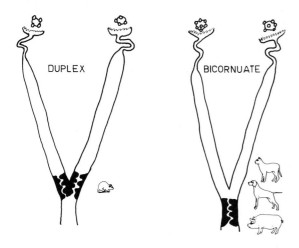

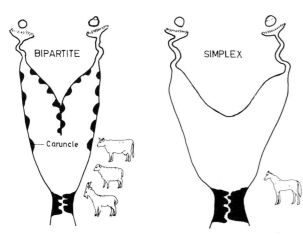

Figure 53–1 Various types of female genital tracts resulting from the development of a portion of the müllerian ducts. In the *duplex* uterus (rodents, rabbit), each müllerian duct is transformed into a separate uterine horn and cervix. The *bicornuate* uterus (pig) has only a small area where the uterine horns have fused into a common lumen and a single cervix. The *bipartite* uterus (ruminants) remains with only a partial septum between the two uterine horns, which constitute an extensive uterine cavity. In the *simplex* uterus (horse), a complete fusion of the two horns creates a vast uterine cavity. The degree of fusion of the uterine horns is associated with a reduction in the number of fetuses that can be carried.

TABLE 53–1   Haploid Number of Chromosomes in the Gametes of Some Animal Species

Cat	19	Mouse	20
Chicken	39	Pigeon	31
Cow	30	Pig	19
Dog	39	Rat	21
Goat	30	Sheep	27
Horse	32	Turkey	41
Mink	15		

luteolysis, and ultimately all that is left is a nodule of cortical ovarian connective tissue.

The adult ovary can be conceived of as an assemblage of three separate functional units, the stroma (connective tissue), the follicles, and the corpus luteum. These structural units are in a constant state of flux, one succeeding to another as the regression of a functional unit creates elements for the formation of another type of unit. The conversion of the follicle into the corpus luteum, and the transformation of the latter into connective tissue, can serve to illustrate this simplified concept.

OVARIAN STEROID HORMONES

The ovarian steroid secretions function as *autocrine* agents, acting on or within the cells in which they are produced; as *paracrine* agents, influencing adjacent cells; and as classic *endocrine* agents, transported via the circulation to remote target cells.

The ability of the ovary to produce steroid hormones depends on the presence of a special collection of enzymes, the mixed function oxidases. These enzymes, involved in several oxidation-reduction reactions, require a system that generates nicotinamide-adenine dinucleotide phosphate (NADPH) and an oxygen-transport system using cytochrome P_{450}. All ovarian steroids are derived from free cholesterol, which enters into the mitochondrion (a rate-limiting reaction) for cleavage and transformation into pregnenolone. Once pregnenolone is returned into the cytosol of follicular or corpus luteum cells, it serves as the precursor to all steroid hormones. The mitochondrial transformation of cholesterol into pregnenolone is a short-term effect of LH, which can act on follicular or luteal cells.

Luteal cells secrete primarily 21-carbon *progestins,* and the interstitial, or theca, cells produce mostly 19-carbon *androgens.* Neither cell type is able to produce 18-carbon *estrogens* de novo, but ovarian aromatase enzymes are found in the follicular granulosa cells and in the large luteal granulosa (granulosa-lutein) cells. These enzymes transform the androgens (androstenedione, testosterone) into estrogens (estrone, estradiol) by aromatization of the A-ring (Fig. 53–2). This effect is stimulated by FSH, the other adenohypophysial gonadotropin, and is limited to the granulosa cells, since all other ovarian cells lack FSH receptors. Androgens must diffuse from the theca cells, across the basement membrane, and into the follicular fluid bathing the aromatizing granulosa cells.

The enzymatic reactions within the theca interstitial cell and the granulosa cell are influenced by a flock of hormones (Fig. 53–3). The stimulating or depressing actions of these various types of hormones modify the relationship between these follicular or luteal cells. In theca cells, the production of androgens from cholesterol can be either stimulated or inhibited. In the granulosa cells, the aromatization of androgens to estrogens can also be enhanced or decreased.

Figure 53-2 Diagram of the two-cell, two-gonadotropin concept of ovarian steroid hormone synthesis. Under the influence of FSH, the granulosa cell can produce progesterone from cholesterol, and estrogens from androgens. The secreted progesterone and estradiol both can appear in the blood capillaries separating the granulosa and theca cells. LH stimulates the theca cell to produce androstenedione from progesterone, which comes from either theca or granulosa cells. Androstenedione must diffuse into the granulosa cell to be converted into testosterone. In the granulosa cell, both androstenedione and testosterone can be aromatized into estrogens, but this transformation is inhibited if progesterone is the dominant secretion of the granulosa cell. When progesterone is used as a precursor to androgens, and the latter are aromatized to estrogens, the end-products are estrone (from androstenedione) and estradiol (from testosterone). Estradiol is the major steroid hormone present in the follicular fluid.

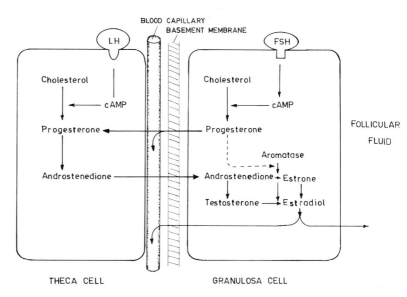

Progesterone

Pregnenolone, the most important progestin and the key precursor of all steroids, is readily converted to *progesterone* (P$_4$). Progesterone is produced as a biosynthetic intermediate by follicles at all growing stages of development and as a secretory end-product in the periovulatory and postovulatory periods. In all animal species, the greatest stimulation of progesterone biosynthesis follows the LH surge and ovulation, as granulosa cells hypertrophy or luteinize to form granulosa-lutein cells.

The general categories of follicles are *primordial,* or nongrowing, follicles; *preantral* follicles characterized mainly by increases in oocyte size and the number of granulosa cells;

and small or large *antral* follicles, featuring the formation of a fluid-filled antrum and further increases in granulosa cell number.

In bovine follicular fluid, pregnenolone secreted by granulosa cells is metabolized to progesterone. In porcine follicular fluid, theca cells transform pregnenolone to aromatizable androgens.

Androgens

Androstenedione and *testosterone* are androgens formed in thecal cells by hydroxylation at the 17-C position, and removal of the 21-C side-chain of either pregnenolone or

Figure 53-3 In the theca cell, the formation of androgen from cholesterol is stimulated mostly by LH, but also by catecholamines, insulin, and prostaglandins (PGs). Hormones that inhibit the synthesis of androgens include epidermal growth factor (EGF), estrogens, glucocorticoids, GnRH, and PRL. In the granulosa cell, the aromatization of androgens is enhanced by FSH, insulin, and LH. The aromatase complex of enzymes is depressed by glucocorticoids, GnRH, and PRL.

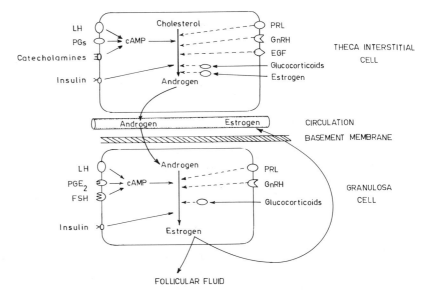

progesterone. LH increases androgen secretion by the theca cells. By enhancing the conversion of cholesterol to pregnenolone, both FSH and androgens independently stimulate theca progesterone biosynthesis in the follicles of cows, ewes, and sows.

These ovarian androgens have an obligatory role as substrate for estrogen biosynthesis by granulosa cells. Androgens also have other roles in follicular function. They exert an antagonistic effect on the growth of preantral follicles, but a facilitatory effect on that of large antral follicles entering their final stage of development. On the other hand, FSH promotes aromatization of androgens and greatly increases the estradiol concentration in bovine antral follicles as they progress from small to large size.

Estrogens

Estrone and *estradiol* (ten times more active biologically) are produced from androgens in granulosa cells. Since the necessary androgens are secreted by the theca cells, the production of ovarian estrogens depends on the participation of two types of cells, theca and granulosa, and also of two gonadotropins, LH and FSH. This has led to the concept of the "two-cell, two-gonadotropin model" of follicular estrogen secretion. Under the stimulus of LH, androstenedione is synthesized in theca interna cells and transported (by diffusion) across the basement membrane to adjacent granulosa cells. Under the impulse of FSH and LH, androstenedione is then converted to testosterone, and later both androgens are aromatized to estrone and estradiol, respectively.

Release and Transport

In contrast with peptidic hormones, ovarian steroid hormones are not stored in granules but are released as soon as they are synthesized by the interstitial (stromal, thecal) and granulosa cells. The increased secretion of steroid hormones is directly reflected by a higher plasma concentration. However, only a small proportion, the unbound or free fraction, of the lipid-soluble steroid hormones found in the plasma is biologically active.

Most of the steroid hormones in the plasma are biologically inactive because of the binding to plasma proteins that occurs during their passage through the liver or because of metabolic conjugation in the same organ. The concentration of free or active steroid hormones regulates the hepatic production of binding or transport proteins, that is, higher levels of free active steroids induce a higher output of proteins by the liver. By protecting hormones from metabolism and renal clearance, these plasma-binding proteins provide a reservoir of hormones, which can be released to target cells. This reservoir significantly extends the circulating half-life of steroid hormones, buffers the increases in steroid hormone production, and constitutes a source when their secretion or synthesis is lowered. In a nonspecific manner, plasma *albumin* (formed in the liver) binds with all steroids, whether they are of gonadic (progesterone, androgens, estrogens), hepatic (vitamin D), or adrenocortical (mineralocorticoids and glucocorticoids) origin.

Several *beta-globulins* (transport proteins), also of hepatic origin, bind with specific steroids. *Corticosteroid-binding globulin* (CBG), also known as *transcortin,* is a 52,000-dalton glycoprotein that contains one high-affinity binding site that accepts specifically cortisol or progesterone. Although CBG binds both steroids with about equal affinity, most of its binding sites are filled by cortisol, since the cortisol blood concentration is usually several times higher than that of progesterone. Estrogens increase the production of CBG, and so do thyroid hormones. *Sex hormone–binding globulin* (SHBG), also known as testosterone-estradiol–binding globulin (TEBG), is a molecule with a single binding site that has more affinity for testosterone than for estradiol. Under most conditions, testosterone occupies the binding site, and estradiol binds nonspecifically to albumin. The concentration of SHBG is increased about ten times by estrogens and somewhat less by thyroid hormones, but it is lowered about twofold by androgens.

Vitamin D–binding globulin (DBG) is a 56,000-dalton glycoprotein that has a single binding site with a higher affinity for 25-hydroxyvitamin D than for 1,25-dihydroxyvitamin D. As for other transport proteins, more DBG is produced in response to estrogens.

Preovulatory Control of Secretion

In the cycling nonpregnant female animal, the secretion of ovarian steroids is regulated by adenohypophysial gonadotropins, which are themselves controlled by the adenohypophysiotropic gonadotropin-releasing hormone (GnRH) from the hypothalamus. Another adenohypophysial hormone, prolactin (PRL), is also implicated in the secretion of progesterone shortly before ovulation. The hypothalamic GnRH influences a single type of adenohypophysial cell, the gonadotrope, which produces both LH and FSH. Neural extrinsic and intrinsic stimuli to hypothalamic nuclei, termed regulators, modulate the output and action of GnRH. The "pulse generator" (for basal, pulsatile, or tonic gonadotropin secretion) appears to be located in the medial basal hypothalamus (arcuate and ventromedial nuclei). The "surge generator" that produces a single massive ovulatory peak of LH coincident with a smaller peak of FSH secretion seems to be be located in the preoptic and suprachiasmatic nuclei.

Basal, *pulsatile,* or tonic gonadotropin secretion, which occurs during most of the reproductive cycle, is kept in check by the negative feedback of gonadal steroids, since gonadectomy results in a great increase in the production of gonadotropins. These sex steroids and other substances (catecholamines, opiate agonists, and antagonists) can alter the amplitude and frequency of LH pulses through interactions with the neuronal pulse generator in the arcuate nucleus. Simultaneous measurements of the levels of GnRH (in the hypothalamo-adenohypophysial portal system) and LH in the peripheral plasma of sheep indicate the excellent concordance between the basal GnRH and LH pulses (Fig. 53–4).

In contrast, the almost simultaneous *surges* of LH and FSH secretions punctuate each reproductive cycle, before ovulation (i.e., the shedding of one or several mature oo-

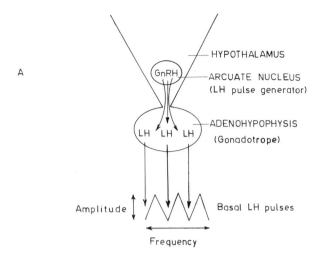

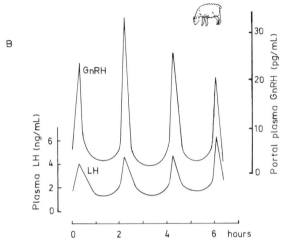

Figure 53–4 **A,** A pulse generator is situated in the arcuate nucleus of the hypothalamus. It induces episodic secretion of GnRH, which enters the hypothalamo-adenohypophysial portal system and reaches its target cells, the gonadotropes. These cells respond by producing corresponding pulses of secretions (i.e., LH and FSH). In the ewe, the amplitude and frequency of the gonadotropin response is reflected in the peripheral plasma levels of LH. **B,** In the ewe, simultaneous measurements of the concentrations of GnRH (in the hypothalamo-adenohypophysial portal blood) and of LH (in the peripheral plasma) reveal an excellent concordance. The pulses occur at about 90-minute intervals, but the amplitude (portal blood levels) of the GnRH oscillations is much less (pg/mL) than that of plasma LH (ng/mL).

cytes). The amplitude of the preovulatory LH surge is such that the massive increase in plasma gonadotropin may be several hundred times higher than the peak concentration measured during the basal or pulsatile (pulse) secretion. The activation of the "surge generator" is the result of a precise and intricate positive-feedback cascade of neural events influencing the hypothalamo-adenohypophysio-ovarian axis. These events or factors originate in the external and the internal environments. Some factors in the external environment include auditory stimuli, availability of food, day length, the sexual receptivity of individuals of the opposite sex, smell (pheromones), and temperature. In contrast, body

metabolism, weight, and fat are considered as factors in the internal environment. In the majority of mammals, the "surges" of LH and of FSH that precede ovulation occur spontaneously and last 12 to 18 hours except in bitches (about 3 to 4 days) and mares (about 1 week).

In spontaneous ovulators, the tonic pulses of LH and FSH that act on the theca and granulosa cells gradually increase the secretion of *estrogens* during the folliculogenesis period of the estrous cycle. When follicles are near maturity, the aromatase enzyme functions maximally to transform androgens into estrogens and to create a sustained elevation in the estradiol concentration in each mature follicle and in the peripheral blood. The follicular estradiol content increases several hundred times above that of plasma. This sustained peak of estradiol exerts a positive-feedback action on the hypothalamic surge generator, which induces a cascade of surges, first of GnRH and then of both gonadotropins (Fig. 53–5). In addition, an increased secretion of PRL by adenohypophysial lactotropes is induced by the elevated estradiol levels and by a paracrine action of the neighboring gonadotropes.

During folliculogenesis, the *progesterone* secretion remains minimal, but the slight preovulatory increase, provoked by PRL, may be significant enough to potentiate the positive feedback of estradiol on the hypothalamic surge generator. PRL increases progesterone accumulation by preventing the transformation of progesterone into androgens, possibly by inhibiting protein (enzyme) synthesis. PRL and FSH both contribute to an effect on the plasma membrane of granulosa cells, inducing the proliferation of LH receptors.

Ovulation

Ovulation—rupture of the follicular wall at the site of the stigma—is caused by enzymatic proteolysis. The LH surge stimulates follicular cells to produce prostaglandins $F_{2\alpha}$ and E_2 ($PGF_{2\alpha}$; PGE_2). $PGF_{2\alpha}$ induces the release of *collagenase enzymes* from lysosomes in the epithelial and theca cells lining each follicle. The proteolytic digestion products provoke an inflammatory reaction, with leukocytic infiltration and production of PGE_2 and histamine, which increases the local blood supply. Also, the FSH surge stimulates granulosa cells to liberate another proteolytic enzyme, *plasminogen activator,* which contributes to weakening of the follicular wall, to rupture of the follicle, and to release of the oocyte.

In most spontaneous ovulators, an interval of about 24 to 36 hours elapses between the end of the LH surge and ovulation. However, in bitches, ovulation happens a few days after the LH surge, whereas in mares, it often coincides with the peak of the prolonged LH surge. In cows, ovulation coincides with the beginning of a wave of anovulatory follicles, termed the first wave. These follicles gradually develop without ever reaching maturity and produce a postovulatory rise in estradiol that is of lesser amplitude than the preovulatory one. A second wave of folliculogenesis starts at about the regression time of the first wave. One of these second-wave follicles is destined to grow, reach maturity, and rupture (ovulation) at the next estrous cycle.

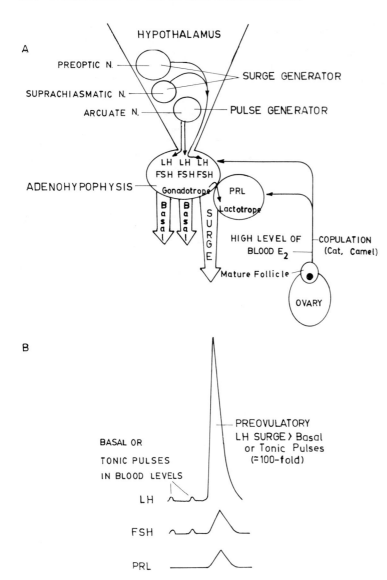

Figure 53–5 **A**, Near the end of folliculogenesis, when the follicle is mature and the estradiol level is high (in spontaneous ovulators) or when copulation occurs (in reflex or induced ovulators), a massive adenohypophysial secretion of LH, FSH, and PRL is induced. **B**, The tonic (basal, intermittent, pulsatile) secretions of LH and FSH recur at about 90 minutes, but the massive surge happens only before ovulation.

In reflex or induced ovulators (e.g., camels, cats, ferrets, minks, rabbits, short-tailed tree shrews, 13-lined ground squirrels, and field voles), mating is the stimulus that initiates the surges of LH and FSH that occur after about 24 to 36 hours. The subsequent reflex or induced ovulation requires an additional 24 to 36 hours—that is, it happens more than 2 days after copulation.

Beside these broad divisions of mammals into spontaneous and reflex ovulators, other classifications exist on the basis of whether the species are seasonal breeders and whether they have estrous or menstrual cycles. Seasonal breeding is determined mainly by day length in the northern or southern hemisphere. The Basenji bitch, deer, goat, and sheep are short-day breeders, that is, their breeding season occurs in the autumn. Cats, hamsters, horses, voles, and wallabies are long-day breeders—their breeding season occurs in the spring and summer.

Multisynaptic pathways, which link the neocortex of the brain with the hypothalamus, appear to mediate the potent effects of visual and auditory stimuli on ovulation.

In addition, light affects ovulation by two other pathways. First, by a direct connection of the retina with the suprachiasmatic nuclei. Second, by another multisynaptic route involving the retina, the suprachiasmatic nuclei, the superior cervical ganglia, and the pineal gland. This retinal–superior cervical ganglion–pineal pathway is important in species such as the deer, goat, hamster, horse, sheep, vole, and wallaby.

Estrous and Menstrual Cycles

The term *estrous* cycle refers to the cyclical occurrence of physical and endocrine events associated with folliculogenesis, ovulation, luteinization, and luteolysis in adult female animals. It should not be confused with the term *estrus,* which refers to a period of increased female sexual receptivity accompanied by greater physical and behavioral activities, and spontaneous or reflex ovulation. Some females (bitches, cows, elephants, red deer hind, sows) secrete pheromones that are shed in their urine to signal estrus and to make them sexually appealing to the male. By using their vomeronasal-olfactory organ, especially when exhibiting the lip-curl response ("flehmen"), male (and female) can detect and savor microosmolal levels of these estrogen-dependent sexual pheromones (e.g., methyl-*p*-hydroxybenzoate in bitches, dimethyl sulfide in the hamster). In some species, termed *polyestrous,* nonbred females have estrous cycles that recur periodically regardless of the season, for example, cows, elephants, guinea pigs, mice, nonhuman primates (except rhesus monkey), rabbits, rats, red kangaroos, sows. Seasonal breeders may be *monoestrous,* that is, they have a single estrous cycle (e.g., bitches), but most species are polyestrous, experiencing several estrous cycles during the season if they are not bred. It is worth mentioning that all induced ovulators are seasonally polyestrous species.

The term *menstrual* cycle refers to the shedding of the uterine endometrium and the concomitant bleeding that occurs at about monthly intervals in primates (human and nonhuman). Women do not show any obvious estrus, but many nonhuman primates show a period of estrus, and seasonal changes in reproductive behavior. During the estrous cycle, some species experience a loss of blood without any desquamation of endometrium. This diapedesis of erythrocytes, which has no relation to menstruation (a pseudomenstruation) occurs during proestrus in bitches and during metestrus in cows.

Postovulatory Control of Secretion

The postovulatory secretion of steroids by the ovary is marked by two phases: luteinization and luteolysis. The first phase, *luteinization,* takes place in the granulosa cells in response to the LH-receptor complex. It is the result of postovulatory binding of LH to plasma membrane receptors, which are acquired by the granulosa cells during late folliculogenesis. The LH-receptor complex induces modifications in the morphology and the function of the granulosa cells remaining in the ruptured follicle and converts them into a distinctive structure, the corpus luteum (CL). The CL then develops into a transient organ that enjoys the richest blood flow in the body.

The second phase, *luteolysis,* terminates the life span of the CL. Within the ovary, somewhat like the follicle, the corpus luteum is a dynamic and transient organ, whose duration can be extended by pregnancy. In most species, the CL regresses (i.e., undergoes necrosis or luteolysis) at the end of the estrous cycle. In marsupials (kangaroo, wallaby) and in the dog, the life spans of the corpora lutea in nonpregnant and pregnant females are similar. In species in which ovulation is induced (cat, ferret, hamster, mouse, rabbit, rat), copulation without fertilization prolongs the life span of the CL of the nonpregnant female. Since the life span of the CL in such an animal may be almost identical to that of the pregnant animal, such a nonpregnant animal is said to be in *pseudopregnancy.*

Luteinization

During the initial part of the process of luteinization, usually termed *metestrus,* the CL has a hemorrhagic appearance (*corpus hemorrhagicum.*) Within a few days, the CL becomes a firmer mass protruding above the surface of the ovary (except in mares), and the female enters the *diestrous* portion of the estrous cycle. In most species, as diestrus progresses, the color of the CL changes gradually from a reddish color to a liver-like, yellow, or pale-cream color (*corpus albicans.*) In cows and mares, the CL remains dark because of a lipochrome (yellow) pigment, lutein.

The luteinization phase of the estrous cycle is highlighted by a greater ovarian secretion of progesterone (Fig. 53–6) and by a reduction (by about 75 percent) in the number of LH pulses issued by the gonadotropes. The accumulation of progesterone is associated with a depression of its conversion into androgens and an inhibition of aromatization of androgens into estrogens.

> In the diestrus of cows and of ewes, a new generation of follicles is signaled by massive production of estradiol. A single peak coincides with this growth of anovulatory follicles in cows, whereas several peaks accompany these anovulatory follicles in ewes.

In ewes, mice, and rats, progesterone synthesis is also increased by PRL, whereas this effect is brought about by a LH-associated mechanism in bitches, cows, mares, and sows. This higher level of circulating progesterone stimulates a hypothalamic network of opioid peptide neurons, which, in turn, inhibit neighboring GnRH-synthesizing neurons. Thus, both the frequency of the intermittent GnRH secretion and the number of LH pulses are reduced by the higher concentration of progesterone.

Luteolysis

Except in cats, dogs, and primates, the uterus initiates the final postovulatory phase of the estrous cycle, luteolysis, which calls for regression of the CL. In the nongravid uterus, locally produced $PGF_{2\alpha}$ passes into the uterine vein, which is encircled by branches of the ovarian artery, and reaches the CL by a countercurrent exchange between the uterine vein and ovarian artery. $PGF_{2\alpha}$ brings about the demise of the CL through several actions. First, $PGF_{2\alpha}$ inhibits the production of progesterone, by interfering with the ability of LH to activate the adenylate cyclase enzyme. Second, it has a vasoconstrictive action on the rich microvasculature of the CL, which then is no longer the transient organ endowed with the best blood supply of the body. Third, in the CL, $PGF_{2\alpha}$ can stimulate the production of oxytocin, which also promotes luteolysis.

By lowering the level of progesterone in the blood, luteolysis breaks the inhibition of the opioidergic neurons on the GnRH-producing neurons and allows more frequent delivery of GnRH to the adenohypophysis. In turn, the LH pulses return to a more frequent rate and stimulate the initiation of a new estrous cycle (i.e., folliculogenesis of a new set of primordial follicles). This is the occurrence in most animals, but in some species (dog, fox), it marks the entrance into a period of anestrus.

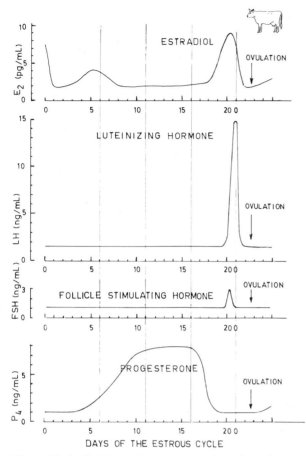

Figure 53-6 Peripheral plasma concentrations of gonadotropin (LH and FSH) and of steroid (estradiol, progesterone) hormones in the estrous cycle of the cow. The tonic levels of the gonadotropins are nearly identical except at the moment of the preovulatory surge, when the LH concentration may be six times higher. The progesterone level (ng/mL) is almost 1,000 times higher than that of the estradiol (pg/mL). The rise in estradiol follows the demise of the corpus luteum and precedes ovulation.

Metabolism

All free (i.e., active) ovarian steroids in the plasma are rapidly catabolized, mostly in the liver. By conjugation with glucuronic acid and sulfates, these steroids become water-soluble and are excreted in bile and urine. The half-life of progesterone, androgens, and estrogens is relatively short, about 10 to 30 minutes.

Biological Action

Bioactive, non–protein-bound, or free ovarian lipid-soluble steroids enter target cells by diffusion. The amount of intracellular ovarian steroids in a given tissue is determined by the plasma concentration of free steroids, since steroids bound to low-affinity (albumin) and high-affinity (beta-globulins) proteins are not available.

Only cells with specific intracellular (intranuclear, on chromatin) steroid-receptor proteins have their activity affected by ovarian steroids. Many synthetic steroid analogues that do not bind to plasma proteins also exert potent biological effects by interacting with the specific intranuclear receptors. The original two-step model of steroid action—that is, the binding of the steroid to cytoplasmic receptor proteins and the transfer of the steroid-receptor complex to the nucleus—has been challenged. The current concept is that receptor-proteins are concentrated in the cell nucleus (Fig. 53–7). The presence of receptors in the cytosol is believed to be an artifact produced during the process of experimental lysis of the target cells.

Tissues or organs made of cells with few or without these intranuclear receptor proteins show little or no response to free ovarian steroids. In their target cells, steroid hormones elicit specific cell responses by inducing the expression of genes that code for enzymes and for other regulatory proteins. These proteins determine the specific metabolic and the secretory activities of the target cells. The ovarian steroid hormones are involved mostly in the regulation of gene expression and growth in reproductive tissues.

Progesterone

The specific *progesterone* receptors present in female tissues such as the oviduct, uterus, vagina, mammary gland, and adenohypophysis are markedly increased by estradiol. The administration of progesterone decreases the number of receptor proteins available (down-regulation). Estradiol and progesterone thus have opposing effects on the ovarian steroid-receptor system. Progesterone receptors can also be occupied by a synthetic derivative of the progestin nor-

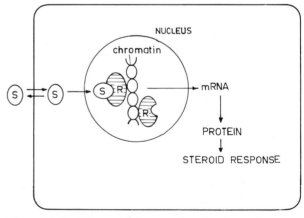

Figure 53-7 Diagram of the general model of steroid hormone action. The free steroid (S) in the blood circulation diffuses across both the plasma membrane and the nuclear membrane of the target cell. The steroid hormone binds to the intranuclear receptor (R) attached to chromatin, and this steroid hormone–receptor protein complex induces gene activation. The resulting mRNA is then transferred to the cytosol, where it directs protein syntheses that are specific for the response of the steroid hormone.

ethindrone, RU 486, that functions as a progesterone antagonist. In addition to its antiprogesterone effect, RU 486 is also an antiglucocorticoid because of its high affinity for glucocorticoid receptors.

The action of progesterone is limited mostly to the reproductive organs and the mammary tissue. Progesterone regulates the egg movement through the oviduct and particularly prepares the uterus to receive the blastocyst by inducing the development of complicated gland structures in the proliferating endometrium.

Progesterone also contributes to the expression of estrus in cows and ewes. In ewes, seasonal breeders, the first estrous cycle of the mating season is usually without manifestation of estrus (silent estrus, silent heat, or silent ovulation). In cows, this also occurs frequently at the first estrus following parturition. In these species, estrogens are unable to cause expression of sexual receptivity in the absence of a previous progesterone priming. The luteal phase of the first estrous cycle provides the progesterone priming required for the proper manifestation of estrus during the second estrous.

During pregnancy, progesterone causes relaxation of the smooth muscles, reduces the excitability of the myometrium, and generates the secretory system of mammary glands. It is also involved in immunosuppressive processes that prevent the "host" organism from rejecting the developing embryo.

Estrogens

The number of specific *estrogen* receptors in the female reproductive organs (ovary, corpus luteum, uterus, vagina) and mammary glands is increased by estradiol. Other estrogen receptors in the hypothalamus, adenohypophysis, and brain (amygdala, cortex, preoptic area, septum) also contribute to significant bioactivities. Antiestrogens such as clomiphene, nafoxidine, and tamoxifen (derivatives of triphenylethylene) reduce the specific uptake of estrogens.

In contrast with progesterone, estrogens display a multiplicity of systemic effects. Estrogens exhibit genital and extragenital biological effects. Associated with cell growth and hyperplasia, the genital actions of estrogens include the development of the vagina, proliferation of vaginal mucosa, development of the cervix and oviducts, ovarian growth, sexual development and receptivity, and proliferation of mammary tissue. The extragenital effects of estrogens encompass the development and maintenance of secondary sex characteristics, as well as the development and maturation of bone. Progesterone also stimulates protein synthesis in hepatic cells (angiotensinogen, steroid-binding globulin) and in target cells of progesterone and of estrogens (steroid intranuclear receptors). Mineral metabolism is also influenced by estrogens (e.g., retention of phosphorus and of sodium, causing water accumulation in tissues, and excretion of potassium).

The bioactive ovarian androgens that are not aromatized into estrogens play some role in stimulating sexual libido in female animals.

OVARIAN NONSTEROID HORMONES

In addition to steroid hormones, the ovary produces several hormones of lipid (eicosanoids) and of peptidic (inhibin, oxytocin, and relaxin) nature.

In the preovulatory follicle, the granulosa cells produce large amounts of *eicosanoids:* PGE_2 and $PGF_{2\alpha}$. These prostaglandins have paracrine (local) actions and participate in inducing the rupture of the mature follicle (i.e., the process of ovulation). In primates, in which the uterus does not participate in luteolysis, prostaglandins seem to be produced within the corpus luteum and contribute to luteal regression.

The follicular fluid, which bathes the granulosa cells, contains large amounts of a substance analogous to *inhibin,* the protein synthesized by Sertoli's cells of the testes. In the cycling female, inhibin may be an inhibitor of FSH secretion, especially after the preovulatory surge, when estrogens rapidly return to basal levels.

During the postovulatory phase of the estrous cycle of ewes, the large luteal cells of the CL secrete $PGF_{2\alpha}$, which has an autocrine action that increases the release of *oxytocin* and neurophysin I. In cows, some antidiuretic hormone (ADH), or vasopressin, and neurophysin II are also produced at a much lower rate than that of oxytocin; the ratio of oxytocin to vasopressin is about 2,000 to 1. Locally, oxytocin binds the receptors and inhibits the secretion of progesterone. Oxytocin thus participates in reducing the frequency of the LH pulses during the postovulatory phase of the estrous cycle and in regulating the life span of the CL by promoting luteolysis. In addition, oxytocin contributes to sexual receptivity and to ovum transport in the oviduct.

Relaxin, a 6,000-dalton peptide (48 amino acids) that shows homologies with insulin-like growth factors, is produced by porcine theca interstitial cells of the corpus luteum. In nonpregnant females, the search for a physiological role of relaxin has not been productive. Preliminary studies suggest a role of relaxin in regulating folliculogenesis during the estrous cycle.

Some reports suggest that the ovary may be the source of a number of other proteins, such as beta-endorphin, follicular regulatory protein, oocyte maturation inhibitor, and plasminogen activator. The granulosa and secondary interstitial cells of the corpus luteum appear to produce *beta-endorphin* and other proopiomelanocortin-derived peptides, which are without known functions but are presumed to exert a paracrine role. The granulosa cell is at the origin of a putative peptide, *follicular regulatory protein,* that suppresses the follicular response to gonadotropin. This substance may be an inter- or intra-ovarian regulator of folliculogenesis. The membrana granulosa cells, which interact with the cumulus—corona radiata—oocyte complex, secrete the *oocyte maturation inhibitor.* This protein arrests the oocyte in the dictyate stage, or dictyotene (i.e., the resting phase, with considerable oocyte growth), of the first meiotic division, and suppresses the resumption of meiotic maturation. The granulosa cell of the preovulatory follicle produces the *plas-*

minogen factor. Under its influence, follicular fluid plasminogen is converted to plasmin, an active proteinase that weakens the follicular wall at the stigma and helps the follicle to rupture (ovulation).

REFERENCES

Barbieri RL, Makris A, Ryan KJ. Effects of insulin on steroidogenesis in cultured porcine ovarian theca. Fertil Steril 1983;40:237.

Bronson RA, Bryant G, Balk MW, Emanuele N. Intrafollicular pressure within preovulatory follicles of the pig. Fertil Steril 1979;31:205.

Bryant-Greenwood GD. Relaxin as a new hormone. Endocr Rev 1982;3:62.

Clarke IJ, Cummins JT. The temporal relationship between gonadotropin-releasing hormone (GnRH) and luteinizing hormone (LH) secretion in ovariectomized ewes. Endocrinology 1982;111:1737.

Conn PM. The molecular basis of gonadotropin-releasing hormone action. Endocr Rev 1986;7:3.

Dejong FH, Sharpe RM. Evidence for an inhibin-like activity in bovine follicular fluid. Nature 1976;263:71.

Eddy EM, Clark JM, Gong D, Fenderson BA. Origin and migration of primordial cells in mammals. Gamete Res 1981;4:333.

Erickson GF, Magoffin D, Dyer CA, Hofeditz C. The ovarian androgen-producing cells: a review of structure/function relationships. Endocr Rev 1985;6:371.

Evans G, Wathes DC, King GJ, et al. Changes in relaxin production by the theca during the preovulatory period of the pig. J Reprod Fertil 1983;69:697.

Flint APF, Sheldrick EL. Ovarian secretion of oxytocin is stimulated by prostaglandin. Nature 1982;297:587.

Flint APF, Sheldrick EL. Evidence for a systemic role for ovarian oxytocin in luteal regression in sheep. J Reprod Fertil 1983;67:215.

Hillier SG. Regulation of follicular oestrogen biosynthesis: a survey of current concepts. J Endocrinol 1981;89:30.

Kawakami M, Kubo K, Yemura T, et al. Involvement of ovarian innervation in steroid secretion. Endocrinology 1981;109:136.

Lim AT, Lolait S, Barlow JW, et al. Immunoreactive beta-endorphin in sheep ovary. Nature 1983;303:709.

Moor RM. Role of steroids in the maturation of ovine oocytes. Ann Biol Anim Biochem Biophys 1978;18:477.

Moore LG, Choy VJ, Elliot RL, Watkins WB. Evidence for the pulsatile release of $PGF_{2\alpha}$ inducing the release of oxytocin during luteolysis in the ewe. J Reprod Fertil 1986;76:159.

Olson PN, Husted PW, Allen TA, Nett TM. Reproductive endocrinology and physiology of the bitch and queen. Vet Clin North Am (Small Anim Pract) 1984;14:927.

Richards JS. Maturation of ovarian follicles: actions and interaction of pituitary and ovarian hormones on follicular cell differentiation. Physiol Rev 1980;60:51.

Strauss JF, Schuler LA, Rosenblum MF, Tanaka T. Cholesterol metabolism in ovarian tissue. Adv Lipid Res 1981;18:99.

Turnbull KE, Braden AWH, Mattner PE. The pattern of follicular growth and atresia in the ovine ovary. Aust J Biol Sci 1977;30:229.

Walters DL, Schallenberger E. Pulsatile secretion of gonadotropins, ovarian steroids and ovarian oxytocin during the periovulatory phase of the oestrous cycle in the cow. J Reprod Fertil 1984;71:503.

Wathes DC. Possible actions of gonadal oxytocin and vasopressin. J Reprod Fertil 1984;71:315.

Wathes DC, Swann RW, Pickering BT. Variations in oxytocin, vasopressin and neurophysin concentrations in the bovine ovary during the estrous cycle and pregnancy. J Reprod Fertil 1984;71:551.

Wildt DE, Chan SYM, Seager SWJ, Chakraborty PK. Ovarian activity, circulating hormones, and sexual behavior in the cat. I. Relationships during the coitus-induced luteal phase and the estrus period without mating. Biol Reprod 1981;25:15.

Wildt DE, Seager SWJ, Chakraborty PK. Behavioural, ovarian and endocrine relationships in the pubertal bitch. J Anim Sci 1981;53:182.

CHAPTER 54

REPRODUCTIVE LIFE AND CYCLES IN ANIMALS

Reproductive life, characterized in general by gametogenesis and by a desire for sexual activity (libido), becomes possible at *puberty* and continues for most of the life span of the animals until senescence. Most male animals have the capacity for a continuous reproductive life throughout the year, whereas the sexual activity of females is governed by estrous cycles that occur nonseasonally (year-round) or seasonally (i.e., during a limited part of the year). In seasonally breeding species, such as caprine and ovine, males and females undergo periodic changes analogous to puberty, at the start, and to senescence, at the end of the season (Fig. 54–1). Some breeds of sheep and goats have a longer breeding season. The ewes of the Dorset, Finnish-Landrace (Finn), Moroccan D'Man, and some Merino strains will breed out of season.

A new breed, the Polypay, will breed as lambs younger than 8 months of age and during the period when other breeds are anestrous. The Polypay, developed in Idaho at the Dubois Station, has genes from the Dorset, Finn, Rambouillet and Targhee breeds.

PUBERTY

Puberty arrives before growth is completed, when animals have reached a critical somatic development (mass or body weight) for each species or for each breed. Females reach this threshold body mass sooner than their male counterparts and show puberty at a younger age, that is, at the lower end of the age range (Table 54–1). It should be noted that involution of the thymus starts with the onset of puberty.

Breed size, quality and quantity of feeding, and season of birth contribute to hastening or to delaying the onset of puberty. Factors that delay the appearance of puberty include large body size in some breeds (e.g., Great Dane dog, beef cattle), malnutrition, and birth at the end of the breeding season. In seasonal breeders (cat, goat, horse, sheep), birth near the beginning of the coming breeding season prevents the onset of puberty inside that season. These animals mature sexually at the following breeding season, and the beginning of their reproductive life occurs more than 6 months later.

Until the young male or female animal reaches puberty, it does not show cyclical interest in sexual activity. Puberty signals the onset of periodic hypothalamo-adenohypophysio-gonadal hormonal processes that cause an interest in sexual activity. These hormonal changes, which are continuous in the male but intermittent in the female, are maintained for the rest of the animal's postpuberal reproductive life. In females, puberty indicates that the progressively developing hypothalamic gonadostat has reached an adequate and sufficiently mature state (i.e., that it is no longer very sensitive to the inhibitory feedback of ovarian estrogens). At puberty, the system for secreting gonadotropins has a decreased sensitivity and allows gonadotropin secretion to increase and to generate the requisite cyclical endocrine pulses and surges of gonadotropin-releasing hormone (GnRH), luteinizing hormone (LH), follicle-stimulating hormone (FSH), and prolactin (PRL). As in males, triggering of the female pubertal hypothalamic activity implicates input from the amygdala, the olfactory bulb, and the pineal gland.

In nonbred females, emergence into postpuberal life is manifested by the so-called *estrous cycles,* during which spontaneous ovulations recur periodically throughout the year in polyestrous species (Fig. 54–2).

In several nonmated seasonal species, a single (*monoestrous, monocyclic*) or periodic (*polyestrous, polycyclic*) spontaneous ovulation occurs during the breeding season (Fig. 54–3). Of course, nonmated seasonal polyestrous species that are reflex or induced ovulators show only a succession of reproductive cycles without ovulation. In seasonal breeders, postpuberal females reaching the end of the breeding period without mating enter into a period of reproductive rest (anestrus), which is a sort of temporary "senescence" between breeding seasons.

In the young male, puberty is signaled by the production and the ejaculation of fertile spermatozoa and also by the nascence of sexual desire. The secretory function of accessory reproductive glands appears earlier than spermatogenesis. Enlargement of the testes marks an important sign of puberty, since it represents an increase in the volume of the seminiferous tubules. The functioning of the seminiferous tubules (i.e., *spermatogenesis*) follows a gradual maturation of the hypothalamic gonadostat, which leads eventually only to the pulsatile (basal) synthesis of GnRH, LH, FSH, and testosterone. Unlike the female, the male does not produce a cyclical massive surge of GnRH, LH, and FSH. In species in which females are continuously polyestrous, the males also have a continuous potential for reproductive activity. In species in which breeding is seasonal, some males (e.g., rams and billy goats) also experience a temporary lack of sexual desire (libido), or temporary senescence, akin to a period of "male anestrus." However, male cats, dogs, and horses remain fertile throughout the year although their testosterone output is reduced.

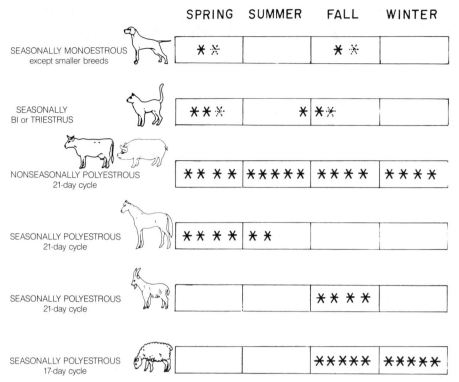

Figure 54–1 The reproductive life of nonmated female animals living under natural-light conditions. The estrous cycles recur throughout the year in females of nonseasonally polyestrous species (e.g., cow, sow), or seasonally in bitches, ewes, mares, and queens. Seasonal breeders may have only a single or several repeated estrous cycles during a part of the year. The reproductive life of bitches and queens perks up in spring and fall, when the bitch exhibits a single (exceptionally two) and the queen two (exceptionally three) estrous cycles. With artificial lighting, dogs and cats may show sexual activity throughout the year. In mares and ewes, the occurrence of the estrous cycles is influenced by the duration of daylight. In mares, the progressively longer illumination of spring induces several estrous cycles that cease in midsummer but that may be extended until the end of fall under artificial lighting. In contrast, ewes are stimulated to reproduction by the shorter days of fall and winter. This can be altered by manipulation of the lighting cycle.

TABLE 54–1 Approximate Age (Months) at Which Puberty Occurs in Large and Small Animals

Buffalo		Goat	4–8
river	15–18	Guinea pig	4
swamp	21–24	Hamster	2
Cat	6–15	Horse	12–20
Chinchilla	4	Mink	10–12
Cow	6–18	Mouse	2
Dog		Pig	5–10
small	4–7	Rabbit	6
large	6–12	Rat	2–3
Ferret	6	Sheep	6–12
Gerbil	2		

SPERMATOGENESIS

Spermatogenesis, the testicular production of spermatozoa, occurs in the seminiferous tubules, which contain the Sertoli's cells, or "nurse cells," and two types of the germ

PHASES AND DURATION OF

THE ESTROUS CYCLE

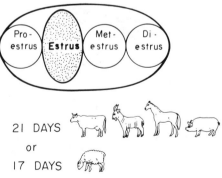

Figure 54–2 The phases (proestrus, estrus, metestrus, and diestrus) of the estrous cycle reappear at intervals of 17 of 21 days in seasonally or nonseasonally polyestrous females that are unmated. The cycles reappear every 17 days in the ewe, whereas the other species experience this event about every 21 days.

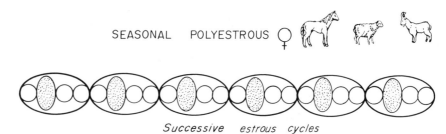

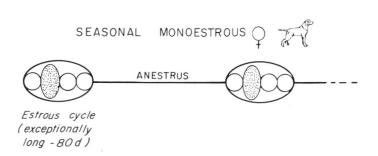

Figure 54–3 In seasonal breeding species, a limited succession of estrous cycles occurs in unmated polyestrous females (ewes, goats, mares). In the seasonally monoestrous bitch, the duration of the single estrous cycle is exceptionally long (about 80 days). This can be explained by the combination of longer proestrous and estrous phases (about 9 days each), with a metestrous phase of average duration and a diestrous phase that continues for as many days as pregnancy (about 60 days).

cells (spermatogonia A and B). Tight junctions between adjacent Sertoli's cells create the *basal compartment*, which holds the spermatogonia, and the *adluminal compartment*, which carries the spermatocytes, spermatids, and spermatozoa.

During postpuberal life, *spermatogonia of the A, or reserve, type* divide and remain in the basal compartment. Those of the *B type* move from the basal compartment to the adluminal compartment, where they remain in intimate association with the Sertoli's cells, augment their number by *mitotic* division, and are termed *primary spermatocytes*. By a *first meiotic* division, the primary spermatocytes form *secondary spermatocytes,* which hold half (haploid) the chromosomal number contained in the original germ cells (diploid). The secondary spermatocyte then undergoes a *second meiotic division* to form the *spermatid,* that is, a small rounded cell that is destined to be gradually transformed into a *spermatozoon* (Fig. 54–4). The fully differentiated, but immature and nonmotile, testicular spermatozoa leave the Sertoli's cells to enter the lumen of the seminiferous tubule.

During their slow transit through the epididymis, the spermatozoa mature (*epididymal maturation*) by changes (addition, masking, removal) in their entire plasma membrane glycoproteins and lipids. In the epididymis, they also acquire motility and an ability to adhere to the zonae pellucidae of the ova. The entire process of spermatogenesis takes about 30 days in the boar, about 50 days in the ram, and about 60 days in the bull, dog, and stallion.

At ejaculation, the *mature* (fully mobile) spermatozoa leave the epididymis and become mixed with the secretions of the accessory males glands (e.g., seminal vesicle, prostate). In many mammals, the freshly ejaculated spermatozoa are *not capable of fertilization* until they have undergone some changes, the capacitation and the acrosome reaction, which usually occur in the female reproductive tract but can be induced in vitro.

Capacitation

The collective term of "*capacitation*" regroups a series of events that occur in spermatozoa and precede the physiological acrosome reaction. These changes include enhanced adenylate cyclase activity related to an intracellular influx of Ca^{++}, higher glycolytic activity and oxygen consumption, as well as increased intracellular Na^+ concentration. During capacitation, sperm surface antigens and glycoproteins are either removed (or masked) or added, and membrane phospholipid composition is changed mostly by lateral migration of plasma membrane lipids and cholesterol.

Physiological, or True Acrosome, Reaction

The acrosome, found in the head of the spermatozoa, is a specialized cap-like lysosome (huge in guinea pigs, small in bulls and rams) that contains a number of acid hydrolases. The plasma membrane of the sperm cell joins and then covers the outer acrosomal membrane to form a fenestrated complex. The thin junction line of both membranes is rich in calcium-binding sites. A massive influx of Ca^{++} triggers the physiological, or true acrosome, reaction, causing rapid disruption of the acrosome and release of its hydrolytic enzymes. This catalyzes the digestion of the materials surrounding the ovum (cumulus and corona cells) and of the thick glycoprotein coat (zona pellucida) of the ovum. After these alterations of the protective layers, a sperm cell is able to fuse with the plasma membrane and to penetrate into the ovum to achieve fertilization. A false acrosome reaction is the

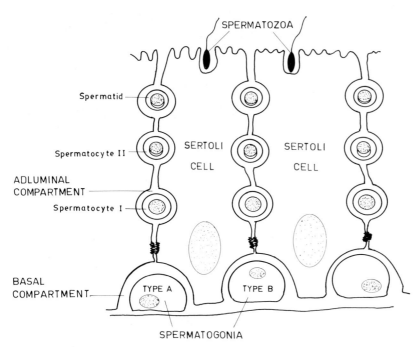

Figure 54–4 Spermatogenesis, the production of spermatozoa, takes place in the seminiferous tubules, in which are found the Sertoli's cells, or "nurse cells," and two kinds of germ cells (spermatogonia A and B). Tight junctions between adjacent Sertoli's cells form the basal compartment, which contains the spermatogonia, and the adluminal compartment, which carries the spermatocytes, spermatids, and spermatozoa. During the postpuberal life, spermatogonia of the the A, or reserve, type divide and remain in the basal compartment. Those of the B type move from the basal compartment to the adluminal compartment, where they stay in intimate association with Sertoli's cells, increase in number through mitotic division, and are called primary spermatocytes. By a first meiotic division, the primary spermatocytes form secondary spermatocytes, which contain half (haploid) the number of chromosomes contained in the original germ cells (diploid). The secondary spermatocyte then undergoes a second meiotic division, forming the spermatid (i.e., a small, rounded cell destined to be gradually transformed into a spermatozoon). The fully differentiated spermatozoa leave the Sertoli's cells, enter the lumen of the seminiferous tubule, and mature and acquire motility during passage through the epididymis.

hydrolytic autodigestion of the acrosome of weakened or dead spermatozoa.

ESTROUS CYCLES

In nonpregnant postpuberal females, estrous cycles or periodic phases in the reproductive life recur to make them sexually receptive to males. The chronological phases of a complete estrous cycle are proestrus, estrus, metestrus, and diestrus (Fig. 54–5).

Estrus, the most specific phase of the estrous cycle, is displayed by females in the presence of a mature male. Its characteristic features vary between animals species. In general terms, it may include arching of the back or raising of the hindquarters, bellowing, frequent urination, immobility, homosexual behavior of females mounting or permitting themselves to be mounted, hyperactivity, and pricking of the ears. In an animal, these overt behavioral signs can be recognized by an informed observer and can be determined in relation to time.

It is customary to consider the first day of estrus as "day 0," so that ovulation usually occurs on "day 1" in cows, ewes, and sows (see Fig. 54–5). The interval between successive estrous cycles is occupied by the remainder of estrus and the other phases: metestrus, diestrus, and proestrus.

Proestrus

The follicular part of the estrous cycle corresponds to the proestrus phase. It lasts about 1 to 2 days in the queen (female cat), about 2 days in the ewe and sow, about 3 to 4 days in the cow and mare, and much longer (about 9 days) in the bitch (Table 54–2).

In proestrus, the hypothalamo-adenohypophysial pulses of GnRH, LH, and FSH recur at their peak frequency and lowest amplitude. At the culmination of folliculogenesis, the follicle and the ovary reach their maximum size,

NONGRAVID   CYCLING   POLYESTROUS   ♀

Figure 54–5 Diagram of the chronological events in two successive estrous cycles in a nonpregnant female. Each estrous cycle comprises four phases: proestrus, estrus, metestrus, and diestrus. Since detection of the estrus is used as a time-marker of the estrous cycle, the onset of estrus is considered to occur at "day 0," and the interval before the return or coming of the next "day 0" includes metestrus, diestrus, and also proestrus of the next cycle if the animal is unmated. The interval between estrous cycles may be as short as 17 days in ewes, but it is usually about 21 days in most domesticated and female animals (cow, goat, mare, sow).

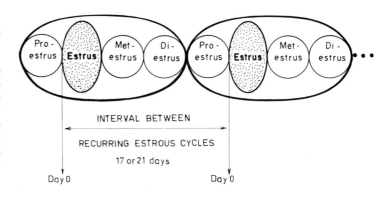

and the female shows increased sexual excitement under the influence of estrogens. The blood flow in the reproductive tract increases, causing a thickening edema and secretion by the epithelium of the oviduct, uterus, cervix, and vagina.

In bitches, the permanent longitudinal folds (plicae) in the caudal vagina become thickened and rounded; in addition, erythrocytes and a few desquamated epithelial cells are present in vaginal smears taken during proestrous. Tumefaction of the vulva, excretion of an abundant production of clear mucus laden with erythrocytes resulting from diapedesis, and frequent urination characterize the last part of proestrus in bitches. In addition, the vaginal epithelium of the bitch in proestrus excretes a pheromone (methylparahydroxybenzoate), which has an odor that attracts males even if the bitch does not permit mating.

Estrus

The most obvious phase of the estrous cycle, estrus, is marked by the female's acceptance of the male, or mating behavior. In species that are spontaneous ovulators, its duration varies considerably: less than 24 hours in buffalo (river, swamp); from 24 to 36 hours in cows, ewes, and goats; from

1 to 3 days in sows; about 6 days in mares; and about 9 days in bitches. In species that are reflex ovulators, it ranges from 1 to 7 days in camels (one-humped, or dromedaries, and two-humped, or Bactrians) and from 4 to 10 days in queens.

The ovary is softened by one or several voluminous follicles. The oviduct is hypertrophic, hyperactive, and hypersecretory. The uterus is increased in size, presents a thickened and hypertonic myometrium, and secretes profuse amounts of a viscous mucus that runs through the relaxed cervix. The vagina is dilated and hyperemic and is coated with an abundant fluid mucus that may hang as a string from the swollen, moistened, and warm ("coming into heat") vulva. Vaginal smears from a bitch in estrus show a predominance of cornified or keratinized (pyknotic, or shrunk nucleus) epithelial cells and much fewer erythrocytes than during the proestrus phase.

In behavioral terms, estrus is characterized by nervousness and the desire of females to allow coitus. Small animals in estrus (*bitches, queens*) respond to lumbar pressure by standing still, arching the back slightly ("lordosis reflex"), deflecting the tail ("flagging"), and rotating the pelvis to facilitate intromission (Fig. 54–6). The queen's estrus is also marked by increased vocalization ("calling"), rolling, rubbing against inanimate objects, and repetitive pawing. The queen assumes the mating stance when she is approached by a tom cat and stands still during neck biting and mounting.

The *sow* in estrus seeks out the male in a much quieter way than the cow, although she emits frequent estrous "grunts." At this time, blood may tint the vaginal mucus. Also, the vaginal secretion and urine contain sex pheromones that are attractive to the boar. In turn, the excited boar secretes androstenol- and androstenone-containing saliva, with an odor that induces a sow in estrus to become immobile. This standing response allows a farmer to press on her back. The standing response can also be obtained by an experienced herdman, since the same androstenol and androstenone pheromones occur in man's sweat and urine, and can be used to detect estrus in a sow that is to be artificially inseminated. The estrus of the *ewe* is difficult to detect, and the only prominent sign seems to be a fluttering of the tail.

TABLE 54–2 Range and Mean Length (in Days) of the Phases of the Estrous Cycle in Some Domestic Animals

Species	Estrous Cycle	Proestrus	Estrus	Metestrus	Diestrus
Bitch	120–390 (180)	9	4–9	2	40–60*
Camel	10–20†		1–7	2	
Cow	14–25 (21)	3–4	1–1.5	2	15
Ewe	3–35 (17)	2–3	1–1.5	2	10–12
Goat	15–21		1–1.5	2	16
Mare	10–35 (21)	3–4	2–30 (6)	2	12–13
Queen	14–28†	1–2	4–10	2	30–50*
Sow	18–24	2	1–3	2	14

*Pseudogestation.
†Nonmated.

ESTRUS   BEHAVIOR   OF   THE   CAT

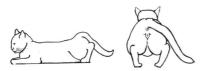

Figure 54–6 Lordosis reflex and flagging of the tail that characterize a reproductive behavior during the estrus of the queen.

The *cow* in estrus may bawl frequently, is usually restless, is without appetite, and produces much less milk. Also, she exhibits homosexual traits by attempting to mount other cows and is shown sexual attention by other cows. The vaginal mucus contains some pheromone, of yet undetermined chemical composition, that sexually stimulates bulls. In *goats,* estrus is also accompanied by increased activity and vocalization, and the tail is maintained erect with vigorous wagging.

The *mare* in estrus does not show any homosexual traits. When she is introduced to a protected "teaser" stallion, she raises her tail, urinates, and "winks" (i.e., rhythmically contracts her vulva, and exposes her clitoris).

Also termed the "period of heat," estrus begins before ovulation when folliculogenesis is nearly completed, and the estrogen level is high. The elevated concentration of estradiol exerts a positive-feedback action on the hypothalamo-adenohypophysial axis to induce a cascade of GnRH, LH, FSH, and PRL surges. The prostaglandins (E_2 and $F_{2\alpha}$) that are produced prior to ovulation, and proteolytic enzymes (plasmin), are thought to contribute to the rupture of the mature follicle. In induced ovulators, copulation soon brings the estrus to an end and causes a cascade of surges similar to the one resulting from the sustained estradiol peak.

During estrus, the LH surge precedes either spontaneous or reflex ovulation by about 30 hours. In bitches, the LH peak anticipates ovulation by about 48 hours and coincides with a rise in progesterone concentration in the peripheral blood. In all species (except the cow), spontaneous ovulation occurs during the estrous phase. The bitch ovulates near midestrus, that is, 3 to 4 days after the beginning of estrus. Ovulation is near the end of estrus in ewes, goats, mares, and sows. Contrary to other species, the cow ovulates spontaneously about 10 to 12 hours after estrus has ended (i.e., during metestrus).

Of course, induced ovulation does not occur in females that remain unmated until the end of estrus. Instead of their experiencing metestrus (followed by pregnancy) at the end of estrus, they enter a short *interestrous* phase, if the breeding season is to continue. This interestrous phase is characterized by a basal estradiol blood level, the regression of unovulated follicles, and the initiation of another wave of folliculogenesis for the following estrus, which occurs when the estradiol blood level suddenly rises. As expected, *anestrus* follows the end of the last estrus of the breeding season in unmated reflex-ovulating females.

Metestrus

Metestrus, the short (2-day) postovulatory phase of the estrous cycle, is used to designate the early luteal function. In the ruptured follicle, the *corpus hemorrhagicum* becomes organized and begins to produce progesterone, oxytocin, and inhibin, while estrogen production decreases to its minimum level. The vaginal smears contain many leukocytes with some noncornified cells.

In heifers some erythrocytes are also added. This bovine endometrial bleeding during metestrus appears to be associated with estrogen withdrawal. In buffalo and cows, ovulation occurs about 12 hours after the end of estrus (i.e., during metestrus). Accordingly, in these species the general definition of metestrus, as the early organization of the corpus luteum, is not exactly applied.

Diestrus

Diestrus constitutes the major or longest phase of the estrous cycle, when the corpus luteum secretes progesterone and oxytocin. The diestrous progesterone level is three times that of the estrous concentration in ewes, about six times in cows and mares, about ten times in bitches, about 20 times in queens, and about 24 times in sows. In cows, ewes, and sows, folliculogenesis can also occur during the luteal phase of the estrous cycle, as evidenced by estradiol peaks in the plasma of venous blood (ovarian or jugular).

In cows, ultrasonic monitoring of the ovaries reveals two waves of follicular activity during the diestrous phase of the estrous cycle. The first wave of this bimodal folliculogenesis, which is anovulatory, appears on the day of ovulation (during metestrus) and continues for about 1 week. Near the middle of diestrus, the dominant follicle of the first wave regresses as the second wave begins. The dominant follicle of the second wave becomes the ovulatory follicle at the next estrous cycle, during metestrus.

The diestrus of the unmated bitch and of the mated but unfertilized rabbit or queen is remarkable. Because it lasts almost as long as pregnancy, the canine, feline, and lagomorph (rabbit) diestrus is termed *pseudopregnancy* (false pregnancy, pseudocyesis) (Fig. 54–7).

The extensive phase of the canine diestrus ends in a phase of reproductive rest, termed *anestrus,* that lasts several months until initiation of proestrus of the next estrous cycle.

RETURN OF ESTROUS CYCLES DURING PREGNANCY AND AFTER PARTURITION

Pregnancy, which may ensue from mating or from artificial insemination, suspends the rhythm of the reproductive cycles in either nonseasonal or seasonal species. However, estrous behavior is occasionally seen during the pregnancy of cows, ewes, mares, queens, and sows, usually without ovulation. However, ovulation can occur in ewes,

SPECIAL ESTROUS CYCLES IN DOGS AND CATS

Figure 54–7 The estrous cycles in bitches and queens differ from those of large animals. In the spontaneously ovulating bitch, because diestrus is nearly as long as pregnancy, it has been designated by various terms, such as false pregnancy, pseudopregnancy, and pseudocyesis. In queens, the estrous cycle is subject to several variations associated with the presence or absence of reflex ovulation. Nonmated queens that do not ovulate have an estrous cycle limited to proestrus and estrus. Metestrus and diestrus are absent and are replaced by an interestrous phase during which the unruptured follicles regress, and a new wave of folliculogenesis begins. Queens that ovulate after copulation have a metestrous phase that is followed by either pregnancy or diestrus of almost identical duration. Pregnancy occurs if the mating is fertile, whereas diestrus (false pregnancy, pseudopregnancy, or pseudocyesis) ensues from an infertile mating.

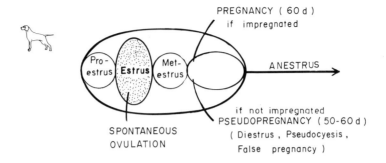

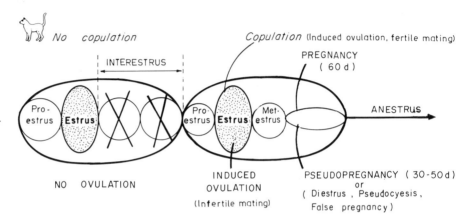

queens, and sows; if so, a fertile mating can initiate a second pregnancy that proceeds with a lag on the continuing first pregnancy. This situation, referred to as *superfetation,* leads to two parturitions separated by a notable interval.

> This concept of superfetation is not universally accepted. Another view is that it results from delayed implantation of blastocysts or embryos, which remain in diapause, that is, an arrested or latent phase of development that occurs normally in badgers, deer, and some other wild species.

In females of most species, except cows and mares, parturition is followed by a period of lactational anestrus (i.e., the estrous cycles are delayed while the female nurses its offspring). The estrous cycles reappear usually about a week after the offspring are weaned (i.e., at about 5 to 6 weeks). However, it is usual for sows to show signs of an anovulatory estrus within the 48 hours that follow parturition. Mares experience a fertile estrus, which is termed the "foal heat," during the 7 to 14 days postpartum. The preparation of this particular estrous cycle is started during the last 2 weeks of the equine pregnancy. Mares are routinely bred during this "foal heat" despite results indicating a reduced fertilization rate and a higher prevalence of abortions. About 21 days after parturition, cows present a fertile ovulation, which is not always preceded by overt estrous signs and is termed "silent heat" because it is seldom detected by herdsmen.

Ewes of most sheep breeds reproduce only during periods of short days. After lambing, because of a decrease in LH secretion, they enter into a long period of seasonal anestrus. The LH decline is associated with the increasing daylength during spring and summer. Manipulation of this problem can be accomplished in one of three ways: artificial regulation of photoperiod, administration of gonadotropins, or administration of exogenous melatonin.

Artificial Regulation of Photoperiod. Ewes are confined in light-free barns, with a regulated lighting program that changes the hours of exposure to light and darkness during each 24-hour period. Alternating every 90 days between long (light: 16 hours; dark: 8 hours) and short (light: 8 hours; dark: 16 hours) day lengths allows the ewes to have two breeding and anestrous seasons per year. Estrous behavior is observed about 6 to 10 weeks after the switch to short days. The effect is induced by the change in the hours of light rather than the absolute duration of the light period. This allows an alternative to light-proof barns via provision of supplemental lighting to confined sheep in the spring.

Administration of Gonadotropins. Follicular growth can be restarted during anestrus, with resultant ovulation. However, these ewes usually fail to exhibit behavioral estrus, perhaps because the centers in the brain have not been primed with progesterone prior to the estradiol of estrus. This can be surmounted by pretreatment with progesterone (via an intravaginal releasing device) or a synthetic progestin (via an ear implant) for 9 days. Then, either a combination of FSH and LH, or of pregnant mare serum gonadotropin ([PMSG] or equine chorionic gonadotropin [eCG]) and human chorionic gonadotropin (hCG), is used to stimulate follicle growth and maturation. Several doses are required if the FSH-LH combination is used (because of the short biological half-life, 6 hours), but one dose of PMSG (long biological half-life, 6 days) after the progestin has been withdrawn will suffice. However, antibodies to PMSG are formed, so it is not fully effective if it is repeated during the following season.

Administration of Exogenous Melatonin. Melatonin is produced by the pineal gland during the hours of darkness. If ewes are treated with melatonin during the spring and summer, the body responds in a manner equivalent to the darkness periods in the fall. It can be fed daily in late afternoon or given as an implant that lasts for 30 days. After this period, LH levels are adequate for follicular development and for ovulation with estrous behavior. This can be repeated each year.

SENESCENCE OF REPRODUCTIVE LIFE

Until the end of their lives, most females retain a reproductive capacity that wanes as their age advances. Then, the length of the interval between the estrous cycles increases, fertility (penetration of the female gamete by the spermatozoon) and fecundity (number of living offspring produced) diminish, and the incidence of stillbirths and neonatal mortality are higher. Also, the prevalence of adenohypophysial hypofunction, of insufficient milk production, and of ovarian and uterine pathological conditions is augmented. Pregnancy tends to be longer in aged females.

In older animals, the age at which this slowing of reproductive activity occurs is not definite and varies with the species. Comparatively, senescence seems to appear sooner in sows than in cows and bitches (at about the eighth year), and it occurs much later (at 10 years) in ewes.

REFERENCES

Bedford JM. Significance of the need for sperm capacitation before fertilization in eutherian mammals. Biol Reprod 1983;28:108.

Chakraborty PK, Panko WB, Fletcher WS. Serum hormone concentrations and their relationships to sexual behavior at the first and second estrous cycles of the Labrador bitch. Biol Reprod 1980;22:227.

Chang MC. The meaning of sperm capacitation. J Androl 1984;5:45.

Cline EM, Jennings LL, Sojka NJ. Analysis of the feline vaginal epithelial cycle. Feline Pract 1980;10:47.

Courot M. Transport and maturation of spermatozoa. Proc Reprod Biol 1981;8:67.

Ginther OJ, Kastelic JP, Knopf L. Composition and characteristics of follicular waves during the bovine estrous cycle. Anim Reprod Sci 1989;20:187.

Hammerstedt RH, Hay SR, Amann RP. Modification of the ram sperm membrane during epididymal transit. Biol Reprod 1982;27:745.

Hansel W, Convey EM. Physiology of estrous cycle. J Anim Sci 1983; (Suppl 2):404.

Levasseur MC. Thoughts on puberty. Initiation of the gonadotrophic function. Ann Biol Anim Biochim Biophys 1977;17:345.

Nett T. The problem of seasonality. National Sheep Reproduction Symposium. Fort Collins: Colorado State University, 1989: p. 87.

Olson PN, Husted PW, Allen TA, Nett TM. Reproductive endocrinology and physiology of the bitch and queen. Vet Clin North Am (Small Anim Pract) 1984;14:927.

Olson PN, Thrall MA, Wijkes PM, et al. Vaginal cytology. Part I. A useful tool for staging the canine estrous cycle. Compendium Continuing Educ Pract Vet 1984;6:288.

Saling PM. Development of the ability to bind zonae pellucidae during epididymal maturation. Biol Reprod 1982;26:429.

Schille VM, Stabenfeldt GH. Current concepts in reproduction of the dog and cat. Adv Vet Sci Comp Med 1980;24:211.

Tilton JE, Foxcroft GR, Ziecik AJ, et al. Time of preovulatory LH surge in the gilt and sow relative to the onset of behavioral estrus. Theriogenology 1982;18:227.

Van Haaften B, Dieleman SJ, Okkens AC, Willemse AH. Timing the mating of dogs on the basis of blood progesterone concentration. Vet Rec 1989;125:524.

Wildt DE, Chan SYW, Seager SWJ, Chakraborty PK. Ovarian activity, circulating hormones, and sexual behavior in the cat. I. Relationships during the coitus-induced luteal phase and the estrus period without mating. Biol Reprod 1981;25:15.

Wildt DE, Seager SWJ, Chakraborty PK. Effect of copulatory stimuli on incidence of ovulation and on serum luteinizing hormone in the cat. Endocrinology 1980;107:1212.

Wildt DE, Seager SWJ, Chakraborty PK. Behavioral, ovarian and endocrine relationships in the pubertal bitch. J Anim Sci 1981;53:182.

CHAPTER 55

COPULATION AND FERTILIZATION

Among animal species, the reproductive behavior of male and female differs greatly. During estrus, which occurs prior to ovulation, the sexually receptive female usually permits mating. Precoital auditory, olfactory, tactile, and visual cues concur to coordinate the critical, dynamic conjunction of the two sexes.

During coitus, the erect and elongated penis is introduced into the mucus-lubricated peripheral organs (vulva and vagina) of the female genital tract, and copulation culminates with ejaculation. Spermatozoa are deposited into the vagina in some animals (cows, ewes, goats, rabbit does). In females of other species (bitches, ferrets, mares, sows, and rodents such as guinea pigs, hamsters, mice, and rats), the spermatozoa are forced through the cervix into the uterus.

PRECOITAL COURTSHIP

The process of arousal of sexual desire (erection, mounting, ejaculation, and withdrawal with dismounting) is complex and requires a great deal of coordination among body systems over time. Intricate neuroendocrine events stimulate as well as synchronize the increases in penile circulation and in vaginocervical mucous secretions of the mating pair. This precopulatory courtship, with its stimuli, leads to the copulatory behavior, which may result in an incomplete or a complete coitus.

Before mating, most ungulate males engage in a characteristic lip-curling behavior, known as *"flehmen,"* to increase the perception of olfactory cues (pheromones) from the female's urine or perineum to his vomeronasal organ.

In goats, monkeys, rats, and sheep, the precopulatory courtship frequently involves only sniffing, nuzzling, or licking the female's genitalia.

In cats, cattle, horses, and pigs, complex multisensory stimuli are added, whereas in dogs and elephants, complex motor patterns are also involved.

At termination of the precopulatory courtship, the penis of the sexually aroused male is in *erection* (except in dogs) and rigid. In males in which the penis is of the *fibroelastic* type (pigs, ruminants), erection is accompanied mostly by changes in the position, length, and stiffness of the penis. In males with a *musculocavernous* type of penis (cats, horses), erection brings more complex modifications of the shape, consistency, volume, and firmness of the penis. The musculocavernous penis of dogs is special, with a central bony part that helps intromission with only a partial erection, which is completed in the female's vagina. The multiphasic erection of the dog reaches its maximum only after intromission, which is possible because of a partial erection and the penile rigidity contributed by the os penis.

In pigs and ruminants, the nonerect, or quiescent, fibroelastic penis is firm or hard and is folded upon itself, forming a sigmoid flexure, which is more caudad in pigs. In this type of penis, erection is essentially the simple temporary tensing of the elastic sigmoid flexure (Fig. 55–1). This is caused by a hydraulic straightening of the localized sigmoid corpus cavernosum that increases its length and causes the penis to protrude from the prepuce.

During erection in bulls and boars, when it is viewed from behind, the free part of the penis is spiraled counterclockwise. This spiral tip of the boar's penis contributes to prolonging coitus by locking into the folds of the cervix.

In billy goats and rams, a urethral process that projects beyond the rounded glands stiffens during erection.

In horses, from a flaccid and compressible state, the penis becomes rigid as blood fills the cavernous erectile tissue of the *corpus cavernosum* and of the *glans.*

Both fibroelastic and musculocavernous types of penises have collapsed cavernous spaces in the *corpus cavernosum* and a coiled network of helicine arteries. The corpus cavernosum penis (CCP) is an erectile tissue encased in, or enmeshed with, thick connective tissue (*tunica albuginea* and *trabeculae*). The helicine arteries are coiled and can be straightened, without changing their inside diameter, to allow a rapid inflow of blood into the cavernous spaces, while the venous outflow is reduced. Arterial relaxation and dilatation of the vessels supplying the crura of the penis (the backward extensions of the corpora cavernosa of the penis) and cavernous bodies of the penis allow for an influx of blood to the penile structures and a rise in the blood pressure inside. Arteriovenous shunts close, to prevent rapid escape of blood, and the CCP fills with blood as its smooth muscle walls relax. The venous bleed valves close as the veins are compressed, and the CCP becomes a closed system.

The process of erection is linked to the parasympathetic and sympathetic portions of the autonomic nervous system and to the activity in the ischiocavernous muscles. The parasympathetic fibers arise from the S2-4 segments of the spinal cord. The synapses and ganglia of this cholinergic system may involve two cotransmitters, acetylcholine and vasoactive intestinal polypeptide (VIP), since intravenous VIP leads to erection. Also a reduction in the activity of sympathetic fibers in T12–L3 may lower the vasoconstrictive tone in the penile arteries. As blood fills the spaces between the trabeculae, the connective-tissue cocoon tightens, the intracavernous pressure increases, and the erectile tissue becomes rigid. The blood pressure in the corpus cavernosum can then rise to more than 7,000 mm Hg in billy goats, to about 14,000 mm Hg in bulls, and above 6,500 mm Hg in stallions. The contractions of the ischiocavernous muscles compress the closed system of the corpus cavern-

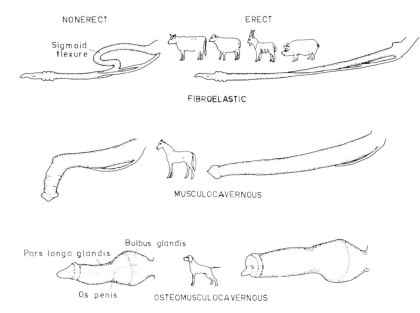

Figure 55-1 Diagrammatic representation of nonerect and erect fibroelastic (bull), musculocavernous (stallion), and osteomusculocavernous (dog) penises. Erection, caused by engorgement of the corpus cavernosum, results in a straightening of the sigmoid flexure, or distention and elongation of the penis. The penises of sheep, goats, and boars are also fibroelastic, with a sigmoid flexure, but the extremity of the glands is shaped differently. Baculum is a term synonymous with os penis.

osum penis and create these extremely high pressures. These striated muscles also compress the crura to occlude completely the blood vessels and to raise the pressure within the CCP to extreme levels, particularly in bulls.

Because the intracavernous pressure can reach a level 100 times that of arterial pressure, hematoma from rupture of the bull's CCP occurs as a frequent cause of inadequate extrusion of the penis.

In *bulls,* control CCP pressure at rest averages about 15 mm Hg. Mean systolic and diastolic carotid artery pressures are about 125/70 mm Hg during the control period, 150/100 mm Hg during the precoital stage. After exposure to a receptive cow, a partial erection increases the pressure in the corpus cavernosum penis to a mean of 75 mm Hg. Then, several oscillations of CCP pressure with peaks over 2,000 mm Hg occur prior to full erection, mounting, and intromission.

In cats, the distal end of the penis is studded with androgen-dependent small cornified papillae, the penile spines. The cat possesses an os penis that is relatively smaller than that of the dog.

COPULATION

During coitus, the systolic and diastolic arterial blood pressures may be double the control values (125/75 mm Hg), peaking near 250/150 mm Hg and falling to 135/80 mm Hg immediately after withdrawal of the penis. However, the CCP pressure far exceeds this arterial pressure for a total of about 8 seconds during the precoital and coital stages. The mean peak pressures within the CCP can reach 4,000 mm Hg in stallions, 7,000 mm Hg in billy goats, and 14,000 mm Hg in bulls (Fig. 55–2). Individual CCP pressures have been recorded at 6,500 mm Hg in Shetland pony stallions, and almost 33,000 mm Hg in a Jersey bull.

A complete copulation includes the *mounting,* the *intromission,* the *ejaculation,* and the *postejaculatory or postcopulatory phases.*

Mounting

The aroused receptive female stands or crouches (the camel sits down), remains immobile, and allows the male to mount her dorsally and from the rear. During this activity, the male fixes his forelimbs around the female's body and suddenly contracts the rectus abdominis muscles to bring his pelvis into direct apposition to the external genitalia of the female. The tom cat and the male ferret also take a firm "neck

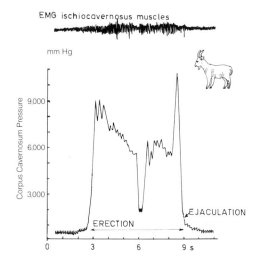

Figure 55–2 Electromyogram of the ischiocavernosus muscles of a billy goat, demonstrating a hyperactivity that coincides with an increase in the blood pressure inside the corpus cavernosum, which is sustained throughout the erection (i.e., about 6 seconds). The peak pressure in the corpus cavernosum is about 7,000 mm Hg.

bite," that is, a neck hold with their teeth for the duration of the copulation. The mating male camel squats behind the sitting and bleating female camel. Bouts of pelvic thrusting, which accentuate the loudness of female bleating, are accompanied by oral gurgling and frothing, with occasional protrusion of the soft palate.

Intromission and Ejaculation

Intromission refers to the skeletal motor patterns associated with penile insertion into the female copulatory organs. Far from being passive in this act, the female adjusts her perineal region toward the male's thrusting penis, contributes vaginal secretions of lubricating mucus, and provides temperature and pressure sensations leading to ejaculation. Receptors on the glans penis may help the male locate the vaginal entrance, and lubricant from the bulbourethral glands may also help achieve intromission.

After penetration of the vagina, within 3 seconds the bull makes about 10 quick thrusts, each of which is accompanied by a sharp peak in CCP pressure. The highest peak is usually attained at the final thrust, when ejaculation occurs.

> Prior anesthesia of the nerves supplying the ischiocavernous muscles results in a much lower peak pressure (mean, 2,200 mm Hg), and the erection is insufficient to permit intromission.

In horses, coitus lasts longer (20 seconds or more), and equine ejaculation involves 5 to 10 jets. The first three ejaculatory jets carry about 80 percent of the total sperm ejaculated, the later jets contain mainly the mucus fraction. In *boars,* intromission lasts as long as 7 minutes and is accompanied by ejaculation of a very large volume of semen.

During coitus in dogs, because of the elasticity of trabeculae in the *bulbus glandis* (a proximal part of the corpus cavernosum), the diameter of the penis increases locally. The local distention and engorgement of the bulbus glandis, prolonged by a physical occlusion of the penile venous return by the female's constrictor (vestibuli and vulvi) muscles, maintains and lengthens the duration of the intravaginal erection. During the immediate 15 to 30 seconds after intromission, the *dog* exhibits pelvic thrusting, a first ejaculation of sperm-rich semen, and intravaginal engorgement with dilation of the penile bulb. The bulb becomes too large to be withdrawn from the vagina, leading to the so-called "tie," or "lock," between the canine sexual partners. A second ejaculatory reflex occurs with rhythmic contractions of the bulbocavernous muscle and expulsion of mainly prostatic fluid. The male dog rotates 180 degrees, facing away from the bitch, and may remain in this awkward position for 10 to 30 minutes.

Ejaculation (i.e., the forceful expulsion of the ejaculate from the urethra to the outside) differs from *seminal emission,* which refers to the movement of the ejaculate into the urethra. Ejaculation of seminal fluid (or of coagulated material, in some species) and sperm involves a very high pressure wave (over 1,000 mm Hg in billy goats) in the periurethral corpus spongiosum (Fig. 55–3). This is accompanied by a

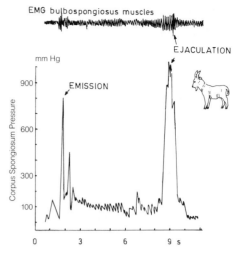

Figure 55–3 Electromyogram of the bulbospongiosus muscles in the billy goat, demonstrating two phases of hyperactivity closely associated with sudden rises in the corpus spongiosum pressure. The first short (1-second) preerection hyperactivity seen in the striated muscles coincides with an abrupt increase in corpus spongiosum pressure, and seminal emission. The longer (2 second) second phase of hyperactivity and highest corpus spongiosum pressure is ejaculatory. The corpus spongiosum pressure peaks associated with emission and ejaculation (about 1,000 mm Hg) are nearly ten times greater than that of arterial blood pressure. However, the highest corpus spongiosum pressures are about seven times less than the pressure recorded during erection in the corpus cavernosum.

number of characteristic spasmodic contractions of skeletal muscles (in the hips, abdominal wall, hindlimbs, and forelimbs) and of striated muscles (bulbospongiosus).

The process of ejaculation, the pumping out of semen, is effected by the sympathetic fibers of the hypogastric nerves and plexus. Electrical stimulation of these nerves per rectum (e.g., via an electroejaculator) causes ejaculation. Ejaculation initially involves contractions of the smooth muscles of the epididymis and vas deferens, of the seminal vesicles (when they are present), and of the prostate gland. This occurs under alpha-adrenergic sympathetic nerve stimulation arising from the T11 to the L2 segments of the spinal cord traveling via the hypogastric plexus to the glandular structures of the genital tract. The mixture of spermatozoa and seminal plasma is expelled into the penile urethra (emission). The bulbocavernous striated muscles also participate to force the semen along the urethra in spurts while thrusting occurs. Contraction of the urethra near the bladder prevents reflux. One component of the afferent trigger for ejaculation may be the pressure receptors in the body of the penis deep to the epithelium. If the dorsal nerve to the penis is severed, ejaculation is blocked in most species. At the end of ejaculation, sympathetic nerve stimuli to the arteries supplying the penis cause vasoconstriction, terminating erection as the blood drains from the CCP to the veins, and the penis returns to a flaccid state.

In some animals (bison, cats, cattle, goats, rabbits, rodents, sheep), vaginal intromission and ejaculation take place quickly, in a matter of a few seconds, after a single pelvic thrust. The urethral orifice of the bull turns counterclockwise through about 300 degrees as ejaculation occurs. In horses, these phases of copulation last about 20 to 30 seconds, and ejaculation is accompanied by up and down movements of the tail that coincide with the contractions of anal and penile muscles. In other animals, intromission and ejaculation occur at a more leisurely pace, involving repeated thrusts of the penis within the vagina. For instance, complete coitus requires about 10 to 30 minutes in dogs and pigs, and hours in the camel.

The erection and ejaculation reflexes utilize the same sensitive or afferent avenues, the internal pudendal nerve, that ramifies to centers in different segments of the spinal cord (erection, between L1 and S3; ejaculation, between L2 and S1). The efferent pathway for erection is parasympathetic, traveling in a relatively well-defined bundle that is called the "nervus erigens." These motor fibers dilate the arteries and restrict the venous drainage of both corpora cavernosa to cause the vascular engorgement responsible for erection.

The stimulus for ejaculation is not the same for all species. In bulls, the slightly higher vaginal temperature induces the ejaculatory reflex. In boars and stallions, pressure rather than temperature is the sensitive stimulus for ejaculation, whereas in the dog, gentle friction initiates ejaculation. The urethral emission part of ejaculation is mediated by sympathetic fibers, whereas ejaculation proper is primarily parasympathetic.

The volume of sperm and the quantity of spermatozoa per ejaculate differ between mammals (Table 55–1).

Postejaculatory, or Postcoital, Reactions

After ejaculation, the male dismounts, and its penis retracts into the prepuce or undergoes detumescence. The CCP pressure declines rapidly after ejaculation, as the bull dismounts. In dogs, because of the special type of erection, detumescence of the bulbus glandis is retarded by occlusion of the venous outflow, causing the so-called "tie." Ejaculation of semen rich in spermatozoa occurs before or during the early phase of this "tie." While he remains attached to the

female, the male dog breaks the ventrodorsal mount and does a 180-degree turn, and both partners face in opposite directions until detumescence of the bulbus glandis releases the sexual lock. After coitus, male dogs and cats either stand or sit and occasionally lick their penile area.

Female postcoital display is discrete in the large domesticated animals, which may simply arch their backs and elevate their tails. Screams or shrieks accompany intromission in the queen, which then breaks the sexual contact by rolling under the male and attempting to strike him with her claws. She then lies on her side, energetically rubs and rolls herself on the ground, and intensely licks her vaginal area, going through the so-called postcoital "after-reaction."

In species in which semen is deposited in the vagina, little or no seminal fluid (plasma) enters the uterus, and only a small percentage of the deposited spermatozoa reaches the uterus. The acid vaginal secretions, which provide an unfavorable environment for the alkaline seminal plasma, shorten the viability of the spermatozoa ejaculated into the vagina. In contrast, when the ejaculate is deposited directly into the uterus, this organ contains a comparatively enormous number of spermatozoa. In the guinea pig and sow, a gelatinous fraction of the seminal fluids even plugs the uterine-side of the cervical opening, to prevent loss of sperm from the uterus. In mice and rats, a "copulation plug" forms in the vagina and persists for about a day.

Whether the place of semen deposition is vaginal or uterine, only a small fraction of all types of ejaculates (a few hundred spermatozoa) arrives in the ampulla. This dilated part of the oviduct, the site of fertilization in most mammals, is the primary destination of both spermatozoa and ova. After fertilization in the ampulla, each spermatozoon-ovum complex, first known as a zygote and after some further growth as an embryo, negotiates the remaining part of the oviduct to reach the uterus.

ARTIFICIAL INSEMINATION

Artificial insemination means the deposition of spermatozoa in the female reproductive tract by means of instruments rather than by normal copulation. It is a method of breeding universally utilized in cattle and turkey reproduction; less widely recognized by breeders of goats, pigs, and sheep; and occasionally accepted by fanciers of companion animals such as cats, dogs, and horses.

Some of the advantages of artificial insemination are breeding of females at selected periods of the year; evaluation of the quality of semen that can be diluted or extended to inseminate several females on the same day; prevention of venereal disease; prolongation of the sexual life of aging, injured, or dead males; and reduction of the chances of injury to, or overuse of, the male.

The semen, previously obtained from the male, is evaluated, extended with diluters, and then used in several receptive females either immediately as fresh sperm or at a later date after it has been frozen.

TABLE 55–1 Approximate Volume of Sperm and Number of Spermatozoa per Ejaculate (Ejaculum)

Species	Volume (mL)	No. of Spermatozoa (10^9)
Cat	0.05	0.01
Cattle	5	6
Dog	5	1.8
Goat	1	2.4
Guinea pig	0.2	0.06
Horse	60	10
Mouse	0.1	0.06
Pig	200	48
Rabbit	0.5	0.03
Rat	0.1	0.06
Sheep	1	3

Collection of Semen

Semen can be collected from the male with an artificial vagina, by electroejaculation, or by manipulation (pressure, massage) of the penis (dog) or the seminal vesicles (bull). All the methods require training in an environment familiar to the male. The artificial vagina and the manipulation techniques require the arousal and response of the male to the sight of a female in estrus or to the pheromones exuding from a "teaser" (a female in estrus or a "dummy" exuding female pheromones). In both instances, the ejaculate is directed into an adequate-sized artificial vagina. Electroejaculation, which does not require sexual arousal, results from intrarectal electrical stimulation with a weak pulsatile electrical current. The collected sperm must be protected from air, heat, cold, and light.

Evaluation and Extension of the Collected Semen

To verify that the collected semen is of good quality and that it is probably able to impregnate the receptive female, it is screened routinely for appearance, volume, sperm-cell concentration (by nephelometry), and motility (microscopic). The viscous component of the stallion's semen is separated and discarded from the rest before dilution. In the boar's ejaculate, the clear accessory fluid first emitted and the filtered gel component are also rejected from the semen.

The appropriate fraction of the semen is then processed with an extender (a diluter that also nourishes and extends the life of the sperm cells) to ensure maximum fertility and is packaged for convenient handling and insemination. For semen that is to be used fresh, usually on the same day, the added extender may be a natural fluid from the same species (e.g., cow's milk) or a composite specially prepared and tested for efficacy (e.g., egg yolk–glucose citrate). The volume and the spermatozoa concentration in a "dose" of semen for fresh use differ between animal species (Table 55–2).

For semen intended for storage and later use, ampules (0.5, 1.0 mL) or straws (0.25, 0.5 mL) of bovine sperm are frozen in liquid nitrogen (− 196° C), which has replaced the originally used dry ice and alcohol or acetone (− 70° C)

TABLE 55–2 Approximate Volume and Number of Spermatozoa in a "Dose" of Extended Semen for Fresh Use

Species	Volume (mL)	No. of Spermatozoa (10^6)
Cat	0.1	0.7
Cattle	1	20
Dog	5–10	50
Goat	0.1	60
Horse	10	100
Pig	50–100	2,000
Sheep	0.05–2	50–150

method. Pellets (0.1 mL) of extended sperm (cattle, goat, horse, sheep), which take even less space than ampules or straws, may also be formed in holes on the surface of dry ice blocks, and then preserved in liquid nitrogen. During the freezing process, glycerol and antibacterial agents are added. Glycerol acts as a protective agent against water crystal formation inside the sperm cells, whereas selected antibiotics (e.g., streptomycin, penicillin), sulfonamides, or both can control bacterial growth.

Insemination

In goats, horses, pigs, and sheep, artificial insemination is usually carried out with fresh semen, although frozen semen may also be used. The nanny goat and ewe are inseminated intracervically, about 12 to 18 hours after the beginning of heat. The intrauterine insemination of mares, with a minimum dose of 10 mL, starts on the third day of heat and is then repeated every 48 hours for the rest of the estrus. For sows, the optimal time of insemination is during the middle of estrus, when the receptive female responds (is immobilized) to pressure on the back. The relatively large dose (about 50 mL) is administered into the uterus through a narrow-tipped spiral rubber catheter that is rotated counterclockwise until it locks in the folds of the cervix, to prevent backward leakage into the vagina.

The artificial insemination of cows, from semen frozen in ampules or straws, is performed during the 24 hours preceding ovulation, which occurs 12 hours after the end of estrus, or heat. An ampule is thawed in an iced-water bath and is dried before the semen is aspirated into a catheter-syringe insemination device (without breaking the liquid column in the catheter). A straw is thawed in a 35° C water bath (for 6 to 12 seconds, depending of the type of straw), dried, cleanly cut at one tip. Then it is inserted and locked into the plastic insemination sheath, and the straw gun (*pistolet*) is armed (plunger in place). Frozen pellets of sperm are thawed, diluted in sodium citrate (cattle), sterile milk (horses), or trisglucose–egg yolk (goats, sheep), and loaded in a syringe-catheter insemination device. Either type of insemination device is immediately inserted into the vagina and then visually or manually guided into the uterus, to discharge accurately the sperm into the posterior portion of the body of the uterus. The visual approach requires a headlight and a heavy-walled Pyrex glass speculum. The manual technique involves transrectal palpation of the cervix and gentle guidance of the catheter-tip, with the thumb and first two fingers, through the cervix.

TRANSPORT OF SPERMATOZOA IN THE FEMALE GENITAL TRACT

Within the reproductive tract of the female, the duration of motility of the spermatozoa varies among species, from a low of about 18 hours in cows to as long as 11 days (264 hours) in bitches. Although it is an important sign of vigor, the intrinsic motility of the spermatozoa does not account for the rapid upward transport of sperm cells within the female reproductive tract (Table 55–3). Transfer of spermatozoa toward the ampulla, with the objective of a chance meeting with an ovum, occurs chiefly because of massive displacement of fluids within the uterotubal environment. These hydraulic waves result from the profuse mucosal secretions, the higher motor activity of smooth muscles (peristalsis and antiperistalsis), and the local eddies created by myriads of beating cilia in the walls of the uterus and of the oviducts. Prostaglandins from the spermatozoa, and oxytocin and estrogen from the ovaries, stimulate these motor and secretory activities of the female reproductive tract. After about 2 or 3 days, except in mares, the spermatozoa in the female reproductive system degenerate and are phagocytized by leukocytes and epithelial cells in the uterus and the oviducts.

TRANSPORT OF OOCYTES IN THE FEMALE GENITAL TRACT

After ovulation, each of the ruptured follicles yields an oocyte (egg) that is set free in the immediate periovarian space, which may be in open communication with the peritoneal cavity. In cows, ewes, and goats, oocytes come mostly from the right ovary, whereas the oocytes of mares and sows originate mostly from the left ovary. Because of a mobility permitting close contact and of a facilitatory ciliary action, the funnel-shaped end (fimbriated infundibulum) of the oviducts (fallopian tubes) takes up the free oocytes. In mares, bitches, queens, and small rodents, the ovarian bursa that surrounds the ovary is an additional insurance against any oocytes' straying into the peritoneal cavity. Once the oocytes are in the lumen of the tubes, they are rapidly propelled toward the ampulla by rushes of peristalsis produced by contractions of the smooth muscles in the walls of the oviducts. In most animals, the oocyte reaches the ampulla within minutes after ovulation (see Table 55–3).

In most species, the oocytes that reach the ampulla are in the resting stage of the second meiosis and are readily fertilizable. However, the freshly ovulated oocytes of dogs and foxes cannot be immediately fertilized, since the first meiosis of the primary oocyte is not completed. It takes about 2 or 3 days after ovulation for the first polar body to be extruded and the arrest of the second meiosis. Meiosis is resumed by penetration of the spermatozoon at fertilization. The oocyte of the mare, which is also immature at ovulation, can be fertilized within a few hours, contrary to that of the bitch. Unfertilized oocytes remain in the ampullary area for about 24 hours, except in mares, in which they persist for months in spite of a subsequent ovulation and fertilization. In most species, the transfer of unfertilized or fertilized oocytes from the ampulla to the uterus requires about 3 days, except in bitches and queens (about 5 to 8 days).

FERTILIZATION

Fertilization, or conception, can take place only after several hours of sustained effort by many spermatozoa, which release proteolytic enzymes from their acrosome. In most species, the acrosomal trypsin-like enzyme (acrosin) participates in softening the layers of cells that cover the zona pellucida. However, in the oviducts of cows, ewes, goats, mares, and sows, an enzyme (acid phosphatase) loosens the coronata cells and denudes the ovum as it is made to tumble down from the infundibulum to the ampulla.

In the ampulla, fertilization is a multistep process that begins with the physical penetration of the zona pellucida of the oocyte by a single vigorous spermatozoon. As it crosses the perivitelline space and reaches the cytoplasm of the egg, the spermatozoon causes the regression of microgranules bordering the endoplasmic surface of the plasma membrane of the oocyte. The evanescence of these microgranules coincides with a reaction that transforms the receptors on the zona pellucida and makes them unresponsive to other spermatozoa. This prevents polyspermy, that is, the fusion of more than one sperm with a single ovum.

In the different animal species, fertilization lasts from 6 to 24 hours. During this time, the ovum is activated from a resting meiosis and merges its cytoplasm with that of the penetrating spermatozoon (amphimixis). After its passage through the plasma membrane, the spermatozoon sheds its tail and midpiece before fusing its plasma membrane with that of the ovum.

The union (syngamy) of both female and male gametes, as each one contributes its haploid number of chromosomes, reestablishes the diploid number of the animal species in the genome of the newly formed zygote. At fertilization, the combination of the X and Y chromosomes also determines the genetic sex of mammals: the union of two X chromosomes (XX) for a female zygote, and a heterogametic union of an X and a Y chromosome (XY) for a male zygote.

In birds and fish, the genetic sex is determined at ovulation. Males are homogametic (ZZ), and females are heterogametic (ZW).

TABLE 55–3 Duration of Spermatozoal Motility and Approximate Travel Time of Spermatozoa and Eggs Within the Reproductive Tract of Domesticated Females

Females	Duration of Motility (hr)	Uteroampullary Travel Time (min)	Ovarioampullary Travel Time (min)
Bitch	144–264	20–120	20
Cow	18–48	15	120
Ewe	48	5–300	1,440
Queen	48		6–15
Mare	72–144		
Sow	48	15	<45

REFERENCES

Baum MJ. Differentiation of coital behavior in mammals: a comparative analysis. Neurosci Biobehav Rev 1979;3:265.

Beach FA. Hormonal modulation of genital reflexes in male and masculinized female dogs. Behav Neurosci 1984;98:325.

Beckett SD, Hudson RS, Walker DF, et al. Blood pressure and penile muscle activity in the stallion during coitus. Am J Physiol 1973;225:1072.

Beckett SD, Hudson RS, Walker DF, et al. Corpus cavernosum penis pressure and external penile muscle activity during erection in the goat. Biol Reprod 1972;7:359.

Beckett SD, Purohit RC, Reynolds TM. The corpus spongiosum penis pressure and external penile muscle activity in the goat during coitus. Biol Reprod 1975;12:289.

Beckett SD, Walker DF, Hudson RS, et al. Corpus cavernosum penis pressure and penile muscle activity in the bull during coitus. Am J Vet Res 1974;35:761.

Bedford JM. Fertilization. In: Austin CR, Short RV, eds. Reproduction in mammals. I. Germ cells and fertilization, 2nd ed. New York: Cambridge University Press, 1982.

Benson GS. Mechanism of penile erection. Invest Urol 1981;19:65.

Beyer C, Velasquez J, Larsson K, Contreras JL. Androgen regulation of the motor copulatory pattern in the male New Zealand white rabbit. Horm Behav 1980;14:179.

Carroll RS, Erskine MS, Doherty PC, et al. Coital stimuli controlling luteinizing hormone secretion and ovulation in the female ferret. Biol Reprod 1985;32:925.

Demick DS, Voss JL, Pickett BW. Effect of cooling, storage, glycerolization and spermatozoal numbers on equine fertility. J Anim Sci 1976; 43:633.

Dewsbury DA. Patterns of copulatory behavior in male mammals. Q Rev Biol 1972;47:1.

Hafez ESE. Reproduction in farm animals, 5th ed. Philadelphia: Lea & Febiger, 1987.

Harper MJK. Sperm and egg transport. In: Austin CR, Short RV, eds. Reproduction in mammals. I. Germ cells and fertilization, 2nd ed. New York: Cambridge University Press, 1982.

Hart BL. Physiology of sexual function. Vet Clin North Am 1974;4:557.

Herman HA, Madden FW. The artificial insemination and embryo transfer of dairy and beef cattle, 7th ed. Danville, IL: The Interstate Printers and Publishers Inc., 1987.

Johnson MH, Everitt BJ. Essentials of reproduction, 2nd ed. Oxford: Blackwell, 1984.

Johnson RD, Kitchell RL, Gilanpour H. Rapidly and slowly adapting mechanoreceptors in the glans penis of the cat. Physiol Behav 1986; 37:69.

Lott DF. Sexual behavior and intersexual strategies in American bisons. Z Tierpsychol 1981;56:97.

McDonald LE. Veterinary endocrinology and reproduction, 4th ed. Philadelphia: Lea & Febiger, 1989.

Pineda MH, Dooley MP, Martin PA. Long-term study of the effects of electroejaculation on seminal characteristics of the domestic cat. Am J Vet Res 1984;45:1038.

Van Haaften B, Dieleman SJ, Okkens AC, Willemse AH. Timing the mating of dogs on the basis of blood progesterone concentration. Vet Rec 1989;125:524.

Wasserman PM. The biology and chemistry of fertilization. Science 1987;235:553.

CHAPTER 56

ZYGOTE AND EMBRYO PERIODS OF PREGNANCY; EMBRYO TRANSFER

Pregnancy is the series of events beginning with fertilization of the ovum and ending with parturition, or delivery of the fetus and its membranes. The process of multiplication and growth of the zygote, a unique cell about 0.1 mm in diameter that combines the genetic material of the parents, is continuous. In females of uniparous species (cows, mares), one fertilized ovum grown to full term gives an offspring that is 8 to 10 percent of the maternal weight. In females of pluriparous species (bitches, ewes, goats, queens, and sows), several fertilized eggs arrive at full term as a litter, each of the offsprings weighing only 1 to 3 percent of the maternal weight.

Females that have not conceived are called *nulliparous*, those that have had one gestation are said to be *primiparous*, and the term *multiparous* is reserved for those that have experienced at least two pregnancies.

The study of pregnancy interests many disciplines. Embryology follows the development of the zygote to a full-term fetus. Anatomy examines the structures of the placenta. Biochemistry and endocrinology consider the neuro-humoral mechanisms. Cellular genetics scrutinizes the chromosomes, and immunology studies antigens and antibodies. Physiology borrows from these specialized fields to present a concise and integrated picture of gestation.

The changes in structures, arrangements, and functions of the continuously growing conceptus are considered in three periods:

1. Blastogenesis: cellular division of the zygote, or cleavage of the fertilized ovum,
2. Embryogenesis: differentiation and organogenesis, or metamorphosis, and
3. Fetal growth.

BLASTOGENESIS, OR ZYGOTE PERIOD

This period, which starts with fertilization and ends with the hatching of the blastocyst, lasts less than a week in small laboratory animals (rats, mice, rabbits), about a week (7 to 8 days) in both cows and mares, and about 2 weeks in other domesticated animals. Nutrition (embryotroph) is provided by uterine secretions (histiotroph, uterine milk) containing proteins (mare, 18 percent; cow, 10 percent) and lipids (ruminants, 1 percent; mare, 0.006 percent) and by the zygote's own cytoplasmic reserves.

Fertilization occurs in the ampulla of the fallopian tube (oviduct). It involves the meeting of the male and female gametes and penetration of the spermatozoon into the ovum. Paternal and maternal chromosomes mingle, each equally

contributing to the chromosomal complement (diploid chromosome number) of the species (Table 56–1). In addition, the fertilized ovum is activated, or stimulated, to develop into a zygote.

The zygote divides about once a day during its passage into the oviduct and the uterus. In most animal species, it leaves the oviduct and reaches the uterus 3 to 5 days after fertilization, usually as a structure composed of 16 cells, or blastomeres (Table 56–2). Exceptions are the pig (2 days, 4 blastomeres), the cat (5 to 6 days, 8 cells), and the dog (5 to 8 days, blastocyst). In nearly all animals, except the horse, the donkey, and the mule, the oviduct transports unfertilized eggs as well as fertilized eggs. In members of Equidae, the oviduct generally delivers only fertilized eggs to the uterus and may retain unfertilized eggs from previous ovulations for as long as 8 months.

In the uterus, cleavages into blastomers proceed until these cells are too numerous to count and form a ball called a *morula* (Fig. 56–1). Further development leads to formation of a cavity (blastocoele) within the mass of cells (morula), which then becomes an early *blastocyst*. Because of the expansion within the unattached blastocyst and of the action of a uterine protease, the acellular zona pellucida ruptures in a process termed "hatching." In the inner cell mass, a clump of cells ultimately grows and gives rise to the embryo and the embryonic membranes the amnion and the allantois, whereas the denuded outer layer of the blastocyst, the *trophoblast,* is made up of large, flattened, negatively charged and very sticky cells. The trophoblast enlarges to form the blastodermic, or chorionic, vesicle, whose cells act first as a pump for active transfers between the blastocyst and the uterine environment. Later, the trophoblastic cells adhere to the epithelium of the endometrium, invade its deeper layers, and become the chorion, which maintains physical and chemical contact with the maternal organism (see Fig. 56–1).

In marsupials (kangaroo, wallaby), the blastocysts have a very thin zona pellucida, and the similarity of the cells prevents any identification of inner mass and outer layer.

Antiluteolysis. The trophoblast, which elongates in most species, also produces proteins that inhibit the local release of a luteolytic substance, prostaglandin $F_{2\alpha}$ ($PGF_{2\alpha}$) from the endometrium. Initially identified as trophoblastins (in cows and sheep) but now recognized as active interferons (IFN) of the IFN-alpha-2 subfamily, these proteins prevent the normal involution of the corpus luteum (CL). In addition, ewes transform $PGF_{2\alpha}$ into PGE_2, which vasodilates the ovarian vessels and is luteotrophic. Thus, the necessary progesterone (P_4) secretion continues for the stimulation of

TABLE 56–1 Chromosomal Complements in Domesticated Animals

Animal Species	Chromosomal Complement (2n)
Cat	38
Cattle	60
Dog	78
Donkey	62
Goat	60
Horse	64
Pig	38
Sheep	54

TABLE 56–2 Stage of Development of Zygotes Collected at Various Times after Onset of Estrus

Day	Cow	Ewe	Goat	Mare
2	2 cells	2–4 cells	1–2 cells	2–4 cells
3	4–8 cells	4–8 cells	4–8 cells	4–8 cells
4	16–32 cells	8–16 cells	16–32 cells	8–16 cells
5	Morula	Morula	Morula	Morula
6	Blastocyst	Morula	Blastocyst	Morula
7	Blastocyst	Blastocyst	Blastocyst	Blastocyst
8	Hatched and hatching blastocysts	Hatched and hatching blastocysts	Hatched spherical blastocysts	Hatched and hatching blastocysts

endometrial development and the production of glandular secretions (histiotroph) to nourish the early embryo.

The antiluteolytic mechanism is different in other species. The trophoblast of mares and the sows produces an increased amount of estrogens (estrone and estradiol). A minimum of four to five pig blastocysts is required to produce the adequate level of luteotropic estrogens. The long life span of the corpus luteum in bitches and queens precludes the need for any special antiluteotropic mechanisms.

Uterine Migration of Blastocysts. While the blastocyst is free in the uterus, it may migrate internally into the

opposite uterine horn, except in cows. Also, during the period of blastogenesis, the blastocyst can tolerate short intervals of exposure to controlled conditions outside the body. This characteristic makes transfer of fertilized eggs (embryo transfer) possible from one female (superovulated donor) to several females (synchronized receivers) of the same species at one moment. Nonsurgical procedures are used in cows and mares, and surgical procedures in ewes, goats, and sows. Blastocysts from cows, ewes, goats, and mares (embryo viability is lost at − 15° C in pigs) can be frozen for short-term or long-term storage and can eventually be transferred to properly prepared (synchronized) receivers (cows, ewes, goats, mares). In each receiver cow, the transferred embryo must be deposited in the horn on the same side of the ovulated ovary (i.e., the one carrying a corpus luteum). By microsurgery, it is possible to separate a blastocyst into two or more units, and to isolate cells that can be immunologically or cytogenetically sexed. In the literature on embryo transfer in farm animals, the term embryo is used interchangeably with fertilized egg, fertilized ovum, morula, blastocyst, and blastodermic vesicle.

In animals that may bear several fetuses in a given pregnancy (pluriparous), such as bitches, ewes, goats, queens, and sows, the blastocysts become almost evenly distributed in both uterine horns. However, the bovine embryo does not migrate. Twin calves are located in both horns only if the ova have originated from both ovaries; bovine twins are carried in the same uterine horn when the two ova are from the same ovary. In contrast, the equine embryo migrates from one horn to the other up to the time when fixation (implantation) begins, at about 40 days.

EMBRYOGENESIS, OR EMBRYO PERIOD

With the disappearance of the zona pellucida, the blastocyst ceases to move freely about in the uterine fluid, and its trophoblast begins to adhere loosely to the endometrium. It

Figure 56–1 Diagrammatic transformation of the fertilized ovum, or zygote, into a blastocyst. Inside the impermeable zona pellucida, the process involves almost daily cell divisions (e.g., 1 cell; 2 cells—4, 8, 16, and 32 cells, or morula) of the zygote, before cavitation of the blastocyst and its differentiation into endoderm and ectoderm. After rupture of the zona pellucida (hatching), the endoderm is destined to become the embryo and the fetal membranes (amnion and allantois), whereas the ectoderm develops as the trophoblast (chorion).

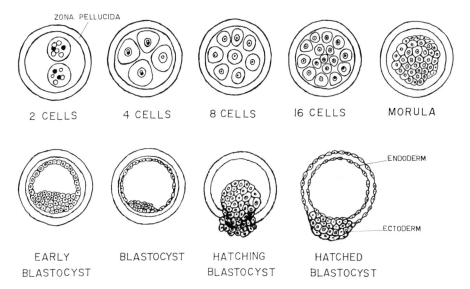

also goes through a stage of elongation (very rapid in ewes and sows) that modifies it from a sphere 1 to 2 mm in diameter to a creamy membranous thread about 100 mm long. Unlike those of other farm animal species, the equine embryo remains more or less spherical in shape until its implantation, when it takes the shape of the whole uterus.

During the embryonic period, the major tissues, organs, and systems are formed but are not growing. Values for the duration of the embryonic period lack precision except in swine and rodents (Table 56–3). In these species, the embryonic period is initiated when the blastocyst begins the gradual process of implantation, which is associated with the combined action of luteal progesterone and minute amounts of estrogen. The embryonic period ends when the primordial nervous, circulatory, excretory, and digestive systems and the limb buds are formed. At the end of this period, the embryo is recognizable as a miniature example of a given animal species.

Implantation is the lasting contact between the embryonic trophoblast and the maternal endometrium epithelium. A gradual process, it is completed in about a week in small animals (cats, dogs, mice, rabbits, rats), in about 2 weeks in pigs and small ruminants, and about a month in cattle and horses (see Table 56–3).

In mice, nonpaternal male sexual odors may inhibit implantation (Bruce effect). In some species (armadillo, badger, bear, deer, kangaroo, otter, wallaby), the period of the embryo is prolonged because of a delay in implantation.

Delayed implantation is related to an embryonic diapause, that is, a temporary pause or suspension in the development of the embryo. Embryonic diapause is a mechanism of adaptation to environmental changes in the seasons (light-darkness, temperature) and in the maternal or fetal nutrition (lactation, availability of food and water). To accommodate to environmental difficulties, the embryo is maintained in a state of suspended animation until uterine or environmental conditions improve. The chances for successful gestation and parturition increase, or the young are born at a time of the year that is more opportune for their survival.

In bears and deer, with midsummer fertilization and relatively short pregnancy, this embryonic diapause is related to the light-darkness cycles. In marsupials (also possible in mice and rats), the embryonic diapause is due to lactation.

Embryonic deaths occur at an important rate in domestic animals. The loss is as high as 15 percent in companion animals (queens, bitches, and mares) and two times higher (up to 30 percent) in cows, ewes, goats, and sows. Much of ruminant embryonic mortality occurs in the preimplantation stage, because of nutritional deficiency, excessive ambient temperature (sheep), and infections (trichomoniasis, vibriosis, and viral infections). Also, the period of embryogenesis is the most vulnerable stage for malformation of the embryo to be initiated by teratogenic agents.

FETAL PERIOD

The fetal period, the longest of the three periods of gestation (blastocyst, embryo, fetus), begins when implantation is completed. The functional fetoplacental unit of the

TABLE 56–3 Approximate Length of the Blastogenesis and Embryogenesis Periods in Domesticated and Laboratory Animals

Species	Blastogenesis (days)	Embryogenesis (days)
Cat	11–17	18–22
Cattle	12–15	14–45
Dog	14–21	20–30
Goat	10–15	15–32
Horse	12–15	15–60
Mouse	4.5	4–9
Rabbit	7–8	9–14
Rat	4–6	6–12
Sheep	17–20	21–32
Swine	10–15	16–35

TABLE 56–4 Length of Gestation in Domesticated Animals

Species and Breed	Duration (days)
Cat	
House	56–65
Siamese	63–69
Cattle	
Beef	
Angus	273–282
Brahman	271–310
Charolais and Simmental	285–287
Hereford	283–286
Limousin	287–290
Dairy	
Ayrshire	277–279
Brown Swiss	288–291
Guernsey	282–285
Holstein	278–282
Jersey	277–280
Shorthorn	275–292
Dog	59–68
Donkey	
Bred to jackass	365–375
Bred to horse: Hinny foal	340–350
Goat	146–155
Horse	
Blood	
Arabian	335–339
Morgan	342–346
Thoroughbred	336–340
Draft	
Belgian	333–337
Clydesdale	334
Percheron	321–345
Pony	
Welsh	365–366
Bred to donkey: Mule foal	355
Sheep	
Corriedale	148–150
Dorset and Southdown	143–145
Hampshire	144–146
Merino	147–151
Rambouillet	149–151
Shropshire	145–147
Swine	111–116

period of the fetus lasts until parturition. *Hemotrophic* nutrition, through allantoic capillaries in close juxtaposition to the maternal capillaries, replaces the initial *histiotrophic* nutrition provided by secretions of the uterine glands. During this period, details in the differentiation of tissues, organs, and systems occur.

The size of the fetus increases in a geometrical fashion, as most of the weight is gained very rapidly during the last third of pregnancy. During this final part of the period of the fetus, maternal nutritive intake must be abundant and of high quality, to ensure optimum growth of the offspring and to decrease neonatal mortality. Also, adequate maternal nutrition preserves the dam's body stores for the stress of parturition, improves the milk output during lactation, and shortens the interval before breeding.

In the larger species (cattle, horse), the fetal period (and the gestation) of the male fetus is slightly longer than that of the female fetus (Table 56–4). Differences are noted also between breeds and types of animals of the same species (e.g., draft < race horse; dairy < beef cattle; house < Siamese cat). Large litters have shorter gestation length, except in the pig. Twins generally have a shorter pregnancy by 3 to 6 days in cattle and by half a day in sheep. Daylight at conception influences the duration of pregnancy in mares. Foals conceived in spring (increasing daylight) are carried more than a week longer than those conceived in summer and fall (declining daylight). In the hybrid members of Equidae, the gestational length seems related to the paternal species. A mare cross-mated to a donkey stallion (jackass) may carry a mule foal for 355 to 375 days, whereas a donkey (ass) bred to a stallion delivers a hinny foal after only 340 to 350 days of gestation. Considerable variation in the duration of pregnancy is also observed in wild and exotic animal species (Table 56–5).

EMBRYO TRANSFER

Embryo transfer is the *collection* of an embryo from a donor female, its short-term or long-term *preservation,* and its *placement* into the oviduct or uterus of a recipient female. Embryo transfer is used mostly in cows to increase rapidly the number of offspring from the best females that have been artificially inseminated with the sperm of the best males. It offers a new research tool for reproduction genetics (birth weight, cloning, identical twins, length of pregnancy, postnatal production) and for uterine physiology (endocrinology of pregnancy, maternal recognition of pregnancy, uterine capacity and environment). It permits an international import-export trade in embryos, for genetic improvement of cattle breeds, with minimal risk of transmitting bacterial or viral diseases such as brucellosis, bluetongue, foot-and-mouth, bovine leukemia, and bovine viral diarrhea.

However, in ewes, goats, mares, and sows, embryo transfer is possible but is limited by greater technical difficulties at some stage of the process. Also, in horses, the breed societies have shown some reluctance to register progeny.

TABLE 56–5   Length of Gestation in Laboratory and Exotic Animals

Species	Duration (days)
Bear	208–240
Buffalo	270–276
Camel (bactrian)	333–430
Chinchilla	111–128
Elephant	615–650
Ferret	42
Fox	51–52
Guinea pig	63–70
Hamster	19–20
Lion	105–112
Mink	42–52
Mouse	19–22
Rabbit	30–32
Rat	22
Tammar wallaby	26
Tiger	105–113
Wolf	63

The successful completion of the major phases of the embryo transfer process is the result of applied knowledge in

1. superovulation (in the donor female),
2. fertilization,
3. surgical or nonsurgical flushing of the embryos from the oviducts or the uterus with a phosphate-buffered saline solution,
4. extracorporeal manipulation of the embryos for selection, division, cryopreservation, thawing of the cryoprotected embryos,
5. induction of estrus in each recipient female to synchronize it with that of the donor (i.e., the stage of development of the dormant embryo), and
6. surgical or nonsurgical placement of each embryo in the recipient female.

Superovulation in the Donor Female

Superovulation or multiple ovulations are caused by an acceleration in the growth of some follicles and an inhibition of the atresia of other follicles, following pharmacological stimulation of the ovaries. An abnormally high rate of folliculogenesis is produced by the administration of gonadotropins during the normal diestrous phase of an estrous cycle. Estrus is induced by administration of analogues of $PGF_{2\alpha}$. Successive superovulations need to be separated by an interval of about 6 to 8 weeks.

In donor *cows,* the regimen to cause superovulation varies with the type of gonadotropin used. With *equine chorionic gonadotropin* (eCG), also known as *pregnant mare serum gonadotropin* (PMSG), which has a long biological half-life (about 5 days), a single intramuscular injection, 2,000 to 3,000 International Units (IU), is given on one day of the period from day 8 to 14 of the cycle. Two days later, an analogue of $PGF_{2\alpha}$ is also injected to cause regression of the midcycle corpus luteum and to induce estrus, which occurs 40 to 60 hours later. To neutralize the biological activity of

PMSG, and to dampen the exuberant ovulatory response (up to 50 eggs), an ovine anti-PMSG serum (1,800 IU) may be injected intravenously on the day of estrus.

With mammalian (bovine, ovine, porcine) pituitary (adenohypophysial) extracts rich in follicle-stimulating hormone (FSH-P) that have short biological half-lives (about 6 hours), several injections, 4 mg intramuscularly (also intravenously or subcutaneously) twice a day for 4 days, are administered, starting on a day of the period from day 8 to 14. A prostaglandin analogue is then given on the third day after the first injection. Estrus appears on the fifth day.

In *ewes* and *goats*, either PMSG or FSH-P (bovine: bFSH-P; porcine: pFSH-P) can be used to induce superovulation. PMSG, 750 to 1,000 IU, is injected subcutaneously or intramuscularly on one day between days 11 and 13 in ewes, and between days 16 and 18 in goats. FSH-P, 20 mg per day over 3 days, is injected on similar days of the estrous cycle of ewes (between day 11 and day 13) or of goats (between day 16 and day 18). An analogue of $PGF_{2\alpha}$ is administered 2 days after either type of gonadotropin so that estrus appears about 36 to 48 hours later.

In *sows*, superovulation is provoked with PMSG, about 1,250 IU, administered on day 15 or 16 of the estrous cycle. Estrus, with about 25 to 30 ovulations, usually occurs after 3.5 to 4 days.

In *mares*, superovulation is not successfully induced by equine or porcine pituitary extracts, and PMSG is ineffective in producing superovulation. In normal breeding, PMSG is produced during pregnancy, from day 45 to 120.

Fertilization of the Superovulated Ova

In cows, inseminations are initiated from 48 to 60 hours after the administration of the $PGF_{2\alpha}$ analogue. To compensate for any asynchrony in the ovulations of the donor, sperm is deposited two or three times, at 12-hour intervals. However, larger but fewer doses of sperm are more successful, probably because the cow's genital tract is then less often manipulated.

Collection of the Embryos

In all species, modified phosphate-buffered saline (PBS) solution or physiological saline solution (PSS) is the medium for collection, manipulation, and preservation of the embryos. Embryo recovery from the donor's reproductive system is done by a nonsurgical procedure in cows and mares, by laparoscopy in ewes and goats, and by surgery in sows. These embryos can be kept alive for up to 24 hours by supplementing PBS with heat-treated serum or serum albumin.

The bovine embryos, which enter the uterus on day 4, are collected on day 7 or 8, by sequential or simultaneous PBS-flushing of the separate uterine horns (Fig 56–2).

After epidural anesthesia, to provide regional anesthesia of the perineal region, or tranquilization with xylazine (25 mg intramuscularly), the front feet of the cow may be elevated about 0.3 m in the large-volume technique. A three-way No. 20 French Foley catheter is passed through the cervix into the uterus, and its cuff is inflated with air from a syringe.

By gravity, through the inlet of the catheter, PSS or PBS is then delivered into the uterine horn (750 mL) or uterus (1,000 mL) and drained from the outlet into a 1-L graduated cylinder. After a settling period of 30 minutes, all but the bottom 150 mL of the PSS column is siphoned out. The remaining 150 mL are poured into Petri dishes, which are scrutinized under a dissecting microscope (magnification of ×10 to ×30) in a search for embryos that do not float and sink to the bottom.

A small-volume technique, where the Foley catheter is placed near the ovarian end of the uterine horn, is also used to collect embryos separately from each horn.

In mares, superovulation is difficult to obtain. A single embryo is usually recovered, 6 to 8 days after ovulation, via the nonsurgical method with a Foley catheter.

In ewes and goats, the tortuous cervix is difficult to negotiate with a catheter during the nonsurgical technique for recovery of the embryos. A nonsurgical technique is being developed for goats, but surgery is the usual method for recovery of embryos from superovulated small ruminants. By laparotomy or by laparoscopy, 3 to 7 days after estrus, the abdominal cavity is invaded to catheterize and to flush embryos from the uterus and the oviducts. In sows, a midventral laparotomy, 3 to 7 days after estrus, is used to gain access to the uterine horns and to recover successfully 90 percent of the embryos.

Extracorporeal Manipulations of the Embryos

Bovine embryos develop according to a predictable pattern (Table 56–6). Day-7 bovine embryos (175 μm) (i.e., blastocysts or late morula) are still within the zona pellucida. They can be micromanipulated with sterile fine glass pipettes to isolate each embryo in a small Petri dish containing PSS in addition to inactivated calf serum and antibiotics (penicillin, streptomycin). Under the microscope (×50 to 100), the quality or viability of each embryo can be evaluated according to the stage of development relative to age, and the appearance of the cells. They are classified on a scale from 1 to 4 (or A to D), with the numbers or letters representing embryos that are good, fair, poor, and unsuitable for successful transfer.

> The equine embryo is generally larger (100 to 4,500 μm) than the bovine embryo at day 6 to 9 after ovulation. On day 4, sheep blastocysts are about 150 μm, whereas those of the pig are only about 50 to 100 μm.

Other practical micromanipulations that can be considered at this time are embryo bisection, cryopreservation of embryos, and sexing of embryos. Studies in embryology and genetics have used micromanipulations for experimental transfers (nuclei, single cells, DNA or genes) into embryos.

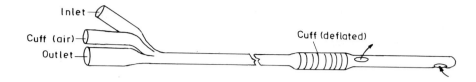

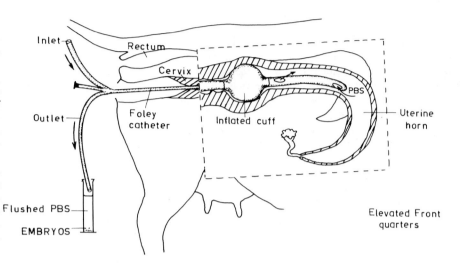

Figure 56–2 Diagram of the nonsurgical large-volume embryo recovery technique, with a three-way Foley catheter in the distal uterine horns of the uterus. The conduits provide for insufflation of the cuff and for infusion and retrieval of the fluid medium (physiological saline solution [PSS] or phosphate-buffered saline [PBS]). Beyond the inflatable cuff, the PSS or the PBS circulates between the two openings on the tip of the catheter. The proximal opening admits the fluid medium, whereas the distal one is the outlet for the embryo-PBS suspension.

Besides producing identical twins, the *bisection of farm animal embryos* (blastocysts, morulae) aims at increasing the supply of viable embryos by as much as 80 percent. Considering the survival rates after transfer, embryo bisection may permit a pregnancy rate of 100 to 120 percent of the number of whole embryos collected.

Cryopreservation or deep-freezing of cattle embryos is a well-established technique for their long-term storage. Each embryo must be packaged in a vial or straw with a cryoprotectant (glycerol, dimethyl sulfoxide [DMSO]) before cooling (Fig. 56–3). The cryopreservative dehydrates the embryo to prevent the formation of deleterious intracellular ice crystals. A rapid method simply consists of plunging the embryo-container system into liquid nitrogen

($-196°/C$) for immediate vitrification. A slower, more conventional freezing technique uses step-wise controlled cooling. The first step is from room temperature to $-6°$ C, followed by a slower gradual loss of $0.4°$ C per minute until $-35°$ C is reached. Then, a final transfer into liquid nitrogen lowers the temperature to $-196°$ C. After rapid thawing and rehydration by removal of the cryoprotectant, the embryo is placed into a recipient female.

A nontraumatic procedure for *sexing of embryos* is based on the immunological detection of a male cell–specific antigen, termed the H-Y antigen, which is not found on the surface (plasma membrane) of female cells. This immunofluorescence assay is about 80 percent accurate in the early embryos (from the 8-cell stage to the blastocyst stage) of

TABLE 56–6   Classic Chronology of Embryonic Development in Cows

Day	Event	Morphology
0	Estrus	Follicular oocyte
1	Ovulation	1 cell
2	In ampulla	2 cells (blastomeres)
3	In oviduct	4, 8 cells
4	In oviduct	16, 32 cells
5	In uterus	Young morula
6		Compact morula
7		Young blastocyst
8		Blastocyst in expansion
9		Hatching of blastocyst
10		Free blastocyst
11		Elongation is initiated
13		Blastocyst is elongated
14–23		Cardiac beats, beginning of implantation

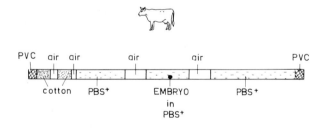

Figure 56–3 A straw (0.25 mL) containing a deep-frozen bovine embryo between two air spaces that are adjacent to columns of phosphate-buffered saline (PBS) with cryoprotectant (glycerol). Polyvinyl caps (PVC) or seals (alcogels of polyvinyl alcohol powder) are present at both ends. One end also carrying a cotton plug that serves as a plunger when the straw is to be emptied of its contents.

cattle, pigs, and sheep and does not affect their survival rate after transfer.

The experimental transfer of nuclei microdissected from embryos into unfertilized oocytes has produced identical ovine or bovine multiplets or genetic clones. The *injection of single cells* of embryos (blastomeres) into the embryonic blastocoele cavity of the same or different animal species has been used to produce *chimeras* (abnormal fetuses with parts of different genetic origin). The development of these nonviable chimeras is of considerable interest in embryology. The introduction of a gene isolated from an animal, and its incorporation into a pronucleus of an embryo, is termed production of *transgenic animals*. Such animals can pass a new trait (e.g., rapid growth, disease resistance) to succeeding generations at a rate of change much faster than by conventional selection or crossing. The transfer of modified growth hormone genes into fish, pigs, rabbits, and sheep is a current theme of research.

Synchronization and Induction of Estrus in Recipient Females

For successful embryo transfer, a synchrony of about 24 hours is necessary between the estrus of the donor and the recipient animals. In ruminant females and in mares, in the presence of an active corpus luteum, the synchronization of estrus is usually obtained by the administration of an analogue of $PGF_{2\alpha}$. The luteolytic eicosanoid induces an estrus within the next 60 to 80 hours in the recipient (but after only 48 hours in the superovulated ruminant donor).

When the phase of the estrous cycle of a normal cow is unknown, and in order to synchronize the appearance of estrus, $PGF_{2\alpha}$ is administered. It obviates problems due to the absence of a functional corpus luteum. Two intramuscular injections are given at an interval of 11 days in cows and goats, of 10 days in ewes, and of 9 days in mares. The last injection in the recipient animals should precede that in the donor animal by about 24 hours.

Placement of the Embryo in the Recipient Female

Before the embryo is deposited, a transrectal examination of the ovaries of the recipient female is indicated to locate the side on which the corpus luteum is developing. The embryo is deposited nonsurgically or surgically in the uterine horn ipsilateral (on the same side) to the corpus luteum.

REFERENCES

Armstrong DT, Evans GL. Factors influencing success of embryo transfer in sheep and goat. Theriogenology 1983;19:31.

Bielanski A, Schneider U, Pawlyshyn VP, Mapletoft RJ. Factors affecting survival of deep frozen bovine embryos in vitro: the effect of freezing container and method of removing cytoprotectant. Theriogenology 1986;25:429.

Elsden RP, Nelson LD, Seidel GE, Jr. Superovulating cows with follicle-stimulating hormone and pregnant mare's serum gonadotrophin. Theriogenology 1978;9:17.

Flint APF, Renfree MB, Weir BJ. Embryonic diapause in mammals. J Reprod Fert 1981; Suppl 29.

Hay JH, Phelps DA, Hanks DR, Foote WD. Sequential uterine horn versus simultaneous total uterine flush to recover bovine embryos nonsurgically. Theriogenology 1990;33:563.

Lindner GM, Wright RW, Jr. Bovine embryo morphology and evaluation. Theriogenology 1983;20:407.

McKelvey WAC, Robinson JJ, Aitken RP, Robertson IS. Repeated recoveries of embryos from ewes by laparoscopy. Theriogenology 1986;25:855.

Pope WF, First NL. Factors affecting the survival of pig embryos. Theriogenology 1985;23:91.

Roberts RM, Schalue-Francis T, Francis H, Keisler D. Maternal recognition of pregnancy and embryonic loss. Theriogenology 1990;33:175.

Saumande J, Procureur R, Chupin D. Effect of injection time of anti-PMSG antiserum on ovulation rate and quality of embryos in superovulated cows. Theriogenology 1984;21:727.

Seidel GE, Jr. Superovulation and embryo transfer in cattle. Science 1981;211:351.

Singh EL. The disease control potential of embryos. Theriogenology 1987;27:9.

Sreenan JM. Embryo transfer: its uses and recent developments. Vet Rec 1988;122:624.

Torres S, Cognie Y, Colas G. Transfer of superovulated sheep embryos obtained with different FSH-P. Theriogenology 1987;27:407.

CHAPTER 57

FETOMATERNAL UNIT OF PREGNANCY

Following intrauterine fixation of the embryo, the placenta maintains a physical contact between the maternal endometrium and the fetus and serves for exchanges between the distinct and separate maternal and fetal circulations. Through its amniotic and allantoic fluids, the placenta also contributes mechanical protection to the fetus. This section presents the physical, biochemical, and neuroendocrine relationships between fetal, placental, and maternal structures.

PLACENTA

Formed from the interaction of the fetal and maternal tissues within the pregnant uterus, the placenta differs from the other organs of the body. Situated outside the body of the fetus, it is a disposable organ, with a limited life span for each animal species. Closely related species have placentas that are functionally and structurally different.

Classification

The various classifications of placentas are based on morphological characteristics such as the shape of the areas of chorionic villi, the histological arrangement of the layers of tissue separating fetal and maternal bloods, and damage to the endometrium at parturition. It is unfortunate that predictions of functions have been made from these structural characteristics, but experimental evidence to correlate the anatomical classifications to the functional interpretation is yet to come, since the placenta is relatively inaccessible for physiological studies in its natural site. For convenience, and to recall the concepts, these anatomical classifications are briefly reviewed.

On the basis of the shape of the area or the distribution of the chorionic villi over the endometrial surface or the fetal membranes, four main placental types are recognized: diffuse; cotyledonary, or multiplex; zonary; and discoid (Fig. 57-1).

In the *diffuse* placenta, most of the chorionic surface is covered with small villi or folds corresponding to depressions or sulci in the endometrium (e.g., camels, mares, sows). The *cotyledonary*, or *multiplex*, placenta has chorionic villi restricted to a number of well-defined circular or oval areas, called *cotyledons*, that overlie similar specialized uterine areas, known as *caruncles*. *Placentomes* are placental units made by the union of fetal cotyledons and uterine caruncles. The usual number of cotyledons is 85 in cows and ewes, 170 in goats, and only six in reindeer. The *zonary* placenta has villi aggre-

gated into a band, completely (cats, dogs) or incompletely (brown bears, ferrets, mink, polar bears, and raccoon) encircling the middle of the chorionic sac. Marginal effusions of maternal blood are found between the uterus and placenta in the cat (brown border) and the dog (green border). Central effusion is seen in the ferret, the mink, and the raccoon. A *discoid* placenta is found in guinea pigs, mice, primates, rabbits, and rats.

Although much debated, but still used for reasons of convenience, another morphological classification relies on the presence or absence of cell layers in the fetomaternal unit. The *epitheliochorial* placenta seen in horses, pigs, and ruminants has a complete set (three maternal and three fetal layers) of layers (Fig. 57-2).

The *endotheliochorial* placenta, with three fetal but only two maternal layers (loss of maternal epithelium) is found in most carnivores (Fig. 57-3). The *hemochorial* placenta, without any maternal layers but retaining the three fetal layers, occurs in primates, rabbits, and rodents.

A gynecological system considering the endometrial damage at birth classifies a placenta as *deciduate* if the chorion carries a substantial amount of maternal tissue in the third phase of parturition, expulsion of the fetal membranes. A *nondeciduate* or *adeciduate* placenta does not damage the endometrium at parturition.

Arrangement of Fetal Membranes

The fetal membranes, amnion and allantois, are arranged differently in the animal species (Fig. 57-4). The placenta is totally chorioallantoic in mares and mostly so in ruminants and sows, in which a part of the chorion is fused with the amnion. The chorioallantoic placenta is supplied with fetal blood through the allantoic vessels.

Placental Circulation

Ewes and goats are the classic animals for studies of the fetal placental circulation and maternal placental circulation. These two separate placental circulations are coupled to the umbilical artery or vein in lambs, and to the uterine artery or vein in ewes. Over 95 percent of the umbilical blood flow goes through the fetal placental circulation, and 85 percent of the uterine blood flow does likewise in the ewe's maternal placental circulation. An even greater proportion of both uterine and umbilical blood passes through the mare's placenta. Fetal placental capillaries are present in all animal species. Maternal placental capillaries, absent in the species

CLASSIFICATION OF PLACENTA

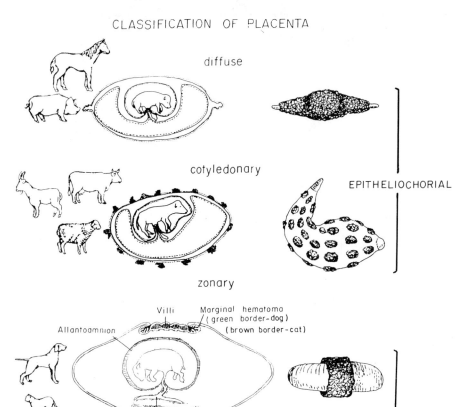

Figure 57–1 Animal species with the disposition of the various membranes inside the chorion; their type of placenta according to distribution of chorionic villi: diffuse, cotyledonary, zonary, and discoid (not represented); and the histological classification according to the number of layers of tissue between the maternal and fetal erythrocytes.

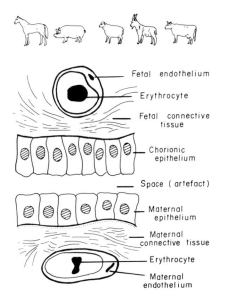

Figure 57–2 Diagrammatic representation of the epitheliochorial placenta (the most common in large animals) with six layers of tissue separating the maternal and fetal erythrocytes, i.e., maternal endothelium, connective tissue, and epithelium; and chorionic epithelium and fetal connective tissue and endothelium.

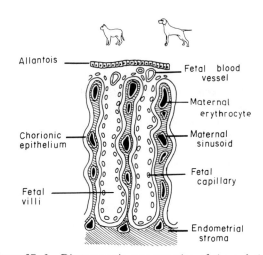

Figure 57–3 Diagrammatic representation of the endotheliochorial placenta in which the maternal endothelium is absent, and maternal erythrocytes are in sinusoids within the maternal connective tissue.

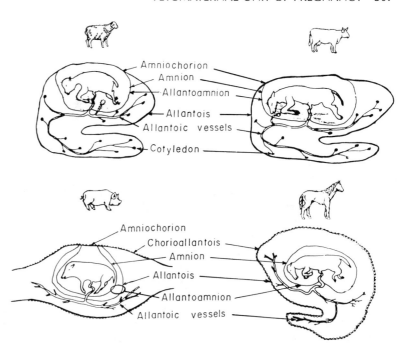

Figure 57–4 Disposition and connections of the various membranes (allantoamnion) containing the amniotic and allantoic fluids, and their adhesion to the most superficial membrane of the placenta (chorion) to form the amniochorion (cows, ewes, sows) or the chorioallantois (mares) sheets.

with hemochorial placenta, have a different arrangement in the epitheliochorial placenta of ewes and mares. The chorionic villi of the mare penetrate depressions in the endometrium known as microcotyledons, which are several times smaller than the smallest ruminant cotyledons or placentomes. In cows, mares, rabbits, and sheep, blood in the maternal and fetal placental circulations moves in opposite directions, creating a countercurrent system most effective for gaseous exchanges.

Blood flow in the fetal placental circulation varies widely according to the size of the conceptus. Most of the blood reaches the cotyledons in lambs, whereas only a minor part (5 percent) is distributed to the intercotyledonary areas. Even if measurements of uterine artery blood volume flow are unreliable in pregnant ewes, it seems that 1 month before full term is reached, 84 percent of the total uterine blood flows to the placentomes, 13 percent to the endometrium (intercotyledonary areas, or paraplacenta), and 3 percent to the myometrium. Total uterine blood flow increases progressively throughout gestation, and at full term 17 percent of the maternal cardiac output goes to the uterus. During labor, uterine blood flow decreases according to the intensity of each myometrial contraction. The flow rate recovers and returns to precontraction levels during uterine diastole. During intense contractions, as recovery is incomplete, uterine blood flow is almost stopped and entails a risk of anoxia for the fetus. After detachment and expulsion of the placenta, uterine blood flow falls sharply as the vascular resistance increases ten times over that of the pregnant uterus.

Transplacental Transport of Substances

The placental transfer of nutrients toward the fetal circulation and of excretory products into the maternal blood is directed by the usual processes of diffusion and of active transport. Carbon dioxide, electrolytes, hormones, oxygen, and water move freely between the maternal and fetal placental circulations by simple diffusion gradients (i.e., from a high concentration to a lower concentration). Substances such as amino acids, glucides, and minerals transfer from areas of low concentration to areas of high concentration by active transport (i.e., with energy expenditure).

The placenta functions as the fetal lungs. In ruminants, the principal sites of gas exchange are the placentomes. Experimental maternal placental circulation hyperoxia (PO_2 above 100 torr) scarcely affects the oxygen level in the ruminant fetal circulation but raises the fetal PO_2 above the maternal levels in mares. However, maternal placental circulation hypoxia (PO_2 below 100 torr) slightly decreases fetal placental circulation oxygenation in calves, foals, and lambs. Ovine and caprine fetal and maternal blood gas levels (PO_2, PCO_2), pH, and hematocrit remain stable during the last third of pregnancy and even during the first stage of labor (cervical dilation).

A transplacental gradient of 20 torr exists normally between the PO_2 levels in the ruminant maternal and fetal veins, whereas in mares the difference is only 2 to 4 torr. The PCO_2 gradient across the placenta is small in both ruminants and mares, about 3 to 4 torr in ruminants and even less in mares. The importance of these gaseous partial pressure gradients may be related to the presence, in late gestation, of greater distances between arterial and venous capillaries in ewes than in mares.

The placenta is an efficient barrier against the transfer of bacteria and viruses. However, some microorganisms can cross the fetal-placental-maternal complex. Examples of such invaders include *Brucella canis*, *Listeria*, *Mycobacterium paratuberculosis*, *Mycobacterium tuberculosis*, *Salmonella*, *Streptococcus*, bovine rhinotracheitis virus, equine and ovine abortion virus, canine herpesvirus, canine distemper virus, and virus of infectious canine hepatitis. The scrapie agent occurs in the placenta of an infected ewe, but the fetus is not always infected. The following parasites can also pass through the placental barrier: *Ancylostoma caninum, Dirofilaria immitis, Neoascaris vitulorum, Strongyloides ransomi, Strongyloides westeri, Toxocara canis,* and *Toxoplasma gondii.*

Placental Endocrine Function

From fertilization to implantation, the ovaries produce the *progesterone* required for maintenance of gestation. In most animals, except cats and dogs, stimuli from the endometrium and the trophoblast exert a luteotrophic effect on the corpus luteum of estrus and assist in its transformation into a structure of pregnancy. The ovaries of dogs, goats, mice, pigs, and rabbits secrete progesterone throughout pregnancy and are essential for maintenance of gestation. The placenta can supplement, or can replace before parturition, the progesterone production of the corpus luteum in cats, cows, guinea pigs, horses, and sheep. In sows, the placental production of progesterone is not enough to maintain gestation after ovariectomy. In cows, the placenta is able to convert progesterone into estrogens, but the placenta in ewes, sows, and mares is unable to do so.

In mares, during the initial half of pregnancy, the high level of progesterone is provided originally from the corpus luteum of ovulation, and afterwards by secondary luteinized follicles. The ovaries of mares are stimulated to produce a series of accessory ovulations, each followed by a corpus luteum (or luteinized follicle) secreting the indispensable progesterone during the first half of gestation. After implantation, the equine *fetoplacental unit* becomes an endocrine organ and a source of steroid (*5-alpha-pregnanes, estrogens*) and protein hormones. During most of the second half of pregnancy, the maternal progesterone level is low, but the fetoplacental unit produces metabolites (progestins) of pro-

gesterone (5-alpha-pregnanes) rather than progesterone. About 2 weeks before parturition, a surge of progestins and progesterone occurs in mares (see Fig. 57–6A).

In most species, secretion of *estrogens* by the placenta usually begins only after the first fifth or quarter of the gestation. From about the eighth week of gestation, the placenta of the mare produces not only the classic estrogens (estrone, 17-alpha-estradiol, and 17-beta-estradiol) but also the unusual estrogens equilenin and equilin (Fig. 57–5), and all are excreted in the urine. The excretion of estrogens at midterm and near parturition is a reflection of correspondingly high plasma concentrations of estrone. In cows and ewes, plasma estrogens remain stable throughout gestation and peak only just before parturition. By contrast, in goats, estrogens increase constantly, reaching levels comparable with those in sows and mares a few days before full term is reached.

Pregnant mare serum gonadotropin (PMSG), also known as *equine chorionic gonadotropin* (eCG), is secreted by the endometrial cups in the fetal part of the placenta, in high concentrations during the first half of gestation. PMSG is a unique glycoprotein molecule having both follicle-stimulating hormone (FSH) and luteinizing hormone (LH) activities at a ratio of 10:1 to 30:1. A single injection of PMSG induces follicular growth and ovulation in domesticated animals (except mares, which only respond to equine adenohypophysial extract and to FSH-rich human menopausal gonadotropin [hMG]). PMSG is widely used in embryo transfer to produce superovulation (larger than normal number of ovulations, multiple ovulations) in donor females and to increase the harvest of fertilized ova.

Human chorionic gonadotropin (hCG), which is widely used in veterinary medicine for its luteinizing activity, is produced by the trophoblast very soon after implantation and may be detected in the urine. *Placental lactogens* (PL), secreted by bovine, caprine, and ovine placentae throughout pregnancy but not found in the plasma a few days before

CLASSIC   ESTROGENS

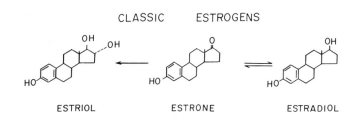

ESTRIOL   ESTRONE   ESTRADIOL

UNUSUAL ESTROGENS

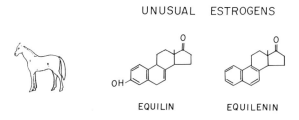

EQUILIN   EQUILENIN

PLACENTAL   ESTROGENS   IN THE URINE   OF THE MARE

Figure 57–5 Structure of the classic estrogens estrone, estradiol, and estriol and of the unusual estrogens unique to the pregnant members of Equidae, equilin and equilenin.

parturition, play a role in the mammary gland growth of ewes and goats but not cows.

Profiles of Hormones in Maternal Plasma during Gestation

Plasma concentrations and secretory patterns of steroid and protein hormones in the plasma of pregnant females vary greatly among and within animal species. Profiles during gestation of the major steroids, progesterone and estrogens, can be sketched for easy comparison in large animals (Fig. 57–6) and in small animals (Fig. 57–7).

Other hormones found in the maternal plasma near parturition are oxytocin, prolactin, PGF, and relaxin. The appearance of PGF in the maternal plasma is preceded by an increase in the corticosteroid levels of the fetal plasma (Fig. 57–8). The levels of relaxin, secreted by the maternal ovary, peak on the day before parturition, while prolactin reaches it maximum concentration at parturition.

AMNIOTIC AND ALLANTOIC FLUIDS

The *amniotic fluid* immediately surrounding the fetus is opalescent as a result of sebum in suspension, straw-colored, and slightly mucoid (saliva and nasopharyngeal secretions). The fetus bathes in a fluid environment similar to a serum ultrafiltrate with a pH on the acidic side of neutrality. It contains desquamated fetal skin cells and leukocytes. By amniocentesis (transvaginal aspiration of amniotic fluid) at days 8 to 120, fetal amniotic cells may be used for prenatal detection of sex and cytogenetic defects in cattle. During gestation, surfactant (dipalmitoyl lecithin) from the developing respiratory tract is added (day 100 in mares) to the amniotic fluid. Tints of meconium (black, brown, or greenish brown), when they are present, indicate the occurrence of fetal stress (anoxia) at some time during gestation. The volume of amniotic fluid surrounding the fetus is 3 to 7 L in horses.

Amniotic plaques or pustules, glycogen-rich local accumulations of ectoderm, are found in cows, horses (day 70), and sheep. These yellowish-white, angular elevations occur mostly on the inner amnion covering the umbilical cord and, to a lesser extent, on the inner surface of the remainder of the amnion. In both cows and sheep, the umbilical cord lies exclusively within the amniotic cavity.

The amniotic fluid has physical and physiological roles. It physically protects the fetus from jolts associated with maternal activity, and it keeps the fetal environment at a constant temperature. It also gives relative freedom of movement to the floating fetus without hindrance from or damage to the amnion. Physiologically, the amniotic fluid is related primarily to fetal nutrition. Exchanges of fluids and solutes occur in the respiratory tract. Also, swallowed amniotic fluid, once it is absorbed by the digestive tract, supplies lipids, essential amino acids, and growth-promoting vitamins (pantothenic, folic acids) to intracellular and extracellular fluids. Small amounts of antibodies are concentrated in

the fetal rat gut by removal of water. Amniotic fluid contributes to the formation of *meconium* (i.e., the mucilaginous material in the intestine of the full-term fetus).

The allantoic sac, a thin-walled sac connected to the fetal bladder by the urachus, is filled with watery (serous) *allantoic fluid.* As gestation progresses, the composition of allantoic fluid steadily increases in electrolytes, total nitrogen, and volume. Near parturition, allantoic fluid volumes are 8 to 18 L in horses, 8 to 15 L in cattle, and about 100 mL per piglet in sows. Its color varies from a clear yellow in early pregnancy to a turbid yellowish-brown or brown near full term. Allantoic fluid contains desquamated epithelium and testosterone.

In cattle, the testosterone contents of allantoic fluid is used for early detection of the fetal sex. The fetus is likely to be male if the testosterone level is more than 320 pg per milliliter; if it is less than 240 pg per milliliter, the fetus is a female.

In horses, the allantoic sac contains (1) small allantoic vesicles or peduncles, that is, pedunculated invaginations of the allantoic membrane; (2) allantochorionic pouches, which are pedunculated invaginations of the chorioallantois containing within their lumen a greenish-brown substance of putty-like consistency; and (3) usually a single hippomane ("colt's tongue"). Occasionally, hippomanes (allantoic calculi) are found in the allantoic fluid of cattle and sheep. *Hippomanes* are amber-colored or mottled-brown, amorphous, flattened, irregularly shaped, pliable, rubber-like, semisolid soft masses or bodies with thin edges, 2.5 to 15 cm in diameter and 0.3 to 3.8 cm in thickness. In fact, they are allantoic calculi consisting of a central nucleus of cell debris surrounded by concentric layers of material deposited from the allantoic fluid.

DETECTION OF PREGNANCY

Early detection of gestation is important in preventing any delay in rebreeding, which results in additional feed and labor expenses, and decreases revenue from milk or progeny. Detection of gestation is accomplished by direct methods, where the conceptus or its environment are examined, and by indirect methods, which evaluate signals from the conceptus and their maternal effects. *Direct methods* include transrectal exploration of the uterus, laparoscopy and laparotomy, radiography, ultrasound, and fetal electrocardiography. *Indirect methods* involve estrus observation, vaginal biopsy, vaginal smears, pregnancy-specific or pregnancy-associated proteins, $PGF_{2\alpha}$, progesterone, and estrone sulfate and total estrogens.

Explorative Palpation of Reproductive Tract

After removal of fecal material, *transrectal palpation* of the cervix, the uterus and its contents, the ovaries, and the uterine blood vessels is the method of choice for pregnancy

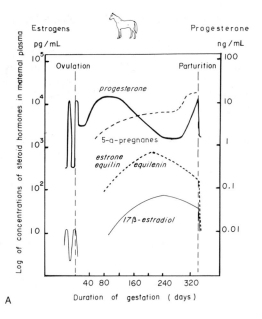

A

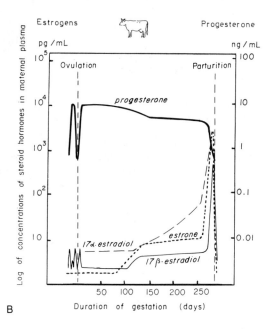

B

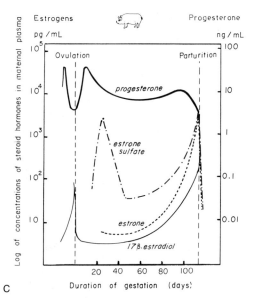

C

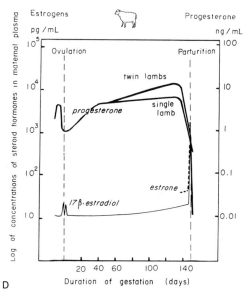

D

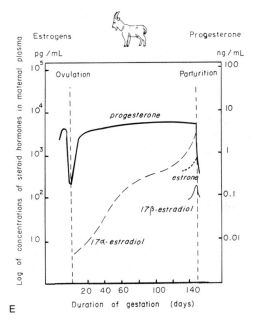

E

Figure 57–6 Profiles of the plasma levels of progesterone, and of estrogens, during the gestation of large animals. (**A**, Mare; **B**, cow; **C**, sow; **D**, ewe; and **E**, goat.)

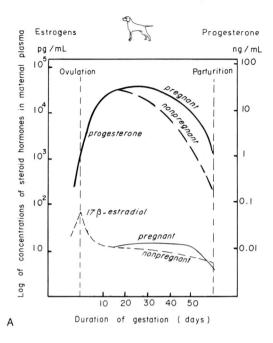

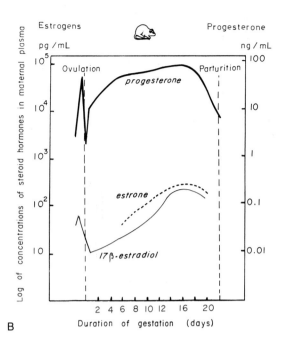

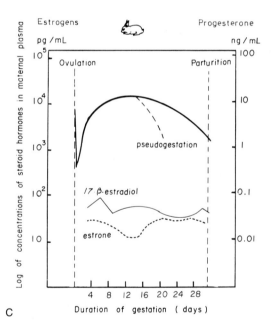

Figure 57–7 Profiles of the levels of plasma progesterone and estrogens during the gestation of small animals. **A,** Bitch; **B,** rat; and **C,** rabbit.

diagnosis and for estimation of the duration of pregnancy in cows. It can be used also in horses, pigs, and water buffaloes.

The accuracy of the transrectal palpation method depends on a methodical approach, proper anatomical orientation, and the skill of the operator in evaluating the different structures in relation to gestation. Palpation of the bovine corpus luteum (CL) is 90 percent accurate at 21 to 24 days after breeding. "Rolling up" the cow's uterus to palpate and to grasp gently the fluid-filled horn, and feeling the chorioallantois and then the uterine wall *slip* between the thumb and forefinger, are possible at 30 to 35 days after breeding. As the bovine gestation progresses, the increased pulse (at 40

to 60 days), the fremitus or thrill (at 3 to 4 months), and the size of the middle uterine arteries in relation to the fingers (6 months = auricular finger; 7 months = major finger; 8 + months = thumb) may be noticed.

A modified *rectal-abdominal*, or *rectoabdominal*, palpation, using a rectal probe, is applied to ewes and goats. With the animal in dorsal recumbency, a well-lubricated 50-cm plastic rod is inserted 35 cm into the rectum, and its tip is moved in an arc from the spine toward the abdominal wall, on each side. From 70 days, the gravid uterus, cranial to the pubis, can be palpated with the other hand. If the animal is not pregnant, the end of the rod is palpated instead.

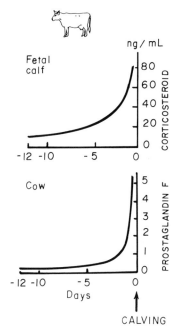

Figure 57–8 Correlation between the increase in fetal corticosteroid and that in maternal prostaglandin during the few days preceding parturition (calving) in the cow.

Abdominal palpation for detection of pregnancy can be performed in bitches, queens, ewes and goats. In bitches, abdominal palpation is done with the animal in a standing position, by grasping the abdomen gently as if one were holding a football. By applying steady pressure upward and then gently bringing the fingers together, the abdominal viscera will slip through the fingers, and the pregnant uterus is detectable from day 18 to day 28 of gestation. Diagnosis of feline pregnancy is improbable prior to day 14. The optimum period is between days 17 and 21, and after 50 days the fetal head of the kitten is the most prominent feature palpated. In small ruminants, abdominal palpation is performed by standing behind the female and attempting to touch both hands together through her body. Another method is to encircle the abdomen and lift it upward. Ballottement in the lower right flank is also used. A fetus can be detected near 100 days, and fetal movements observed in the right flank a month before full term.

Digital palpation of the cervix can be applied to the standing goat by inserting one or two sterile, lubricated, gloved fingers into the vagina after cleansing the vulva. The nonpregnant anestrous cervix projects into the vagina and is very firm and conical with distinct folds. After day 30 of gestation, the cervix begins to soften. After 50 days, the weight of the gravid uterus pulls the soft cervix forward and over the brim of the pelvis, where it remains out of reach.

Laparoscopy, Laparotomy, and Radiology

Laparoscopy or peritoneoscopy has been used in cows, ewes, queens, bitches, and several other animals. The technique requires local anesthesia or tranquilization, a laparoscope inserted through a trocar cannula, and Verres's needle probes (calibrated in millimeters) traversing the skin to reach the abdomen laterally to the trocar. In large animals (ewes, cows), abdominal insufflation with 5 percent carbon dioxide in air or nitrogen allows more rapid location of the uterus and ovaries and forces intestinal structures away from the pelvic inlet. Gestation status is determined by the degree of distention of the uterus and by the vascularization pattern.

With the patient under local or general anesthesia, through paramedian (ewe) or midline (goat) *laparotomy* just anterior to the udder, digital (2 or 3 fingers) palpation of the uterus, placenta, fetus, and ovaries is possible after 42 days of gestation.

Radiographic pregnancy diagnosis has been used in queens (38 days), bitches (42 days), ewes and goats (70 days), and rarely in sows.

Ultrasonic Methods

Instruments for ultrasonic pregnancy detection are based either on the amplitude-depth technique or on the Doppler technique.

The *amplitude-depth technique* (also called the A-mode, B-mode, pulse mode, echo pulse technique, or real-time ultrasound echography with multicrystal scanner probe) may be compared with a ship searching for fish or a submarine by sonar. When a target is spotted, a "blip" (trace, or echo) shows up on the scope and gives an indication of its distance from the transabdominal or intrarectal emitting and receiving device. The fluid-surrounded fetus produces a characteristic trace on the right half of the scope's screen (static transducer) or an image that can be frame-frozen on the scope (scanner) for study or photography (Fig. 57–9).

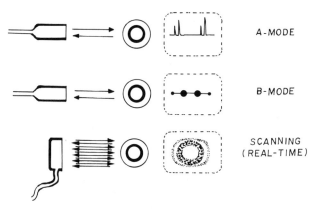

Figure 57–9 Types of ultrasonic probes used for echography of pregnant reproductive tracts. The configuration of the A-mode and B-mode probes limits their use to the transabdominal approach, whereas the real-time probe can be used for both transabdominal and transrectal techniques.

The method is efficient from day 14 of gestation in mares (scanner), day 22 (with scanner) or day 30 (with a static sensor) in sows, day 29 in bitches, day 55 in cows, and day 60 in ewes and goats. Intrarectal real-time ultrasonic echography has been used to detect twinning in mares after 2 weeks of gestation, and in ewes and goats after 35 days of gestation.

The *Doppler technique* detects the faster fetal pulse or blood circulation by a change in the frequency of an emitted sound wave detected by a transducer placed intrarectally. It provides definite evidence that the fetus is alive and also indicates multiple pregnancies. It is efficient from day 25 in sows, day 55 in goats, day 56 in mares, day 60 in ewes (more than 200 cardiac pulsations per minute), and day 80 in cows.

Fetal Electrocardiography

From electrodes on the maternal body surface, fetal electrocardiograms may be obtained in mares, cows, ewes, and goats (50 days).

Observation for Estrus

In farm animals, estrus is normally absent during gestation. Estrus with ovulation may occur in mares, and exceptionally in sows. Occasionally, pregnant cows (2 to 6 percent) and ewes exhibit sexual receptivity (estrus behavior without ovulation) that is associated with excessive estrogen production by the corpus luteum of pregnancy. As a rule, observation of estrus at intervals corresponding to the length of the estrous cycle (i.e., 17 days in ewes or 21 days in cows, sows, buffalo, goats, mares) after service or artificial insemination indicates the absence of gestation.

In sows, intramuscular injection of a mixture of testosterone (500 mg) and estradiol (200 mg) on day 21 following breeding stimulates hypothalamic secretion of gonadotropin-releasing hormone (GnRH) and of adenohypophysial gonadotropins (FSH and LH) in 2 to 4 days. Signs of estrus and ovulation occur in nonpregnant sows, which may be rebred immediately, but the absence of such signs in gravid sows confirms gestation.

Vaginal Biopsy and Vaginal Smears

Vaginal biopsy for pregnancy diagnosis can be performed at the interval of a normal estrous cycle (21 days in pigs and 17 days in sheep). The result of a vaginal biopsy test is positive when the sample from the dorsocranial epithelium (5 cm caudad to the cervix) shows two to four cell layers parallel to the basal membrane (instead of one in the nonpregnant animal). Near the end of gestation, the high levels of estrogens increase vaginal epithelium thickness to as many as 20 to 25 cell layers in sows, and 10 to 12 in ewes.

Cytological examination of *vaginal smears* for gestation testing is reported to be efficient in sows (days 22 to 60) and in ewes (days 23 to 146).

Pregnancy-Specific or Pregnancy-Associated Proteins

Proteins (hormones or not) of placental, fetal, or maternal origin such as equine chorionic gonadotropin (eCG) or pregnant mare serum gonadotropin (PMSG), pregnancy-specific antigen, early pregnancy factor (EPF), and placental lactogen (PL) are used for gestation testing.

PMSG, or eCG, of placental origin (the endometrial cups), is detectable in the mare's blood plasma between days 35 to 40 and 130 of gestation, by methods based on bioassay and immunoassay.

Bioassay methods include the Aschheim-Zondek test (A-Z) on a sexually immature mouse or rat, Friedman's test on a sexually immature rabbit, and the Galli-Mainini test on the male frog (fastest). The A-Z mouse or rat test requires a subcutaneous injection (0.5 mL) of the test serum in two animals, which are killed by chloroform or ether after 48 hours. By comparison with two control animals, criteria for a positive test result are a five-fold increase in uterine volume; ovaries with mature, hemorrhagic, or luteinized follicles; and tumefaction of vagina and vulva. Friedman's rabbit test uses 15 mL of test serum injected intravenously into a sexually immature rabbit, which is laparotomized 48 hours later. The rabbit test uses the same criteria as the A-Z test: hemorrhagic or luteinized follicles and uterine hypertrophy. The male frog test demands an injection of the test serum into the lymphatic dorsal sac; collection (by pipette) of urine at the cloaca after 4 to 6 hours; and microscopic examination of the urine for spermatozoa, which may be colored with 1 percent methylene blue.

Immunoassay methods for PMSG include immunochemical or immunoelectrophoretic determination of as little as 1 IU, hemagglutination inhibition, direct latex agglutination (DLA), radioreceptor assay (RA), and radioimmunoassay (RIA). As a field test, giving accurate results within a few hours, the hemagglutination inhibition is outstanding (PMSG inhibiting agglutination of PMSG-coated sheep erythrocytes in the presence of PMSG-antiserum for rabbits). Rapid microenzymoimmunoassays or microELISAs (enzyme-linked immunosorbent assays) of PMSG or eCG with monoclonal or polyclonal antibody seem promising for easy detection of early pregnancy.

A *pregnancy-specific antigen* of fetal origin has been detected, by immunoagglutination of heterogenous erythrocytes, in the maternal plasma a few days after conception. It has been reported in mares (day 6), ewes (day 8), cows (day 14), and sows (day 17).

Early pregnancy factor (EPF), produced by the ovaries and the oviduct, is considered to play an important role in the maternal nonrejection of the conceptus. It has been found in the maternal circulation within a few hours after mating in sows (4 hours), cows, and ewes (24 hours). EPF is detected by inhibition of the rosette formation between lymphocytes and heterologous erythrocytes, which is the very tedious, time-consuming, and complicated rosette-inhibition test (RIT). The RIT might be helpful in embryo transfer to select viable embryos and monitor the successful outcome of the procedure.

Placental lactogen (PL) has been detected by RIA in ewes (after day 64), in cows (after day 160), and goats (during late pregnancy). Elevated maternal plasma concentrations of this mammotrophic, lactogenic, and growth-promoting protein are related to multiple gestation.

Prostaglandin F$_{2\alpha}$

Measured by RIA, a PGF metabolite (PGFM, or 15-keto-13,14-dihydro-PGF$_{2\alpha}$) in maternal plasma has been proposed as an early pregnancy test in sows (day 14 or 15) and mares (day 15). Gestation is confirmed when the maternal plasma levels of PGFM are near the limit of detection and are not pulsatile, in sharp contrast with the high and pulsatile PGFM levels that occur during the luteal phase of the estrous cycle.

Progesterone Concentration in Plasma or in Milk

Early pregnancy testing by RIA measurements of progesterone in blood samples is used in all farm animals (cows, beef cows, sows, buffalo, mares, ewes, goats). Between day 18 and day 23 after insemination, the plasma progesterone values in nongravid and gravid animals are as follows:

	Nongravid Level	Gravid Level
Cow	0.5 ng/mL	>2 ng/mL
Ewe	<0.5 ng/mL	>1.5 ng/mL
Goat*	<0.5 ng/mL	>4 ng/mL
Mare	0.5 ng/mL	>2 ng/mL
Sow	0.5 ng/mL	9 ng/mL

In milk and milkfat samples taken during days 23 to 24, the progesterone contents in nongravid and gravid cows are as follows:

	Nongravid Level	Gravid Level
Milk	8 ng/mL	>11 ng/mL
Milkfat	<1 ng/mL	>1 ng/mL

A positive correlation between plasma progesterone content and multiple pregnancies is reported in cows and in ewes; in the latter, each nanogram per milliliter above 2 ng per milliliter represents an additional lamb.

As an alternative to the laboratory RIA of hormones, the enzyme immunoassay (EIA) techniques are being developed for their potential use as "on the farm" tests for pregnancy diagnosis. *EIA for progesterone,* with results observed by the naked eye, has been tested in milk, milkfat, and blood plasma of cows, and in the plasma of pigs and water buffaloes.

Levels of Estrone Sulfate and Total Estrogens in Plasma, Milk, Urine, and Feces

Conjugated estrone sulfate (E$_1$S) has been measured, usually by RIA, in the blood plasma, milk, urine, and feces of various pregnant farm animals. Levels adequate for positive pregnancy testing have been found in the urine and the plasma of sows at days 24 to 32; in the milk and plasma of goats at day 50; in the plasma and feces of mares at day 105; in the plasma, milk, and feces of cows after days 105 to 112; and in the plasma of buffalo during late pregnancy.

An enzyme immunoassay (EIA) for estrone sulfate is being developed for pregnancy testing of pig plasma. A liquid-phase EIA for E$_1$S is accurate at days 22 to 27, whereas a solid-phase EIA for E$_1$S gives valid results at days 25 to 31 after mating.

Total estrogens in the urine of pregnant mares can also be qualitatively identified between the fourth and ninth months of gestation with the *Cuboni* test (*Cuboni reaction*). The basis of the test is that estrogens treated with sulfuric acid develop a green fluorescence. When the test is negative, the urine–sulfuric acid mixture is colored burgundy-red. To perform this simple and inexpensive procedure,

1. Mix 15 mL of filtered urine with 3 mL of concentrated HCl,
2. Heat the mixture over boiling water for 10 minutes,
3. Cool, filter, and place it in a separation flask,
4. Add 18 mL of benzol, and shake it well,
5. Purge the urine, and add 10 mL of concentrated sulfuric acid,
6. Shake it well, collect the acid in a test tube, and heat it at 80° C for 10 minutes,
7. Cool the tube under tap water,
8. Observe it for green fluorescence (positive result) or for a burgundy color (negative result) under a Wood's lamp or indirect lighting.

In pregnant cows, mostly because of an elevation in the levels of conjugated estrogen (sulfate), the plasma levels of total estrogens increase slightly from day 100 to day 220. During the last month of gestation (days 250 to 280), the levels of total estrogens rise from 11 to 30 ng/mL in cows with one fetus, from 14 to 45 ng/mL with twins, and from 15 to 161 ng/mL with triplets.

REFERENCES

Abbitt B, Ball L, Kitto GP, et al. Effect of three methods of palpation for pregnancy diagnosis per rectum on embryonic and fetal attrition in cows. J Am Vet Med Assoc 1978;173:973.

Allen WR. Aspects of early embryonic development in farm animals. Proc Int Congr Anim Rep AI 1984;10:XIII-1.

Allen WE, Meredith MJ. Detection of pregnancy in the bitch: a study of abdominal palpation, A-mode ultrasound and Doppler ultrasound techniques. J Small Anim Pract 1981;22:609.

Cameron RDA. Pregnancy diagnosis in the sow by rectal examination. Aust Vet J 1977;53:432.

Chaplin VM, Holdsworth RJ. Oestrone sulphate in goat's milk. Vet Rec 1982;111:224.

Concannon PW, Hansel W, Visek WJ. The ovarian cycle in the bitch: plasma estrogen, LH, and progesterone. Biol Reprod 1975;13:112.

Davidson AP, Nyland TG, Tsutsui T. Pregnancy diagnosis with ultrasound in the domestic cat. Vet Radiol 1986;27:109.

Findlay JK. Blastocyst-endometrial interactions in early pregnancy in the sheep. J Reprod Fertil (Suppl) 1981;30:171.

Fukui Y, Kimura T, Ono H. Multiple pregnancy diagnosis in sheep using an ultrasonic Doppler method. Vet Rec 1984;114:145.

Godkin JD, Bazer FW, Moffatt RJ, et al. Purification and properties of a major low molecular weight protein released by the trophoblast of sheep blastocysts at day 13 to 21. J Reprod Fertil 1982;65:141.

Holtan DW, Nett TM, Estergreen VL. Plasma progestins in pregnant, post partum and cycling mares. J Anim Sci 1975;40:251.

Holtan DW, Squires EL, Lapin DR, Ginther OJ. Effect of ovariectomy on pregnancy in mares. J Reprod Fertil (Suppl) 1979;27:457.

Hunt B, Lein DH, Foote RH. Monitoring of plasma and milk progesterone for evaluation of postpartum estrous cycles and early pregnancy in mares. J Am Vet Med Assoc 1978;172:1298.

Inaba T, Nakazima Y, Matsui N, Imori T. Early pregnancy diagnosis in sows by ultrasonic linear electronic scanning. Theriogenology 1983;20:97.

Jackson GH. Pregnancy diagnosis in the sow by real-time ultrasonic scanning. Vet Rec 1986;119:90.

Madel AJ. Detection of pregnancy in ewe lambs by A-mode ultrasound. Vet Rec 1983;112:11.

Martal J, Lacroix MC, Lourdis C, et al. Trophoblastin, an antiluteolytic protein present in early pregnancy in sheep. J Reprod Fertil 1979;56:63.

Moss GE, Estergreen VL, Becker SR, Grant BD. Source of the 5-alpha-pregnanes that occur during gestation in mares. J Reprod Fertil 1979;Suppl 27.

Pierson RA, Ginther OJ. Ultrasonography of the bovine ovary. Theriogenology 1984;21:495.

Plant JW. Pregnancy diagnosis in sheep using a rectal probe. Vet Rec 1980;106:305.

Reeves JJ, Rantanen NW, Hauser M. Transrectal real-time ultrasound scanning of the cow reproductive tract. Theriogenology 1984;21:485.

Reimers TJ, Phemister RD, Niswender GD. Radioimmunological measurement of follicle-stimulating hormone and prolactin in the dog. Biol Reprod 1978;19:673.

Robertson HA, King GJ, Dyck GW. The appearance of estrone sulphate in the peripheral plasma of the pig early in pregnancy. J Reprod Fertil 1978;52:337.

Stabenfeldt GH. Physiologic, pathologic and therapeutic roles of progestins in domestic animals. J Am Vet Med Assoc 1974;164:311.

Tainturier D, Moysan F. Diagnostic de gestation chez la chienne par échotomographie. Revue de Med Vet 1984;135:525.

Van de Wiel DFM. Evaluation of pregnancy status. Proc Int Congr Anim Reprod AI 1984;10:X-26.

Verhage HG, Beamer NB, Brenner RM. Plasma levels of estradiol and progesterone in the cat during polyestrus, pregnancy and pseudopregnancy. Biol Reprod 1976;14:579.

Voss JL, Villahoz MD, Squires EL. Comparison of diagnostic tests for early pregnancy detection in mares. Proc Int Congr Anim Rep AI 1984;10:99.

White IR, Russel AJF, Fowler DG. Real-time ultrasonic scanning in the diagnosis of pregnancy and the determination of fetal numbers in sheep. Vet Rec 1984;115:140.

CHAPTER 58

PARTURITION

Parturition is the process of expelling each fetus and its placenta from the uterus. A complicated process, it ends gestation and starts lactation in the mother, while it marks the beginning of an independent existence for one (in uniparous animals) or several offspring (in multiparous animals).

Normal parturition involves endocrinological, mechanical, and behavioral factors from maternal and fetal origins (Fig. 58–1). The complexity of interaction among these factors is made more difficult by important differences existing among animal species.

Observations made on domestic animals do not lead to generalized extrapolations, as exemplified by the following:
1. Foaling is manifestly a more painful process than farrowing,
2. Maternal progesterone and estrogen profiles are quite different at foaling and at lambing,
3. The bitch and the sow readily accept foster offspring, whereas the ewe and the doe reject even their own offspring unless they are able to lick them immediately after delivery,
4. Duration of parturition is longer in primigravid (first gestation) then in multigravid (nth gestation) females.

SIGNS OF IMPENDING PARTURITION

Cow and Mare

In large animals such as cows and mares, the main criteria to consider are mammary development, secretion of colostrum, and relaxation of the pelvic ligaments. *Enlargement of the udder* begins during the fourth month of gestation in heifers, whereas it may not show until 2 or 3 weeks before labor in cows. Mares at full term present edema of the udder and of the ventral body wall, and a substantial increase in size of the two mammary glands.

Just prior to calving, the sticky serum that can be discharged from the udder is replaced by *colostrum,* a fluid that is thick, yellowish, and opaque. In mares, mammary secretions pass from a straw or an amber color, to a cloudy straw color in the weeks preceding foaling, and then to yellow or yellowish-white and become viscous. In most mares, colostrum dries as beads of wax at the end of each teat 1 to 4 days before parturition.

A slight *relaxation of the pelvic ligaments* (sacroiliac and sacrosciatic) may be palpated, and a slight dropping of the muscles over this region slightly raises the tailhead in some cows near full term. Calving usually occurs within 12 hours, when relaxation of the caudal border of the ligaments is

complete. Relaxation of the pelvic ligaments is a much less obvious sign of impending parturition in mares than in cows. Some mares may show hollowing and softening of the area, accompanied by relaxation and lengthening of the vulva. About 4 hours before foaling, sweating may occur at the elbows and on the flanks.

A weak predictor of parturition, because of considerable individual variability, is the rectal temperature decrease during the last 48 hours of gestation (about $0.5°$ C in cows and 2 to $3°$ C in mares).

Bitches, Ewes, Goats, Queens, and Sows

In smaller animals (bitches, ewes, goats, queens, sows), important behavioral changes accompany the modifications in the mammary glands' size and secretion, the softening of the pelvic ligaments, and the enlargement of the vulva.

Bitches and *queens* often try to find a quiet place in the house, and quite frequently they establish their nest under furniture or in a bed. Some bitches may dig a large hole as wolves do. In the primiparous bitch, milk may be present up to 7 days prior to parturition, but in the multiparous, lactation usually occurs 24 hours prior to whelping. Mammary development begins in the queens several days prior to parturition, with visible growth evident during the last 72 hours. Milk can usually be expressed from the nipples 24 hours prior to queening. A drop in body temperature (at least 1 to $2°$ C) generally occurs within 24 hours before whelping, but its transient nature makes it difficult to detect.

Expectant *ewes* develop a premature maternal instinct and an increasing interest in the lambs of other ewes. During the last 2 to 3 days of pregnancy, the previously relatively quiescent ovine uterus and cervix show dramatic changes. Infrequent (2 to 3 contractions per hour) phases of contractions of low amplitude (20 g), lasting longer than 5 minutes, occur about 72 hours before full term. About 48 hours before parturition, uterocervical motor activity decreases for the next 12 to 24 hours. An accelerated softening of the cervix, to increase its compliance (distensibility), coincides with this motor inhibition. In the last 12 to 24 hours before delivery, after this momentary depression, uterocervical motor activity resumes and increases progressively to become almost continuous shortly before parturition. In 80 percent of the ewes, body temperature drops about $0.5°$ C (below $39.4°$ C) during the last 48 hours prior to lambing.

As kidding approaches, the *goat's* udder may need to be milked to relieve mammary pressure, the vulva enlarges, and the expectant nanny goat is restless and hollows out a nest.

During the last week prior to farrowing, reddening of the *sow's* vulva increases as parturition approaches. The mammary glands are prominent and distended during the last 1

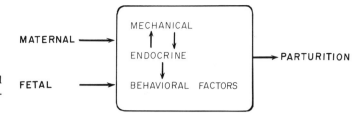

Figure 58–1   General outline of the maternal and fetal factors implicated in ending pregnancy and initiating parturition.

to 3 days of gestation, especially in gilts. A few drops of clear or straw-colored fluid can then be obtained by manual pressure. Most sows will usually farrow within 6 to 12 hours after free milk flow is established, but some may need up to 24 hours. On the day before farrowing, sows show nervousness and nest-building. In confinement, they are restless, urinate and defecate frequently, have an accelerated respiration rate, bite the walls or surrounding objects, scratch the floor, and rearrange the bedding material. Gradually, this physical exertion subsides, and the sows settle into a recumbent position as farrowing becomes imminent. About 12 hours before delivery of the first piglet, the body temperature of sows or gilts *increases* by about 1° C, irrespective of the ambient conditions.

MECHANICAL ASPECTS OF PARTURITION IN MOTHERS

For descriptive purposes, on the basis of mechanical events, it is convenient to divide parturition into three stages. The first stage starts with increasingly frequent uterine contractions, which raise the intrauterine pressure and cause *dilation of the cervix*, and ends before rupture of the allantoic membrane. The second stage (*fetal expulsion*) marks the escape of the allantoic and then of the amniotic fluids, and some vigorous straining leading to the eventual delivery of each offspring. The birth canal includes the cervix, vagina, and vulva, each of which can expand sufficiently to accommodate the fetus. The third stage is highlighted by the rupture of the umbilical cord and the expulsion of the fetal membranes from the uterus (Fig. 58–2). The second and third stages of whelping are repeated for the delivery of each fetus in the litter.

Any event occurring before the onset of the second stage of parturition is regarded as *prepartum,* whereas any event occurring after completion of the second stage of labor is termed *postpartum.* The interval between the end of the third stage of parturition and the return of the female reproductive system to its normal cyclical (nonpregnant) state is known as the *puerperium.* The puerperal period usually extends from parturition to first copulation or fertile insemination.

The electromechanical events during the traditional three stages of parturition in females of several uniparous (cows, mares, and ewes) and multiparous (bitches and sows) species present considerable differences.

About every 50 minutes, the cervix and the uterus of the prepartum pregnant ewe exhibit rhythmic bursts of

regular spiking activity (RSA), which are accompanied by contractions (Fig. 58–3). About 2 days before parturition, the cervical electromechanical activity decreases as the wall tension is reduced (increased compliance, or "softening"). Subsequently, the uterocervical activity returns to its previous level and then increases progressively over the next 30 hours or so, with a large rise in irregular spiking activity (ISA). The lamb is delivered over a period of 0.5 to 3.8 hours. In this final phase, in which the RSA and ISA become almost continuous and indistinguishable, forceful contractions of the uterus and dilation of the cervix are aided by an abdominal press. Expulsion of the lamb is followed by even stronger contractions that are propagated from the uterus toward the cervix, unlike those occurring prior to delivery. This stage lasts for several hours and usually results in passage of the placenta.

Cows (Calving)

Stage 1.   Calving occurs most frequently during the night. It begins when smooth muscle fibers of the uterus contract about every 15 minutes, and it ends when the ripened cervix dilates to let fetal parts enter the birth canal, which undergoes changes in its diameters (Fig. 58–4). The cervix is dilated sufficiently to admit a hand, and slight dorsal arching of the back is apparent at this time. The

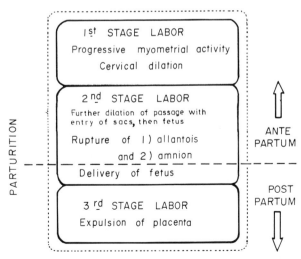

Figure 58–2   Diagrammatic representation of the major mechanical antepartum and postpartum events highlighting the three stages of parturition.

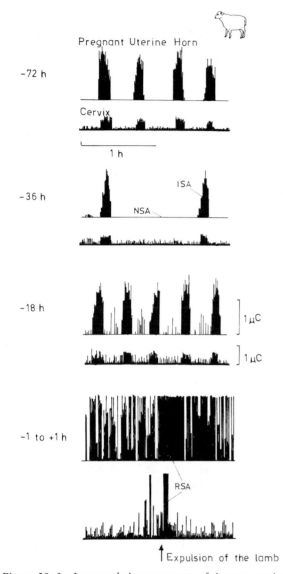

Figure 58–3 Integrated electromyogram of the pregnant horn and cervix during late pregnancy (− 72, − 36, − 18, and − 1 hr), during lambing (0 hr), and during early puerperium (+ 1 hr). At − 72 hours of full term, two coincident bursts of regular spiking activity (RSA), separated by nonspiking activity (NSA), occur during each hour. At − 36 hours of full term, the electromyographical activity is halved (1 burst per hour). At − 18 hours of full term, the bursts return to a slightly faster frequency and are separated by some irregular spiking activity (ISA). Before full term, the almost continuous and intense RSA and ISA cannot be separated in the uterine horn. At full term, and after expulsion of the lamb, intense RSA continues in the horn but not in the cervix (μC, microcoulomb).

duration of stage 1 labor is 2 to 6 hours, but may be longer in heifers, which may also show signs of colic.

A stringy vaginal discharge increases at the edematous vulva (Fig. 58–5), with liquefaction and expulsion of the cervical plug. Visible signs of first-stage labor are scanty or absent. Signs of discomfort and restlessness, with a frequent tendency for the animal to lie down and get up, are often observed.

Stage 2. Uterine contractions now occur at about every 3 to 5 minutes. The allantois gets nearer the vulva, the cervix becomes completely effaced, and fetal parts enter the birth canal and stretch the vagina to provoke definite straining. Contractions of the abdominal muscles, coordinated with the rib cage and diaphragm at the position of maximum inspiration (abdominal press), soon bring the unruptured allantoic sac (first water bag) to the vulva. The abdominal press becomes weaker or quiescent after expulsion of the allantoic sac, with liberation of the allantoic fluid, but it resumes its action as the amnion nears the vulva.

The unbroken amniotic sac ("second water bag") is often forced through the vulva after the cow has been in labor for a short time (Fig. 58–6). The feet of the fetus, seen through the amniotic sac, may cause the rupture of the sac, either just before or just after it appears at the vulva. Escape of the lubricating amniotic fluid is followed by a brief rest period. The mean interval between rupture of the allantois and the amnion may reach about 1 hour. Delivery of the fetus should be completed within 2 hours after the amniotic (second water bag or foot bag) sac appears at the vulva.

As parturition progresses, the action of the abdominal press is exerted more frequently and for longer periods, until it occurs every 1.5 to 2.5 minutes, with a short period of rest following a series of presses. In heifers, stretching of the vulva requires more time, and because little outward progression takes place during each of these contractions the calf frequently recedes into the vagina between bouts. Nearly continuous straining, with the greatest frequency and force of the abdominal press, is seen when the fetal head is passed through the vulva.

Following passage of the head, a short period of rest may ensue before strong expulsive efforts are needed again to force the thorax through the birth canal. Afterwards, delivery of the hips and hindlegs is usually uneventful, except where the calf has an unusually wide pelvis and the heifer or cow a narrow one. The cow may stop straining for a short time following delivery of the thorax, allowing the rear legs to stay in the birth canal.

The umbilical cord may remain intact throughout most of the delivery process, supplying some oxygen to the fetus, and the calf may even breathe while maintaining placental circulation. The cord eventually ruptures spontaneously at a preformed spot (about 6 cm from the umbilicus).

The bovine fetus can live in utero for 8 to 10 hours after stage 2 begins, but it is usually expelled within 2 to 4 hours. The birth canal of heifers is slower to dilate than that of cows, and parturition progresses more slowly.

Stage 3. The fetal membranes are usually expelled within 0.5 to 8 hours following delivery of the fetus. The cow may eat the placenta and sometimes the bedding contaminated by parturition fluids. If the fetal membranes are retained, *manual removal should not be practiced,* and broadspectrum antibiotics should be administered ideally between the endometrium and the placental membranes.

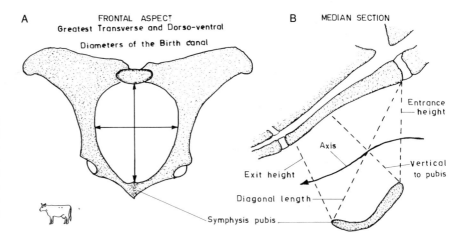

Figure 58–4 Aspects of the bovine birth canal. **A,** Frontoventral view, with the transverse and dorsoventral diameters. **B,** Median section, with the general axis of the birth canal, and the different descriptive lengths (entrance, exit, diagonal, and vertical to pecten or pubic bone).

To reduce the possibility of uterine prolapse and to assess the extent of possible pelvic nerve damage during delivery, the cow should be made to stand after the calf is born.

Mares (Foaling)

Stage 1. More than 70 percent of mares give birth at night between 22:00 and 02:00 hours. Increasingly frequent and painful uterine waves of contraction with marked signs of distress, and loss of milk and colostrum that may drip or spurt from the teats, characterize the first-stage labor. During these painful bouts, the mare may be restless, showing an anxious facial expression, pawing the ground, looking at her flank and raising her tail, rubbing her hindquarters against a wall, and yawning or curling her upper lip in a *flehmen-like* manner. First-stage labor terminates just before rupture of the placenta and escape of the allantoic fluid.

The signs of first-stage labor may be premature and may not lead to second-stage labor in thoroughbred mares. In such instances, after a postponement period (cool off),

which may be a matter of hours or days, a fresh first-stage labor is repeated and is followed by second-stage labor.

Stage 2. Rupture of the placenta (chorioallantois) at its weak spot near the cervix (cervical star) and passage at the lengthened vulva of a yellow-brown allantoic fluid mark the onset of second-stage labor. Within 5 minutes after this event, the amnion usually appears at the vulva, and the profusely sweating mare usually lies down.

Straining efforts seem more successful when the mare is lying on her side or in a sternal recumbency. The mare is attracted to and even licks allantoic fluid fallen on the straw bedding, on her hair, or on clothes of attendants. She often turns her head toward her hindquarters and neighs. Once the head of the fetus is past the vulva, and until complete delivery, the mare remains recumbent and appears to be under a strong tranquilizing influence.

The second stage of foaling lasts 5 to 60 minutes (mean, about 20 minutes), multiparous requiring the longest time. Mares experiencing a prolonged first-stage labor often have a short second-stage labor.

Stage 3. The umbilical cord normally ruptures at a predetermined weak point (about 3 cm from the abdomen) either when the foal attempts to stand for the first time or when the mare rises to her feet. It is customary to tie the amnion to the ruptured cord.

Generally, the placenta is expelled after rupture of the cord, but it may occur with the cord still intact, then manual rupture is required. Mares may lick but do not eat the afterbirth. Signs of pain (rolling, sweating, pawing the ground, restlessness, and *flehmen*) are seen during the third-stage of foaling, which has a mean duration of about 60 minutes (0.5 to 3 hours).

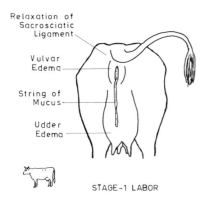

Relaxation of
Sacrosciatic
Ligament

Vulvar
Edema

String of
Mucus

Udder
Edema

STAGE-1 LABOR

Figure 58–5 In the cow, edema of the vulva and of the udder, relaxation and sinking of the ligaments around the tail head and the pelvis (sacrosciatic, sacroiliac), and a stringy mucous vulvar discharge are the prominent visible signs of the first stage of parturition.

Ewes (Lambing)

Stage 1. At about 2 to 8 hours before lambing, in advanced first-stage labor, uterine contractions and relaxations occur without pause, and the intrauterine pressure

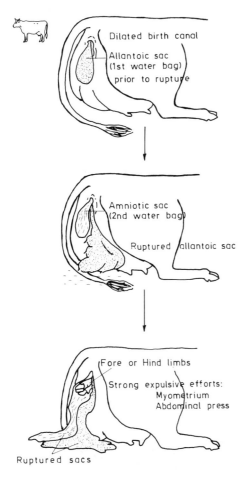

Dilated birth canal

Allantoic sac
(1st water bag)
prior to rupture

Amniotic sac
(2nd water bag)

Ruptured allantoic sac

Fore or Hind limbs

Strong expulsive efforts:
Myometrium
Abdominal press

Ruptured sacs

STAGE-2 LABOR

Figure 58–6 The expulsion of the fetus—the second stage of bovine parturition—often occurs while the cow is lying down. Physical dilation of the birth canal is caused by the placental fluids in their sacs, which act as a penetrating but malleable wedge. The unruptured allantochorion (first water bag) seen at the vulva often heralds this second stage. This is followed by the amniotic sac (second water bag), through which the extended front legs may be seen. The amnion, usually ruptured by the front legs, provides a lubricating sheet that prevents contact of the fetus with the mucosa lining the birth canal. In the final stage (stage 2) of labor, the contraction of the myometrium and the abdominal press concur to produce strong expulsive efforts.

rises to an amplitude of 20 mm Hg. Parturient pain is evidenced by the animal's lying down, getting up, paddling with the hind feet, and restlessness. In twin pregnancies, the larger horn is dominant in initiating contractions. The lamb in that horn engages into the distended and semirelaxed cervix, which yields to the pressure exerted by the fluid-distended placental membranes.

Stage 2. Most ewes remain recumbent until the fetus is partially or completely expelled. Birth follows in a few minutes, as stretch receptors in the cervix and the vagina are activated, and expulsive pressure is increased by two reflexes. The first one, by causing release of oxytocin (mostly in the

goat) and prostaglandins, raises the intrauterine pressure to 40 mm Hg. The second one operates through contractions of the abdominal press, which are precisely superimposed on uterine contractions. Fetuses of twin and multiple lambings follow each other within a matter of minutes. Lambing is considered to be a relatively swift process (30 to 120 minutes), the mean joint duration of the two first stages is less than 90 minutes.

The ewe accepts its lamb only after licking off fetal fluids containing olfactory substances to which she is especially sensitive immediately after birth.

Stage 3. Immediately after delivery of the lamb, powerful rhythmic contractions continue and placentomes gradually begin to separate into their placental cotyledons and endometrial caruncle components. Most of the placenta is finally delivered after a few hours, and often the ewe will chew and eat parts of the fetal membranes (placentophagia). For 2 to 3 days afterwards, myometrial activity is maintained in order to discharge the final necrotic placental shreds and the lochia (secretions made of blood, desquamated epithelial cells, and mucus).

Induction of Parturition in Ewes. Parturition in ewes can be induced reliably by infusion of adrenocorticotropic hormone (ACTH) in the fetus. The fetus then matures in utero, and the ewe delivers a viable lamb even if parturition is induced prior to day 135 of gestation. Surgical cesarian delivery at that stage results in a premature lamb with a low chance of survival. Large doses of dexamethasone successfully induce labor, but the interval is highly variable. Oxytocin or prostaglandins are effective only after labor is initiated. A new experimental approach involves inhibition of 3-beta-hydroxysteroid dehydrogenase (3β-HSD) by injecting 50 mg of epostane, an inhibitor of this enzyme.

> Epostane reduces the formation of progesterone from pregnenolone, resulting in induction of parturition with delivery in 33 to 36 hours of viable lambs. Maternal plasma progesterone levels fall precipitously within 15 minutes of injection, accompanied by a lesser fall in cortisol.

Bitches (Whelping)

Stage 1. The expectant bitch may show anorexia, restlessness, apprehension, trembling, and occasional vomiting. Some bitches engage in nest-making (dig a hole or scratch the floor), others seek a closed and secluded spot, or others will have a special dependence on the help of the owner.

The pelvic ligaments and the lower tract relax, and myometrial contractions gradually increase the intrauterine pressure. The waves of contraction start just cranial to the rearmost fetus in the uterine horns.

This first-stage labor lasts 6 to 12 hours, but may extend over 36 hours in the nulliparous (first whelping) bitch.

Stage 2. During this stage of whelping, an apparent tenesmus coincides with uterine contractions to further raise intrauterine pressure. The force exerted is such that the fetus is propelled through the birth canal and to the exterior.

Each fetus is covered by the amnion at birth. The allantois has ruptured under the expulsive efforts or is opened by the dam's teeth at the vulva. The bitch, which thoroughly licks the fetus on delivery, bites through the umbilical cord, removes the amnion, cleans the puppy, and stimulates its cardiovascular and respiratory functions.

Generally, fetuses are delivered from each horn alternately. The second-stage labor is repeated to deliver each fetus of the litter. The mean time between delivery of successive puppies varies greatly but is usually about 30 minutes. By contrast, the delivery of kittens may be spaced minutes or hours or even days apart; several kittens may be born, with others appearing days later.

Stage 3. This stage is repeated after the delivery of each fetus of the litter or after the delivery of two fetuses from different horns. It is a period of uterine contractions leading to expulsion of the fetal membranes within 15 minutes after the birth of a puppy.

The fetal fluids of whelping have a greenish stain (uteroverdin) that is due to the breakdown products of extravasated maternal blood.

Normally, the bitch eats the expulsed fetal membranes, which may produce vomiting. Similarly, after birth, the kittens are cleaned by the queen. A dead puppy may also be eaten or buried. In fear, the bitch may eat the litter.

Sows (Farrowing)

Stage 1. Farrowing, a function accomplished with a minimum of physical activity, more often occurs during the night. The sow is usually lying on her side, occasionally changing to a ventral position or standing. Initial uterine contractions are indicated by leg and abdominal movements.

Stage 2. The sow shows very little abdominal straining, a minimal fluid loss trickling from the vulva, and frequently only a switch of her tail as each fetus enters the birth canal.

Piglets are delivered with ease at intervals of about 15 minutes. The time that elapses between delivery of the first and the last piglet ranges from less than 1 hour to as long as 8 hours, but usually only 1 to 4 hours are required to deliver the complete litter.

The order of birth is related to the location of the fetus in the uterine horn. The piglet closest to the uterine body is the first one to be delivered from the uterine horn. The remaining fetuses follow in sequence, from an entire uterine horn before any are delivered from the contralateral horn, or from each horn in a random fashion.

The newborn pig remains immobile for a few seconds before respiration is initiated. Afterwards, it immediately struggles to rupture the intact umbilical cord, which is still attached to the intrauterine placental membranes. Piglets late in the farrowing order may be delivered with the umbilical cord already ruptured. When the duration of the farrowing is extremely long, many of the piglets in the last third of the birth order are stillbirths, because of intrapartum anoxia. Each piglet's hepatic stores of glycogen are depleted progressively with time during parturition. Those born last are less viable as a result. Rupture of the umbilical cord and the necessity of traveling a longer length of uterine horn are deleterious factors contributing to these intrapartum deaths. The time interval between deliveries of a normal and a stillborn piglet is increased by 5 minutes, amounting to 20 minutes instead of 15 minutes.

Stage 3. The fetal membranes are usually expelled in batches of two to four after the birth of the last piglet. Some of the fetal membranes may be ejected before the birth of all the piglets. If these membranes are not removed immediately from the farrowing site, sows will eat at least a part of the placental membranes. The time that elapses between delivery of the last fetus and expulsion of the placental membranes may range from a few minutes to longer than 8 hours.

MECHANICAL ASPECTS OF PARTURITION ASSOCIATED WITH THE FETUS

The terms presentation, position, and posture are used to describe the disposition of the fetus at the time of birth. *Presentation* is either anterior or posterior, depending on whether the head or the hindquarters of the fetus appear first in the pelvic inlet (Fig. 58–7). In most species, anterior presentation is the norm, but in bitches and sows about 40 percent are posterior (breech) presentations. In a posterior presentation, compression of the umbilical cord against the maternal pelvis may stimulate the fetus to attempt breathing, with consequent inhalation of fetal fluids.

Position refers to the orientation of the fetal vertebral column in the birth canal in relation to the dorsal surface of the uterus or the maternal vertebral column. Position can be dorsal, ventral, or lateral. The norm is the dorsal position, with the spine of the fetus facing the dorsal wall of the birth canal.

Posture denotes the disposition (flexed or extended) of the fetal head, neck, and extremities in relation to the body of the fetus. Usually, the head and forelegs are extended in front of the fetus, and the hindlegs are stretched behind.

In the final stages of gestation, the equine and bovine fetuses assume an anterior presentation. The fetal calf is in the proper dorsal position; in contrast, the fetal foal is in the ventral position and must undertake its own rotational correction to the dorsal position before birth. The posture of general flexion changes prior to birth (1 week in calves and foals, 4 days in lambs, kids, and piglets). Stretching and full extension of the fetus are required for proper delivery without dystocia. Provided that the extended feet precede the head or the rump, both anterior and posterior presentations can be considered normal. Anterior presentation occurs in 70 to 90 percent of kidding. With either anterior (head) or posterior (breech) presentations, the position is dorsosacral, and the posture is with extension of the extremities.

A

B

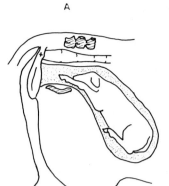
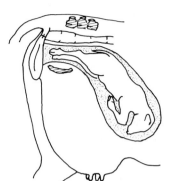

ANTERIOR PRESENTATION
DORSAL POSITION
POSTURE: Extended forelegs
and head

POSTERIOR PRESENTATION
DORSAL POSITION
POSTURE: Extended hind legs

Figure 58–7 Examples of presentations, positions, and postures in bovine fetuses. **A,** A normal anterior presentation, in a dorsal position (fetal spine toward the dorsal endometrium, or dorsal aspect of fetal vertebral column toward the ventral aspect of maternal vertebral column), with a posture showing extended head and forelegs. **B,** A normal posterior presentation, in a dorsal position, with a posture displaying extension of the hind limbs.

Many lambs have meconium (orange to ochre color) staining on their hair coat following birth, which indicates that fetal defecation has occurred near full term into the amniotic fluid.

During the course of farrowing, the uterine horn is transformed into a slippery tube by rupture of the ends of the chorionic sacs, while the individual placental connections remain intact. Piglets can be moved in either direction of the horn, the limiting factors are the length of the umbilical cords and the placental connections. Despite a considerable retraction of the uterine wall near the end of farrowing, the last fetal piglets of the litter must be transported over a longer distance than the previous fetuses. An intact umbilical cord and proper placental connections are not always ensured to fetal piglets from the ovarian ends of the horns. A higher number of broken umbilical cords and prepartum dead piglets (stillbirths) occur during the last third of farrowing.

ENDOCRINE ASPECTS OF PARTURITION

Initiation of parturition is dominated by fetal and placental (chorion) mechanisms in the various animal species. In pregnant cows, ewes, goats, and sows, parturition is preceded by a fall in maternal progesterone (P_4) level, which is triggered by a rise in the level of cortisol in fetal blood. Higher outputs of hypothalamic corticotropin-releasing factor (CRF) and adenohypophysial ACTH are the causes of this higher level of cortisol in the fetal circulation (Fig. 58–8). The increased production of fetal corticosteroids near full term is also important for the formation of surfactant material in the pulmonary alveoli of the fetus.

In preparturient females of most species (cows, ewes, goats, and sows), an increase in the *fetal corticosteroids* stimulates placental aromatization enzyme systems to transform progesterone into estrogens, via androgens. The prepartum concentration of *estrogen* is much higher in does than in ewes. Generally, an increase in the estrogen:progesterone ratio stimulates the release of prostaglandins (PGE_2 and $F_{2\alpha}$) from the uterine wall, by a positive feedback. In fetal vascular mechanics, PGE is especially important for maintenance of a patent ductus arteriosus during the latter part of gestation. Neurohypophysial release of oxytocin is linked to production of prostaglandins, mostly $PGF_{2\alpha}$, into the uterine venous blood. Both compounds are considered to be the major stimuli to the strong uterine contractions of second-stage labor.

Prostaglandins, especially PGE, are more abundant in the cervical vein of ewes during parturition. In most species, PGE is involved in the process of cervical dilation, by increasing the proportion of collagen in the tissues of the body of the uterus and of the cervix.

Beside their effects on ovarian luteolysis, on inhibition of placental progesterone production, on stimulation of neurohypophysial oxytocin release, on cervical relaxation, and on myometrial contractions, prostaglandins also favor an ovarian and a placental production of *relaxin,* a nonsteroid hormone. Relaxin may be important in bitches, ewes, and sows for relaxation of the pelvic ligaments and may also contribute to softening of the cervix as well as the rest of the birth canal at the time of delivery of the fetuses. Relaxin is associated with the myometrial quiescence during preterm.

In mares and fetal foals, different endocrine changes occur near full term. Knowledge of fetal hormones in horses is still incomplete, but the evidence available points to initiation of parturition from the fetal side of the placenta (chorion). Relatively high levels of progestagens, and low levels of estrogens of fetoplacental origin, are seen in the maternal plasma before foaling. The rise in progestagens is due mainly to an increase in 5-alpha-pregnane metabolites rather than to a rise in progesterone itself. Cortisol levels in fetal foals remain constant near full term, whereas maternal plasma corticosteroid levels undergo a significant rise only during foaling and reflect the stress and pain of labor. Also,

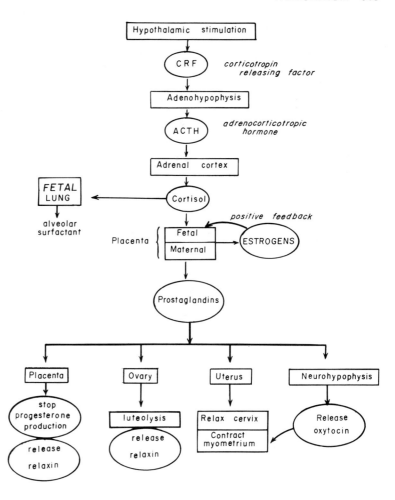

Figure 58–8 Endocrine initiation of parturition through uterine production of prostaglandins, which are induced by fetal cortisol and by a positive-feedback effect of placental estrogens. The alveolar surfactant-producing fetal hypercortisolemia results from a sudden drop in progesterone, in most of the species, but of progestins (5-alpha-pregnanes) in the mare-foal unit. The prostaglandins have effects on the placenta (release of relaxin, inhibition of progesterone production), on the ovaries (release of relaxin), on the uterus (relaxation of the cervix, contraction of the myometrium), and on the neurohypophysis (release of oxytocin).

$PGF_{2\alpha}$ increases only during the second stage of foaling, from movement and stretching of the cervix and vagina and from the displacement of the fetal foal through the birth canal. The factors influencing cervical dilation and changes in cervical collagen at the time of foaling have not been identified in mares.

Oxytocin is released in a similar pattern in mares, goats, ewes, and cows. Small amounts of oxytocin begin to be released during the first stage (dilation of the cervix), and maximum levels occur at the time when the fetal head emerges from the vulva during the second stage of labor. In mares, oxytocin seems concerned largely with expulsion of the uterine contents (fetal and placental) and possibly with subsequent involution of the uterus. It appears that stimulation of stretch receptors in the cervix of all these species is the prime stimulus for oxytocin release. Vaginal distention in cows and ewes also results in a brisk increase in plasma oxytocin levels, reflected in milk let down (Ferguson's neurohumoral reflex). Secretion of oxytocin is also modulated by plasma levels of steroid hormones: estrogen-potentiating and progesterone-inhibiting release. Estrogens also sensitize the myometrium to the action of oxytocin.

Neurophysins I and II, carrier proteins stored in the neurosecretory granules together with the neurohypophysial hormones, are released with oxytocin (neurophysin I) and vasopressin, or antidiuretic hormone (neurophysin II). During and after parturition, the pattern of neurophysin I release is very similar to that of oxytocin in the plasma of cows, mares, goats, and ewes during the first and second stages of labor.

REFERENCES

Arthur GH, Noakes DE, Pearson H. Veterinary reproduction and obstetrics (theriogenology) 6th ed. London: Baillière Tindall, 1989.

Challis JRG. Endocrinology of late pregnancy and parturition. Int Rev Physiol 1980;22:277.

Challis JRG, Olson DM. Parturition. In: Knobil E. Neil J, eds. The physiology of reproduction. New York: Raven Press Ltd, 1988.

Constantin A, Meissonnier E. L'utérus de la vache. Anatomie, physiologie, pathologie. Paris: Société française de buiatrie, Alfort, 1981.

Derivaux J, Ectors F. Physiopathologie de la gestation et obstétrique vétérinaire. Paris: Editions du Point Vétérinaire, 1980.

Ellendorff F, Taverne M, Smidt D. Physiology and control of parturition in domestic animals. New York: Elsevier, 1979.

Ginther OJ. Reproductive biology of the mare. Cross Plaines, WI: OJ Ginther, 1979.

Hammond D, Matty G. A farrowing management system using cloprostenol to control the time of parturition. Vet Rec 1980;106:72.

Hennessy DP, Coghlan JP, Hardy KJ, et al. The origin of cortisol in the blood of fetal sheep. J Endocrinol 1982;95:71.

Lagercrantz H, Slotkin TA. The "stress" of being born. Sci Am 1986;254:100.

Lickliter RE. Behavior associated with parturition in the domestic goat. App Anim Biol Sci 1984;13:335.

Liggins GC, Fairclough RJ, Grieve SA, et al. The mechanism of initiation of parturition in the ewe. Recent Progr Horm Res 1973;29:111.

McDonald LE. Veterinary endocrinology and reproduction. 4th ed. Philadelphia: Lea & Febiger, 1989.

Rees LH, Jack PMB, Thomas AL, Nathanielsz PW. Role of foetal adrenocorticotrophin during parturition in sheep. Nature (Lond) 1985;253:274.

Rossdale PD, Ricketts SW. Equine stud farm medicine. 2nd ed. London: Baillière Tindall, 1980.

Rowlands IW, Allen WR, Rossdale PD. Equine reproduction III. J Reprod Fert 1982;Suppl 32.

Silver M. Effect on maternal and fetal steroid concentrations of induction of parturition in the sheep by inhibition of 38-hydroxy-steroid dehydrogenase. J Reprod Fert 1988;82:457.

Steven DH. Comparative placentation. Essays in structure and function. New York: Academic Press, 1975.

Thorburn GD, Challis JRG. Endocrine control of parturition. Physiol Rev 1979;59:863.

Toutain PL, Gargia-Villar R, Hanzen C, Ruckebusch V. Electrical and mechanical activity of the cervix in the ewe during pregnancy and parturition. J Reprod Fertil 1983;68:195.

CHAPTER 59

LACTATION

The aim of postpartum lactation is to supply nutrients in fluids of maternal origin (colostrum and milk) until the offspring is able to cope with solid food. The composition of mammary fluids varies among species, according to the needs of the young.

The study of lactation can be considered from the aspects of growth and structure of the mammary glands, lactogenesis (initiation of milk secretion), and galactopoiesis (maintenance of milk production).

GROWTH AND STRUCTURES OF THE MAMMARY GLANDS

Mammary development or mammary growth, which refers to the growth of the glandular tissue (parenchyma), is similar in males and females during embryonic and fetal life. After birth, prior to puberty the mammary gland is only slightly more developed in the female than in the male. However, in cats, guinea pigs, and horses, a transient burst of growth may occur in neonates of both sexes as a result of hormonal influences associated with parturition. Because a suitable fatty pad is lacking in relation to the mammary gland in most males, further development from hormone stimulation is impossible, exept in guinea pigs and humans.

The mammary gland of the female is an organ made of specialized skin glands that are able to secrete a form of nourishment to immature offspring. Mammary development begins during fetal life with a simple primary duct structure. After birth, this simple primary duct system elongates and branches, mostly after puberty, with each hormonal surge (estrogens and progesterone) of the recurring estrous cycles. At the onset of gestation in most species, the mammary gland already possesses an advanced duct system. During gestation, the ducts proliferate into grape-like clusters (lobules) of epithelial alveolar cells organized into hollow spherical structures (alveoli). This lobuloalveolar system continues to grow at least up to midgestation in most animal species or during pseudogestation (after ovulation in bitches, hamsters, mice, and rats; and ovulation after an infertile mating in queens and rabbits). Separated by connective tissue, the lobules are regrouped into lobes.

The protruding structure, which is ultimately used by the offspring to harvest milk, may be called a nipple, a teat, a thelium (thelia), or a papilla (papillae). Generally, the term teat is reserved for species whose mammary gland has support and results in an udder (e.g., camel, cattle, donkey, elephant, giraffe, goat, horse, and sheep). Species with mammary glands without support have nipples rather than teats (e.g., bears, cats, chinchillas, dogs, gerbils, hamsters, mice, pigs, primates, raccoons, and rats). A significant proportion of females may have more than the normal number of teats or nipples (polythelia). In cattle, supernumerary teats may be located behind the normal four (caudal, 93 percent), between the normal teats (intercalary, 5 percent), or in association with a normal teat (ramal, 2 percent). The males of some species lack mammary nipples (athelia), for example, beaver, mouse, and rat, or teats (horse).

Mammary glands may be at different positions on the ventral or lateral aspects of the body. Ventral mammary glands are found in the region of the neck (cervical), the chest (thoracic, or pectoral), the abdomen, the groin (inguinal), or the thigh (crural). Lateral mammary glands are placed mostly on the thorax. The smallest number of mammary glands is 2, for example, goat, guinea pig, horse, and sheep (inguinal), primates (thoracic), and seals (abdominal). Two pairs of mammary glands exist in cattle and camel (inguinal), lion and leopard (abdominal), and beaver (thoracic). Three pairs of nipples (thoracic, abdominal, and inguinal) occur in brown bears, chinchillas, and raccoon. Species with four pairs of nipples include the house cat, small breeds of dogs, fox, gerbil, lemming, mole, and squirrel. Five pairs of nipples are observed in the large breeds of dogs, rabbits, and weasels. Animals with six pairs of mammary glands comprise the domestic pig, the laboratory rat, and the ground squirrel; the golden hamster has seven pairs.

Galactophores, or streak canals, are the channels by which milk travels from the mammary gland to the sucking neonate. Species with a single galactophore per teat include cattle, gerbil, goat, guinea pig, hamster, mouse, rat, and sheep. Two streak canals are found in the horse and in swine, which may have from 1 to 3. Many animals besides the pig have a variable number of galactophores per papilla; e.g., domestic cat, three to seven openings; the domestic dog, 8 to 14 ducts; and humans, 15 to 25 ducts (Table 59–1).

The total weight of the udder of a high-producing dairy cow may exceed 50 kg before milking. Support to this mass is provided mainly by a median (fibro-elastic) and a lateral suspensory (nonelastic) ligament. These ligaments project into the udder to form a framework of connective tissue that gives support without compressing the glandular tissue and interfering with the circulation of the blood. The udder of the cow also has smooth muscles, some forming a sphincter around the papillary duct, whereas others are in blood vessels and large milk ducts. The smooth muscles forming the teat sphincter are very important in the lactating cow and in the dry cow. The sphincter minimizes entrance of harmful materials (bacteria, dirt) into the enlarged terminal portion of the ducts (sinus, or cistern, in cattle, goats, horses, pigs, and sheep) of the mammary gland and controls the rate of milk removal from the gland. Myoepithelial (basket) cells surrounding the alveolus contract in response to oxytocin, the

TABLE 59–1 Locations, Numbers, and Nipple or Teat Openings of Mammary Glands of Some Animals

| NAME | | POSITION OF GLANDS | | | | NO. OF |
Common	Scientific	Thor	Abd	Ing	TOTAL	OPENINGS
Camel	Camelus dromedarius			4	4	3
Cat (house)	Felis domestica	2	6	—	8	3–7
Cattle	Bos taurus, Bos indicus	—	—	4	4	1
Chinchilla	Chinchilla laniger	2	2	2	6	1–2
Domestic dog	Canis familiaris	2	6	2	10	8–20
Gerbil	Meriones unguiculatus	4	—	4	8	1
Goat	Capra hircus	—	—	2	2	1
Ground squirrel	Spermophilus tridecemlineatus	4	4	4	12	4–5
Guinea pig	Cavia porcellus	—	—	2	2	1
Hamster (golden)	Mesocricetus auratus	4	8	2	14	1
Horse	Equus caballus	—	—	2	2	2–3
Monkey (rhesus)	Macaca mulatta	2	—	—	2	2–10
Pig	Sus scrofa	4	6	2	12	2
Rabbit	Oryctolagus cuniculus	4	4	2	10	8–10
Raccoon	Procyon lotor	2	4	2	8	10
Sheep	Ovis aries	—	—	2	2	1

Thor, Thoracic; Abd, abdominal; Ing, inguinal.

neurohypophysial hormone released by neurohumoral reflexes. Oxytocin thus raises the intramammary pressure inside the alveoli and the large milk ducts and initiates milk let-down.

The large mammary vessels are conventional, but the smaller arteries and arterioles carry sensory and efferent adrenergic sympathetic nerves. As a consequence, in the conscious animal, a very mild stress or disturbance (e.g., venipuncture in the goat, or lifting a rat from the nest) reduces the mammary blood flow. Sensory receptors are confined essentially to the base of the teat, just where the gums of the suckling neonate will assume maximum stimulation. Blood vessels in the teats are specialized: arteries run straight along the length of the teat, and thick-walled veins form a network throughout the teat. Lymphatics are not found inside the lobules, and excess tissue fluid is drained by fine lymphatics surrounding the lobules.

LACTOGENESIS

The term lactogenesis is used to describe the initiation of milk secretion after parturition (delivery of the fetus), when the mammary glands have reached a suitable degree of development. The process of lactogenesis at parturition encompasses the hormones involved in its initiation, milk secretion by the epithelial cells of the alveolus, and removal of milk stored in the mammary gland. It should not be confused with pharmacological hormone-induced lactation in barren, nonlactating cows and heifers.

Secretions by the Epithelial Alveolar Cells

Alveolar cells of the lactating (postparturient) mammary gland synthesize and secrete milk proteins (casein, serum albumin, alpha-lactalbumin, beta-lactoglobulin, immunoglobulins, and glycoproteins), fats, and lactose. Junctions between these cells enable them to carry on functions of

adhesion (desmosomes), occlusion (tight junctions), and communication (gap junctions).

At about midgestation, the epithelial alveolar cells begin to secrete appreciable quantities of specific milk products, which frequently accumulate in the mammary gland as precolostrum. This lactogenesis stage I is a prerequisite for lactogenesis stage II, which is the onset of copious colostrum and milk secretions at parturition.

Lactogenesis I

The onset of lactogenesis I, that is, secretory activity in the mammary alveoli, is marked by production of precolostrum. The appearance of lactose in the precolostrum is of physiological importance, since it indicates that the intracellular apparatus for milk synthesis is functionally differentiated. It occurs at midgestation in goats, in the last third of pregnancy in rabbits, a month before parturition in ewes, 15 days before foaling in mares, at 10 days before calving in cows, and a day before delivery in mice and rats. During this period of late pregnancy, when the mammary gland remains unmilked, a local factor maintains "leaky" tight junctions to keep the epithelial paracellular pathway open, and the ducts permeable. Transfers between extracellular fluid and precolostrum ar then possible. The precolostrum contains some large molecules such as immunoglobulins, and its aqueous phase shows fluctuating levels of chloride, sodium, potassium, and lactose. Fat globules, protein granules, desquamated epithelial cells, and leukocytes also accumulate in the lumen of the alveoli. Disappearance of this factor, with removal of precolostrum (sucking or milking), results in closure of the paracellular pathways in the alveolar epithelium and duct system.

Lactogenesis II

Lactogenesis II usually begins shortly before parturition, when the mammary gland first releases colostrum, then normal milk, which are not identical in all animal species. For

TABLE 59–2 Approximate Composition of Colostrum in Some Domestic Animals (g/L)

Constituents	Cow	Ewe	Goat	Mare	Sow
Ash	10	10	9	6	6
Lactose	22	22	34	47	24
Lipids	51	177	82	24	72
Proteins	176	201	57	72	188
Water	733	588	812	851	698

instance, the colostrum of some animals (cows, bitches, ewes, goats, mares, and sows) contains globulin antibodies, which are essential for transmitting passive immunity to their offspring. The milk of carnivores, with high-protein and low-sugar contents, is noticeably different from the milk of equidae (protein-poor and sugar-rich).

Colostrum

Colostrum, the transitional fluid between precolostrum and normal milk, is the first food of the neonate. In addition to its rich nutritive value, it transfers passive immunity, and it has a slight laxative effect to aid in clearing the intestine of meconium (greenish mucilaginous material in the intestine of the full-term fetus).

Secreted and stored in the mammary gland during the last 2 to 7 days of gestation and the first 2 or 3 days postpartum, colostrum contains more proteins (including immunoglobulins), lipids, and ash (sodium, and chloride) and less lactose than milk (except in mares). It also contributes fat-soluble and water-soluble vitamins and all the essential amino acids to the rapidly growing neonate (Table 59–2). In the colostrum of sows, a trypsin inhibitor offers protection to the immunoglobulins in the gut of piglets.

Colostrum is essential for supplying immunoglobulins to the neonates from females of species (cows, ewes, goats, mares, and sows) in which antibodies are not transferred from maternal to fetal blood (Fig. 59–1). During their first 2 days of life, kittens and puppies need colostrum to supplement the immunoprotection conferred through the placenta during gestation. A calf should ingest about 6 percent of its body weight in colostrum within 6 hours after delivery. A dairy cow produces about 50 kg of colostrum during the first six milkings after parturition (the first milking is the richest in immunoglobulins). After fermentation (souring), refrigeration, or freezing, colostrum can be fed to calves until the age of 3 weeks, as a source of energy. Colostrum can be frozen in cartons and kept for several months.

In the newborn lamb, bovine colostrum is a satisfactory substitute for natural ovine colostrum. A synthetic ovine colostrum, adequate for its nutritive value but without protective antibodies, can be made with one beaten egg, 1 teaspoon (10 mL) of cod liver oil, and 2 teaspoons (20 g) of sucrose added to 750 mL of cow's milk. Commercial preparations containing concentrated immunoglobulins are available for calves, lambs, and piglets.

Equine colostrum (300 to 500 mL) must be administered within 6 hours to foals born to mares with anticipated lactogenesis II (running milk), that is, mares producing only milk, without any colostrum, at parturition.

During the first 3 days of lactogenesis II, the composition of colostrum, far from being static, changes, with the gradual modification of colostrum into normal milk (Table 59–3).

The immunological experiences of the mother determine the mix of antibodies available to the fetus and the neonate. Domestic carnivores and primates deliver antibodies to their fetuses across the placenta. Important additional immunoglobulins (Igs), mostly IgA, and lesser amounts of IgG and IgM, particularly significant for protection against viral diseases, are also provided in colostrum.

Domestic herbivores and swine have placentas that allow very little transfer of maternal antibodies to the fetus. These species are very dependent upon the immunoglobulins

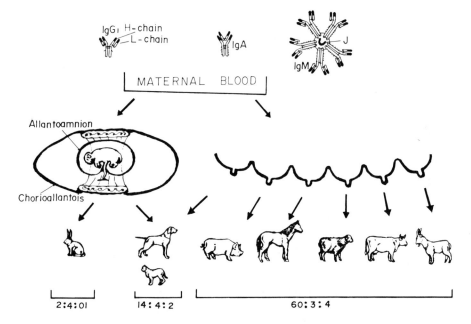

Figure 59–1 Diagrammatic structure of immunoglobulins (IgG$_1$, IgA, and IgM) in maternal blood. In the rabbit and also in the cat and the dog, the placenta is permeable to these immunoglobulins, which reach the fetal blood with a 2:4:1 ratio in the rabbit and 14:4:2 in the cat and the dog. The kitten and the puppy also receive some immunoglobulins via the colostrum. In sows, mares, ewes, cows, and nanny-goats, because their placenta is impermeable to immunoglobulins, colostrum produced during the first 24 hours following parturition is the only way of transmitting antibodies to their offspring.

TABLE 59–3 Average Composition of Bovine Precolostrum, Colostrum, and Milk (%)

Constituents	Colostrum (1st day)	Colostrum (2nd day)	Milk
Immunoglobulins	13.0	1.0	1.0
Lactose	2.5	4.0	4.5
Lipids	6.0	3.5	3.5
Nonfat solids	22.0	12.5	9.0
Proteins	19.0	7.5	3.3

in colostrum to provide passive immunity to protect the newborn for the first few weeks of life. Their colostrum is particularly rich in IgG (Fig. 59–2). Substantial amounts of IgA and IgM are also present. The neonatal animal has little proteolytic activity in the gut, and colostrum contains trypsin inhibitors. Consequently, the Igs pass intact to the ileum, where they are absorbed via pinocytosis for a limited time only.

Permeability to and absorption of the Igs in the digesta is at a peak during the first few hours after birth and starts to decline after about 6 hours. Often, by 24 hours, because of a phenomenon known as "closure," little further absorption of proteins occurs. In species that have nearly protein-impermeable placentas, it is imperative that the newborn receive an adequate supply of colostrum within the first 24 hours after birth.

For example, calves are born with very low plasma levels of Igs. These levels rise rapidly after a colostrum meal, peaking during the first day. This rise is accompanied by a transient proteinuria, resulting from renal filtration of smaller milk proteins, such as beta-lactoglobulin, that are also absorbed. The plasma IgG levels persist for several weeks, providing passive immunity until the young animal's immune system becomes activated. Some IgA is protected from digestion by a protein called secretory component, which also reduces its absorption. Lymphocytes, which may also be absorbed from colostrum, convey cell-mediated immunity, but also some infectious agents such as viruses may be absorbed.

The IgA protects against adhesion of pathogenic bacteria and viruses to the mucosa.

Confined to the vascular system because of its large size, IgM promotes phagocytosis and neutralizes antigens.

In contrast, as it readily escapes from capillaries, IgG is involved in antigen neutralization and in inflammatory reactions in the tissues.

Normal Milk

Normal milk contains proteins derived from amino acids taken up by, and synthesized in, the alveolar epithelium of the mammary gland. In the lactating mammary gland, the entire duct system is impermeable and acts as a storage region. The epithelium of the alveolus is also impermeable, blocking all paracellular (between cells) transfers, and all transport is via the transcellular route across epithelial cells. This holds even for the aqueous phase of milk, which constitutes 88 percent of cow's milk and contains the main ions (potassium, sodium, and chloride) and other substances (citrate, phosphate, calcium, urea) that make milk isoosmolar to blood plasma (Fig. 59–3). After synthesis in the endoplasmic reticulum, milk proteins for secretion pass to the Golgi vesicles, where caseins undergo phosphorylation and associate with calcium to form micelles. The Golgi vesicles move to the apical surface, and their protein contents are released by reverse pinocytosis (exocytosis, exopinocytosis, merocrine secretion).

Lactose, the predominant milk sugar, is synthesized from glucose, enters the Golgi apparatus as a complex (since the Golgi is impermeable to lactose), and is released into the alveolar lumen by exocytosis, together with milk proteins. In humans, intolerance to lactose, a deficiency in lactase (enzyme) within the small intestine mucosa, causes diarrhea and upsets the gastrointestinal tract in certain populations (e.g., Eskimos, American Indians, blacks, Asians, and New Guinea and Australian aborigines) after weaning.

Triglycerides constitute over 95 percent of milk lipids. Fatty acids are either derived from the diet or synthesized in the mammary gland. Lipid droplets migrate to the apical

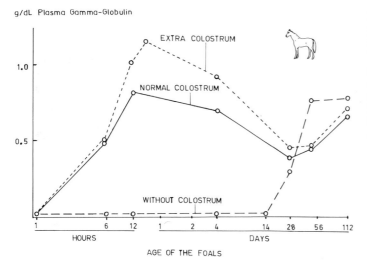

g/dL Plasma Gamma-Globulin

EXTRA COLOSTRUM

NORMAL COLOSTRUM

WITHOUT COLOSTRUM

HOURS   DAYS

AGE OF THE FOALS

Figure 59–2 In foals, illustration of the effects on plasma gamma-globulins of feeding an extra quantity, feeding a normal quantity, and a deprivation of colostrum. The deprived foals are without immunoglobulins until the second week, when they begin to produce their own, at initiation of active immunity. In contrast, the foals fed a normal or an extra quantity of colostrum within the first 6 hours possess immunoglobulins from passive immunity. In all foals, active immunity starts from about the second to the fourth week.

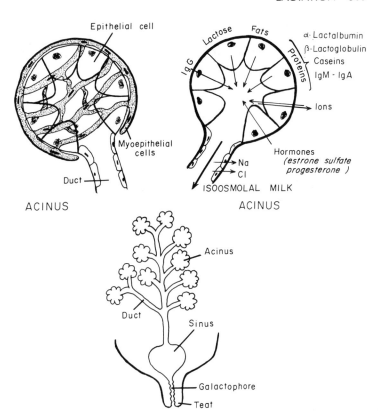

Figure 59–3 The general structure of an acinus of the mammary gland, outlining the epithelial and the myoepithelial types of cells, the milk components secreted by the alveolar cells (IgG, lactose, fats, proteins, ions, and hormones), and the reabsorption of ions in the duct. The isoosmolal milk remains stored in a converging system of ducts and in the sinus.

membrane, are enveloped, and then extruded from the cell into the lumen of the alveolus.

The composition of milk varies with the animal species, and within a given species the composition of secreted milk is not static but changes with the stage of lactogenesis and the level of nutrition. Usually, toward the end of lactogenesis, when milk production is declining, the concentrations of proteins, milk fat, and sodium (600 mg per liter) steadily increase, whereas lactose and potassium (1450 mg per liter) decrease. In mare's milk, except for sodium and potassium, the concentrations of calcium, phosphorus, magnesium, copper, and zinc decrease during the course of lactation. In 16 weeks, the content of total solids in mare's milk can pass from 12 to 10 percent, and that of ash can be halved from 0.6 to 0.3 percent. Milk is isoosmotic to plasma and has a pH near 6.8 (Table 59–4).

Epithelial cells, macrophages, mononuclear leukocytes, and cell fragments are normal elements in milk, but not polynuclear neutrophils associated with a diseased or infected mammary gland. The number of cells considered as normal in average bovine milk (0.2 × 10^6 cells per milliliter) varies with the time of day, the stage of lactogenesis, and the quarter of the udder. Equine milk usually contains very few leukocytic cells (8,000 cells per milliliter). A high-quality bovine milk must meet the major standards of low counts of somatic cells and of viable bacteria.

Certain plant alkaloids (colchicine, vincristine, vinblastine) and some plant lectins (concanavalin A) interfere with the transport and discharge phases of the secretory process, and bring a retention of the synthesized milk within the alveolar cells. Ergot derivatives (e.g., bromocriptine) can depress or stop lactogenesis II in sows by inhibiting release of prolactin (PRL) from the adenohypophysis.

Removal of Milk Stored in the Mammary Gland

Milk secreted into the lumen of the alveoli dilates and fills the alveoli, the duct system of the mammary gland, and, depending on the species, the enlarged terminal portion of the ducts (the sinus, or cistern). In ruminants, only the milk present in the larger ducts and sinus, or cistern, can be removed by cannulation of the teat (Fig. 59–4). The mammary glands of the sow do not have a sinus or cistern.

The bulk of the milk is retained in the alveoli and small ducts until the neuroendocrine milk-ejection reflex occurs. The neurohumoral reaction is activated by sensory receptors in the teat, at suckling or milking, and by conditioned responses to sound and sight at milking or suckling. The

TABLE 59–4   Average Composition of Milk in Domestic Species

Components	Bitch	Cow	Doe	Ewe	Mare	Queen	Sow
Calcium (mg/L)	2,300	1,250	1,300	1,925	1,025	350	2,100
Lactose (g/L)	35	50	45	45	45	50	45
Lipids (g/L)	85	35	40	55	15	50	95
Phosphorus (mg/L)	1,600	975	1,050	1,000	650	700	1,500
Proteins (g/L)	75	35	35	55	25	70	60
Water (mL/L)	800	875	875	825	900	800	800

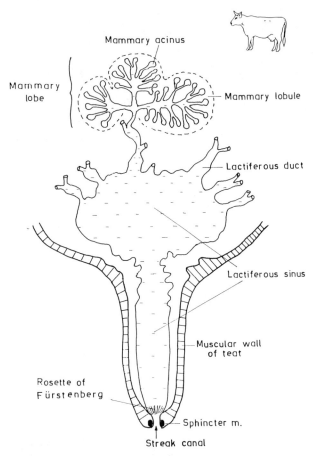

Figure 59–4 Diagrammatic representation of a bovine mammary quarter to show lobe, lobule, lactiferous duct, cisterna, and teat with its single duct, the Fürstenberg rosette, and sphincter.

nervous signals finally reach the neurohypophysis through still-unknown paths and result in oxytocin release. Oxytocin causes myoepithelial cells surrounding the alveoli to contract and to increase milk pressure in the duct system and also causes stored milk to be forced down the galactophore (Fig. 59–5). Oxytocin, released in a single spurt, has a half-life of 2 to 3 minutes.

In lambs and kids, the tongue and mouth of the sucking ruminant acts on the teat like the hand of a milker with suction added. The milk is trapped in the teat cistern by compressing the base of the teat and is then expressed through the teat canal at the tip of the teat.

> By cineradiography, with milk rendered radiopaque in the doe's udder, it has been possible to get the following description of the sucking sequence in the kid's mouth.
>
> The kid compresses the base of the teat between its upper gum and the tip of the tongue resting on the lower gum. Then, it raises its tongue to indent the teat from the base toward the tip, closing the lumen of the teat sinus and expressing the milk to be swallowed. At the same time, it lowers its jaw and tongue to allow the teat sinus to fill again with milk, and the cycle begins again.

Emotional stress, pain, fright, and epinephrine interfere with milk removal through inhibition of oxytocin release from the neurohypophysis. The inhibitory effects of epinephrine on milk ejection are also mediated by vasoconstriction of the mammary blood vessels, reducing access of oxytocin to the myoepithelial cells, and by competition for receptor sites on the myoepithelium. Some ergot derivatives (alpha-ergocryptine, ergotamine, ergocornine) are also potent inhibitors of the milk-ejection reflex.

In postparturient sows, oxytocin administration may correct some forms of a condition of agalactia, which is considered part of a syndrome also involving mastitis and metritis.

Hormonal Control

The initiation of lactogenesis is controlled mainly by lactogenic hormones from the adenohypophysis (PRL and growth hormone [GH]) and the placenta (placental mammogenic hormones or placental lactogens [PL] in cattle, sheep, and goats). PRL, GH, and PL have similar structures, but within a given species each hormone is believed to have a distinct biological role, not yet precisely characterized. Adenohypophysial lactogenic hormones can partly replace their placental counterparts in studies on initiation of lactogenesis, but they cannot do so completely. A growing body of experimental evidence gives a role to PLs in the normal growth of the udder. The metabolic hormones, such as adrenal corticoids (corticosteroids), insulin, and glucagon from the pancreas, and thyroid hormones, also directly affect the mammary gland; these same hormones exert an indirect effect on the metabolic precursors needed for milk synthesis.

In most periparturient females, the levels of progesterone and of PL decrease. These declines are followed by a rise in levels of PRL, estrogens, $PGF_{2\alpha}$, oxytocin, and adrenal corticoids. Two basic hormonal concepts are invoked to explain the triggering of lactogenesis stage II at parturition:

1. The release of the mammary gland from the inhibitory effect of progesterone, and
2. A rise in the levels of some lactogenic hormones (PRL and GH) to overcome the progesterone inhibition.

In beagle bitches, PRL levels rise steadily from midpregnancy to early lactation, decline slowly as lactation progresses, and fall abruptly upon weaning. PRL levels are not significantly lower in pseudopregnant (diestrous) bitches.

During the last week of pregnancy, the mare shows a major increase in plasma PRL concentration, which fluctuates but stays high during early lactation, then declines to basal levels in 1 to 2 months. If the foal dies shortly after birth, plasma PRL falls rapidly, and estrus occurs as early as 4 days postpartum, rather than a week after parturition, as the usual "foal heat." PRL appears to be important for the completion of mammary development and the initiation of milk secretion. Suckling triggers increases in postpartum PRL secretion.

In ruminants, after lactation is established, PRL secretion can be completely suppressed without arresting milk secretion. The release of PRL and GH, episodic in ruminants, is mostly spontaneous and due only in part to stimuli

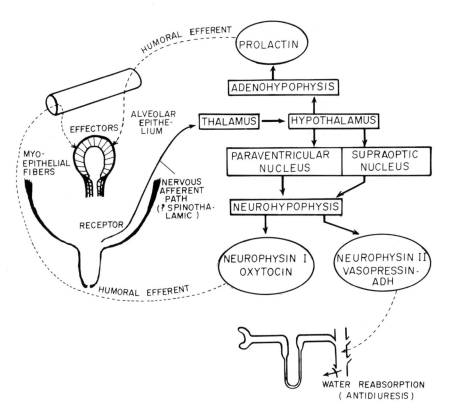

Figure 59–5 Schematic efferent actions of adenohypophysial prolactin (PRL), and neurohypophysial peptidic hormones (oxytocin and vasopressin, or antidiuretic hormone [ADH]), following the arrival of nervous afferent stimuli in the thalamus and in the hypothalamus. From the hypothalamus, the signal directly leads to release of PRL. The signal to the neurohypophysis involves either the paraventricular nucleus (for oxytocin release) or the supraoptic nucleus (for ADH release). Oxytocin contributes to galactopoiesis by contracting the myoepithelial cells for expulsion of milk stored in the alveolar cells. It also contributes to lactogenesis by accelerating the transfer of milk constituents into the alveolar cells and loosening the tight junction between the alveolar cells.

such as suckling or stress. In cows and goats, PRL plays a decisive role only for establishment of milk secretion. Although PRL release is not related to the short ruminant sleep, and to circadian activity, morning and afternoon milkings cause an immediate release of PRL and initiate a gradually decreasing chronic release of the hormone. The concentrations of PRL in blood, dependent on season (day length), are highest during summer and lowest during winter in cows, goats, and sheep. This PRL periodicity is maintained from birth to maturity in heifers and bulls, in rams, in pregnant cows, and in response to milking in cows and goats and to suckling in ewes. Goats and ewes, pregnant during the winter months, have an increase in PRL levels only a few days before parturition. Similarly, PRL levels rise sharply in the last 2 days of bovine gestation and, because of seasonal variations, are higher in autumn calving than in spring calving cows. PRL release is inhibited by PRL-inhibiting factor (PIF, or dopamine) and is stimulated by a PRL-releasing factor (PRF), which may well be thyrotropin-releasing hormone (TRF).

Growth hormone is more important than PRL for galactopoiesis in ruminants. Levels of GH are low in pregnant ewes and cows but are somewhat higher and more fluctuating in ewes carrying twins or triplets. Lactating or not, goats do not liberate GH in association with sleep, air temperature, time of day or night, or husbandry routines, or in response to plasma levels of PRL, insulin, glucose, or free fatty acids. The final release of GH is thought to be the result of a balance between the opposing effects of two hypothalamic peptides: GHRF (growth hormone–releasing factor, or somatoliberin) and somatostatin (growth hormone release–inhibiting hormone). Bovine GH produced by biotechnology, that is, by fermentation in bacteria from recombinant DNA, is known as recombinant somatotropin (rbST).

In lactating cows receiving supplemental bovine GH (bovine somatotropin, or bST), milk production is increased by 10 to 25 percent, and the feed efficiency also becomes 5 to 15 percent higher.

Sustained-release formulations have been developed that are effective for over 2 weeks.

Industrial production of bovine somatotropin made by recombinant DNA technology in bacteria (rbST) has made possible the manipulation of bovine lactation physiology. It seems that bST produces an increase in insulin-like growth factor I (IGF-I) and that this agent increases milk synthesis. A large increase in milk production, on the order of 5 to 25 percent, depending on the standard of herd management, occurs after the first 2 to 3 months of lactation. Given daily injections of rbST, the increased yield persists throughout the remainder of the lactation. New sustained-release preparations, lasting over 14 days, avoid the undesirable feature of daily injections. The only negative effect of rbST treatment is an increase in the average number of services (from about 2 to 2.5) required to achieve conception, which causes the cows to remain open (unbred) for about 21 days longer.

In one trial, the milk yield ($\bar{x}$: 20 % = 3.7 kg per day) increased promptly (2 to 3 days) after initiation of bST injection, at 9 weeks after calving (Fig. 59–6).

After a lag of about 8 weeks, dry matter intake increased by 1.7 kg per day. Feed efficiency improved by 6 percent, because of the reduced contribution of the maintenance requirements per gallon (about 4 L) of milk.

In the treated cows, an initial negative energy balance was then compensated for, through the delayed increase in food intake.

Plasma PL levels rise to a plateau of highest values during the last third of gestation in goats and cows but only 10 days before full term in ewes. Concentrations of ovine PL in peripheral plasma begin to fall 5 days before parturition and disappear rapidly after delivery.

GALACTOPOIESIS

The term galactopoiesis refers to the maintenance or stimulation of an already established milk production (lactogenesis II). Galactopoiesis is related to the removal of milk from the mammary gland by either milking or suckling. It is a commonly known fact that lactogenesis II slows or ceases altogether if the frequency and the extent of milk removal is reduced. The secretory activity of the mammary gland declines slowly and eventually ceases, even though milk is removed regularly. The natural decline in lactogenesis often coincides with weaning of the young. A negative-feedback mechanism operating locally within the gland may participate in this slow, direct, and *gradual involution* of the alveolar epithelium during the later stages of lactogenesis. In marsupials, suckling is continuous during the first part of pouch life, which is equivalent to the fetal period of placental animals (the "fetus" is firmly anchored to a nipple).

In some animals, milk is produced during a period far exceeding the weaning period of the offspring. These main milk-producing species are the goat, water buffalo, sheep, reindeer, and cattle. As a result of genetic selection for milk-producing ability, the typical modern cow produces more than four times the milk required to raise her calf, and top producers yield milk that would suffice for more than 20 times the physiological needs of the normal calf. Postpartum anestrus occurs in cows and ewes. In ewes, the duration of the postpartum anestrus is related to the degree of mammary stimulation during suckling. In cows, which are usually pregnant for most of the period of lactation, the degree of udder stimulation does not influence the duration of postpartum anestrus. In the absence of a new pregnancy, and with continual suckling or milking, lactation may be prolonged far beyond the normal weaning period (e.g., as long as several years in cows).

Hormones

Prolactin (PRL), growth hormone (GH), thyroxine (T_4), insulin, corticosteroids, and oxytocin are the hormones recognized as also associated with maintenance of lactogenesis (galactopoiesis). However, adenohypophysial release of PRL at milking or suckling is essential for galactopoiesis in most animal species, except the goat and cattle. In these two ruminants, PRL has a decisive role only in establishing lactogenesis II. The conditioned stimuli of events preceding milking, and the tactile sensations at the

EFFECTS OF BOVINE SOMATOTROPIN

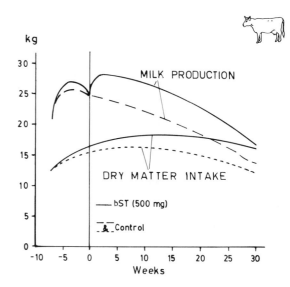

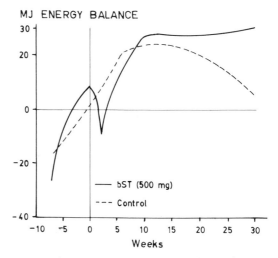

Figure 59–6 Over a period of 30 weeks, results are compared in lactating cows receiving and not receiving bovine somatotropin. The effects of injecting bovine somatotropin (bST) are an increase in milk production and a slight increase in dry matter intake. After slightly decreasing it during the first 10 weeks, bST improves and maintains the energy balance during the remaining 20 weeks (MJ).

udder and teat during milking or suckling, normally increase maternal plasma *prolactin* and *oxytocin* levels in all species. In most dams, except the cow and the nanny goat, failure to empty the milk from a producing mammary gland leads to lower levels of PRL and consequent hypogalactia, whereas inhibition of circulating PRL with an ergot alkaloid derivative (bromocriptine) induces agalactia. Besides its classic role in the milk-ejection reflex, oxytocin also influences lactogenesis and galactopoiesis. Oxytocin injected into lactating animals without immediate milking generally inhibits lactogenesis, whereas lactogenesis is stimulated if the ejected milk is removed immediately. Oxytocin would contribute to galactopoiesis by loosening the tight junctions between epithelial alveolar cells and by accelerating the transfer of milk constituents into the alveoli.

Suckling or milking causes the release of *growth hormone* in nanny goats and rats but not in cows and bitches. In nanny goats, the release of GH is unpredictable and may not be entirely related to the tactile stimulation of the mammary gland. In contrast with the situation in nonruminants, in which PRL is more important for lactogenesis, GH assumes a more prominent galactopoietic role in ruminants (cows and goats). GH is required for maintenance of galactopoiesis in cows and goats and increases milk yield in cattle without requiring a proportionate increase in food intake or a proportionate reduction in body tissue reserves in the short term.

A normally functioning thyroid gland is required for maintenance of lactogenesis. Lowered milk yield and reduced milk fat percentage resulting from thyroid deficiency are reversed by prolonged iodinated protein feeding. The role of *thyroxine* in maintaining ruminant lactogenesis is not clear, since there is less hormone in lactating cows than in nonlactating cows, and the levels are negatively correlated with milk yield.

Insulin is recognized as essential for the maintenance of normal lactogenesis, but its exact mammary gland action is difficult to distinguish from its general anabolic role. Insulin treatment decreases milk yield and milk lactose in lactating cows and goats and increases milk protein and milk fat. In goats, exogenous insulin favors synthesis of milk fat containing more C_{12} to C_{18} fatty acids.

Intact adrenal glands are essential for the maintenance of lactogenesis in both ruminant and nonruminant species, and replacement therapy is best effected by a combination of mineralocorticoids and glucocorticoids. In cattle, plasma *corticosteroids* are higher in lactating animals than in nonlactating ones, and high-yielding cows have more corticosteroids than low-yielding ones. A disagreement remains to be resolved on the relationship between plasma level of corticosteroids and the stage of lactogenesis in cattle. Some claim that the basal postpartum level increases as lactation progresses, whereas others support the opposite view, that is, a high postpartum level that decreases with progressing lactogenesis.

Cessation of Galactopoiesis by Involution of the Mammary Gland

In animals, involution of the mammary gland may be "initiated" or "gradual." *Initiated involution* refers to the regression of the gland as a result of sudden cessation of milk removal during galactopoiesis. *Gradual involution* is the regression of the mammary gland during the normal course of galactopoiesis.

Initiated involution is of practical value in sows, since the production objectives aim at increasing the annual number of piglets per dam, rather than the annual milk yield. Regression of the mammary gland by early and sudden weaning of piglets (i.e., at 3 weeks instead of at 6 weeks) is recommended in order to decrease the length of lactogenesis

and the interval between farrowing. In this sow-breeding system, sudden stoppage of milk removal ends lactogenesis II at 3 weeks postpartum, when it is actually reaching its peak. Withholding feed for the first 2 or 3 days after withdrawal of the piglets reduces the milk flow, and gonadotropins (pregnant mare serum gonadotropin and human chorionic gonadotropin) are then injected to speed up and synchronize the onset of estrus after early weaning. Complete involution of the gland occurs after 8 days in sows.

Sudden weaning of animals in full lactogenesis usually results in gross distention of the mammary gland for 3 or 4 days. The interstitial fluid is laden with milk constituents (milk edema). During initiated involution, milk secretion is unaffected for 16 hours in cows, and for 12 hours in ewes. Distention is concomitant with neutrophilic infiltration, which is followed by the appearance of macrophages (foamy cells, bodies of Donné) before lymphocytic dominance sets in, usually from the fourth day in ewes.

Gradual involution does not proceed uniformly throughout the gland. Areas adjacent to the abdominal walls are the last to involute. Even at the height of lactogenesis II, as much as 20 percent of the mammary gland of the cow shows areas of alveoli without secretory activity. These areas resemble those of a nonlactating gland, with prominent interalveolar and interlobular connective tissue. Stilbestrol (unauthorized drug) fed to cows, and injections of GH or of small doses of estradiol to nonpregnant cows, prolong galactopoiesis or decrease the gradual involution of the mammary gland. Gestation stops galactopoiesis in goats and reduces milk production in cows. In mares and bitches, large doses of estrogens are used to put a sudden end to lactogenesis.

In the involuting gland, lactoferrin production by mammary epithelial cells increases (as in acute mastitis) to exert a bacteriostatic effect. Lactoferrin, the major iron-binding protein of milk, is a natural protective factor. By binding to iron, lactoferrin withholds an essential nutrient from pathogenic bacteria.

REFERENCES

Akers RM. Lactogenic hormones: binding sites, mammary growth, secretory cell differentiation, and milk biosynthesis in ruminants. J Dairy Sci 1985;68:501.

Bauman DE, Currie WB. Partitioning of nutrients during pregnancy and lactation: a review of mechanisms involving homeostasis and homeorrhesis. J Dairy Sci 1980;63:1514.

Bauman DE, Epperd PJ, DeGeeter MJ, Lanza GM. Responses of high-producing dairy cows to long-term treatment with pituitary somatotropin and recombinant somatotropin. J Dairy Sci 1985;68:1352.

Brandon MR, Watson DL, Lascelles AK. The mechanism of transfer of immunoglobulins into mammary secretions of cows. Aust J Biol Med Sci 1971;49:613.

Campbell SG, Siegel MJ, Knowlton BJ. Sheep immunoglobulins and their transmission to the lamb. NZ Vet J 1977;25:361.

Collier RJ, McNamara JP, Wallace CR, Dehoff MH. A review of endocrine regulation of metabolism during lactation. J Anim Sci 1984;59:498.

Cowie AT, Forsyth IA, Hart IC. Hormonal control of lactation. New York: Springer-Verlag, 1980.

DeLouis C, Dijane J, Houdebine LM, Terqui M. Relation between hormones and mammary gland function. J Dairy Sci 1980;63:1492.

Forsyth IA. Variation among species in the endocrine control of mammary growth and function: the roles of prolactin, growth hormone, and placental lactogen. J Dairy Sci 1986;69:886.

Houdebine LM, Dijane J, Dusanter-Fourt I, et al. Hormonal action controlling mammary activity. J Dairy Sci 1985;68:489.

Jeffcott LB. Studies on passive immunity in the foal. I. γ-Globulin and antibody variations associated with the maternal transfer of immunity and the onset of active immunity. J Comp Pathol 1974;84:93.

Larson BL. Lactation. A comprehensive treatise. IV. The mammary gland—Human lactation—Milk synthesis. New York: Academic Press, 1978.

Larson BL, Smith VR. Lactation. A comprehensive treatise. I. The mammary gland—Development and maintenance. New York: Academic Press, 1974.

Larson BL, Smith VR. Lactation. A comprehensive treatise. II. Biosynthesis and secretion of milk—Diseases. New York: Academic Press, 1974.

Larson BL, Smith VR. Lactation. A comprehensive treatise. III. Nutrition and biochemistry of milk—Maintenance. New York: Academic Press, 1974.

Logan EF, Penhale WJ. Studies on the immunity of the calf to colibacillosis. Vet Rec 1971;88:222.

Mepham TB, Lawrence SE, Peters AR, Hart IC. Effect of exogenous growth hormone on mammary function in lactating goats. Horm Metab Res 1985;16:248.

Phipps RH. A review of the influence of somatotropin on health, reproduction, and welfare in lactating dairy cows. In: Sejrsen K, Vestergaard M, Neimann-Sørensen A, eds. Use of somatotropin in livestock production. New York: Elsevier Science Pub., 1989.

Schryver HF, Oftedal OT, Williams J, et al. Lactation in the horse: the mineral composition of mare milk. J Nutr 1986;116:2142.

Swanson EW, Poffenbarger JI. Mammary gland development of dairy heifers during their first gestation. J Dairy Sci 1979;62:702.

Weber AF. The bovine mammary gland: structure and function. J Am Vet Med Assoc 1977;170:1133.

Winters WD. Time-dependent decreases of maternal canine virus antibodies in newborn pups. Vet Rec 1981;108:295.

CHAPTER 60

PERIPARTURIENT, PUERPERAL, AND NEONATAL PERIODS

The periparturient period, particularly well-known in the cow, describes the time of parturition and the events that occur a few weeks prior to and following parturition. This period generally includes the dry period (from the seventh to the eighth month of pregnancy) through the first 3 to 4 weeks after calving.

The puerperal (maternal) period is more limited, including an interval from parturition until the resumption of the estrous cycles. The puerperium includes the involution of the uterus, the restoration of the endometrium, and the return of estrous cyclical activity. In mares, the puerperium is much shorter than that in ruminants, whereas it is very similar in length in cows, ewes, and goats.

The neonatal (newborn) period is very short, extending only from parturition to up to 96 hours after birth. The perinatal period encompasses the initiation of parturition, the puerperium, and the neonatal period.

PERIPARTURIENT PERIOD

In cows, complex synchronous hormonal changes occur during the periparturient period. These hormones regulate lactogenesis, parturition, postpartum milk production, and reproduction performances.

In the periparturient cow, during the last 10 prepartum days, the peripheral blood plasma concentration of progesterone continuously declines, whereas that of estrone and estrone sulfate first increases then decreases gradually. The fall in the plasma progesterone level is precipitated by a slow rise in the level of 13, 14-dihydro 15-keto prostaglandin $F_{2\alpha}$, the prostaglandin metabolite also termed PGFM (Fig. 60–1).

A rapid postpartum increase in plasma prostaglandin $F_{2\alpha}$, which is produced by the uterine caruncles, coincides with the rapid uterine involution during days 3 to 4 following parturition. The plasma prolactin concentration, which peaks prior to parturition, follows an isometric curve that straddles the prepartum and postpartum periods for about a week. The rise in prolactin, which is involved in lactogenesis, correlates with the reduction in the C19 (estrone) and C21 (progesterone) steroids, which rapidly reach postpartum basal levels (Fig. 60–2).

Periparturient lactogenesis is associated with intense mammary growth, copious synthesis and secretion (carbohydrates, fats, and proteins), rapid differentiation of secretory parenchyma, and marked accumulation of colostrum and milk. Prior to and during parturition, the mammary gland is very susceptible to infections, particularly to ubiquitous environmental bacteria (e.g., coliforms, *Streptococcus dysgalactiae, S. uberis, S. faecalis*), which are then less susceptible to antibiotic therapy. In addition, the periparturient cow is at risk for common reproductive disorders, which include abnormal health status, anovulation, cystic ovaries, dystocia, infections of the reproductive tract, metritis, retained placenta, stillbirth, and twinning. The relative incidence of these periparturient reproductive disorders is variable (Table 60–1).

Abnormal health status includes abnormal parturition and other abnormal periparturient problems that reduce milk yield, reproductive performance, and overall productivity.

Anovulation in a dairy cow is defined as a prolonged or delayed interval (i.e., beyond 4 weeks, between parturition and the first postpartum estrus or ovulation).

Cystic ovaries contain either thin-walled (follicular) cysts or thick-walled (luteal) cysts.

Dystocia generally includes any calving in which assistance is required. It occurs more frequently with the heavier male offspring, which requires a prolonged gestation.

Infections of the reproductive tract include various abnormal or purulent discharges from the genitalia (cervicitis, endometritis, metritis, pyometra, vaginitis).

Metritis is an inflammation limited to the uterus.

Retained placenta is the nondelivery of the fetal membranes after 8 to 12 hours and up to 24 hours. It increases the risk for uterine infections, and for metabolic disorders such as ketosis and left displaced abomasum.

Stillbirth refers to the birth of a dead fetus or calf.

Twinning occurs in a cow bearing two offspring. The risks of retained placenta, stillbirth, and left displaced abomasum are increased.

In addition, in the periparturient high-milk-producing cow, some metabolic disorders (clinical ketosis, downer cow syndrome, hypomagnesemic tetany, left displaced abomasum, milk fever, and udder edema) seem "associated" with each other. In this association, milk fever would link these clinical disorders together (Fig. 60–3).

Clinical ketosis (acetonemia, lactation ketosis) is a condition manifested by a lack of appetite (negative energy balance) for concentrates within 5 weeks of calving, in a high-producing cow. The "ketone bodies" (acetone, acetoacetate, beta-hydroxybutyrate) level in blood increases and they overflow into urine, milk, or both.

Downer cow complex (alert downer, atypical milk fever, creeper cow, downer cow syndrome, downer, fat cow syndrome) is applied to any cow with milk fever that does not get up within 10 minutes to 24 hours of first treatment with intravenous calcium. The cow is generally alert with no forelimb problems, but a hindlimb paresis keeps her from

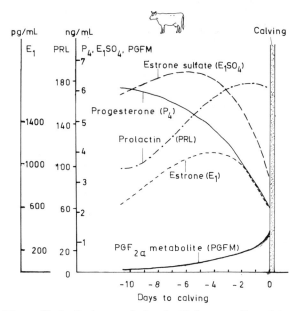

Figure 60–1 In the cow, during the 10 days preceding calving, the plasma levels of estrone (E_1), estrone sulfate (E_1SO_4), and progesterone (P_4) decrease. The rise in prolactin (PRL) is linked to the increase and decline in E_1 and E_1SO_4. The concentration of PGFM (metabolite of prostaglandin F) increases slightly and correlates with the decline in progesterone.

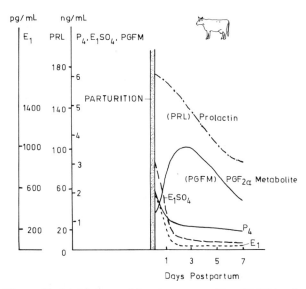

Figure 60–2 After parturition, the estrogens (E_1 and E_1SO_4) and progesterone return to basal levels. Over a week, the concentration of prolactin gradually declines from its preparturition peak. In contrast, the postparturient plasma level of a metabolite of prostaglandin F (PGFM) suddenly undergoes about a four-fold surge, which is maintained for roughly 2 days before it begins gradually to subside to the basal level.

TABLE 60–1 Relative Incidence (%) of Reproductive Disorders in Periparturient Cows

Abnormal health status	37
Anovulation	6
Cystic ovaries	12
Dystocia	6
Metritis	21
Reproductive tract infections	17
Retained placenta	9
Stillbirth	4
Twinning	3

rising for at least 24 hours, for no apparent reason. The sequelae from recumbency are ischemic myonecrosis and neuropathy from pressure on the muscles and sciatic nerve.

Hypomagnesemic tetany (clinical hypomagnesemia, grass tetany, "Kopziekte") affects cattle, sheep, and goats not receiving adequate available magnesium. It can be of the spring (grass), winter (hay), or out-winter (sparse pasture) type.

Left displaced abomasum is a condition in which the fundus and greater curvature of the atonic abomasum creep from the midline to the left side, between the dorsal sac of the rumen and the left abdominal wall.

Milk fever (eclampsia, parturient apoplexy, parturient hypocalcemia, parturient paresis, parturient puerperalis) is an afebrile hypocalcemic disease associated with parturition and initiation of lactation.

Udder edema is an increased volume of extracellular fluid in the supporting tissue (stroma) of the mammary gland starting 2 to 4 days before calving, peaking at calving, and declining within 1 to 2 weeks of calving.

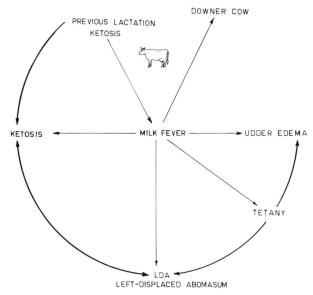

Figure 60–3 A diagrammatic representation of the loose "associations" between the postparturient metabolic dysfunctions, which are not cause-related or cause-dependent. It is convenient to place parturient paresis (milk fever) in a central position and relate it to six periparturient metabolic problems: downer cow, ketosis, left displaced abomasum, hypomagnesemic tetany, previous lactation ketosis, and udder edema.

PUERPERAL EVENTS

The principal areas of placental exchanges in ruminants, the *placentomes,* are the functional units formed by the maternal caruncles and the fetal cotyledons. During the third stage of parturition and during the postpartum periods, an undisturbed loosening process in the placentomes is essential for timely spontaneous expulsion of the placenta in cows, ewes, and goats.

A normal *separation of the bovine placenta* requires

1. a preterm final collagenous maturation of the placentomes by a high-estrogen secretion, maintained for at least 5 days to break down lysosomes and release hydrolases;
2. intrapartum uterine contractions to increase and decrease alternately the size of the fetomaternal interface at the placentomes, to expand the caruncular connective tissue stalk sidewards, and to press the maternal caruncle against the fetus;
3. local efflux of blood after rupture of the umbilical cord to decrease the size of the fetal cotyledons; and
4. postpartum uterine contractions to decrease and invert the fetal sac, to reduce the size of the caruncular stalk, to dilate the caruncular crypts, and to separate the fetoplacental unit.

In the early phase of parturition in cows, hormonal influences (prostaglandin E) start the placental detachment mechanism by imbibition for expansion and softening of the collagenous tissues of the placentomes. During labor, alternating anemic and congestive conditions are created at the *fetal cotyledons* by forcible contractions of the uterine wall and by great oscillations in uterine pressure. Gradually diminishing uterine contractions persist for the first 2 or 3 days postpartum.

Following delivery of the fetus, the shape of the softened cotyledons changes, and their contact area with the caruncles shrinks after rupture of the umbilical cord owing to lack of blood in the fetal capillaries (Fig 60–4). After impairment of the attachment of the cotyledons to the maternal caruncles, physiological *expulsion of the fetal membranes* can proceed.

From the onset of the postpartum period, the *maternal caruncles* then regress, and the endometrium undergoes an important double process of degeneration and regeneration. Necrosis sets in, in the caruncular arteries, and on the surface of the caruncles. The epithelium of the intercaruncular and glandular endometriun also degenerates and is shed in the lochia near the tenth day postpartum. In the meantime, a new epithelial surface is gradually generated to cover the entire uterus, caruncles included, within 30 days.

The term *lochia* is applied to fluids of changing characteristics and abundance (about 1,000 mL in the cow) normally discharged from the vulva after parturition. Of uterine origin, the lochia consist mostly of gestation fluids, with some blood at first, together with some placental and uterine epithelial cells, and blood or reticuloendothelial system macrophages and polynuclear cells associated with bacteria. The elimination of lochia is irregular: profuse for the first 2 or 3 days, it then regresses to reappear abundantly on the tenth to

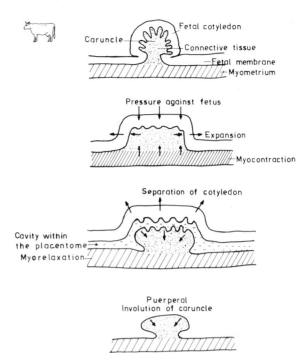

Figure 60–4   Diagrammatic changes in the mushroom-shaped bovine placentomes that are associated with separation of the fetoplacental units. The reduction in the size of the cotyledons combined with widening of the stalk of the caruncles leads to the third stage of parturition, the delivery of the fetal membranes.

twelfth days and completely disappears after 21 days postpartum. In ewes and goats, the discharge of lochia (dark red, odorless) persists for about 3 weeks.

The species with noncotyledonary placentation have a relatively slight lochial discharge compared with that of ruminants. In the postparturient bitch, after normal completion of the third stage of labor, the green-tinted (uteroverdin) lochia disappears from the vulva within about 24 hours, after changing gradually from opaque to clear mucus with a tinge of blood. In the mare, the slight lochial discharge usually ceases in less than 3 days.

Involution of the Uterus.   Immediately after parturition, the bovine uterus is a large, flabby sac nearly a meter long by 40 cm across and weighs about 9 kg. However, the uterus decreases in size rapidly, and these values are reduced by 50 percent in 5 days for the diameter, in 7 days for the weight, and in 10 days for the length (Fig. 60–5). The size of myometrial fibers rapidly shrinks (from 700 to 200 μm) without any evidence of necrotic or degenerative change in the muscular cells. Complete involution of the postparturient cow's uterus is completed between the 25th and 45th days.

In ewes and goats, uterine involution proceeds more rapidly, as the length of the delivered horn is reduced by 50 percent in the first 24 hours postpartum. In general, the bitch, ewe, nanny goat, and sow complete the involution of the postparturient uterus within 4 weeks, whereas it only requires about 2 weeks in the mare.

POSTPARTUM UTERINE INVOLUTION

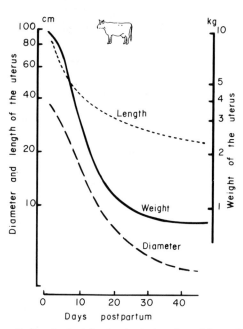

Figure 60–5 Gradual decrease in the length, weight, and diameter of the uterus of the cow during the puerperium, that is, from parturition to return of the cyclical reproduction pattern. During the first 2 weeks of the puerperal period, the decrease in uterine mass and diameter is more rapid than the reduction in length.

In the bitch, when postpartum involution of the uterus is abnormal, the retained blood, placental fluids, and placental debris are broken down into products that are ultimately excreted into the canine milk. In the nursing puppies, these products induce restlessness and signs of digestive troubles. However, an abnormal involution of the uterus is not a serious hazard to the health of the bitch.

At parturition, the uterine cavity is a sterile environment, without *bacteria*. Within a short time-span after parturition, bacteria (*Escherichia coli, Proteus, Staphylococcus, Actinomyces pyogenes*) migrate into the uterus of the cow and the mare by an ascending process from the outer anogenital regions. In the cow, the bacteria multiply in the anaerobic uterus during the postpartum period, reach a maximum number at about day 9, and subside near the 21st day following delivery (Fig. 60–6). Almost all cows (about 90 percent) acquire some nonspecific postpartum genital tract infections. In the mare, these organisms usually disappear at the foal estrus (i.e., about 1 week after parturition).

Although signs of *estrus* may be seen in some sows 3 to 5 days following parturition, this estrus is without ovulation and is infertile. A normal estrus usually occurs 1 week after weaning of the piglets. In the mare, a fertile postpartum estrus (foal heat) is ordinarily seen during the 7 to 10 days following foaling. In contrast, in bitches, ewes, goats, and queens, the seasonal period of anestrus follows the puerperium.

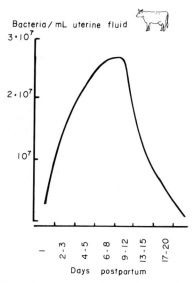

Figure 60–6 In the cow, during the first 2 weeks of puerperium, the number of bacteria (number per milliliter of uterine fluid) rapidly progresses to a summit. A faster regression in the uterine bacterial count occurs during the following week.

Hormonal Changes in the Puerperium. In the puerperal cow, the secretion of FSH soon increases to stimulate the development of follicles. The adenohypophysis gradually responds to gonadotropin-releasing hormone (GnRH) with more frequent release of pulses of luteinizing hormone (LH). Follicular growth results in the production of estradiol and inhibin. The positive-feedback response to estradiol is gradually restored, enabling the release of a surge of preovulatory gonadotropins. The entire process may be completed in about 3 weeks after parturition. The short, and often unnoticed, first behavioral postpartum estrus is said to be "silent," because of a reduced progesterone concentration in the blood and milk.

In mares and sows, the influence of follicle-stimulating hormone (FSH) seems more pronounced (Fig. 60–7), as within a week after parturition, the mare has a fertile estrus, and the sow exhibits signs of an infertile estrus.

NEONATAL EVENTS

After parturition, the passive fetal existence in a temperature-controlled aquatic environment is no longer possible, and the nervous system of the mature newborn must quickly adapt to challenges in the seemingly hostile surroundings. The *immediate neonatal changes* include discrete modifications of the circulatory system, the mother-offspring bond, thermoregulation, the intestinal epithelium, and the evident onset of respiration.

Circulatory Changes. The *circulatory changes* consist of the closure of the *ductus venosus*, the *ductus arteriosus*, and the *foramen ovale*. The ductus venosus closure is secondary to a

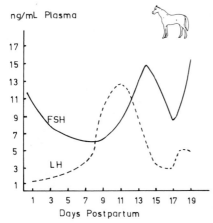

Figure 60–7 Approximate plasma concentration of FSH and LH in puerperal mares. At parturition, the level of FSH is higher than that of LH. In about 7 days, the level of LH rises to equal that of FSH and then peaks at ovulation. The peak of FSH follows the foal heat.

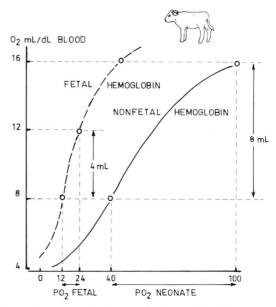

Figure 60–8 Range of PO_2 in fetal and neonatal calves, that is, before and after transformation of the fetal hemoglobin into nonfetal hemoglobin. The transformation makes double the volume of oxygen (from 4 to 8 mL per deciliter of blood) available to the tissues of the animal.

drop in blood pressure in the umbilical cord. In contrast, the closure of the ductus arteriosus and that of the foramen ovale are associated with pulmonary vasodilation and the entrance of air to dilate the alveoli. Simultaneous to the pulmonary vasodilation, tachycardia (increased frequency of the heartbeat) occurs. A jugular vein refill time of less than 5 seconds indicates an adequate or normal circulatory venous pressure, whereas a longer refill time points to hypotension or circulatory shock. When the pulmonary vasoconstriction is maintained after birth, marked hypoxia rapidly causes death of the newborn. During the neonatal period, the fetal hemoglobin is changed for nonfetal hemoglobin, which operates within a wider spectrum of partial pressure of oxygen (PO_2) and allows blood to deliver more oxygen to the tissues (Fig. 60–8).

Respiratory Changes. The calf is able to breathe as soon as the nose passes the vulva, but the expansion of the chest is restricted by the narrow birth canal. When the calf is completely delivered, and is released from peripheral and central inhibitory respiratory reflexes, respiration is established after a short period of "gasping." The warm liquid in the oropharynx and over the surface of the skin maintains the peripheral respiratory inhibition. Efficient physical means to counteract this peripheral inhibition and to stimulate the respiration are the pouring of cold water over the head, brisk rubbing to dry the skin, or the tickling of the nasal mucosa of the calf with a piece of straw. An increase in arterial PCO_2, in concert with the declining blood pH and PO_2, neutralizes the central reflex inhibition of respiration and activates arterial chemoreceptors that stimulate breathing.

Once the offspring are released from the inhibitory respiratory reflexes, they must generate a negative intrathoracic pressure of about 70 cm H_2O, which is about five times higher than that required for a normal inspiration. This high pressure is necessary to displace the remaining pulmonary fluids and to accelerate their absorption into the

pulmonary capillaries (venous and lymphatic). The decrease in pulmonary fluids begins during the 24 to 48 hours preceding parturition, continues during parturition (stage 2 of parturition) as the thorax is compressed, and is completed with the first inspirations. Now dilated with air, the alveoli are prevented from collapsing by phospholipids (surfactant) from granular pneumocytes (type II alveolar cells), which are stimulated by a higher parturient and neonatal output of catecholamines (norepinephrine, 4-fold; epinephrine, 100-fold). Surfactant also keeps interstitial fluid from entering the alveoli.

Mother-Offspring Bond. The *bond between mother and offspring* results from exchange of tactile, auditory, olfactory, and visual stimuli during the first 2 hours following parturition, when maternal behavior (licking, grooming) and offspring care-seeking behavior develop. Some offspring, born with considerable maturity (foal, piglet, young of ruminants) can see, vocalize (kid, lamb, piglet) with their mother, stand, and walk. In some species, the offspring are blind and are only able to crawl (kitten, puppy). Sucking movements with the tongue and the lips may be present within minutes after birth. The piglets that are born first take longer to locate the udder than those born later, which benefit from a social facilitation. The mature calf, foal, kid, lamb, and piglet show thigmotaxis (searching for udder) soon after standing.

Intestinal Epithelium. During the period immediately following birth, the *permeability of the small intestine* is greater than a few days later. This period of increased permeability to compounds (proteins, drugs) corresponds to the time during which the gastrointestinal mucosa is immunologically naive. Only those cells of the intestinal epithelium produced prenatally are able to absorb large amounts of protein. The cells slowly migrating out, from the crypts up the villi, that eventually replace these prenatal cells have more limited absorption capacities.

Because the newborn calf, foal, lamb, kid, and piglet have a low level of blood immunoglobulins at birth, they must ingest colostrum within 6 hours of birth. The small intestine is permeable to the colostral immunoglobulins (IgG, IgA, and IgM) for only a short time after birth; afterwards this pinocytotic absorption of large proteins decreases with time. In the calf, each class of Ig has a different "shut down": 27 hours for IgG, 22 hours for IgA, and 16 hours for IgM. In the foal, the small intestine's permeability to immunoglobulins (Igs) is estimated to be less than 36 hours, and more like 24 hours. Not only does colostrum provide protection via immediate passive humoral immunity that persists for several weeks, but also colostrum has a high nutritive value (rich in fat, protein, and vitamins) that is important in thermoregulation. Colostrum also has some laxative effect for evacuation of meconium.

Intestinal Absorption of Drugs. During the first 2 days of life, the intestine absorbs compounds (proteins) or drugs not absorbed normally from the gut (sulfonamides, neomycin, streptomycin, carbenicillin, and some nitrofurans). In the neonate, such substances may cause systemic effects because of large quantities in the blood, due to increased absorption and to a slower hepatic biological transformation that may last for as long as 3 to 5 weeks in the calf. Ingestion of milk-containing drugs, pesticides, or plant alkaloids by a nursing neonate represents a real threat, since renal function is deficient until 1 or 2 months. Antimicrobial drugs used for treatment of neonatal diarrhea can perturb the flora of the gut of suckling animals. Intoxication in the neonate can occur in the absence of signs in the dam.

Thermoregulation of the Newborn. At birth, the body temperature of the newborn rapidly declines from that of the comfortable uterine environment (a drop of 5 °C in the neonatal puppy and kitten). Several factors contribute to lowering the body temperature of the newborn: cooling evaporation from the wet skin, poor hair coat (piglet), lack of subcutaneous fat for insulation, and a high surface area per unit of body mass in small individuals. With an immediate and adequate provision of energy (colostrum), the neonate increases its metabolic rate about three-fold and attempts to produce heat to regulate its body temperature. The neonate uses this metabolic mechanism and shivering, with physical means to reduce their heat loss (thermoneutral environment, insulation by dry bedding, drying of hair coat, huddling) and control their body temperature. The mature newborns usually return their body temperature to normal in a few hours (calf, foal, kid, lamb) or in about 24 hours (piglets). The less mature neonates (kitten, puppy) need about a week to recover a normal body temperature.

In foals, an important digestive activity that occurs between 0.5 and 3 days is the *voiding of meconium* (fetal digestive glandular secretions, digestive amniotic fluid, and cell debris). It appears as brown, greenish-brown, or black, hard pellets or a paste-like mass covered by semiviscous mucus. The first micturition occurs after between 5 hours (colt) and 9 hours (filly). A transient proteinuria following administration of colostrum to foals is due to renal excretion of small proteins (alpha-lactalbumin and beta-lactoglobulin) absorbed together with the larger Ig. Renal function, usually reduced in the neonate, is exceptional in the newborn calf, in which it is comparable to that of adult cattle.

Development of the Nervous System. In foals and ruminant offspring, the maturity of the nervous system is evaluated by the presence of several physiological nervous reflexes. The major ones that are used clinically are the leg retraction reflex (nociception: pinching of the digits), the sucking reflex (finger in the mouth), the ocular reflex (vibration, in response to slight pressure on the ocular globe), and the pupillary reflex (light induces a reduction in the size of the pupil).

Puppies and kittens are less mature offspring than calves, foals, kids, lambs, and piglets. The offspring of carnivores are born blind, since about 5 to 6 days elapse before their eyelids separate. However, more resistant to anoxia, puppies and kittens can endure about 10 minutes without breathing, whereas the more mature calves, foals, kids, lambs, and piglets can only withstand less than 5 minutes of apnea.

At the time of birth, the generation of neurons and pathways is complete, and even excessive, in the mammalian nervous system. Postnatally and throughout life, only olfactory neurons are subject to regeneration and turnover. Other types of neurons do not regenerate. However, a lack of stimulation during a critical period of postnatal development can lead to the elimination of neurons and pathways, which are then presumed or considered to be extraneous or redundant. With the monocularly deprived neonatal kitten as an experimental model, this has been demonstrated on the visual geniculostriate neurons. From this has evolved a concept stressing the importance of early treatment of visual disorders.

As a model of physiological sensory (visual, light) depression, monocularly deprived kittens are raised to adulthood after neonatal suture-closing of the eyelids over one cornea.

The eyelids can be reopened (at 4 to 6 months) to evaluate the long-term influence of a lack of light stimulation on the development of sight in that eye.

With this model, subtle changes in the postnatal development of the visual nervous system have been discovered. For instance, absence of light stimulation during a critical period, which extends from 3 weeks to 6 months and peaks at about 3 to 4 months, results in permanent defects in geniculostriate neurons. Before or after this critical period, deprivation of light sensation does not induce regression of these visual neurons and pathways.

Premature newborns are weak, emaciated, and smaller than normal, can stand only after an abnormally long delay (over 2 hours for a foal), and their skin and mucosa are meconium stained (orange-red). *Dysmaturity* is a term applied to newborns that are smaller than expected because of deprivation due to placental dysfunction or insufficiency. Deterioration (weakness, emaciation, inability to stand and to suck) is quite dramatic and disappointing on the second and third days of life of these newborns. Specialized technologies for life support of premature neonates have been developed.

REFERENCES

Bureau MA, Begin R. Postnatal maturation of the respiratory response to O_2 in awake newborn lambs. J Appl Physiol 1982;52:428.

Da Rosa GO, Wagner WC. Adrenal-gonad interactions in cattle. Corpus luteum function in intact and adrenalectomized heifers. J Anim Sci 1981;52:1098.

Easter SS Jr. Birth of olfactory neurons: life-long neurogenesis. Trends Neurosci 1984;7:105.

Edquist JE, Kindahl H, Stabenfelt G. Release of prostaglandin $F_{2\alpha}$ during the bovine perinatal period. Prostaglandins 1978;16:111.

Edwards S, Foxcraft GR. Endocrine changes in sows weaned at two stages of lactation. J Reprod Fertil 1983;67:163.

Eley DS, Thatcher WW, Head HH, et al. Periparturient and postpartum endocrine changes of conceptus and maternal units in Jersey cows bred for milk yield. J Dairy Sci 1981;64:312.

Erb HN, Grohn YT. Symposium: health problems in the periparturient cow. J Dairy Sci 1988;71:2557.

Foster JP, Lamming GE, Peters AR. Short-term relationships between plasma LH, FSH, and progesterone concentrations in post-partum dairy cows and the effect of Gn-RH injection. J Reprod Fertil 1980;59:321.

Fowden AL, Ellis L, Rossdale PD. Pancreatic beta cell function in the neonatal foal. J Reprod Fertil 1982;Suppl 32:p.529.

Garcia M, Larsson K. Clinical findings in postpartum dairy cows. Nordisk Vet Med 1982;34:255.

Gygax AP, Ganjam VK, Kennedy RM. Clinical, microbiological, and histological changes associated with uterine involution in the mare. J Reprod Fertil 1979;Suppl 27:p.571.

Jeffcott LB, Rossdale PD, Leadon DP. Haematological changes in the neonatal period of induced premature foals. J Reprod Fertil 1982;Suppl 32:p.537.

Lamming GE, Foster JP, Bulman DC. Pharmacological control of reproduction cycles. Vet Rec 1979;104:156.

Leslie KE. The events of normal and postpartum reproductive endocrinology and uterine involution in dairy cows: a review. Can Vet J 1983;24:67.

Loy RG, Evans MJ, Pemstein R, Taylor TB. Effects of injection of ovarian steroids on reproductive patterns and performance in postpartum mares. J Reprod Fertil 1982;Suppl 32:p.199.

Mather EC, Melancon JJ. The periparturient cow—a pivotal entity in dairy production. J Dairy Sci 1981;64:1422.

Oliver SP, Sordillo LM. Udder health in the periparturient period. J Dairy Sci 1988;71:2584.

Olson JD, Ball L, Mortimer RG, et al. Aspects of bacteriology and endocrinology of cows with pyometra and retained fetal membranes. Am J Vet Res 1984;45:2251.

Pearson RC, Hallowell AL, Bayly WM, Perryman LE. Times of appearance and disappearance of colostral IgG in the mare. Am J Vet Res 1984;45:186.

Peters AR, Lamming GE. Regulation of ovarian function in the postpartum cow: an endocrine model. Vet Rec 1986;118:236.

Petrie L. Maximizing the absorption of colostral immunoglobulins in the newborn diary calf. Vet Rec 1984;114:157.

Rose RJ, Rossdale PD, Leadon DP. Blood gas and acid-base status in spontaneously delivered, term-induced and induced premature foals. J. Reprod Fertil 1982;Suppl 32:p.521.

Rossdale PD. Clinical studies on the newborn thoroughbred foal. Br Vet J 1967;123:470.

Schmidt PM, Chakraborty PK, Wildt DE. Ovarian activity, circulating hormones, and sexual behavior in the cat. Relationships during pregnancy, parturition, lactation, and the postpartum estrus. Biol Reprod 1983;28:657.

Sherman SM, Spear PD. Organization of visual pathways in normal and visually deprived cats. Physiol Rev 1982;62:738.

Stevenson JS, Call EP. Reproductive disorders in the periparturient dairy cow. J Dairy Sci 1988;71:2572.

Svajgr AJ, Hays VM, Cromwell GL, Dutt RH. Effect of lactation on reproductive performance of sows. J Anim Sci 1974;38:100.

Wright PJ, Geytenbeek PE, Clarke IJ, Findlay JK. Evidence for a change in oestradiol negative feedback and LH pulse frequency in post-partum ewes. J Reprod Fertil 1981;61:97.

APPENDIX I

SYMBOLS AND ABBREVIATIONS OF TERMS USED IN RESPIRATORY PHYSIOLOGY

Primary Symbols* for Blood and Gas

C	Concentration of gas in blood
D	Diffusion capacity of gas
f_R	Respiratory frequency
F	Fractional concentration in dry gas phase
M	Mass or quantity of substance
$\dot{M}$	Quantity of substance per unit of time
P	Gas pressure or partial pressure
$\bar{P}$	Mean gas pressure
Q	Volume of blood
$\dot{Q}$	Volume of blood per unit of time
R	Respiratory exchange ratio or $\dot{V}CO_2/\dot{V}O_2$
S	Percentage saturation of hemoglobin with O_2 or CO_2
torr	Partial gas pressure equivalent to 1 mm Hg, 13.6 mm H_2O, or 133.3 Pa; note that 1 KPa = 7.5 mm Hg = 10 cm H_2O
V	Volume of gas
$\dot{V}$	Volume per unit of time

Secondary Symbols* for Blood

a	Arterial blood
b	Blood in general
c	Capillary blood
c′	End capillary
i	Ideal
v	Venous
$\bar{v}$	Mixed venous blood

Secondary Symbols* for Gases

A	Alveolar gas
B	Barometric
D	Dead space gas
E	Expired gas
I	Inspired gas
L	Pulmonary
T	Tidal gas
ATPS	Ambient temperature and pressure, saturated with water vapor

*The symbols are generally as follows: the FIRST LETTER, the primary symbol (a large capital), represents variables such as pressure and volume; the SECOND LETTER, the secondary symbol (a lowercase letter or a small capital on the same line), qualifies the primary variable (e.g., stands for venous or arterial; inspiration or expiration); and, in capitals and subscript, the gas considered (O_2, CO_2, N_2).

BTPS	Body (37° C) temperature and pressure saturated with water vapor
STPD	Standard temperature and pressure (0° C, 760 torr), and dry

Examples

CaO_2	mL oxygen per 100 mL arterial blood or O_2 concentration in arterial blood
$(CaO_2 \div C\bar{v}O_2)$	Arteriovenous difference in O_2 concentration
$(C\bar{v}CO_2 \div CaCO_2)$	Venoarterial difference in CO_2 concentration
DO_2	Diffusing capacity for O_2 (mL O_2 per minute per torr)
FEN_2	Fractional concentration of N_2 in expired gas
$FICO_2$	Fractional concentration of CO_2 in inspired gas
FIO_2	Fractional concentration of O_2 in inspired gas
$\dot{M}CO_2$	Mass of CO_2 produced per unit of time
$\dot{M}O_2$	Mass of O_2 consumed per unit of time
PA	Alveolar pressure
PB	Barometric pressure
$PaCO_2$	Partial pressure of CO_2 in arterial blood
PAO_2	Partial pressure of O_2 in alveolar gas
$PcCO_2$	Partial pressure of CO_2 in pulmonary capillary blood
$\bar{P}cCO_2$	Mean partial pressure of CO_2 in pulmonary capillary blood
PO_2	Partial pressure of oxygen
$P\bar{v}O_2$	Partial pressure of O_2 in mixed venous blood
Qc	Volume of blood in pulmonary capillaries
$\dot{Q}c$	Blood flow through pulmonary capillaries per unit of time
$S\bar{v}O_2$	Saturation of hemoglobin with O_2 in mixed venous blood
VA	Volume of alveolar gas
VD	Volume of dead space gas
VE	Volume of expired gas
$\dot{V}E$	Volume of expired gas per unit of time
$\dot{V}O_2$	O_2 consumption per minute
VT	Tidal volume

Abbreviations for Lung Volumes

ERV	Expiratory reserve volume
FRC	Functional residual capacity
IC	Inspiratory capacity
IRV	Inspiratory reserve volume
RV	Residual volume
TLC	Total lung capacity
V$_D$	Vital capacity
V$_T$	Tidal volume

Symbols for Respiratory Mechanics

C	Compliance
E	Elastance (the reciprocal of C)
Gaw	Airway conductance (the reciprocal of Raw)
Ppl	Pleural pressure (intrathoracic pressure)
P$_m$	Pressure at the mouth
Raw	Airway resistance
R$_L$	Pulmonary resistance
R$_T$	Total resistance

Note: Page numbers in italics refer to illustrations; those followed by (t) indicate tables.